THOMPSON & THOMPSON

# GENETICS IN MEDICINE

THOMPSON & THOMPSON

# GENETICS IN MEDICINE

Sixth Edition

**Robert L. Nussbaum, MD**
Chief, Genetic Diseases Research Branch
Acting Chief, Inherited Disease Research Branch
National Human Genome Research Institute
Executive Faculty
Johns Hopkins/NHGRI Joint Genetic Counseling Graduate Program
National Institutes of Health
Bethesda, Maryland

**Roderick R. McInnes, MD, PhD, FRS(C)**
Scientific Director, Institute of Genetics
Canadian Institutes of Health Research
Anne and Max Tanenbaum Chair in Molecular Medicine
Professor of Pediatrics and Molecular and Medical Genetics
University of Toronto and The Hospital for Sick Children
Toronto, Ontario, Canada

**Huntington F. Willard, PhD**
President and Director
The Research Institute of University Hospitals of Cleveland
Henry Willson Payne Professor and Chairman
Department of Genetics
Case Western Reserve University School of Medicine
Director, Center for Human Genetics
University Hospitals of Cleveland
Cleveland, Ohio

With Clinical Case Studies prepared by
**Cornelius F. Boerkoel III, MD, PhD**
Assistant Professor
Department of Molecular and Human Genetics
Baylor College of Medicine
Houston, Texas

**W.B. SAUNDERS COMPANY**
A Harcourt Health Sciences Company
Philadelphia London New York St. Louis Sydney Toronto

**W.B. SAUNDERS COMPANY**
*A Harcourt Health Sciences Company*
The Curtis Center
Independence Square West
Philadelphia, Pennsylvania 19106

**Library of Congress Cataloging-in-Publication Data**

Nussbaum, Robert L.
Thompson & Thompson genetics in medicine.–6th ed. / Robert L. Nussbaum, Roderick R. McInnes, Huntington F. Willard.

p.; cm.

Rev. ed. of: Thompson & Thompson genetics in medicine / Margaret W. Thompson, Roderick R. McInnes, Huntington F. Willard. 5th ed. c1991.
Includes bibliographical references and index.

ISBN 0–7216–6902–6

1. Medical genetics. I. Title: Thompson and Thompson genetics in medicine. II. Title: Genetics in medicine. III. McInnes, Roderick R. IV. Willard, Huntington F. V. Thompson, Margaret W. (Margaret Wilson), Thompson & Thompson genetics in medicine. VI. Title.

[DNLM: 1. Genetics, Medical. QZ 50 N975t 2001]
RB155 .T52 2001
616'.042—dc21 2001020324

*Acquisitions Editor:* William Schmitt
*Designer:* Marie Gardocky-Clifton
*Production Manager:* Peter Faber
*Manuscript Editor:* Linda Lewis Grigg
*Illustration Coordinator:* Rita Martello

THOMPSON & THOMPSON GENETICS IN MEDICINE ISBN 0–7216–6902–6



Printed in the United States of America

Last digit is the print number: 9 8 7 6 5 4 3 2 1

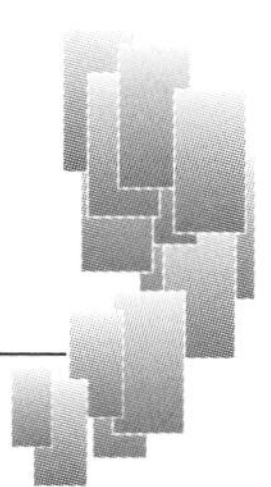

# Preface

In their preface to the first edition of *Genetics in Medicine*, published 35 years ago, James and Margaret Thompson wrote

> Genetics is fundamental to the basic sciences of preclinical medical education, and has important applications to clinical medicine, public health and medical research. With recognition of the role of genetics in medicine has come the problem of providing a place for it in the undergraduate curriculum, a problem which is as yet only partly solved in most medical schools. This book has been written to introduce the medical student to the principles of genetics as they apply to medicine, and to give him (her) a background for his own reading of the extensive and rapidly growing literature in the field. If his (her) senior colleagues also find it useful, we shall be doubly satisfied.

What was true then is even more so now as our knowledge of genetics and of the genome is rapidly becoming an integral part of public health and the practice of medicine. This new edition of *Genetics in Medicine*, the sixth in the series, has the same goal as did the previous five: to provide an accurate exposition of the fundamental principles of human genetics, with an emphasis on the genes and molecular mechanisms operating in human diseases. The concepts presented within the text are illustrated with examples drawn from medicine. A new, additional feature of this edition of *Genetics in Medicine* is a set of cases designed to demonstrate and reinforce general principles of disease inheritance, pathogenesis, diagnosis, management, and counseling. The book is not intended to be a compendium of genetic diseases nor is it an encyclopedic treatise on human genetics in general. Rather, the authors hope that the sixth edition of *Genetics in Medicine* will provide students with a framework for understanding the field of medical genetics while giving them a basis on which to establish a program of continuing education in this area. Any medical or genetic counseling student, advanced undergraduate, graduate student in genetics, resident in any field of clinical medicine, practicing physician, or allied medical professional in nursing or physical therapy should find this book to be a thorough but not exhaustive (or exhausting!) presentation of the fundamentals of human genetics as applied to health and disease.

ROBERT L. NUSSBAUM, MD
RODERICK R. MCINNES, MD, PhD
HUNTINGTON F. WILLARD, PhD

# Acknowledgments

The authors wish to express their appreciation and gratitude to their many colleagues who, through their ideas, suggestions, and criticisms, improved this revised edition of *Genetics in Medicine.* In particular, we are grateful to Gregory Barsh of Stanford University School of Medicine for his extraordinary contribution to Chapter 17 on Developmental Genetics and to Cheryl Shuman and Riyana Babul of The Hospital for Sick Children in Toronto for assistance with Chapter 18 on Prenatal Diagnosis. We also thank Donald Hadley and Sara Hull at the National Human Genome Research Institute; Richard Spielman of the University of Pennsylvania; Terry Hassold, Pat Hunt, and Stuart Schwartz of Case Western Reserve School of Medicine; Eric Fearon of the University of Michigan; David Ledbetter of the University of Chicago; Huda Zoghbi and Lisa Shaffer of the Baylor College of Medicine; George Stamatoyannopoulos and Peter Byers of the University of Washington; Aravinda Chakravarti, David Valle, and Garry Cutting of Johns Hopkins School of Medicine; Mark Kay of Stanford University; Michael Hershfield of Duke University; Charles Scriver and Paula Waters of McGill University; Alex Levine, Joe Clarke, David Chitayet, Peter Ray, and Donald Mahuran of The Hospital for Sick Children, Toronto; Ants Toi of the University Health Network, Princess Margaret Hospital, Toronto; Peter St. George-Hyslop of the University of Toronto; Joseph Goldstein of the University of Texas Southwestern Medical Center; Robert Desnick of the Mount Sinai School of Medicine, New York; Diane Cox of the University of Alberta; and Douglas C. Wallace and John M. Shoffner of Emory University.

Our deepest thanks go to our colleague and friend Dr. Margaret Thompson, not only for her help in reviewing new material but also for her trust and guidance during the revision process. Finally, we thank our families for their patience and understanding during the many hours of writing and revising that went into the sixth edition of *Genetics in Medicine.*

# Contents


**Chapter 1**
Introduction . . . . . . . . . . . . . . . . . . . . . . . . .1
The Role of Genetics in Medicine 1
Classification of Genetic Disorders 2
Onward 2

**Chapter 2**
Chromosomal Basis of Heredity . . . . . . . .4
The Human Chromosomes 5
The Life Cycle of a Somatic Cell 5
Meiosis 9
Human Gametogenesis and Fertilization 12
Medical Relevance of Mitosis and Meiosis 15

**Chapter 3**
The Human Genome: Structure and Function of Genes and Chromosomes . . . . . . . . . . . . . . . . . . . . . .17
DNA Structure: A Brief Review 17
The Central Dogma: DNA → RNA → Protein 18
Fundamentals of Gene Expression 22
Structure of Human Chromosomes 27
Organization of the Human Genome 30
Variation in Gene Expression and its Relevance to Medicine 31

**Chapter 4**
Tools of Human Molecular Genetics . . .33
Analysis of Individual DNA and RNA Sequences 33
Methods of Nucleic Acid Analysis 41
The Polymerase Chain Reaction 44
In Situ Hybridization to Chromosomes 46
DNA Sequence Analysis 48
Methods of Protein Analysis 49

**Chapter 5**
Patterns of Single-Gene Inheritance 51
Terminology 51
Genetic Disorders with Classical Mendelian Inheritance 53
Autosomal Recessive Inheritance 56
Patterns of Autosomal Dominant Inheritance 61
X-linked Inheritance 65
Patterns of Pseudoautosomal Inheritance 71
Atypical Patterns of Inheritance 72
Summary 77

**Chapter 6**
Genetic Variation in Individuals: Mutation and Polymorphism . . . . . . . . . .79
Mutation 79
The Molecular Basis of Mutations and Their Detection 81
Human Genetic Diversity 87
Inherited Variation and Polymorphism in Proteins 87
Inherited Variation and Polymorphism in DNA 90
Uses of Polymorphisms in Medical Genetics 93

**Chapter 7**
Genetic Variation in Populations . . . . . .95
Genetic Diversity in Human Populations 95
Phenotypes, Genotypes, and Gene Frequencies 96
The Hardy-Weinberg Law 97
Frequency of X-Linked Genes and Genotypes 98
Factors That Disturb Hardy-Weinberg Equilibrium 99
Conclusion 108

**Chapter 8**
Gene Mapping and the Human Genome Project . . . . . . . . . . . . . . . . . . . . . . . . . .111
Physical Mapping of Human Genes 111
Mapping Human Genes by Linkage Analysis 118
Applications of Human Gene Mapping 125
The Human Genome Project 132

**Chapter 9**
Principles of Clinical Cytogenetics .......................135
Introduction to Cytogenetics 135
Chromosome Abnormalities 140
Parent-of-Origin Effects 151
Studies of Chromosomes in Human Meiosis 153
Mendelian Disorders with Cytogenetic Effects 153
Cytogenetic Analysis in Cancer 154

**Chapter 10**
Clinical Cytogenetics: Disorders of the Autosomes and the Sex Chromosomes .................157
Autosomal Disorders 157
The Sex Chromosomes and Their Abnormalities 165

**Clinical Case Studies Illustrating Genetic Principles**

**Chapter 11**
Principles of Molecular Disease: Lessons from the Hemoglobinopathies ...............181
The Effect of Mutation on Protein Function 181
How Mutations Disrupt the Formation of Biologically Normal Proteins 183
Hemoglobins and Their Diseases 184
Genetic Disorders of Hemoglobin 187
Conclusion 201

**Chapter 12**
The Molecular and Biochemical Basis of Genetic Disease ............203
Diseases Due to Mutations in Different Classes of Proteins 203
Enzyme Defects 206
Defects in Receptor Proteins 218
Transport Defects 222
Disorders of Structural Proteins 225
Neurodegenerative Disorders 234
Pharmacogenetic Diseases 249
Conclusion 253

**Chapter 13**
The Treatment of Genetic Disease 255
The Current State of Treatment of Genetic Disease 255
Special Considerations in Treating Genetic Disease 257
Treatment Strategies 258

**Chapter 14**
Genetics of the Immune System ......277
The Major Histocompatibility Complex 277
Immunoglobulins 281
The T-Cell Antigen Receptor 284
Single-Gene Disorders of the Immune System 285

**Chapter 15**
Genetics of Disorders with Complex Inheritance ...............289
Genetic Analysis of Qualitative Disease Traits 289
Genetic Analysis of Quantitative Traits 293
Genetic Mapping of Complex Traits 297
Diseases with Complex Inheritance 299
Conclusion 309

**Chapter 16**
Genetics and Cancer ...............311
Cancer Biology 311
Genetic Basis of Cancer 312
Oncogenes 313
Tumor-Suppressor Genes 320
Tumor Progression by Clonal Evolution 330
Cancer and the Environment 331
Conclusion 332

**Chapter 17**
Genetic Aspects of Development ....335
(*With the assistance of Gregory* S. *Barsh*, MD, *PhD*.)
Introduction to Developmental Biology 335
Genes in Development 336
Early Development: Fertilization to Gastrulation 339
Gene Expression During Development 341
Developmental Genetics in Clinical Practice 350
Recent Advances in Developmental Genetics and Potential Applications 355

**Chapter 18**
Prenatal Diagnosis .................359
Indications for Prenatal Diagnosis 359
Genetic Counseling for Prenatal Diagnosis 360
Methods of Prenatal Diagnosis 360

Emerging Technologies for Prenatal Diagnosis 368
Laboratory Studies 369
The Effect of Prenatal Diagnosis on the Prevention and Management of Genetic Disease 372
Conclusion 372

**Chapter 19**
Genetic Counseling and Risk Assessment .....................375
Genetic Counseling 375
Case Management in Genetic Counseling 377
Determining Recurrence Risks 379
Conclusion 388

**Chapter 20**
Genetics and Society ..............391
Population Screening for Genetic Disease 391
Ethical Issues in Medical Genetics 393
Eugenic and Dysgenic Effects on Gene Frequencies 396
Conclusion 397

Glossary .........................399

Answers to Problems ..............415

Index ............................427

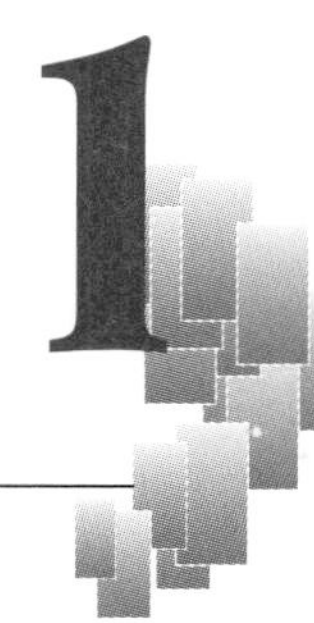

# Introduction

## THE ROLE OF GENETICS IN MEDICINE

### Genetics as a Medical Specialty

This is an especially exciting time in medical and human genetics. Medical genetics has achieved a recognized role as *the* specialty of medicine that deals with the diagnosis, treatment, and management of hereditary disorders. The idea that medical genetics is concerned only with the inheritance of trivial, superficial, and rare characteristics has given way to an understanding of the fundamental role of the **gene** in basic life processes. Medical and human geneticists are at the forefront of investigations into human variability and human heredity while also participating in and benefiting from rapid progress in molecular biology, biochemistry, and cell biology. In particular, the last decade of the 20th century and the beginning of the 21st century have seen the initiation of the **Human Genome Project**, an international effort to determine the complete content of the human genome, defined simply as the sum total of the genetic information of our species, encoded within each nucleated cell of the body. In partnership with all the other disciplines of modern biology, the Human Genome Project is already revolutionizing human and medical genetics by providing fundamental insights into many diseases and promoting the development of far better diagnostic tools, preventive measures, and therapeutic methods in the near future. When completed, the Human Genome Project will make available the complete sequence of all human DNA; knowledge of the complete sequence will, in turn, allow the identification of all human genes and, ultimately, make it possible to determine how variation in these genes contributes to health and disease.

### Relevance of Genetics to All Medical Practice

Although medical genetics has become a recognized specialty, it has also become abundantly clear that human genetics provides important unifying concepts that illuminate and unify all medical practice. To give patients and their families the full benefit of expanding genetic knowledge, all physicians and their colleagues in the health professions need to understand the underlying principles of human genetics. The existence of alternative forms of a gene (**alleles**) in the population; the occurrence of similar **phenotypes** developing from mutation and variation at different loci; the importance of gene-gene and gene-environmental interactions in disease; the role of somatic mutation in cancer and aging; the feasibility of prenatal diagnosis, presymptomatic testing, and population screening; and the promise of powerful gene therapies are concepts that now permeate all medical practice and will become only more important in the future. Thus, genetic principles and approaches are not restricted to any one medical subspecialty.

One aspect of medical genetics practice relevant to all of medicine deserves special emphasis: it focuses not only on the patient but also on the entire family. A comprehensive family history is an important first step in the analysis of any disorder, whether or not the disorder is known to be genetic. As pointed out by Childs, "to fail to take a good family history is bad medicine. . . ." A family history is important because it can be critical in diagnosis, may show that a disorder is hereditary, can provide information about the natural history of a disease and variation in its expression, and can clarify the pattern of inheritance. The diagnosis of a hereditary condition allows the risk in other family members to be estimated, so that proper management, prevention, and counseling can be offered to the patient *and* the family.

### Disciplines within Human and Medical Genetics

**Genetics** is a diverse subject concerned with variation and heredity in all living organisms. Within this broad field, **human genetics** is the science of variation and heredity in human beings, whereas **medical**

**genetics** deals with the subset of human genetic variation that is of significance in the practice of medicine and in medical research.

Within human and medical genetics, there are many fields of interest, as indicated by the various directions in which genetics has developed. Major recognized areas of specialization are the study of chromosomes (**cytogenetics**); the study of the structure and function of individual genes (**molecular and biochemical genetics**); the study of the genome, its organization, and functions (**genomics**); the study of genetic variation in human populations and the factors that determine allele frequencies (**population genetics**); the study of the genetic control of development (**developmental genetics**); and the application of genetics to diagnosis and patient care (**clinical genetics**). The literal meaning of *clinical* is *bedside* (*klinikos*, Greek for "bedside"), and a clinical geneticist is an appropriately qualified physician-geneticist directly involved in the diagnosis of genetic diseases and the care of patients with such diseases. **Genetic counseling**, which combines the provision of risk information while providing psychological and educational support, has matured into a new health profession with a whole cadre of genetic professionals dedicated to the care of patients and their families.

In addition to direct patient contact, medical geneticists provide care to individuals, through the provision of laboratory diagnosis, and to the population at large, through screening programs designed to identify persons at risk of developing or transmitting a genetic disorder. The diagnosis of genetic disease in patients, carrier testing, prenatal diagnosis, and the identification of individuals at risk of developing disease later in life are rapidly expanding specialties in clinical laboratories. Population screening for genetic disease is also becoming increasingly widespread.

## CLASSIFICATION OF GENETIC DISORDERS

In clinical practice, the chief significance of genetics is in elucidating the role of genetic variation and mutation in the etiology of a large number of disorders. Virtually any disease is the result of the combined action of genes and environment, but the relative role of the genetic component may be large or small.

Among disorders caused wholly or partly by genetic factors, three main types are recognized:

1. Single-gene disorders
2. Chromosome disorders
3. Multifactorial disorders

**Single-gene defects** are caused by individual mutant genes. The mutation may be present on only one chromosome of a pair (matched with a normal allele on the homologous chromosome) or on both chromosomes of the pair. In a few cases, the mutation is in the mitochondrial rather than the nuclear genome. In any case, the cause is a critical error in the genetic information carried by a single gene. Single-gene disorders usually exhibit obvious and characteristic pedigree patterns. Most such defects are rare, with a frequency that may be as high as 1 in 500 but is usually much less. Although individually rare, as a group single-gene disorders are responsible for a significant proportion of disease and death. Taking the population as a whole, single-gene disorders affect 2 percent of the population sometime over an entire life span. In a population study of more than 1 million live births, the incidence of serious single-gene disorders in the pediatric population was estimated to be 0.36 percent; among hospitalized children, 6 to 8 percent probably have single-gene disorders.

In **chromosome disorders**, the defect is due not to a single mistake in the genetic blueprint but to an excess or a deficiency of the genes contained in whole chromosomes or chromosome segments. For example, the presence of an extra copy of one chromosome, chromosome 21, produces a specific disorder, Down syndrome, even though no individual gene on the chromosome is abnormal. As a group, chromosome disorders are quite common, affecting about 7 per 1000 liveborn infants and accounting for about half of all spontaneous first-trimester abortions.

**Multifactorial inheritance** is responsible for a number of developmental disorders resulting in congenital malformations and for many common disorders of adult life. There appears to be no single error in the genetic information in many of these conditions. Rather, the disease is the result of a combination of small variations in genes that together can produce or predispose to a serious defect, often in concert with environmental factors. Multifactorial disorders tend to recur in families but do not show the characteristic pedigree patterns of single-gene traits. Estimates of the impact of multifactorial disease range from 5 percent in the pediatric population to more than 60 percent in the entire population.

## ONWARD

During the 40-year professional life of today's medical and genetic counseling students, extensive changes are likely to take place in appreciating—and acting on—the role of genetics in medicine. It is hard to imagine that any period could encompass changes greater than those seen over the past 50 years, during which the field has gone from first recognizing the identity of DNA as the active agent of inheritance, to uncovering the molecular structure of DNA and chromosomes, to determining the complete code of the human genome. And yet, judging from the quickening pace of discovery within only the past decade, it is virtually certain that we are just at the beginning of a revolution in integrating knowledge of genetics and the genome into public health and the practice of medicine.

An introduction to the language and concepts of human and medical genetics and an appreciation of the genetic and genomic perspective on health and disease will form a framework for lifelong learning that is part of any health professional's career.

## General References

Childs B (1982) Genetics in the medical curriculum. Am J Med Genet 13:319–324.
King RA, Rotter JI, Motulsky AG (1992) The Genetic Basis of Common Diseases. Oxford University Press, Oxford, England.
McKusick VA (1998) Mendelian Inheritance in Man: Catalogs of Autosomal Dominant, Autosomal Recessive, and X-Linked Phenotypes, 12th ed. Johns Hopkins University Press, Baltimore. See online version at *http://www3.ncbi.nlm.nih.gov*.
Rimoin DL, Connor JM, Pyeritz RE (1997) Emery and Rimoin's Principles and Practice of Medical Genetics, 3rd ed. Churchill Livingstone, Edinburgh.
Scriver CR, Beaudet AL, Sly WS, Valle D (eds) (2000) The Metabolic and Molecular Bases of Inherited Disease, 8th ed. McGraw-Hill, New York.
Vogel F, Motulsky AG (1997) Human Genetics: Problems and Approaches, 3rd ed. Springer-Verlag, New York.

# 2

# Chromosomal Basis of Heredity

Appreciation of the importance of genetics to medicine requires an understanding of the nature of the hereditary material, how it is packaged into the human genome, and how it is transmitted from cell to cell during cell division and from generation to generation during reproduction. The human genome consists of large amounts of the chemical deoxyribonucleic acid (**DNA**) that contains within its structure the genetic information needed to specify all aspects of embryogenesis, development, growth, metabolism, and reproduction—essentially all aspects of what makes a human being a functional organism. The genome contains, by current estimates, about 50,000 **genes**, which at this point we define simply as units of genetic information. Genes are encoded in the DNA that makes up a number of rod-shaped organelles called **chromosomes** in the nucleus of each cell. The influence of genes and genetics on states of health and disease is widespread, and its roots are the information encoded in the DNA found in the human genome.

Within each cell, the genome is packaged as **chromatin**, in which genomic DNA is complexed with several classes of chromosomal proteins. Some of the proteins found in chromatin perform structural roles, whereas others serve to regulate the expression of individual genes. Except during cell division, chromatin is distributed throughout the nucleus and is relatively homogeneous in appearance under the microscope. When a cell divides, however, its nuclear material condenses to appear as microscopically visible chromosomes. Chromosomes are thus visible as discrete structures only in dividing cells, but they nevertheless retain their integrity between cell divisions.

Each species has a characteristic chromosome complement (**karyotype**) in terms of the number and the morphology of its chromosomes. The genes are in linear order along the chromosomes, each gene having a precise position or **locus**. The **gene map** is the map of the chromosomal location of the genes and is also characteristic of each species and the individuals within a species.

The study of chromosomes, their structure, and their inheritance is called **cytogenetics**. The science of modern human cytogenetics dates from 1956, when Tjio and Levan developed effective techniques for chromosome analysis and established that the normal human chromosome number is 46. Since that time, much has been learned about human chromosomes, their normal structure, their molecular composition, the locations of the genes that they contain, and their numerous and varied abnormalities.

Chromosome analysis has become an important diagnostic procedure in clinical medicine. As described more fully in subsequent chapters, some of these applications include the following:

**Clinical Diagnosis.** Numerous medical disorders, including some that are quite common, such as Down syndrome, are associated with microscopically visible changes in chromosome number or structure and require chromosome analysis for diagnosis and genetic counseling (see Chapters 9 and 10).

**Gene Mapping.** A major goal of medical genetics today is the mapping of specific genes to chromosomes as part of the Human Genome Project. This topic is referred to repeatedly but is discussed in detail in Chapter 8.

**Cancer Cytogenetics.** Chromosomal changes in somatic cells are involved in the initiation and progression of many types of cancer (see Chapter 16).

**Prenatal Diagnosis.** Chromosome analysis is an essential procedure in prenatal diagnosis (see Chapter 18).

The ability to interpret a chromosome report and some knowledge of the methodology, the scope, and the limitations of chromosome studies are essential skills for physicians and others working with patients with birth defects, mental retardation, disorders of sexual development, and many types of cancer.

## THE HUMAN CHROMOSOMES

With the exception of cells in the germline, all cells that contribute to one's body are called **somatic cells** (*soma*, body). The 46 chromosomes of human somatic cells constitute 23 pairs. Of those 23 pairs, 22 are alike in males and females and are called **autosomes**, numbered in decreasing order from the largest (chromosome 1) to the smallest (chromosomes 21 and 22). The remaining pair comprises the **sex chromosomes**: XX in females and XY in males. Each chromosome carries a different subset of genes that are arranged linearly along its DNA. Members of a pair of chromosomes (described as **homologous chromosomes** or **homologs**) carry matching genetic information; that is, they have the same genes in the same sequence. At any specific locus, however, they may have either identical or slightly different forms of the same gene, called **alleles**. One member of each pair of chromosomes is inherited from the father, the other from the mother. Normally, the members of a pair of autosomes are microscopically indistinguishable from each other. In females, the sex chromosomes, the two **X chromosomes**, are likewise largely indistinguishable. In males, however, the sex chromosomes differ. One is an X, identical to the Xs of the female, inherited by a male from his mother and transmitted to his daughters; the other, the **Y chromosome**, is inherited from his father and transmitted to his sons. In Chapter 10, we look at some exceptions to the simple and almost universal rule that human females are XX and human males are XY.

There are two kinds of cell division: mitosis and meiosis. **Mitosis** is ordinary somatic cell division, by which the body grows, differentiates, and effects tissue regeneration. Mitotic division normally results in two daughter cells, each with chromosomes and genes identical to those of the parent cell. There may be dozens or even hundreds of successive mitoses in a lineage of somatic cells. In contrast, **meiosis** occurs only in cells of the germline. Meiosis results in the formation of reproductive cells (**gametes**), each of which has only 23 chromosomes: one of each kind of autosome and either an X or a Y. Thus, whereas somatic cells have the **diploid** (*diploos*, double) or the 2n chromosome complement (i.e., 46 chromosomes), gametes have the **haploid** (*haploos*, single) or the n complement (i.e., 23 chromosomes). Abnormalities of chromosome number or structure, which are usually clinically significant, can arise in either somatic cells or cells of the germline by errors in cell division.

## THE LIFE CYCLE OF A SOMATIC CELL

A human being begins life as a fertilized ovum (**zygote**), a diploid cell from which all the cells of the body (estimated at about 100 trillion in number) are derived, by a series of dozens or even hundreds of mitoses. Mitosis is obviously crucial for growth and differentiation, but it takes up only a small part of the life cycle of a cell. What goes on in **interphase**, the period between two successive mitoses?

As Figure 2–1 shows, mitosis is the shortest of the four stages of the cell cycle. Immediately after mitosis, the cell enters a phase, called $G_1$, in which there is no DNA synthesis. Some cells spend a very long time, days or even years, in $G_1$; others pass through this stage in hours. Although the molecular mechanisms controlling cell-cycle progression are incompletely understood, the cell cycle is governed by a series of **checkpoints** that determine the timing of each step in mitosis. In addition, checkpoints monitor and control the accuracy of DNA synthesis, as well as the assembly and attachment of an elaborate network of microtubules that facilitate chromosome movement. If damage to the genome is detected, these mitotic checkpoints halt cell-cycle progression until repairs are made or, if the damage is excessive, until the cell is instructed to die by programmed cell death (a process called **apoptosis**).

$G_1$ is followed by the **S phase**, the stage of DNA synthesis. During this stage, each chromosome, which in $G_1$ has been a single DNA molecule (whose exact structure we examine in Chapter 3), replicates to become a bipartite chromosome consisting of two **sister chromatids** (see Fig. 2–1), each of which contains an identical copy of the original linear DNA molecule. The ends of each chromosome (or

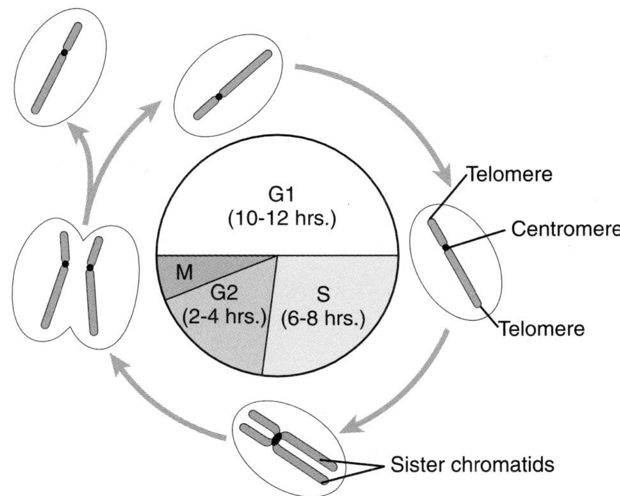


**Figure 2–1.** A typical mitotic cell cycle, described in the text. The telomeres, the centromere, and sister chromatids are indicated.

chromatid) are marked by **telomeres**, which consist of specialized DNA sequences that ensure the integrity of the chromosome during cell division. The two sister chromatids are held together physically at the **centromere**, a region of DNA that associates with a number of specific proteins to form the **kinetochore**. This complex structure serves to attach each chromosome to the microtubules of the mitotic spindle and to govern chromosome movement during mitosis. DNA synthesis during S phase is not synchronous throughout all chromosomes or even within a single chromosome; rather, along each chromosome, it begins at hundreds to thousands of sites, called **origins of DNA replication**. Individual chromosome segments have their own characteristic time of replication during the 6- to 8-hour S phase.

By the end of S phase, the DNA content of the cell has doubled, and the cell enters a brief next stage, called $G_2$. Throughout the whole cell cycle, ribonucleic acids and proteins are produced and the cell gradually enlarges, eventually doubling its total mass before the next mitosis. $G_2$ is ended by mitosis, which begins when individual chromosomes begin to condense and become visible under the microscope as thin, extended threads, a process that is considered in greater detail in the following section and in Chapter 3.

The $G_1$, S, and $G_2$ phases together constitute interphase. In typical dividing human cells, the three phases take a total of 16 to 24 hours, whereas mitosis lasts only 1 to 2 hours (see Fig. 2–1). There is great variation, however, in the length of the cell cycle, which ranges from a few hours in rapidly dividing cells, such as those of the dermis of the skin or the intestinal mucosa, to months in other cell types. In fact, some cell types, such as neurons and red blood cells, do not divide at all once they are fully differentiated; rather, they are permanently arrested during $G_1$ in a phase known as $G_0$. Other cells, such as liver cells, may enter $G_0$ but, following organ damage, eventually return to $G_1$ and continue through the cell cycle.

## Mitosis

During the mitotic phase of the cell cycle, an elaborate apparatus is brought into play to ensure that each of the two daughter cells receives a complete set of genetic information. This result is achieved by a mechanism that distributes one chromatid of each chromosome to each daughter cell and is illustrated schematically in Figure 2–2. The process of distributing a copy of each chromosome to each daughter cell is called **chromosome segregation**. The importance of this process for normal cell growth is illustrated by the observation that many tumors are invariably characterized by a state of genetic imbalance that results from mitotic errors in distributing chromosomes to daughter cells.

The process of mitosis is continuous, but five stages are distinguished: prophase, prometaphase, metaphase, anaphase, and telophase.

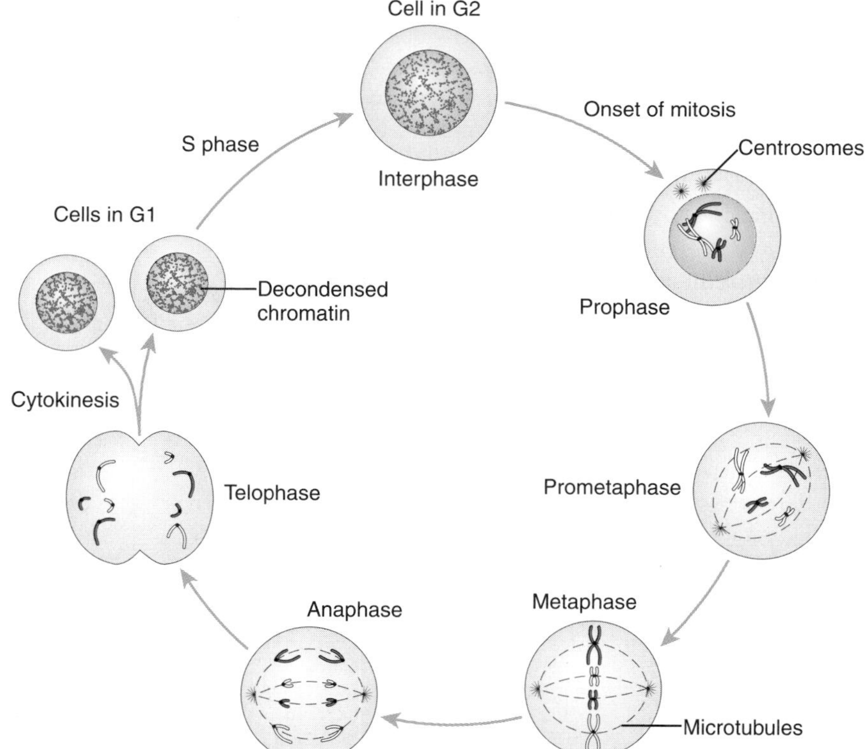


**Figure 2–2.** Mitosis. Diagrammatic representation, showing only two chromosome pairs. For further details, see text.

**Prophase.** This stage initiates mitosis and is marked by gradual condensation of the chromosomes, disintegration and eventual disappearance of the nucleolus, and the beginning of the formation of the **mitotic spindle**. A pair of microtubule organizing centers, also called **centrosomes**, form foci from which microtubules radiate. The centrosomes gradually move to take up positions at the poles of the cell.

**Prometaphase.** The cell enters prometaphase when the nuclear membrane breaks up, allowing the chromosomes to disperse within the cell and to attach, via their kinetochores, to microtubules of the mitotic spindle. The chromosomes begin to move toward a point midway between the spindle poles, a process called **congression**. The chromosomes continue to condense throughout this stage.

**Metaphase.** At metaphase, the chromosomes reach maximal condensation. They become arranged at the equatorial plane of the cell, balanced by the equal forces exerted on the kinetochore of each chromosome by microtubules emanating from the two spindle poles. The chromosomes of a dividing human cell are most readily analyzed at the metaphase or the prometaphase stage of mitosis (see later discussion and Chapter 9).

**Anaphase.** Anaphase begins abruptly when the chromosomes separate at the centromere. The sister chromatids of each chromosome now become independent **daughter chromosomes**, which move to opposite poles of the cell (see Fig. 2–2).

**Telophase.** In telophase, the chromosomes begin to decondense from their highly contracted state, a nuclear membrane begins to reform around each of the two daughter nuclei, and each nucleus gradually resumes its interphase appearance.

To complete the process of cell division, the cytoplasm cleaves by a process known as **cytokinesis**, which begins as the chromosomes approach the spindle poles. Eventually there are two complete daughter cells, each with a nucleus containing all the genetic information of the original cell.

There is an important difference between a cell entering mitosis and one that has just completed the process. The parent cell's chromosomes in $G_2$ each have a pair of chromatids, but the chromosomes of the daughter cell each consist of only one copy of the genetic material. This copy will not be duplicated until the daughter cell in its turn reaches the S phase of the next cell cycle (see Fig. 2–1). The entire process of mitosis thus ensures the orderly duplication and distribution of the genome through successive cell divisions.

## The Human Karyotype

The condensed chromosomes of a dividing human cell are most readily analyzed at metaphase or prometaphase. At these stages, the chromosomes are visible under the microscope as a **chromosome spread**, and each chromosome can be seen to consist of its sister chromatids, joined at the centromere.

Most chromosomes can be distinguished not only by their length, but also by the location of the centromere. The centromere is apparent as a **primary constriction**, a recognizable cytogenetic landmark, dividing the chromosome into two **arms**, a short arm designated **p** (for *petit*) and a long arm designated **q**. The staining methods originally available for human cytogenetic analysis, however, did not allow all 24 types of chromosome (22 autosomes, X, and Y) to be individually identified. Instead, the chromosomes could be classified only into seven groups, named by the letters A to G, on the basis of their overall length and the position of the centromere. These designations are no longer in general use but are seen in the literature. With techniques now in common use, all the chromosomes can be individually identified.

Figure 2–3 shows a prometaphase cell in which the chromosomes have been stained by the Giemsa-staining (**G-banding**) method, the technique most

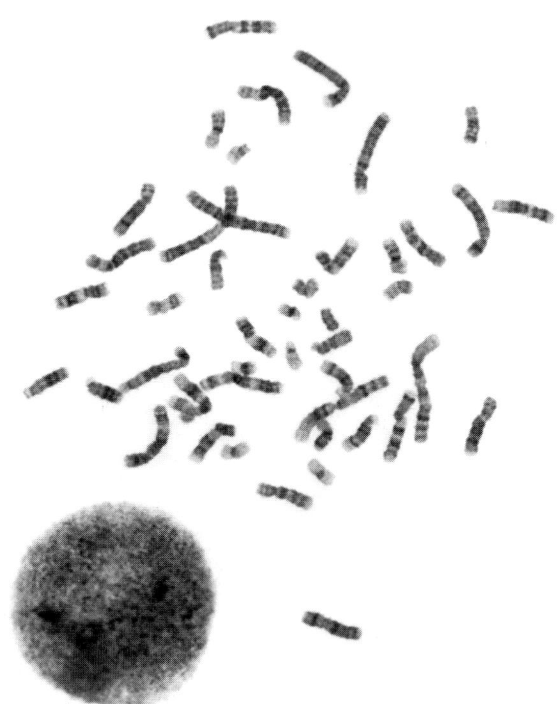

**Figure 2–3.** A chromosome spread prepared from a lymphocyte culture which has been stained by the Giemsa-banding (G-banding) technique. The darkly stained nucleus adjacent to the chromosomes is from a different cell in interphase, when chromosomal material is diffuse throughout the nucleus. (Photomicrograph courtesy of Stuart Schwartz, University Hospitals of Cleveland.)

widely used in clinical cytogenetics laboratories. The chromosomes are treated first with trypsin to digest the chromosomal proteins and then with Giemsa stain. Each chromosome pair stains in a characteristic pattern of light and dark bands (G bands). Using this method and other so-called banding techniques, all of the chromosomes can be individually distinguished. Further, the nature of any structural or numerical abnormalities can be readily determined, as we examine in greater detail in Chapters 9 and 10.

Although experts can often analyze metaphase chromosomes directly under the microscope, a common procedure is to cut out the chromosomes from a photomicrograph and arrange them in pairs in a standard classification, as shown in Figure 2–4. The completed picture is called a **karyotype**. The word *karyotype* is also used to refer to the standard chromosome set of an individual ("a normal male karyotype") or of a species ("the human karyotype") and, as a verb, to refer to the process of preparing such a standard figure ("to karyotype").

Unlike the chromosomes seen in stained preparations under the microscope or in photographs, the chromosomes of living cells are fluid and dynamic structures. During mitosis, for example, the chromatin of each interphase chromosome condenses substantially (Fig. 2–5). At prophase, when chromosomes become visible under the light microscope, chromosome 1 has condensed to an overall length of about 50 $\mu$m. When maximally condensed at metaphase, DNA in chromosomes is about 1/10,000 of its fully extended state. When chromosomes are prepared to reveal bands (see Figs. 2–3 and 2–4), as many as 1000 or more bands can be recognized in stained preparations of all the chromosomes, and each cytogenetic band therefore contains as many as 50 or more genes. After metaphase, as cells complete mitosis, chromosomes decondense and return to their relaxed state as chromatin in the interphase nucleus, ready to begin the cycle again (see Fig. 2–5).

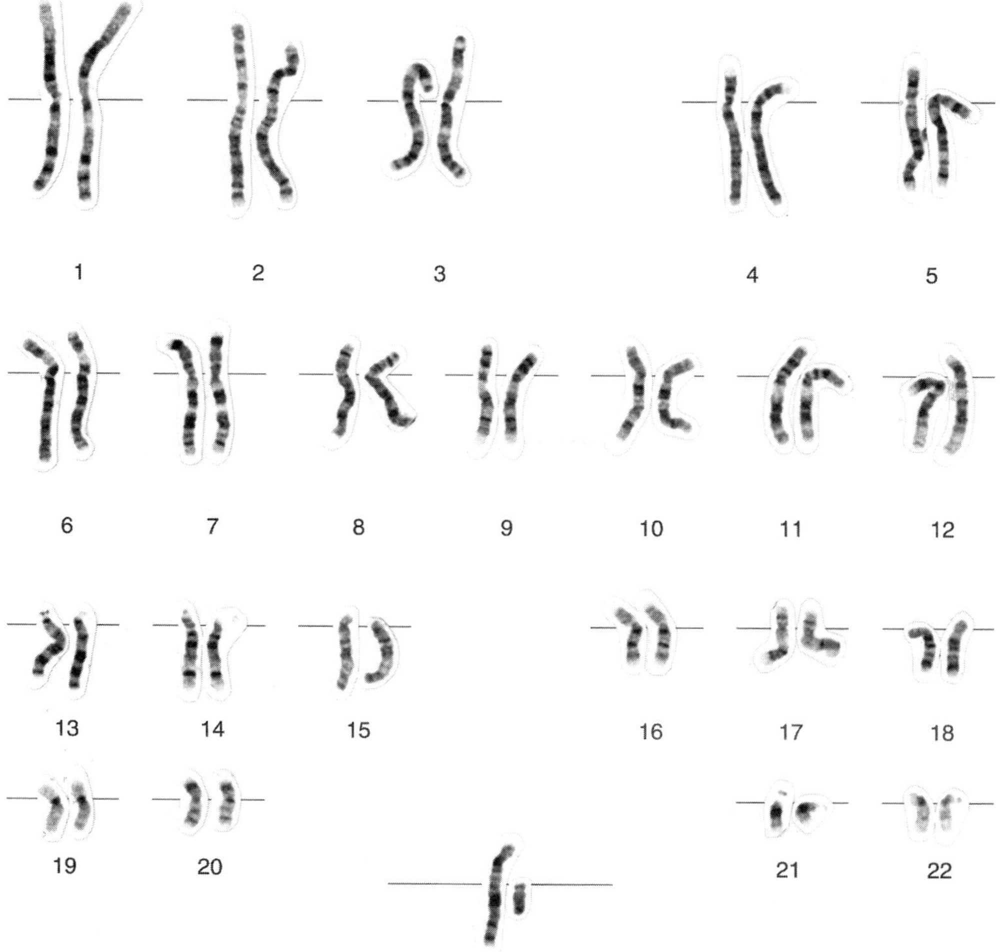


**Figure 2–4.** A human male karyotype with Giemsa banding (G banding). The chromosomes are at the prometaphase stage of mitosis and are arranged in a standard classification, numbered 1 to 22 in order of length, with the X and Y chromosomes shown separately. (Photomicrograph courtesy of Stuart Schwartz, University Hospitals of Cleveland.)

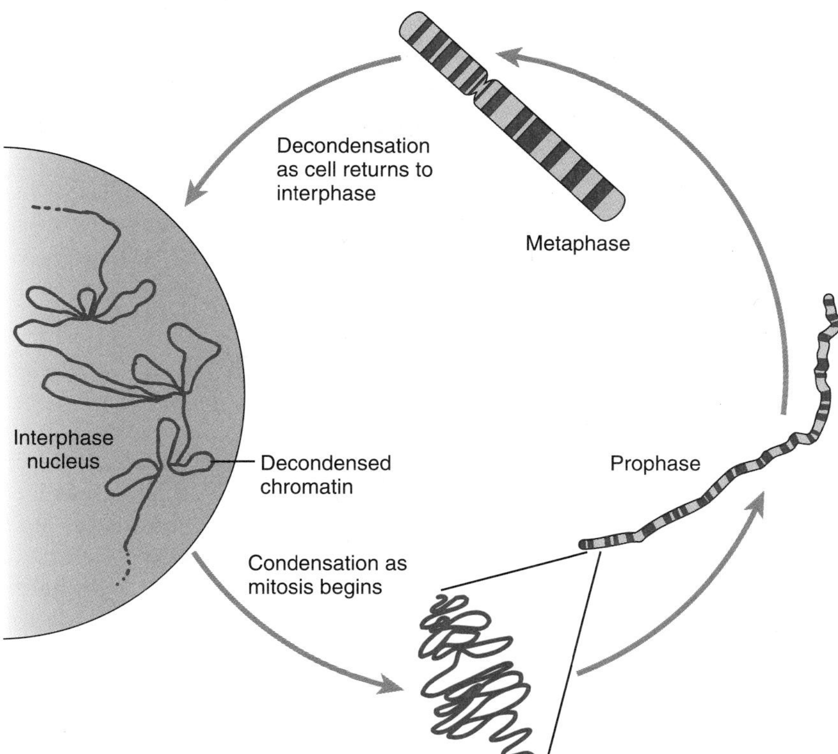


**Figure 2–5.** Cycle of condensation and decondensation as a chromosome proceeds through the cell cycle.

## MEIOSIS

Meiosis is the type of cell division by which the diploid cells of the germline give rise to haploid gametes. Meiosis consists of one round of DNA synthesis followed by two rounds of chromosome segregation and cell division (Fig. 2–6). The cells in the germline that undergo meiosis, primary spermatocytes or primary oocytes, are derived from the zygote by a long series of mitoses before the onset of meiosis.

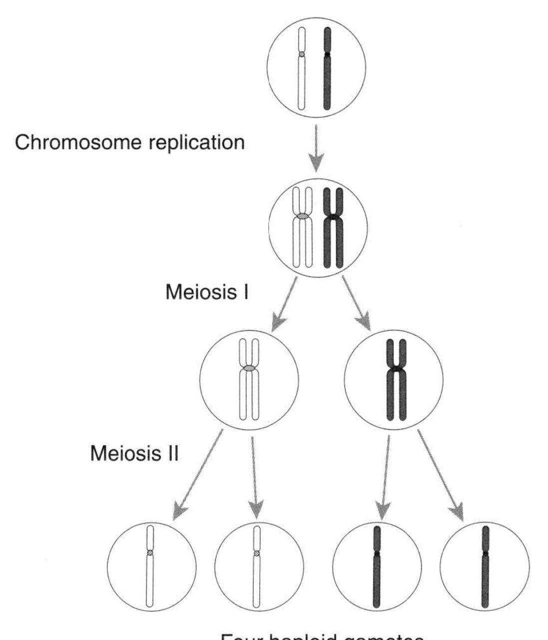


**Figure 2–6.** A simplified representation of the essential steps in meiosis, consisting of one round of DNA replication, followed by two rounds of chromosome segregation, meiosis I and meiosis II.

Male and female gametes have different histories, but the sequence of events is the same, although their timing is very different. The two successive meiotic divisions are called meiosis I and meiosis II. Meiosis I is also known as the **reduction division** because it is the division in which the chromosome number is reduced from diploid to haploid by the pairing of homologs in prophase and by their segregation to different cells at anaphase of meiosis I. The X and Y chromosomes are not homologs in a strict sense but do have homologous segments at the ends of their short and long arms, and they pair in both regions.

Meiosis I is also notable because it is the stage at which genetic **recombination** (also called **meiotic crossing over**) occurs. In this process, homologous segments of DNA are exchanged between nonsister chromatids of a pair of homologous chromosomes, thus ensuring that none of the gametes produced by meiosis is identical to another. The concept of recombination is fundamental to the process of mapping genes responsible for inherited disorders, as we discuss at length in Chapter 8. Because recombination involves the physical intertwining of the two homologs until the appropriate point during meiosis I, it is also critical for ensuring proper chromosome segregation during meiosis. Failure to recombine properly can lead to chromosome missegregation in meiosis I and is a frequent cause of chromosome abnormalities like Down syndrome (see Chapter 9).

Meiosis II follows meiosis I without an intervening step of DNA replication. As in ordinary mitosis, the chromatids separate, and one chromatid of each chromosome passes to each daughter cell. Some of the stages distinguished in meiosis, as well as the process of crossing over, are shown in Figure 2–7.

## The First Meiotic Division (Meiosis I)

### Prophase I

The prophase of meiosis I is a complicated process that differs from mitotic prophase in a number of ways, with important genetic consequences. Several stages are defined. Throughout all the stages, the chromosomes continually condense and become shorter and thicker.

**Leptotene.** The chromosomes, which have already replicated during the preceding S phase, become visible as thin threads that are beginning to condense. At this early stage, the two sister chromatids of each chromosome are so closely aligned that they cannot be distinguished.

**Zygotene.** At this stage, homologous chromosomes begin to pair closely along their entire length. The process of pairing or **synapsis** is normally very precise, bringing corresponding DNA sequences into alignment along the length of the entire chromosome.

Although the molecular basis of synapsis is not completely understood, electron microscopy reveals that the chromosomes are held together by a **synaptonemal complex,** a ribbon-like protein-containing structure (Fig. 2–8). The synaptonemal complex is essential to the process of recombination.

**Pachytene.** During this stage, the chromosomes become much more tightly coiled. Synapsis is complete, and each pair of homologs appears as a **bivalent** (sometimes called a **tetrad** because it contains four chromatids). Pachytene is the stage at which meiotic crossing over takes place (see Fig. 2–7).

**Diplotene.** Following recombination, the synaptonemal complex disappears, and the two components of each bivalent now begin to separate from each other. Although the homologous chromosomes separate, each of their centromeres remains intact, so that each set of sister chromatids initially remains joined. Eventually the two homologs of each bivalent are held together only at points called **chiasmata** (crosses), which are believed to mark the locations of crossovers. The average number of chiasmata seen in human spermatocytes is about 50, that is, several per bivalent.

**Diakinesis.** In this stage, the chromosomes reach maximal condensation.

### Metaphase I

Metaphase I begins, as in mitosis, when the nuclear membrane disappears. A spindle has formed, and the paired chromosomes align themselves on the equatorial plane with their centromeres oriented toward different poles.

### Anaphase I

The two members of each bivalent move apart, and their respective centromeres with the attached sister chromatids are drawn to opposite poles of the cell, a process termed **disjunction**. Thus, the chromosome number is halved, and each cellular product of meiosis I has the haploid chromosome number. The different bivalents assort independently of one another, and as a result, the original paternal and maternal chromosome sets are sorted into random combinations. The possible number of combinations of the 23 chromosome pairs that can be present in the gametes is $2^{23}$ (more than 8 million). In fact, the variation in the genetic material that is transmitted from parent to child is actually much greater than this because of the process of crossing over. As a result of this process, each chromatid typically contains segments derived from each member of the parental chromosome pair; for example, at this stage a typical chromosome 1 is composed of three to five segments, alternately paternal and maternal in origin. (See further discussion in Chapter 8.)

Many errors can occur in cell division. Anaphase of meiosis I is the most error-prone step, the error resulting in both homologs of a chromosome pair going to the same, rather than opposite, poles. This pathogenic process is termed **nondisjunction**. Some of the consequences of meiotic irregularities are discussed in Chapters 9 and 10.

### Telophase I

By telophase, the two haploid sets of chromosomes have normally grouped at opposite poles of the cell.

## Cytokinesis

After telophase I, the cell divides into two haploid daughter cells and enters meiotic interphase. In spermatogenesis, the cytoplasm is more or less equally divided between the two daughter cells (Fig. 2–9), but in oogenesis, one product (the secondary oocyte) receives almost all the cytoplasm, and the reciprocal

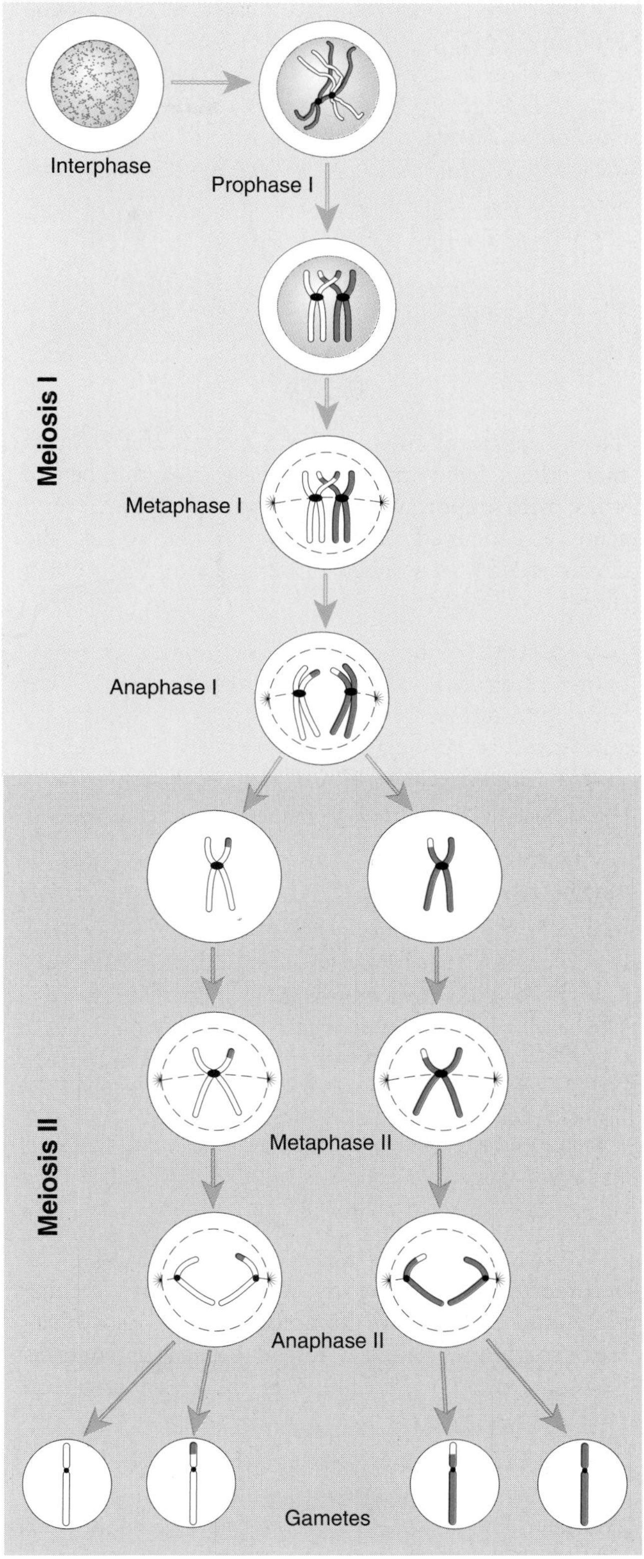

**Figure 2–7.** Diagrammatic representation of meiosis and its consequences. A single chromosome pair and a single crossover are shown, leading to formation of four distinct gametes. The chromosomes replicate during interphase and begin to condense as the cell enters prophase of meiosis I. In meiosis I, the chromosomes synapse and recombine. Chiasmata are visible as the homologs align at metaphase I, with the centromeres oriented toward opposite poles. In anaphase I, the exchange of DNA between the homologs is apparent as the chromosomes are pulled to opposite poles. After completion of meiosis I and cytokinesis, meiosis II proceeds with a mitosis-like division. The sister kinetochores separate and move to opposite poles in anaphase II, yielding four haploid products.

product becomes the first polar body (Fig. 2–10). In contrast to mitosis, interphase is brief, and meiosis II begins. The notable point that distinguishes meiotic and mitotic interphase is that there is no S phase (i.e., no DNA synthesis) between the first and second meiotic divisions.

## The Second Meiotic Division (Meiosis II)

The second meiotic division is similar to an ordinary mitosis except that the chromosome number of the cell entering meiosis II is haploid. The end result is four

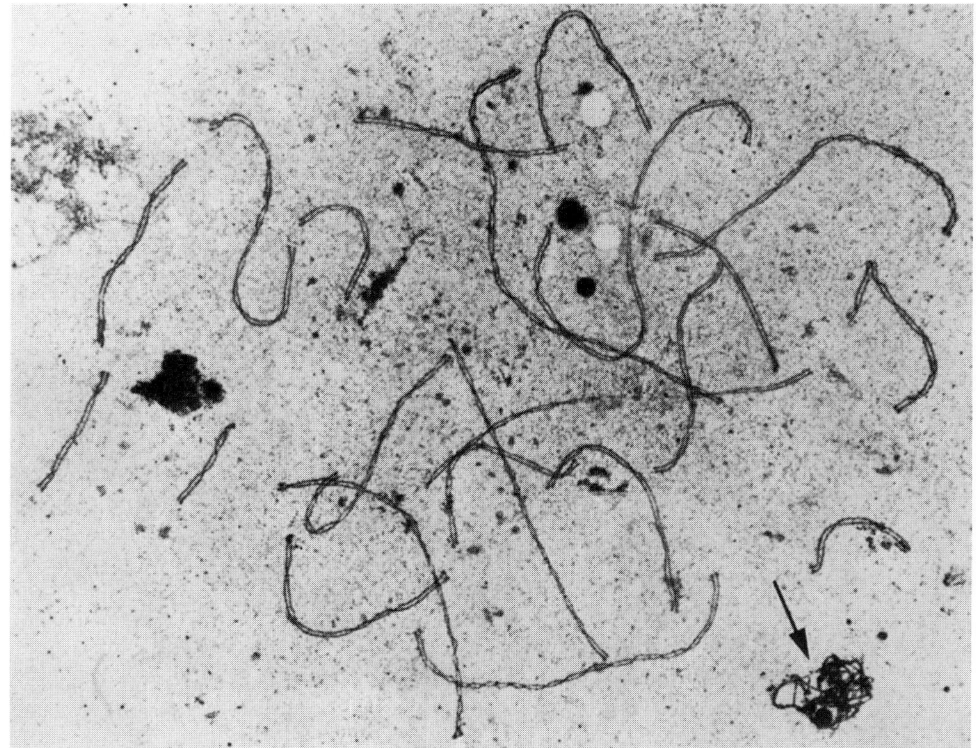

Figure 2–8. Electron micrograph of a human primary spermatocyte in meiosis, showing the 22 autosomal synaptonemal complexes and the XY pair *(arrow)*. The DNA of each bivalent is not visible, but extends laterally on each side of the synaptonemal complexes. (Photomicrograph courtesy of A. C. Chandley, Western General Hospital, Edinburgh.)

haploid cells, each containing 23 chromosomes (see Fig. 2–7). As mentioned earlier, because of crossing over in meiosis I, the chromosomes of the resulting gametes are not identical. Segregation of the different paternal and maternal alleles of each gene takes place during either the first or the second meiotic division (see box), depending on whether they have been involved in a crossover event in meiosis I.

### Genetic Consequences of Meiosis

1. **Reduction of the chromosome number** from diploid to haploid, the essential step in the formation of gametes.
2. **Segregation of alleles**, at either meiosis I or meiosis II, in accordance with Mendel's first law.
3. Shuffling of the genetic material by **random assortment of the homologs**, in accordance with Mendel's second law.
4. Additional shuffling of the genetic material by **crossing over**, which is thought to have evolved as a mechanism for substantially increasing genetic variation, but is, in addition, critical to ensure normal chromosome disjunction.

## HUMAN GAMETOGENESIS AND FERTILIZATION

The human primordial germ cells are recognizable by the fourth week of development outside the embryo proper, in the endoderm of the yolk sac. From there, they migrate during the sixth week to the genital ridges and associate with somatic cells to form the primitive gonads, which soon differentiate into testes or ovaries, depending on the cells' sex chromosome constitution (XY or XX), as we examine in greater detail in Chapter 10. Both spermatogenesis and oogenesis require meiosis but have important differences in detail and timing that may have clinical and genetic consequences for the offspring. Female meiosis is initiated once, early during fetal life, in a limited number of cells. In contrast, male meiosis is initiated continuously in many cells from a dividing cell population, throughout the adult life of a male.

It is difficult to study human meiosis directly. In the female, successive stages of meiosis take place in the fetal ovary, in the oocyte near the time of ovulation, and after fertilization. Although postfertilization stages can be studied in vitro, access to the earlier stages is limited. Testicular material for the study of male meiosis is less difficult to obtain, inasmuch as testicular biopsy is included in the assessment of many men attending infertility clinics. Much remains to be learned about the cytogenetic, biochemical, and

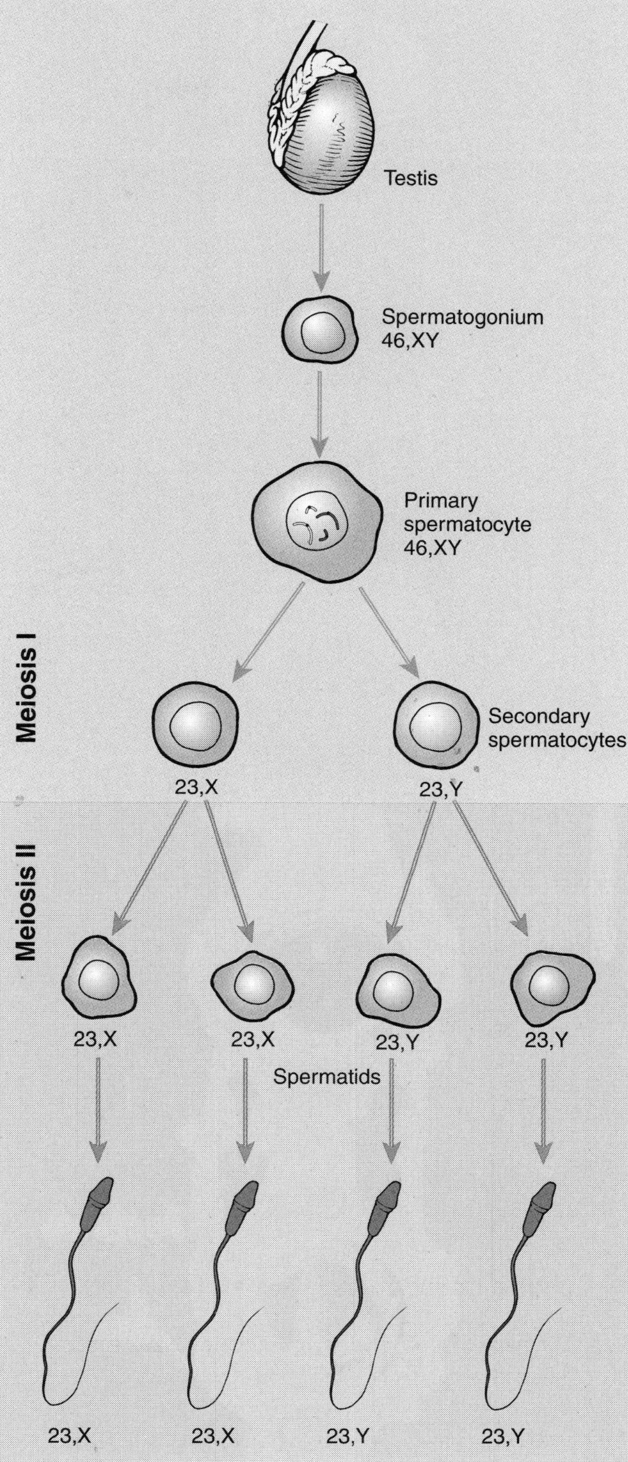


**Figure 2–9.** Diagram to illustrate human spermatogenesis in relation to the two meiotic divisions. The sequence of events begins at puberty and takes about 64 days to complete. The chromosome number (46 or 23) and the sex chromosome constitution (X or Y) of each cell are shown. (Modified from Moore KL and Persaud TVN [1998] The Developing Human: Clinically Oriented Embryology, 6th ed. WB Saunders, Philadelphia.)

molecular mechanisms involved in normal meiosis and about the causes and consequences of meiotic irregularities.

## Spermatogenesis

The stages of spermatogenesis are shown in Figure 2–9. **Sperm** (spermatozoa) are formed in the seminiferous tubules of the testes after sexual maturity is reached. The tubules are lined with **spermatogonia**, which are in different stages of differentiation. These cells have developed from the primordial germ cells by a long series of mitoses. The last cell type in the developmental sequence is the **primary spermatocyte**, which undergoes meiosis I to form two haploid **secondary spermatocytes**. Secondary spermatocytes rapidly undergo meiosis II, each forming two **spermatids**, which

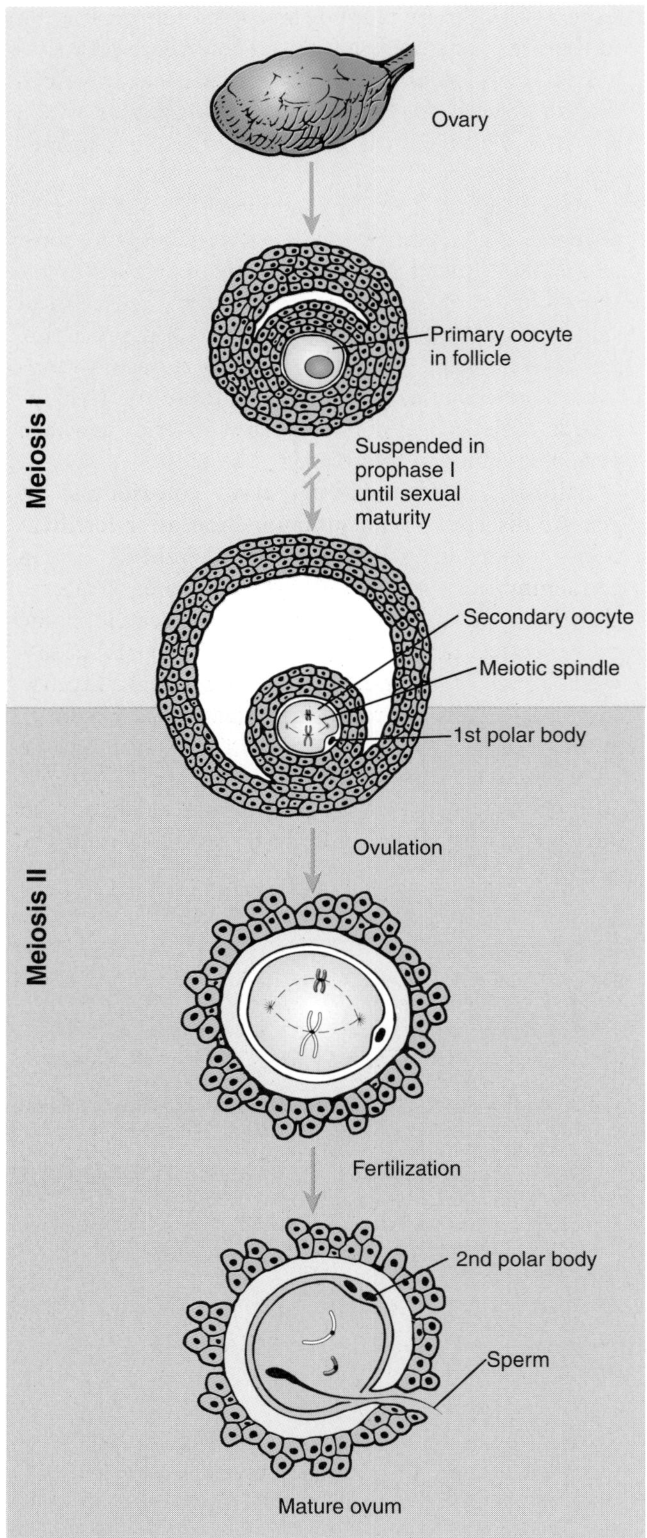


**Figure 2–10.** Diagram to illustrate human oogenesis and fertilization in relation to the two meiotic divisions. The primary oocytes are formed prenatally and they remain suspended in prophase of meiosis I for decades until the onset of puberty. An oocyte completes meiosis I as its follicle matures, resulting in a secondary oocyte and the first polar body. After ovulation, each oocyte continues to metaphase of meiosis II. Meiosis II is completed only if fertilization occurs, resulting in a fertilized mature ovum and the second polar body.

differentiate without further division into **sperm**. In humans, the entire process takes about 64 days. The enormous number of sperm produced, typically about 200 million per ejaculate and an estimated $10^{12}$ in a lifetime, requires several hundred successive mitoses.

## Oogenesis

In contrast to spermatogenesis, which is ongoing throughout adult life, oogenesis is largely confined to prenatal development. The process is shown in Figure 2–10. The ova develop from **oogonia**, cells in the ovarian cortex that have descended from the primordial germ cells by a series of about 30 mitoses. Each oogonium is the central cell in a developing follicle. By about the third month of prenatal development, the oogonia of the embryo have begun to develop into **primary oocytes**, most of which have already entered prophase of meiosis I. The process of oogenesis is not synchronized, and both early and late stages coexist in the fetal ovary. There are about 2.5 million oocytes at the time of birth, but most degenerate, and only about 400 eventually mature. The primary oocytes have all reached prophase I by the time of birth, and those that do not degenerate remain in that stage for decades.

After a woman has reached sexual maturity, each individual follicle matures and ovulation occurs. Each oocyte rapidly completes meiosis I, dividing in such a way that one cell becomes the secondary oocyte (an egg or **ovum**), containing most of the cytoplasm with its organelles, and the other becomes the first polar body (see Fig. 2–10). Meiosis II begins promptly and proceeds to the metaphase stage during ovulation, but it is completed only if fertilization occurs.

### Fertilization

Fertilization of the egg usually takes place in the fallopian tube within a day or so of ovulation. Although very large numbers of sperm may be present, the penetration of a single sperm into the ovum sets up a series of biochemical events that prevent the entry of other sperm.

Fertilization is followed by the completion of meiosis II, with the formation of the second polar body (see Fig. 2–10). The chromosomes of the fertilized egg and sperm become **pronuclei**, each surrounded by a nuclear membrane. The chromosomes of the diploid **zygote** replicate soon after fertilization, and the zygote divides by mitosis to form two diploid daughter cells. This mitosis is the first of the series of cleavage divisions that initiate the process of embryonic development (see Chapter 17).

Although development begins with the formation of the zygote (conception), in clinical medicine, the stage and duration of pregnancy are usually measured as the "menstrual age," dating from the beginning of the mother's last menstrual period, about 14 days before conception.

## MEDICAL RELEVANCE OF MITOSIS AND MEIOSIS

The biological significance of mitosis and meiosis lies in ensuring the constancy of chromosome number from one cell to its progeny and from one generation to the next. The medical relevance of these processes lies in errors of one or the other mechanism of cell division, leading to formation of an individual or of a cell lineage with an abnormal number of chromosomes.

As we see in detail in Chapter 9, meiotic nondisjunction, particularly in oogenesis, is the most common mutational mechanism in our species, responsible for chromosomally abnormal fetuses in at least several percent of all recognized pregnancies. Among pregnancies that survive to term, chromosome abnormalities are a leading cause of developmental defects, failure to thrive in the newborn period, and mental retardation.

Mitotic nondisjunction also contributes to genetic disease. Nondisjunction soon after fertilization, either in the developing embryo or in extraembryonic tissues like the placenta, leads to chromosomal mosaicism that can underlie some medical conditions, such as a proportion of patients with Down syndrome. Further, abnormal chromosome segregation in rapidly dividing tissues, such as in cells of the colon, is frequently a step in the development of chromosomally abnormal tumors, and, thus, evaluation of chromosome balance is an important diagnostic and prognostic test in many cancers.

## *General References*

Handel MA (ed) (1998) Meiosis and Gametogenesis. Academic Press, San Diego.

Moore KL, Persaud TVN (1998) The Developing Human: Clinically Oriented Embryology, 6th ed. WB Saunders, Philadelphia.

Murray A, Hunt T (1993) The Cell Cycle: An Introduction. Oxford University Press, Oxford, England.

Therman E, Susman M (1993) Human Chromosomes: Structure, Behavior, Effects, 3rd ed. Springer-Verlag, New York.

## *Problems*

1. At a certain locus, a person has two alleles $A$ and $a$.
   a) What are the genotypes of this person's gametes?
   b) When do $A$ and $a$ segregate (i) if there is no crossing over between the locus and the centromere of the chromosome? (ii) if there is a single crossover between the locus and the centromere?
2. What is the main cause of numerical chromosome abnormalities in humans?
3. Disregarding crossing over, which increases the amount of genetic variability, estimate the probability that all your chromosomes have come to you from your father's mother and your mother's mother. Would you be male or female?

4. A chromosome entering meiosis is composed of two chromatids, each of which is a single DNA molecule.
   a) In our species, at the end of meiosis I, how many chromosomes are there per cell? How many chromatids?
   b) At the end of meiosis II, how many chromosomes are there per cell? How many chromatids?
   c) When is the diploid chromosome number restored? When is the two-chromatid structure of a typical metaphase chromosome restored?

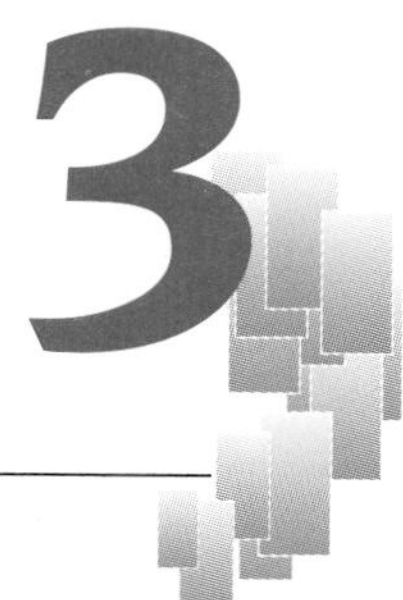

# The Human Genome: Structure and Function of Genes and Chromosomes

Over the past 20 years, remarkable progress has been made in our understanding of the structure and function of genes and chromosomes at the molecular level. More recently, this has been supplemented by an in-depth understanding of the organization of the human genome at the level of its DNA sequence. These advances have come about in large measure through the applications of molecular genetics and genomics to many clinical situations, thereby providing the tools for a distinctive new approach to medical genetics. In this chapter, we present an overview of the organization of the human genome and the aspects of molecular genetics that are required for an understanding of the genetic approach to medicine. This chapter is not intended to provide an extensive description of the wealth of new information about gene structure and regulation. To supplement the information discussed here, Chapter 4 describes many experimental approaches of modern molecular genetics that are becoming critical to the practice and understanding of human and medical genetics.

The increased knowledge of genes, and of their organization in the genome, has had an enormous impact on medicine and on our perception of human physiology. As Nobel laureate Paul Berg stated presciently at the dawn of this new era:

> Just as our present knowledge and practice of medicine relies on a sophisticated knowledge of human anatomy, physiology, and biochemistry, so will dealing with disease in the future demand a detailed understanding of the molecular anatomy, physiology, and biochemistry of the human genome. . . . We shall need a more detailed knowledge of how human genes are organized and how they function and are regulated. We shall also have to have physicians who are as conversant with the molecular anatomy and physiology of chromosomes and genes as the cardiac surgeon is with the structure and workings of the heart.

## DNA STRUCTURE: A BRIEF REVIEW

DNA is a polymeric nucleic acid macromolecule composed of three types of units: a five-carbon sugar, deoxyribose; a nitrogen-containing base; and a phosphate group (Fig. 3–1). The bases are of two types, purines and pyrimidines. In DNA, there are two purine bases, adenine (A) and guanine (G), and two pyrimidine bases, thymine (T) and cytosine (C). Nucleotides, each composed of a base, a phosphate, and a sugar moiety, polymerize into long polynucleotide chains by 5′–3′ phosphodiester bonds formed between adjacent deoxyribose units (Fig. 3–2). In the human genome, these polynucleotide chains (in their double-helix form) are hundreds of millions of nucleotides long, ranging in size from approximately 50 million base pairs (for the smallest chromosome, chromosome 21) to 250 million base pairs (for the largest chromosome, chromosome 1).

The anatomical structure of DNA carries the chemical information that allows the exact transmission of genetic information from one cell to its daughter cells and from one generation to the next. At the same time, the primary structure of DNA specifies the amino acid sequences of the polypeptide chains of proteins, as described later in this chapter. DNA has elegant features that give it these properties. The native state of DNA, as elucidated by James Watson and Francis Crick in 1953, is a double helix (Fig. 3–3). The helical structure resembles a right-handed spiral staircase in which its two polynucleotide chains run in opposite directions, held together by hydrogen bonds between pairs of bases: A of one chain paired with T of the other, and G with C (see Fig. 3–3). Consequently,

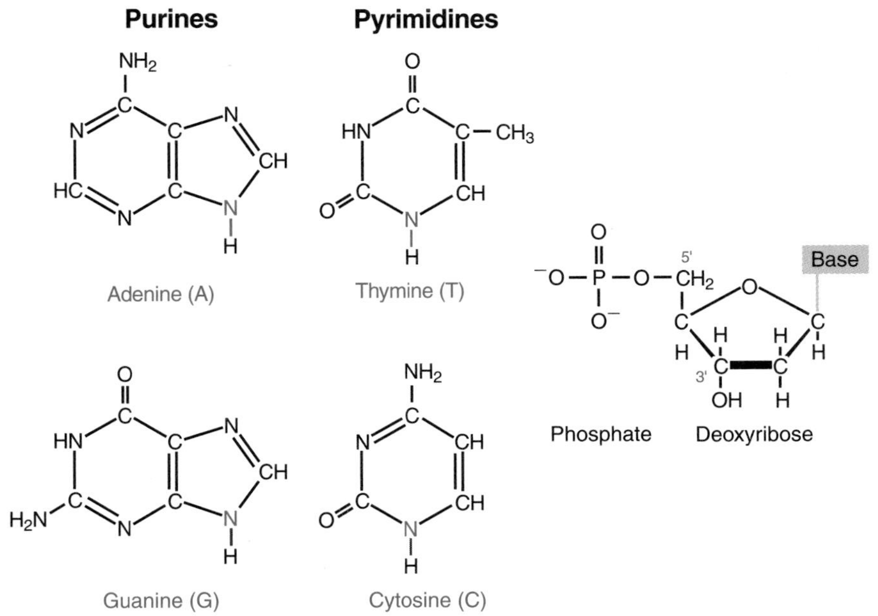

**Figure 3–1.** The four bases of DNA and the general structure of a nucleotide in DNA. Each of the four bases bonds with deoxyribose (through the nitrogen shown in red) and a phosphate group to form the corresponding nucleotides.

knowledge of the sequence of nucleotide bases on one strand automatically allows one to determine the sequence of bases on the other strand. The double-stranded structure of DNA molecules allows them to replicate precisely by separation of the two strands, followed by synthesis of two new complementary strands, in accordance with the sequence of the original template strands (Fig. 3–4). Similarly, when necessary, the base complementarity allows efficient and correct repair of damaged DNA molecules.

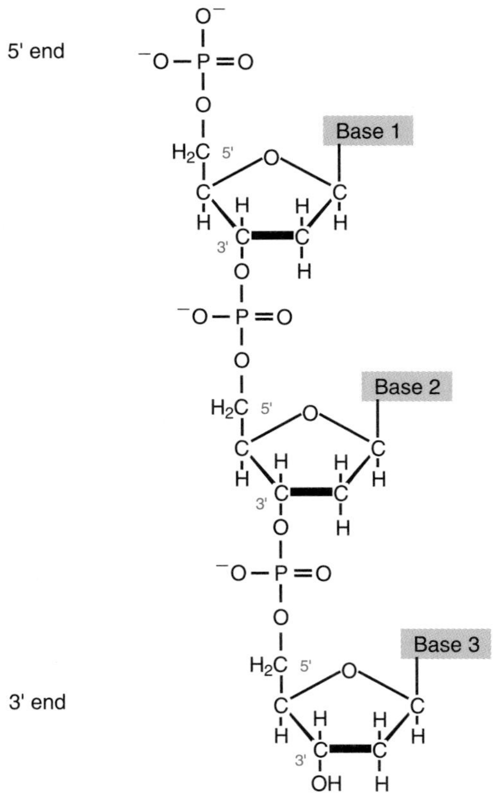

**Figure 3–2.** A portion of a DNA polynucleotide chain, showing the 3′–5′ phosphodiester bonds that link adjacent nucleotides.

## THE CENTRAL DOGMA: DNA → RNA → PROTEIN

Genetic information is contained in DNA in the chromosomes within the cell nucleus, but protein synthesis, during which the information encoded in the DNA is used, takes place in the cytoplasm. This compartmentalization reflects the fact that the human organism is a **eukaryote**. This means that human cells have a genuine nucleus containing the DNA, which is separated by a nuclear membrane from the cytoplasm. In contrast, in prokaryotes like the intestinal bacterium *Escherichia coli*, DNA is not enclosed within a nucleus. Because of the compartmentalization of eukaryotic cells, information transfer from the nucleus to the cytoplasm is a very complex process that has been a focus of attention among molecular and cellular biologists.

The molecular link between these two related types of information (the DNA code of genes and the amino acid code of proteins) is **ribonucleic acid (RNA)**. The chemical structure of RNA is similar to that of DNA, except that each nucleotide in RNA has a ribose sugar component instead of a deoxyribose; in addition, uracil (U) replaces thymine as one of the pyrimidines of RNA (Fig. 3–5). An additional difference between RNA and DNA is that RNA in most organisms exists as a single-stranded molecule, whereas DNA exists as a double helix.

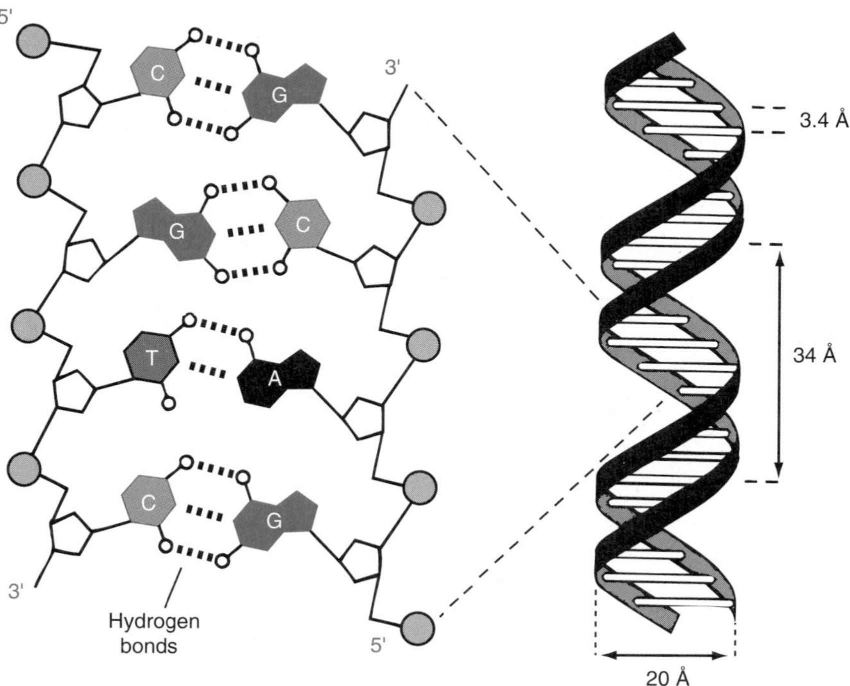


**Figure 3–3.** The structure of DNA. *Left*, A two-dimensional representation of the two complementary strands of DNA, showing the AT and GC base pairs. Note that the orientation of the two strands is antiparallel. *Right*, The double-helix model of DNA, as proposed by Watson and Crick. The horizontal "rungs" represent the paired bases. The helix is said to be right-handed because the strand going from lower left to upper right crosses over the opposite strand. (Based on Watson JD, Crick FHC [1953] Molecular structure of nucleic acids—A structure for deoxyribose nucleic acid. Nature 171:737–738.)

The informational relationships among DNA, RNA, and protein are intertwined: DNA directs the synthesis and sequence of RNA, RNA directs the synthesis and sequence of polypeptides, and specific proteins are involved in the synthesis and metabolism of DNA and RNA. This flow of information is referred to as the "central dogma" of molecular biology.

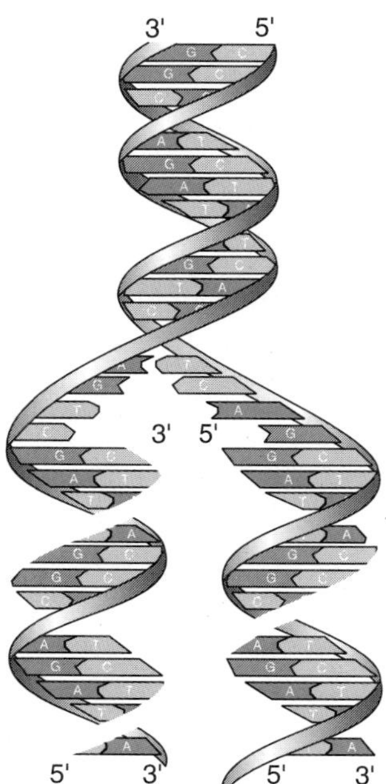


**Figure 3–4.** Replication of a DNA double helix, resulting in two identical daughter molecules, each composed of one parental strand (*black*) and one newly synthesized strand (*red*).

Genetic information is stored in DNA by means of a code (the **genetic code**, discussed later) in which the sequence of adjacent bases ultimately determines the sequence of amino acids in the encoded polypeptide. First, RNA is synthesized from the DNA template through a process known as **transcription**. The RNA, carrying the coded information in a form called **messenger RNA (mRNA)**, is then transported from the nucleus to the cytoplasm, where the RNA sequence is decoded, or translated, to determine the sequence of amino acids in the protein being synthesized. The process of **translation** occurs on **ribosomes**, which are cytoplasmic organelles with binding sites for all of the interacting molecules, including the mRNA, involved in protein synthesis. Ribosomes are themselves made up of many different structural proteins in association with a specialized type of RNA known as **ribosomal RNA (rRNA)**. Translation involves yet a third type of RNA, **transfer RNA (tRNA)**, which provides the molecular link between the coded base sequence of the mRNA and the amino acid sequence of the protein.

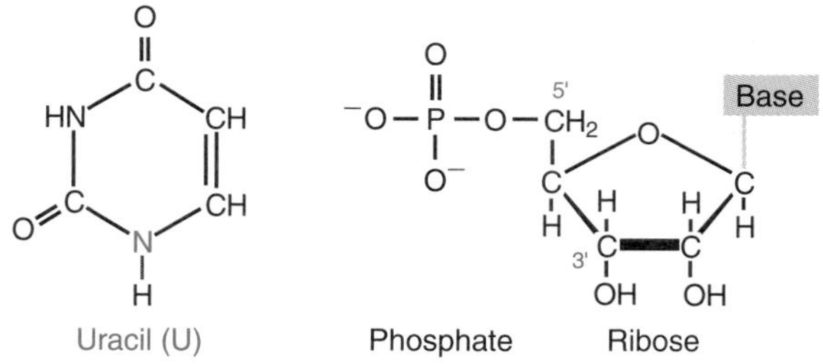


**Figure 3–5.** The pyrimidine uracil and the structure of a nucleotide in RNA. Note that the sugar ribose replaces the sugar deoxyribose of DNA. Compare with Figure 3–1.

Because of the interdependent flow of information represented by the central dogma, one can begin discussion of the molecular genetics of gene expression at any of its three informational levels: DNA, RNA, or protein. We begin by examining the structure of genes as a foundation for discussion of the genetic code, transcription, and translation.

## Gene Structure and Organization

In its simplest form, a gene can be visualized as a segment of a DNA molecule containing the code for the amino acid sequence of a polypeptide chain and the regulatory sequences necessary for expression. This description, however, is inadequate for genes in the human genome (and indeed in most eukaryotic genomes), because few genes exist as continuous coding sequences. Rather, the vast majority of genes are interrupted by one or more noncoding regions. These intervening sequences, called **introns**, are initially transcribed into RNA in the nucleus but are not present in the mature mRNA in the cytoplasm. Thus, information from the intronic sequences is not normally represented in the final protein product. Introns alternate with coding sequences, or **exons**, that ultimately encode the amino acid sequence of the protein (Fig. 3–6). Although a few genes in the human genome

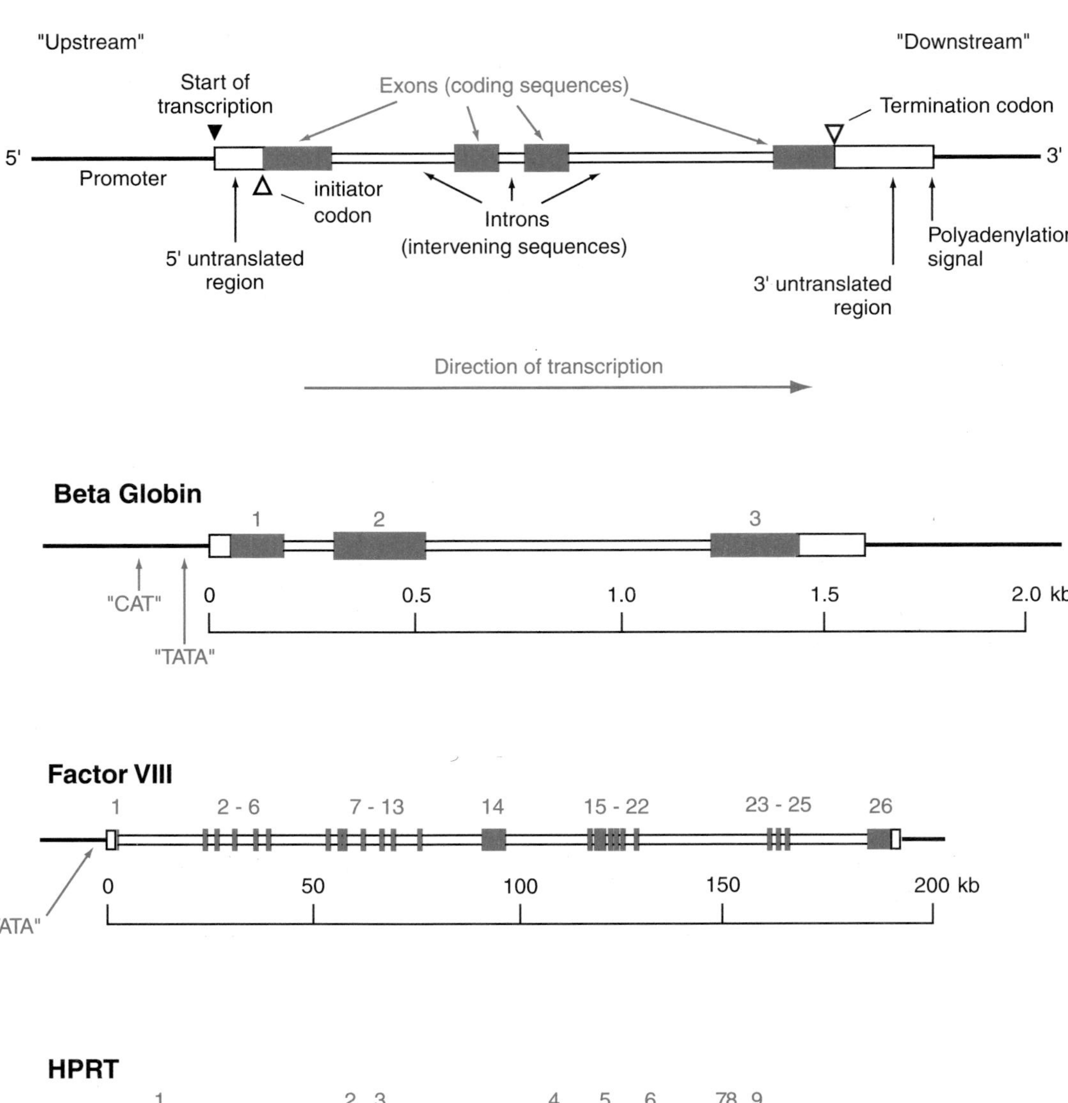


**Figure 3–6.** General structure of a typical human gene. Individual features are labeled in the figure and discussed in the text. Examples of three medically important human genes are presented at the bottom of the figure. Individual exons are numbered. Different mutations in the β-globin gene cause a variety of important hemoglobinopathies. Mutations in the factor VIII gene cause hemophilia A. Mutations in the hypoxanthine phosphoribosyltransferase (*HPRT*) gene lead to Lesch-Nyhan syndrome.

have no introns, most genes contain at least one and usually several introns. Surprisingly, in many genes, the cumulative length of introns makes up a far greater proportion of a gene's total length than do the exons. Whereas some genes are only a few kilobases (kb, where 1 kb = 1000 base pairs) in length, others, like the factor VIII gene shown in Figure 3–6, stretch on for hundreds of kb. There are a few exceptionally large genes, including the X-linked dystrophin gene (mutations in which lead to Duchenne muscular dystrophy) that spans more than 2 million base pairs (2000 kb), of which less than 1 percent consists of coding exons.

## Structural Features of a Typical Human Gene

A schematic representation of a portion of chromosomal DNA containing a typical gene is shown in Figure 3–6, along with the structure of several medically relevant genes. Together, they illustrate the range of features that characterize human genes. In Chapters 1 and 2, we briefly defined "gene" in general terms. At this point, we can provide a molecular definition of a gene. In typical circumstances, we define a gene as *a sequence of chromosomal DNA that is required for production of a functional product*, be it a polypeptide or a functional RNA molecule. As is clear from Figure 3–6, a gene includes not only the actual coding sequences but also adjacent nucleotide sequences required for the proper expression of the gene—that is, for the production of a normal mRNA molecule, in the correct amount, in the correct place, and at the correct time during development or during the cell cycle.

The adjacent nucleotide sequences provide the molecular "start" and "stop" signals for the synthesis of mRNA transcribed from the gene. At the 5′ end of the gene lies a **promoter** region, which includes sequences responsible for the proper initiation of transcription. Within the 5′ region are several DNA elements whose sequence is conserved among many different genes. This conservation, together with functional studies of gene expression in many laboratories, indicates that these particular sequence elements play an important role in regulation. There are several different types of promoter found in the human genome, with different regulatory properties that specify the developmental patterns, as well as the levels of expression, of a particular gene in different tissues. The roles of individual conserved promoter elements, identified in Figure 3–6, are discussed in greater detail in the section on "Fundamentals of Gene Expression." Both promoters and other regulatory elements (located either 5′ or 3′ of a gene or in its introns) can be sites of mutation in genetic disease that can interfere with the normal expression of a gene. These regulatory elements, including **enhancers, silencers**, and **locus control regions** (LCRs), are discussed more fully later in this chapter.

At the 3′ end of the gene lies an untranslated region of importance that contains a signal for addition of a sequence of adenosine residues (the so-called polyA tail) to the end of the mature mRNA. Although it is generally accepted that such closely neighboring regulatory sequences are part of what is called a "gene," the precise dimensions of any particular gene will remain somewhat uncertain until the potential functions of more distant sequences are fully characterized.

## Gene Families

Many genes belong to families of closely related DNA sequences, recognized as families because of similarity of the nucleotide sequence of the genes themselves or of the amino acid sequence of the encoded polypeptides.

One small, but medically important gene family is composed of genes that encode the protein chains found in hemoglobins. The α-globin and β-globin gene clusters, on chromosomes 16 and 11, respectively, are shown in Figure 3–7 and are believed to have arisen by duplication of a primitive precursor gene about 500 million years ago. These two clusters contain genes coding for closely related globin chains expressed at different developmental stages, from embryo to adult. The individual genes within each cluster are more similar in sequence to one another

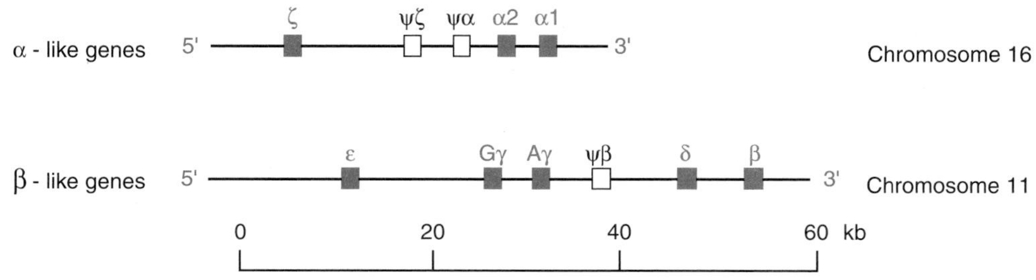


**Figure 3–7.** Chromosomal organization of the two clusters of human globin genes. Functional genes are indicated in red. Pseudogenes are indicated by the open boxes. (Redrawn from Nienhuis AW, Maniatis T [1987] Structure and expression of globin genes in erythroid cells. *In* Stamatoyannopoulos G, Nienhuis AW, Leder P, Majerus PW [eds] The Molecular Basis of Blood Diseases. WB Saunders, Philadelphia, pp. 28–65.)

than to genes in the other cluster; thus, each cluster is believed to have evolved by a series of sequential gene duplication events within the past 100 million years. The exon-intron patterns of the globin genes appear to have been remarkably conserved during evolution; each of the functional globin genes shown in Figure 3–7 has two introns at similar locations, although the sequences contained within the introns have accumulated far more nucleotide base changes over time than have the coding sequences of each gene. The control of expression of the various globin genes, in the normal state as well as in the many inherited hemoglobinopathies, is considered in more detail both later in this chapter and in Chapter 11.

Several of the globin genes do not produce any RNA or protein product and therefore are unlikely to have any function. DNA sequences that closely resemble known genes but are nonfunctional are called **pseudogenes**. Pseudogenes are widespread in the genome and are thought to be byproducts of evolution, representing genes that were once functional but are now vestigial, having been inactivated by mutations in coding or regulatory sequences. In some cases, as in the pseudo-α-globin and pseudo-β-globin genes, the pseudogenes presumably arose through gene duplication, followed by the introduction of numerous mutations into the extra copies of the once-functional gene. In other cases, pseudogenes have been formed by a process, called **retrotransposition**, that involves transcription, generation of a DNA copy of the mRNA, and, finally, integration of such DNA copies back into the genome. Pseudogenes created by retrotransposition lack introns and are called **processed pseudogenes**. They are not necessarily or usually on the same chromosome (or chromosomal region) as their progenitor gene.

The largest known gene family in the human genome is the so-called **immunoglobulin superfamily**, which includes many hundreds of genes involved in cell surface recognition events in the immune and nervous system, such as genes on chromosomes 2, 14, and 22 that encode the immunoglobulin heavy and light chains themselves; genes on chromosome 6 that make up the major histocompatibility complex; genes on chromosomes 7 and 14 whose products make up the T-cell receptor; and genes that are expressed primarily in neural tissues, such as genes for cell adhesion molecules or for myelin-associated glycoproteins. The structure and function of many of these genes are examined in detail in Chapter 14.

## FUNDAMENTALS OF GENE EXPRESSION

The flow of information from gene to polypeptide involves several steps (Fig. 3–8). Initiation of transcription of a gene is under the influence of promoters and other regulatory elements, as well as specific proteins known as **transcription factors** that interact with specific sequences within these regions. Transcription of a gene is initiated at the transcriptional "start site" on chromosomal DNA just upstream from the coding sequences and continues along the chromosome, for anywhere from several hundred base pairs to more than a million base pairs, through both introns and exons and past the end of the coding sequences. After modification at both the 5′ and 3′ ends of the primary RNA transcript, the portions corresponding to introns are removed, and the segments corresponding to exons are spliced together. After RNA splicing, the resulting mRNA (now colinear with only the coding portions of the gene) is transported from the nucleus to the cytoplasm, where the mRNA is finally translated into the amino acid sequence of the encoded polypeptide. Each of the steps in this complex pathway is prone to error, and mutations that interfere with the individual steps have been implicated in a number of inherited genetic disorders (see Chapters 5, 11, and 12).

### Transcription

Transcription of protein-coding genes by RNA polymerase II (one of several classes of RNA polymerases) is initiated upstream from the first coding sequence at the transcriptional start site, the point corresponding to the 5′ end of the final RNA product (see Figs. 3–6 and 3–8). Synthesis of the primary RNA transcript proceeds in a 5′-to-3′ direction, whereas the strand of the gene being transcribed is actually read in a 3′-to-5′ direction with respect to the direction of the deoxyribose phosphodiester backbone (see Fig. 3–2). Because the RNA synthesized corresponds both in polarity and in base sequence (substituting U for T) to the 5′-to-3′ strand of DNA, this nontranscribed DNA strand is sometimes called the "coding," or "**sense**," DNA strand. The 3′-to-5′ transcribed strand of DNA is then referred to as the "noncoding," or "**antisense**," strand. Transcription continues through both intron and exon portions of the gene, beyond the position on the chromosome that eventually corresponds to the 3′ end of the mature mRNA. Whether transcription ends at a predetermined 3′ termination point is unknown.

The primary RNA transcript is processed by addition of a chemical "cap" structure to the 5′ end of the RNA and cleavage of the 3′ end at a specific point downstream from the end of the coding information. This cleavage is followed by addition of a polyA tail to the 3′ end of the RNA; the polyA tail appears to increase the stability of the resulting polyadenylated RNA. The location of the polyadenylation point is specified in part by the sequence AAUAAA (or a variant of this), usually found in the 3′ untranslated

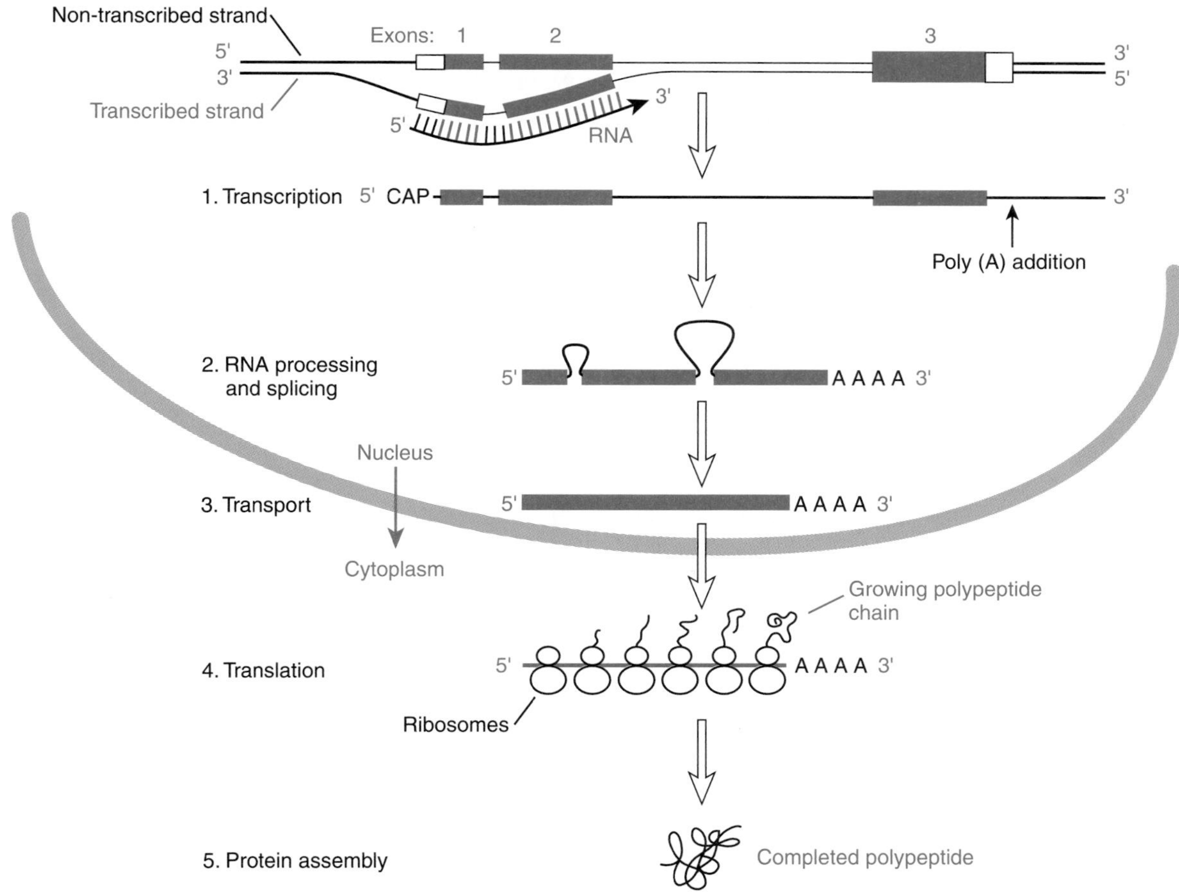


**Figure 3–8.** Flow of information from DNA to RNA to protein for a hypothetical gene with three exons and two introns. Steps include transcription, RNA processing and splicing, RNA transport from the nucleus to the cytoplasm, and translation.

portion of the RNA transcript. These post-transcriptional modifications take place in the nucleus, as does the process of RNA splicing. The fully processed RNA, now called mRNA, is then transported to the cytoplasm, where translation takes place (see Fig. 3–8).

## Translation and the Genetic Code

In the cytoplasm, mRNA is translated into protein by the action of a variety of tRNA molecules, each specific for a particular amino acid. These remarkable molecules, each only 70 to 100 nucleotides long, have the job of transferring the correct amino acids to their positions along the mRNA template, to be added to the growing polypeptide chain. Protein synthesis occurs on ribosomes, macromolecular complexes made up of rRNA (encoded by the 18S and 28S rRNA genes) and several dozen ribosomal proteins (see Fig. 3–8).

The key to translation is a code that relates specific amino acids to combinations of three adjacent bases along the mRNA. Each set of three bases constitutes a **codon**, specific for a particular amino acid (Table 3–1). In theory, almost infinite variations are possible in the arrangement of the bases along a polynucleotide chain. At any one position, there are four possibilities (A, T, C, or G); thus, there are $4^n$ possible combinations in a sequence of $n$ bases. For three bases, there are $4^3$, or 64, possible triplet combinations. These 64 codons constitute the **genetic code**.

Because there are only 20 amino acids and 64 possible codons, most amino acids are specified by more than one codon; hence the code is said to be **degenerate**. For instance, the base in the third position of the triplet can often be either purine (A or G) or either pyrimidine (T or C) or, in some cases, any one of the four bases, without altering the coded message (see Table 3–1). Leucine and arginine are each specified by six codons. Only methionine and tryptophan are each specified by a single, unique codon. Three of the codons are called **stop** (or **nonsense**) **codons** because they designate termination of translation of the mRNA at that point.

Translation of a processed mRNA is always initiated at a codon specifying methionine. Methionine is therefore the first encoded (amino-terminal) amino acid of each polypeptide chain, although it is usually removed before protein synthesis is completed. The

TABLE 3–1

**The Genetic Code**

| First Base | Second Base: U | | C | | A | | G | | Third Base |
|---|---|---|---|---|---|---|---|---|---|
| U | UUU | phe | UCU | ser | UAU | tyr | UGU | cys | U |
| | UUC | phe | UCC | ser | UAC | tyr | UGC | cys | C |
| | UUA | leu | UCA | ser | UAA | stop | UGA | stop | A |
| | UUG | leu | UCG | ser | UAG | stop | UGG | trp | G |
| C | CUU | leu | CCU | pro | CAU | his | CGU | arg | U |
| | CUC | leu | CCC | pro | CAC | his | CGC | arg | C |
| | CUA | leu | CCA | pro | CAA | gln | CGA | arg | A |
| | CUG | leu | CCG | pro | CAG | gln | CGG | arg | G |
| A | AUU | ile | ACU | thr | AAU | asn | AGU | ser | U |
| | AUC | ile | ACC | thr | AAC | asn | AGC | ser | C |
| | AUA | ile | ACA | thr | AAA | lys | AGA | arg | A |
| | AUG | met | ACG | thr | AAG | lys | AGG | arg | G |
| G | GUU | val | GCU | ala | GAU | asp | GGU | gly | U |
| | GUC | val | GCC | ala | GAC | asp | GGC | gly | C |
| | GUA | val | GCA | ala | GAA | glu | GGA | gly | A |
| | GUG | val | GCG | ala | GAG | glu | GGG | gly | G |

Abbreviations for amino acids:

| | | | |
|---|---|---|---|
| ala (A) | alanine | leu (L) | leucine |
| arg (R) | arginine | lys (K) | lysine |
| asn (N) | asparagine | met (M) | methionine |
| asp (D) | aspartic acid | phe (F) | phenylalanine |
| cys (C) | cysteine | pro (P) | proline |
| gln (Q) | glutamine | ser (S) | serine |
| glu (E) | glutamic acid | thr (T) | threonine |
| gly (G) | glycine | trp (W) | tryptophan |
| his (H) | histidine | tyr (Y) | tyrosine |
| ile (I) | isoleucine | val (V) | valine |

Other abbreviation:

stop — termination codon

Codons are shown in terms of messenger RNA, which are complementary to the corresponding DNA codons.

codon for methionine (the initiator codon, AUG) establishes the **reading frame** of the mRNA; each subsequent codon is read in turn to predict the amino acid sequence of the protein.

The molecular links between codons and amino acids are the specific tRNA molecules. A particular site on each tRNA forms a three-base **anticodon** that is complementary to a specific codon on the mRNA. Bonding between the codon and anticodon brings the appropriate amino acid into the next position on the ribosome for attachment by formation of a peptide bond to the carboxyl end of the growing polypeptide chain. The ribosome then slides along the mRNA exactly three bases, bringing the next codon into line for recognition by another tRNA with the next amino acid. Thus, proteins are synthesized from the amino terminus to the carboxyl terminus, which corresponds to translation of the mRNA in a 5′-to-3′ direction.

As mentioned earlier, translation ends when a stop codon (UGA, UAA, or UAG) is encountered in the same reading frame as the initiator codon. (Stop codons in either of the other two, unused reading frames are not read and therefore have no effect on translation.) The completed polypeptide is then released from the ribosome, which becomes available to begin synthesis of another protein.

## Post-Translational Processing

Many proteins undergo extensive post-translational modifications. The polypeptide chain that is the primary translation product is folded and bonded into a specific three-dimensional structure that is determined by the amino acid sequence itself. Two or more polypeptide chains, products of the same gene or of different genes, may combine to form a single mature protein complex. For example, two α-globin chains and two β-globin chains associate noncovalently to form the tetrameric $\alpha_2\beta_2$ hemoglobin molecule. The protein products may also be modified chemically by, for example, addition of phosphate or carbohydrates at specific sites. Other modifications may involve cleavage of the protein, either to remove specific amino-terminal sequences after they have functioned to direct a protein to its correct location within the cell (e.g., proteins that function within the nucleus or mitochondria) or to split the molecule into smaller polypeptide chains. For example, the two chains that make up mature insulin, one 21 and the other 30 amino acids long, are originally part of an 82 amino-acid primary translation product, called proinsulin.

## Gene Expression in Action: The Beta-Globin Gene

The flow of information outlined in the preceding sections can best be appreciated by reference to a particular well-studied gene, the β-globin gene. The β-globin chain is a 146 amino-acid polypeptide, encoded by a gene that occupies approximately 1.6 kb on the short arm of chromosome 11. The gene has three exons and two introns (see Fig. 3–6). The β-globin gene, as well as the other genes in the β-globin cluster (see Fig. 3–7), is transcribed in a centromere-to-telomere direction. This orientation, however, is different for other genes in the genome and depends on which strand of the chromosomal double helix is the coding strand for a particular gene.

DNA sequences required for accurate initiation of transcription of the β-globin gene are located in the promoter within approximately 200 base pairs upstream from the transcription start site. The double-stranded DNA sequence of this region of the β-globin gene, the corresponding RNA sequence, and the translated sequence of the first 10 amino acids are depicted in Figure 3–9 to illustrate the relationships among these three information levels. As mentioned previously, it is the 3′-to-5′ strand of the DNA that serves as template and is actually transcribed, but it is the 5′-to-3′ strand of DNA that most directly corresponds to the 5′-to-3′ sequence of the mRNA (and, in fact, is identical to it except that U is substituted for T). Because of this correspondence, the 5′-to-3′ DNA strand of a gene (i.e., the strand that is *not* transcribed) is the strand generally reported in the scientific literature or in databases.

In accordance with this convention, the complete sequence of approximately 2.0 kb of chromosome 11 that includes the β-globin gene is shown in Figure 3–10. (It is sobering to reflect that this page of nucleotides represents only 0.000067 percent of the sequence of the entire human genome!) Within these 2.0 kb are contained most, but not all, of the sequence elements required to encode and regulate the expression of this gene. Indicated in Figure 3–10 are many of the important structural features of the β-globin gene, including conserved promoter sequence elements, intron and exon boundaries, RNA splice sites, the initiator and termination codons, and the polyadenylation signal, all of which are known to be mutated in various inherited defects of the β-globin gene (see Chapter 11).

### Initiation of Transcription

The β-globin promoter, like many other gene promoters, consists of a series of relatively short functional elements that are thought to interact with specific proteins (generically called **transcription factors**) that regulate transcription, including, in the case of the globin genes, those proteins that restrict expression of these genes to erythroid cells, the cells in which hemoglobin is produced. One important promoter sequence is the "TATA box," a conserved region rich in adenines and thymines that is approximately 25 to 30 base pairs upstream of the start site of transcription (see Figs. 3–6 and 3–10). The TATA box appears to be important for determining the position of the start of transcription, which in the β-globin gene is approximately 50 base pairs upstream from the translation initiation site (see Fig. 3–9). Thus, in this gene there are about 50 base pairs of sequence that are transcribed but are not translated. In other genes, this 5′ transcribed but untranslated region (called the 5′ UTR) can be much longer and can, in fact, be interrupted by one or more introns. A second conserved region, the so-called CAT box (actually CCAAT), is a few dozen base pairs farther upstream (see Fig. 3–10). Both experimentally

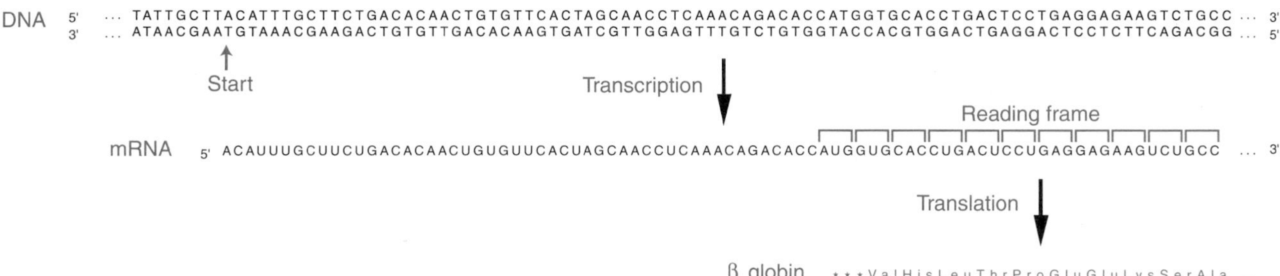


**Figure 3–9.** Structure and nucleotide sequence of the 5′ end of the human β-globin gene on the short arm of chromosome 11. Transcription of the 3′- to-5′ (*lower*) strand begins at the indicated start size to produce β-globin mRNA. The translational reading frame is determined by the AUG initiator codon (***); subsequent codons specifying amino acids are indicated in red. The other two potential frames are not used.

```
          5'....agccacaccctagggttggccaatctactcccaggagcagggagggcaggagccagggctgggcataaaa
                                                                                    ***
          gtcagggcagagccatctattgcttACATTTGCTTCTGACACAACTGTGTTCACTAGCAACCTCAAACAGACACCATG

          ValHisLeuThrProGluGluLysSerAlaValThrAlaLeuTrpGlyLysValAsnValAspGluValGlyGlyGlu
Exon 1    GTGCACCTGACTCCTGAGGAGAAGTCTGCCGTTACTGCCCTGTGGGGCAAGGTGAACGTGGATGAAGTTGGTGGTGAG

          AlaLeuGlyAr-
          GCCCTGGGCAGgttggtatcaaggttacaagacaggtttaaggagaccaatagaaactgggcatgtggagacagagaag

                                                                       -gLeuLeuValValTyr
Intron 1  actcttgggtttctgataggcactgactctctctgcctattggtctattttcccacccttagGCTGCTGGTGGTCTAC

          ProTrpThrGlnArgPhePheGluSerPheGlyAspLeuSerThrProAspAlaValMetGlyAsnProLysValLys
          CCTTGGACCCAGAGGTTCTTTGAGTCCTTTGGGGATCTGTCCACTCCTGATGCTGTTATGGGCAACCCTAAGGTGAAG
Exon 2
          AlaHisGlyLysLysValLeuGlyAlaPheSerAspGlyLeuAlaHisLeuAspAsnLeuLysGlyThrPheAlaThr
          GCTCATGGCAAGAAAGTGCTCGGTGCCTTTAGTGATGGCCTGGCTCACCTGGACAACCTCAAGGGCACCTTTGCCACA

          LeuSerGluLeuHisCysAspLysLeuHisValAspProGluAsnPheArg
          CTGAGTGAGCTGCACTGTGACAAGCTGCACGTGGATCCTGAGAACTTCAGGgtgagtctatgggacccttgatgtttt

          ctttccccttcttttctatggttaagttcatgtcataggaaggggagaagtaacagggtacagtttagaatgggaaac

          agacgaatgattgcatcagtgtggaagtctcaggatcgttttagtttcttttatttgctgttcataacaattgttttc

          ttttgtttaattcttgctttctttttttttcttctccgcaatttttactattatacttaatgccttaacattgtgtat

Intron 2  aacaaaaggaaatatctctgagatacattaagtaacttaaaaaaaaactttacacagtctgcctagtacattactatt

          tggaatatatgtgtgcttatttgcatattcataatgtccctactttattttcttttatttttaattgatacataatca

          ttatacatatttatgggttaaagtgtaatgttttaatatgtgtacacatattgaccaaatcagggtaattttgcatt

          tgtaattttaaaaaatgctttcttcttttaatatacttttttgtttatcttatttctaatactttccctaatctcttt

          ctttcagggcaataatgatacaatgtatcatgcctctttgcaccattctaaagaataacagtgataatttctgggtta

          aggcaatagcaatatttctgcatataaatatttctgcatataaattgtaactgatgtaagaggtttcatattgctaa

          tagcagctacaatccagctaccattctgcttttattttatggttgggataaggctggattattctgagtccaagctag

                                                      LeuLeuGlyAsnValLeuValCysValLeuAla
          gccctttgctaatcatgttcatacctcttatcttcctcccacagCTCCTGGGCAACGTGCTGGTCTGTGTGCTGGCC

          HisHisPheGlyLysGluPheThrProProValGlnAlaAlaTryGlnLysValValAlaGlyValAlaAsnAlaLeu
Exon 3    CATCACTTTGGCAAAGAATTCACCCCACCAGTGCAGGCTGCCTATCAGAAAGTGGTGGCTGGTGTGGCTAATGCCCTG

          AlaHisLysTyrHisTer
          GCCCACAAGTATCACTAAGCTCGCTTTCTTGCTGTCCAATTTCTATTAAAGGTTCCTTTGTTCCCTAAGTCCAACTAC

          TAAACTGGGGGATATTATGAAGGGCCTTGAGCATCTGGATTCTGCCTAATAAAAAACATTTATTTTCATTGCaatgat

          gtatttaaattatttctgaatattttactaaaaagggaatgtgggaggtcagtgcatttaaaacataaagaaatgatg

          agctgttcaaaccttgggaaaatacactatatcttaaactccatgaaagaaggtgaggctgcaaccagctaatgcaca

          ttggcaacagcccctgatgcctatgccttattcatccctcagaaaaggattcttgtagaggcttga....   3'
```

**Figure 3–10.** Nucleotide sequence of the complete human β-globin gene. The sequence of the 5′-to-3′ strand of the gene is shown. Capital letters represent sequences corresponding to mature mRNA. Lowercase letters indicate introns and flanking sequences. The CAT and TATA box sequences in the 5′ flanking region are boxed. The ATG initiator codon (AUG in mRNA) and the TAA stop codon (UAA in mRNA) are shown in red. The amino-acid sequence of β-globin is shown above the coding sequence; the three-letter abbreviations in Table 3–1 are used here. The GT and AG dinucleotides important for RNA splicing at the intron/exon junctions are boxed. (From Lawn RM, Efstratiadis A, O'Connell C, et al [1980] The nucleotide sequence of the human β-globin gene. Cell 21: 647–651.)

induced and naturally occurring mutations in either of these sequence elements, as well as in other regulatory sequences even farther upstream, lead to a sharp reduction in the level of transcription, thereby demonstrating the importance of these elements for normal gene expression. Many mutations in these regulatory elements have been identified in patients with the disorder β-thalassemia (see Chapter 11).

Not all gene promoters contain the two specific elements described. In particular, genes that are constitutively expressed in most or all tissues (called "housekeeping" genes) often lack the CAT and TATA boxes that are more typical of tissue-specific genes. Promoters of many housekeeping genes often contain a high proportion of cytosines and guanines in relation to the surrounding DNA (see the promoter of the hypoxanthine phosphoribosyltransferase gene in Fig. 3–6). Such CG-rich promoters are often located in regions of the genome called **CG** (or **CpG**) **islands**, so named because of the unusually high concentration of the dinucleotide 5′-CG-3′ that stands out from the more general AT-rich chromosomal landscape. Some of the CG-rich sequence elements found in these promoters are thought to serve as binding sites for specific transcription factors.

In addition to the sequences that constitute a promoter itself, there are other sequence elements that can markedly alter the efficiency of transcription. The best characterized of these "activating" sequences are called **enhancers**. Enhancers are sequence elements that can act at a distance (often several kb) from a gene to stimulate transcription. Unlike promoters, enhancers are both position- and orientation-independent and can be located either 5′ or 3′ of the transcription start site. Enhancer elements function only in certain cell types and thus appear to be involved in establishing the tissue specificity and/or level of expression of many genes, in concert with one or more transcription factors. In the case of the β-globin gene, several tissue-specific enhancers are present within both the gene itself and in its flanking regions. The interaction of enhancers with particular proteins leads to increased levels of transcription.

Normal expression of the β-globin gene during development also requires more distant sequences called the **locus control region (LCR)**, located upstream of the ε-globin gene (see Fig. 3–7), which is required for appropriate high-level expression. As expected, mutations that disrupt or delete either enhancer or LCR sequences interfere with or prevent β-globin gene expression (see Chapter 11).

### RNA Splicing

The primary RNA transcript of the β-globin gene contains two exons, approximately 100 and 850 base pairs in length, that need to be spliced together. The process is exact and highly efficient; 95 percent of β-globin transcripts are thought to be accurately spliced to yield functional globin mRNA. The splicing reactions are guided by specific DNA sequences at both the 5′ and the 3′ ends of introns. The 5′ sequence consists of nine nucleotides, of which two (the dinucleotide GT located in the intron immediately adjacent to the splice site) are virtually invariant among splice sites in different genes (see Fig. 3–10). The 3′ sequence consists of about a dozen nucleotides, of which, again, two, the AG located immediately 5′ to the intron/exon boundary, are obligatory for normal splicing. The splice sites themselves are unrelated to the reading frame of the particular mRNA. In some instances, as in the case of intron 1 of the β-globin gene, the intron actually splits a specific codon (see Fig. 3–10).

The medical significance of RNA splicing is illustrated by the fact that mutations within the conserved sequences at the intron/exon boundaries commonly impair RNA splicing, with a concomitant reduction in the amount of normal, mature β-globin mRNA; mutations in the GT or AG dinucleotides mentioned earlier invariably eliminate normal splicing of the intron containing the mutation. A number of splice site mutations, identified in patients with β-thalassemia, are discussed in detail in Chapter 11.

### Polyadenylation

The mature β-globin mRNA contains approximately 130 base pairs of 3′ untranslated material (the 3′ UTR) between the stop codon and the location of the polyA tail (see Fig. 3–10). As in other genes, cleavage of the 3′ end of the mRNA and addition of the polyA tail is controlled, at least in part, by an AAUAAA sequence approximately 20 base pairs before the polyadenylation site. Mutations in this polyadenylation signal in patients with β-thalassemia (as well as mutations in the corresponding polyadenylation signal in the α-globin gene in patients with α-thalassemia) document the importance of this signal for proper 3′ cleavage and polyadenylation (see Chapter 11). The 3′ untranslated region of some genes can be quite long, up to several kb. Other genes have a number of alternative polyadenylation sites, selection among which may influence the stability of the resulting mRNA and thus the steady-state level of each mRNA.

## STRUCTURE OF HUMAN CHROMOSOMES

The composition of genes in the human genome, as well as the determinants of their expression, is specified in the DNA of the 46 human chromosomes. As we saw in an earlier section, *each human chromosome is believed to consist of a single, continuous DNA double helix*; that is, each chromosome in the nucleus is a long, linear double-stranded DNA molecule. Chromosomes are not naked DNA double helices, however. The DNA molecule of a chromosome exists as a complex with a family of basic chromosomal proteins called histones and with a heterogeneous group of acidic, nonhistone proteins that are much less well characterized, but that appear to be critical for establishing a proper environment to ensure normal chromosome behavior and appropriate gene expression. Together, this complex of DNA and protein is called **chromatin**.

There are five major types of histones that play a critical role in the proper packaging of the chromatin fiber. Two copies each of the four core histones H2A, H2B, H3, and H4 constitute an octamer, around which a segment of DNA double helix winds, like thread around a spool (Fig. 3–11). Approximately 140 base pairs of DNA are associated with each histone core, making just under two turns around the octamer. After a short (20 to 60 base-pair) "spacer" segment of DNA, the next core DNA complex forms, and so on, giving chromatin the appearance of beads on a string. Each complex of DNA with core histones is called a **nucleosome**, which is the basic structural unit of chromatin. The fifth histone, H1, appears to bind to DNA at the edge of each nucleosome, in the internucleosomal spacer region. The amount of DNA associated with a core nucleosome, together with the spacer region, is about 200 base pairs.

During the cell cycle, as we saw in Chapter 2, chromosomes pass through orderly stages of condensation and decondensation (see Fig. 2–5). In the interphase nucleus, chromosomes and chromatin are quite decondensed in relation to the highly condensed state of chromatin in metaphase. Nonetheless, even in interphase chromosomes, DNA in chromatin is substantially more condensed than it would be as a native, protein-free double helix.

The long strings of nucleosomes are themselves further compacted into a secondary helical chromatin structure that appears under the electron microscope as a thick, 30-nm-diameter fiber (about three times thicker than the nucleosomal fiber) (see Fig. 3–11). This cylindrical "solenoid" fiber (from the Greek *solenoeides*, "pipe-shaped") appears to be the fundamental unit of chromatin organization. The solenoids are themselves packed into **loops** or domains attached at intervals of about 100 kb or so to a nonhistone protein **scaffold** or matrix. It has been speculated that loops are, in fact, functional units of DNA replication or gene transcription, or both, and that the attachment points of each loop are fixed along the chromosomal DNA. Thus, one level of control of gene expression may depend on how DNA and genes are packaged into chromosomes and on their association with chromatin proteins in the packaging process.

The various hierarchical levels of packaging seen in an interphase chromosome are illustrated schematically in Figure 3–11. The enormous amount of DNA packaged into a chromosome can be appreciated when chromosomes are treated to remove most of the chromatin proteins in order to observe the protein scaffold (Fig. 3–12). When DNA is released from chromosomes treated this way, long loops of DNA can be visualized, and the residual scaffolding can be seen to reproduce the outline of a typical metaphase chromosome.

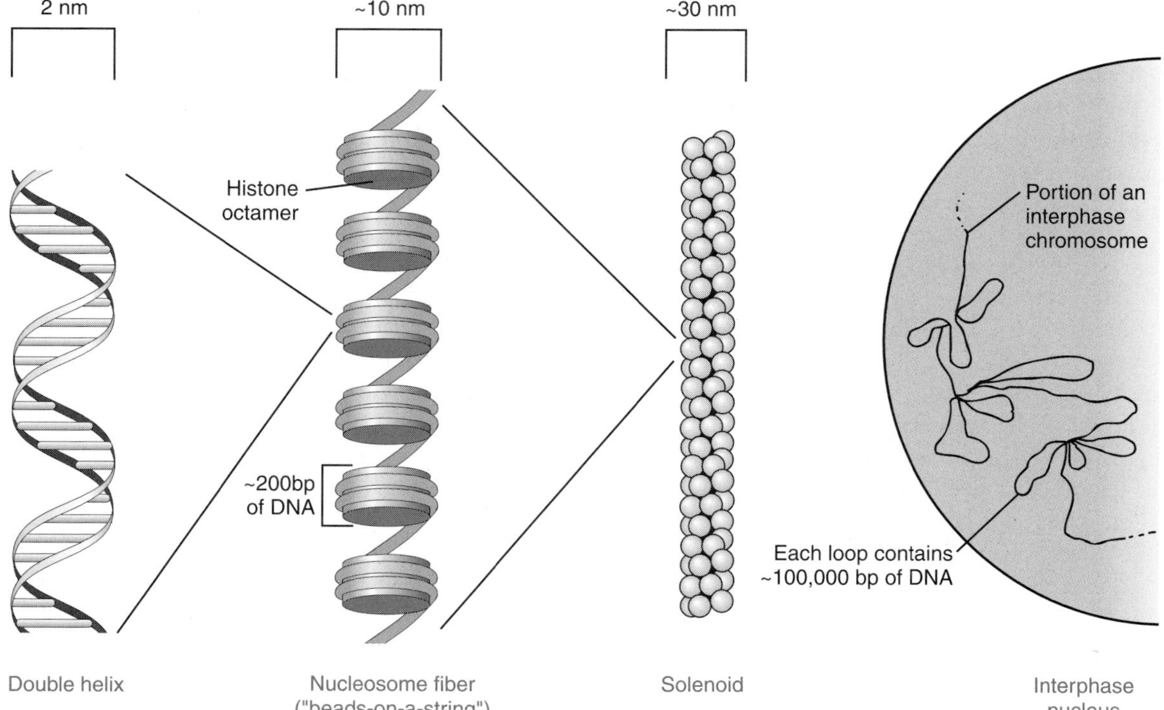


**Figure 3–11.** Hierarchical levels of chromatin packaging in a human chromosome.

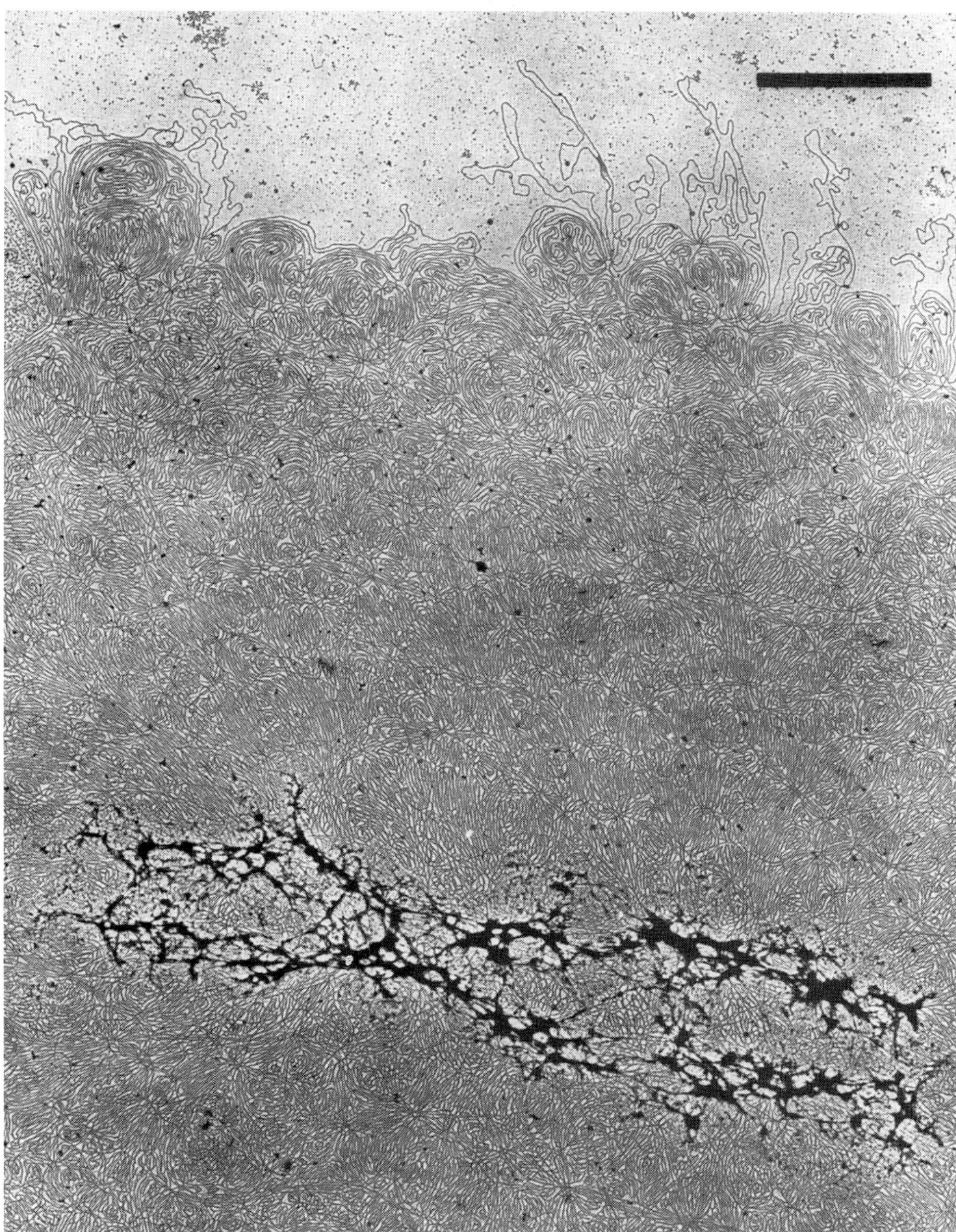

**Figure 3–12.** Electron micrograph of a protein-depleted human metaphase chromosome, showing the residual chromosome scaffold and loops of DNA. Individual DNA fibers can be best seen at the edge of the DNA loops. Bar = 2 μ. (From Paulson JR, Laemmli UK [1977] The structure of histone-depleted metaphase chromosomes. Cell 12:817–828. Reprinted by permission of the authors and Cell Press.)

## The Mitochondrial Chromosome

A small but important subset of genes encoded in the human genome resides in the cytoplasm in the mitochondria. Mitochondrial genes exhibit exclusively maternal inheritance (see Chapter 5). Human cells have hundreds of mitochondria, each containing a number of copies of a small circular molecule, the mitochondrial chromosome. The mitochondrial DNA molecule is only 16 kb in length (less than 0.03

percent of the length of the smallest nuclear chromosome!) and encodes only a few dozen genes. Although the products of these genes function in mitochondria, it should be emphasized that the vast majority of proteins found in mitochondria are, in fact, the products of nuclear genes. Mutations in mitochondrial genes have been demonstrated in several maternally inherited, as well as sporadic, disorders (see Chapter 12).

## ORGANIZATION OF THE HUMAN GENOME

Regions of the genome with similar characteristics or organization, replication, and expression are not arranged randomly but, rather, tend to be clustered together. This functional organization of the genome correlates remarkably well with its structural organization as revealed by metaphase chromosome banding (introduced in Chapter 2 and discussed in detail in Chapter 9). The overall significance of this functional organization is that chromosomes are not just a random collection of different types of genes and other DNA sequences. Some chromosome regions, or even whole chromosomes, are quite high in gene content ("gene-rich"), whereas others are low ("gene-poor"). Certain types of sequence are characteristic of the different physical hallmarks of human chromosomes. The clinical consequences of abnormalities of genome structure reflect the specific nature of the genes and sequences involved. Thus, abnormalities of gene-rich chromosomes or chromosomal regions tend to be much more severe clinically than similar-sized defects involving gene-poor parts of the genome.

As the Human Genome Project nears completion, it is apparent that the organization of DNA in the human genome is far more complex than was anticipated, as illustrated in Figure 3–13 for the fully characterized region of chromosome 17 in the vicinity of the *BRCA1* gene, mutations in which are responsible for some forms of familial breast cancer (see Chapter 16). Of the DNA in the genome, less than 10 percent actually encodes genes. Only about one half to three quarters of the total linear length of the genome consists of so-called **single-copy** or **unique DNA**—that is, DNA whose nucleotide sequence is represented only once (or at most a few times) per haploid genome. The rest of the genome consists of several classes of **repetitive DNA** and includes DNA whose nucleotide sequence is repeated, either perfectly or with some variation, hundreds to millions of times in the genome. Whereas most (but not all) of the estimated 50,000 genes in the genome are represented in single-copy DNA, sequences in the repetitive DNA fraction contribute to maintaining chromosome structure.

### Single-Copy DNA Sequences

Although single-copy DNA makes up most of the DNA in the genome, much of its function remains a mystery because, as mentioned, sequences actually encoding proteins (i.e., the coding portion of genes) constitute only a small proportion of all the single-

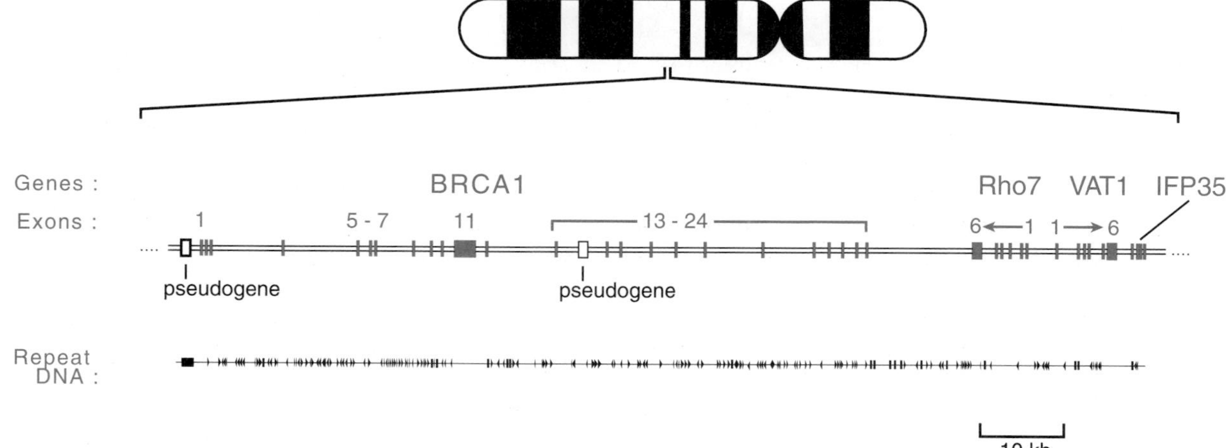


**Figure 3–13.** Sequence organization of the region of the human genome near the *BRCA1* gene that is responsible for some cases of familial, early-onset breast cancer. Four genes and two pseudogenes are found in this 117-kb sequence from chromosome 17, and their locations and structures are indicated above the chromosome. Nearly half of the sequence consists of various interspersed repetitive elements, including 170 copies of *Alu* repeats and 8 copies of L1 repeats that are indicated below the chromosome. *BRCA1* contains a GC-rich promoter, with a number of specific transcription-factor binding sites. The *RHO7* gene encodes a member of a GTP-binding protein family. *VAT1* encodes a membrane protein found in synaptic vesicles. Both *RHO7* and *VAT1* also have GC-rich promoters. *IFP35* encodes a protein whose expression can be induced by interferon. (Based on Smith TM, Lee MK, Szabo CI et al [1996] Complete genomic sequence and analysis of 117 kb human DNA containing the gene *BRCA1*. Genome Research 6:1029–1049.)

copy DNA. Long stretches of unique DNA sequences ($>$ 25 kb) are quite rare in the genome. Most single-copy DNA is found in short stretches (several kb or less), interspersed with members of various repetitive DNA families (see Fig. 3–13).

## Repetitive DNA Families

Several different categories of repetitive DNA are recognized. A useful distinguishing feature is whether the repeated sequences ("repeats") are clustered in one or a few locations or whether they are dispersed throughout the genome, interspersed with single-copy sequences along the chromosome. Clustered repeated sequences constitute an estimated 10 to 15 percent of the genome and consist of arrays of various short repeats organized tandemly in a head-to-tail fashion. The different types of such tandem repeats are collectively called **satellite DNAs**, so named because many of the original tandem repeat families could be purified by density centrifugation from the rest of the genome as "satellite" fractions of DNA.

Satellite DNA families vary with regard to their location in the genome, the total length of the tandem array, and the length of the constituent repeat units that make up the array. In general, satellite arrays can stretch several million base pairs or more in length and constitute up to several percent of the DNA content of an individual human chromosome. Many satellite sequences are important as molecular tools that have revolutionized clinical cytogenetic analysis because of their relative ease of detection (see Chapter 9). Some human satellite sequences are based on repetitions (with some variation) of a short sequence such as a pentanucleotide. Long arrays of such repeats are found in heterochromatic regions on the proximal long arms of chromosomes 1, 9, and 16 and on nearly the entire long arm of the Y chromosome (see Chapter 9). Other satellite DNAs are based on somewhat longer basic repeats. For example, the α-satellite family of DNA is composed of tandem arrays of different copies of an approximately 171 base-pair unit, found at the centromeric region of each human chromosome. This repeat family is believed to play a role in centromere function, ensuring proper chromosome segregation in mitosis and meiosis.

In addition to satellite DNAs, another major class of repetitive DNA in the genome consists of related sequences that are dispersed throughout the genome rather than localized (see Fig. 3–13). Although many small DNA families meet this general description, two in particular warrant discussion because together they make up a significant proportion of the genome and because they have been implicated in genetic diseases. The best-studied dispersed repetitive elements belong to the so-called ***Alu* family**. The members of this family are about 300 base pairs in length and are recognizably related to each other although not identical in sequence. In total, there are about 500,000 *Alu* family members in the genome, making up at least several percent of human DNA. In some regions of the genome, however, including near the *BRCA1* gene as seen in Figure 3–13, they make up a much higher percentage of the DNA. A second major dispersed, repetitive DNA family is called the **L1 family**. L1 elements are long, repetitive sequences (up to 6 kb in length) that are found in about 100,000 copies per genome. They are plentiful in some regions of the genome but relatively sparse in others.

Families of repeats dispersed throughout the genome are clearly of medical importance. Both *Alu* and L1 sequences have been implicated as the cause of mutations in hereditary disease through the process of retrotransposition, introduced in an earlier section. At least a few copies of the L1 and *Alu* families are still transpositionally active and generate copies of themselves that can integrate elsewhere in the genome, occasionally causing insertional inactivation of a medically important gene. The frequency of retrotransposition events causing genetic disease in humans is unknown currently, but they may account for as many as 1 in 500 mutations. In addition, aberrant recombination events between different copies of dispersed repeats can also be a cause of mutation in some genetic diseases (see Chapter 6).

# VARIATION IN GENE EXPRESSION AND ITS RELEVANCE TO MEDICINE

The regulated expression of the estimated 50,000 genes encoded in human chromosomes involves a set of complex interrelationships among different levels of control, including proper gene dosage (controlled by mechanisms of chromosome replication and segregation), gene structure, and, finally, transcription, mRNA stability, translation, protein processing, and protein degradation. For some genes, fluctuations in the level of functional gene product, due either to inherited variation in the structure of a particular gene or to changes induced by nongenetic factors such as diet or the environment, are of relatively little importance. For other genes, changes in the level of expression can have dire clinical consequences, reflecting the importance of those gene products in particular biological pathways. The nature of inherited variation in the structure and function of chromosomes and genes, and the influence of this variation on the expression of specific traits, is the very essence of medical and molecular genetics and is dealt with in subsequent chapters.

## General References


Abel T, Maniatis T (1994) Mechanisms of eukaryotic gene regulation. *In* Stamatoyannopoulos G, Nienhuis AW, Majerus PW, Varmus H, (eds) The Molecular Basis of Blood Diseases. WB Saunders, Philadelphia. pp. 33–70.

Alberts B, Bray D, Lewis J, et al. (1994) Molecular Biology of the Cell, 3rd ed. Garland Publishing, New York.

Bernardi G (1995) The human genome, organization, and evolutionary history. Ann Rev Genet 29:445–476.

Lewin B (2000) Genes VII, 7th ed. Oxford University Press, Oxford, England.

Semenza G (1999) Transcription Factors and Human Disease. Oxford University Press, New York.

Singer M, Berg P (1997) Exploring Genetic Mechanisms. University Science Books, Sausalito, California.

Wolffe A (1998) Chromatin Structure and Function, 3rd ed. Academic Press, San Diego.


## References Specific to Particular Topics


Berg P (1981) Dissections and reconstructions of genes and chromosomes (Nobel Prize lecture). Science 213:296–303.

Kazazian HH, Moran JV (1998) The impact of L1 retrotransposons on the human genome. Nature Genetics 19:19–24.

Lawn RM, Efstratiadis A, O'Connell C, et al (1980) The nucleotide sequence of the human β-globin gene. Cell 21:647–651.

Smith TM, Lee MK, Szabo CI, et al (1996) Complete genomic sequence and analysis of 117 kb of human DNA containing the gene *BRCA1*. Genome Research 6:1029–1049.

Wallace DC (1999) Mitochondrial diseases in man and mouse. Science 283:1482–1488.


## Problems

1. The following amino acid sequence represents part of a protein. The normal sequence and four mutant forms are shown. By consulting Table 3–1, determine the double-stranded sequence of the corresponding section of the normal gene. Which strand is the strand that RNA polymerase "reads"? What would the sequence of the resulting mRNA be? What kind of mutation is each mutant protein most likely to represent?

   Normal -lys-arg-his-his-tyr-leu-
   Mutant 1 -lys-arg-his-his-cys-leu-
   Mutant 2 -lys-arg-ile-ile-ile-
   Mutant 3 -lys-glu-thr-ser-leu-ser-
   Mutant 4 -asn-tyr-leu-

2. The following items are related to each other in a hierarchical fashion. What are these relationships? Chromosome, base pair, nucleosome, G-band, kb pair, intron, gene, exon, chromatin, codon, nucleotide.

3. The following schematic drawing illustrates a chromosome 5 in which the most distal band (band p15) on the short arm is deleted. This deleted chromosome is associated with the cri du chat syndrome (see Chapters 9 and 10). Given what you know about the organization of chromosomes and the genome, approximately how much DNA is deleted? How many genes?

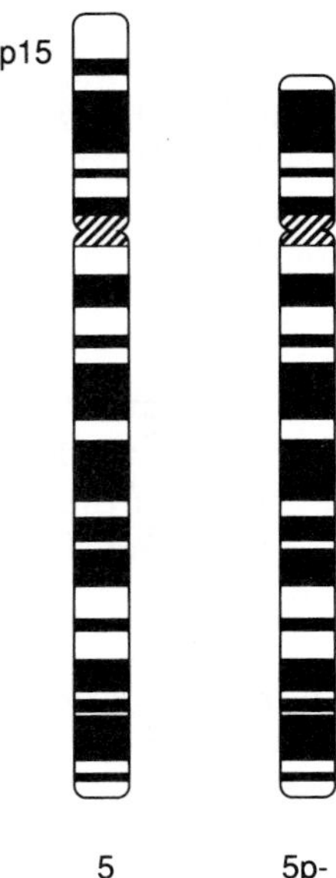


4. Most of the human genome consists of sequences that are not transcribed and do not directly encode gene products. For each of the following, consider ways in which these genome elements can contribute to human disease: introns, *Alu* or L1 repetitive sequences, locus control regions, pseudogenes.

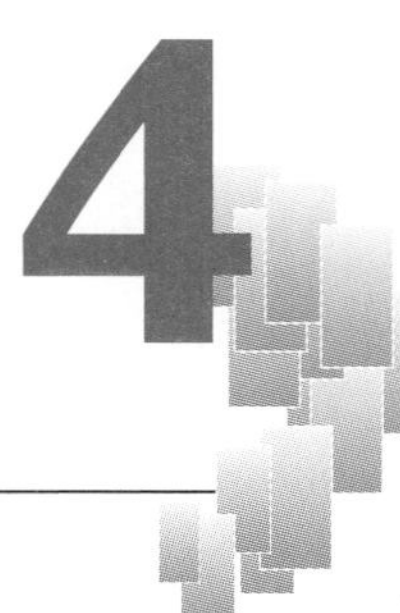

# Tools of Human Molecular Genetics

One of the principal aims of modern medical genetics is to understand the molecular basis of mutations that lead to genetic disease and to use that information to improve methods of diagnosis and treatment. Advances in our understanding of molecular genetics have been aided considerably by the development of revolutionary new technologies that permit the detailed analysis of both normal and abnormal genes. The application of these techniques has both increased the understanding of molecular processes at all levels, from the gene to the whole organism, and supported the development of a wide array of laboratory procedures for the detection and diagnosis of genetic diseases.

This chapter is not intended to be a "cookbook" of recipes for genetic experiments or of laboratory diagnostic methods. Rather, it serves only as an introduction to the techniques that have been and continue to be largely responsible for advances in both basic and applied genetic research. The contents of this chapter supplement the basic material presented in Chapters 3 and 5 and provide a basis for understanding much of the molecular information contained in the chapters that follow. Readers who have had a course or laboratory experience in molecular human genetics may use this chapter as review or skip over it entirely without interfering with the continuity of the text. For others who find the material in this chapter too brief, far more detailed accounts of modern techniques, along with complete references, can be found in the General References listed at the end of this chapter.

## ANALYSIS OF INDIVIDUAL DNA AND RNA SEQUENCES

Molecular geneticists face two fundamental obstacles to carrying out their investigations of the molecular basis of hereditary disease. The first obstacle is that of obtaining a sufficient quantity of a DNA or RNA sequence of interest to allow it to be analyzed, because each cell generally has only two copies of a gene and some genes may be transcribed only in a subset of tissues or only at low levels, or both, providing only a small number of messenger RNA (mRNA) molecules. The second obstacle is that of purifying the sequence of interest from all the other segments of DNA or mRNA molecules present in the cell. The past 3 decades have witnessed a technological revolution that solved both the problems of quantity and of purification. These two complementary technologies are **molecular cloning** and the **polymerase chain reaction (PCR)** (Fig. 4–1).

Like many technological advances, these come with their own jargon, the mastery of which may seem more imposing than the concepts involved (see box).

### Molecular Cloning

The process of **molecular cloning** involves the transfer of a DNA sequence of interest into a single cell of a microorganism. The microorganism is subsequently grown in culture so that it reproduces the DNA sequence along with its own complement of DNA. Large quantities of the sequence of interest can be isolated in pure form for detailed molecular analysis (see Fig. 4–1).

### Restriction Enzymes

One of the key advances in the development of molecular cloning was the discovery in the early 1970s of bacterial **restriction endonucleases** (often referred to as restriction enzymes), enzymes that recognize specific double-stranded sequences in DNA and cleave the DNA at or near the recognition site. For example, the restriction enzyme *Eco*RI recognizes the

## The Language of Recombinant DNA Technology

**Complementary DNA (cDNA):** a synthetic DNA made by a special DNA polymerase enzyme known as reverse transcriptase, which uses messenger RNA (mRNA) as a template. Used to refer either to a single-stranded copy or to its double-stranded derivative. Usage: "a cDNA clone," "a cDNA library," or "to isolate a cDNA."

**Clone:** a recombinant DNA molecule containing a gene or other DNA sequence of interest. Also, the act of generating such a molecule. Usage: "to isolate a clone" or "to clone a gene."

**Host:** the organism used to isolate and propagate a recombinant DNA molecule. Usually a strain of the bacterium *Escherichia coli* or the yeast *Saccharomyces cerevisiae.* Usage: "What host did they clone in?"

**Hybridization:** the act of two complementary single-stranded nucleic acid molecules forming bonds according to base-pairing rules (A with T or U, G with C) and becoming a double-stranded molecule. Usage: "The probe hybridized to a gene."

**Insert:** a fragment of foreign DNA cloned into a particular vector. Usage: "They purified the insert."

**Library:** a collection of recombinant clones from a source known to contain the gene, cDNA, or other DNA sequences of interest. In principle, a library may contain all the DNA or cDNA sequences represented in the original cell, tissue, or chromosome. Usage: "a muscle cDNA library" or "a human genomic library."

**Ligation:** the act of forming phosphodiester bonds to join two double-stranded DNA molecules with the enzyme DNA ligase. Usage: "The fragments were ligated together."

**Northern blot:** a filter to which RNA has been transferred after gel electrophoresis to separate the RNA molecules by size, named for the compass point, as a pun on Southern blot (see later); also, the act of generating such a filter and hybridizing it to a specific probe. Usage: "to probe a Northern blot" or "they did a Northern."

**Oligonucleotide:** a short strand of nucleic acid, ranging in length from a few base pairs to a few dozen base pairs, often synthesized chemically. Often referred to as an "oligo."

**Polymerase chain reaction (PCR):** enzymatic amplification of a fragment of DNA located between a pair of primers. Usage: "I PCR'd the fragment" or "I isolated the fragment using PCR."

**Primers (for PCR):** two oligonucleotides, one on each side of a target sequence, designed so that one of the primers is complementary to a segment of DNA on one strand and the other is complementary to a segment of DNA on the other strand of a double-stranded DNA molecule. A specific pair of primers serves to prime synthesis of DNA in a PCR reaction. Usage: "I designed primers for PCR."

**Probe:** a cloned DNA or RNA molecule, labeled with radioactivity or another detectable tracer, used to identify its complementary sequences by molecular hybridization; also, the act of using such a molecule. Usage: "the $\beta$-globin probe" or "to probe a patient's DNA."

**Restriction endonucleases (restriction enzymes):** enzymes that recognize specific double-stranded DNA sequences and cleave the DNA at or near the recognition site. Usage: "a restriction enzyme digest" (or just "a restriction digest") or "the restriction enzyme *Eco*RI."

**Southern blot:** a filter to which DNA has been transferred, usually after restriction enzyme digestion and gel electrophoresis to separate DNA molecules by size (named after the developer of the technique, Ed Southern); also, the act of generating such a filter and hybridizing it to a specific probe. Usage: "to probe a Southern blot" or "they did a Southern."

**Vector:** the DNA molecule into which the gene or other DNA fragment of interest is cloned, capable of replicating in a particular host. Examples include plasmids, bacteriophage lambda, cosmids, and yeast or bacterial artificial chromosomes. Usage: "a cloning vector" or "the cosmid vector."

**Western blot:** a filter to which protein molecules have been transferred after gel electrophoresis to separate the protein molecules by size (named, tongue in cheek, for a direction on a compass other than Southern or Northern); also, the act of generating such a filter and exposing it to a specific antibody. Usage: "to probe a Western blot" or "they did a Western."

specific six base-pair sequence 5′-GAATTC-3′ wherever it occurs in a double-stranded DNA molecule. The enzyme cleaves the DNA at that site by introducing a nick on each strand between the G and the adjacent A. Cleavage generates two fragments, each with a four-base, single-stranded overhang at the end (Fig. 4–2). Such "sticky" ends are useful for subsequent joining reactions in the construction of recom-

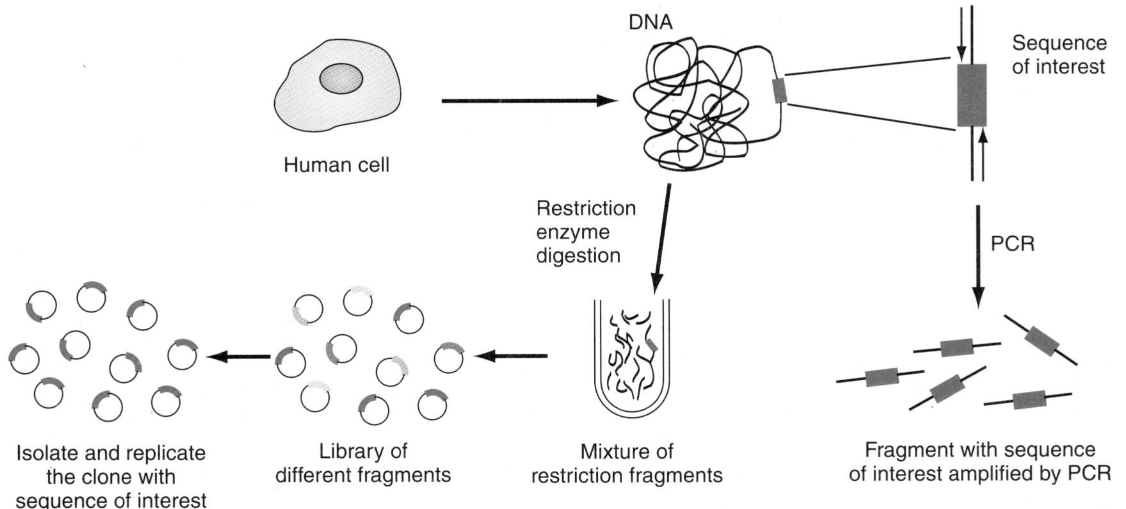


**Figure 4–1.** The use of molecular cloning and the polymerase chain reaction (PCR) to isolate arbitrarily large quantities of a particular desired DNA sequence of interest in pure form.

binant DNA molecules. Other restriction enzymes recognize different sequences of nucleotides that are specific for each particular enzyme. More than 1000 such enzymes are now known; some of the ones most commonly used are listed in Table 4–1. Most restriction enzymes have recognition sites that consist of four or six base pairs, although a few have longer sites. Usually, the sequences are **palindromes**; that is, the sequence of bases in the recognition site, read 5′ to 3′, is the same on both strands.

Cleavage of a DNA molecule with a particular restriction enzyme digests the DNA into a characteristic and reproducible collection of fragments, which reflect the frequency and the location of specific cleavage sites. This property of restriction enzymes has two important implications central to their role in recombinant DNA technology and its application to medical genetics. First, digestion of genomic DNA samples with, for example, the enzyme *Eco*RI generates a collection of approximately 1 million *Eco*RI fragments, each from a particular location in the genome. Because *Eco*RI cleaves double-stranded DNA specifically at each and every 5′-GAATTC-3′ that it encounters, and because even a single base change in a potential cleavage site abolishes its recognition and cleavage by the enzyme, such digestion allows one to examine, in effect, this particular sequence of six nucleotides at approximately 1 million locations in the genome. (On average, an enzyme with a six base-pair recognition site should cleave human DNA every $4^6$ base pairs, or once every 4 kb. In reality, however, such sites are located nonrandomly, reflecting the particular base composition and sequence of different regions of the genome, and *Eco*RI fragments ranging in size from a few base pairs to well over 1 million base pairs are observed.)

Second, all DNA molecules digested with *Eco*RI, regardless of their origin, have identical single-stranded sticky ends, independent of the nature of the DNA sequences flanking a particular *Eco*RI site. Therefore, *any* two DNA molecules that have been generated by *Eco*RI digestion can be joined together in vitro by interaction of their complementary four-base overhangs, which is followed by completion of the phosphodiester backbones on each strand by an enzyme called **DNA ligase.** This ligation step creates a "recombinant" DNA molecule, one end derived from one DNA source and the other end derived from a different source (see Fig. 4–2). Many restriction enzymes, such as *Eco*RI, generate short overhangs; others, however, cut both strands at the same location, leaving blunt ends. DNA ligase can join blunt ends created by any restriction enzyme that cuts DNA without leaving an overhang.

## Vectors

A vector is a DNA molecule that can replicate autonomously in a host such as bacterial or yeast cells, from which it can be subsequently isolated in pure form for analysis. Cloning of human DNA fragments into a vector by means of restriction enzymes and DNA ligase, as just described, allows for the propagation of the cloned fragment along with the vector molecule. Because replicating vectors can often achieve a high number of copies per cell and because the bacterial or yeast hosts can be grown indefinitely

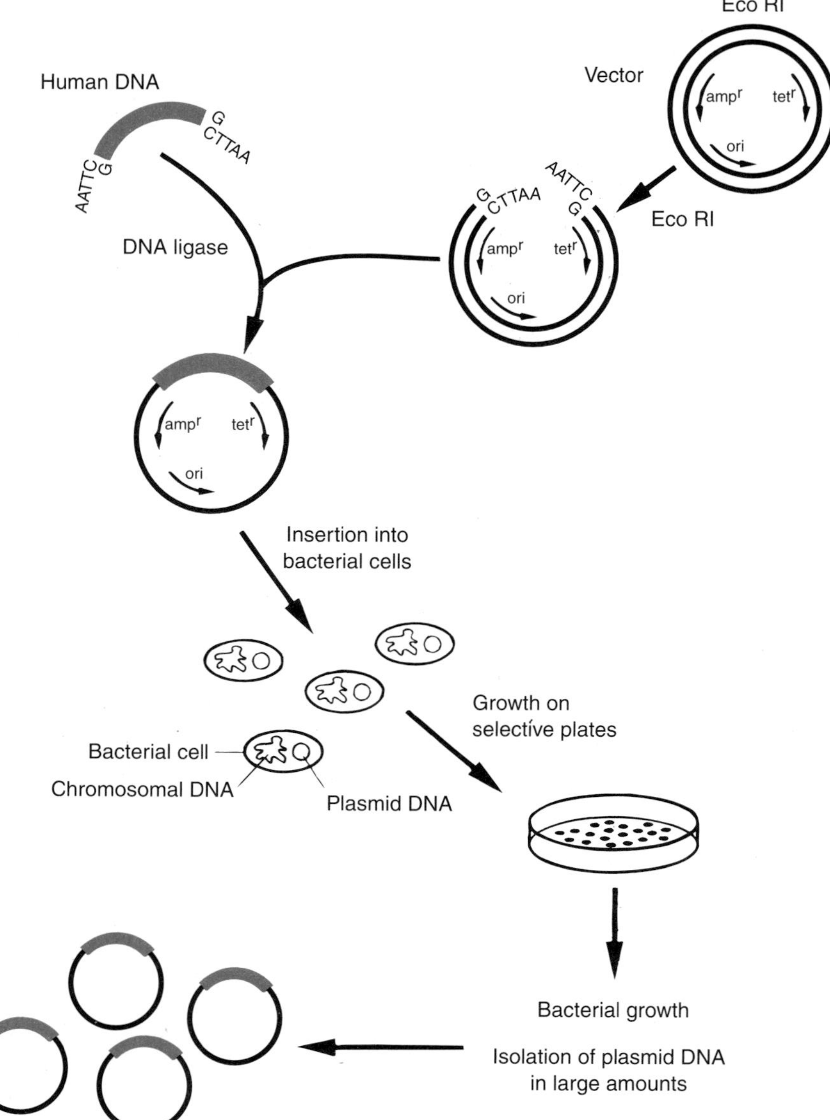


**Figure 4–2.** The process of cloning a segment of human DNA (between two *Eco*RI sites) into a plasmid cloning vector. "ori" denotes an origin of DNA replication for replicating the plasmid in bacterial cells. "amp$^r$" and "tet$^r$" denote bacterial genes conferring resistance to ampicillin and tetracycline. Growth of bacteria on plates containing antibiotics selects for those cells that contain copies of the plasmid, with its cloned human insert. (Modified from Fritsch EF, Wozney JM [1994] Methods of molecular genetics. *In* Stamatoyannopoulos G, Nienhuis AW, Majerus PW, Varmus H [eds] The Molecular Basis of Blood Diseases, 2nd ed. W.B. Saunders, Philadelphia.)

in the laboratory, vast quantities of the DNA sequences of interest can be obtained. The ability to generate any desired number of identical copies (clones) of a particular sequence is a product of **recombinant DNA technology**. The name "recombinant DNA" refers to novel combinations of DNA created in vitro between human (or other) DNA sequences of interest and bacterial (or other) vector molecules capable of indefinite duplication within a laboratory strain of a microorganism. A number of vectors are commonly used for this purpose, each with its own set of advantages and limitations (Table 4–2).

### PLASMIDS

Plasmids are circular double-stranded DNA molecules that replicate extrachromosomally in bacteria or yeast. The plasmids used as vectors are derived from naturally occurring circular molecules that were first discovered in bacteria because they carried antibiotic resistance genes and could be passed easily from one bacterium to another, thereby spreading antibiotic resistance rapidly throughout the microbial population. Plasmids specifically designed for molecular cloning are usually small (several kb in size) and contain an origin of replication

TABLE 4–1

**Examples of Restriction Enzymes and Their Recognition Sequences**

| Restriction Enzymes | Source | Recognition Sequences* |
|---|---|---|
| *Bam*HI | *Bacillus amyloliquefaciens* H | 5′-G ^ GATC C-3′<br>3′-C CTAG ^ G-5′ |
| *Eco*RI | *Escherichia coli* RY 13 | G ^ AATT C<br>C TTAA ^ G |
| *Hae*III | *Haemophilus aegyptius* | GG ^ CC<br>CC ^ GG |
| *Hind*III | *Haemophilus influenzae* $R_d$ | A ^ AGCT T<br>T TCGA ^ A |
| *Not*I | *Nocardia otitidis-cavarium* | GC ^ GGCC GC<br>CG CCGG ^ CG |
| *Sau*3A | *Staphylococcus aureus* 3A | ^ GATC<br>CTAG ^ |
| *Sst*II | *Streptomyces stanford* | CC GC ^ GG<br>GG ^ CG CC |

*All recognition sequences are given in the 5′ → 3′ polarity, as shown for *Bam*HI. Cleavage sites on each strand are indicated by the small circumflexes.

(for replication either in *Escherichia coli* or in yeast), one or more selectable markers (such as a gene that confers resistance to antibiotics), and one or more restriction sites that can be cut and used for the ligation of foreign DNA molecules. A schematic drawing of the important steps involved in cloning of foreign DNA into the *Eco*RI site of a plasmid is shown in Figure 4–2. Identification of colonies that contain the desired recombinant plasmid, followed by mass growth and isolation of pure plasmid DNA, allows the isolation of large amounts of the cloned insert. Cloning into plasmids is a standard procedure for the analysis of short DNA molecules (see Table 4–2).

### Bacteriophage Lambda

Another commonly used vector is bacteriophage lambda, a bacterial virus with a relatively large (approximately 45 kb) double-stranded DNA molecule. After infecting an *E. coli* cell, lambda replicates to produce huge numbers of infectious viruses, eventually bursting the bacterial cells (lysis) and releasing 1 million or so bacteriophages. Approximately one third of the bacteriophage genome is nonessential (labeled "internal fragments" in Fig. 4–3) for growth and lysis and can be replaced by other DNA sequences; thus, lambda phage is highly suitable for cloning pieces of human DNA up to 20 kb.

### Cosmids and Bacterial Artificial Chromosomes

One drawback of standard plasmids as vectors is that they are inefficient for introducing recombinant DNA molecules into bacteria if the inserts are larger than approximately 20 kb. One method of overcoming this inefficiency was the development of cosmid vectors. Cosmids are essentially plasmids that use the ability of bacteriophage lambda infectious particles to efficiently "package" large linear pieces of DNA into protein shells that then attach to the surface of bacterial cells and inject their DNA contents. The limitation on cosmid insert size is that lambda is not capable of packaging its DNA (or a cosmid), whether or not there is an insert, if the bacteriophage chromosome exceeds approximately 50 kb in length. After infection of bacteria in a manner similar to that of a lambda virus, the cosmid recircularizes and replicates as a large plasmid. Fragments of foreign DNA twice the size of lambda phage inserts can be cloned in cosmid vectors.

In the late 1990s, technology has become available to clone, in bacteria, fragments of DNA much larger than cosmids. Such huge plasmids are termed

TABLE 4–2

**Examples of Vector Commonly Used in Molecular Cloning**

| Vector | Host | Type of Cloning | Insert Size Range |
|---|---|---|---|
| Plasmids | Bacteria, yeast | Genomic, cDNA | Up to ~15 kb |
| Bacteriophage lambda | Bacteria | Genomic, cDNA | Up to ~20 kb |
| Cosmids | Bacteria | Genomic | Up to ~45 kb |
| BACs | Bacteria | Genomic | 100 to 300 kb |
| YACs | Yeast | Genomic | 100 to 2000 kb |

BAC = bacterial artificial chromosome; YAC = yeast artificial chromosome.

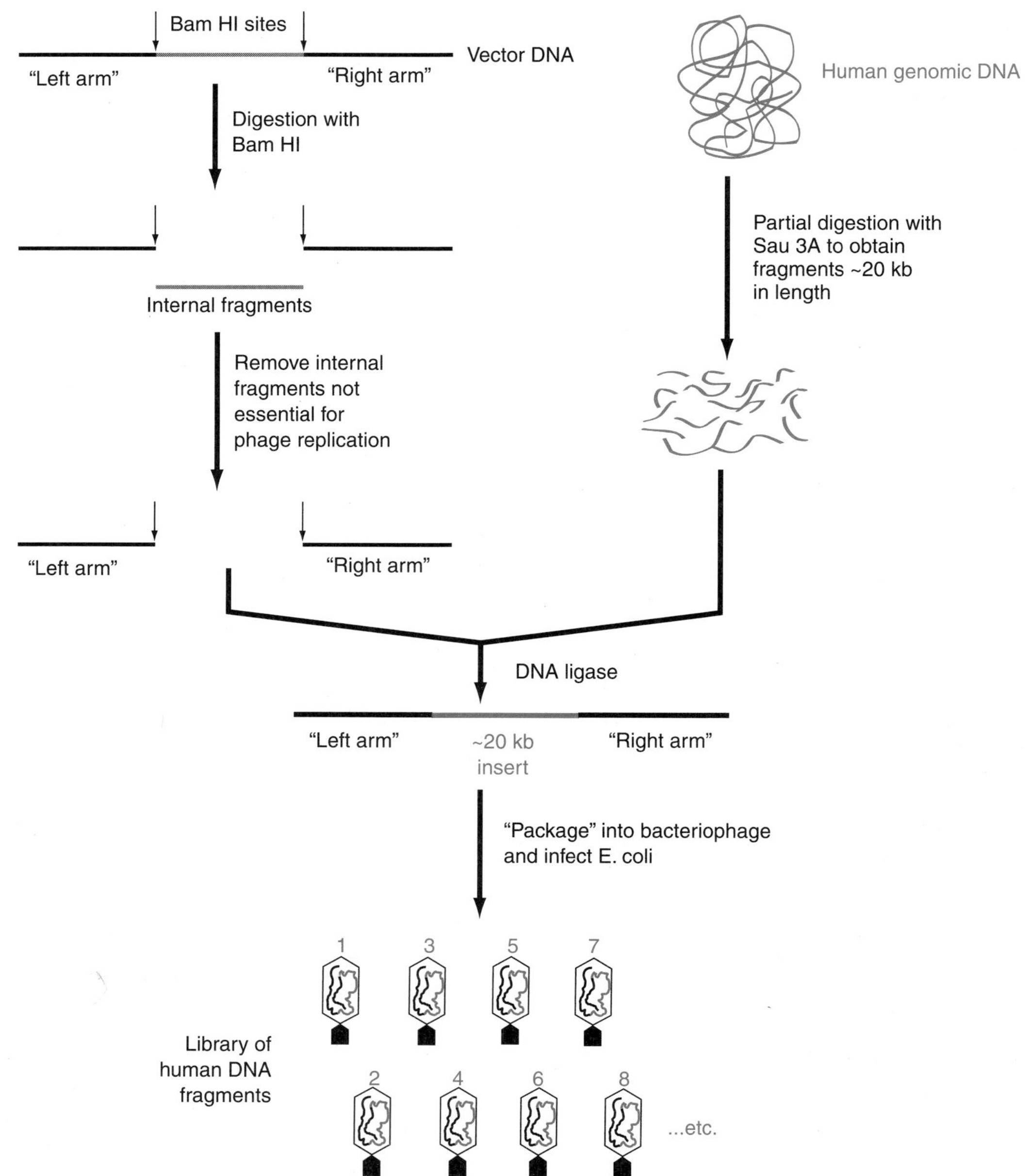


**Figure 4–3.** Construction of a "library" of DNA from the human genome in a bacteriophage vector. Each of the recombinant phage particles at the bottom contains a different fragment of human DNA. A collection of several hundred thousand such phages would represent all the DNA from the human genome.

bacterial artificial chromosomes (BACs). BACs can carry inserts of human DNA from 100 to 300 kb in size.

The use of cosmid or BAC vectors for cloning is essentially the same as shown for plasmids in Figure 4–2. The difference between plasmids, cosmids, and BACs is in how the vectors carrying these large inserts are introduced into bacteria.

### YEAST ARTIFICIAL CHROMOSOMES

For many approaches to gene cloning and gene mapping, illustrated in Chapter 8, it is advantageous to isolate the largest piece of human chromosomal DNA possible. The cloning vector with the largest capacity by far is the yeast artificial chromosome (YAC). Two arms, one containing a yeast telomere, a centromere, and a selectable marker and the other containing a telomere and a second selectable marker, are ligated onto the ends of large human restriction fragments generated by partial digestion of genomic DNA, thereby creating an artificial chromosome (Fig. 4–4). These fragments are transferred into a host, *Saccharomyces cerevisiae* (common baker's yeast), where they replicate and segregate like normal linear yeast chromosomes. YACs allow cloning and isolation of fragments of DNA up to 1000 to 2000 kb in length, much smaller than a normal human chromosome but approximately the same size as a normal yeast chromosome.

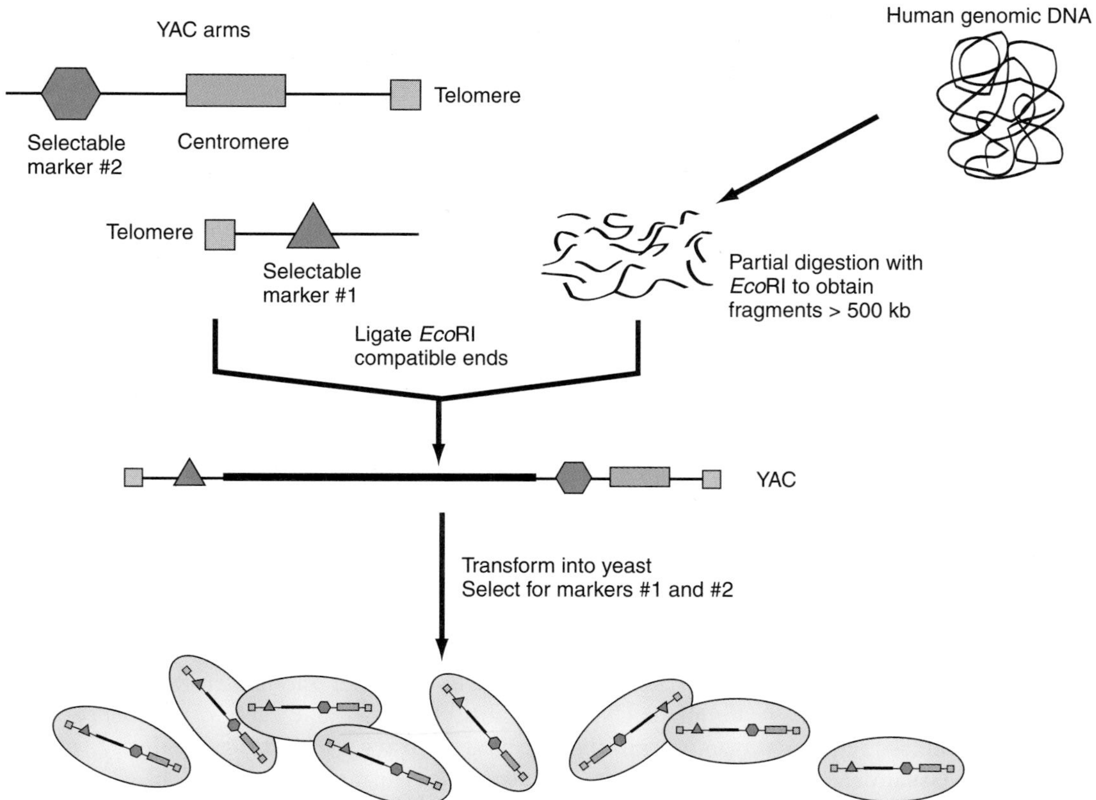


**Figure 4–4.** Construction of a genomic library in yeast artificial chromosomes (YACs). Large fragments ( >500 kb) of human DNA are generated by partial *Eco*RI digestion of human genomic DNA. Each vector arm contains a telomere at one end and an *Eco*RI compatible overhang at the other end. Each also carries a different selectable marker, and one arm also contains a centromere. Vector arms are ligated to the human DNA fragments to generate an artificial linear chromosome with yeast telomeres and selectable markers at each end and a yeast centromere at one end. The YACs are transferred into yeast, and the selectable markers are used to select only those yeasts that contain a properly constructed YAC.

## Construction of Libraries

The purpose of molecular cloning, of course, is to isolate a particular gene or other DNA sequence in large quantities for further study. A common approach to generating large quantities of a sequence is to construct a set of clones of bacteria or yeast that contain a vector into which fragments of DNA have been inserted. Such a collection of clones is called a **library**, which at least theoretically contains all of the sequences found in the original source, including your sequence of interest. One then has to identify the clone or clones of interest in the library by using sensitive screening methods that are capable of finding, in some cases, even a single copy of the clone of interest in a collection of up to 10 million starting clones.

### Genomic Libraries

One approach to constructing a library of genomic DNA is shown in Figure 4–3. Human genomic DNA is *partially* digested with a restriction enzyme like *Sau*3A in such a way that some of the sites are cleaved and others are not. In this way, if random cleavage of such sites occurs, a collection of overlapping fragments of length suitable for cloning can be obtained and ligated into bacteriophage lambda "arms" prepared so that the *Sau*3A ends of human DNA fragments can be ligated into the vector (see Fig. 4–3). After packaging of the recombinant lambda chromosome into infectious bacteriophage particles, the library, containing 1 million or more fragments of genomic DNA, can be stored for the future isolation of many genes. Genomic libraries containing much larger fragments of genomic DNA have been made by making YACs containing DNA partially digested with, for example, *Eco*RI (see Fig. 4–4).

### Complementary DNA Libraries

Another common type of library used to isolate genes is a cDNA library, which represents **complementary DNA** (hence cDNA) copies of the mRNA population present within a particular tissue. Such cDNA libraries are often preferable to genomic libraries as a source of cloned genes (1) because the obtained clone is a direct representation of the coding sequences, without introns or other noncoding sequences found in genomic DNA, and (2) because the use of a particular mRNA source often enriches substantially for the sequences derived from a given gene known to be expressed selectively in that tissue. For example, the β-globin gene is represented at only one part per million in a human genomic library, but it is a major mRNA transcript in red blood cells. Thus, a cDNA library prepared from red blood cells represents an excellent cloning source to isolate β-globin gene cDNAs. Similarly, a liver or muscle cDNA library is a good source of clones for genes known to be expressed preferentially or exclusively in those tissues. A cDNA, however, contains only the exons of a gene but not the introns or promoter sequences. In addition, a cDNA does not provide any indication of the size or number of exons or the sequence of the 5′ and 3′ splice sites.

A number of methods have been developed to clone cDNAs, all of which rely on the enzyme **reverse transcriptase**, an RNA-dependent DNA polymerase derived from retroviruses that can synthesize a cDNA strand from an RNA template (Fig. 4–5). Reverse transcriptase requires a primer to initiate DNA synthesis. Usually, an oligonucleotide consisting of thymidines (oligo-dT) is used; this short homopolymer binds to the polyA tail at the 3′ end of mRNA molecules (see Chapter 3) and thus primes synthesis of a complementary copy. This single-stranded cDNA is then converted to a double-stranded molecule by one of several available methods, and the double-stranded cDNA can then be ligated into a suitable vector, usually a plasmid or a bacteriophage, to create a cDNA library representing all of the original mRNA transcripts found in the starting cell type or tissue (see Fig. 4–5). Some cleverly engineered vectors, called **expression vectors**, contain transcription and translation signals adjacent to the site of insertion of the cDNA to facilitate expression of the protein encoded by the cloned cDNA in *E. coli* or in yeast.

Representative cDNA libraries from many different tissues or different times of development are valuable resources for gene cloning. Hundreds of such libraries are now widely available and are the source of clones used for sequencing to generate huge databases of **expressed sequence tags** as part of the Human Genome Project (see Chapter 8).

## Nucleic Acid Probes

Once a library is made, the next step is to identify the clone carrying a sequence of interest among the millions of other clones carrying other fragments. Identifying the clone carrying an insert of interest is called **library screening**. Library screening is usually performed with a widely used technique in molecular genetics known as **nucleic acid hybridization**. In a hybridization reaction, single-stranded nucleic acids are mixed under conditions of temperature and salt concentration that permit only correct base pairing (A with T, G with C) between the DNA strands. Only those strands that are correctly base-paired can form a stable *double-stranded* nucleic acid; no stable double-stranded molecules

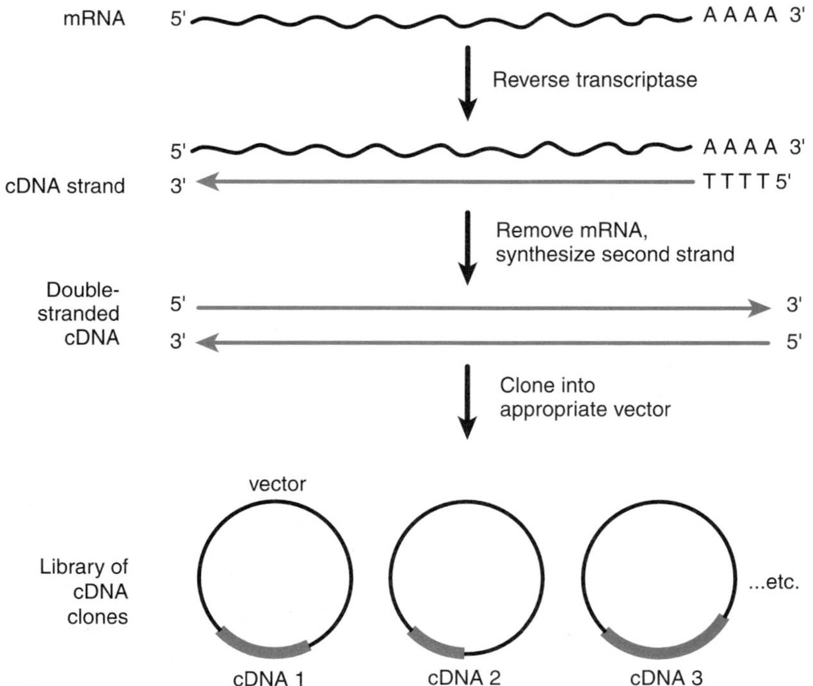


**Figure 4–5.** Construction of a cDNA library in a plasmid vector. RNA from a particular tissue source is copied into DNA by the enzyme reverse transcriptase. After synthesis of the complementary second strand, the double-stranded cDNA is then cloned.

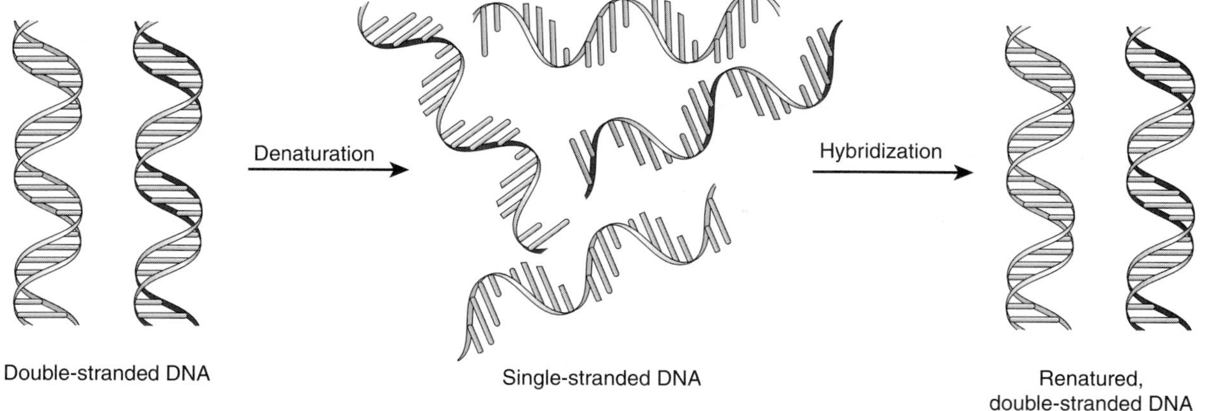


**Figure 4–6.** The principle of nucleic acid hybridization. The two complementary strands of a Watson-Crick double helix can be "denatured" by a variety of treatments (such as high temperature, high pH, or very low salt conditions) to yield a collection of single-stranded DNA molecules. Under conditions that favor formation of renatured double-stranded DNA, complementary strands will "hybridize" to each other, but not to other fragments of DNA that have a different nucleotide sequence.

will form between noncomplementary sequences in the mixture (Fig. 4–6).

The specificity of nucleic acid hybridization for complementary strands makes the use of nucleic acid **probes** possible. One sequence (the "target") in a mixture of nucleic acids is tested for its complementarity to a DNA or RNA fragment of known sequence (the "probe"), which has been tagged with a radioactive tracer, a histochemical compound, or a fluorescent dye to allow the probe to be subsequently detected. For example, a common way to tag a probe is to label it with phosphorus-32 ($^{32}$P) whose high energy exposes x-ray film. One can introduce $^{32}$P into a probe by a variety of methods that substitute $^{32}$P into the phosphodiester backbone of a strand of DNA. If the probe is complementary to the target, it will form a stable double-stranded molecule. The target sequence in the original DNA or RNA sample is now identified by the tag on the probe, thus facilitating its subsequent detection and analysis or isolation.

Probes can be cloned genomic or cDNA molecules obtained by use of recombinant DNA technology, DNA fragments generated by PCR (see later discussion), or synthetic nucleic acid (usually DNA) molecules. Probes derived from cloned DNA or generated by PCR are usually several hundred to several thousand nucleotides in length. One can also use as probes chemically synthesized single-stranded DNA molecules, typically 15 to 60 nucleotides in length, known as **oligonucleotide probes** or, simply, **oligonucleotides**.

Nucleic acid hybridization is a fundamental concept in molecular biology. The technique is used not only for screening libraries of cloned DNA but also more generally for the analysis of DNA or RNA in cells and tissues, as described in the following section of this chapter.

## METHODS OF NUCLEIC ACID ANALYSIS

The analysis of RNA or DNA, or both, requires the detection of one particular DNA or RNA sequence among all the many other sequences present in a sample of cells or tissue. When analyzing genomic DNA, the problem is to find and examine the specific DNA fragment one is interested in from a complex mixture of genomic DNA containing several million DNA fragments. For example, one might use a probe for the $\beta$-globin gene to examine a sample of patient DNA by Southern analysis (see later) for a specific mutation thought to be responsible for sickle cell anemia. With RNA samples, the problem is to detect and measure the amount and the quality of a particular mRNA in an RNA sample from a tissue in which the desired mRNA might account for only 1/1000 or less of the total RNA transcripts. For example, one might wish to use a probe for the X-linked dystrophin gene to carry out Northern analysis (see later) of a sample of muscle RNA obtained from a patient with X-linked Duchenne muscular dystrophy for dystrophin mRNA transcripts. The solution to this problem of detecting one rare sequence among many involves using gel electrophoresis to separate the molecules of DNA or RNA by size and then carrying out nucleic acid hybridization with a probe to identify the molecule of interest.

### Southern Blotting

The Southern blotting technique, developed in the mid-1970s, is the standard method for analyzing the structure of DNA cleaved by restriction enzymes. In this procedure, diagrammed in Figure 4–7 for a genomic DNA sample, DNA is first isolated from an

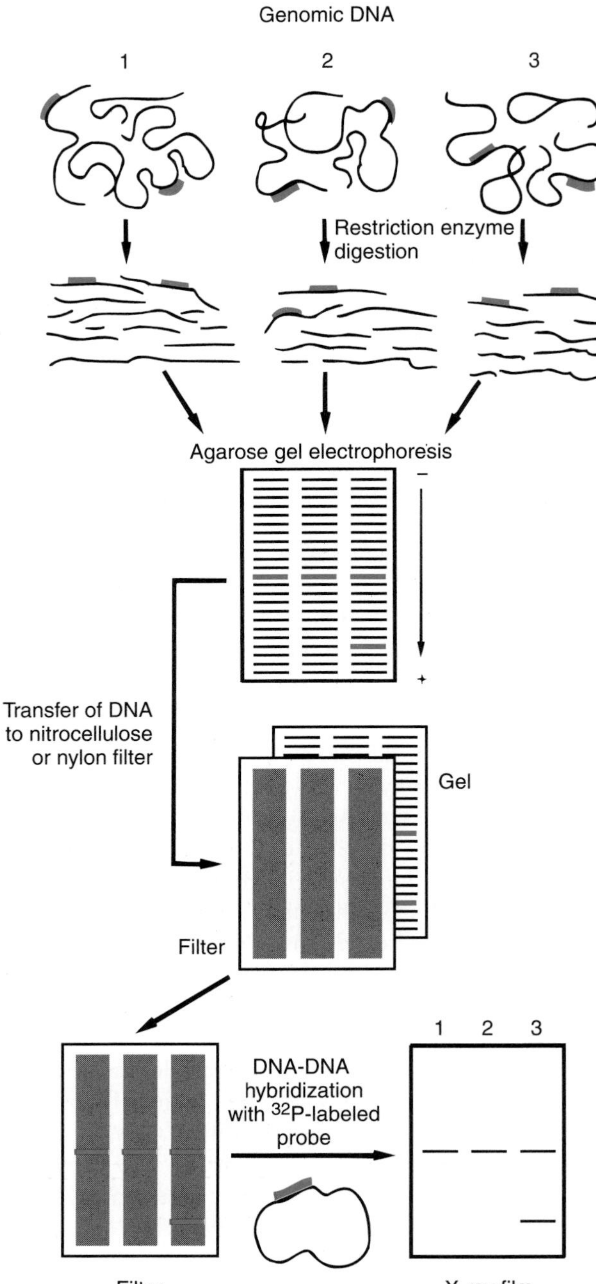


**Figure 4–7.** The Southern blotting procedure for analyzing specific DNA sequences in a complex mixture of different sequences, such as genomic DNA. In this example, sample 3 has a different restriction enzyme pattern for the DNA sequence detected by the probe. This variation might be due to a restriction fragment length polymorphism (see Chapter 6) or to a deletion of DNA near the detected sequence.

accessible source. Any cell in the body can be used as the source of DNA, except for mature red blood cells, which have no nuclei. For analysis of patient DNA samples, one typically prepares genomic DNA from lymphocytes obtained by routine venipuncture. A 10-ml sample of peripheral blood contains approximately $10^8$ white blood cells and provides more than 100 $\mu$g of DNA, enough for dozens of restriction enzyme digestions. Genomic DNA can also be prepared from other tissues, however, including cultured skin fibroblasts, amniotic fluid or chorionic villus cells for prenatal diagnosis (see Chapter 18), or any organ biopsy specimen (e.g., liver, kidney, placenta). The approximately 1 million distinct DNA fragments generated by restriction enzyme cleavage of a genomic DNA sample are separated on the basis of size by agarose gel electrophoresis, in which small fragments move through an electric field more rapidly than do larger ones. When digested DNA separated in this way is stained with a fluorescent DNA dye such as ethidium bromide, the genomic DNA fragments appear as a smear of fluorescing material because there are usually far too many DNA fragments for any one to stand out from the others (Fig. 4–8, *left*). The Southern blotting technique allows one to find and examine, at a gross level, the one or two DNA fragments of interest in this seemingly uninformative collection of a million or so restriction enzyme fragments.

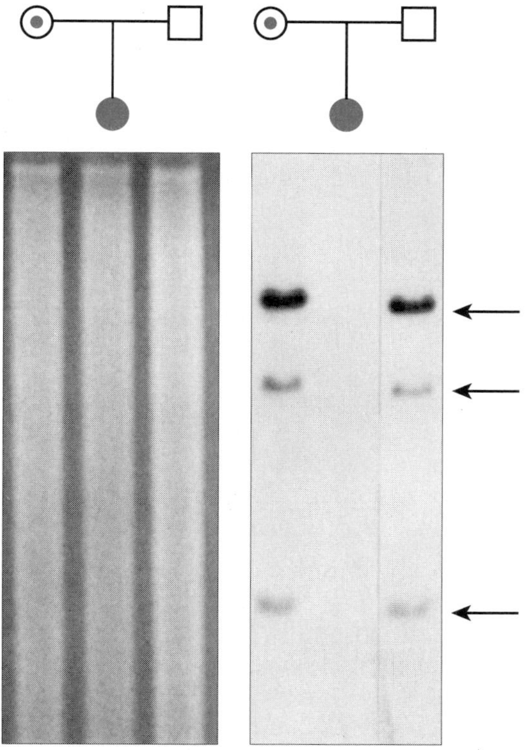

Figure 4–8. Detection of a gene deletion by Southern blotting. When genomic DNA from family members is digested with a restriction enzyme and the DNA stained with a fluorescent DNA dye (such as ethidium bromide) after electrophoresis, all samples appear the same (*left*). After Southern blotting and hybridization to a cDNA probe for the human X-linked androgen receptor gene, the individual with androgen insensitivity syndrome can be seen to be deleted for this gene (*right, middle lane*). The individual with androgen insensitivity has a 46,XY karyotype but is phenotypically female. (Figure courtesy of R. Lafreniere, Stanford University.)

Double-stranded DNA fragments are first denatured with a strong base to separate the two complementary DNA strands (see Fig. 4–6). The now single-stranded DNA molecules are then transferred from the gel to a piece of nitrocellulose or nylon filter paper by blotting and capillarity (hence, the name "Southern blot" or "Southern transfer").

To identify the one or more fragments of interest among the millions of fragments on the filter, a specific labeled probe is used. As described earlier, the probe is usually a piece of cloned DNA that has been radioactively labeled and itself denatured to become single-stranded. The labeled probe and the filter are incubated together in solution under conditions that favor formation of double-stranded DNA molecules (as in Fig. 4–6). Because of the exquisite specificity of DNA basepairing, the probe anneals and forms stable hydrogen bonds only to its complementary strand on the filter and not to all of the other DNA fragments. If the probe is itself a piece of cloned genomic DNA, it usually hybridizes to one or two fragments on the filter, depending on how the gene or genes in the original DNA sample were cut by the specific restriction enzyme used. If the probe is a cloned cDNA, however, many fragments may hybridize because genomic DNA is usually not colinear with a gene's mRNA transcript due to the presence of introns (see Chapter 3). After being washed to remove unbound probe, the filter (with its bound radioactive probe) is exposed to x-ray film to reveal the position of the one or more fragments to which the probe hybridized. Thus, as shown in Figure 4–8 (*right*), specific radioactive bands are detectable on the x-ray film for each lane of human DNA on the original agarose gel. In this example, the Southern blotting technique shows that the gene for the X-linked androgen receptor, which is responsible for male secondary sex characteristics (see Chapter 10), is absent from a genomic DNA sample of a patient with X-linked androgen-insensitivity syndrome (also known as testicular feminization). Southern blotting remains a standard procedure for the diagnosis of many genetic diseases in molecular diagnostic laboratories around the world, but it has frequently been replaced by PCR-based methods.

## Analysis with Allele-Specific Oligonucleotide Probes

When a particular mutation is known in at least some cases of a genetic disease, one can refine the analysis of mutations to ask whether that mutation is present or absent in a DNA sample from a particular patient. The best probe to use for detection of a particular single base mutation is a synthetic oligonucleotide because its shorter length makes it much more sensitive to even single base-pair mismatches between the probe and the sample to be analyzed. Thus, an oligonucleotide probe synthesized to match precisely the normal DNA sequence in a gene (an **allele-specific oligonucleotide**, or **ASO**) hybridizes only to the normal complementary sequence but not to an imperfect complementary sequence in which there are one or more mismatches between target and probe (Fig. 4–9). Similarly, an ASO made to the sequence corresponding to a mutant gene hybridizes only to the mutant complementary sequence but not to the sequence in a normal gene.

It is important to recognize the distinction between ASO analysis and conventional Southern blot analysis with cloned DNA probes. In the case of cloned DNA probes, the analysis cannot usually reveal a single base change unless, by chance, the single base change creates or destroys a restriction enzyme site near the region of complementarity to the probe, thereby altering the size of the fragment detected by the probe. In the vast majority of cases, mutant genes due to single base changes or to similar small changes in the DNA (small deletions or insertions,

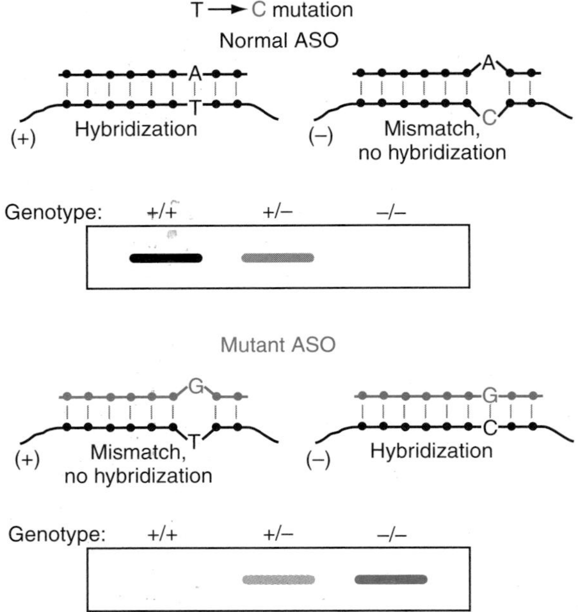


**Figure 4–9.** Detection of single base-pair mutations using allele-specific oligonucleotide probes. The "normal" probe will base-pair only to DNA sequences that are identical to the probe (*top*). The "mutant" probe will pair only to DNA sequences that differ from the "normal" sequence by a specific single base-pair mutation (*bottom*). Individuals of all three genotypes can be distinguished by this method.

for example) are indistinguishable from normal genes by Southern blot analysis done using standard, cloned DNA probes. Only short ASO probes have the ability to reliably detect single nucleotide changes.

ASO analysis permits precise identification of a particular DNA sequence and can distinguish among individuals who carry the normal DNA sequence on both chromosomes, the mutant sequence on both chromosomes, or individuals with the normal sequence on one chromosome and the mutant sequence on the other (see Fig. 4–9). Care must be taken, however, in interpreting results from ASO analysis because not all mutant genes at a given locus share exactly the same DNA sequence alteration. Thus, failure to hybridize to the mutant gene ASO does not necessarily mean that the patient's gene is normal throughout its entire sequence; there may be a mutation elsewhere in the gene at a location other than that examined by a particular ASO. ASO analysis is used primarily in cases for which there is a strong probability, based on other lines of evidence, that a family or an individual is at risk for a specific known mutation. The use of ASO analysis is therefore restricted to situations in which the particular mutation in a family is known or for genetic disorders that are characterized by a finite number of different mutations. Specific examples of such diseases are considered in Chapters 5, 11, and 12.

### Northern Blotting

The counterpart of the Southern blotting technique for analysis of RNA samples is called "Northern" or RNA blotting. Northern blotting is the standard approach for determining the size and abundance of the mRNA from a specific gene in a sample of RNA. RNA cannot be cleaved by the restriction enzymes used for DNA analysis. Different RNA transcripts are of different lengths, however, depending on the size and number of exons within a transcribed gene (see Chapter 3). Thus, total cellular RNA (or purified mRNA) obtained from a particular cell type is separated according to size by agarose gel electrophoresis and transferred to nitrocellulose or nylon filters. As in the Southern blotting procedure, the filter is then incubated with a denatured, labeled probe that hybridizes to one or more specific RNA transcripts. After exposure of the washed filter to x-ray film, one or more bands may be apparent, revealing the position and abundance of the specific transcript of interest.

## THE POLYMERASE CHAIN REACTION

The **polymerase chain reaction (PCR)** is an alternative to cloning for generating essentially unlimited amounts of a sequence of interest (see Fig. 4–1). PCR can selectively amplify a single molecule of DNA or RNA several billion-fold in a few hours and has revolutionized both molecular diagnosis and the molecular analysis of genetic disease. PCR is an enzymatic amplification of a fragment of DNA (the target) located between two oligonucleotide "primers." These primers are designed so that one is complementary to one strand of a DNA molecule on one side of the target sequence and the other primer is complementary to the other strand of the DNA molecule on the opposite side of the target sequence. Because the 3′ end of each oligonucleotide primer (see Fig. 3–2) points toward the target sequence to be amplified and the primers flank the target sequence, the primers are extended by the synthesis by DNA polymerase of the sequence between them. As diagrammed schematically in Figure 4–10, the primers are oriented so that they prime two new strands of DNA that are themselves complementary and essentially form a second copy of the original target sequence. Repeated cycles of heat denaturation, hybridization of the primers, and enzymatic DNA synthesis result in the exponential amplification (2, 4, 8, 16, 32, . . . copies) of the target DNA sequence (see Fig. 4–10). With the use of specifically designed "PCR machines," a round of amplification takes only a few minutes. In only a few hours, many billions of copies of a starting sequence can be created.

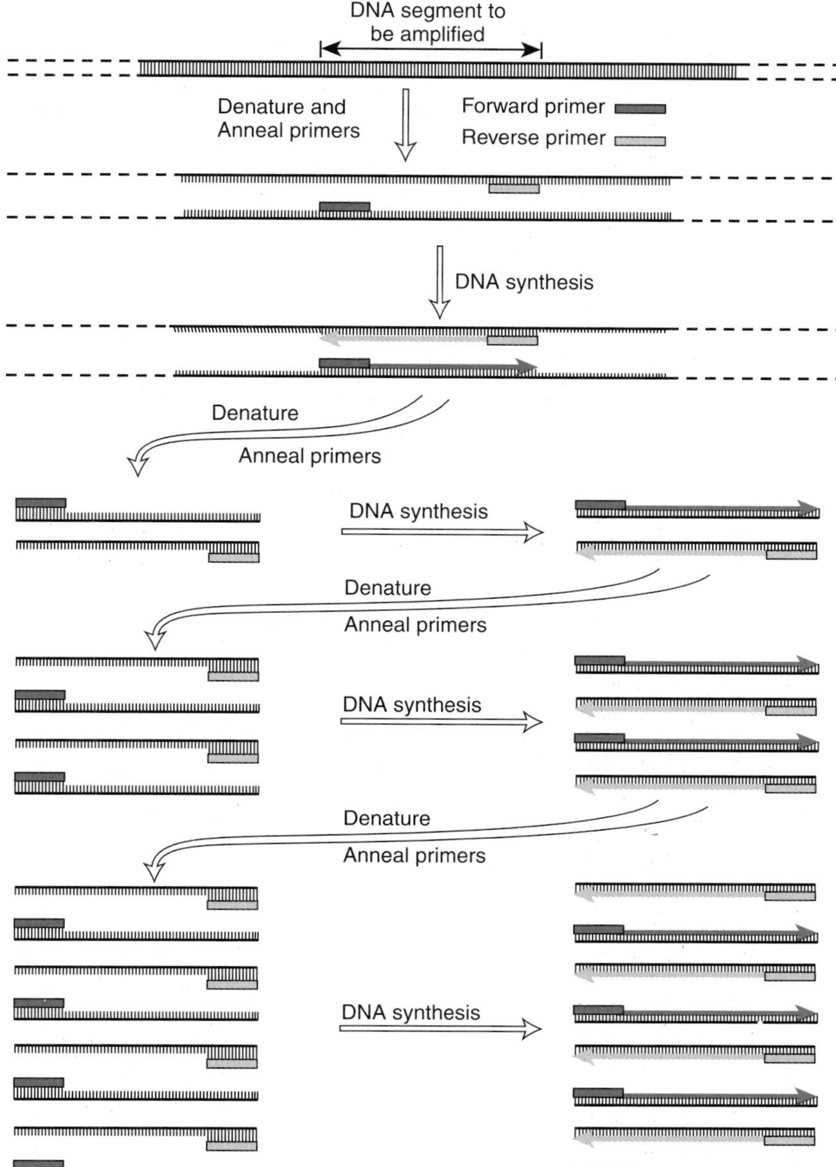


**Figure 4–10.** The polymerase chain reaction. By repeatedly synthesizing a region of DNA located between two DNA primers, this region of DNA is specifically and selectively amplified in an exponential fashion. Three successive rounds of amplification are shown, resulting in a total of eight copies of the targeted sequence. After 30 rounds of amplification, more than a billion copies of the sequence are created.

Rapid PCR amplification of specific sequences can be used to facilitate cloning of specific genes from DNA samples for the analysis of mutation (see Fig. 4–1). Particular portions of a gene (usually the exons) from DNA can be rapidly amplified using primers known to be specific to the normal gene. The mutant gene can then be either sequenced easily (see later discussion) or tested by ASO hybridization methods. What used to be a very laborious procedure, involving construction of a genomic or cDNA library from a patient's DNA or RNA followed by screening for the gene of interest, now can be carried out in less than a day. PCR has greatly facilitated the development and clinical application of many DNA diagnostic tests.

PCR can also be applied to the analysis of small samples of RNA, a procedure often referred to as reverse transcriptase PCR. A single-stranded cDNA is first synthesized from the mRNA of interest with the same reverse transcriptase enzyme that is used to prepare cDNA clone libraries (see Fig. 4–5). PCR primers are then added, along with DNA polymerase, as in the case of DNA PCR. One of the oligonucleotides primes synthesis of the second strand of the cDNA, which in its double-stranded form then serves as a target for PCR amplification.

PCR is an extremely sensitive technique. It allows the detection and analysis of specific gene sequences in a patient's sample without cloning and without the need for Southern or Northern blotting. Analyses can even be performed on a single cell obtained from a hair root, from the few buccal cells present in mouth rinses, from a single blastomere removed from an embryo at the four-cell stage, from the sperm in a vaginal swab obtained from a rape victim, or from a drop of dried blood at a crime scene. PCR thus eliminates the need to prepare large amounts of DNA or RNA from tissue samples.

PCR is rapidly becoming a standard method for analysis of DNA and RNA samples in research laboratories, in clinical molecular diagnostic laboratories, and in forensic and law enforcement laboratories. PCR is faster, less expensive, more sensitive, and less demanding of patients' samples than any other method for nucleic acid analysis. Specific examples of its use for the detection of mutations in genetic disorders are presented in Chapter 19.

## IN SITU HYBRIDIZATION TO CHROMOSOMES

Just as nucleic acid probes can be hybridized to samples of restriction enzyme–digested DNA or purified RNA immobilized on filters for Southern and Northern blot analysis, probes can also be hybridized to the DNA contained within chromosomes immobilized on microscope slides (see Chapter 3). This technique is called **in situ hybridization** because the DNA in metaphase chromosomes fixed on slides is denatured in place (hence "in situ") to expose the two strands of DNA, thus allowing a labeled probe to hybridize to the chromosomal DNA. The most common method of labeling probes for in situ hybridization to chromosomes is with a fluorescent dye. The hybridized probe fluoresces when the chromosomes are viewed with a wavelength of light that excites the fluorescent dye. The location of the hybridization signal, and, thus, the location of the DNA segment to which the probe hybridizes, is then determined under a microscope (see Figs. 8–8 and 9–4). This technique, known as **fluorescence in situ hybridization (FISH)**, is used widely in diagnostic clinical cytogenetics (see Chapters 9 and 10) as well as in gene mapping (see Chapter 8).

### The Molecular Analysis of a Human Mutation

How does one proceed to identify a mutation in a gene in a patient with a genetic disorder known or suspected to be due to defects in that gene? For example, consider a patient with a diagnosis of $\beta$-thalassemia, an autosomal recessive defect in the $\beta$-globin gene (see Chapter 11). The initial diagnosis is generally made on the basis of clinical and hematological findings alone. It is important to examine the gene itself, however, first to confirm the clinical diagnosis and second, to determine the specific mutation in the $\beta$-globin locus both for future use in carrier testing and possible prenatal diagnosis in the patient's family. In addition, identifying the mutation increases our understanding of the relationship between specific mutations in a gene and the resulting pathophysiology.

Several tests can be used initially to examine the gross integrity of the $\beta$-globin gene itself and its mRNA. Are both copies of the gene present in the patient, and is their structure normal? Or is one or both copies of the gene deleted, as has been described in some cases of $\beta$-thalassemia? Southern blotting of the $\beta$-globin gene can address the question of whether the gene is present and whether it is grossly normal in structure. By this method, one can detect large molecular defects (e.g., deletions, rearrangements) that are well below the level of sensitivity of chromosome analysis. Southern blotting cannot reveal the presence of most single mutations, however, such as base-pair changes or very small deletions of only a few base pairs, unless they disrupt a restriction endonuclease site.

If the gene is present, is it transcribed? To determine whether a specific transcript is present, **Northern blotting** is used. This approach also enables one to detect major changes in mRNA levels or structure of a specific gene, but not to detect minor alterations (e.g., a mutation that changes a codon in an exon).

Having asked whether there are gross changes in the gene or in its mRNA, one can proceed to examine gene structure and expression at increasingly finer levels of analysis. In $\beta$-thalassemia, as in many other genetic disorders, many mutations are already known that are responsible for the disease. To determine whether one of the known mutations is responsible for a particular case of $\beta$-thalassemia, one can use **allele-specific oligonucleotides (ASOs)** that enable one to detect specific single base-pair mutations (see main text). If ASO analysis fails to reveal a known mutation, it may be necessary to compare the sequence of the mutant $\beta$-globin gene (or cDNA) from the patient for comparison with a normal $\beta$-globin gene by using the **polymerase chain reaction (PCR)** to specifically generate many millions of copies of a particular gene fragment, and sequencing it. In this way, the specific mutation responsible for the genetic disorder in the patient can be identified and used to develop direct screening tests for that mutation in the patient's family.

A commonly used type of probe for FISH is a single contiguous genomic sequence, cloned as an insert in a cosmid, BAC, or YAC vector that hybridizes to the location of the probe sequence on a pair of homologous chromosomes. A FISH probe can also be a complex mixture of DNA from one part of a chromosome arm, an entire chromosome arm, or even an entire chromosome. Depending on how the probe is constituted, a large portion of a chromosome arm, the whole arm, or an entire chromosome will stain with the fluorescent hybridized probe. Such probe mixtures are known as **chromosome "painting" probes** (see Chapter 9 for examples).

Two recently developed techniques expand even more dramatically the power of FISH technology for human chromosome analysis. The first of these techniques, **comparative genome hybridization**, is used to measure differences in copy number or dosage of a particular chromosomal segment between two different DNA samples. Total DNA from one sample is labeled with a red fluorescent dye, and the other sample is labeled with a green dye. The two labeled DNA samples are mixed in equal amounts and used as a painting probe for FISH with *normal* human metaphase chromosomes. The ratio of red-to-green fluorescence emitted by the probe along each chromosome is then measured. If the DNA from a particular region of a chromosome is represented equally in the two samples that make up the probe, the ratio of red-to-green fluorescence in the FISH signal will be 1:1 (Fig. 4–11). If, however, the DNA labeled with green is from a normal cell line and the DNA labeled with red comes from cells that are either lacking material (**monosomy**; see Chapter 9) or have additional material (**trisomy**; see Chapter 9) from all or part of a chromosome, the ratio of red-to-green fluorescence will shift from 1:1 to either less than 1 in the case of monosomy or more than 1 in the case of trisomy in the region of the chromosome with the abnormal gene dosage. For example, as shown in Figure 4–11, DNA labeled with red from the tissues of an individual with partial trisomy for the tip of chromosome 18p results in a ratio of red-to-green of 1.5:1 over distal 18p. Similarly, if the individual were monosomic for 18p, the ratio of red-to-green fluorescence along 18p will be 0.5:1. Comparative genome hybridization is particularly useful for finding changes in gene dosage in tissues that can serve as a source of DNA for making a probe but cannot be easily karyotyped (see Chapter 3), such as solid tumors and soft tissue sarcomas. The technique is finding its widest application in the study of chromosomal aberrations in cancer cells (see Chapter 16).

A second, powerful FISH technique is **spectral karyotyping (SKY)**. An essential reagent for SKY is to have 24 different chromosome-painting probes, one for each of the 24 human chromosomes. These chromosome-specific probes are obtained by separating each chromosome on the basis of size and banding characteristics from all of the other chromosomes

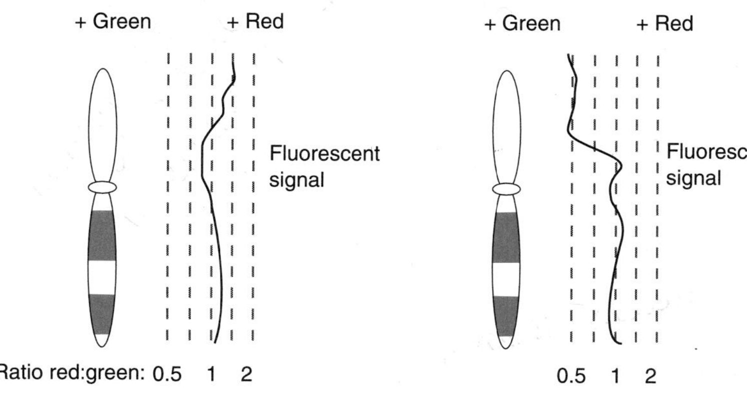


**Figure 4–11.** Results of comparative genome hybridization, typically reported by a graph of fluorescence intensity running along the length of a chromosome. DNA from two different sources is purified, each labeled with a different fluorescent dye, the probes mixed, and used as a total chromosome paint for normal metaphases. The intensity of hybridization with each dye will be equal over all regions of the metaphase chromosomes that are present in equal amounts in the two different DNA sources. If one segment of a chromosome is duplicated or deleted in one cell line versus the other, the relative intensity of hybridization with each dye will shift from 1:1.

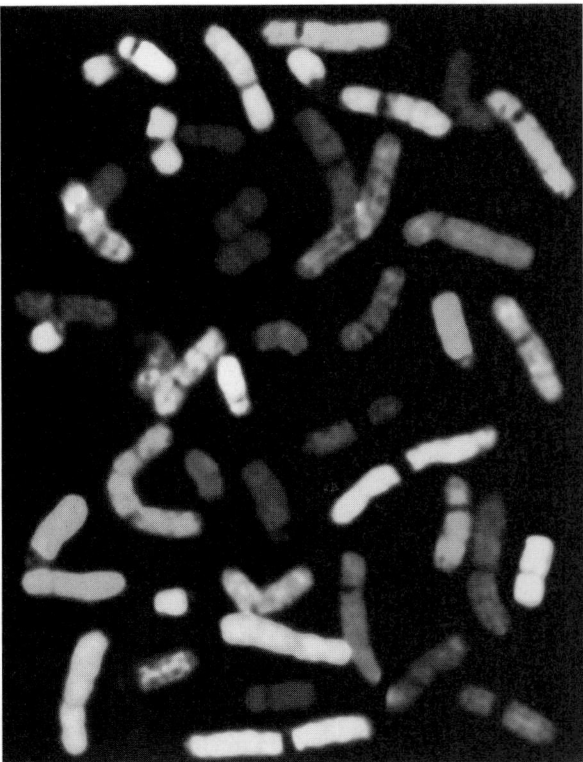

Figure 4–12. Spectral karyotyping (SKY). Twenty-four individual chromosome painting probes are labeled with different fluorescent dyes and used as a total genome chromosome paint. The fluorescent signals are analyzed by sophisticated imaging software and stored in a computer. To generate the photograph, the computer assigns a different color to each of the 24 different fluorescence spectra generated by the individual chromosome painting probes. In this metaphase from a 46, XX female, only 23 colors are present; the unique spectrum generated by the Y chromosome painting probe is not seen. (See Fig. 9–5*B*, *color insert*.) (Figure courtesy of Dr. Amalia Dutra, National Human Genome Research Institute.)

using fluorescence-activated chromosome sorting. Each chromosome-specific DNA sample is labeled with a different combination of fluorescent dyes that emit at different wavelengths. In this way, each human chromosome is represented by a probe with its own characteristic spectra of wavelengths of fluorescence. All 24 probes for the human chromosomes are then combined and used for FISH of metaphase chromosomes (see Fig. 9–5*B*, *color insert*). Because each chromosome-specific probe emits its own signature wavelength of fluorescence, structural rearrangements are easily seen, and the chromosomes involved can be readily identified.

## DNA SEQUENCE ANALYSIS

The most widely used approach for DNA sequence analysis is Sanger sequencing (named after Fred Sanger, who, with Walter Gilbert, received the Nobel prize in 1980 for developing DNA sequencing). The sequence of virtually any purified DNA segment can now be determined, whether it be a cloned fragment or a target sequence amplified by PCR. Sanger sequencing takes advantage of chemical analogs of nucleotides to inhibit the enzyme DNA polymerase as it synthesizes the strand complementary to the original template being sequenced (Fig. 4–13). To carry out the sequencing reaction, DNA synthesis is primed by a short oligonucleotide and the DNA polymerase proceeds along the template sequence, extending the primer and incorporating either radioactively labeled nucleotides or nucleotides carrying fluorescent tags into the newly synthesized sequence. One obtains sequence information by adding one of the inhibitory analogs along with all four normal nucleotides into each of four sequencing reactions. Thus, in a reaction to define the location of G residues, a G analog is included in the reaction, so that the extension of a proportion of individual molecules will stop when DNA polymerase incorporates the analog. The relative amounts of the normal G nucleotide and the G analog in this reaction are adjusted so that the polymerase incorporates the analog of G in some newly synthesized strands the very first time it incorporates a G, whereas in other strands, a G analog is incorporated the next time a G is incorporated, some at the third, and so forth. When this sample is then analyzed by gel electrophoresis, a series of bands is observed at lengths corresponding to the locations of each G residue. Similar reactions for the A, T, and C residues provide corresponding series of fragments. The set of four reactions can then be read as a directional sequencing "ladder" to determine the nucleotide sequence of the DNA fragment being analyzed (see Fig. 4–13).

Machines now automate the procedure of DNA sequencing, which is routinely applied for analysis of both normal and mutant genes. DNA sequence information is critical for predicting the amino acid

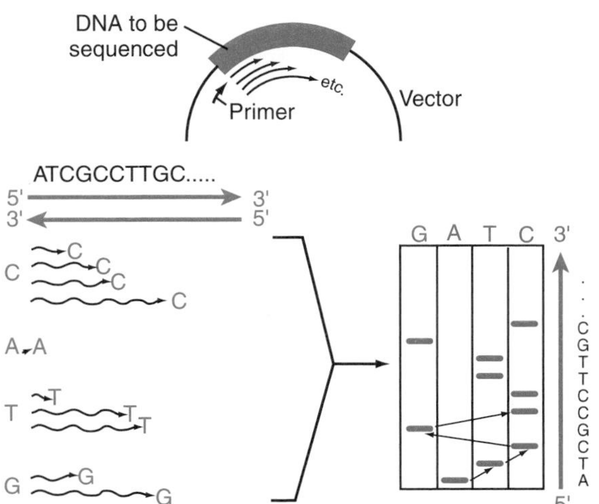


Figure 4–13. The Sanger method of determining the nucleotide sequence of a cloned DNA fragment. See text for description.

sequence encoded by a newly isolated gene, for detecting individual mutations in genetic disease, and for designing either ASO probes or PCR primers used in molecular diagnostic procedures. Automated sequencing is also being massively applied in the Human Genome Project to obtain the nucleotide sequence of all 3 billion bases of the entire human genome (see Chapter 8), as well as the complete sequence of other organisms of medical and scientific importance including *E. coli*, the yeast *S. cerevisiae*, the worm *Caenorhabditis elegans*, the fruitfly *Drosophila melanogaster*, the mouse, and many pathogenic microorganisms.

## METHODS OF PROTEIN ANALYSIS

The analysis of both normal and abnormal gene function often requires an examination of the protein encoded by a normal or mutant gene of interest. In most instances, one wants to know not only the molecular defect in the DNA, but also how that defect alters the encoded protein to produce the clinical phenotype.

### Western Blotting

Shortly after development of Southern and Northern blotting for DNA and RNA, a conceptually related procedure for the detection of specific proteins was described and dubbed **Western blotting**. This technique can be used to obtain information on the size and amount of mutant protein in cell extracts from patients with genetic diseases. In this method, proteins isolated from a cell extract are separated according to size by polyacrylamide gel electrophoresis and then transferred to a membrane. The membrane containing the separated proteins is then incubated with antibodies that specifically recognize the protein to be analyzed. The specific interaction between the antibody and its antigen can then be detected by a second antibody against the first, tagged with a detectable histochemical, fluorescent, or radioactive substance. An example of a Western blot used to detect the presence or absence and, if present, the size of the muscle protein dystrophin in patients with X-linked muscular dystrophy is shown in Figure 4–14.

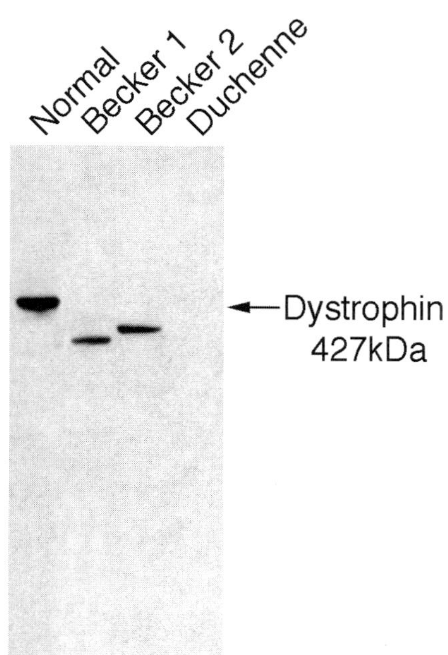


**Figure 4–14.** A Western blot demonstrating the presence or absence of the muscle protein dystrophin (*arrow*) in protein extracts from patients with the severe Duchenne or mild Becker form of X-linked muscular dystrophy. See Chapter 12 for further description. (Original photograph courtesy of P. Wray, Hospital for Sick Children, Toronto.)

## General References

Davies K (1995) Human Genetic Disease Analysis: A Practical Approach, 2nd ed. IRL Press, Oxford, England.

Dieffenbach C, Dveksler G (1995) PCR Primer: A Laboratory Manual. Cold Spring Harbor Laboratory, Cold Spring Harbor, New York.

Fritsch EF, Wozney JM (1994) Methods of molecular genetics. *In* Stamatoyannopoulos G, Nienhuis AW, Majerus PW, Varmus H (eds) The Molecular Basis of Blood Diseases, 2nd ed. W.B. Saunders, Philadelphia.

Sambrook J, Russell D (2001) Molecular Cloning: A Laboratory Manual, 3rd ed. Cold Spring Harbor Laboratory, Cold Spring Harbor, New York.

## References Specific to Particular Topics

Handyside AH (1998) Clinical evaluation of preimplantation genetic diagnosis. Prenat Diagn 18:1345–1348.

Monaco AP, Larin Z (1994) YACs, BACs, PACs and MACs: Artificial chromosomes as research tools. Trends Biotechnol 12:280–286.

Vnencak-Jones CL (1999) Molecular testing for inherited diseases. Am J Clin Pathol 112 (suppl 1): S19–S32.

Weedn VW (1996) Forensic DNA tests. Clin Lab Med 16:187–196.

## Problems

1. Consider the following diagnostic situations. What laboratory method or methods would be most appropriate?
   (a) Prenatal diagnosis of a male fetus at risk for Duchenne muscular dystrophy (DMD). Previous studies in this family have already documented a complete gene deletion.
   (b) You want to estimate the amount of dystrophin mRNA present in a muscle specimen from a mildly affected obligate carrier of DMD.
   (c) Prenatal diagnosis of a male fetus at risk for DMD. Previous studies have already documented a particular nucleotide base change that is responsible for the defect in this family.
2. What are some of the advantages or disadvantages of PCR for diagnosis of genetic defects in comparison with

Southern blotting? With biochemical assays of enzyme levels to diagnose enzyme deficiencies?

3. From which of the following tissues can DNA be obtained for diagnostic procedures: tissue biopsy specimens, white blood cells, cultured amniotic fluid cells, red blood cells?

4. Why is cloning of a gene considered such a significant advance for the field of medical genetics? What does the availability of a cloned gene allow one to do that one could not do before?

5. You want to clone a gene that is expressed in liver and is suspected to be involved in a genetic disease. Both a human genomic DNA library and a liver cDNA library are available to you. Which would you choose and why?

6. A patient with a genetic disease has a mutation (**C** to **T**, underlined) in exon 18 of a gene. The normal sequence is:

   CTGTGCCGTATGAAAAGACCAATC**C**GA-
   GAAGTTCCTGTTACCAAACTCATAGAC

   The sequence in the patient is:

   CTGTGCCGTATGAAAAGACCAATC**T**GA-
   GAAGTTCCTGTTACCAAACTCATAGAC

   (a) What is the consequence of this mutation on gene function? (The first three nucleotides in each sequence constitute a codon of the gene.)
   (b) You need to develop an ASO assay for the mutation in genomic DNA. Which of the following oligonucleotide(s) would be useful in an ASO for the normal sequence? For the mutant sequence? Give your reasons for selecting or rejecting each oligonucleotide.

   1. 5′ GCCGTATGAAAAGACCAATCTG
   2. 5′ GACCAATCCGAGAAGTTCC
   3. 5′ GACCAATCTGAGAAGTTCC
   4. 5′ GGAACTTCTCAGATTGGTC
   5. 5′ ATCTGAG

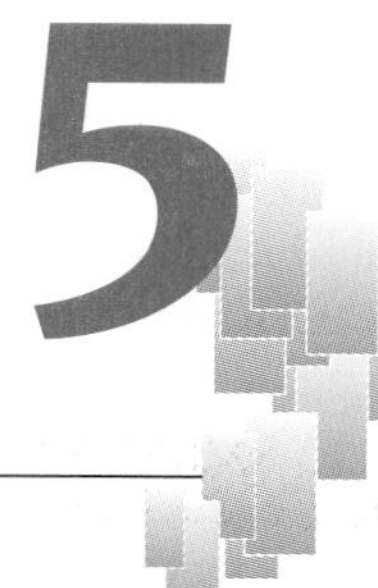

# Patterns of Single-Gene Inheritance

In Chapter 1, the three main categories of genetic disorders—single-gene, chromosomal, and complex—were named and briefly characterized. In the first section of this chapter, the typical patterns of transmission of single-gene disorders are discussed in further detail; the emphasis is on the molecular and genetic mechanisms by which mutations in genes result in recessive, dominant, and X-linked inheritance patterns. In the next section, we describe how gene imprinting and mosaicism can alter or obscure typical single-gene inheritance patterns.

Single-gene traits are often called **mendelian** because, like the characteristics of garden peas studied by Gregor Mendel, they occur on average in fixed proportions among the offspring of specific types of matings. The single-gene phenotypes known so far are listed in Victor A. McKusick's classic reference *Mendelian Inheritance in Man* (12th edition, 1998), which has been indispensable to medical geneticists for decades. The online version of *Mendelian Inheritance in Man* (OMIM) is continually updated and is available through the World Wide Web. OMIM lists more than 9300 genes, of which more than 1400 are established gene loci at which mutations are associated with a clinically significant disorder. Thus, of the estimated 50,000 human genes, more than 3 percent have already been identified as contributing in a major way to human disease. The 3 percent figure is likely a great underestimate. The pace of new gene discovery is high, and it appears certain to accelerate because of international efforts dedicated to mapping and sequencing the entire human genome and the genes expressed in differentiated human tissues.

Single-gene disorders are primarily, but by no means exclusively, disorders of the pediatric age range; less than 10 percent manifest after puberty, and only 1 percent occur after the end of the reproductive period. Although individually rare, as a group they are responsible for a significant proportion of childhood diseases and deaths. In a population study of more than 1 million live births, the incidence of serious single-gene disorders was estimated to be 0.36 percent; among hospitalized children, 6 to 8 percent are thought to have single-gene disorders.

## TERMINOLOGY

Even though the principles of medical genetics are relatively easy to understand, the unfamiliar terminology may make the subject seem inaccessible at first. To help address the language problem, we review some terms and introduce others that have not been defined previously.

Inherited variation in the genome is the cornerstone of human and medical genetics. As introduced in Chapter 2, alternative variants of genetic information at a particular locus are called **alleles**. For many genes, there is a single prevailing version, present in the majority of individuals, which geneticists call the **wild-type** or normal allele. The other versions of the gene are **mutant** alleles that differ from the wild-type allele by **mutation**, a permanent change in the nucleotide sequence or arrangement of DNA. If there are at least two relatively common alleles at the locus in the population, the locus is said to exhibit **polymorphism** (literally "many forms"), as is discussed in detail in subsequent chapters. In addition to a normal allele or to common polymorphic alleles, loci may also have one or more rare, variant alleles; some of these rare alleles were originally identified because they cause genetic disease, whereas others are of no known significance to health.

The **genotype** of a person is the set of alleles that make up his or her genetic constitution, either collectively at all loci or, more typically, at a single locus. In contrast, the **phenotype** is the observable expression of a genotype as a morphological, clinical, biochemical, or molecular trait. A phenotype may, of course, be either normal or abnormal in a given individual, but in this book, which emphasizes disorders of medical significance, the focus is on abnormal phenotypes—that is, genetic disorders.

A **single-gene disorder** is one that is determined by the alleles at a single locus. A variant allele, which arose by mutation at some time in the recent or remote past and is usually relatively rare, replaces a wild-type allele on one or both chromosomes. When a person has a pair of identical alleles, he or she is said to be **homozygous** (a **homozygote**); when the alleles are different, he or she is **heterozygous** (a **heterozygote** or carrier). The term **compound heterozygote** is used to describe a genotype in which two different mutant alleles of the same gene are present, rather than one normal and one mutant. These terms (homozygous, heterozygous, and compound heterozygous) can be applied either to a person or to a genotype. The term **mutation** is used in medical genetics in two senses: sometimes to indicate a new genetic change that has not been previously known in a kindred and sometimes merely to indicate a disease-causing allele. Mutation and mutant, however, are not used to refer to the human beings who carry mutant alleles that arose by mutation.

Single-gene disorders are characterized by their patterns of transmission in families. To establish the pattern of transmission, a usual first step is to obtain information about the family history of the patient and to summarize the details in the form of a **pedigree**, a graphical representation of a family tree, using standard symbols (Fig. 5–1). The member through whom a family with a genetic disorder is first brought to attention (ascertained) is the **proband** (synonyms **propositus** or **index case**) if he or she is affected. The person who brings the family to attention by consulting a geneticist is referred to as the **consultand**; the consultand may be an affected individual or an unaffected relative of a proband. A family may have more than one proband, if ascertained through more than one source. Brothers and sisters are called **sibs**, and a family of sibs forms a **sibship**. The entire family is called a **kindred** (Fig. 5–2). Relatives are classified as **first-degree** (parents, sibs, and offspring of the proband); **second-degree** (grandparents and grandchildren, uncles and aunts, nephews and nieces, and half-sibs); **third-degree** (e.g., first cousins), and so forth, depending on the number of steps (in other words, the number of meioses) in the pedigree between the two relatives. The offspring of first cousins are second cousins, and a child is a "first cousin once removed" of his or her parents' first cousins. Couples who have one or more ancestors in common are **consanguineous**. If there is only one affected member in a family, he or she is an **isolated** case or, if the disorder is determined to be due to new mutation in the propositus, a **sporadic** case (see Fig. 5–2).

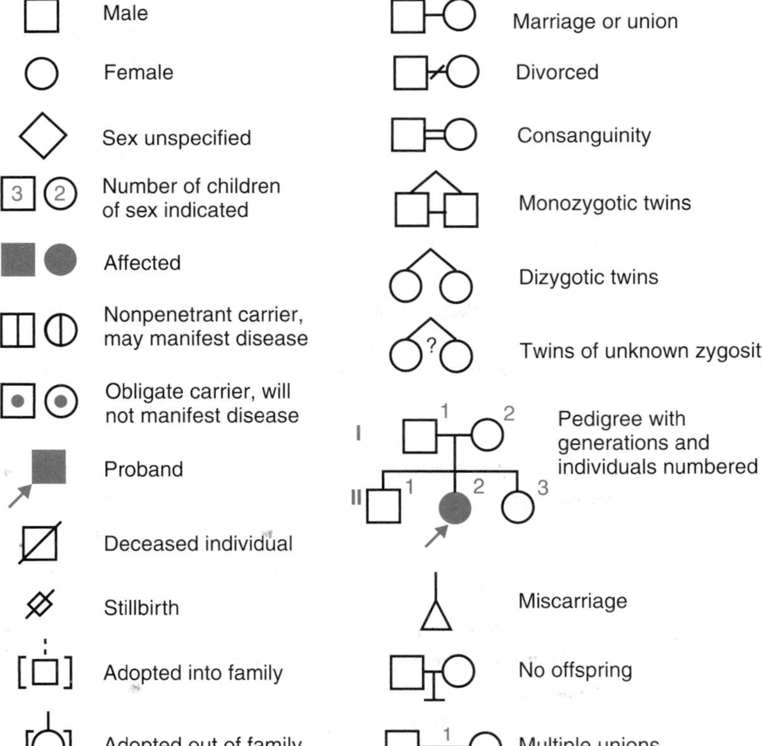


**Figure 5–1.** Symbols commonly used in pedigree charts. Although there is no uniform system of pedigree notation, the symbols used here are according to recent recommendations made by professionals in the field of genetic counseling. (From Bennett RL, Steinhaus KA, Uhrich SB et al (1995) Recommendations for standardized pedigree nomenclature. J Genet Counsel 4:267–279.)

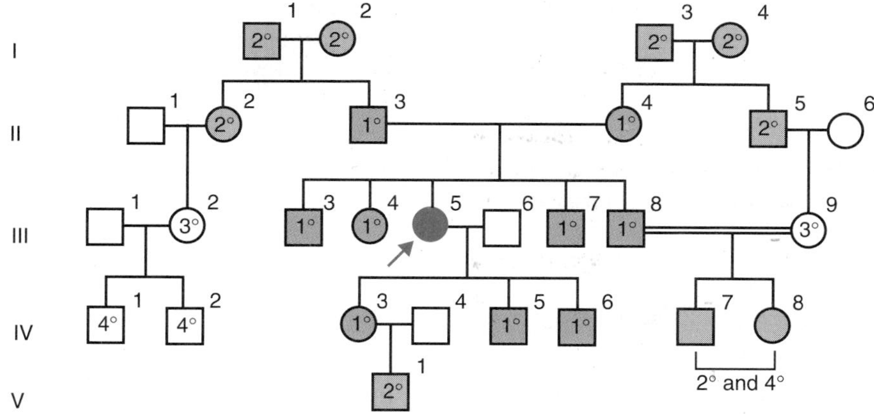


**Figure 5–2.** Relationships within a kindred. Arrow indicates the **proband**, III-5, who represents an **isolated case** of a genetic disorder. She has four **sibs**, III-3, III-4, III-7, and III-8. Her partner/spouse is III-6, and they have three children (their **F1** progeny). The proband has nine **first-degree** relatives (her parents, siblings, and offspring), nine **second-degree** relatives (grandparents, uncles/aunts, nieces/nephews, grandchildren), two **third-degree** relatives (first cousins), and four **fourth-degree** relatives (first cousins once removed). IV-3, IV-5, and IV-6 are **second cousins** of IV-1 and IV-2. IV-7 and IV-8, whose parents are **consanguineous**, are doubly related to the proband: second-degree relatives through their father and fourth-degree relatives through their mother.

## GENETIC DISORDERS WITH CLASSICAL MENDELIAN INHERITANCE

The patterns shown by single-gene disorders in pedigrees depend chiefly on two factors: (1) the chromosomal location of the gene locus, which may be **autosomal** (located on an autosome) or **X-linked** (located on the X chromosome), and (2) whether the phenotype is **dominant** (expressed when only one chromosome of a pair carries the mutant allele, despite there being a normal allele on the other chromosome of the pair) or **recessive** (expressed only when both chromosomes of a pair carry a mutant allele). Thus, there are four basic patterns of single-gene inheritance:

| | Dominant | Recessive |
|---|---|---|
| **Autosomal** | Autosomal dominant | Autosomal recessive |
| **X-linked** | X-linked dominant | X-linked recessive |

### Autosomal and X-Linked Inheritance

The distinction between autosomal and X-linked inheritance is obvious, because it depends solely on the chromosomal location of the gene. The clinical expression of an abnormal gene also depends on whether it is autosomal or X-linked, however. There are two considerations, which are discussed in more detail later: (1) Males have only a single X and therefore are said to be **hemizygous** with respect to X-linked genes, rather than homozygous or heterozygous; 46,XY males are never heterozygous for X-linked traits. (2) To compensate for the double complement of X-linked genes in females, alleles for most X-linked genes are expressed from only one of the two X chromosomes in any given cell of a female (see **X chromosome inactivation**, later), whereas both alleles of most, but not all autosomal loci are active (see **imprinting**, later).

### Dominant and Recessive Inheritance

By definition, a phenotype expressed in the same way in both homozygotes and heterozygotes is dominant, whereas a phenotype expressed only in homozygotes (or, for X-linked traits, hemizygotes) is recessive. In medical genetics, however, this definition is too rigid to be useful in practice; instead, any phenotype expressed in heterozygotes is classified as dominant, whether or not heterozygotes and homozygotes for the mutant allele have the same phenotype. In fact, autosomal dominant disorders are typically more severe in homozygotes than in heterozygotes, and so far only two autosomal dominant disorders, Huntington disease (see Chapter 12) and multiple endocrine adenomatosis I, are known to be equally severe in both genotypes. When the phenotype due to a heterozygous genotype is different from the phenotype seen in both homozygous genotypes and its severity is intermediate between them, the phenotype may be described more precisely as **incompletely dominant**. If expression of each allele can be detected even in the presence of the other, the two alleles are termed **codominant**.

Strictly speaking, it is the phenotype rather than the allele that is dominant or recessive; however, alleles are often classified as dominant or recessive on the basis of whether they can cause a change in phenotype when in the heterozygous or homozygous state, respectively, and so the terms "dominant allele or gene" and "recessive allele or gene" are widely, albeit loosely, used.

The distinction between dominant and recessive inheritance is not absolute; rather, it is an arbitrary designation, based on clinical phenotypes, that may be without significance at the level of gene action. Although a recessive phenotype is defined as being clinically undetectable in heterozygotes, many traits classified as recessive do have heterozygous manifestations when examined at the cellular, biochemical, or molecular level. For example, the well-known disorder of hemoglobin, **sickle cell disease** (or anemia), is inherited as an autosomal recessive disease (see Chapter 11 for further discussion). Patients with the disease are homozygous for a defective allele at the $\beta$-globin locus and consequently produce the abnormal hemoglobin S (Hb S) rather than the normal adult hemoglobin A (Hb A) in their red blood cells, which become sickle-shaped under conditions of low oxygen tension. Heterozygotes produce both Hb A and Hb S, a proportion of their red blood cells show the sickling phenomenon, and they have mild anemia. Thus, at the level of hemoglobin synthesis, the normal $\beta$-globin allele and the defective allele are expressed as codominant alleles; at the level of physiological function, the normal allele is incompletely dominant (and the abnormal allele is incompletely recessive); and at the clinical level, sickle cell disease behaves as a recessive trait.

Many of the autosomal recessive disorders described to date are enzyme defects, in which there appears to be a margin of safety wide enough to allow normal function in heterozygotes even though only one of a pair of alleles is fully functional and the other (abnormal) allele is defective or nonfunctional. In contrast, in autosomal dominant disorders, disease occurs despite the presence of the normal gene product made from the remaining normal allele. Broadly speaking, there are at least four different situations in which one normal copy of the gene does not suffice to prevent disease:

1. Normal physiology requires more than 50% of fully active gene product to prevent disease. There is no margin of safety wide enough to allow normal function in heterozygotes even though only one of the pair of alleles is fully functional. When loss of half of the normal activity of a protein causes disease, the situation is referred to as **haploinsufficiency**. Haploinsufficiency has been shown to occur with mutations in genes encoding certain transcription factors, structural proteins, and cell surface receptors.
2. Instead of simple deficiency or dysfunction of the protein product, an abnormal protein may be synthesized that causes an abnormal phenotype by interfering with the function of the product of the normal allele (**dominant negative effect**), as is seen with collagen mutations in osteogenesis imperfecta ("brittle-bone disease") (see Chapter 12).
3. The mutant protein may be enhanced in one or more of its normal properties through mutation (**simple gain of function**), as in the dwarfing condition achondroplasia, or become toxic to the cell through acquisition of a novel property, as in Huntington disease (see Chapter 12).
4. An inherited dysfunction of one copy of certain autosomal genes may result in pedigrees with dominantly inherited cancers (e.g., retinoblastoma; see Chapter 16). Random loss of the other, normal allele, even if an extremely rare event occurring in only a very few cells, eliminates both copies of the gene in those cells and renders them cancerous. Thus, although the predisposition to cancer is inherited as a dominant trait, the mutations that lead to cancer are recessive at the cellular level, because both copies of the gene must be rendered dysfunctional for cancer to develop.

In summary, the distinction between a dominant and a recessive mutant allele is really a simple one: in heterozygotes, with one normal and one mutant allele, is the half-normal amount of gene product from the normal allele sufficient to perform its designated function? If the answer is yes, the mutant allele (and its associated disorder) is termed recessive. If the mutant allele causes disease regardless of whether there is a normally functioning wild-type allele, however, the answer must be no, and the allele (and the disease) are called dominant.

## Other Pedigree Patterns

Sometimes a pedigree pattern simulates a single-gene pattern even though the disorder does not have a single-gene basis. It is easy to be misled in this way by teratogenic effects; by certain types of inherited chromosomal disorders, such as balanced translocations or microdeletions that cause rare **contiguous gene syndromes** (or **microdeletion syndromes**) in which there is deletion of multiple genes at closely linked loci (see Chapter 10); or by environmental exposures shared among family members. Inherited single-gene disorders can usually be distinguished from other types of familial disorders by their typical mendelian segregation ratios within kindreds. Confirmation that a disease is due to mutations in a single gene may eventually require demonstration of defects at the level of the gene product or the gene.

Many patients with genetic disorders have no similarly affected relatives, but it may still be possible to recognize that the disorder is genetic. Because of the remarkable similarity of phenotype among different families with the same defect, well-established patterns of inheritance in other families with the same disorder can often be used as a basis for diagnosis and counseling even if the patient is an isolated case in the family.

## Age of Onset and Other Factors Affecting Pedigree Patterns

### Age of Onset

Not all genetic disorders are congenital; many are not expressed until later in life, some at a characteristic age and others at variable ages. Because the terms "genetic" and "congenital" are frequently confused, it is important to keep in mind that a genetic disorder is one that is determined by genes, whereas a congenital disorder is merely one that is present at birth and may or may not have a genetic basis.

Many genetic disorders develop prenatally and thus are both genetic and congenital. Dysmorphic phenotypes of many kinds originate during development and are recognized at birth (or even prenatally, in some cases, by ultrasonography; see Chapter 18) as "birth defects." Some genetic disorders may be lethal in prenatal life. Others are expressed as soon as the infant begins its independent life. Still others appear even later or make their clinical appearance at a variety of ages extending from birth to the postreproductive years.

### Other Factors Affecting Pedigree Patterns

Although as a general rule pedigrees of single-gene disorders can be readily classified as autosomal or X-linked and as dominant or recessive, the inheritance pattern of an individual pedigree may be obscured by a number of other factors that may make the mode of inheritance difficult to interpret. The segregation of genes from parents to children through the gametes is a random process and, especially with the small family size typical of most developed countries today, the patient may be the only affected family member; the inheritance pattern, if any, may not be immediately apparent. Some other points to keep in mind are the following: new mutation is not an infrequent cause of dominant and X-linked disease; diagnostic difficulties may occur owing to absent or variable expression of the gene concerned; other genes and environmental factors may affect gene expression; persons of some genotypes may fail to survive to the time of birth; accurate information about the presence of the disorder in relatives or about family relationships may be lacking.

## Genetic Heterogeneity

When a genetic disorder that appears to be a single entity is thoroughly analyzed, it is frequently found to be genetically heterogeneous; that is, it includes a number of phenotypes that are similar but are actually determined by different genotypes. Genetic heterogeneity may be the result of different mutations at the same locus **(allelic heterogeneity)**, mutations at different loci **(locus heterogeneity)**, or both. Recognition of genetic heterogeneity is an important aspect of clinical diagnosis and genetic counseling (see Chapter 12, Table 12-2).

### Locus Heterogeneity

For many phenotypes, pedigree analysis alone has been sufficient to demonstrate genetic heterogeneity. For example, **retinitis pigmentosa**, a common cause of visual impairment due to photoreceptor degeneration associated with abnormal pigment distribution in the retina, has long been known to occur in autosomal dominant, autosomal recessive, and X-linked forms. In recent years, the heterogeneity has been shown to be even more extensive; DNA analysis has demonstrated that there are probably at least 3 X-linked forms, 12 autosomal dominant forms, and 5 autosomal recessive forms of retinitis pigmentosa that are not associated with other phenotypic abnormalities. If one includes disorders in which retinitis pigmentosa is found in conjunction with other defects such as mental retardation or deafness, the number of different genetic diseases manifesting retinitis pigmentosa is well over 30! **Ehlers-Danlos syndrome,** in which skin and other connective tissues may be excessively elastic or fragile because of an underlying defect of collagen structure, may also have autosomal dominant, autosomal recessive, or X-linked inheritance, and analysis at the clinical and molecular levels has shown that there are more than 10 different loci associated with this disorder.

### Allelic Heterogeneity

Allelic heterogeneity is an important cause of clinical variation. Many loci possess more than one mutant allele; in fact, at a given locus there may be several or many mutations. Sometimes, these different mutations result in clinically indistinguishable or closely similar disorders. In other cases, different mutant alleles at the same locus result in very different clinical presentations. For example, some mutations in the *RET* gene, which encodes a receptor tyrosine kinase, can cause dominantly inherited failure of development of colonic ganglia leading to defective colonic motility and severe chronic constipation **(Hirschsprung disease)** (see Chapter 15), whereas other mutations in the same gene result in dominantly inherited cancer of the thyroid and adrenal glands **(multiple endocrine neoplasia type IIa and IIb)** (see Chapter 16). A third group of mutations in *RET* causes both Hirschsprung disease and multiple endocrine neoplasia in the same individuals.

Unless they have consanguineous parents, most people with autosomal recessive disorders are more likely to have compound rather than truly homozygous genotypes, although for most purposes they are still usually referred to as homozygotes if they have a pair of abnormal alleles at a locus. Because different allelic combinations may have somewhat different clinical consequences, clinicians must be aware of allelic heterogeneity as one possible explanation for variability among patients considered to have the same disease.

## AUTOSOMAL RECESSIVE INHERITANCE

We begin with autosomal recessive phenotypes because, although they are less common than autosomal dominants, their inheritance pattern and mechanism of disease are generally better understood in molecular terms. As discussed in the previous section, autosomal recessive disease occurs only in homozygotes, individuals with two mutant alleles and no normal allele, because in these diseases, one normal gene copy in a heterozygote is able to compensate for the mutant allele and prevent the disease from occurring. Because an individual inherits only one of the two alleles at any locus from one parent, homozygotes must have inherited a mutant allele from each parent (barring the rare new mutation). A typical pedigree illustrating autosomal recessive inheritance is shown in Figure 5–3. Both parents of an affected person are heterozygotes (**carriers**). Their children's risk of receiving a recessive allele is one half from each parent, and so the chance of inheriting two recessive alleles and therefore being affected is $1/2 \times 1/2$ or 1 in 4. The proband may be the only affected family member, but if any others are affected, they are usually in the same sibship and not elsewhere in the kindred, unless the family is highly inbred.

Although any mating in which each parent has at least one recessive allele can produce homozygous affected offspring, the most common one by far is the mating of two unaffected carriers. The three types of matings, with the risk to the offspring in each case, are listed here. The mutant recessive allele is symbolized as *r* and its normal dominant allele as *R*.

| Parents | Risk to Offspring |
|---|---|
| Carrier × carrier: *R/r* × *R/r* | 1/4 *R/R*, 1/2 *R/r*, 1/4 *r/r*<br>3/4 unaffected, 1/4 affected |
| Carrier × affected: *R/r* × *r/r* | 1/2 *R/r*, 1/2 *r/r*<br>1/2 unaffected, 1/2 affected |
| Affected × affected: *r/r* × *r/r* | *r/r* only<br>All affected |

### Gene Frequency and Carrier Frequency

Carriers of autosomal recessive genes are not clinically recognizable but are far more common than homozygous affected individuals. The mutant allele responsible for a recessive disorder is generally rare, and so the chance that an individual has two copies of a rare mutant allele is much lower than the chance that he or she inherits one normal and one mutant allele. (We discuss how to calculate actual carrier and disease frequencies in Chapter 7). Because an autosomal recessive disorder must be inherited *through both parents*, the risk that any carrier will have an affected child depends partly on the chance that his or her mate is also a carrier of the condition. Thus, knowledge of the carrier frequency of a disease is clinically important for genetic counseling.

The most common autosomal recessive disorder in Caucasian children is **cystic fibrosis (CF)** (see Chap-

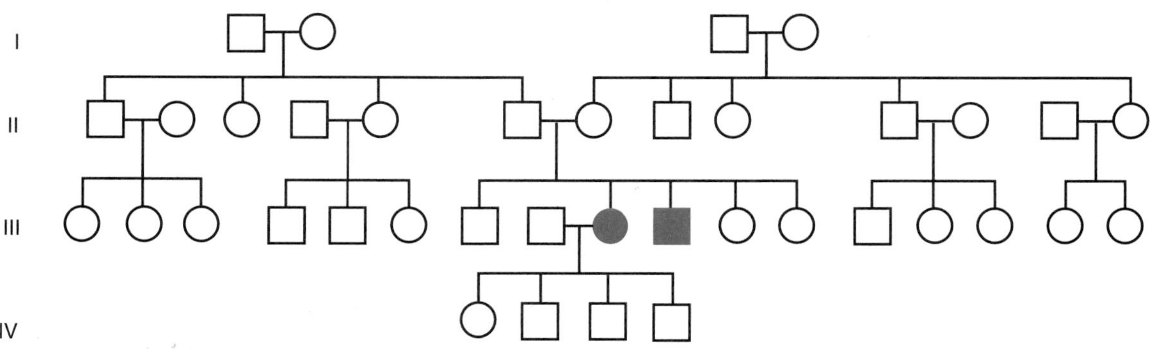


**Figure 5–3.** Typical pedigree showing autosomal recessive inheritance.

ter 12). CF is virtually unknown in Asian populations and is relatively rare in African-American populations, but in Caucasian populations, about 1 child in 2000 has two mutant CF alleles and has the disease. The frequency of carriers can be calculated to be approximately 1/22 (see Chapter 7). In a population of 2000 Caucasians, then, one expects 1 CF patient, 90 unaffected carriers of the CF mutation, and 1909 normal homozygotes. Because a patient has two CF alleles and a carrier has only one, 90/92 (about 98 percent) of all the CF genes in this population of 2000 individuals are hidden in carriers (who usually are unaware that they are carriers), and only 2 percent are in patients.

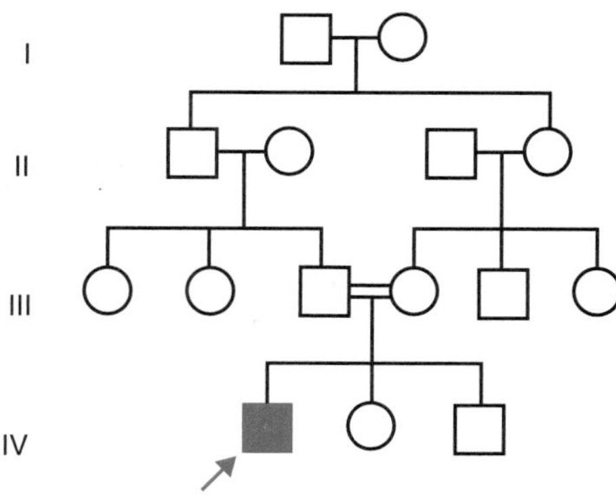


**Figure 5–4.** Pedigree in which parental consanguinity suggests autosomal recessive inheritance.

## Consanguinity and Inbreeding

As just discussed, the vast majority of the mutant alleles responsible for autosomal recessive disorders are in carriers rather than in homozygotes. Mutant alleles can be handed down in families for numerous generations without ever appearing in homozygous form; the presence of such hidden recessive genes is not revealed unless the carrier happens to mate with someone who also carries a mutant allele at the same locus and the two deleterious alleles are both inherited by a child. It is believed from studies of the offspring of incestuous matings that everyone carries at least eight to ten mutant alleles for well-known, easily recognizable autosomal recessive disorders. The total number of recessive deleterious gene mutations carried by any individual is certainly greater than this minimal estimate.

### Consanguinity

The chance that both parents are carriers of a mutant allele at the same locus is increased substantially if the parents are related and could each have inherited the mutant allele from a single common ancestor, a situation called **consanguinity**. Consanguinity of the parents of a patient with a genetic disorder is strong evidence (though not proof) for the autosomal recessive inheritance of that condition. For example, the disorder in the pedigree in Figure 5–4 is likely to be an autosomal recessive trait, even though other information in the pedigree may seem insufficient to establish this inheritance pattern. Even if the parents consider themselves unrelated, they may have common ancestry within the past few generations, especially if they are of closely similar ethnic or geographic origin. Thus, in taking a family history, it is important to ask about consanguinity and background.

Although in most populations in Western societies today the incidence of cousin marriage is low, it had been relatively common in some ethnic groups, for example, in Japan, southern India, and the Middle East. In recent times, the rate of first-cousin marriages, and consanguinity in general, is declining in many traditional societies.

A note of caution: it is important to recognize that consanguinity is not the most common explanation for an autosomal recessive trait. The mating of unrelated persons, each of whom happens by chance to be a carrier, accounts for most cases of autosomal recessive disease, particularly if a recessive trait has a high frequency in the population. Thus, most affected persons with a relatively common disorder, such as CF, are *not* the result of consanguinity, because the mutant allele is so common in the general population. Consanguinity is more frequently found in the background of patients with very rare conditions, however. In xeroderma pigmentosum, a rare autosomal recessive condition of DNA repair (see Chapter 16 and Table 9–6), for example, more than 20 percent of cases are reported to result from marriages between first cousins.

Although genealogical research casts light on the history of the human species as a single family, the genetic risk to the offspring of marriages between related people is not as great as is sometimes imagined. The absolute risks of abnormal offspring (stillbirth, neonatal death, and congenital malformations) for marriages between first cousins is 3 to 5 percent, about double the overall background risk of 2 to 3 percent for offspring born to any unrelated couple (see Chapter 19). Consanguinity at the level of third cousins or more remote relationships is not considered to be genetically significant, and the increased risk of abnormal offspring is negligible in such cases. Even so, many people who are homozygous for a rare allele may well have inherited it through both parents from a remote common ancestor who was heterozygous.

### The Measurement of Consanguinity

The measurement of consanguinity is relevant in medical genetics because the risk of a child's being homozygous for some rare recessive allele is propor-

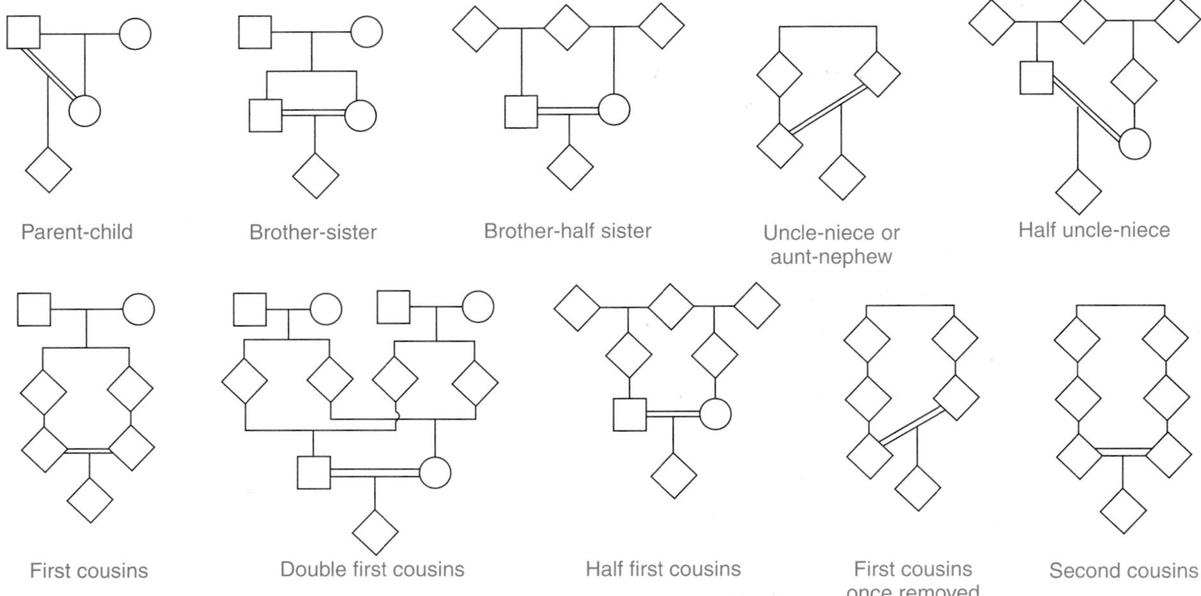


**Figure 5–5.** Types of consanguineous mating. The probability that the offspring in each of these matings is homozygous by descent at any one locus is equal to the coefficient of inbreeding, F.

tional to how related the parents are. Some types of consanguineous mating that carry an increased risk are shown in Figure 5–5.

The **coefficient of inbreeding** (F) is the probability that a homozygote has received both alleles at a locus from the same ancestral source; it is also the proportion of loci at which a person is homozygous or **identical by descent.** In Figure 5–6, person IV–1 is the offspring of a first-cousin mating. For any specific allele that his father possesses, the chance that his mother has also inherited that same allele *from the same source* is 1/8. Thus, for any gene the father passes to his child, the chance that the mother transmits the same allele is 1/8 (the chance that she carries that allele) × 1/2 (the chance that she will transmit it) = 1/16. This is the coefficient of inbreeding for the child of first cousins. It means that a child of a first-cousin mating has a 1/16 chance of being homozygous by descent at any one locus or, alternatively, that the child is homozygous at 1/16 (about 6 percent) of his or her loci. An alternative way of reaching the same conclusion (and the same F coefficient) is to consider that each of the four alleles at locus A in generation I has a 1/64 chance of being homozygous in IV–1; thus, the probability that IV–1 is homozygous for any one of the four alleles is 4 × 1/64 = 1/16. Table 5–1 shows the coefficients of inbreeding for the offspring of a number of consanguineous matings. If a person is inbred through more than one line of descent, the separate coefficients are summed to find his or her total coefficient of inbreeding.

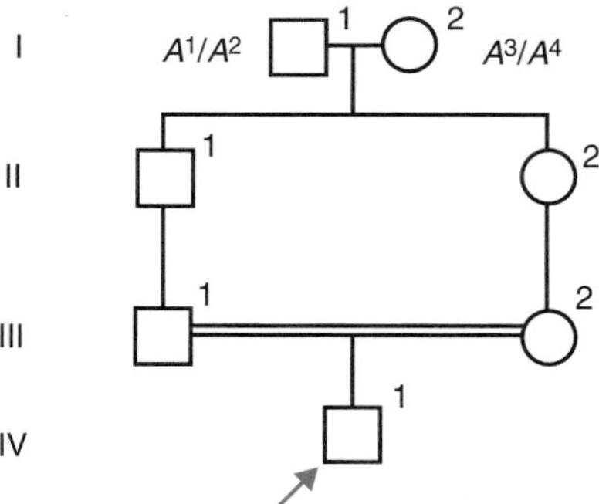


**Figure 5–6.** A cousin marriage, used in the text to demonstrate how to calculate the coefficient of inbreeding, F, of the child IV-1.

## Rare Recessive Disorders in Genetic Isolates

There are many small groups in which the frequency of certain rare recessive genes is quite different from that in the general population. Such groups, **genetic isolates,** may have become separated from their neighbors by geographic, religious, or linguistic barriers. Although such populations are not, strictly speaking, consanguineous, the chance of mating with another carrier of a particular recessive condition may be as high as that observed in cousin marriages.

For example, among Ashkenazic Jews in North America, the gene for **Tay-Sachs disease** ($GM_2$ gangliosidosis) is very common. Tay-Sachs disease is an autosomal recessive, neurological degenerative disorder that develops when a child is about 6 months old. Affected children develop blindness and regress mentally and physically (see Chapter 12). The disease is fatal in early childhood. The frequency of Tay-Sachs disease is 100 times higher in Ashkenazic Jews (1 in

TABLE 5–1
**Consanguineous Matings**

| Type | Degree of Relationship | Proportion of Genes in Common | Coefficient of Inbreeding of Child (F) |
|---|---|---|---|
| MZ twins | — | 1 | — |
| Parent-child | 1st | 1/2 | 1/4 |
| Brother-sister (including dizygotic twins) | 1st | 1/2 | 1/4 |
| Brother-half sister | 2nd | 1/4 | 1/8 |
| Uncle-niece or aunt-nephew | 2nd | 1/4 | 1/8 |
| Half uncle-niece | 3rd | 1/8 | 1/16 |
| First cousins | 3rd | 1/8 | 1/16 |
| Double first cousins | 2nd | 1/4 | 1/8 |
| Half first cousins | 4th | 1/16 | 1/32 |
| First cousins once removed | 4th | 1/16 | 1/32 |
| Second cousins | 5th | 1/32 | 1/64 |

Coefficients of inbreeding for the offspring of a number of consanguineous matings. If a person is inbred through more than one line of descent, the separate coefficients are summed to find his or her total coefficient of inbreeding.

3600) than in most other populations (1 in 360,000). Thus, the Tay-Sachs carrier frequency among Ashkenazic Jews is approximately 3 percent (calculated as described in Chapter 7).

When a recessive trait has a high frequency in a population, consanguinity is generally not a striking feature of pedigrees with the trait. Consequently, among Ashkenazic Jews, the parents of affected children are usually not closely consanguineous, whereas in the other populations in which the frequency of carriers is very low, such as in Quebec, Canada, the consanguinity rate in the parents of Tay-Sachs patients is high.

Although we make a distinction between consanguinity occurring within a family and inbreeding, which occurs between unrelated individuals in a genetic isolate, an increased risk for mating between heterozygote carriers of autosomal recessive disorders exists in both situations. To measure the risk in inbred populations, the concept of coefficients of inbreeding can be expanded to include populations as well as related individuals in families, and some examples are given in Table 5–2. Thus individuals from a fairly restricted population may have a significant F coefficient, even though they may not think of themselves as consanguineous. For some highly inbred populations, the average value of the F coefficient is as high as or higher than the value for children of second cousins; for example, F = 0.04 for Samaritans, a group numbering only about 500 people that has been genetically isolated for more than 3000 years, in comparison with 0.016 for offspring of second cousins. In Japan, F is about 0.005 (0.5 percent), meaning that, on the average, a Japanese person is homozygous by descent at as many as 250 loci.

TABLE 5–2
**Examples of Coefficient of Inbreeding (F) for Some Human Populations**

| Population | F |
|---|---|
| Canada | |
| Roman Catholic | .00004–.0007 |
| United States | |
| Roman Catholic | 0–.0008 |
| Hutterites | .02 |
| Dunkers (Pennsylvania) | .03 |
| Latin America | 0–.003 |
| Southern Europe | .001–.002 |
| Japan | .005 |
| India (Andhra Pradesh) | .02 |
| Samaritans | .04 |

## Sex-Influenced Disorders

Although autosomal recessive disorders ordinarily occur with equal frequency in males and females, some autosomal recessive phenotypes are sex-influenced, that is, expressed in both sexes but with different frequencies. Among autosomal disorders, **hemochromatosis** is an example of a phenotype more common in males. In this common autosomal recessive disorder of iron metabolism, there is enhanced absorption of dietary iron, which leads to iron overload with serious pathological consequences. The lower incidence of the clinical disorder in females (one tenth that of males) is believed to be related to lower dietary intake of iron and increased iron loss through menstruation.

## Segregation Analysis

It is not always obvious by inspection whether a pedigree reflects autosomal recessive inheritance or some other form of inheritance. **Segregation analysis** is a statistical method that uses the frequency and distribution of affected and unaffected individuals in families to determine the most likely mode of inheritance. Inheritance patterns result from the transmission of alleles from one generation to the next. Much of genetics is therefore the result of discrete probabilities: one has a certain probability of inheriting one allele versus another allele or a certain probability of developing one phenotype or another phenotype. To study such processes, geneticists rely on a mathematical formulation that is often used to describe such discrete processes: the **binomial theorem**. The next section provides a basic introduction to the binomial theorem and applies it to a simple example of segregation analysis; it is also used in population genetics (see Chapter 7) and in gene mapping by linkage (see Chapter 8).

### Binomial Theorem

Suppose there are two alternative outcomes of an experiment, "success" occurring with probability $p$ and "failure" occurring with probability $q$. Because there are only two possible outcomes, $p + q$ must equal 1; therefore, $q = 1 - p$. The first time the experiment is performed, the probability of a success is $p$, and the probability of a failure is $q$. If the experiment is performed twice, the probability of two successes is $p \times p = p^2$, of two failures is $q^2$, and of one success and one failure is $2 \times p \times q$ (the factor 2 comes from there being two ways of having a success and failure: the success can come in the first experiment and failure in the second, or vice versa). With three experiments, the chance of three successes is $p \times p \times p = p^3$; three failures is $q^3$; success and two failures is $3 \times pq^2$ (because the success could come from the first, the second, or the third experiment); and, similarly, two successes and one failure is $3p^2q$. In general terms, when there are two alternative events, one with probability $p$ and the other with probability $1 - p = q$, the frequencies of the possible combinations of $p$ and $q$ in a series of $n$ trials are given by the individual terms of the expansion of $(p + q)^n$. This formulation of probabilities of a series of experiments based on the probability of the outcomes from a single experiment is the **binomial theorem**.

### Application of the Binomial Theorem to Segregation Analysis

We now examine a simple example of the use of the binomial theorem in segregation analysis for a clinically relevant problem. Suppose one seeks to determine whether a particular disorder whose pattern of inheritance has not been previously established is autosomal recessive. We do this by examining whether the disease occurs in sibships in proportions that fit the 25 percent expectation for autosomal recessive inheritance.

Assuming recessive inheritance, what proportion of three-child families would have 0, 1, 2, and 3 affected children? According to the approach used earlier, $p$ (chance of clinically normal child) = 3/4, $q$ (chance of affected child) = 1/4, $n = 3$, and $(p + q)^3 = p^3 + 3p^2q + 3pq^2 + q^3$. Thus, the theoretical expectation, based on autosomal recessive inheritance, is that

27/64 (42 percent) of all such families have no affected child;
27/64 (42 percent) have 1 affected child;
9/64 (14 percent) have 2 affected children;
1/64 (2 percent) have 3 affected children.

We have determined the expected proportions of affected children in three-child families of parents who are carriers for an autosomal recessive disorder. Suppose, however, that we only know to include ("ascertain") a family in our study when it has at least one affected child. Then 27 of the 64 families at risk (42 percent) will not be included in the study because we would not even know the parents were carriers. Of the remaining 37 families that we can ascertain,

27 (73 percent) have 1 affected child;
9 (24 percent) have 2 affected children;
1 (3 percent) has 3 affected children.

In the ascertained group, then, the total number of affected children among 111 children in 37 families is $27 \times 1$ affected + ($9 \times 2$ affected) + ($1 \times 3$ affected) = 48 affected out of 111 children or 43 percent, far greater than the theoretical 25 percent expected for autosomal recessive inheritance. This is an example of **bias of ascertainment**, a bias to avoid in medical research, especially in medical genetics. In tests for autosomal recessive inheritance, sibships with no affected members are inevitably missed. The problem may be made even worse if, as may occasionally happen, the chance of ascertaining a sibship may be higher when it has two or more affected members than when it has only one. A number of statistical methods to correct for bias under different conditions of ascertainment are known and are described in many statistics texts.

#### Characteristics of Autosomal Recessive Inheritance

1. An autosomal recessive phenotype, if it appears in more than one member of a kindred, typically is seen only in the sibship of the proband, not in parents, offspring, or other relatives.
2. For most autosomal recessive diseases, males and females are equally likely to be affected.
3. Parents of an affected child are asymptomatic carriers of mutant alleles.
4. The parents of the affected person may in some cases be consanguineous. This is especially likely if the gene responsible for the condition is rare in the population.
5. The recurrence risk for each sib of the proband is 1 in 4.

## PATTERNS OF AUTOSOMAL DOMINANT INHERITANCE

Among the 6000 or so known mendelian phenotypes, more than half are autosomal dominant traits. The incidence of some autosomal dominant disorders is quite high, at least in specific geographic areas: for example, 1 in 500 for familial hypercholesterolemia in populations of European or Japanese descent; more than 1 in 1000 for myotonic dystrophy in some parts of North America; and about 1 in 2500 to 3000 for several conditions such as Huntington disease (in populations of Northern European origin), neurofibromatosis, and polycystic kidney disease. Although many autosomal dominant disorders are individually much less common, they are so numerous that, in the aggregate, their total incidence is appreciable. The burden of autosomal dominant disorders is further increased because of their hereditary nature; they may be transmitted through families and become problems not only for individuals but for whole kindreds, often through many generations. In some cases the burden is compounded by social difficulties resulting from physical or mental disability.

In typical autosomal dominant inheritance, every affected person in a pedigree has an affected parent, who also has an affected parent, and so on as far back as the disorder can be traced or until the occurrence of an original mutation. This is also true, as discussed later, of X-linked dominant pedigrees. Autosomal dominant inheritance can readily be distinguished from X-linked dominant inheritance, however, by **male-to-male transmission**, which is obviously impossible for X-linked inheritance because males transmit the Y chromosome, not the X, to their sons.

Most mutations that cause disease are rare in the population, in comparison with normal alleles. Denoting *A* as the mutant allele and *a* as the normal allele, matings that produce children with an autosomal dominant disease are therefore usually between a heterozygote for the mutation (*A*/*a*) and a homozygote for a normal allele (*a*/*a*). The offspring expected from an *A*/*a* × *a*/*a* mating are given in the table here.

**Progeny of A/*a* × *a*/*a* Mating**

| | | Normal Parent *a*/*a* | |
|---|---|---|---|
| | | *a* | *a* |
| **Affected Parent** *A*/*a* | *A* | *A*/*a* Affected | *A*/*a* Affected |
| | *a* | *a*/*a* Normal | *a*/*a* Normal |

Each child of this mating has a 50 percent chance of receiving the affected parent's abnormal allele *A* and thus being affected (*A*/*a*) and a 50 percent chance of receiving the normal allele *a* and thus being unaffected (*a*/*a*). (The unaffected parent can transmit only a normal *a* allele to each child.) Statistically speaking, each pregnancy is an "independent event," not governed by the outcome of previous pregnancies; thus, within a family the distribution of affected and unaffected children may be quite different from the theoretical 1:1, although in the population as a whole the offspring of *A*/*a* × *a*/*a* parents are approximately 50 percent *A*/*a* and 50 percent *a*/*a*. Typical autosomal dominant inheritance can be seen in the pedigree of a family with hereditary deafness (Fig. 5–7).

### New Mutation in Autosomal Dominant Disorders

In any population, new alleles arise by mutation and are maintained or removed by selection. After a new mutation has arisen, its survival in the population depends on the **fitness** of persons carrying it, in comparison with that of persons carrying other alleles at the locus concerned.

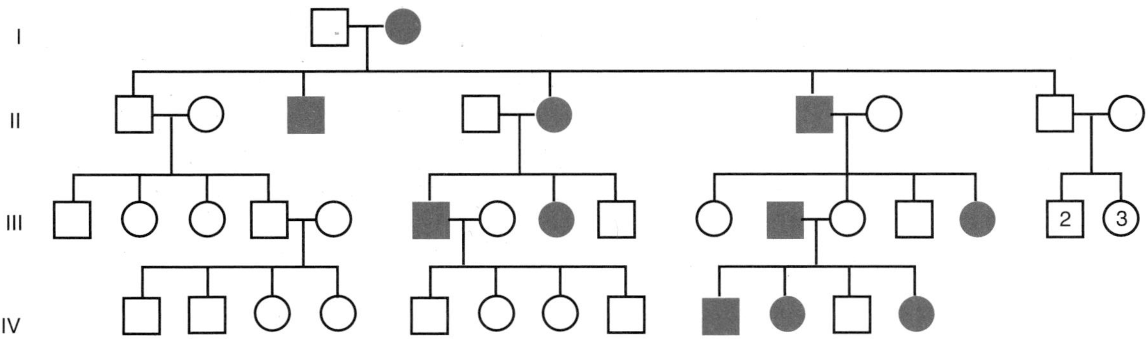


**Figure 5–7.** Pedigree showing typical inheritance of a form of progressive sensorineural deafness (DFNA1) inherited as an autosomal dominant trait.

The fitness of a condition is measured by the number of offspring of affected persons who survive to reproductive age, in comparison with an appropriate control group. Many autosomal dominant disorders are associated with reduced fitness. There is an inverse relation between the fitness of a given autosomal dominant disorder and the proportion of all patients with that disorder who have new mutant genes. When a disorder reduces the reproductive fitness of affected persons, a proportion of all those affected are likely to have received the defective gene as a new mutation in a gamete from a genotypically normal parent. Some disorders have a fitness of zero; in other words, patients with such disorders never reproduce. Essentially all observed cases of a disorder with zero fitness are therefore due to new mutations, because mutations cannot be inherited. Other disorders have virtually normal reproductive fitness because of the late age of onset in typical cases. If the fitness is normal, the disorder is rarely seen as a result of fresh mutation; a patient is much more likely to have inherited the disorder than to have a new mutant gene. The measurement of mutation frequency and the relation of mutation frequency to fitness are discussed further in Chapter 7.

## Variability in the Phenotypic Manifestations of Mutant Genes: Penetrance, Expressivity, and Pleiotropy

Many genetic conditions segregate sharply within families; that is, the abnormal phenotype can be distinguished clearly from the normal one. In clinical experience, however, some disorders are not expressed at all in genetically predisposed persons, and others have extremely variable expression in terms of clinical severity or age of onset, or both. Expression of an abnormal genotype may be modified by the effects of aging, other genetic loci, and the effects of environment. These differences in expression, which are particularly characteristic of autosomal dominant disorders though by no means restricted to them, can often lead to difficulties in diagnosis and pedigree interpretation. There are three distinct ways in which such differences in expression can occur: **reduced penetrance**, **variable expressivity**, and **pleiotropy**.

**Penetrance** is the probability that a gene will have any phenotypic expression at all. When the frequency of expression of a phenotype is less than 100 percent—that is, when some of those who have the appropriate genotype completely fail to express it—the gene is said to show **reduced penetrance**. Penetrance is an all-or-none concept. In statistical terms, it is the percentage of people with a particular genotype who are actually affected, at least to some degree.

**Expressivity** is the severity of expression of the phenotype. When the severity of disease differs in people who have the same genotype, the phenotype is said to have **variable expressivity**. Even within a kindred, a disorder may vary in the severity of any one manifestation.

When a single abnormal gene or gene pair produces diverse phenotypic effects, such as which organ systems are involved and which particular signs and symptoms occur, its expression is said to be **pleiotropic**. Each gene has only one primary effect: it directs the synthesis of a polypeptide chain or an RNA molecule. From this primary effect, however, there may be multiple consequences. Even in the same kindred, two individuals carrying the same mutant genes may have some signs and symptoms in common, whereas other disease manifestations may be quite different, depending on which tissues or organs happen to be affected in the two related individuals. For most pleiotropic disorders, the connection between the various manifestations is neither obvious nor well understood.

Some of the difficulties in understanding the inheritance of a disease phenotype in families are demonstrated by the autosomal dominant disease **neurofibromatosis** (NF1). NF1 is a common disorder of the nervous system, shown in one of its typical clinical presentations in Figure 5–8. NF1 is characterized by (1) the growth of multiple benign fleshy tumors, neurofibromas, in the skin; (2) the presence of multiple flat, irregular pigmented skin lesions known as café-au-lait spots; (3) the growth of small benign tumors (hamartomas) on the iris of the eye

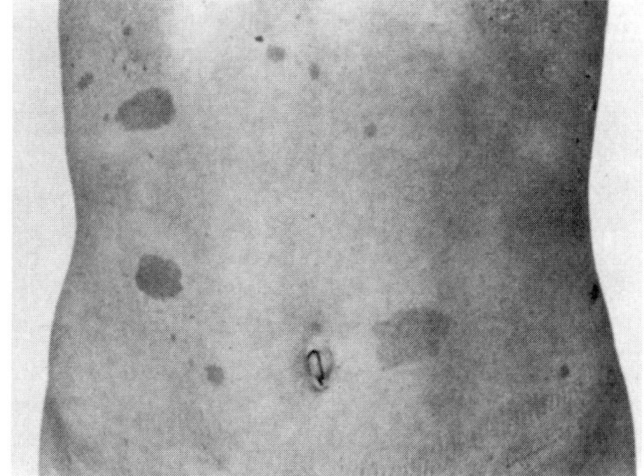

Figure 5–8. Neurofibromatosis, type 1: café-au-lait spots, hyperpigmented spots on the skin, are a useful diagnostic sign in family members who otherwise may appear unaffected. Most patients have six or more spots at least 15 mm in diameter, usually on the trunk. (Photograph courtesy of Rosanna Weksberg, The Hospital for Sick Children, Toronto.)

called Lisch nodules; and (4) less frequently, mental retardation, central nervous system tumors, diffuse plexiform neurofibromas, and the development of cancer of the nervous system or muscle.

NF1 was first fully described by the physician Von Recklinghausen in 1882, but the disease has probably been known since ancient times. Although adult heterozygotes almost always demonstrate some sign of the disease (penetrance is therefore said to be 100 percent in adults), some may have only café-au-lait spots, freckles on the axillary skin, and Lisch nodules, whereas others may have life-threatening benign tumors involving the spinal cord or malignant sarcomas of an extremity. Thus, there is frequently great variability in disease expression; even within a kindred, some individuals are severely affected and others only mildly so. Diagnosis is further complicated in children because the signs develop only over time during childhood. For example, in the newborn period, less than half of all affected newborns show even the most subtle signs of the disease, an increased incidence of café-au-lait spots. Penetrance, therefore, is age-dependent. Approximately half the cases of NF1 result from a new, rather than inherited, mutation. In the family shown in Figure 5–9, the proband (indicated by an arrow) appears to have a new mutant gene, because his parents and their parents are all unaffected.

The chief genetic problem in counseling families of patients with NF1 is to decide between two equally likely possibilities: Is the disease in this family due to new mutation, or has the patient inherited a clinically significant form of the disorder from a parent in whom the gene is present but only mildly expressed? If the patient has inherited the defect, the risk that any of his or her sibs will also inherit it is 50 percent, but if the child has a new mutant gene, there is very little risk that any sib will be affected. Significantly, in either case, the risk that the patient will pass the gene on to any one of his or her offspring is 50 percent. The unpredictability of the severity of the manifestations of NF1, a characteristic of many autosomal dominant disorders, is an added complication for genetic counseling. In view of these uncertainties, it is reassuring to families of patients with NF1 to know that the disorder can be detected presymptomatically and even prenatally by molecular genetic analysis (see Chapter 18). Unfortunately, there is no way to predict the large proportion of cases that are due to new mutation.

Another example of an autosomal dominant malformation with reduced penetrance is the **split-hand deformity** or lobster-claw malformation, a type of ectrodactyly (Fig. 5–10). The malformation originates in the sixth or seventh week of development, when the hands and feet are forming. Failure of penetrance in pedigrees of split-hand malformation can lead to apparent skipping of generations, and this complicates genetic counseling because an at-risk person with normal hands may nevertheless possess the gene for the condition and thus be capable of having children who are affected.

Figure 5–11 is a pedigree of split-hand deformity in which the person shown by the arrow is the consultand (the person who asks for genetic counseling). Her mother is a nonpenetrant carrier of the split-hand mutation. Review of the literature on split-hand deformity suggests that the disorder has about 70 percent penetrance (i.e., only 70 percent of the people who have the gene exhibit the defect). Using this information in Bayesian analysis, a mathematical method for determining conditional probabilities in pedigrees (see further discussion in Chapter 19), one can calculate the risk that the consultand might have a child with the abnormality.

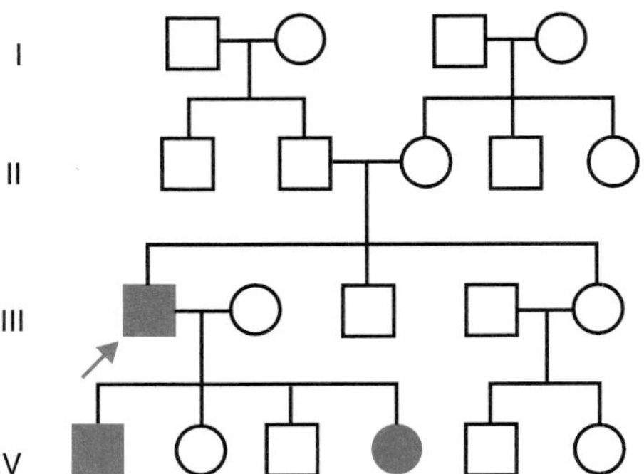


Figure 5–9. Pedigree of family with neurofibromatosis, type 1, apparently originating as a new mutation in the proband (*arrow*).

## Homozygotes for Autosomal Dominant Traits

In medical practice, homozygotes for rare dominant phenotypes are not often seen because matings that could produce homozygous offspring are rare. Again denoting the mutant allele as *A* and the normal allele as *a*, the parents of a homozygote might theoretically be $A/a \times A/a$, $A/A \times A/a$, or $A/A \times A/A$, or the patient might, in exceedingly rare instances, have received a new mutation from a genetically unaffected parent. Practically speaking, however, only the mating of two heterozygotes need be considered, and even that is an unusual event for most autosomal dominant conditions.

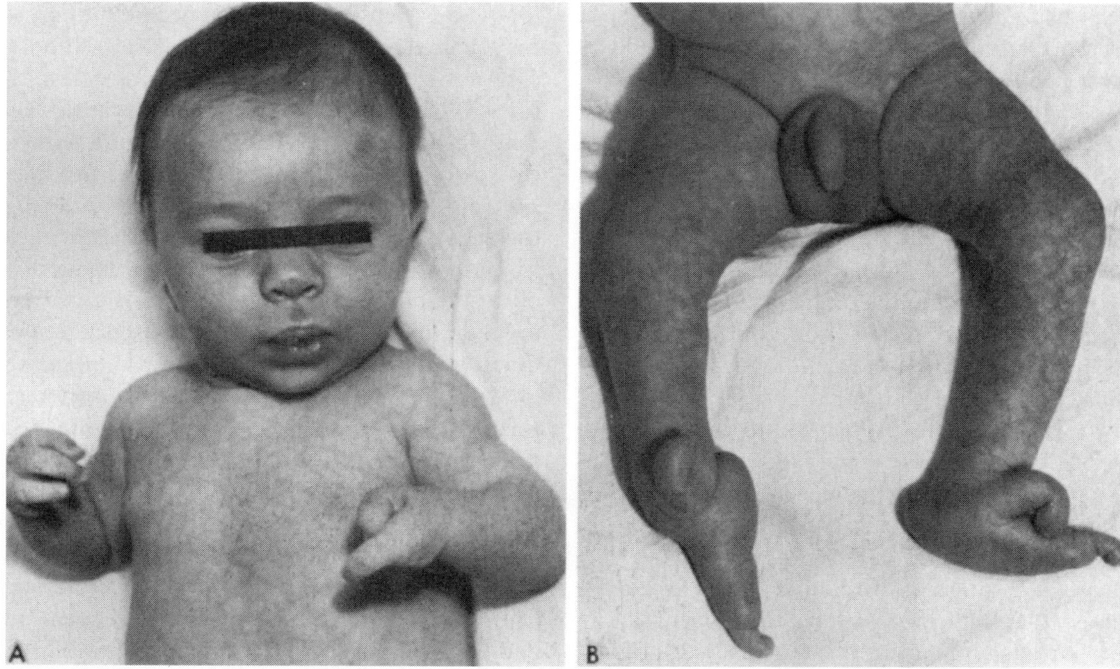


Figure 5–10. Split-hand deformity, an autosomal dominant trait involving the hands and feet, in a 3-month-old boy. *A*, upper part of body; *B*, lower part of body. (From Kelikian H [1974] Congenital deformities of the hand and forearm. WB Saunders, Philadelphia.)

**Progeny of *A*/*a* × *A*/*a* Mating**

| | | Affected Parent *A*/*a* | |
|---|---|---|---|
| | | *A* | *a* |
| **Affected Parent *A*/*a*** | *A* | *A*/*A* Homozygous Affected | *A*/*a* Affected |
| | *a* | *A*/*a* Affected | *a*/*a* Normal |

Clinically, the distinction between affected heterozygotes and homozygotes can be made with considerable certainty in many cases because autosomal dominant disorders are usually much more severe in homozygotes than in heterozygotes. Figure 5–12 shows a child with the typical heterozygous form of **achondroplasia**, a skeletal disorder of short-limbed dwarfism and large head size. Most achondroplastic individuals have normal intelligence and lead normal lives within their physical capabilities. It is understandable that marriages between two achondroplastic individuals are not uncommon. A homozygous child of two heterozygotes is often recognizable on clinical grounds alone; homozygous achondroplastic patients are much more severely affected than are heterozygotes and commonly do not survive early infancy.

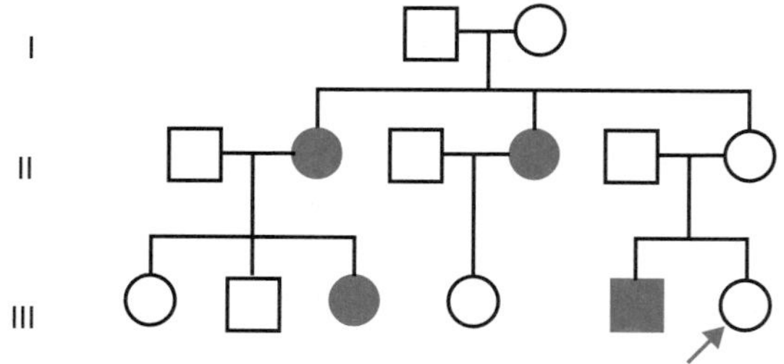


Figure 5–11. Pedigree of split-hand deformity demonstrating failure of penetrance in the mother of the consultand. Consultand is indicated by the arrow. Reduced penetrance must be taken into account in genetic counseling.

Another example is **familial hypercholesterolemia** (see Chapter 12), an autosomal dominant disorder leading to premature coronary heart disease, in which the rare homozygous patients have a much more severe disease, with much shorter life expectancy, than do the relatively common heterozygotes (Fig. 5–13).

In fact, in virtually every reported example, homozygosity for a defective allele results in a more severely abnormal phenotype than does heterozygosity. One well known exception is **Huntington disease** (HD), a neurodegenerative disease characterized by progressive dementia and abnormal movements (see Chapter 12). HD homozygotes can be distinguished from the far more common heterozygotes by molecular analysis of the mutant gene, and the clinical expression appears to be the same in both genotypes.

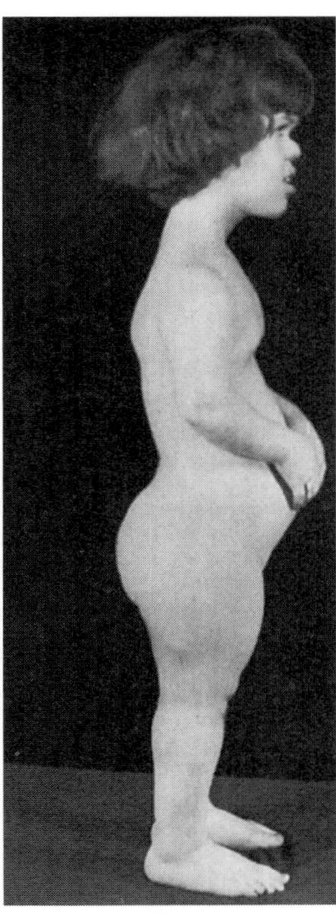

**Figure 5–12.** Achondroplasia, an autosomal dominant disorder that often occurs as a new mutation. Note small stature with short limbs, large head, low nasal bridge, prominent forehead, lumbar lordosis. (From Tachdjian MO [1972] Pediatric Orthopedics, vol 1. WB Saunders, Philadelphia, p. 284.)

### Sex-Limited Phenotype in Autosomal Disease

As discussed earlier for autosomal recessive conditions, autosomal dominant phenotypes may demonstrate a sex ratio that differs significantly from 1:1. Extreme divergence of the sex ratio is seen in sex-limited phenotypes, in which the defect is autosomally transmitted but expressed in only one sex. An example is **male-limited precocious puberty** (familial testotoxicosis), an autosomal dominant disorder in which affected boys develop secondary sexual characteristics and undergo an adolescent growth spurt at about 4 years of age (Fig. 5–14). In some families, the defect has been traced to a mutation in the gene that encodes the receptor for luteinizing hormone that constitutively activates the receptor's signaling action even in the absence of its hormone. The defect is nonpenetrant in heterozygous females. Figure 5–15, part of a much larger pedigree, shows that although the disease can be transmitted by unaffected females, it can also be transmitted directly from father to son, showing that it is autosomal, not X-linked.

Males with precocious puberty have normal fertility, and numerous multigeneration pedigrees are known. For disorders in which affected males do not reproduce, however, it is not always easy to distinguish sex-limited autosomal inheritance from X-linkage because the critical evidence, absence of male-to-male transmission, cannot be provided. Other lines of evidence, especially gene mapping to learn whether the responsible gene maps to the X chromosome or to an autosome (see Chapter 8), can determine the pattern of inheritance and the consequent recurrence risk.

## X-LINKED INHERITANCE

The X and Y chromosomes, which are responsible for sex determination (see Chapter 10), are distributed unequally to males and females in families. For this reason, phenotypes determined by genes on the X have a characteristic sex distribution and a pattern of inheritance that is usually easy to identify. About 500 genes have already been mapped to the X chromosome, 70 percent of which are known to be associated with disease phenotypes.

Consider a mutant X-linked gene, $X_h$ (for example, hemophilia A due to a mutation in the gene for coagulation factor VIII), in comparison with a normal

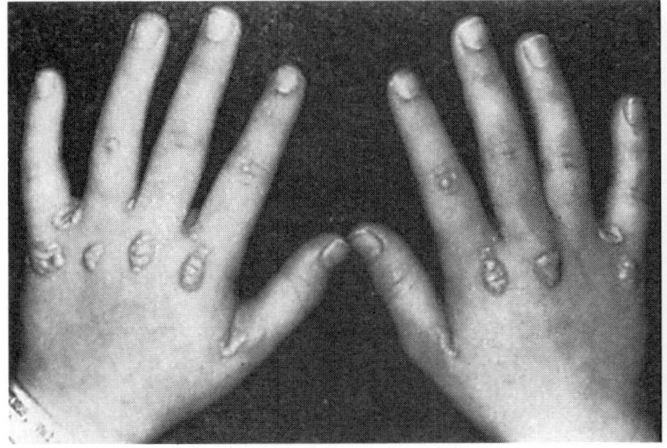

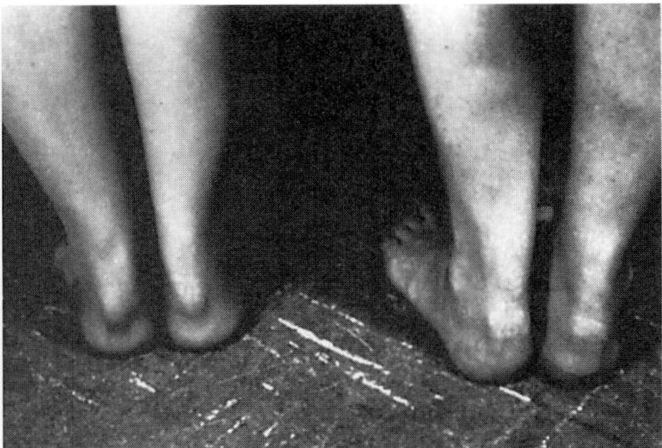

**Figure 5–13.** Comparison of severity of symptoms in familial hypercholesterolemia (FH): cutaneous xanthomas in an FH homozygote (*left*) and tendon xanthomas in FH heterozygotes (*right*). (Photographs courtesy of JL Goldstein, University of Texas Southwestern Medical Center, Dallas.)

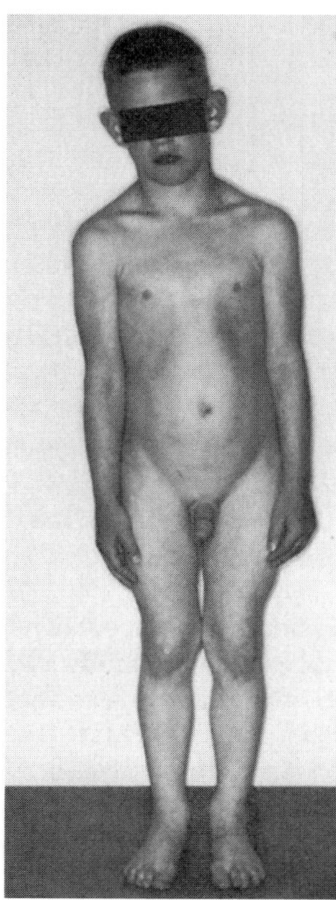

**Figure 5–14.** Male-limited precocious puberty (familial testotoxicosis), an autosomal dominant disorder expressed exclusively in males. This child, at 4.75 years, is 120 cm in height (above the 97th percentile for his age). Note the muscle bulk and precocious development of the external genitalia. Epiphyseal fusion occurs at an early age, and affected persons are relatively short as adults.

allele, $X_H$. Because males have one X chromosome but females have two, there are two possible genotypes in males but three in females; males are hemizygous with respect to X-linked genes, whereas females may be homozygous for either allele or may be heterozygous.

| | Genotypes | Phenotypes |
|---|---|---|
| **Males** | $X_H$ | Unaffected |
| | $X_h$ | Affected |
| | $X_H/X_H$ | Homozygous unaffected |
| **Females** | $X_H/X_h$ | Heterozygous |
| | $X_h/X_h$ | Homozygous affected |

## Characteristics of Autosomal Dominant Inheritance

1. The phenotype usually appears in every generation, each affected person having an affected parent.

   Exceptions or apparent exceptions to this rule in clinical genetics: (1) cases originating by fresh mutation in a gamete of a phenotypically normal parent; (2) cases in which the disorder is not expressed (nonpenetrant) or is expressed only subtly in a person who has inherited the responsible gene.
2. Any child of an affected parent has a 50 percent risk of inheriting the trait.

   This is true for most families, in which the other parent is phenotypically normal. Because statistically each family member is the result of an "independent event," wide deviation from the expected 1:1 ratio may occur by chance in a single family.
3. Phenotypically normal family members do not transmit the phenotype to their children.

   Failure of penetrance or very subtle expression of a condition may lead to apparent exceptions to this rule.
4. Males and females are equally likely to transmit the phenotype, to children of either sex. In particular, male-to-male transmission can occur, and males can have unaffected daughters.
5. A significant proportion of isolated cases are due to new mutation. The less the fitness is, the greater is the proportion due to new mutation.

# X Inactivation, Dosage Compensation, and the Expression of X-Linked Genes

### Lyon Hypothesis

Although males have only one copy or "dose" of each X-linked gene, whereas females have two, the quantity of product formed by a single allele in the male or

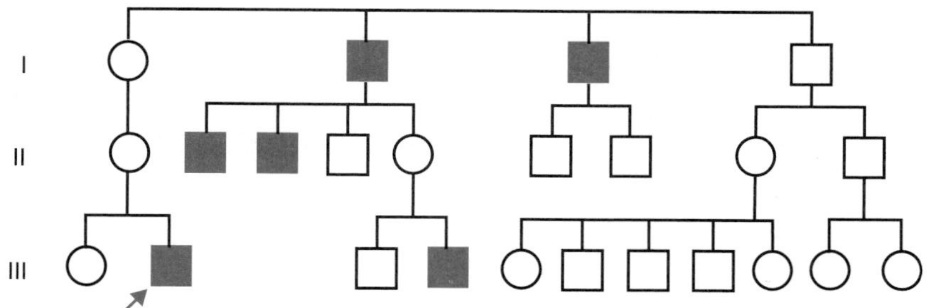


**Figure 5–15.** Pedigree pattern of male-limited precocious puberty in the family of the child shown in Figure 5–14. This autosomal dominant disorder can be transmitted by affected males or by unaffected carrier females. Male-to-male transmission shows that the inheritance is autosomal, not X-linked. Because the trait is transmitted through unaffected carrier females, it cannot be Y-linked.

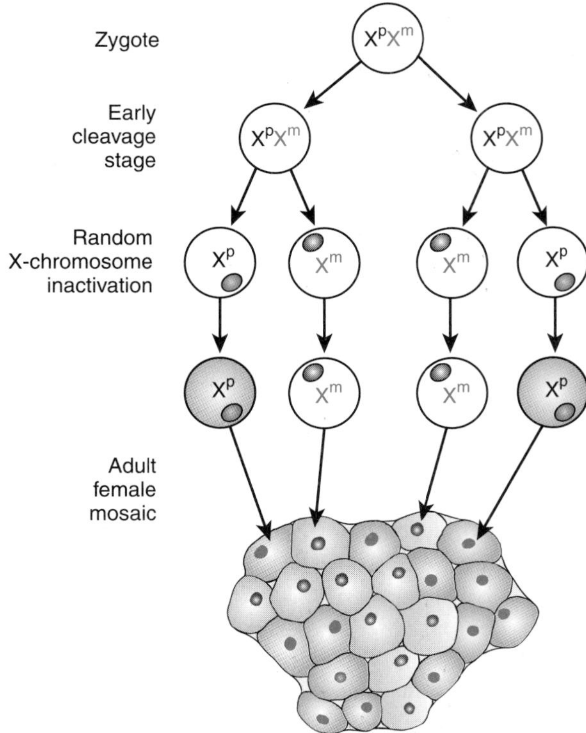


**Figure 5–16.** The Lyon hypothesis of random X chromosome inactivation in female somatic cells. $X^p$ = paternally inherited X chromosome. $X^m$ = maternally inherited X chromosome. Gray or red ovals represent Barr bodies formed by the inactivated paternal or maternal X chromosome, respectively. Adult tissues (*bottom*) are a mosaic of clonal populations expressing alleles from either $X^p$ or $X^m$. (Modified from Rosenberg LE [1980] Inborn errors of metabolism. *In* Bondy PK, Rosenberg LE [eds] Metabolic control and disease, 8th ed. WB Saunders, Philadelphia, pp. 73–102.)

by a pair of alleles in the female is usually equivalent. The mechanism by which this "dosage compensation" is achieved can be explained by the principle of X inactivation (Fig. 5–16), which is often called the **Lyon hypothesis** because it was originally put forward in detail by the mouse geneticist Mary Lyon. In brief, the principle has three points:

1. In the somatic cells of female mammals, only one X chromosome is transcriptionally active. The second X is heterochromatic and inactive and appears in interphase cells as sex chromatin, the Barr body.
2. Inactivation occurs early in embryonic life, beginning soon after fertilization, but is not complete in the inner cell mass, which forms the embryo, until about the end of the first week of development. At this stage of development, placental implantation is occurring, there is differentiation of trophoblast into cytotrophoblast and syncytiotrophoblast, and the epiblast, consisting of perhaps only 100 cells, is poised to undergo gastrulation (see Chapter 17).
3. In any one female somatic cell, the inactive X may be either the paternal or the maternal X ($X^p$ or $X^m$); it is entirely a matter of chance which of the pair becomes inactivated in any one cell. After one X chromosome has become inactivated in a cell, however, all cells descended from that cell have the same inactive X. In other words, inactivation is randomly determined, but once made, the decision is permanent.

In this section, we describe three consequences of X inactivation that are significant both genetically and clinically: dosage compensation, variability of expression in heterozygous females, and mosaicism. The implications of X inactivation for clinical cytogenetics are discussed in greater detail in Chapter 10.

### Dosage Compensation

X inactivation provides an explanation for dosage compensation, because the inactive X chromosome is almost entirely silenced and, with some exceptions, its genes appear not to be transcribed. The basic features of the Lyon hypothesis have been firmly established; the details of how it occurs are not completely known. Our current understanding of the mechanism of X inactivation is presented in Chapter 10.

### Escape from X Inactivation

Although in female somatic cells much of one X is inactivated, several regions of the short arm and at least one on the long arm contain genes that escape inactivation and continue to be expressed from both X chromosomes in females. X-linked genes that escape inactivation fall into three classes. One class are the genes located in the **pseudoautosomal region**, on the very distal short and long arms of the X, in which there are matching sequences on the Y chromosome by means of which the X and Y pair in meiosis and exchange material by crossing over. Genes in the pseudoautosomal segment remain active, and both females (two X copies) and males (one X and one Y copy) have two expressed doses of such genes. Alleles for genes in the pseudoautosomal region can show male-to-male transmission by crossing over from the X to the Y, which can then be passed on to male offspring and therefore mimic autosomal inheritance. A second class of X-linked genes that escape inactivation are located outside the pseudoautosomal region on the short arm and on the long arm; these genes have related copies on the Y chromosome, and so both males and females have two active copies of these genes. The X-linked copies of these genes do not show pseudoautosomal inheritance because they do not participate in crossing over with the Y chromosome in male meiosis. A third class of genes that also escape inactivation are located outside the pseudoautosomal region of the X chromosome and do *not* have a copy on the Y; for example, the gene for steroid sulfatase (deficiency of which causes an X-linked form of the skin disease ichthyosis) lies not within the pseudoautosomal region on the X chromosome but just proximal to it and remains partially active, even on the inactive X. Because no active copy exists on the Y chromosome in humans, copy number and expression levels are higher in females than in males.

The clinical relevance of most genes that escape inactivation is uncertain, but for at least one noninactivated gene, steroid sulfatase, an X-linked clinical disorder is associated with loss of function of this gene. These genes are also candidates to explain clinical symptoms in cases of numerical abnormalities of the X chromosome, such as 45,X Turner syndrome (See Chapter 10) because their gene products would not show appropriate dosage in comparison with normal females carrying two normal X chromosomes.

### Variable Expression of X-Linked Genes in Heterozygotes

Because inactivation is random but is established at a stage of embryonic development when the developing embryo has fewer than 100 cells, the fraction of cells in carrier females in which the normal or mutant allele happens to remain active can be quite variable. As a result, clinical variation in expression of X-linked disorders is seen commonly in heterozygotes and can be extreme, ranging from entirely normal to fully manifesting the defect, with all gradations in between. A **manifesting heterozygote**, in whom the deleterious allele is located on the active X and the normal allele is located on the inactive X in all or most cells, is an extreme example of highly unbalanced or "skewed" X-inactivation. Manifesting heterozygotes have been described for many X-linked disorders, including color blindness; hemophilia A (classic hemophilia, factor VIII deficiency); hemophilia B (Christmas disease, factor IX deficiency); Duchenne muscular dystrophy (DMD); Wiskott-Aldrich syndrome (an X-linked immunodeficiency); and several X-linked eye disorders.

In addition to manifesting heterozygotes, the opposite pattern of **unbalanced inactivation** (that is, with the mutant allele preferentially on the inactive X in some or all tissues of the heterozygous female) can also occur and is characteristic of several X-linked disorders. In general, skewed inactivation of this type is seen in asymptomatic heterozygotes and is believed to reflect a cell survival or proliferative disadvantage for those cells that originally had the mutant allele on the active X (see Chapter 10). Patterns of skewed inactivation in relevant tissues have been used to diagnose the carrier state for some X-linked conditions, including several forms of X-linked mental retardation, certain X-linked immunodeficiencies (see Chapter 14), dyskeratosis congenita (an X-linked form of skin disease and bone marrow failure), and incontinentia pigmenti (an X-linked condition affecting skin and teeth).

### Functional Mosaicism Resulting from X Inactivation

Females have two cell populations, in which one or the other X chromosome is the active one (see Fig. 5–16); in other words, females are mosaics with respect to their X-linked genes. Mosaicism in human females is readily detected for some disorders. For example, in DMD, female carriers exhibit typical mosaic expression, allowing carriers to be identified by dystrophin immunostaining (Fig. 5–17). In addition, heterozygosity for a number of X-linked disorders can be demonstrated experimentally by culture of single cells to provide clones, which can then be analyzed to show that some clones have an active paternal X, whereas others have an active maternal X.

X inactivation accounts for an important difference between autosomal and X-linked inheritance. In females, as in males, there is only one functional X in any cell. Consequently, although X-linked "dominant" and "recessive" patterns of inheritance are distinguished on the basis of the phenotype in heterozygous females, the distinction breaks down in practice. This difficulty occurs because in a female heterozygous for either a dominant or a recessive disorder, the mutant allele is the only functional allele in about half (but sometimes far more or less than half) of her somatic cells. In males, the inherited allele is inevitably expressed whether its expression in heterozygotes is dominant or recessive. Some medical geneticists prefer not to classify X-linked phenotypes as dominant or recessive, but others believe that the distinction is useful because some X-linked phenotypes are consistently expressed in carriers (dominant), whereas others are usually not expressed in carriers (recessive) unless there is a highly unbalanced inactivation pattern. In the following discussion, X-linked dominance and recessiveness are examined separately.

## X-Linked Recessive Inheritance

The inheritance of X-linked recessive phenotypes follows a well-defined and easily recognized pattern (Fig. 5–18). An X-linked mutation is typically expressed phenotypically in all males who receive it but only in those females who are homozygous for the mutation. Consequently, X-linked recessive disorders are generally restricted to males and, with the

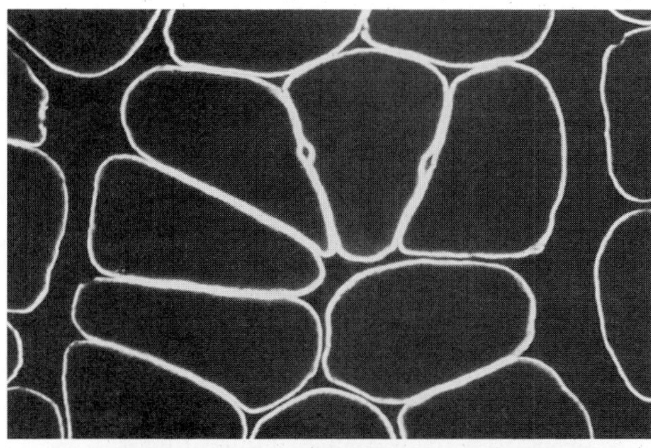

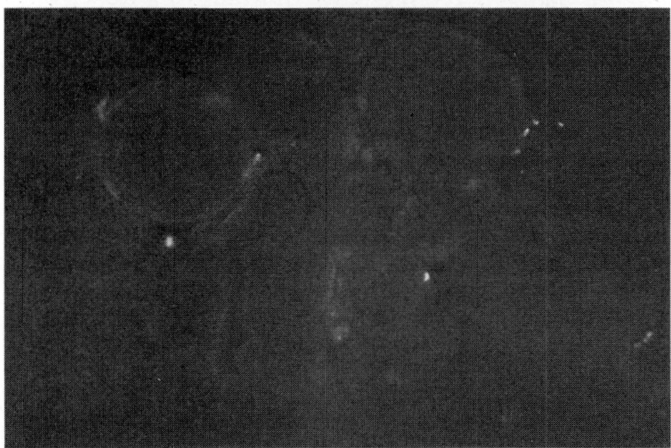

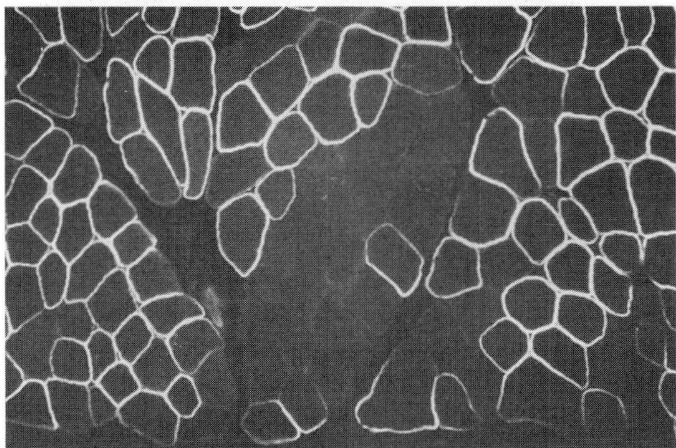

**Figure 5–17.** Immunostaining for dystrophin in muscle specimens from (*top*) a normal female (×480), (*middle*) a male with Duchenne muscular dystrophy (×480), and (*bottom*) a carrier female (×240). Muscle from DMD patients lacks dystrophin staining. Muscle from DMD carriers exhibits both positive and negative patches of dystrophin immunostaining, reflecting X inactivation. (Photographs courtesy of K Arahata, National Institute of Neuroscience, Tokyo.)

exception of the rare manifesting heterozygotes discussed earlier, are hardly ever seen among females.

**Hemophilia A** is a classic X-linked disorder in which the blood fails to clot normally because of a deficiency of factor VIII, a protein in the clotting cascade. The hereditary nature of hemophilia and even its pattern of transmission have been recognized since ancient times, and the condition became known as

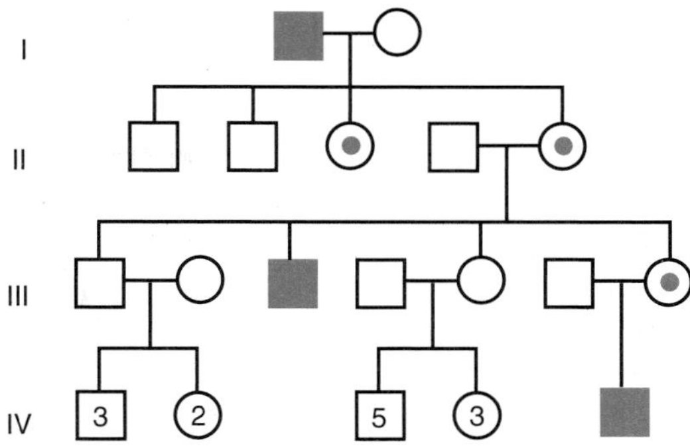


**Figure 5–18.** Pedigree pattern demonstrating an X-linked recessive disorder such as hemophilia A, transmitted from an affected male through females to an affected grandson and great-grandson.

the "royal hemophilia" because of its occurrence among descendants of Britain's Queen Victoria, who was a carrier.

As in the earlier discussion, $X_h$ represents the mutant factor VIII allele causing hemophilia A, and $X_H$ represents the normal allele. If a hemophiliac mates with a normal female, all the sons receive their father's Y chromosome and a maternal X and are unaffected, but all the daughters receive the paternal X chromosome with its hemophilia allele and all are obligate carriers.

**Affected Male × Normal Female: $X_h/Y \times X_H/X_H$**

| | $X_H$ | $X_H$ | |
|---|---|---|---|
| $X_h$ | $X_H/X_h$ | $X_H/X_h$ | Daughters: ALL carriers |
| Y | $X_H/Y$ | $X_H/Y$ | Sons: ALL unaffected |

Now assume that a daughter of the affected male mates with an unaffected male. Four genotypes are possible in the progeny, with equal probabilities.

**Normal Male × Carrier Female: $X_H/Y \times X_H/X_h$**

| | $X_H$ | $X_h$ | |
|---|---|---|---|
| $X_h$ | $X_H/X_H$ | $X_H/X_h$ | Daughters: 1/2 normal, 1/2 carriers |
| Y | $X_H/Y$ | $X_h/Y$ | Sons: 1/2 normal, 1/2 affected |

The hemophilia of an affected grandfather, which did not appear in any of his own children, has a 50 percent chance of appearing in any son of any of his daughters. It will not reappear among the descendants of his sons, however.

A daughter of a carrier has a 50 percent chance of being a carrier herself (see Fig. 5–18). By chance, an X-linked recessive allele may be transmitted undetected through a series of female carriers before it is expressed in a male descendant.

### Homozygous Affected Females

A gene for an X-linked disorder is occasionally present in both a father and a carrier mother, and female offspring can then be homozygous affected, as shown in the pedigree of X-linked color blindness, a relatively common X-linked disorder. Most X-linked diseases are so rare, however, that it is very unusual for a female to be homozygous unless her parents are consanguineous (Fig. 5–19).

**Affected Male × Carrier Female: $X_h/Y \times X_H/X_h$**

| | $X_H$ | $X_h$ | |
|---|---|---|---|
| $X_h$ | $X_H/X_h$ | $X_h/X_h$ | Daughters: 1/2 carriers, 1/2 affected |
| Y | $X_H/Y$ | $X_h/Y$ | Sons: 1/2 normal, 1/2 affected |

### New Mutation in X-Linked Disorders

In males, genes for X-linked disorders are exposed to selection. The selection is complete for some disorders, partial for others, and absent for still others, depending on the fitness of the genotype. Hemophiliacs have only about 70 percent as many offspring as unaffected males; that is, the fitness of affected males is about 0.70. Selection against mutant alleles is more dramatic for X-linked disorders such as DMD, a disease of muscle that affects young boys (see Chapter 12). The disorder is usually apparent by the time the child begins to walk and progresses inexorably, so that the child is confined to a wheelchair by about the age of 10 and usually does not survive his teens. Although the situation may change as a result of advances in research aimed at therapy for affected boys, DMD is said to be a **genetic lethal** because affected males usually fail to reproduce. It may, of course, be transmitted by carrier females, who themselves rarely show any clinical manifestation of the disease.

New mutations constitute a significant fraction of isolated cases of many X-linked diseases. When patients are affected with a very severe X-linked recessive disease, such as DMD, they cannot reproduce (i.e., selection is complete), and, therefore, the mutant alleles they carry are lost from the population. Because the incidence of DMD is not changing, mutant alleles lost through failure of the affected males to reproduce have to be continually replaced by new mutations. For hemophilia, in which reproduction is reduced but not eliminated, a proportionately smaller fraction of cases will be due to new mutation. The balance between new mutation and selection is discussed more fully in Chapter 7.

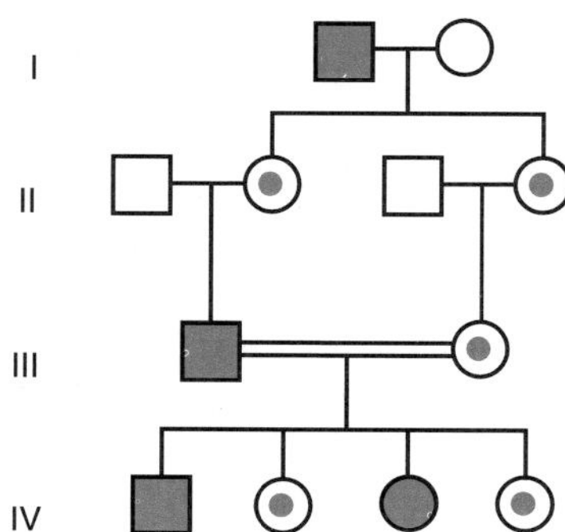


**Figure 5–19.** Consanguinity in an X-linked recessive pedigree for red-green color blindness, resulting in a homozygous affected female.

**Characteristics of X-Linked Recessive Inheritance**

1. The incidence of the trait is much higher in males than in females.
2. Heterozygous females are usually unaffected, but some may express the condition with variable severity as determined by the pattern of X inactivation.
3. The gene responsible for the condition is transmitted from an affected man through all his daughters. Any of his daughters' sons has a 50 percent chance of inheriting it.
4. The gene is ordinarily never transmitted directly from father to son, but it is transmitted by an affected male to all his daughters.
5. The gene may be transmitted through a series of carrier females; if so, the affected males in a kindred are related through females.
6. A significant proportion of isolated cases are due to new mutation.

## X-Linked Dominant Inheritance

An X-linked phenotype is described as dominant if it is regularly expressed in heterozygotes. The distinguishing feature of a fully penetrant X-linked dominant pedigree (Fig. 5–20) is that *all* the daughters and *none* of the sons of affected males are affected; if any daughter is unaffected or any son is affected, the inheritance must be autosomal, not X-linked. The pattern of inheritance through females is no different from the autosomal dominant pattern; because females have a pair of X chromosomes just as they have pairs of autosomes, each child of an affected female has a 50 percent chance of inheriting the trait, regardless of sex. As a general rule, rare X-linked dominant phenotypes are about twice as common in females as in males, although the expression is usually much milder in females, who are almost always heterozygotes.

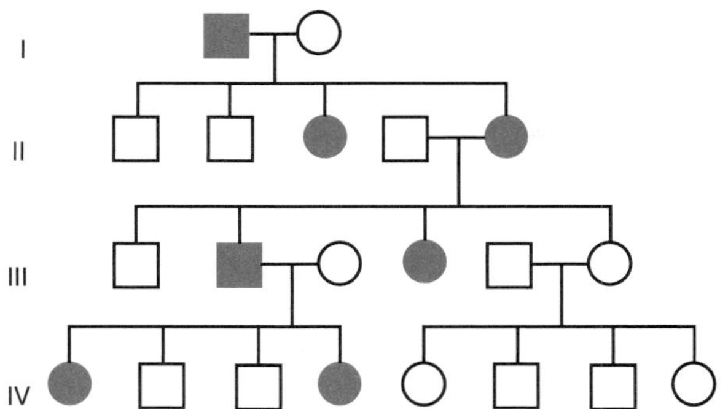


**Figure 5–20.** Pedigree pattern demonstrating X-linked dominant inheritance.

Only a few genetic disorders are classified as X-linked dominants. One example is X-linked **hypophosphatemic rickets** (also called vitamin D–resistant rickets), in which the ability of the kidney tubules to reabsorb filtered phosphate is impaired. This disorder fits the criterion of an X-linked dominant disorder in that, although both sexes are affected, the serum phosphate level is less depressed and the rickets less severe in heterozygous females than in affected males. The defective gene product appears to be a member of a family of endopeptidases that activate or degrade a variety of peptide hormones. The pathogenic mechanism by which a deficiency of this endopeptidase results in a disorder of phosphate metabolism and rickets is not known.

Some of the rare genetic defects expressed exclusively or almost exclusively in females appear to be X-linked dominant conditions that are lethal in males before birth. Typical pedigrees of these conditions show transmission by affected females, who produce affected daughters, normal daughters, and normal sons in equal proportions (1:1:1) (Fig. 5–21). **Incontinentia pigmenti type 2** (IP2) (Fig. 5–22) is a striking disorder that meets all criteria for being an X-linked dominant disorder that is lethal in hemizygous males. The disorder occurs exclusively in females. It is characterized by a skin rash that begins in infancy as a swirling pattern of skin erythema, vesicles, and pustules that then progress to thickening and hyperpigmentation and, eventually, scarring and thinning. Microcephaly, mental retardation, small or absent teeth, and loss of hair are also frequently seen. The hypothesis that IP2 is lethal in males is supported by the fact that only one or two severely affected males are known and the ratio of males to females in the offspring of female heterozygotes for the disorder is only 1:2 instead of the expected 1:1. Furthermore, female heterozygotes are remarkable in that they have a nearly totally nonrandom pattern of X inactivation, which can be explained by assuming that a female heterozygote survives only because the X chromosome carrying the mutation responsible for IP2 is inactive in nearly 100 percent of her cells.

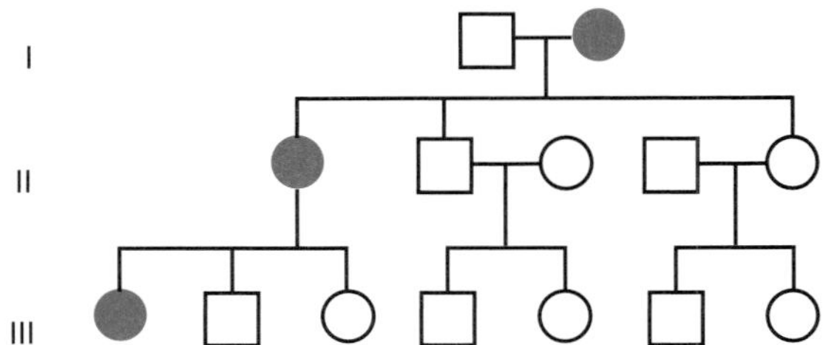


**Figure 5–21.** Pedigree pattern demonstrating an X-linked dominant disorder, lethal in males during the prenatal period.

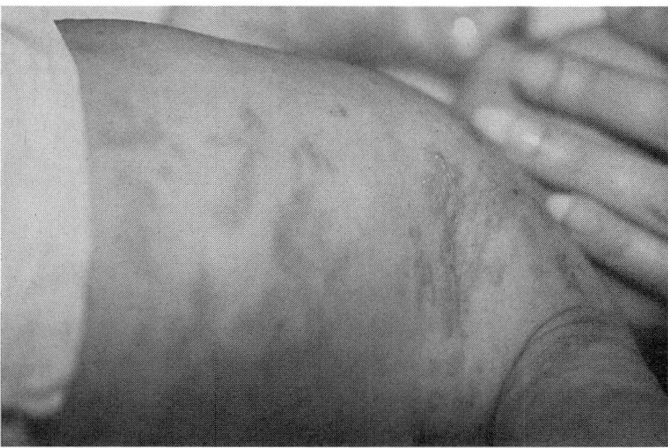

**Figure 5–22.** Typical linear erythema and blistering in a female infant with incontinentia pigmenti. As the child grows older, the skin lesions will become flattened, pigmented streaks. (Photograph courtesy of Virginia Sybert, University of Washington, Seattle.)

### Characteristics of X-Linked Dominant Inheritance

1. Affected males with normal mates have no affected sons and no normal daughters.
2. Both male and female offspring of female carriers have a 50 percent risk of inheriting the phenotype. The pedigree pattern is the same as that seen with autosomal dominant inheritance.
3. For rare phenotypes, affected females are about twice as common as affected males, but affected females typically have milder (though variable) expression of the phenotype.

## PATTERNS OF PSEUDOAUTOSOMAL INHERITANCE

Pseudoautosomal inheritance describes the inheritance pattern seen with genes in the pseudoautosomal region of the X and Y chromosome that can

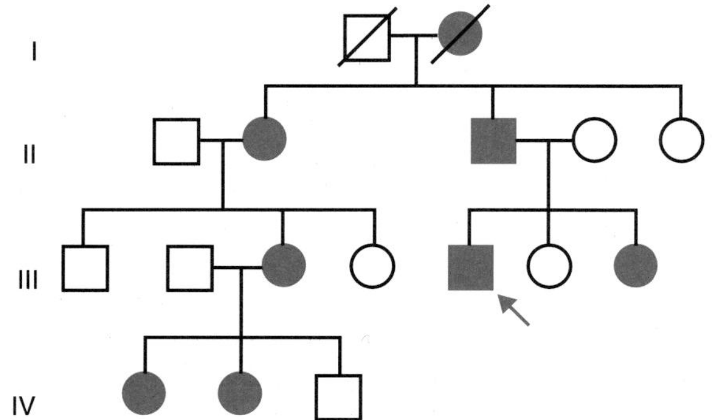


**Figure 5–23.** Pedigree showing inheritance of dyschondrosteosis due to mutations in a pseudoautosomal gene on the X and Y chromosomes. Arrow shows a male who inherited the trait on his Y chromosome from his father. His father, however, inherited the trait on his X chromosome from his mother. (From Shears DJ et al [1998] Mutation and deletion of the pseudoautosomal gene SHOX cause Leri-Weill dyschondrosteosis. Nat Genet 19:70–73.)

exchange regularly between the two sex chromosomes, thus mimicking autosomal inheritance. **Dyschondrosteosis**, a dominantly inherited skeletal dysplasia with disproportionate short stature and deformity of the forearm, is an example of a pseudoautosomal condition. A greater prevalence of the disease was seen in females as compared with males, suggesting an X-linked dominant disorder, but the presence of male-to-male transmission clearly ruled out strict X-linked inheritance (Fig. 5–23). The gene responsible for this dwarfism syndrome is a pseudoautosomal gene that escapes X inactivation and encodes a transcription factor likely involved in the regulation of stature. Either deletion of or mutations in this gene result in dyschondrosteosis in both heterozygous males and females.

## ATYPICAL PATTERNS OF INHERITANCE

As a general rule, the patterns of inheritance and segregation ratios of single-gene disorders are in accord with the principles of mendelian inheritance. Throughout the 20th century, since Garrod and Bateson first applied Mendel's laws to inborn errors of metabolism, few exceptions to mendelian inheritance have been observed. However, close examination of certain unusual disorders and the analysis of mutations in molecular detail have shown that exceptions to mendelian inheritance do occur in single-gene disorders and must be considered in genetic medicine. In this section, we briefly describe situations in which the inheritance of single-gene disorders diverges from typical mendelian patterns.

### Unusual Inheritance Patterns Due to Genomic Imprinting

On the basis of mendelian principles, a mutant allele of an autosomal gene is equally likely to be transmitted from a parent, of either sex, to an offspring of either sex; similarly, a female is equally likely to transmit a mutated X-linked gene to a child of either sex. Originally, little attention was paid to whether the sex of the parent had any effect on the *expression* of the genes each parent transmits. We now know, however, that in some genetic disorders, the expression of the disease phenotype depends on whether the mutant allele has been inherited from the father or from the mother. Differences in gene expression between the allele inherited from the mother and the allele inherited from the father are the result of **genomic imprinting**. Imprinting is caused by an incompletely understood alteration in chromatin that affects the expression of a gene but not its DNA sequence. Thus, it is a reversible form of gene inactivation but is not a mutation.

One important type of imprinting takes place during gametogenesis, before fertilization, and marks certain genes as having come from the mother or father. After conception, the imprint suppresses expression of the imprinted allele in some or all of the somatic tissues of the embryo and even postnatally into adulthood through hundreds of cell divisions. Yet, imprinting must be reversible: an imprinted paternally derived allele, when inherited by a female, must be converted in her germline so that she can then pass it on with a maternal imprint to her offspring. Likewise, an imprinted maternally derived allele, when inherited by a male, must be converted in his germline so that he can pass it on as a paternally imprinted allele to his offspring (Fig. 5–24). Control over this conversion process appears to be governed by a DNA element called the **imprinting center**, located within the imprinted region itself.

#### PRADER-WILLI AND ANGELMAN SYNDROMES

Perhaps the best studied examples of the role of genomic imprinting in human disease are **Prader-Willi syndrome** (PWS) and **Angelman syndrome** (AS). PWS is a relatively common dysmorphic syndrome characterized by obesity, excessive and indiscriminate eating habits, small hands and feet, short stature, hypogonadism, and mental retardation (Fig. 5–25). In approximately 70 percent of cases of the syndrome, there is a cytogenetic deletion (illustrated in Chapter 9, Figure 9-5C) involving the proximal long arm of chromosome 15 (15q11-q13), occurring

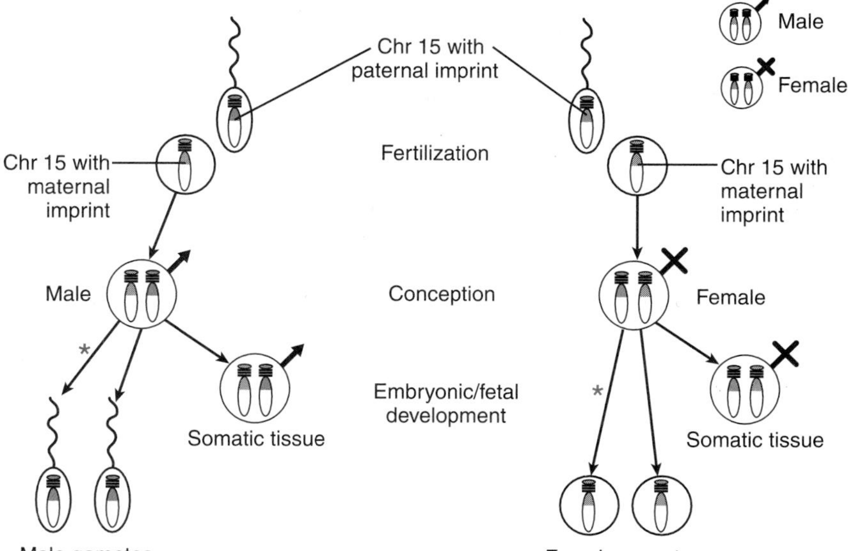


**Figure 5–24.** Diagram of conversion of maternal and paternal imprinting during passage through the germline to make male or female gametes. Erasure of uniparental imprint on one chromosome and conversion to imprint of the other sex is marked by *.

on the chromosome 15 inherited from the patient's father (Table 5–3). Thus, the genomes of these patients have genetic information in 15q11-q13 that derives only from their mothers. In contrast, in approximately 70 percent of patients with the rare AS, characterized by unusual facial appearance, short stature, severe mental retardation, spasticity, and seizures (Fig. 5–26), there is a deletion of approximately the same chromosomal region but on the chromosome 15 inherited from the mother. Patients with AS, therefore, have genetic information in 15q11-q13 derived only from their fathers. This unusual circumstance demonstrates strikingly that the parental origin of genetic material (in this case, on chromosome 15) can have a profound effect on the clinical expression of a defect.

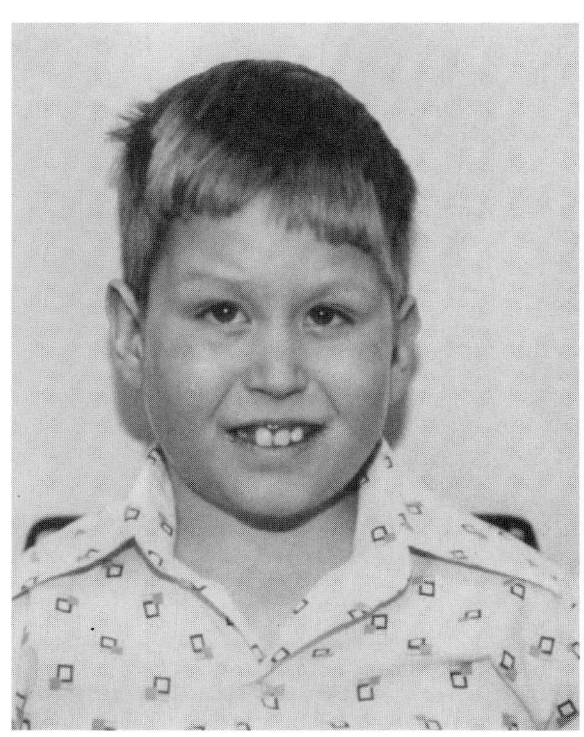

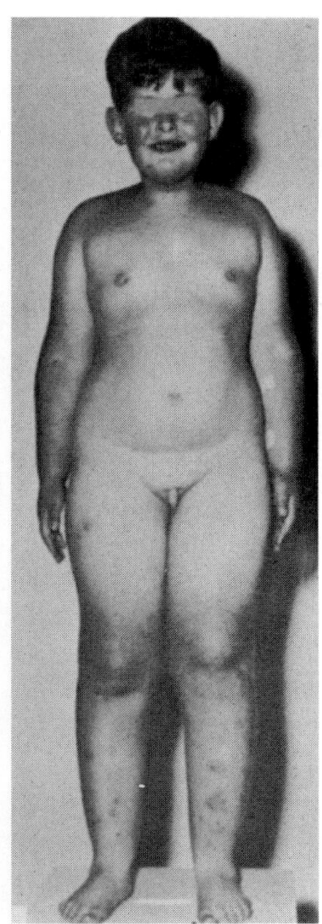

**Figure 5–25.** Prader-Willi syndrome. *Left*, Typical facies in a 9-year-old affected boy. (From Pettigrew AL, Gollin SM, Greenberg F, et al [1987] Duplication of proximal 15q as a cause of Prader-Willi syndrome. Am J Med Genet 28:791–802. Copyright © 1990, Wiley-Liss, Inc. Reprinted by permission of John Wiley and Sons, Inc.) *Right*, Obesity, hypogonadism, and small hands and feet in a 9.5-year-old affected boy who also has short stature and developmental delay. (From Jones KL [1988] Smith's Recognizable Patterns of Human Malformation, 4th ed. WB Saunders, Philadelphia, p. 173.)

TABLE 5–3

**Molecular Mechanisms Causing Prader-Willi and Angelman Syndromes**

| | Prader-Willi Syndrome | Angelman Syndrome |
|---|---|---|
| 15q11-q13 deletion | ~70 percent (paternal) | ~70 percent (maternal) |
| Uniparental disomy | ~30 percent (maternal) | ~3–5 percent (paternal) |
| Single-gene mutation | ND | E6-AP ubiquitin-protein ligase (2–4 percent of total but seen only in familial cases) |
| Imprinting center mutation | 1–2 percent | 7–9 percent |
| Other | ND | 10–20 percent |

ND = none detected.

Data from Jiang Y, Tsai TF, Bressler J, Beaudet AL (1998) Imprinting in Angelman and Prader-Willi syndromes. Curr Opin Genet Dev 8:334–342 and Nicholls RD, Saitoh S, Horsthemke B (1998) Imprinting in Prader-Willi and Angelman syndromes. Trends Genet 14:194–200.

Large deletions are not the only cause of AS. In particular, mutations in the maternal copy of a single gene, the E6-AP ubiquitin-protein ligase gene, have been found to cause AS. The E6-AP ubiquitin-protein ligase gene is located in 15q11-q13 and is normally expressed only from the maternal allele in the central nervous system. Mutations in a single imprinted gene have not yet been found in PWS.

A minority (approximately 30 percent) of patients with PWS do not have cytogenetic deletions; instead, they have an intact pair of chromosome 15s, both of which were inherited from the mother (see Table 5–3). By contrast, only a very small minority of patients with AS (approximately 3 to 5 percent) have two intact chromosome 15s of paternal origin. This unusual situation, termed **uniparental disomy** (see next section), confirms that PWS and AS result from loss of the paternal and maternal contribution of genes in 15q11-q13, respectively.

In addition to chromosomal deletion and uniparental disomy, a few patients with PWS and AS appear to have a defect in the imprinting center itself (see Table 5–3). As a result, the switch from female-to-male imprinting during spermatogenesis or from male-to-female imprinting during oogenesis (see Fig. 5–24) fails to occur. Fertilization by a sperm carrying an abnormally persistent female imprint would produce a child with PWS; fertilization of an egg that bears an inappropriately persistent male imprint would result in AS.

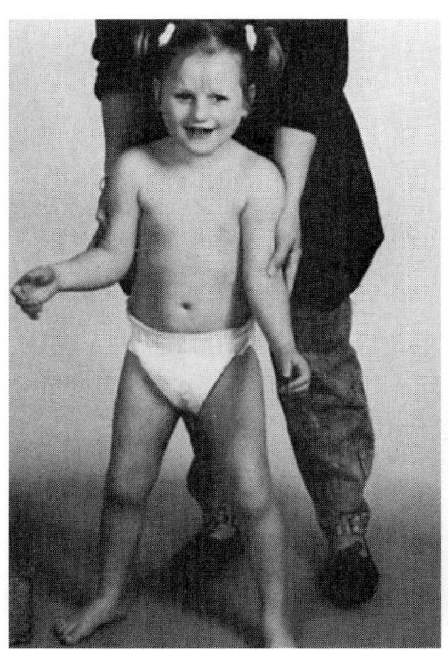

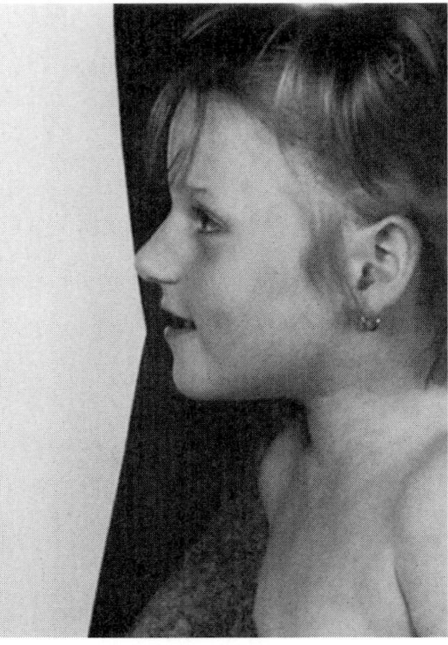

Figure 5–26. Angelman syndrome in a 4-year-old affected girl. Note wide stance and position of arms. Compare with phenotype of Prader-Willi syndrome in Figure 5–25. See text for discussion. (Photograph courtesy of Jan M. Friedman. From Magenis RE, Toth-Fejel S, Allen LJ, et al [1990] Comparison of the 15q deletions in Prader-Willi and Angelman syndromes: specific regions, extent of deletions, parental origin, and clinical consequences. Am J Med Genet 35:333–349. Copyright © 1990, Wiley-Liss, Inc. Reprinted by permission of John Wiley and Sons, Inc.)

### Uniparental Disomy

Uniparental disomy is defined as the presence of a disomic cell line containing two chromosomes, or portions thereof, inherited from only one parent. If the identical chromosome is present in duplicate, the situation is described as **isodisomy**; if both homologs from one parent are present, the situation is **heterodisomy**.

Until the late 1980s, uniparental disomy was unknown, but now that molecular genetic techniques allow the parental source of chromosomes to be readily identified, it has been documented in several clinical disorders in addition to PWS and AS. For example, two patients with CF and short stature have been described with two identical copies of most or all of their maternal chromosome 7. In both cases, the mother happened to be a carrier for CF, and because the child received two maternal copies of the mutant CF gene and no paternal copy of a normal CF gene, the child developed the disease. The growth failure was unexplained but might be related to loss of unidentified paternally imprinted genes on chromosome 7. Uniparental disomy for a portion of chromosome 11 (11p15) is implicated in the **Beckwith-Wiedemann syndrome**. Affected children are very large at birth and have an enlarged tongue and frequent protrusion of the umbilicus. Severe hypoglycemia is a life-threatening complication as are the development of malignancies of kidney, adrenal, and liver. The condition results from an excess of paternal or a loss of maternal contribution of genes, or both, on chromosome 11p15, including the insulin-like growth factor 2 gene. Uniparental disomy can also involve the sex chromosomes, as shown by a reported case of father-to-son transmission of hemophilia A, in which an affected boy inherited both his X and Y chromosomes from his father with no sex chromosome contribution from his mother.

Although it is too early to tell whether uniparental disomy is an interesting rarity or a relatively common phenomenon, there are a number of regions in the genome that show evidence of genomic imprinting (see Fig. 9–13). Physicians and genetic counselors must keep imprinting in mind as a possible cause of genetic disorders, especially in cases of autosomal recessive disorders in patients who have only one documented carrier parent or in cases of X-linked disorders transmitted from father to son or expressed in homozygous form in females.

## Mosaicism

Mosaicism is defined as the presence in an individual or a tissue of at least two cell lines that differ genetically but are derived from a single zygote. Although we are used to thinking of ourselves as being composed of cells that all carry exactly the same complement of genes and chromosomes, this is in reality an oversimplified concept. We already introduced the concept of mosaicism due to X inactivation that generates two different populations of somatic cells in females, those in which the paternal X is the active chromosome and those in which the maternal X is the active chromosome. More generally, mutations arising in single cells in either prenatal or postnatal life can give rise to clones of cells genetically different from the original zygote (Fig. 5–27). Mosaicism is a clinically important phenomenon in chromosomal disorders (see Chapter 9), and somatic mutation is recognized as a major cause of many types of cancer (see Chapter 16). Mosaicism for mutations in single genes, in either somatic or germline cells, seems to be a likely explanation for a number of unusual clinical observations.

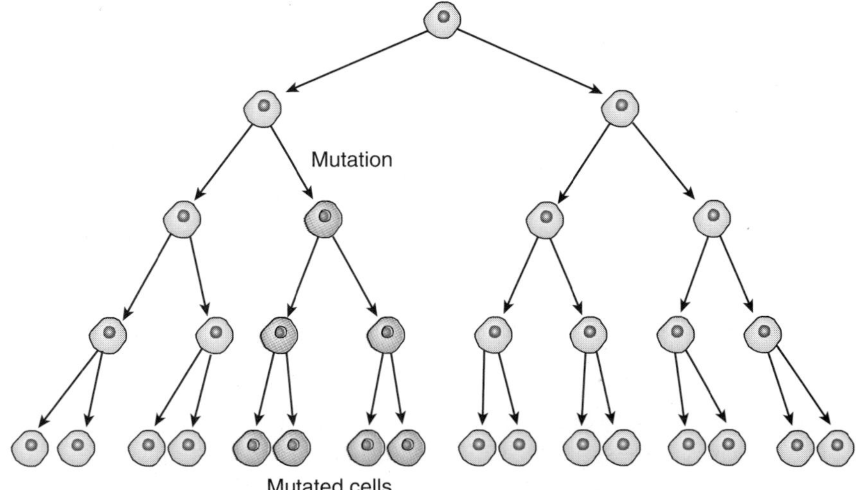


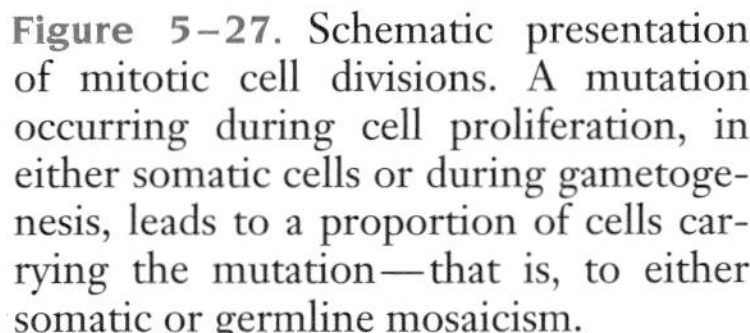
**Figure 5–27.** Schematic presentation of mitotic cell divisions. A mutation occurring during cell proliferation, in either somatic cells or during gametogenesis, leads to a proportion of cells carrying the mutation—that is, to either somatic or germline mosaicism.

### Somatic Mosaicism

A mutation affecting morphogenesis and occurring during embryonic development might be manifested as a segmental or patchy abnormality, depending on the stage at which the mutation occurred and the lineage of the somatic cell in which it originated. If it occurs at an early stage before the separation of germline cells from somatic cells, it is present in both somatic and germline cell lines and thus is transmissible to the offspring in its complete form, as well as being expressed somatically in mosaic form.

NF1 is sometimes segmental, affecting only one part of the body. In such cases, the patient has normal parents, but if he or she has an affected child, the child's phenotype is typical for NF1—that is, not segmental. The possible cause of segmental NF1 is mutation in a somatic cell ancestral to the affected segment. In cases in which NF1 is transmitted genetically by a patient who has the segmental form, however, the mutation must have occurred before separation of germline cells from the somatic cell line that carries the mutation.

Somatic mosaicism has also been documented in a number of X-linked disorders in both males and females. A striking example is a case of dysfunction of the hepatic urea cycle due to a deficiency of the enzyme ornithine transcarbamylase (OTC) in a boy with an unusually mild form of the disorder. Molecular studies demonstrated that the boy had somatic mosaicism for a deletion mutation in the OTC gene. Somatic mosaicism has also been reported for hemophilia A and DMD in females who transmitted the mutation and therefore must have had germline, as well as somatic, mosaicism.

### Germline Mosaicism

As discussed earlier in this chapter, the chance that a disorder due to a new autosomal dominant mutation could occur more than once in a sibship is very low because mutations are generally rare (on the order of 1 chance in $10^5$ to $10^6$; see Chapter 6), and having two occur independently in the same gene in the same family is very unlikely. It used to be customary, therefore, to advise parents of a child who apparently carried a new mutation that the chance of the same defect in a subsequent child was negligible, equivalent to the population risk. There are, however, rare exceptions in which parents who are phenotypically normal have more than one affected child. Assuming the parents have not been diagnosed incorrectly as phenotypically normal homozygotes because of variable expressivity or reduced penetrance of the disease, such unusual pedigrees may be explained by **germline mosaicism**. During the early development of the parent, a somatic mutation has occurred in a germline cell or precursor, has persisted in all the clonal descendants of that cell, and has eventually reached a proportion of the gametes (see Fig. 5–27). There are about 30 mitotic divisions in the cells of the germline before meiosis in the female and several hundred in the male, allowing ample opportunity for mutations to occur during the mitotic stages of gamete development (see Chapter 2).

Now that the phenomenon of germline mosaicism has been recognized, geneticists are aware of the potential inaccuracy of predicting that a specific autosomal dominant phenotype that appears by every test to be a new mutation must have a negligible recurrence risk within the sibship. Germline mosaicism is well documented in as many as 6 percent of severe, lethal forms of the autosomal dominant disorder **osteogenesis imperfecta** (Fig. 5–28) (see Chapter 12), in which mutations in type I collagen genes lead to abnormal collagen, brittle bones, and frequent fractures. Pedigrees that could be explained by germline mosaicism have been reported for several other well-known disorders, such as hemophilia A and B and DMD, but have not been seen in other dominant diseases, such as achondroplasia. Accurate measurement of the frequency of germline mosaicism is difficult, but estimates suggest that the highest incidence found to date is in DMD, in which up to 14 to 15 percent of the mothers of isolated cases show no evidence of the mutation in their somatic tissues and yet carry the mutation in their germline. Thus, in diseases known to show germline mosaicism, phenotypically normal parents of a child whose disease is believed to be due to a new mutation should be informed that the recurrence risk is not negligible. The exact recurrence risk is, however, difficult to assess because it depends on what proportion of gametes contains the mutation. More generally, apparently noncarrier parents of a child with an autosomal dominant or X-linked disorder in which the occurrence of mosaicism is unknown, may also have some recurrence risk that may be as high as 3 to 4 percent; these couples should be offered whatever prenatal diagnostic tests are appropriate.

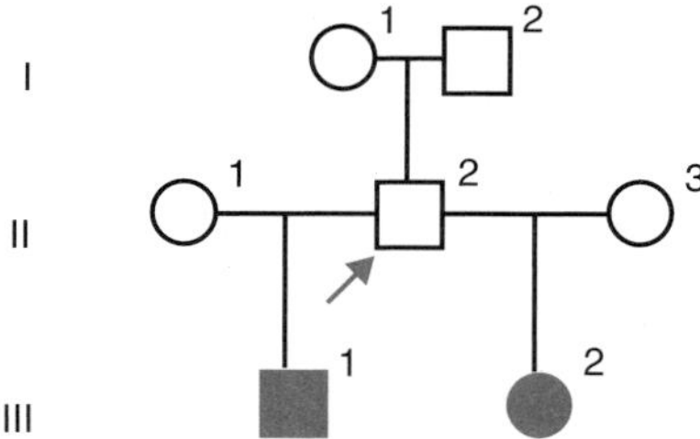


**Figure 5–28.** Pedigree demonstrating recurrence of the autosomal dominant disorder osteogenesis imperfecta. Both affected children have the same point mutation in a collagen gene. Their father (*arrow*) is unaffected and has no such mutation in DNA from examined somatic tissues. He must have been a mosaic for the mutation in his germline.

## Maternal Inheritance of Mitochondrial Mutations

The mitochondrial chromosome is an approximately 16.5 kb circular DNA molecule (mtDNA) located inside the mitochondrial organelle, not in the nucleus, as described in Chapter 3. Two unusual features of mitochondria result in a distinctive inheritance pattern for diseases caused by mutations in mtDNA. First, the ovum, and not the sperm, supplies the zygote with all of its mitochondria. As a consequence, a mother carrying a mutation in mtDNA will pass the mutation on to *all* her offspring, whereas a father carrying the same mutation passes it to none. Defects in mtDNA therefore demonstrate **maternal inheritance**. Another unique feature of the mitochondrial chromosome is the absence of the tightly controlled segregation seen with chromosomes in the nuclear genome. At cell division, the mtDNA replicates and sorts randomly among newly synthesized mitochondria, which are in turn distributed randomly between the two daughter cells. Each daughter cell may receive very different proportions of mitochondria carrying normal and mutant mtDNA (see Figure 12–33). Because mitochondrial function is essential to nearly all cells and the phenotypic expression of a mutation in mtDNA depends on the relative proportions of normal and mutant mtDNA in the cells making up different tissues, reduced penetrance, variable expression, and pleiotropy are typical features of pedigrees of mitochondrial disorders. Diseases caused by mutations in mtDNA are discussed in detail in Chapter 12.

## SUMMARY

An accurate determination of the family pedigree is an important part of the workup of every patient. Pedigrees may demonstrate a straightforward, typical mendelian inheritance pattern or one that is more atypical as is seen with imprinting, mitochondrial mutations, and germline mosaicism. A determination of the inheritance pattern is not only important for making a diagnosis in the proband, it also identifies other individuals in the family who may be at risk and in need of evaluation and counseling. Despite the sophisticated cytogenetic and molecular testing available to geneticists, an accurate family history, including the family pedigree, is still a fundamental tool for physicians and genetic counselors to use in the care of their patients.

### General References

Jones KL (1996) Smith's Recognizable Patterns of Human Malformation, 5th ed. WB Saunders, Philadelphia.

McKusick VA (1998) Mendelian Inheritance in Man: Catalogs of Human Genes and Genetic Disorders, 12th ed. Johns Hopkins University Press, Baltimore. See online version at *http://www.ncbi.nlm.nih.gov/omim/*.

Rimoin DL, Connor JM, Pyeritz RE (1997) Emery and Rimoin's Principles and Practice of Medical Genetics, 3rd ed. Churchill Livingstone, Edinburgh.

Scriver CR, Beaudet AL, Sly WS, Valle D (eds) (2000) The Metabolic and Molecular Bases of Inherited Disease, 8th ed. McGraw-Hill, New York.

Vogel F, Motulsky AG (1997) Human Genetics: Problems and Approaches, 3rd ed. Springer-Verlag, New York.

### References Specific to Particular Topics

Baird PA, Anderson TW, Newcombe HB, Lowry RB (1988) Genetic disorders in children and young adults: A population study. Am J Hum Genet 42:677–693.

Cassidy SB, Schwartz S (1998) Prader-Willi and Angelman syndromes, disorders of genomic imprinting. Medicine 77:140–151.

Costa T, Scriver CR, Childs B (1985) The effect of mendelian disease on human health: A measurement. Am J Med Genet 21:231–242.

Jiang Y, Tsai TF, Bressler J, Beaudet AL (1998) Imprinting in Angelman and Prader-Willi syndromes. Curr Opin Genet Dev 8:334–342.

Nicholls RD, Saitoh S, Horsthemke B (1998) Imprinting in Prader-Willi and Angelman syndromes. Trends Genet 14:194–200.

Shoffner JM, Wallace DC (1992) Mitochondrial genetics: Principles and practice. Am J Hum Genet 51:1179–1186.

Smahi A, Courtois G, Vabres P, et al (2000) Genomic rearrangement in NEMO impairs NF-kappaB activation and is a cause of incontinentia pigmenti. Nature 405:466–472.

Zlotogora J (1998) Germ line mosaicism. Hum Genet 102:381–386.

### Problems

1. Cathy is pregnant for the second time. Her first child, Donald, has CF. Cathy has two brothers, Charles and Colin, and a sister, Cindy. Colin and Cindy are unmarried. Charles is married to an unrelated woman, Carolyn, and has a 2-year-old daughter, Debbie. Cathy's parents are Bob and Betty. Betty's sister Barbara is the mother of Cathy's husband, Calvin, who is 25. There is no previous family history of CF.
   (a) Sketch the pedigree, using standard symbols.
   (b) What is the pattern of transmission of CF, and what is the risk of CF for Cathy's next child?
   (c) How does the risk of CF in Donald's first cousins compare with the population risk of 1/2000?
   (d) Which people in this pedigree are obligate heterozygotes?

2. George and Grace, who have normal hearing, have 8 children. Two of their 5 daughters and 2 of their 3 sons are congenitally deaf. Another couple, Harry and Helen, both with normal hearing, also have 8 children; 2 of their 6 daughters and one of their 2 sons is deaf. A third couple, Gilbert and Gisele, who are congenitally deaf, have 4 children, also deaf. Their daughter Hedy marries Horace, a deaf son of George and Grace, and Hedy and Horace in turn have 4 deaf children. Their eldest son Isaac marries Ingrid, a daughter of Harry and Helen; although both Isaac and Ingrid are deaf, their 6 sons all have *normal* hearing. Sketch the pedigree, and answer the following questions. (Hint: how many different types of congenital deafness are segregating in this pedigree?)

(a) State the probable genotypes of the children in the last generation.
(b) Why are all the children of Gilbert and Gisele and of Hedy and Horace deaf?

3. Consider the following situations:
(a) Retinitis pigmentosa occurs in X-linked and autosomal forms.
(b) Two parents each have a typical case of familial hypercholesterolemia diagnosed on the basis of hypercholesterolemia, arcus corneae, tendinous xanthomas, and demonstrated deficiency of LDL receptors, together with a family history of the disorder; they have a child who has a very high plasma cholesterol level at birth and within a few years develops xanthomas and generalized atherosclerosis.
(c) A couple with normal vision, from an isolated community, have a child with autosomal recessive gyrate atrophy of the retina. The child grows up, marries another member (with normal vision) of the same community, and has a child with the same eye disorder.
(d) A child has severe neurofibromatosis (NF1). Her father is phenotypically normal; her mother seems clinically normal but has several large café-au-lait spots and areas of hypopigmentation, and slit-lamp examination shows that she has a few Lisch nodules (hamartomatous growths on the iris that are common in persons with NF1).
(e) Parents of normal stature have a child with achondroplasia.
(f) An adult male with myotonic dystrophy has cataracts, frontal balding, and hypogonadism, in addition to myotonia.
(g) A man with vitamin D–resistant rickets transmits the condition to all his daughters, who have a milder form of the disease than their father; none of his sons is affected. The daughters have approximately equal numbers of unaffected sons, affected sons, unaffected daughters, and affected daughters, the affected sons being more severely affected than their affected sisters.
(h) A boy has progressive muscular dystrophy with onset in early childhood and is wheelchair bound by the age of 12 years. An unrelated man also has progressive muscular dystrophy but is still ambulant at age 30. Molecular analysis shows that both patients have large deletions in the dystrophin gene, which encodes the protein that is deficient or defective in the Duchenne and Becker types of muscular dystrophy.
(i) A patient with a recessive disorder is found to have inherited both copies of one chromosome from the same parent and no representative of that chromosome from the other parent.
(j) A child with maple syrup urine disease is born to parents who are first cousins.

Which of the concepts listed here are illustrated by the situations described above?

Variable expressivity
Uniparental disomy
Consanguinity
Inbreeding
X-linked dominant inheritance
New mutation
Allelic heterogeneity
Locus heterogeneity
Homozygosity for an autosomal dominant trait
Pleiotropy

4. Don and his maternal grandfather Barry both have hemophilia A. Don's partner Diane is his maternal aunt's daughter. Don and Diane have one son, Edward, and two daughters, Elise and Emily, all of whom have hemophilia A. They also have an unaffected daughter, Enid.
(a) Draw the pedigree.
(b) Why are Elise and Emily affected?
(c) What is the probability that a son of Elise would be hemophilic? What is the probability that her daughter would be hemophilic?
(d) What is the probability that a son of Enid would be hemophilic? A daughter?

5. A boy is born with a number of malformations but does not have a recognized syndrome. The parents are unrelated, and there is no family history of a similar condition. Which of the following conditions could explain this situation? Which are unlikely? Why?
(a) Autosomal dominant inheritance with new mutation
(b) Autosomal dominant inheritance with reduced penetrance
(c) Autosomal dominant inheritance with variable expressivity
(d) Autosomal recessive inheritance
(e) X-linked recessive inheritance
(f) Autosomal dominant inheritance, misattributed paternity
(g) Maternal ingestion of a teratogenic drug at a sensitive stage of embryonic development

6. A couple has a child with NF1. Both parents are clinically normal, and neither of their families shows a positive family history.
(a) What is the probable explanation for NF1 in their child?
(b) What is the risk of recurrence in other children of this couple?
(c) If the husband has another child by a different mother, what would the risk of NF1 be?
(d) What is the risk that any offspring of the affected child will also have NF1?

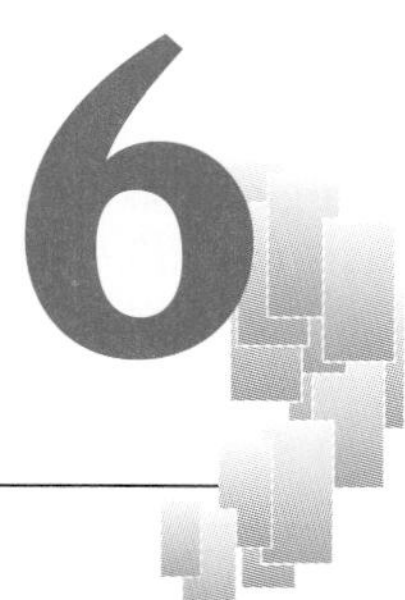

# Genetic Variation in Individuals: Mutation and Polymorphism

This chapter is one of several in which we explore the nature of genetically determined differences among individuals. Although the basis of phenotypic differences can be either genetic changes encoded in the DNA or nongenetic differences in the environment, we deal in this chapter with permanent differences among individuals in the nucleotide sequence of their genomes and the effect of these differences, if any, on phenotype. The sequence of nuclear DNA is nearly 99.9 percent identical between any two humans. Yet it is precisely the small fraction of DNA sequence that is different among individuals that is responsible for the genetically determined variability among humans. Of course, some DNA sequence differences have little or no effect on phenotype, whereas other differences are directly responsible for causing disease. Between these two extremes is the variation responsible for genetically determined phenotypic variability in anatomy, physiology, dietary intolerances, therapeutic responses or adverse reactions to medications, susceptibility to infection, predisposition to cancer, and even variability in various personality traits, athletic aptitude, and artistic talent. One of the important concepts of human and medical genetics is that genetic disease is only the most obvious, and often the most extreme, manifestation of genetic differences, superimposed on a background of entirely normal genetic variability.

## MUTATION

### The Nature of Human Mutation

A mutation is defined as any change in the nucleotide sequence or arrangement of DNA. In broad terms, mutations can be classified into three categories: mutations that affect the number of chromosomes in the cell (**genome mutations**), mutations that alter the structure of individual chromosomes (**chromosome mutations**), and mutations that alter individual genes (**gene mutations**) (Table 6–1). Genome mutations are alterations in the number of intact chromosomes (called **aneuploidy**) arising from errors in chromosome segregation during meiosis or mitosis. Chromosome mutations are imbalances involving only a part of a chromosome, such as duplications, deletions, inversions, and translocations, which can occur spontaneously or may result from abnormal segregation of translocated chromosomes during meiosis. Gene mutations are changes in DNA sequence, ranging from a

TABLE 6–1

**Types of Mutation and Their Estimated Frequencies**

| Class of Mutation | Mechanism | Frequency (Approximate) | Examples |
|---|---|---|---|
| Genome mutation | Chromosome missegregation | $10^{-2}$/cell division | Aneuploidy |
| Chromosome mutation | Chromosome rearrangement | $6 \times 10^{-4}$/cell division | Translocations |
| Gene mutation | Base-pair mutation | $10^{-10}$/base pair/cell division<br>$10^{-5}-10^{-6}$/locus/generation | Point mutations |

Based on Vogel F, Motulsky AG (1997) Human Genetics, 3rd ed. Springer-Verlag, Berlin.

change in as little as a single nucleotide to changes that may affect many thousands of base pairs, but always on a scale too small to be seen even with high-resolution cytogenetic analysis.

A genome mutation that deletes or duplicates an entire chromosome alters the dosage and thus the expression levels of hundreds or thousands of genes. Similarly, a chromosome mutation that deletes or duplicates large portions of one or more chromosomes may also affect the expression of hundreds of genes. Even a small gene mutation can have large effects depending on which gene has been altered and what effect the alteration has on expression of the gene. A gene mutation consisting of a change in a single nucleotide in the coding sequence of a given gene may lead to complete loss of expression of the gene or to the formation of a variant protein with altered properties. The phenotypic changes produced by gene mutations are considered in detail in Chapters 11 and 12.

Some DNA changes, however, may have no phenotypic effect. A chromosome mutation may not affect a critical portion of the genome and may have no phenotypic effect whatsoever. A mutation within a gene may have no effect, either because the change does not alter the primary amino acid sequence of a polypeptide or because, even if it does, the resulting change in the encoded amino acid sequence does not alter the functional properties of the polypeptide. Not all mutations, therefore, have clinical consequences.

All three types of mutation occur at appreciable frequencies in many different cells. If a mutation occurs in the DNA of cells that will populate the germline, the mutation will be a heritable change that can be passed on to future generations. In contrast, some mutations—**somatic mutations**—occur by chance only in a subset of cells from only certain tissues and result in somatic mosaicism as seen, for example, in many instances of cancer. Somatic mutations cannot be transmitted to the next generation.

## The Origin of Mutations

### Genome Mutations

As we discuss at length in Chapter 9, missegregation of a chromosome pair during meiosis causes genome mutations responsible for conditions such as trisomy 21 (Down syndrome). Genome mutations produce chromosomal aneuploidy and are the most common mutation seen in humans (see Table 6–1), with a rate of one missegregation event per 25 to 50 meiotic cell divisions (see Chapter 9). This estimate is clearly a minimal one because the developmental consequences of many such events may be so severe that the resulting aneuploid fetuses are spontaneously aborted shortly after conception without being detected. Genome mutations are also very common in cancer cells (see Chapter 16).

### Chromosome Mutations

Chromosome mutations happen much less frequently than do genome mutations, occurring at a rate of approximately one rearrangement per 1700 cell divisions. Although the frequencies of genome and chromosome mutations may seem high, these mutations are rarely perpetuated from one generation to the next because they are usually incompatible with survival or normal reproduction. Chromosome mutations are also frequently seen in cancer cells (see Chapter 16).

### Gene Mutations

Gene mutations, including base-pair substitutions, insertions, and deletions (Fig. 6–1), can originate by either of two basic mechanisms: errors introduced during the normal process of DNA replication or mutations arising from a failure to repair DNA damage. Some mutations are spontaneous, whereas others are induced by physical or chemical agents, called **mutagens** because these agents greatly enhance the frequency of mutations.

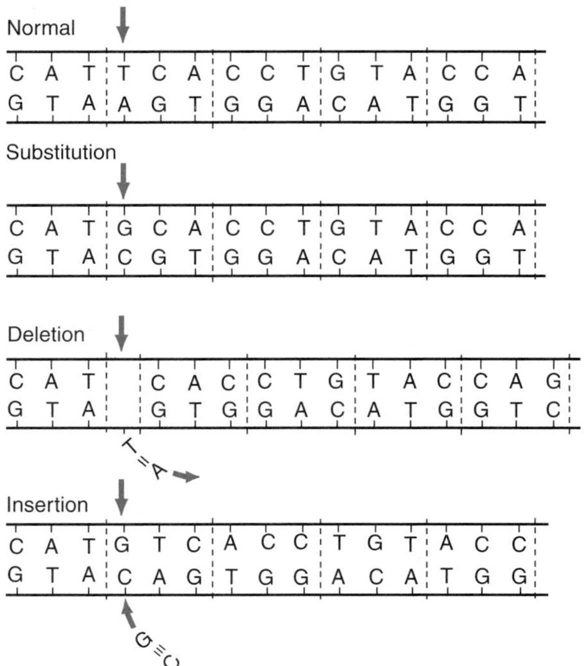


**Figure 6–1.** Examples of gene mutation. The first base of the second codon is mutated by a base substitution, deletion, or insertion. Both the single base-pair deletion and insertion lead to a frameshift mutation in which the translational reading frame is altered. See text for discussion.

**DNA Replication Errors.** The vast majority of replication errors are rapidly removed from the DNA and corrected by a series of DNA repair enzymes that first recognize which strand in the newly synthesized double helix contains the incorrect base, and then replace it with the proper complementary base, a process termed "proofreading." DNA replication (see Fig. 3–4) needs to be a remarkably accurate process, because even if mutations were introduced only once in every million base pairs, the burden of mutation on the organism would be intolerable, and our species would cease to exist. In fact, the DNA replication machinery does considerably better than generating one mutation every million bases. Through a combination of strict base-pairing rules (A pairs with T, C with G) and molecular proofreading, the enzyme DNA polymerase faithfully duplicates the double helix while introducing an incorrect nucleotide into one of the growing daughter strands only once every 10 million base pairs (all this while moving along a human chromosome at a rate of about 20 base pairs per second!). Additional replication error checking then corrects more than 99.9 percent of errors of DNA replication. Thus, the overall mutation rate as a result of replication errors is a remarkably low $10^{-10}$ per base pair per cell division. Because the human diploid genome contains approximately $6 \times 10^9$ base pairs of DNA, replication errors introduce less than one new base-pair mutation per cell division.

**Mutation during Repair of DNA Damage.** In addition to replication errors, mutations can be caused by spontaneous chemical processes, such as depurination, demethylation, or deamination; by reaction with chemical mutagens (natural or otherwise) in the environment; and by exposure to ultraviolet or ionizing radiation. In contrast to replication-related DNA changes, which are usually corrected through proofreading mechanisms, nucleotide changes introduced by DNA damage often remain as permanent mutations.

## THE MOLECULAR BASIS OF MUTATIONS AND THEIR DETECTION

Many types of mutation are represented among the diverse alleles detected at individual loci. Underlying both normal variation in the population and examples of inherited disease, mutations ranging from single base-pair changes to deletion of many millions of base pairs have been documented. With the now seemingly routine application of molecular techniques to mutation detection and elucidation, a large number of specific mutations are being discovered in scores of different genetic disorders. The description of different mutations not only increases awareness of human genetic diversity and of the fragility of human genetic heritage but also, more significantly, contributes information needed for the detection and screening of genetic disease in particular families at risk, as well as, for some diseases, in the population at large.

Here we consider the nature of different mutations, their underlying mechanisms, and their effect on the genes involved. In Chapters 11 and 12, we turn to the ways in which mutations cause disease. Each type of mutation discussed here is illustrated by one or more disease examples; it should be remembered, however, that mutations in most genetic diseases are quite heterogeneous. Different cases of a particular disorder will therefore usually be caused by different underlying mutations (see Box).

### Types of Mutation in Human Genetic Disease

**Nucleotide Substitutions (Point Mutations)**

Missense mutations (amino acid substitutions)
Nonsense mutations (premature stop codons)
RNA processing mutations (destroy consensus splice sites, cap sites, polyadenylation sites, or create cryptic sites). Abnormal splicing often leads to frameshift mutations and premature stop codons.
Regulatory mutations affecting transcription factor binding, transcriptional control, or other aspects of gene expression

**Deletions and Insertions**

Addition or deletion of small number of bases
- If number of bases involved is not a multiple of 3, causes frameshift
- If number of bases involved is a multiple of 3, causes loss or gain of codons and, subsequently, amino acids in translated product.

Larger gene deletions, inversions, fusions, and duplications (may be mediated by DNA sequence homology either within or between DNA strands)
Insertion of L1 or *Alu* element (disrupts transcription or interrupts the coding sequence)
Expansion of trinucleotide repeat sequences

## Nucleotide Substitutions

A single nucleotide substitution (or **point mutation**) in a DNA sequence can alter the code in a triplet of bases and cause the replacement of one amino acid by another in the gene product. Such mutations are called **missense mutations** because they alter the "sense" of the coding strand of the gene by specifying a different amino acid. In many disorders, such as the hemoglobinopathies described in Chapter 11, the vast majority of detected mutations are missense mutations. Overall, missense mutations account for almost half of all mutations reported to cause genetic disease in humans.

Other base substitutions occurring either within or outside the coding sequences of a gene can also have extensive effects on the gene product or interfere directly with the transcription process itself. As discussed in detail in Chapter 11, a number of mutations in the 5′ promoter region or the 3′ untranslated region of the $\beta$-globin gene lead to a sharp decrease in the amount of mature, processed $\beta$-globin mRNA produced. Indeed, such mutations have been critical for elucidating the importance for gene expression of particular nucleotides in these regions.

## Chain Termination Mutations

Normally, translation of mRNA ceases when a termination codon is reached (see Chapter 3). A mutation that creates a termination codon can cause premature cessation of translation, whereas a mutation that destroys a termination codon allows translation to continue until the next termination codon is reached. A mutation that generates one of the three "stop" codons is called a **nonsense mutation**. In general, such mutations have no effect on transcription. However, the mRNA carrying a premature mutation is often unstable—if the mRNA is stable enough to be translated, the truncated translation product is usually so unstable that it is rapidly degraded within the cell (**nonsense-mediated mRNA decay**). Premature termination mutations constitute approximately 12 percent of all disease-causing mutations.

## RNA Splicing Mutations

As described in Chapter 3, the normal mechanism by which introns are excised from unprocessed RNA and exons spliced together to form a mature mRNA is dependent on particular nucleotide sequences located at or near the intron/exon (acceptor site) and exon/intron (donor site) boundaries. Two general classes of splicing mutations have been described. Mutations that affect the required bases at either the splice donor or acceptor site interfere with (and in some cases abolish) normal RNA splicing at that site (see Chapters 11 and 12). A second class of splicing mutations involves intron base substitutions that do not affect the donor or acceptor site sequences themselves. Such mutations create alternative donor or acceptor sites that compete with the normal sites during RNA processing. Thus, at least a proportion of the mature mRNA in such cases may contain improperly spliced intron sequences. Examples of this mechanism of mutation are also presented in Chapter 11. Overall, mutations affecting splicing are responsible for 10 percent of mutations reported to cause human genetic disease.

## "Hotspots" of Mutation

Nucleotide changes that involve the substitution of one purine for the other (A⟷G) or one pyrimidine for the other (T⟷C) are called **transitions**. In contrast, the replacement of a purine for a pyrimidine (or vice versa) is called a **transversion**. If nucleotide substitutions were random, there should be twice as many transversions as transitions, because every base can undergo two transversions but only one transition. Different mutagenic processes may preferentially cause one or the other type of substitution, however. Thus, the finding of a higher frequency of transitions than is expected among a collection of mutant alleles has been taken as evidence of a favored mechanism of mutation rather than of spontaneous or random base substitution.

Insight into the excess of transitions among single base-pair substitutions causing genetic disease has come with the finding that the major form of DNA modification in the human genome involves **methylation** of cytosine residues (to form 5-methylcytosine), specifically when they are located immediately 5′ to a guanine (i.e., as the dinucleotide 5′-CG-3′). Spontaneous deamination of 5-methylcytosine to thymidine (compare the structures of cytosine and thymine in Fig. 3–1) in the CG doublet gives rise to C→T or G→A transitions (depending on in which strand of DNA the 5-methylcytosine is mutated). More than 30 percent of all single nucleotide substitutions are of this type, and they occur at a rate 25 times greater than does any other single nucleotide mutation. Thus, the CG doublet represents a true "hotspot" for mutation in the human genome.

## Deletions and Insertions

Mutations can also be caused by the insertion, inversion, fusion, or deletion of DNA sequences. Some deletions and insertions involve only a few nucleotides and can generally be detected only through molecular analysis involving nucleotide sequencing.

In other cases, a substantial segment of a gene or an entire gene is deleted, inverted, duplicated, or translocated to create a novel hybrid gene. Such mutations are usually detected at the level of Southern blotting of a patient's DNA or by polymerase chain reaction (PCR) analysis of the junction. In rare instances, deletions are large enough to be visible at the cytogenetic level. To be detected even with high-resolution prometaphase banding, these mutations generally must delete at least 2 to 4 million base pairs of DNA. In many instances, such deletions remove more than a single gene and are associated with a **contiguous gene syndrome** (see Chapter 10).

### SMALL DELETIONS OR INSERTIONS

Some deletions and insertions affect only a small number of base pairs. When the number of bases involved is not a multiple of three (i.e., is not an integral number of codons), and when it occurs in a coding sequence, the reading frame is altered beginning at the point of the insertion and deletion. A different sequence of amino acids is thereby generated at the carboxyl terminus. These mutations are called **frameshift mutations**. Other small insertions or deletions do not cause a frameshift because the number of base pairs involved is a multiple of three; instead, they will produce an insertion or deletion of the corresponding amino acid in the translated gene product. Deletions or insertions of just a few base pairs constitute nearly one quarter of all mutations responsible for human genetic disease.

### LARGE DELETIONS AND INSERTIONS

Alterations of gene structure large enough to be detected by Southern blotting are uncommon (approximately 6 percent of disease-causing mutations) but have been described in many inherited disorders. The frequency of such mutations differs markedly among different genetic diseases; some disorders are characterized by a high frequency of detectable deletions, whereas in others, deletion is a very rare cause of mutation. For example, deletions within the large dystrophin gene on the X chromosome in Duchenne muscular dystrophy are present in more than 60 percent of cases (see Chapter 12). Many cases of $\alpha$-thalassemia are due to deletion of one of the two $\alpha$-globin genes on chromosome 16, whereas $\beta$-thalassemia is only rarely due to deletion of the $\beta$-globin gene (see Chapter 11). In some cases, the basis for gene deletion is well understood and is probably mediated by aberrant recombination between multiple copies of similar or identical DNA sequences. In other cases, the basis for deletion is unknown.

Insertion of large amounts of DNA is a cause of mutation that is much rarer than is deletion. A novel mechanism of mutation, however, has been described in two unrelated, sporadic cases of hemophilia A. As discussed in Chapter 3, the L1 family of interspersed repetitive sequences represents a class of repeated DNA that may be transcribed into an RNA that, when reverse transcribed, generates a DNA sequence that can insert itself into different sites in the genome. In a few patients with hemophilia A, L1 sequences several kb long were found to be inserted into an exon in the factor VIII gene, interrupting the coding sequence and inactivating the gene. This finding suggests that at least some of the estimated 100,000 copies of the L1 family in the human genome are capable of causing disease by insertional mutagenesis.

### DELETIONS AND DUPLICATIONS CAUSED BY RECOMBINATION

An important cause of mutation in some disorders involves deletion or duplication mediated by recombination among highly similar or identical DNA sequences. Many genes exist as members of multigene families (see Chapter 3). When the members of such a gene family are located in a head-to-tail tandem fashion in the same chromosomal region, they sometimes misalign and pair out of register either in meiosis (when two homologs pair) or in mitosis after replication (when the two sister chromatids often exchange DNA). Recombination occurring between mispaired chromosomes or sister chromatids can lead to gene deletion or duplication. The mechanism of **unequal crossing over** is believed to be responsible for deletion of one of the $\alpha$-globin genes in $\alpha$-thalassemia (see Chapter 11) and for variation in the copy number of green visual pigment genes in the red and green visual pigment gene cluster on the X chromosome, both in persons with normal color vision and in males with X-linked defects in green or red color perception (Fig. 6–2*A*). Abnormal pairing and recombination between two similar sequences repeated on a single strand of DNA may also occur; depending on the orientation of these sequences, such recombination may lead to deletion or inversion. For example, nearly half of all severe hemophilia A is due to recombination that inverts a number of exons, thereby disrupting gene structure (see Fig. 6–2*B*).

Recombination between homologous noncoding DNA sequences can also cause genetic disease. Recombination between different members of the *Alu* family class of interspersed repeated DNA (see Chapter 3) has been documented as the cause of a duplication of several exons in the low-density lipoprotein receptor gene in familial hypercholesterolemia (see Chapter 12).

Finally, a newly described class of mutations has been seen in disorders such as **Huntington disease**

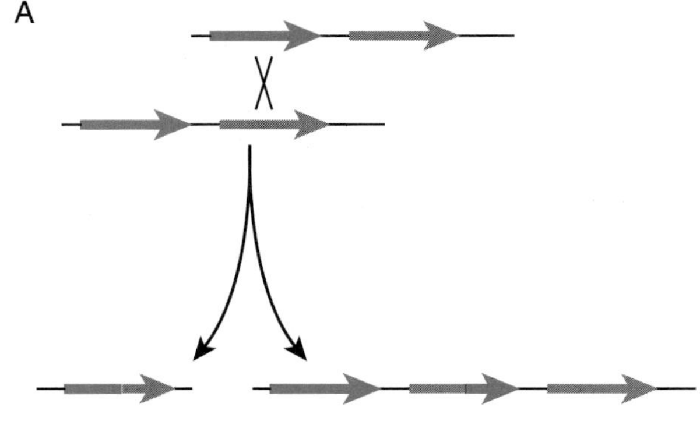


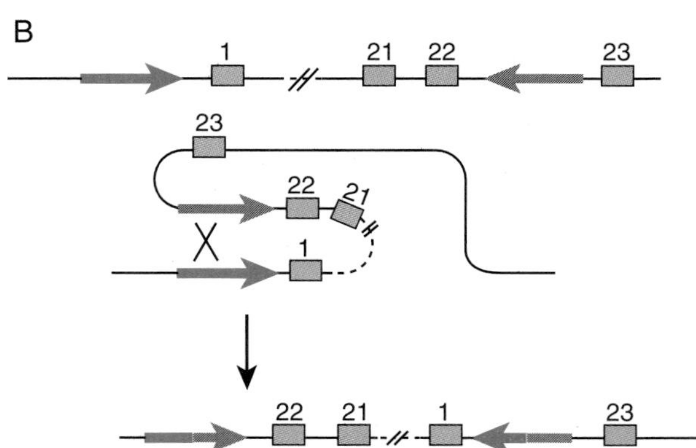


**Figure 6–2.** *A*, Unequal but homologous recombination between misaligned sister chromatids or homologous chromosomes containing highly homologous sequences (*gray and red arrows*) leads to two products, one with only a single copy and one with three copies of the sequence. In *B*, recombination between inverted homologous sequences located 500 kb apart on the same strand (one upstream of the factor VIII gene, the other in intron 22 of the gene) results in inversion of exons 1 through 22 of the gene, thereby disrupting the gene and causing hemophilia.

and **fragile X syndrome** (Chapter 12). In these diseases, a simple trinucleotide repeat, located either in the coding region (in the case of Huntington disease) or in a transcribed but untranslated region of a gene (in the case of fragile X syndrome) may expand and interfere with normal gene expression. A repeat in the coding region will generate an abnormal protein product, whereas repeat expansion in transcribed but untranslated parts of a gene may interfere with transcription or mRNA processing (see Chapter 12).

As researchers identify and catalog literally thousands of mutations in genes causing disease, there is an obvious need for uniform nomenclature to describe any mutation unambiguously in databases designed as repositories of all this information (see Box).

## Estimates of Germline Gene Mutation Rates in Humans

The mutation rate of a gene is usually expressed as the number of new mutations per locus per generation. The most direct way of estimating the rate is to measure the incidence of new, sporadic cases of an autosomal dominant or X-linked genetic disease that is fully penetrant with a clearly recognizable phenotype at birth or shortly thereafter. **Achondroplasia** is one such disease that meets the requirements for directly estimating a mutation rate. In one study, 7 achondroplastic children were born in a series of 242,257 consecutive births. All 7 were born to parents of normal stature, and because achondroplasia is fully penetrant, these 7 cases were considered to represent new mutations. Assuming accurate diagnoses, the new mutation rate can be calculated as 7 new mutations in a total of $2 \times 242{,}257$ alleles, or approximately $1.4 \pm 0.5 \times 10^{-5}$ mutations per locus per generation.

The mutation rate has been estimated for a number of inherited disorders, as shown in Table 6–2. The median gene mutation rate is approximately $1 \times 10^{-6}$ mutations per locus per generation, but the rates vary over a 1000-fold range, from $10^{-4}$ to $10^{-7}$ mutations per locus per generation. The basis for these differences may be related to gene size, the fraction of mutant alleles that give a particular observable phenotype, the mutational mechanism, or the presence or absence of mutational "hotspots," such as methylated CG dinucleotides, in the gene. The **Duchenne muscular dystrophy** and the **neurofibromatosis** genes are both very large, 2000 kb in length; thus, it is not surprising that the mutation rates at these loci are quite high. **Achondroplasia**, on the other hand, results almost exclusively from mutation at one hotspot, a nucleotide change in a glycine codon that substitutes an arginine at position 380 (Gly380Arg) in a fibroblast growth factor receptor. The estimates in Table 6–2 reflect measurements made of very visible and deleterious mutations; less severe or obvious mutations would have escaped detection, as would have more severe, lethal mutations. Thus, the overall new mutation rate may be considerably higher.

Mutation rates have also been estimated using electrophoresis to screen blood serum proteins for alterations of charge and size, a method that is independent of the severity of the mutation. The appearance in a child of a new electrophoretic variant that is not present in either parent suggests a gene mutation that altered either the charge or the size of the encoded protein. Such variants are detected at a frequency of approximately $2 \times 10^{-6}$ per locus per generation. Because only about one third of all amino acid changes produce a change detectable by electrophoresis, the true rate of new mutation in serum proteins using this approach can be estimated to be $3 \times 2 \times 10^{-6}$ or $6 \times 10^{-6}$ per locus per generation.

Despite the limitations of these and other approaches for determining the average gene mutation rate, all methods yield essentially the same range of values for germline mutation rates: approximately $10^{-4}$ to $10^{-6}$ per locus per generation. Because there are

## Mutation Nomenclature

1. The position of a mutation is designated as being either in genomic DNA or in a cDNA sequence by the prefix g. or c., respectively.
2. The A of the translational start ATG is designated +1. The next base upstream is −1; there is no 0.
3. A nucleotide change is noted first by the original base, the nucleotide number of that base, a greater than symbol (>), and the new nucleotide at that position. For example, a mutation responsible for a particular missense mutation causing Tay-Sachs disease can be designated as c.G1444>A in the cDNA.
4. If the full genomic sequence is not known, the nucleotides in an intron (referred to by the expression "intervening sequence," or IVS) are counted as +1, +2, etc., in which +1 is the invariant G of the GT in the 5′ splice donor site, or as −1, −2, etc., counting back from the highly invariant G of the AG 3′ splice acceptor site. A mutation substituting an A for the highly conserved T in a splice donor site of intron 33 of a gene is designated g.IVS33+2T>A, whereas a mutation substituting a T for an A in the highly conserved A of a splice acceptor site in the same intron would be designated g.IVS33−2A>T.
5. Small deletions are indicated by the term "del" written after the nucleotide numbers deleted (1524–1527del).
6. Small insertions are designated similarly by the term "ins" after the two nucleotides between which the insertion occurred, followed by the actual nucleotides inserted. For example, c.1277–1278insTATC denotes a four-base insertion between nucleotides 1277 and 1278 in the cDNA for hexosaminidase A, a common mutation causing Tay-Sachs disease.
7. If a missense mutation is described at the level of the protein, the amino acid residues (single or three-letter code; see Table 3–1) are numbered so that the initiator methionine is assigned number 1. The missense mutation in $\beta$-globin at residue number 6 that causes sickle cell anemia converts a glutamate to valine and is designated Glu6Val (E6V). A premature termination mutation causing $\beta^0$–thalassemia, such as the mutation that changes a glutamine residue at position 39 in $\beta$-globin into a stop codon, is designated Gln39X (Q39X).

about 50,000 genes in the genome, this suggests that, at a minimum, *at least 1 in 20 persons is likely to have received a newly mutated gene from one or the other parent.*

### Inherited Mutation in Humans: Sex Differences

New mutations can occur in the germline during any of the mitotic divisions or during the meiotic division in spermatogenesis or oogenesis. There are, however, marked differences between the sexes in both the number and timing of the mitotic and meiotic divisions, differences that can affect the frequency and types of mutation in paternal versus maternal gametes.

In oogenesis, as we saw in Chapter 2, each haploid ovum is the product of an estimated 22 mitotic divisions in fetal life, after which it enters meiosis I and remains suspended there, for years or even decades, until meiosis I is finally completed at the time of ovulation. There is speculation that the longer oocytes

TABLE 6–2

**Estimates of Mutation Rates for Selected Human Genes**

| Disease | Inheritance | Locus (protein) | Mutation Rate* |
|---|---|---|---|
| Achondroplasia | AD | *FGFR3* (fibroblast growth factor receptor 3) | $0.6–1.4 \times 10^{-5}$ |
| Aniridia | AD | *AN2* (Pax6) | $2.9–5 \times 10^{-6}$ |
| Duchenne muscular dystrophy | X-linked | *DMD* (dystrophin) | $3.5–10.5 \times 10^{-5}$ |
| Hemophilia A | X-linked | *F8* (factor VIII) | $3.2–5.7 \times 10^{-5}$ |
| Hemophilia B | X-linked | *F9* (factor IX) | $2–3 \times 10^{-6}$ |
| Neurofibromatosis, type 1 | AD | *NF1* (neurofibromin) | $4–10 \times 10^{-5}$ |
| Polycystic kidney disease, type 1 | AD | *PKD1* (polycystin) | $6.5–12 \times 10^{-5}$ |
| Retinoblastoma | AD | *RB* (Rb) | $5–12 \times 10^{-6}$ |

* Expressed as mutations/locus/generation.
AD = autosomal dominant.
Based on data in Vogel F, Motulsky AG (1997) Human Genetics, 3rd ed. Springer-Verlag, Berlin.

remain in meiosis I, the greater the chance of an error occurring when the cells finally do complete meiosis. These characteristics of oogenesis may help explain why meiotic nondisjunction leading to genome mutations such as autosomal trisomies of chromosomes 13, 18, and 21 occurs much more frequently in the maternal rather than the paternal germline, and increases in frequency with increasing age of the mother and not the father (see Chapter 10).

Spermatogenesis, on the other hand, involves a continuous series of cell divisions throughout life, resulting in a total of approximately 1 trillion sperm. These cells are the result of about 30 mitotic divisions from the embryo stage to the time of puberty and about 20 to 25 replication cycles per year thereafter. Given a frequency of $10^{-10}$ replication errors per base of DNA per cell division, each diploid spermatogonium, which contains $6 \times 10^9$ base pairs of DNA, will accumulate about one new mutation each time it replicates before meiosis. As an example, each sperm in a 27-year-old man is the product of about 300 rounds of replication, and so each sperm will contain an estimated $3 \times 10^2 \times 6 \times 10^9 \times 10^{-10} = 180$ new mutations as a result of DNA replication errors. Although the vast majority of these mutations will not be deleterious (or will be recessive or lethal to the sperm and thus not phenotypically apparent in a resulting conception and birth), some will be. According to calculated rates of deleterious mutations at individual loci, one can estimate that *approximately 1 in 10 sperm carries a new deleterious mutation.*

Because the DNA in sperm has undergone far more replication cycles than has the DNA in ova, one might expect that gene mutations arising from errors in replication might be more often paternal, rather than maternal, in origin. Furthermore, the older a man is, the more rounds of replication have preceded the meiotic divisions, and thus the frequency of paternal new mutations might be expected to increase with the age of the father. In fact, an excess of gene mutations of paternal origin has been observed for some disorders, notably **neurofibromatosis, achondroplasia**, and **hemophilia B** (where the maternal grandfather is the source of a new mutation). In other diseases, however, new mutations are not more frequently of paternal origin, and, even when there is a bias toward a paternal origin, there is not always an increase in mutation rate with advanced paternal age. The reason why mutations in some disorders show a parental origin bias or an age effect, whereas others do not, is not known.

In trinucleotide repeat disorders (see Chapter 12), a marked parent-of-origin effect is well known. For example, the very large expansions of the CAG repeat that cause juvenile Huntington disease is generally of paternal origin. On the other hand, the massive expansions of the CGG repeat in fragile X syndrome nearly always occur during female gametogenesis. Such differences may be due to fundamental biological differences between oogenesis and spermatogenesis but may also result from selection against gametes carrying repeat expansions, as has been shown for sperm carrying extremely large CGG repeat expansions associated with the fragile X syndrome.

## Somatic Mutation and Cancer

Mutations can occur in any cell, both in germline cells and in somatic cells. Only germline mutations are passed from one generation to the next and are the ones responsible for inherited disease. This is not to say, however, that somatic cell mutations are not medically important. Indeed, the vast majority of cell divisions that produce an adult organism of an estimated $10^{14}$ cells from a single-cell zygote occur in somatic lineages; consequently, most mutations occur in somatic cells. Given a frequency of $10^{-10}$ replication errors per base of DNA per cell division and an estimated $10^{15}$ cell divisions during the lifetime of an adult, replication errors result in thousands of new mutations in the genome in each cell of the organism. The overall magnitude of the human mutational load is clearly enormous. The overwhelming majority of mutations occur in somatic cells and are therefore not heritable. Depending on the nature of the mutation, however, its location in the genome, and the tissue involved, the phenotypic effect of a somatic mutation may have a devastating impact on an individual if it leads to cancer. Chromosomal mutations such as translocations and inversions are responsible for many forms of **leukemia** and **malignant lymphoma**. Somatic gene mutations are believed to be implicated in most if not all forms of cancer; for example, most **colorectal cancer** in adults and **retinoblastoma** and **Wilms' tumor** in children, to name just a few, are known to result from somatic gene mutations. In this sense, cancer is fundamentally a "genetic" disease, and mutations are central to its etiology or progression, as is presented in Chapter 16.

## Generalized Defects in DNA Repair

As expected from the important role that DNA replication and repair enzymes play in mutation surveillance and prevention, inherited defects that alter the function of such enzymes can lead to a dramatic increase in the frequency of mutations of all types. Autosomal recessive disorders such as **xeroderma pigmentosum, ataxia telangiectasia, Fanconi anemia**, and **Bloom syndrome** are due to loss of function of proteins required for normal DNA repair or replication. Patients with these conditions have a high frequency of chromosome and gene mutations that predispose affected persons to cancer (see Chapters 9 and 16). Patients with **hereditary nonpolyposis colon cancer**, an autosomal dominant familial colon cancer, are heterozygous for an abnormal copy of one of a class of genes required for repair of base-pair mismatches introduced during DNA replication or repair; if the other remaining normal copy of the gene is lost or mutated in an intestinal epithelial cell, the cell lacks the ability to repair DNA base mismatches, gene mutations accumulate, and the cell becomes cancerous (see Chapter 16).

## HUMAN GENETIC DIVERSITY

Most of the estimates of mutation rates described involve detection of deleterious mutations with an obvious effect on phenotype. Many mutations, however, are not deleterious but are thought to be selectively neutral. On the basis of information presented earlier in this chapter, each new zygote would be expected to contain 100 or so base-pair changes not present in the genome of either parent. Most of this variation is not in coding sequence but is found in extragenic sequences or in noncoding regions of the chromosomes. During the course of evolution, the steady influx of new nucleotide variation has ensured a high degree of genetic diversity and individuality. This theme extends through all fields in human and medical genetics; genetic diversity may manifest as changes in the staining pattern of chromosomes (see Chapter 9), as protein variation, as nucleotide changes in DNA, or as disease.

### The Concept of Genetic Polymorphism

If the sequence of exactly the same region of DNA located at a particular position on a chromosome is determined in a large number of chromosomes carried by many different individuals from around the world, a remarkably high level of similarity is observed. In fact, any given segment of human DNA about 1000 base pairs in length contains, on average, only one base pair that varies between two individuals in the population. As we have seen previously, different versions of a particular DNA sequence at one particular chromosomal location (**locus**) are called **alleles**. When alleles are so common that they are found in more than 1 percent of chromosomes in the general population, the alleles constitute what is known as **genetic polymorphism**. In contrast, alleles with frequencies of less than 1 percent are, by convention, called **rare variants**. Some alleles represent a change in the sequence of the DNA located between genes or within introns, are inconsequential to the functioning of any gene, and can be detected only by direct DNA analysis. Other sequence changes are located in the coding sequence of genes themselves and may result in different protein variants that may lead in turn to sharply distinct phenotypes. Most (but not all) deleterious mutations that lead to genetic disease are rare variants. Mutant alleles that lead to severe genetic disease are often only the most obvious form of genetic diversity; on examination, many proteins have been found to exist in different populations in several relatively common, distinguishable forms.

Although all polymorphism is ultimately the result of differences in DNA sequence, some polymorphic loci have been studied by examining the variation in the proteins encoded by the alleles rather than by examining the differences in DNA sequence of the alleles themselves. We discuss in detail later a few polymorphisms of medical significance: the ABO and Rh blood groups important in determining compatibility for blood transfusions and, to some degree, tissue transplantation, and the serum alpha$_1$-antitrypsin ($\alpha_1$-AT) system implicated in severe lung disease. Studying variation in proteins rather than studying the DNA that encodes them has real utility: after all, it is the protein product of a polymorphic allele, rather than the DNA sequence change itself, that is often responsible for different phenotypes and, therefore, is likely to dictate how some genetic variation affects the interaction between an individual and the environment. Polymorphic alleles in regulatory regions may also be important in determining phenotype by affecting transcriptional regulation of genes.

It is estimated that any one individual is likely to be heterozygous for alleles determining structurally different polypeptides at approximately 20 percent of all loci; when comparing individuals from different ethnic groups, an even greater fraction of proteins has been found to exhibit detectable polymorphism. Thus, a striking degree of biochemical individuality exists within the human species in its makeup of enzymes and other gene products. Furthermore, because the products of many of the encoded biochemical pathways interact, one may plausibly conclude that each individual, regardless of his or her state of health, has a unique, genetically determined chemical makeup and thus responds in a unique manner to environmental, dietary, and pharmacological influences. This concept of **chemical individuality,** first put forward nearly a century ago by the remarkably foresighted British physician Sir Archibald Garrod, remains true today.

## INHERITED VARIATION AND POLYMORPHISM IN PROTEINS

### Blood Groups and Their Polymorphisms

The first instances of genetically determined protein variation were detected on antigens found in blood, the so-called **blood group antigens**. Numerous

TABLE 6–3
**ABO Genotypes and Serum Reactivity**

| Red Blood Cell Phenotype | Reaction with anti-A | Reaction with anti-B | Antibodies in Serum |
|---|---|---|---|
| O | – | – | anti-A, anti-B |
| A | + | – | anti-B |
| B | – | + | anti-A |
| AB | + | + | Neither |

– represents no reaction; + represents reaction.

polymorphisms are known to exist in the components of human blood, especially in the ABO and Rh antigens of red blood cells (Table 6–3). In particular, the ABO and Rh systems are important in blood transfusion, tissue and organ transplantation, and the treatment of hemolytic disease of the newborn.

### The ABO System

Landsteiner and colleagues found that human blood can be assigned to one of four types according to the presence of two antigens, A and B, on the surface of red blood cells, and the presence of the two corresponding antibodies, anti-A and anti-B, in the plasma.

There are four major phenotypes: O, A, B, and AB. Type A persons have antigen A on their red blood cells, type B persons have antigen B, type AB persons have both antigens A and B, and type O persons have neither. One feature of the ABO groups not shared by other blood group systems is the reciprocal relationship, in an individual, between the antigens present on the red blood cells and the antibodies in the serum. When the red blood cells lack antigen A, the serum contains anti-A; when the cells lack antigen B, the serum contains anti-B. The reason for this reciprocal relationship is uncertain, but formation of anti-A and anti-B is believed to be a response to the natural occurrence of A-like and B-like antigens in the environment (for example, in bacteria). The reaction of the red blood cells of each type with anti-A and anti-B antisera is shown in Table 6–3.

#### Molecular Genetic Basis of the ABO System

The ABO blood groups are determined by a locus on chromosome 9. The *A*, *B*, and *O* alleles at this locus are a classic example of multiallelism in which three alleles, two of which (*A* and *B*) are codominant and the third (*O*) is recessive, determine four phenotypes. The A and B antigens are made by the action of the *A* and *B* alleles on a red-blood-cell surface protein called H antigen. The *B* allele codes for a glycosyltransferase that preferentially recognizes the sugar D-galactose and adds it to the H protein. The *A* allele codes for a slightly different form of the enzyme that preferentially recognizes *N*-acetylgalactosamine instead of D-galactose and adds *N*-acetylgalactosamine to the precursor, thereby creating the A antigen. A third allele, *O*, codes for a mutant version of the transferase that lacks transferase activity and does not detectably affect H substance at all. The antigenic specificity is therefore conferred by which specific terminal sugars, if any, are added.

The molecular differences in the glycosyltransferase gene that are responsible for the *A*, *B*, and *O* alleles have been determined. Four nucleotide sequence differences are found between the *A* and *B* alleles that result in amino acid changes that alter the specificity of the glycosyltransferase encoded by the *ABO* gene. The *O* allele has a single base-pair deletion in the *ABO* gene coding region, which causes a frameshift mutation that eliminates the transferase activity in type O individuals. Now that the DNA sequences are available, ABO blood group typing is being performed directly at the genotype, rather than phenotype, level, especially when there are technical difficulties in serological analysis, as is often the case in forensic investigations or paternity testing.

The primary medical importance of the ABO blood group is in blood transfusion and tissue or organ transplantation. In the ABO blood group system, there are compatible and incompatible combinations. A compatible combination is one in which the red blood cells of a donor do not carry an A or a B antigen that corresponds to the antibodies in the recipient's serum. Although theoretically there are universal donors (group O) and universal recipients (group AB), a patient is given blood of his or her own ABO group, except in emergencies. The regular presence of anti-A and anti-B explains the failure of many of the early attempts to transfuse blood, because these antibodies can cause immediate destruction of ABO-incompatible cells. In tissue and organ transplantation, ABO compatibility of donor and recipient, as well as human leukocyte antigen (HLA) compatibility (described in Chapter 14), is essential to graft survival.

### The Rh System

The Rh system ranks with the ABO system in clinical importance because of its role in hemolytic disease of the newborn and in transfusion incompatibilities. The name Rh comes from Rhesus monkeys that were used in the experiments that led to the discovery of the system. In simplest terms, the population is separated into Rh-positive individuals, who express, on their red blood cells, the antigen Rh-D, a polypeptide encoded by a gene on chromosome 1, and Rh-negative individuals who do not express this antigen. The Rh-negative phenotype usually originates from homozygosity for a nonfunctional allele of the *Rh-D* gene itself. The frequency of Rh-negative individuals varies enormously in different ethnic groups. For example 17 percent of English people are Rh-negative whereas the frequency among Japanese is 0.5 percent.

**Hemolytic Disease of the Newborn.** Clinically, the chief significance of the Rh system is that Rh-negative persons can readily form anti-Rh antibodies after exposure to Rh-positive red blood cells. This is especially a problem when an Rh-negative pregnant woman is carrying an Rh-positive fetus. Normally during pregnancy, small amounts of fetal blood cross the placental barrier and reach the maternal blood stream. If the mother is Rh-negative and the fetus Rh-positive, the mother will form antibodies that return to the fetal circulation and damage the fetal red blood cells, causing hemolytic disease of the newborn with consequences that can be severe if not treated.

The discovery of the Rh system and its role in hemolytic disease of the newborn has been a major contribution of genetics to medicine. At one time ranking as the most common human genetic disease, hemolytic disease of the newborn is now relatively rare because of preventive measures that have become routine practice in obstetrical medicine. When Rh-negative girls or women of child-bearing age require transfusions, they must be given only Rh-negative blood. In pregnant Rh-negative women, the risk of immunization by Rh-positive fetal red blood cells can be minimized with injections of Rh immune globulin during and after pregnancy or after termination of pregnancy, to clear any Rh-positive cells from the mother's circulation before she mounts an immune response.

Most cases of hemolytic disease of the newborn recognized clinically are due to Rh incompatibility, but ABO incompatibility may also occur, and, although difficult to diagnose, it tends to be mild and to require no treatment.

## Serum Protein Polymorphism: Alpha$_1$-Antitrypsin Deficiency

$\alpha_1$-AT is a major serum protein that inhibits the activity of a number of specific proteolytic enzymes, such as trypsin, chymotrypsin, and pancreatic elastase. Its major target is leukocyte elastase, an enzyme that, if not inactivated by $\alpha_1$-AT, destroys lung connective tissue proteins (particularly elastin) leading to alveolar wall damage. Deficiency of $\alpha_1$-AT causes a very severe, early onset emphysema. The gene for $\alpha_1$-AT is on chromosome 14 and is highly polymorphic: there are several relatively common alleles with frequencies of 10 to 75 percent in different populations, and 25 or so rare alleles (Table 6–4). Each of the three most common alleles (*M1*, *M2*, and *M3*) encodes a structurally different version of a functionally normal protein, as do at least some of the rare alleles. Some alleles cause disease because they encode $\alpha_1$-AT molecules with clinically significantly reduced protease inhibitor activity; others do so because their secretion from the liver is impaired and abnormal $\alpha_1$-AT accumulates in the hepatocytes.

The principal medical significance of $\alpha_1$-AT polymorphisms lies in alleles whose products lead to deficiency of serum $\alpha_1$-AT activity. The most common and important of these is the *Z* allele, which has a frequency of 1 to 2 percent in Caucasian populations. Persons with the *Z/Z* genotype have less than 15 percent of the normal plasma concentration of $\alpha_1$-AT and have a high risk of obstructive lung disease in early adult life, as discussed in detail in Chapter 12. $\alpha_1$-AT deficiency is seen at a frequency of 1/2000 to 1/8000 in Caucasian populations but only rarely in African-American or Asian populations.

Genetic polymorphism at the $\alpha_1$-AT locus leads to a several-fold variation in $\alpha_1$-AT activity among apparently "normal" persons. Some of this variation may be highly significant from a public health standpoint because there is a suggestion of predisposition to a number of disorders, such as lung disease

TABLE 6–4
**Selected Alleles at the Alpha$_1$-Antitrypsin Locus in Different Populations**

| Population | Allele Frequencies | | | | | |
|---|---|---|---|---|---|---|
| | *M1* | *M2* | *M3* | *S* | *Z* | Other |
| U.S., Caucasian | .724 | .137 | .095 | .023 | .014 | .007 |
| U.S., African American | .981 | – | – | .015 | .004 | – |
| Denmark | .728 | .136 | .082 | .022 | .023 | .009 |
| Portugal | .510 | .260 | .053 | .150 | .009 | .018 |
| China (average of 5 populations) | .709 | .209 | .070 | – | – | .012 |
| Japan | .785 | .153 | .062 | – | – | – |

Based on data summarized by Cox DW (2000) $\alpha_1$-Antitrypsin deficiency. *In* Scriver CR, Beaudet AL, Sly WS, Valle D (eds) The Metabolic and Molecular Bases of Inherited Disease, 8th ed. McGraw-Hill, New York.

(particularly in smokers), asthma, and rheumatoid arthritis (as well as other immune disorders) among persons heterozygous for either the *Z* or the *S* allele (estimated at approximately 3 to 5 percent of Caucasian populations).

## INHERITED VARIATION AND POLYMORPHISM IN DNA

The previous sections have concentrated on mutations and polymorphism in portions of the genome encoding proteins, an estimated 5 percent of the total genomic DNA. What about genetic diversity in the remaining 95 percent of the human genome? From a number of large surveys in which the same fragments of DNA were sequenced from many individuals, as mentioned earlier, the total proportion of polymorphic base positions has been estimated to be about 1 in 1000 base pairs for any randomly chosen piece of DNA in the genome. This figure is about 2.5 times higher than the proportion of heterozygous nucleotides estimated for protein-coding regions of the genome (about 1 in 2500 base pairs). The difference is not altogether surprising, because it seems intuitively likely that protein-coding regions are under more rigid selective pressure, and thus the incidence of mutations in those regions throughout evolution should be lower.

### Restriction Fragment Length Polymorphisms

Restriction enzymes have specific recognition sequences in DNA (see Chapter 4), and, consequently, sequence changes in genomic DNA lead to the creation or abolition of particular cleavage sites, thereby altering the size of one or more DNA fragments apparent after Southern blotting and hybridization to a cloned DNA probe (Fig. 6–3). Soon after the application of Southern blotting to genome analysis in the late 1970s, it was discovered that not all persons have exactly the same distribution of restriction enzyme sites. Although the existence of some nucleotide variation could be predicted by what was known about mutation and protein polymorphisms, the degree of variation as detected by Southern blotting came as a surprise.

DNA-based variations at restriction sites detected by Southern blotting are called **restriction fragment length polymorphisms (RFLPs)**. The different fragment lengths constitute codominant alleles at a DNA locus (see Fig. 6–3). Thus, one can easily examine a Southern blot and read off the different fragment lengths directly as a reflection of the genotype (the DNA sequence) at a particular restriction site (Fig. 6–4). RFLPs may also arise from deletion or insertion of DNA rather than from single nucleotide changes. If a segment of DNA between two restriction sites is deleted or inserted, the size of the resulting restriction fragment is different (see Fig. 6–3).

RFLPs due to changes in particular restriction endonuclease cleavage sites are a small subset of a more general class of polymorphisms known as **single nucleotide polymorphisms (SNPs)**. Modern methods of DNA sequence detection allow the detection of any SNP, not just ones that alter a restriction enzyme site. SNPs are several orders of magnitude more frequent than are VNTRs or microsatellite polymorphisms (see later) and are uniformly distributed throughout the genome; these characteristics make them excellent markers for generating very dense genetic maps (see Chapter 8), such as those needed for evaluating the potential contribution of a particular gene to a complex genetic disorder (see Chapter 15). RFLPs (and SNPs more generally) usually have only two alleles corresponding to the two different bases occupying a particular position.

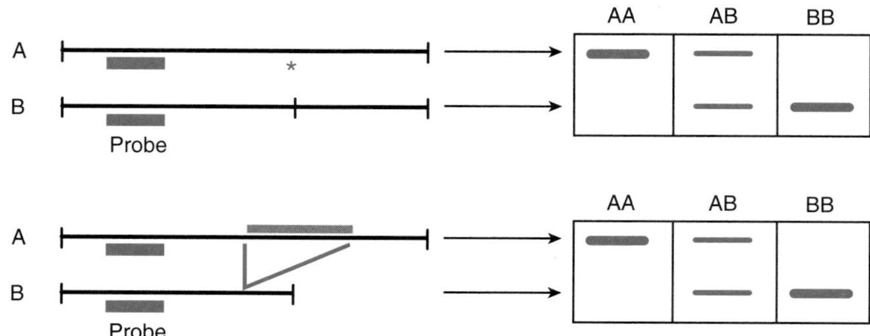


Figure 6–3. Restriction fragment length polymorphisms (RFLPs) detected by DNA hybridization (Southern blotting). At the top, polymorphism is due to variation at a specific cleavage site for a restriction enzyme; in the *A* allele, the site is absent (*asterisk*), and the resulting restriction fragment detected by the probe is larger than in the *B* allele. At the bottom, polymorphism is due to insertion (allele *A*) or deletion (allele *B*) of a DNA segment (*gray bar*) within a particular restriction fragment detected by the probe. For both types of polymorphism, Southern blotting patterns observed in DNA from persons with the three possible genotypes at this locus are indicated.

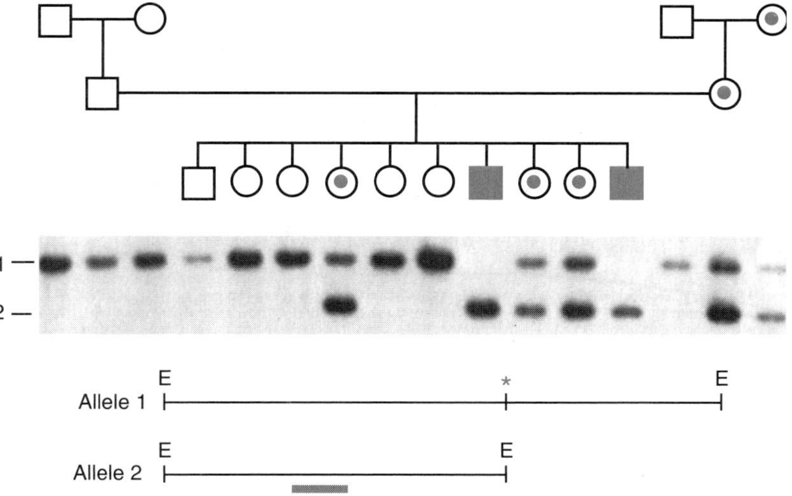


**Figure 6–4.** Codominant inheritance of an X-linked restriction fragment length polymorphism (RFLP). Alleles 1 and 2 differ by variation at a recognition site for the restriction enzyme *Eco*RI (E). Red symbols indicate inheritance of allele 2.

The discovery of SNPs has greatly increased the extent to which individual copies of particular genes are recognized as being truly unique. Conceptually, however, DNA polymorphisms are nothing new; they are simply the molecular manifestation of variation in the genome that has long been apparent from the study of protein polymorphisms.

As an illustration, consider again variation at the $\alpha_1$-*AT* locus. As discussed earlier and presented in Table 6–4, extensive polymorphism has been documented at the protein level in population studies and in studies of patients with inherited $\alpha_1$-AT deficiency. A similar degree of sequence variation is indicated from analysis of DNA at the $\alpha_1$-*AT* locus. Figure 6–5 depicts the structure of the $\alpha_1$-*AT* gene, including the positions and frequencies of some of the most common sites of DNA variation: SNPs (identified originally as RFLPs), a microsatellite polymorphic locus in 5′ flanking DNA, two normal variants in the coding region of the gene, and two pathological mutations. It is worth noting in Figure 6–5 that single base mutations responsible for the SNPs located in the introns or flanking DNA are conceptually identical to the changes responsible for the normal *M2* and *M3* alleles as well as the pathological *Z* and *S* alleles seen in patients with $\alpha_1$-AT deficiency. The only differences among the various types of polymorphism lie in their allelic frequencies, their location within the gene, and their pathological consequences, if any.

## Minisatellite and Microsatellite Polymorphisms

### VNTR Polymorphisms

Some RFLPs are based on the insertion or deletion of a varying amount of DNA rather than on the loss or gain of a restriction endonuclease recognition site.

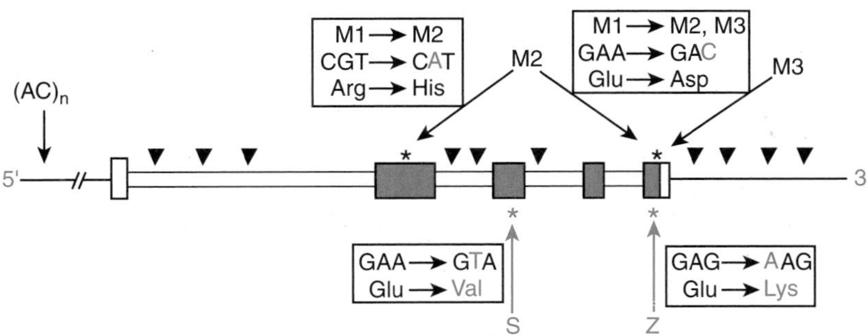


**Figure 6–5.** Schematic of the $\alpha_1$-*AT* gene and the location of DNA polymorphic sites, normal protein variants, and two disease mutations in and around the gene. Exons are boxed; coding exons in red. The black triangles indicate sites of single nucleotide polymorphisms, each consisting of two alleles, located in noncoding portions of the gene. Black asterisks above the gene indicate the sites of mutations in exons resulting in the *M2* and *M3* alleles, whereas red asterisks below the gene are mutations in exons resulting in the *S* and *Z* alleles, respectively. The actual DNA mutations and amino acid substitutions in the *M2*, *M3*, *S*, and *Z* alleles are indicated. Note that the *M2* allele has a mutation in common with the *M3* allele in exon 5 as well as one in exon 2. The position of a highly polymorphic microsatellite $(AC)_n$ locus with 18 different alleles is shown in the 5′ flanking region.

For example, one special class of polymorphisms results from the insertion, in tandem, of multiple copies of a DNA sequence 10 to 100 base pairs in length, known as a **minisatellite**, in the DNA between two restriction sites. This class of RFLP, known as a **variable number of tandem repeat (VNTR)** polymorphism, is characterized by many alleles (Fig. 6–6), because the size of a restriction fragment containing minisatellite sequences differs depending on how many copies of the minisatellite are present. The most informative markers have several dozen or more alleles, and so no two unrelated individuals are likely to share the same alleles.

The minisatellite repeat sequences found in many different VNTR-type polymorphisms are often sufficiently similar to make possible the detection of many different loci simultaneously using one minisatellite fragment as probe in a single Southern blot hybridization. Only identical twins show an indistinguishable pattern (Fig. 6–7), and, therefore, the simultaneous detection of a number of VNTR polymorphisms has been referred to as **DNA fingerprinting**. VNTR markers have been largely superseded by microsatellite markers (see later) for genetic linkage analyses (see Chapter 8) but are still widely used for individual identification, as in comparing the DNA of a suspect with that of the perpetrator of a crime, identifying the remains of crime victims and military personnel, and testing for paternity.

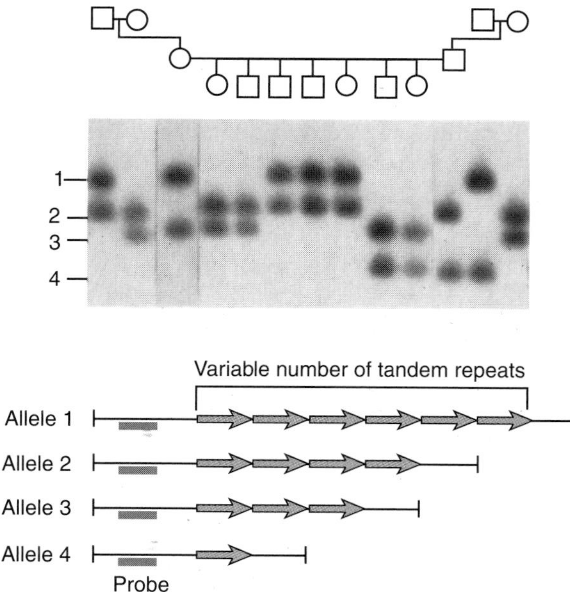


**Figure 6–6.** Codominant inheritance of a hypervariable autosomal DNA polymorphism caused by a variable number of tandem repeats (VNTR). Alleles 1 to 4 are related to one other by a variable number of identical (or nearly so), short DNA sequences (*arrows*). Size variation can be detected after restriction enzyme digestion and hybridization with a unique probe that lies outside the VNTR sequences themselves but inside the restriction sites used to define the allelic fragments. (Original photograph courtesy of A. Bowcock, Washington University, St. Louis.)

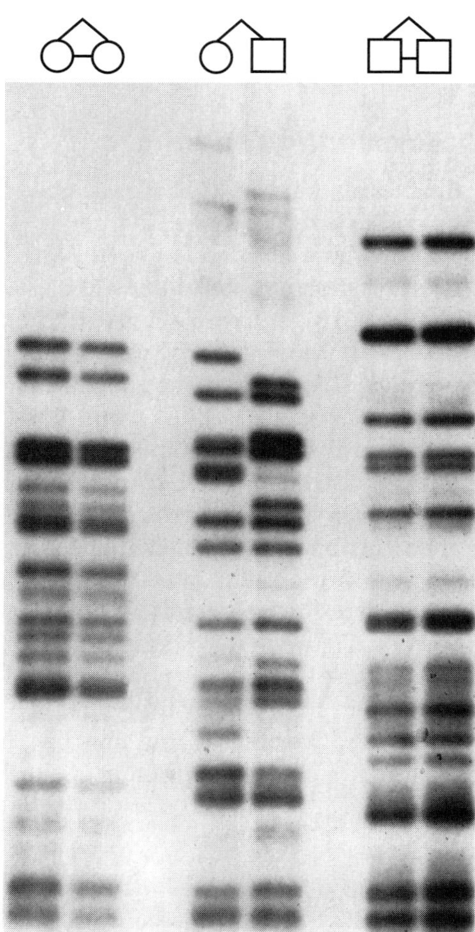

**Figure 6–7.** DNA fingerprinting of twins by means of a probe that detects variable number of tandem repeat (VNTR) polymorphisms at many loci around the genome. Each pair of lanes contains DNA from a set of twins. The twins of the first set (as well as the twins of the third set) have identical DNA fingerprints, indicating that they are identical (monozygotic) twins. The set in the middle have clearly distinguishable DNA fingerprints, indicating that they are fraternal twins. (Southern blot provided courtesy of Alec Jeffreys, University of Leicester, United Kingdom.)

## MICROSATELLITE MARKERS

Even more frequent and polymorphic than the VNTR minisatellite loci are the **microsatellite** loci. Microsatellites are stretches of DNA consisting of repeating units of two, three or four nucleotides, such as TGTG····TG, CAACAA····CAA, or AAATAAAT········AAAT. The number of repeated nucleotide units contained within any one microsatellite may differ between the two homologous chromosomes in an individual and among individuals in the population; a particular microsatellite is therefore a polymorphic locus, and the different numbers of repeat units in a particular microsatellite constitute the alleles at that locus. Three characteristics of microsatellite markers make them very useful for genetic linkage studies (see Chapter 8). First, a microsatellite locus often has many alleles (repeat

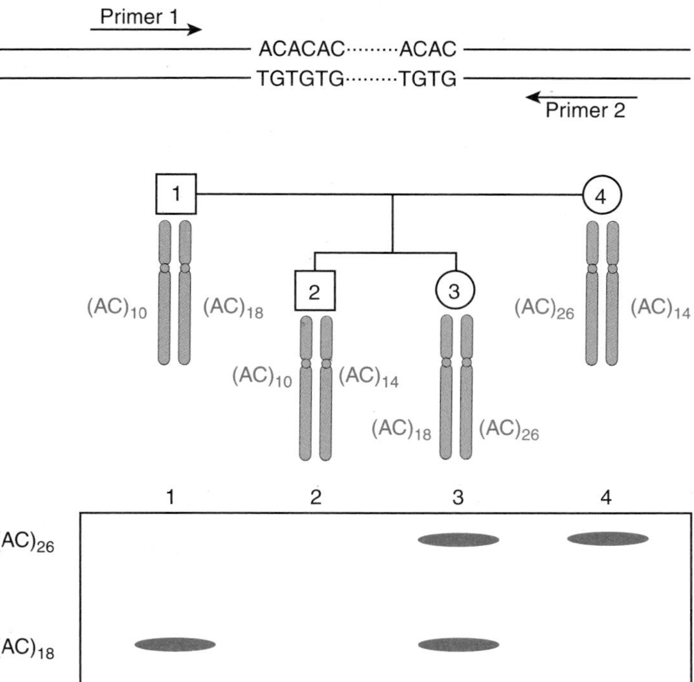


**Figure 6–8.** Microstatellite markers in human DNA. At top is the DNA containing an $(AC)_n$ microsatellite marker on one chromosome; primers 1 and 2 are polymerase chain reaction (PCR) primers complementary to unique sequences that flank the dinucleotide repeat. Below is a pedigree demonstrating codominant inheritance of a microsatellite polymorphism due to variable numbers of the dinucleotide AC. The genotype of each individual is shown below his or her symbol in the pedigree. The different-sized fragments are amplified using PCR and primers 1 and 2 flanking the stretch of AC dinucleotides, and their relative lengths determined by separating them using gel electrophoresis.

lengths) present in the population, making the probability that an individual will be heterozygous usually greater than 70 percent (see Chapter 8 for a discussion of the importance of being heterozygous for linkage studies). Second, unlike RFLP or VNTR analysis, genotyping microsatellite alleles does not require the use of cumbersome Southern blot techniques. PCR using primers complementary to unique DNA sequences flanking the microsatellite generates fragments that differ in length depending on how many repeats are present (Fig. 6–8). Finally, tens of thousands of microsatellite polymorphic loci have already been identified throughout the human genome, so that few if any regions of the genome cannot be mapped by genetic linkage methods using these markers.

## USES OF POLYMORPHISMS IN MEDICAL GENETICS

Polymorphisms are key elements in all human genetics research. The ability to distinguish different inherited forms of a gene or different segments of the genome provides tools that are crucial for a wide array of applications. We have witnessed an explosion in the number and utility of DNA polymorphisms. As illustrated in subsequent chapters, genetic markers are of enormous practical use in medical genetics for the following: mapping a gene to a particular region of a chromosome by linkage analysis (see Chapter 8); prenatal diagnosis of genetic disease (see Chapter 18); detection of heterozygous carriers of genetic disease (see Chapter 19); evaluation of high- and low-risk persons with a predisposition to common adult disorders, such as coronary heart disease, cancer, and diabetes (see Chapter 15); paternity testing and forensic applications in identifying remains of crime victims or matching a suspect's DNA to the perpetrator's; and tissue typing for organ transplantation.

## General References

Crow JF, Denniston C (1985) Mutation in human populations. Adv Hum Genet 14:59–124.

Harris H (1980) The Principles of Human Biochemical Genetics, 3rd ed. Elsevier-North Holland, Amsterdam.

Vogel F, Motulsky AG (1997) Human Genetics, 3rd ed. Springer-Verlag, Berlin.

## References Specific to Particular Topics

Antonarakis SE (1998) Recommendations for a nomenclature system for human gene mutations. Nomenclature Working Group. Hum Mutat 11:1–3.

Cox DW (2000) $\alpha_1$-Antitrypsin deficiency. *In* Scriver CR, Beaudet AL, Sly WS, Valle D (eds) The Metabolic and Molecular Bases of Inherited Disease, 8th ed. McGraw-Hill, New York.

Dunnen JT and Antonarakis SE (2000) Mutation nomenclature extensions and suggestions to describe complex mutations: A discussion. Hum Mutat 15:7–12.

Gardner RJ (1977) A new estimate of the achondroplasia mutation rate. Clin Genet 11:31–28.

Jeffreys AJ (1993) DNA typing: Approaches and applications. J Forensic Sci Soc 33:204–211.

Lowe JB (1994) Red cell membrane antigens. *In* Stamatoyannopoulos G, Nienhuis AW, Majerus PW, Varmus H (eds) Molecular Basis of Blood Diseases, 2nd ed. WB Saunders, Philadelphia, pp. 293–330.

Sheffield VC, Weber JL, Buetow KH, et al (1995) A collection of tri- and tetranucleotide repeat markers used to generate high quality, high resolution human genome-wide linkage maps. Hum Mol Genet 4:1837–1844.

Wang DG, Fan J, Siao C, et al (1998) Large-scale identification, mapping, and genotyping of single-nucleotide polymorphisms in the human genome. Science 280:1077–1082.

Weber JL (1990) Informativeness of human $(dC\text{-}dA)_n \cdot (dG\text{-}dT)_n$ polymorphisms. Genomics 7:524–530.

## URLs *for* Human Mutation Databases

Human Genome Organization (HUGO) database
*http://ariel.ucs.unimelb.edu.au:80/~cotton/mdi.htm*

Institute of Medical Genetics in Cardiff
*http://archive.uwcm.ac.uk/uwcm/mg/hgmd0.html*

Comprehensive databases of mutations in hundreds of different human disease genes. Both also include links to locus-specific and disease-specific mutation databases maintained by researchers around the world.

## *Problems*

1. Among 4.5 million births in one population during a period of 40 years, 41 children diagnosed with the autosomal dominant condition aniridia were born to normal parents. Assuming that these cases were due to new mutations, what is the estimated mutation rate at the aniridia locus? On what assumptions is this estimate based, and why might this estimate be either too high or too low?

2. The following patterns are observed for a DNA polymorphism after digestion of genomic DNA with a particular restriction enzyme; in males, a fragment at either 9 or 11 kb; in females, a fragment at 9 or 11 kb, or both.
   (a) What is the likely origin of these patterns?
   (b) What would you predict if the DNA samples were digested with a different restriction enzyme?

3. A VNTR-type DNA polymorphism detects five different alleles, each with a frequency of 0.20. What proportion of individuals would be expected to be heterozygous at this locus?

4. A woman who is Rh-negative marries a man who is Rh-positive. Are the children at risk for hemolytic disease of the newborn? If their children are at risk, is the risk for disease greater or less during the first pregnancy or subsequent pregnancies? Can the disease be prevented? What if the man were also Rh-negative?

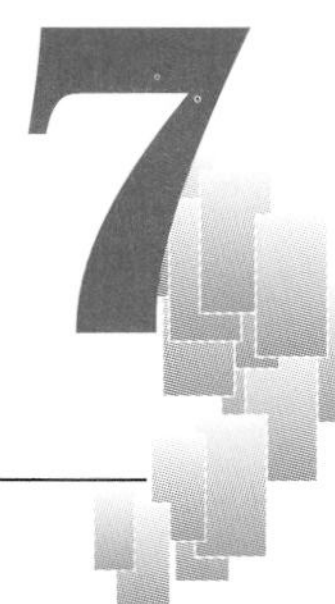

# Genetic Variation in Populations

In genetics more than in any other medical specialty, the patient is a reflection of the family and the population to which he or she belongs. Medical genetics is concerned not only with making the correct diagnosis in a particular case but with determining the genotypes of other family members and estimating recurrence risks both for the parents of an affected person and for his or her sibs, as well as for more distant relatives. Knowledge about the different disease genes that are common in different populations and about their role in health and disease can be a valuable asset in clinical diagnosis and in genetic counseling. Genetics is unique among the various disciplines in medicine because of its emphasis both on the individual patient and the family.

**Population genetics** is the study of the distribution of genes in populations and of how the frequencies of genes and genotypes are maintained or changed. Population genetics is concerned both with genetic factors, such as mutation and reproduction, and with environmental and societal factors, such as selection and migration, that in concert determine the frequency and distribution of genetic diseases in families and communities.

In this section, we describe the underlying principle of population genetics, Hardy-Weinberg equilibrium; we consider its assumptions and the factors that may cause true or apparent deviation from equilibrium in real as opposed to idealized populations; and we also consider how to determine the frequencies and mutation rates of specific genes of clinical importance, both autosomal and X-linked. Finally, the chapter provides some insight into how differences in disease gene frequencies arise among members of different, more or less genetically isolated groups.

## GENETIC DIVERSITY IN HUMAN POPULATIONS

The human species of close to 5 billion members is separated into many distinguishable subpopulations. Although the human chromosomes and the loci that they contain are identical throughout the species, the nature of different alleles and their frequencies at many loci vary widely among population groups. Some variants are virtually restricted to members of a single group, although they are not necessarily present in all members of the group. More often, variant alleles may be found in many population samples but have different frequencies in different populations.

Current anthropological studies suggest that human ancestors arose approximately 1.5 million years ago in Africa and then spread out over the rest of the world in successive, widening waves of migration. Small, scattered human settlements were geographically and thus genetically isolated from one another and developed into **ethnic groups**, with their own characteristic sets of gene frequencies. The selection of favorable mutations in response to environmental conditions or the chance survival of specific neutral or even harmful mutations, together with a degree of reproductive isolation among the groups, allowed genetic differences among population groups to become established. There are often dramatic differences in allele frequencies among population groups, both for alleles that cause genetic disease (Table 7–1) and for presumably selectively neutral genetic markers, such as certain blood group and protein polymorphisms and some DNA polymorphisms (Table 7–2). Although alleles that cause genetic disease are highly significant for determining disease risks in specific population groups, selectively neutral genetic markers are also important as markers of recent human evolution.

TABLE 7–1

**Selected Examples of Disease Alleles with Different Frequencies in Different Populations**

| Allele/Disease | Population Variation |
|---|---|
| $\beta^s$ allele of β-globin gene (sickle cell anemia) | Higher in Africa, less common elsewhere. Allele frequency 1/20 among African Americans; <1/200 among Hispanic Americans |
| $\beta^c$ allele of β-globin gene | High in West Africa (specifically Ghana and Burkina Faso) where allele frequency is 1/6. Allele frequency 1/100 among African Americans |
| Cystic fibrosis (all disease alleles) | High in European and U.S. Caucasian populations (allele frequency 1/40–1/50); low in Finnish, Asian, and African populations |
| Phenylketonuria (all disease alleles) | Higher among Europeans of Celtic and Northern European background (allele frequency 1/67–1/90). Allele frequency 1/125 in Switzerland and Italy, 1/223 among African Americans, 1/330 in Japan, 1/500 in Finland |
| Tay-Sachs disease | High frequency in Ashkenazi Jews (allele frequency 1/60); hundred-fold lower in other groups |
| Familial hypercholesterolemia | High in certain regions of Quebec (allele frequency 1/244) and in Afrikaners in South Africa (allele frequency 1/140). Allele frequency 1/1000 in Europe and United States |
| Myotonic dystrophy | Allele frequency 1/50,000 in Europe and nonexistent in sub-Saharan Africa. Allele frequency 1/950 in certain regions of Quebec |

## PHENOTYPES, GENOTYPES, AND GENE FREQUENCIES

### Deriving Allele Frequencies from Genotype Frequencies

If we could know the actual genotype at every pertinent locus in every individual in every family seeking genetic counseling, we could provide highly accurate determination of recurrence risks. Unfortunately, in many instances, the genotype responsible for the disease is unknown, and it is only the disease phenotype that one can observe and measure. Thus, there is a need to be able to use incidence figures for an inherited disease or other genetic trait to determine the frequency of particular genotypes and then to infer the frequencies of the particular alleles responsible for the different genotypes.

### The Genetics of Human Immunodeficiency Virus Resistance

An important example of a common autosomal trait governed by a single pair of alleles can be used to illustrate the basic principles that determine gene frequencies in populations. Consider the gene *CCR5*, which encodes a cell-surface cytokine receptor that serves as an entry point for certain strains of the human immunodeficiency virus (HIV) that causes the acquired immunodeficiency syndrome (AIDS). A 32 base-pair deletion in this gene results in an allele (*ΔCCR5*) that encodes a nonfunctional protein due to a frameshift and premature termination. Individuals homozygous for the *ΔCCR5* allele do not express the receptor on their cell surface and, as a consequence, are resistant to HIV infection. Loss of function of *CCR5* appears to be a benign trait, and its only known phenotypic consequence is resistance to HIV infec-

TABLE 7–2

**Examples of Polymorphic Loci with Different Allele Frequencies in Different Populations**

| Locus | Allelic Variation |
|---|---|
| ABO blood group system | Wide variation; e.g., *B* allele common in Asians but absent in Native American populations |
| Alpha$_1$-antitrypsin | Frequencies of three major *M* alleles vary between populations (e.g., *M1* from 0.51 to 0.98; *M2* from 0 to 0.26) |
| Alcohol dehydrogenase | Three loci: *ADH1*, *ADH2*, *ADH3*. Variant of *ADH2* much more common in Japanese (90%) than in Europeans (15%) |
| Aldehyde dehydrogenase | Deficiency of *ALDH1* in 50% of Asians, <5% of Native North Americans |
| HLA system | Numerous alleles at each locus making up the entire complex, with wide variation in frequency (see Chapter 14) |
| Debrisoquin metabolism (CYP2D6 4-hydroxylase) | Numerous alleles encoding enzymatic activities ranging from complete deficiency to extremely rapid metabolism. Deficiency due to homozygosity or compound heterozygosity for very slow metabolism alleles is seen in 30% of Hong Kong Chinese, 8% of European Caucasians, 1% of Arab populations |
| Lactase activity (lactose intolerance) | Two major alleles, for high and low activity. Low activity after early childhood common in Africans and Asians (allele frequency 0.8–0.95), less common in Northern Europeans and U.S. Caucasians (allele frequency 0.17–0.48) |

TABLE 7–3

**Genotype Frequencies for Normal CCR5 Allele and the Deletion ΔCCR5 Allele**

| Genotype | Number of People | Observed Relative Genotype Frequency | Allele | Derived Allele Frequencies |
|---|---|---|---|---|
| *CCR5/CCR5* | 647 | 0.821 | | |
| *CCR5/ΔCCR5* | 134 | 0.1682 | *CCR5* | 0.906 |
| *ΔCCR5/ΔCCR5* | 7 | 0.0108 | *ΔCCR5* | 0.094 |
| Total | 788 | 1.000 | | |

Data from Martinson JJ, Chapman NH, Rees DC, et al (1997) Global distribution of the *CCR5* gene 32 basepair deletion. Nat Genet 16:100–103.

tion. The normal allele and the 32 base-pair deletion allele, *ΔCCR5*, are easily distinguished by polymerase chain reaction analysis of the gene. A sampling of 788 individuals from Europe provides absolute numbers of individuals who were homozygous for either allele or heterozygous, as shown in Table 7–3.

On the basis of the observed genotype frequencies, we can directly determine the allele frequencies by simply counting the alleles. In this context, when we refer to the population frequency of an allele, we are considering a hypothetical **gene pool** as a collection of all the alleles at a particular locus for the entire population. For autosomal loci, the size of the gene pool at one locus is twice the number of individuals in the population because each autosomal genotype consists of two alleles, that is, *ΔCCR5/ΔCCR5* individual has two *ΔCCR5* alleles, and a *CCR5/ΔCCR5* individual has one of each. In this example, then, the observed frequency of the *CCR5* allele is

$$\frac{(2 \times 647) + (1 \times 134)}{788 \times 2} = 0.906$$

Similarly, one can calculate the frequency of the *ΔCCR5* allele as 0.094, either by adding up the number of *ΔCCR5* alleles directly ($(2 \times 7) + (1 \times 134) = 148$ of a total of 1576 alleles) or simply by subtracting the frequency of the normal *CCR5* allele, 0.906, from 1 (therefore, the frequency of *ΔCCR5* = $1 - 0.906 = 0.094$), because the frequencies of the two alleles must add up to 1.

## THE HARDY-WEINBERG LAW

As we have shown with the *CCR5* cytokine receptor gene example, we can use a sample of individuals in a population to derive estimates of the relative frequency of the two alleles in the population as a whole by simply counting the alleles in individuals with each genotype. How about the converse? Can we calculate the proportion of the population with various genotypes once we know the allele frequencies? Deriving genotype frequencies from allele frequencies is not as straightforward as counting because we actually do not know in advance how the alleles are distributed among homozygotes and heterozygotes. If a population meets certain assumptions, however, there is a simple mathematical relationship known as the **Hardy-Weinberg law** for calculating genotype frequencies from allele frequencies. This law, the cornerstone of population genetics, was named for Geoffrey Hardy, an English mathematician, and Wilhelm Weinberg, a German physician, who independently formulated it in 1908.

Suppose $p$ is the frequency of allele $A$ and $q$ is the frequency of allele $a$ in the gene pool and alleles combine into genotypes randomly; that is, mating in the population is completely at random with respect to the genotypes at this locus. The chance that two $A$ alleles will pair up to give the $AA$ genotype is $p^2$, the chance that two $a$ alleles will come together to give the $aa$ genotype is $q^2$, and the chance of having one $A$ and one $a$ pair, resulting in the $Aa$ genotype, is $2pq$ (the factor 2 comes from the fact that the $A$ allele could be inherited from the mother and the $a$ allele from the father, or vice versa). *The first important property of the Hardy-Weinberg law is that the frequency of the three genotypes AA, Aa, and aa are given by the terms of the binomial expansion of* $(p + q)^2 = p^2 + 2pq + q^2$.

A second and crucial implication of the Hardy-Weinberg law is that the proportions of the genotypes do not change from generation to generation; that is, the population genotype frequencies will remain constant, at equilibrium, if the allele frequencies $p$ and $q$ remain constant. More specifically, when there is random mating in a population in which the genotypes $AA$, $Aa$, and $aa$ are present in the proportions $p^2{:}2pq{:}q^2$, genotype frequencies in the next generation will remain in the same relative proportions, $p^2{:}2pq{:}q^2$. Proof of this equilibrium is shown in Table 7–4. It is important to note that Hardy-Weinberg equilibrium does not specify any particular values for $p$ and $q$: *whatever allele frequencies happen to be present in the population will result in genotype frequencies of* $p^2{:}2pq{:}q^2$, *and these relative genotype frequencies will remain constant from generation to generation as long as the allele frequencies remain constant.*

Applying the Hardy-Weinberg formula to the *CCR5* example given earlier, with relative frequencies of the two alleles in the gene pool of 0.906 (for the normal allele *CCR5*) and 0.094 (for *ΔCCR5*), then the Hardy-Weinberg law states that the relative

TABLE 7–4

**Frequencies of Mating Types and Offspring for a Population in Hardy-Weinberg Equilibrium with Parental Genotypes in the Proportion $p^2$:$2pq$:$q^2$**

| Mating Types | | | Offspring | | |
|---|---|---|---|---|---|
| *Mother* | *Father* | *Frequency* | *AA* | *Aa* | *aa* |
| *AA* | *AA* | $p^2 \times p^2 = p^4$ | $1(p^4)$ | | |
| *AA* | *Aa* | $p^2 \times 2pq = 2p^3q$ | $1/2\ (2p^3q)$ | $1/2\ (2p^3q)$ | |
| *Aa* | *AA* | $2pq \times p^2 = 2p^3q$ | $1/2\ (2p^3q)$ | $1/2\ (2p^3q)$ | |
| *AA* | *aa* | $p^2 \times q^2 = p^2q^2$ | | $1\ (p^2q^2)$ | |
| *aa* | *AA* | $p^2 \times q^2 = p^2q^2$ | | $1\ (p^2q^2)$ | |
| *Aa* | *Aa* | $2pq \times 2pq = 4p^2q^2$ | $1/4\ (4p^2q^2)$ | $1/2\ (4p^2q^2)$ | $1/4\ (4p^2q^2)$ |
| *Aa* | *aa* | $2pq \times q^2 = 2pq^3$ | | $1/2(2pq^3)$ | $1/2(2pq^3)$ |
| *aa* | *Aa* | $2pq \times q^2 = 2pq^3$ | | $1/2(2pq^3)$ | $1/2(2pq^3)$ |
| *aa* | *aa* | $q^2 \times q^2 = q^4$ | | | $1(q^4)$ |
| Genotypes resulting from all possible matings | | | $p^2$ | $2pq$ | $q^2$ |

Sum of *AA* offspring $= p^4 + 2p^3q + p^2q^2 = p^2(p^2 + 2pq + q^2) = p^2(p + q)^2 = p^2$. (Remember that $p + q = 1$)
Sum of *Aa* offspring $= 2p^3q + 4p^2q^2 + 2pq^3 = 2pq(p^2 + 2pq + q^2) = 2pq(p + q)^2 = 2pq$.
Sum of *aa* offspring $= p^2q^2 + 2pq^3 + q^4 = q^2(p^2 + 2pq + q^2) = q^2(p + q)^2 = q^2$.

proportions of the three combinations of alleles (genotypes) are $p^2 = 0.906 \times 0.906 = 0.821$ (for drawing two *CCR5* alleles from the pool), $q^2 = 0.094 \times 0.094 = 0.009$ (for two *ΔCCR5* alleles), and $2pq = (0.906 \times 0.094) + (0.094 \times 0.906) = 0.170$ (for one *CCR5* and one *ΔCCR5* allele). When these genotype frequencies, which were *calculated* using the Hardy-Weinberg law, are applied to a population of 788 individuals, the derived numbers of people with the three different genotypes (647:134:7) are, in fact, identical to the actual, *observed* numbers in Table 7–3.

As we have seen, Hardy-Weinberg distributions of genotypes in populations are simply a binomial distribution $(p + q)^n$ where symbols $p$ and $q$ represent the frequencies of two alternative alleles at a locus (where $p + q = 1$), and $n = 2$, representing the pair of alleles at any autosomal locus or any X-linked locus in females. (Because males are unique in having only a single X chromosome, frequencies of X-linked genes in males are considered separately later.) If a locus has three alleles, with frequencies $p$, $q$, and $r$, the genotypic distribution can be determined from $(p + q + r)^2$. In general terms, the genotypic frequencies for any known number of alleles $a_n$ with allele frequencies $p_1, p_2, \ldots p_n$ can be derived from the terms of the expansion of $(p_1 + p_2 + \ldots p_n)^2$.

### Use of the Hardy-Weinberg Law

The major, practical application of the Hardy-Weinberg law in medical genetics is in genetic counseling for autosomal recessive disorders. For a disease such as **phenylketonuria** (PKU) (see Chapter 12), the frequency of affected homozygotes in the population can be accurately determined because the disease is identified through newborn screening programs. Heterozygotes, however, are asymptomatic, silent carriers, and their population incidence is impossible to measure directly from phenotype. The Hardy-Weinberg law allows an estimate of heterozygote frequency to be made and used subsequently for counseling. For example, the frequency of PKU is approximately 1/4500 in Ireland. Because all affected individuals are homozygous for a mutant allele, $q^2 = 1/4500$ and therefore $q = \sqrt{1/4500} = 0.015$, and $2pq = 0.029$ or approximately 3 percent. The carrier frequency in the Irish population is therefore 3 percent, and there would be an approximately 3 percent chance that a parent known to be a carrier of PKU through the birth of an affected child would find that a new mate of Irish ethnicity would also be a carrier. If the new mate were from Finland, however, where the frequency of PKU is much lower (~1/200,000), his or her chance of being a carrier would be only 0.6 percent.

## FREQUENCY OF X-LINKED GENES AND GENOTYPES

Recall that for X-linked genes, there are only two possible male genotypes but three female genotypes. To illustrate gene frequencies and genotype frequencies when the gene of interest is X-linked, we use the trait known as red-green color blindness, which is caused by mutations in the series of red and green visual pigment genes on the X chromosome. We use color blindness as an example because, as far as we know, it is not a deleterious trait (except for possible difficulties with traffic lights), and color-blind persons are not subject to selection. As discussed later, allowing for the effect of selection complicates estimates of gene frequencies.

We use the symbol *cb* for the mutant color-blindness allele and the symbol + for the normal allele, with frequencies $q$ and $p$, respectively, as shown in Table 7–5. The frequencies of the normal and

TABLE 7–5

**X-Linked Genes and Genotype Frequencies (Color-Blindness)**

| Sex | Genotype | Phenotype | Incidence (Approximate) |
|---|---|---|---|
| Male | $X^+$ | Normal color vision | $p = 0.92$ |
| | $X^{cb}$ | Color blind | $q = 0.08$ |
| Female | $X^+/X^+$ | Normal (homozygote) | $p^2 = (0.92)^2 = 0.8464$ |
| | $X^+/X^{cb}$ | Normal (heterozygote) | $2pq = 2(0.92)(0.08) = 0.1472$ |
| | | Normal (total) | $p^2 + 2pq = 0.9936$ |
| | $X^{cb}/X^{cb}$ | Color blind | $q^2 = (0.08)^2 = 0.0064$ |

mutant alleles can be determined directly from the incidence of the corresponding phenotypes in *males* by simply counting the alleles. Because females have two X chromosomes, their genotypes are distributed binomially, exactly like autosomal genotypes, but because color-blindness alleles are recessive, the normal homozygotes and heterozygotes are not distinguishable. As shown in Table 7–5, the frequency of color blindness in females is much lower than that in males, even though the allele frequencies are, of course, the same in both sexes. Less than 1 percent of females are color blind, but nearly 15 percent are carriers of a mutant color-blindness allele and are therefore at risk of having color-blind sons.

## FACTORS THAT DISTURB HARDY-WEINBERG EQUILIBRIUM

Formulating the Hardy-Weinberg law requires several fundamental assumptions listed in Table 7–6. In the real world of medical genetics involving human populations and disease alleles, these assumptions often do not hold true, and the genotypes in a population may not be in Hardy-Weinberg equilibrium. As shown in the sections that follow, violating the assumption of random mating can cause large deviations from the frequency of disease based on allele frequencies. On the other hand, changes in allele frequency due to mutation, selection, or migration cause more minor and subtle deviations from Hardy-Weinberg equilibrium. If Hardy-Weinberg equilibrium does not hold at a particular locus, it is instructive to investigate *why* a particular disease allele and its associated genotypes are not in Hardy-Weinberg equilibrium in a given population. Which of the underlying assumptions are being violated, and what does this teach us about the population being studied, the mutation rate for this locus, and the effect of the disease allele on survival and reproduction?

TABLE 7–6

**The Hardy-Weinberg Law Rests on Several Assumptions**

1. The population is large, and matings are random with respect to the locus in question.
2. Allele frequencies remain constant over time because:
   (a) There is no appreciable rate of mutation.
   (b) Individuals with all genotypes are equally capable of mating and passing on their genes, i.e., there is no selection against any particular genotype.
   (c) There has been no significant immigration of individuals from a population with allele frequencies very different from the endogenous population.

### Exceptions to Random Mating

The principle of random mating is that, for any locus, an individual of a given genotype has a purely random probability of mating with an individual of any other genotype, the proportions being determined only by the relative frequencies of the different genotypes in the population. Simple observation, however, shows that a number of factors, some genetically significant and others probably genetically neutral, enter into one's choice of mate. These factors are **stratification**, **assortative mating**, and **consanguinity**.

#### STRATIFICATION

A stratified population is one that contains a number of subgroups that have remained, for the most part, genetically distinct during modern evolution. Worldwide, there are numerous stratified populations; for example, the U.S. population is stratified into two major subgroups, Caucasians and African Americans, as well as several other subgroups, including Native Americans, Asians, and Hispanics. Similarly, gene frequencies may vary significantly among countries across Europe or Asia. When mate selection in a population is restricted to members of one particular subgroup within that population, the result for any locus with more than one allele is an excess of homozygotes in the population as a whole and a corresponding deficiency of heterozygotes.

Suppose a population contains a minority group constituting 10 percent of the population in which a mutant allele for an autosomal recessive disease has a frequency $q_{min} = 0.05$. In the remaining majority 90 percent of the population, $q_{maj}$ is nearly 0. An example of just such a situation is the African-American population of the United States and the mutant allele at the β-globin locus responsible for sickle cell anemia. The overall frequency of the disease allele in the total population, $q_{pop}$, is therefore equal to 0.05/10 = 0.005, and, simply applying the Hardy-Weinberg law, the frequency of the disease in the population as a whole would be $q^2_{pop}$ = 0.000025 if mating were perfectly random throughout the entire population. In many instances, however, a minority group mates nearly exclusively with other members of the minority group. Then the frequency of affected individuals in the minority group would be ($q^2_{min}$) = 0.0025 and, because the minority group is one 10th of the entire population, the true frequency of disease in the total population is 0.0025/10 = 0.00025, 10-fold higher than one would expect from applying the Hardy-Weinberg law to the population as a whole without consideration of stratification. By way of comparison, stratification has no effect on the frequency of autosomal dominant disease and would have only a very minor effect on the frequency of X-linked disease by increasing the small number of females homozygous for the mutant allele.

Because subgroups are likely to have different frequencies of a number of autosomal recessive disease genes, their characteristic diseases are likely to differ. Well-known examples include Tay-Sachs disease in people of Ashkenazi Jewish ancestry, characteristic types of thalassemia in people of Mediterranean or East Asian descent, sickle cell anemia in African Americans, and cystic fibrosis and PKU in Caucasians (see Tables 7–1 and 7–7). Each subgroup seems to have its own profile of disorders that are more common and others that are less common than in the species as a whole.

### STRATIFICATION AFFECTS THE FREQUENCY OF SPECIFIC DISEASE ALLELES

Many genetic disorders are characterized by specific allelic mutations that vary in frequency among different population groups, probably because a small number of ancestral mutations became prevalent in particular populations and did not spread to the population as a whole because of stratification. The existence of population-specific mutant alleles has significance for understanding the origins of genetic disease and also provides opportunities for diagnosis of specific alleles in an at-risk population. For example, studies of β-thalassemia have led to the identification of specific molecular defects in the β-globin gene and recognition of their population distributions (see Chapter 11). Even though dozens of different alleles can cause β-thalassemia, certain alleles tend to be far more common in some populations than in others, so that each population has only a few common alleles (Table 7–8). For example, the most common β-thalassemia alleles responsible for more than 90 percent of the disease in Mediterranean people are very rare in people from Southeast Asia or the Asian subcontinent; the most common alleles in Southeast Asians and Asian Indians are similarly quite rare in the other two unrelated ethnic groups. This information is of great practical value in genetic counseling and prenatal diagnosis. For example, in North America, when persons of Mediterranean descent are at risk of having a child with β-thalassemia, testing of parental DNA for just seven mutant alleles has a more than 90 percent probability of providing the information needed for prenatal diagnosis. A

TABLE 7–7
**Incidence, Gene Frequency, and Heterozygote Frequency for Selected Autosomal Recessive Disorders in Different Populations**

| Disorder | Population | Incidence ($q^2$) | Gene Frequency ($q$) | Heterozygote Frequency ($2pq$) | Heterozygotes/Homozygotes ($2pq/q^2$) |
|---|---|---|---|---|---|
| Sickle cell anemia (*S/S* genotype) | African American | 1 in 400 | .05 | 1 in 11 | 38 |
| | Hispanic American | 1 in 40,000 | .005 | 1 in 101 | 396 |
| Alpha$_1$ antitrypsin deficiency (*Z/Z* genotype) | Denmark | 1 in 2000 | .023 | 1 in 22 | 90 |
| | U.S. African American | 1 in 100,000 | .004 | 1 in 125 | 800 |
| Cystic fibrosis | U.S. Caucasians | 1 in 2000 | .023 | 1 in 22 | 90 |
| Phenylketonuria | Scotland | 1 in 5300 | .014 | 1 in 30 | 175 |
| | Finland | 1 in 200,000 | .002 | 1 in 250 | 800 |
| | Japan | 1 in 109,000 | .003 | 1 in 166 | 657 |
| Tay-Sachs disease | U.S. Ashkenazic Jewish | 1 in 3900 | .016 | 1 in 30 | 130 |
| | U.S. non–Ashkenazic Caucasian | 1 in 112,000 | .003 | 1 in 170 | 660 |

Figures are approximate. Data are from Online Mendelian Inheritance in Man (< *http://www3.ncbi.nlm.nih.gov/Omim/*>) and Scriver CR, Beaudet AL, Sly WS, Valle D (eds) (2000) The Metabolic and Molecular Basis of Inherited Disease, 8th ed. McGraw-Hill, New York.

TABLE 7–8

**β-Thalassemia Alleles in Different Ethnic Groups**

| Population | Number of β-Thalassemia Alleles |
|---|---|
| Mediterranean | 15 (7 comprise 92% of the total) |
| Chinese/Southeast Asian | 9 (8 comprise 91% of total) |
| Asian Indian | 10 (5 comprise 90% of the total) |

similar increased frequency of certain mutant alleles has been observed in specific populations for many other genetic diseases (Table 7–9).

### Assortative Mating

Assortative mating is the choice of a mate because the mate possesses some particular trait. Assortative mating is usually positive; that is, people tend to choose mates who resemble themselves (e.g., in native language, intelligence, stature, skin color, musical talent, or athletic ability). Negative assortative mating, the selection of a mate with characteristics different from those of oneself, is less common. To the extent that the characteristic shared by the partners is genetically determined, the overall genetic effect of positive assortative mating is an increase in the proportion of the homozygous genotypes at the expense of the heterozygous genotype.

TABLE 7–9

**Ethnicity of Genetic Disease**

| | |
|---|---|
| $\alpha^0$-thalassemia | Different deletion mutations in the Mediterranean and Southeast Asia. |
| Gyrate atrophy | Single predominant mutation in the ornithine aminotransferase gene in Finland. Different mutations found in other populations. |
| Tay-Sachs disease | 4 base-pair insertion in exon 11 and a G-to-C substitution in the first nucleotide of intron 12 are the two common mutations in Ashkenazi Jews; a 7.6-kb deletion mutation at the 5′ end of the gene is the most common mutation in French Canadians. Other alleles are seen in other populations. |
| Hereditary breast cancer (*BRCA1* and *BRCA2*) | Mutational heterogeneity in most populations, but 2 base-pair deletion at position 185 and 1 base-pair insertion at position 5382 in *BRCA2* and a single base-pair deletion at 6174 in *BRCA1* constitute most of the mutant alleles in Ashkenazi Jews. |
| Familial hypercholesterolemia | Mutational heterogeneity in most populations, but French Canadians have a predominant mutation, a deletion of the promoter and exon 1; a premature termination codon at amino acid 660 is very frequent in Lebanese but infrequent elsewhere. |

A clinically important aspect of assortative mating is the tendency to choose partners with similar medical problems, such as congenital deafness or blindness or exceptionally short stature (dwarfism). In such a case, the expectations of Hardy-Weinberg equilibrium do not apply because the genotype of the mate at the disease locus is not determined by the allele frequencies found in the general population. For example, in the case of two parents with achondroplasia, a dominant disorder, offspring homozygous for the achondroplasia gene have a severe, lethal form of dwarfism that is almost never seen unless both parents are achondroplasia heterozygotes.

When mates have autosomal recessive disorders caused by the same mutation or by allelic mutations in the same gene, all of their offspring will also have the disease. Of course, not all blindness, deafness, or short stature has the same genetic basis; many families have been described, for example, in which two albino parents have had children with normal pigmentation or two deaf parents have had hearing children because of locus heterogeneity (discussed in Chapter 5). Even if there is genetic heterogeneity, however, with assortative mating, the chance that two individuals are carrying mutations in the same disease locus is increased over what it would be under true random mating, and, therefore, the risk of the disorder in their offspring is also increased. Although the long-term population effect of this kind of positive assortative mating on disease gene frequencies is insignificant, a specific family may find itself at very high genetic risk.

### Consanguinity

**Consanguineous mating** or **inbreeding**, like stratification and positive assortative mating, brings about an increase in the frequency of autosomal recessive disease by increasing the frequency with which carriers of an autosomal recessive disorder mate. Unlike the disorders in stratified populations, in which each subgroup is likely to have a high frequency of a few alleles, the kinds of recessive disorders seen in the offspring of related parents may be very rare and unusual because consanguineous mating allows uncommon alleles to become homozygous.

## Exceptions to Constant Allele Frequency

In contrast to nonrandom mating, which can substantially upset Hardy-Weinberg equilibrium, changes in allele frequency due to selection, mutation, or migration usually occur slowly, in small increments, and cause much less deviation from Hardy-Weinberg equilibrium. Mutation and migration both usually occur at rates that are well below the carrier frequency, and so they also have little effect in the short term on overall allele frequency. As we will see later, selection also has little effect on allele frequencies in autosomal recessive disease because the vast majority of mutant alleles are protected from negative selection in heterozygotes. For dominant or X-linked disease, however, and in the case when heterozygotes for recessive diseases have a selective advantage over homozygotes for the normal allele, selection can significantly perturb allele frequencies from what would be expected under Hardy-Weinberg equilibrium by substantially reducing or increasing certain genotypes.

## Mutation and Selection

The molecular basis for mutation was considered in detail in Chapter 6. In the present context, we introduce the concept of **fitness**, the chief factor that determines whether a mutation is lost immediately, becomes stable in the population, or even becomes, over time, the predominant allele at the locus concerned. The frequency of an allele in a population represents a balance between the rate at which mutant alleles appear through mutation and the effects of selection. If either the mutation rate or the effectiveness of selection is altered, the allele frequency is expected to change.

Whether an allele is transmitted to the succeeding generation depends on its fitness ($f$), which is a measure of the number of offspring of affected persons who survive to reproductive age, when compared with an appropriate control group. If a mutant allele is just as likely as the normal allele to be represented in the next generation, $f$ equals 1. If an allele causes death or sterility, selection acts against it completely, and $f$ equals 0. A related parameter is the **coefficient of selection,** $s$, which is a measure of the loss of fitness and is defined as $1 - f$. In the genetic sense, a mutation that prevents reproduction by an adult is just as lethal as one that causes a very early miscarriage of an embryo, because in neither case is the mutation transmitted to the next generation. Fitness is thus the outcome of the joint effects of survival and fertility. In the biological sense, fitness has no connotation of superior endowment except in a single respect: comparative ability to contribute to the gene pool of the next generation.

## Selection against Autosomal Dominant Mutations

Dominant mutant alleles are openly exposed to selection, in contrast to recessive mutant alleles, most of which are "hidden" in heterozygotes. Consequently, the effects of selection and mutation are more obvious and can be more readily measured for dominant traits. A genetic lethal dominant allele, if fully penetrant, is exposed to selection in heterozygotes, removing all alleles responsible for the disorder in a single generation. Several human diseases are thought or known to be autosomal dominant traits with zero or near-zero fitness and thus always result from new, rather than inherited, autosomal dominant mutations (Table 7–10). In some, the genes and specific mutant alleles are known, and family studies show new mutations in the affected individuals that were not inherited from the parents. In other conditions, the genes are not known, but paternal age effect (see Chapter 6) has been seen, suggesting (but not proving) a new mutation in the paternal germline as a possible cause of the disorder. The implication for genetic counseling is that the parents of a child with an autosomal dominant, genetic lethal condition have a low risk of recurrence because the condition would generally require another independent mutation to recur (except in the rare circumstances of germline mosaicism for the condition; see Chapter 5).

If a dominant disease is deleterious but not lethal, affected persons may reproduce but will nevertheless contribute fewer than the average number of offspring to the next generation; that is, their fitness, $f$, may be

TABLE 7–10

**Examples of Disorders Occurring as Sporadic Conditions Due to Autosomal Dominant Genes with Zero Fitness**

| Disorder | Description |
|---|---|
| Acrodysostosis | Multiple congenital abnormalities, especially short hands with peripheral dysostosis, small nose, mental deficiency. |
| Apert syndrome | Craniosynostosis, broad thumb and great toe, shallow orbits, hypertelorism, frequent but variable mental deficiency. Mutation in fibroblast growth factor receptor-2 gene. Very rarely, a person with this dysmorphic syndrome has offspring; if so, about 50% of the offspring are affected. |
| Atelosteogenesis | Early lethal form of short-limbed dwarfism. |
| Cornelia de Lange syndrome | Mental retardation, micromelia, synophrys, and other abnormalities. |
| Lenz-Majewski hyperostosis syndrome | Dense, thick bone; symphalangism; cutis laxa. |
| Osteogenesis imperfecta, type 2 | Perinatal lethal type, with a defect in type 1 collagen (see Chapter 12). |
| Thanatophoric dysplasia | Early lethal form of short-limbed dwarfism due to mutations in fibroblast growth factor receptor-3 gene. |

reduced. Such a mutation is lost through selection at a rate proportional to the loss of fitness of heterozygotes. For example, achondroplastic dwarfs have only about one fifth as many children as do people of normal stature in the population. Thus, their average fitness, *f*, is 0.20, and the coefficient of selection, *s*, is 0.80. In the subsequent generation, only 20 percent of current achondroplasia alleles are passed on from the current generation to the next. Because the frequency of achondroplasia is not decreasing, new mutations must be responsible for replacing the 80 percent of mutant genes in the population lost through selection.

### The Balance between Mutation and Selection in Dominant Diseases

The mutation rate of autosomal dominant disorders can be measured either directly or indirectly. As we saw in Chapter 6, direct measurement is accurate only when all cases of a disorder in the population are correctly diagnosed and ascertained and those patients with unaffected parents are identified. One can also measure the incidence of new mutation at a disease locus indirectly if an accurate measurement of fitness is available: the mutation rate per generation at a disease locus must be sufficient to account for the proportion of mutant alleles lost by selection from each generation. Thus, the mutation rate, $\mu$, must equal the coefficient of selection, *s*, times the allele frequency, *q*.

The observed allele frequency in any one generation represents a balance between loss of mutant alleles through the effects of selection and gain of mutant alleles through recurrent mutation. A stable allele frequency is reached at whatever level balances the two opposing forces: one (selection) that removes mutant alleles from the gene pool and one (new mutation) that adds new ones back. Thus, if the fitness of affected persons suddenly improved (because of medical advances, for example), the observed incidence of the disease in the population would increase and reach a new equilibrium. Retinoblastoma and certain other dominant embryonic tumors with childhood onset are examples of conditions that now have a greatly improved prognosis, with a predicted consequence of increased disease frequency in the population. On the other hand, if affected persons elected to have no children at all (thus effectively reducing the fitness of the mutant allele to zero), the disease incidence would immediately fall, not to zero, but to a level maintained by the introduction of new mutations to the gene pool in each generation. Allele frequency, mutation rate, and fitness are related; thus, if any two of these three characteristics are known, the third can be estimated.

### Selection against Autosomal Recessive Mutations

Selection against harmful recessive mutations has far less effect on the population frequency of the mutant allele than does selection against dominant mutations because, as discussed earlier, only a small proportion of the genes are present in homozygotes and are therefore exposed to selective forces. Even if there were complete selection against homozygotes ($f = 0$), as in many lethal autosomal recessive conditions, it would take many generations to reduce the gene frequency appreciably because most of the mutant alleles are carried by heterozygotes with normal fitness. For example, the frequency of mutant alleles causing PKU, *q*, is approximately 1 percent in many Caucasian populations. Two percent of the population ($2 \times p \times q$) is heterozygous, with one mutant allele, whereas only 1 individual in 10,000 ($q^2$) is a homozygote with two mutant alleles. The proportion of mutant alleles in homozygotes is given by

$$\frac{2/10000}{(2/10000) + (1/100)} = \sim 0.02$$

Thus, only approximately 2 percent of all the mutant alleles in the population are in affected homozygotes and therefore are exposed to selection if dietary treatment were not available. Removing selection against an autosomal recessive disorder such as PKU by successful medical treatment would have just as slow an effect on increasing the gene frequency over many generations. *Thus, as long as mating is random, genotypes in autosomal recessive diseases can be considered to be in Hardy-Weinberg equilibrium, despite selection against homozygotes for the recessive allele. The mathematical relationship between genotype and allele frequencies described in the Hardy-Weinberg law holds for most practical purposes in medical genetics.* Selected examples of the relationships among incidence, gene frequency, and carrier (heterozygote) frequency for autosomal recessive diseases in various ethnic groups are shown in Table 7–7.

### Selection against X-Linked Recessive Mutations

Almost all X-linked phenotypes of medical interest are recessive, and therefore, as a general rule, selection occurs in hemizygous males and not in heterozygous females, except for the small proportion of females who are manifesting heterozygotes with low fitness. In this brief discussion, however, we assume that heterozygous females have normal fitness.

If an X-linked phenotype is benign and if affected males have normal fitness, one third of the corresponding mutant alleles are in males and two thirds in females, as shown earlier in the discussion of color blindness. In clinically severe X-linked disorders such as Duchenne muscular dystrophy (DMD), in which affected males do not reproduce, only the genes present in carrier females are transmitted to the next generation (see Table 7-11). Thus, in diseases like DMD in which there is a selective disadvantage operating only against hemizygous males (and therefore only against one third of the mutant alleles), the mutation rate must equal the coefficient of selection, $s$, times $q/3$. When $s = 1$, such diseases are called X-linked **genetic lethals**, and one third of all copies of such a mutant gene are lost each generation. As we saw in the case of autosomal dominant mutations, mutant alleles lost through selection must be replaced by recurrent new mutations to maintain the observed disease incidence. Therefore, one third of all persons who have such X-linked lethal disorders are predicted to carry a new mutation, and their genetically normal mothers have very little risk of having subsequent children with the same disorder (barring mosaicism).

In less severe disorders such as hemophilia A, the proportion of affected individuals representing new mutations is less than one third (currently about 15 percent). Because the treatment of hemophilia is improving rapidly, the total frequency of mutant alleles can be expected to rise relatively rapidly and to reach a new equilibrium, as we saw in the case of autosomal dominant conditions. Assuming that the mutation rate at this locus stays the same, the *proportion* of hemophiliacs who result from a new mutation will decrease, even though the incidence of the disease increases. Such a change would have significant implications for genetic counseling for this disorder (see Chapter 19).

### Selection for Heterozygotes (Heterozygote Advantage)

The considerations in the preceding sections explain the present-day frequencies of rare mutant alleles as a balance between loss by selection and gain by new mutation. However, how then can we explain disorders in which the mutant allele achieves quite high frequencies despite reduced fitness in affected individuals who carry these alleles? For example, carrier frequencies in cystic fibrosis are 5 percent among Caucasians, whereas the carrier frequency of the sickle cell anemia mutation in African Americans is 9 to 10 percent. Given the substantial selection against homozygotes for these mutant alleles, the only two possible explanations are the following: (1) The mutant allele is at a higher than expected frequency because of a phenomenon known as **genetic drift**: the population, although reasonably large now, is, in fact, derived from a very small group of individuals in whom, by chance alone, the frequency of the disease allele started out quite high. The frequency of the mutant allele is actually not stably elevated, but sufficient time has not elapsed for selection in the homozygotes to lower the disease allele frequency. The role of genetic

TABLE 7-11

**Incidence and Heterozygote Prevalence for Selected X-Linked Disorders**

| Disorder | Population | Incidence Affected Males (Male Live Births) | Heterozygote Prevalence (In Female Population) | Comments |
|---|---|---|---|---|
| Duchenne muscular dystrophy | Europe, North America, Japan | 1/3650 | 1/2740 | Heterozygote prevalence calculated assuming fitness $f = 0$ and equal male and female mutation rates |
| Hemophilia A | United States | 1/5000 | 1/2500 | Heterozygote prevalence calculated assuming fitness $f = 0.7$ and male mutation rate >> female mutation rate (15:1) |
| Ornithine transcarbamylase deficiency | Japan | 1/80000 | 1/62500 | Heterozygote prevalence calculated assuming fitness $f = 0$ and equal male and female mutation rates |
| Fragile X syndrome | Australia, United States, Finland, Taiwan, Netherlands | 1–2/6000 | 1/3200 (with ~one-half affected)<br>1–2/500 premutation carriers | Heterozygote prevalence (full mutation carriers) is estimated.<br>Heterozygote prevalence (premutation carriers) is measured. |

Figures are approximate. Data are from On-line Mendelian Inheritance in Man (< *http://www3.ncbi.nlm.nih.gov/Omim/*); Scriver CR et al (1997) The Metabolic and Molecular Bases of Inherited Disease, CD-ROM; deVries BB et al (1997) Screening and diagnosis for the fragile X syndrome among the mentally retarded: An epidemiological and psychological survey. Am J Hum Genet 61:660–667; Morton JE et al (1997) Fragile X syndrome is less common than previously estimated. J Med Genet 34:1–5; Reiss AL et al (1994) Frequency and stability of the fragile X premutation. Hum Mol Genet 3:393–398; Rousseau F (1995) Prevalence of carriers of premutation-size alleles of the FMR1 gene—and impications for the population genetics of the fragile X syndrome. Am J Hum Genet 57:1006–1018; Ryynanen M et al (1999) Feasibility and acceptance of screening for fragile X mutations in low-risk pregnancies. Eur J Hum Genet 7:212–216; Turner G et al (1996) Prevalence of fragile X syndrome. Am J Med Genet 64:196–197; Tzeng CC et al (1999) Pilot fragile X screening in normal population of Taiwan. Diagn Mol Pathol 8:152–156.

drift is dealt with in the next section. (2) The frequency of the mutant allele is stably elevated at a higher than expected level that is maintained either by an extraordinarily high mutation rate or by increased fitness of heterozygous carriers over that of normal homozygotes in particular environments.

An elevated mutation rate could theoretically maintain the high frequency of a deleterious allele that is efficiently lost through selection in homozygous recessive persons. There is, however, no evidence of increased mutation rates in disorders such as sickle cell anemia or cystic fibrosis; instead, there are environmental situations in which heterozygotes for some diseases have increased fitness over both homozygous genotypes, a situation termed **heterozygote advantage**. Even a slight heterozygote advantage can lead to an increase in frequency of an allele that is severely detrimental in homozygotes, because heterozygotes greatly outnumber homozygotes in the population.

A well-known example of heterozygote advantage, although not the only one, is resistance to malaria in heterozygotes for the sickle cell anemia mutation. The sickle cell allele has reached its highest frequency in certain regions of West Africa, where heterozygotes are more fit than either type of homozygote because heterozygotes are resistant to the malarial organism. In regions where malaria is endemic, normal homozygotes are susceptible to malaria; many become infected and are severely, even fatally, affected, leading to very reduced fitness. Sickle cell homozygotes are even more seriously disadvantaged, with a fitness approaching zero, because of their severe hematological disease (see Chapter 11). Heterozygotes for sickle cell anemia have red cells that are inhospitable to the malaria organism but do not undergo sickling under normal environmental conditions; the heterozygotes are relatively more fit than either homozygote and reproduce at a higher rate. Thus, over time, the sickle cell mutant allele has reached a frequency as high as 0.15 in some areas of West Africa that are endemic for malaria, far higher than could be accounted for by recurrent mutation.

The heterozygote advantage in sickle cell disease demonstrates how violating one of the fundamental assumptions of Hardy-Weinberg equilibrium—that allele frequencies are not significantly altered by selection—causes the mathematical relationship between allele and genotype frequencies to diverge from what is expected under the Hardy-Weinberg law. Consider two alleles, the normal *A* allele and the mutant *S* allele, which give rise to three genotypes: *A/A* (normal), *A/S* (heterozygous carriers), and *S/S* (sickle cell disease). In a sample of 12,387 individuals from an adult West African population, the three genotypes were detected in the following proportions: 9365 *A/A*:2993 *A/S*:29 *S/S*. By counting the *A* and *S* alleles in these three genotypes, one can determine the allele frequencies to be $p = 0.877$ for the *A* allele and $q = 0.123$ for the *S* allele. Under Hardy-Weinberg equilibrium, the ratio of genotypes should be $A/A:A/S:S/S = p^2:2pq:q^2 =$ 9527:2672:188. The observed ratios, however, $A/A:A/S:S/S =$ 9365:2993:29, differ significantly from expectations. The example of the sickle cell allele illustrates how the forces of selection, operating not only on the relatively rare *S/S* genotype but also on the other two, much more frequent, *A/A* and *A/S* genotypes, distorts the transmission of the *A* and *S* alleles and causes a deviation from Hardy-Weinberg equilibrium in a population.

A situation in which selective forces operate both to maintain a deleterious allele and to remove it from the gene pool is described as a **balanced polymorphism**. Change in the selective pressures would be expected to lead to a rapid change in the relative frequency of the allele. Today, many sickle cell heterozygotes live in nonmalarial regions, and even in malarial areas, major efforts are being made to eradicate the mosquito responsible for transmitting the disease. There is evidence that, in the African-American population in the United States, the frequency of the sickle cell gene may already be falling from its high level in the original immigrant African population of several generations ago, although other factors, such as the introduction of genes from non-African populations into the African-American gene pool, may also be playing a role.

Some other deleterious alleles, including genes for hemoglobin C, the thalassemias, and glucose-6-phosphate dehydrogenase deficiency (see Chapter 12), as well as the benign *FY* allele of the Duffy blood group system, are also thought to be maintained at their present high frequencies in certain populations because of the protection that they provide against malaria.

Heterozygote advantage has also been proposed to explain the high frequencies of cystic fibrosis in Caucasians and of Tay-Sachs disease and other disorders affecting sphingolipid metabolism in the Ashkenazi Jewish population. However, genetic drift (discussed later), is another powerful mechanism for the alteration of gene frequencies and may adequately account for the unusually high frequencies that some deleterious genes achieve in some environments. For cystic fibrosis and Tay-Sachs disease, the question remains unresolved.

## Genetic Drift

Another cause of high frequencies for deleterious disease alleles in a population is a phenomenon known as **genetic drift**, the fluctuation in allele frequency due to chance operating on the small gene pool contained within a small population. For example, when a new mutation occurs, its frequency is represented by only one copy among all the copies of that gene in the population. If the population is small, random factors, such as increased fertility or survival, or both, of the carrier of the mutation, *occurring for reasons unrelated to his carrying the mutant allele*, may cause the allele frequency to rise for reasons that have nothing to do with the mutation itself. In a large population, such random effects would tend to average out but, in a small population, allele frequencies may fluctuate from generation to generation by chance. Similarly, when a small subpopulation breaks off from a larger population, the gene frequencies in the small population may be rather different from those of the population from which it originated because the new group contains a small, random sample of the parent group and, by chance, may not have the same gene frequencies as the parent group. Over the next few generations, although the population size of the new group remains small, there may be considerable fluctuation in gene frequency. These changes are likely to smooth out as the population increases in size.

One form of genetic drift is the **founder effect**: if one of the original founders of a new group just happens to carry a relatively rare allele, that allele will have a far higher frequency than it had in the larger group from which the new group was derived. One example is the high incidence of Huntington disease in the region of Lake Maracaibo, Venezuela (see Chapter 12), but there are numerous other examples of founder effect involving other disease alleles in genetic isolates throughout the world.

The founder effect is well illustrated by the Old Order Amish, a religious isolate of European descent that settled in Pennsylvania and gave rise to a number of small, genetically isolated subpopulations throughout the United States and Canada. The Old Order Amish tend to have large families and a high frequency of consanguineous marriage. The incidence of specific rare autosomal recessive syndromes such as **Ellis–van Creveld syndrome** (Fig. 7–1) in some Amish communities, but not in others, is an illustration of the founder effect.

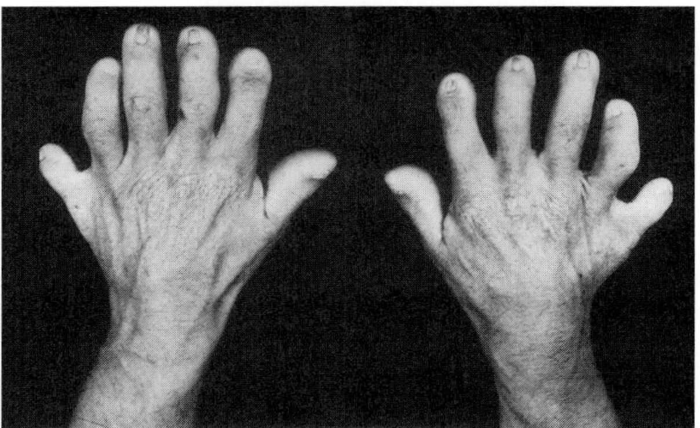

Figure 7–1. The hands of a patient with Ellis–van Creveld syndrome, a very rare disorder seen with increased frequency in some Amish groups. (Photograph courtesy of David Rimoin, Cedars-Sinai Medical Center, Los Angeles.)

Another striking example of founder effect is provided by the Afrikaner population of South Africa. The population was established by 20 original couples, mainly from the Netherlands, over a few decades beginning in 1652, and it underwent explosive growth in its early years. Today, nearly 1 million of the 2,500,000 living Afrikaners bear the names of only 20 original settlers. One early settler brought the gene for **variegate porphyria** (VP), an autosomal dominant disorder of relatively late onset. VP results from deficiency of the enzyme protoporphyrinogen oxidase, which is in the heme synthesis pathway. Heterozygotes develop photosensitivity and neurovisceral symptoms, induced by barbiturates and other factors. Homozygotes have a more severe disorder, with earlier onset and retardation of growth and mental development. Today the incidence of VP in South Africa is approximately 1/333; the incidence of VP in the Netherlands is unknown, but it has been determined to be approximately 1/100,000 in Finland.

The French-Canadian population of Canada also has high frequencies of certain disorders that are rare elsewhere. One disease characteristic of the relatively isolated Lac Saint Jean region of Quebec is hereditary **type I tyrosinemia**; this autosomal recessive condition causes hepatic failure and renal tubular dysfunction due to deficiency of fumarylacetoacetase, an enzyme in the degradative pathway of tyrosine. The disease has an overall frequency of about 1/100,000 in other parts of Quebec and in Norway and Sweden, but its frequency is 1/685 in Lac Saint Jean, where the founder effect has been demonstrated.

The population of Finland, long isolated genetically by geography, language, and culture, has expanded in the past 300 years from 400,000 to about 5 million. The isolation and population expansion have allowed the Finnish population to develop a distinctive pattern of single-gene disorders. There is a high frequency of at least 20 diseases that are rare elsewhere. For example, **choroideremia**, an X-linked degenerative eye disease, is very rare worldwide; only about 400 cases have been described. Fully one third of the total number of patients, however, are from a small region in Finland, populated by a large extended family descended from a founding couple born in the 1640s (Fig. 7–2). Another Finnish genetic disease is hyperornithinemia with **gyrate atrophy** of the choroid and retina, an autosomal recessive condition caused by deficiency of ornithine aminotransferase and leading to loss of vision in young

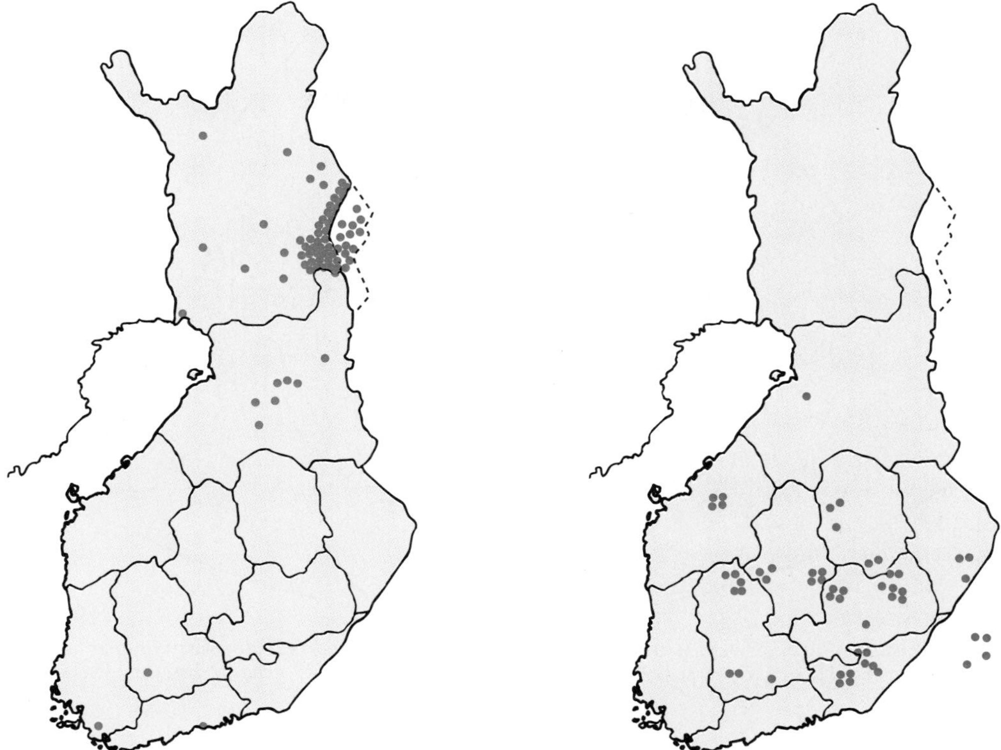

Figure 7–2. The geographical origin of cases of two genetic disorders prevalent in Finland: X-linked choroideremia (*left*) and hyperornithinemia with gyrate atrophy of the choroid and retina (*right*). Most cases of each disease originate from particular communities in Finland, but the distributions of the diseases differ. (Based on Mitchell GA, Brody LC, Sipila I, et al [1989] At least two mutant alleles of ornithine-δ-aminotransferase cause gyrate atrophy of the choroid and retina in Finns. Proc Natl Acad Sci USA 86:197–201; and Nario R, Nevanlinna HR, Perheentupa J [1973] Hereditary diseases in Finland: Rare flora in rare soil. Ann Clin Res 5:109–141.)

adulthood (see Fig. 7–2). As one might expect with a founder effect, one mutation was found in homozygous form in the vast majority of apparently unrelated cases of gyrate atrophy in Finland, but it was not observed at all in non-Finnish cases. Conversely, disorders that are common in other European populations, such as PKU, are quite rare in Finland.

Thus, one of the outcomes of the founder effect and genetic drift is that each population may be characterized by its own particular molecular mutations as well as by an increase or decrease in specific diseases. As these examples show, genetic drift can favor the establishment at high incidence of alleles that are not favorable or even neutral but are actually harmful. The relative mobility of most present-day populations, in comparison with their ancestors of only a few generations ago, may reduce the effect of genetic drift in the future.

## Gene Flow

In contrast to genetic drift, which leads to random variation in allele frequencies in small populations, **gene flow** is defined as the slow diffusion of genes across a barrier, a process that involves a large population and a gradual change in gene frequencies. The genes of migrant populations with their own characteristic gene frequencies are gradually merged into the gene pool of the population into which they have migrated. (The term "migrant" is used here in the broad sense of crossing a reproductive barrier, which may be racial, ethnic, or cultural, and not necessarily geographical and requiring physical movement from one region to another.) Whereas the mechanism of genetic drift is chance, the mechanism of gene flow is population admixture.

The frequencies of the 32 base-pair deletion allele of the *CCR5* cytokine receptor gene, *ΔCCR5*, have been studied in many populations all over the world. The frequency of the *ΔCCR5* allele declines from approximately 10 percent in Western Europe and Russia to a few percent in the Middle East and the Indian subcontinent. The *ΔCCR5* allele is virtually absent from Africa and the Far East, suggesting that the mutation originated in Caucasians and diffused into the more easterly populations (Fig. 7–3).

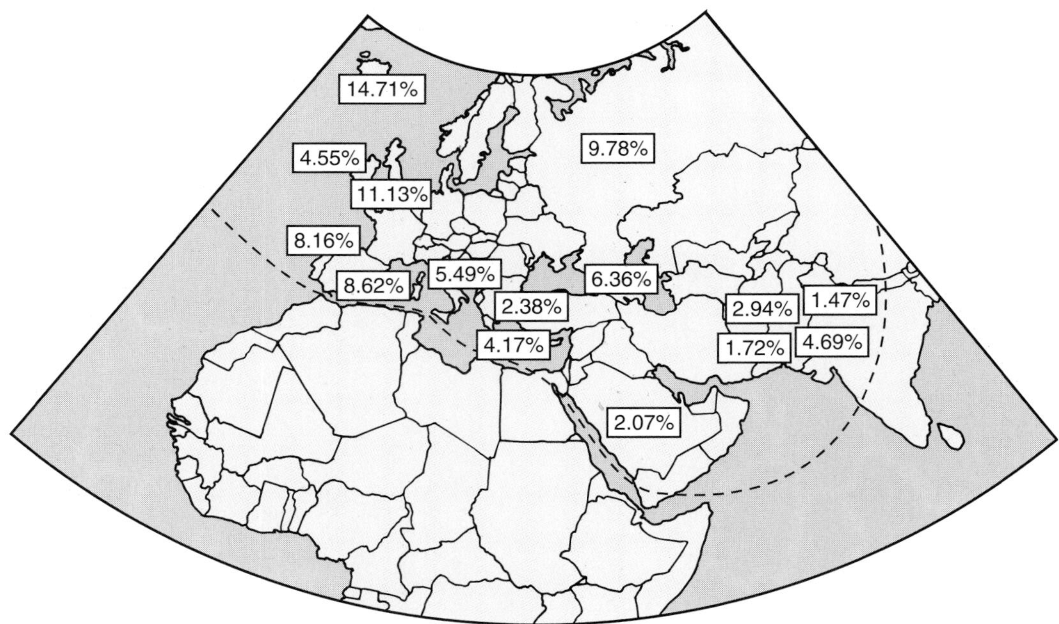


**Figure 7–3.** Frequency of $\Delta$*CCR5* alleles in populations in Europe, Africa, and Asia. (Reproduced with permission from Martinson JJ, Chapman NH, Rees DC, et al [1997] Global distribution of the *CCR5* gene 32 basepair deletion. Nat Genet 16:100–103.)

The north-west to south-east gradient in the frequency of the $\Delta$*CCR5* allele, of course, does not explain why the allele frequency is as high as it is in Northwestern Europe. For example, the highest frequency of the $\Delta$*CCR5* allele is 21 percent, seen among Ashkenazic Jews, and nearly that high in Iceland and the British Isles. The current AIDS pandemic is too recent to have affected gene frequencies through selection; the variation in allele frequencies in Europe itself is most consistent with genetic drift acting on a neutral polymorphism, although it is possible that another selective factor (perhaps another infectious disease such as bubonic plague) may have elevated the frequency of the $\Delta$*CCR5* allele in Northern European populations during an intense period of selection.

Another example of gene flow between population groups is reflected in the frequency of specific mutant alleles causing PKU. There is strong evidence that the most common mutations were of Celtic origin. These same mutations have now turned up in many populations around the world. The presence of the same PKU alleles in different populations reflects the geographical migration of the Celts. Thus, the frequency of PKU is approximately 1/4500 in Ireland, but the disorder is progressively less prevalent across Northern and Southern Europe. There has been considerably less gene flow to East Asia; the incidence of PKU in Japan is only about 1/109,000.

## CONCLUSION

A mathematical description of the behavior of genes in populations is an important element of many disciplines, including anthropology, evolutionary biology, and human genetics. In medical genetic practice, the application of population genetics has been primarily a practical one: providing allele frequencies for risk calculations. At present, serious students of human genetics are using the principles and methods of population genetics to address many unanswered questions concerning the genetic structure of human populations, the flow of genes between populations and between generations, and the optimal methods for identifying the genetic contributions to common disease (see Chapter 15). An understanding of the principles of population genetics will become more and more important as genetic testing and therapeutic technologies magnify the impact of medical genetics care on public health and on the risk for genetic disease in future generations (see Chapter 20).

### *General References*

Cavalli-Sforza LL (1998) The DNA revolution in population genetics. Trends Genet 14:60–65.

de la Chapelle A (1993) Disease gene mapping in isolated human populations: The example of Finland. J Med Genet 30:857–865.

Emery AEH (1986) Methodology in Medical Genetics, 2nd ed. Churchill Livingstone, Edinburgh.

Hartl DL, Clark AG (1997) Principles of Population Genetics, 3rd ed. Sinauer Associates, Sunderland, England.

Li CC (1975) First Course in Population Genetics. Boxwood Press, Pacific Grove, California.

Morton NE (1982) Outline of Genetic Epidemiology. Karger, Basel.

Peltonen L, Uusitalo A (1997) Rare disease genes—lessons and challenges. Genome Res 7:65–767.

## References Specific to Particular Topics

Lorey FW, Arnopp J, Cunningham GC (1996) Distribution of hemoglobinopathy variants by ethnicity in a multiethnic state. Genet Epidemiol 13:501–512.

Martinson JJ, Chapman NH, Rees DC, et al (1997) Global distribution of the *CCR5* gene 32 basepair deletion. Nat Genet 16:100–103.

Nagel RL, Ranney H (1990) Genetic epidemiology of structural mutations of the β-globin gene. Semin Hematol 27:342–359.

Sachse C, Brockmoller J, Bauer S, Roots I (1997) Cytochrome P450 2D6 variants in a caucasian population: Allele frequencies and phenotypic consequences. Am J Human Genet 60:284–295.

Stephens JC, Reich DE, Goldstein DB, et al (1998) Dating the origin of the CCR5-delta32 AIDS-resistance allele by the coalescence of haplotypes. Am J Human Genet 62:1507–1515.

Tada K, Tateda H, Arashima S, et al (1984) Follow-up study of a nation-wide neonatal metabolic screening program in Japan. A collaborative study group of neonatal screening for inborn errors of metabolism in Japan. Eur J Pediatr 142:204–207.

## Problems

1. In a population at equilibrium, three genotypes are present in the following proportions: *A/A*, 0.81; *A/a*, 0.18; *a/a*, 0.01.
   (a) What are the frequencies of *A* and *a*?
   (b) What will their frequencies be in the next generation?
   (c) What proportion of all matings in this population are *A/a* × *A/a*?
2. In a screening program to detect carriers of β-thalassemia in an Italian population, the incidence was found to be about 4 percent. Calculate
   (a) the frequency of the β-thalassemia allele (assuming that there is only one common β-thalassemia mutation in this population);
   (b) the proportion of matings in this population that could produce an affected child;
   (c) the incidence of affected fetuses or newborns in this population;
   (d) the incidence of β-thalassemia among the offspring of couples both found to be heterozygous.
3. Which of the following populations is in Hardy-Weinberg equilibrium?
   (a) *A/A*, 0.70; *A/a*, 0.21; *a/a*, 0.09.
   (b) MN blood groups: (i) M, 0.33; MN, 0.34; N, 0.33. (ii) 100% MN.
   (c) *A/A*, 0.32; *A/a*, 0.64; *a/a*, 0.04.
   (d) *A/A*, 0.64; *A/a*, 0.32; *a/a*, 0.04.
   What explanations could you offer to explain the frequencies in those populations that are *not* in equilibrium?
4. You are consulted by a couple, Abby and Andrew, who tell you that Abby's sister Anna has Hurler syndrome (a mucopolysaccharidosis) and that they are concerned that they themselves might have a child with the same disorder. Hurler syndrome is an autosomal recessive condition with a population incidence of about 1 in 90,000 in your community.
   (a) If Abby and Andrew are not consanguineous, what is the risk that Abby and Andrew's first child will have Hurler syndrome?
   (b) If they are first cousins, what is the risk?
   (c) How would your answers to these questions differ if the disease in question were cystic fibrosis, instead of Hurler syndrome?
5. In a certain population, three disorders—autosomal dominant retinoblastoma, autosomal recessive Friedreich ataxia (a neuromuscular disorder), and X-linked choroideremia (a cause of loss of vision in males at an early age)—each have a population frequency of approximately 1/25,000.
   (a) What are the gene frequency and the heterozygote frequency for each of these?
   (b) Suppose that each one could be successfully treated, so that all selection against it was removed. What would be the effect on the gene frequency in each case? Why?
6. As discussed in this chapter, the autosomal recessive condition tyrosinemia type I has an observed incidence of 1/685 individuals in one population in the province of Quebec but an incidence of about 1/100,000 elsewhere. What is the frequency of the mutant tyrosinemia allele in these two groups?
7. For the population in Quebec in question 6, would you expect the mutant tyrosinemia alleles to be homogeneous or heterogeneous? How about for cases of autosomal dominant neurofibromatosis I in the same French-Canadian population? X-linked Duchenne muscular dystrophy? X-linked color blindness?

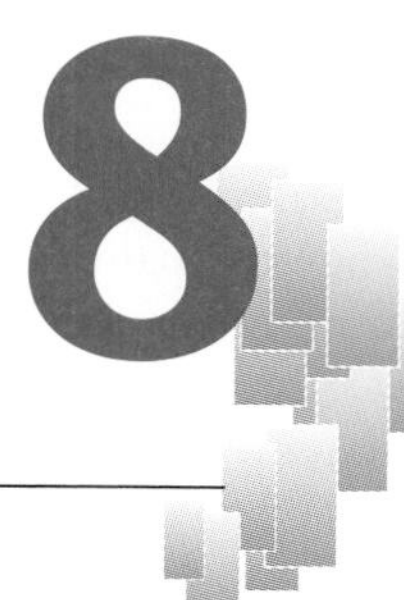

# Gene Mapping and the Human Genome Project

Human gene mapping is one of the most rapidly expanding areas of study in medical genetics today. To have a complete human gene map is to know the location of the approximately 50,000 genes on the 24 chromosomes, their positions relative to one another, and the distances between them. Such map information is extremely valuable not only because it can be applied to disease diagnosis and genetic counseling, but also because it provides a direct route for identifying the genes responsible for genetic diseases.

Early on, chromosomal assignment was accomplished exclusively with family studies in large pedigrees to ascertain the mode of inheritance. In this way, genes for X-linked traits could be assigned to the X chromosome because the traits showed a unique pattern of transmission. In addition, a few autosomal dominant or codominant traits were assigned to individual autosomes because of the fortuitous discovery that the trait phenotype was inherited through many generations in tandem with a particular blood group or with a chromosome with a cytogenetically detectable structural variant (**heteromorphism;** see Chapter 9).The vast majority of human genes, however, could not be mapped in this or any other way until the advent of physical and genetic mapping methodology, the subject of this chapter.

There are two fundamentally different approaches for assembling gene maps of human chromosomes: physical mapping and genetic mapping. **Physical mapping** assigns genes to particular locations along a chromosome using measurements that are a reflection of the physical distance between the genes. At low resolution, physical maps place genes on chromosomes or regions of a chromosome according to cytogenetic bands on metaphase chromosomes; at the highest resolution, physical mapping provides locations and distances between genes in actual physical measurements such as DNA length (in units of base pairs). **Genetic mapping**, on the other hand, uses a completely different method—called **linkage analysis**—to determine the distance between genes. Linkage analysis is based on measuring the frequency with which two genes remain together (remain linked) through meiosis as they are passed from one generation to the next. In this chapter, we discuss both types of mapping and examine several of their applications for identifying and isolating particular human genes and for providing diagnostic information in medical genetics.

## PHYSICAL MAPPING OF HUMAN GENES

Physical mapping of genes encompasses a variety of different methods, each of which uses different units of measurement and provides different levels of resolution, ranging from an entire chromosome to a single base pair.

### Somatic Cell Genetics

Somatic cell genetics is the study of gene organization, expression, and regulation in cultured cells obtained from somatic, as opposed to germline, tissues. Somatic cell genetics takes advantage of the ability of a number of different cell types to grow, sometimes indefinitely, in cell culture. Successful maintenance of cultures for long periods requires the development of media that satisfy the strict nutritional requirements of cells as well as the initiation of precautions to avoid contamination by microorganisms, yeasts, or other cultured cell lines.

Cell culture has proved useful in many situations. The technique allows the propagation of a single cell of defined genetic make-up to make large numbers of cells (clones), genetically identical to the original cell, available for study. A cell line can be established from a patient with a rare disorder or an unusual karyotype when the patient is available and can be stored frozen more or less permanently in liquid nitrogen for study at any convenient time, even decades after the patient's death.

Fibroblasts, usually propagated from small skin biopsy specimens, are among the most useful cell types for somatic cell genetic studies. Fibroblasts have a characteristic spindle shape, grow in monolayers attached to plastic or glass surfaces, and divide for approximately 30 to 100 generations until they become incapable of further cell division (**senescence**). Some cell lines in culture undergo **transformation**, which means that the cells come to resemble cancer cells in their ability to grow indefinitely. Transformation can be spontaneous or induced by viruses such as the Epstein-Barr virus. This virus is now used routinely to transform peripheral blood lymphocytes to create immortalized lymphoblastoid cell lines because blood samples are relatively easy to obtain and the transformation process is rapid and efficient. Transformed lines do not senesce and may retain some of the differentiated characteristics of the cells from which they were derived, but, with the notable exception of lymphoblastoid cells, the majority of transformed lines do not maintain a normal euploid karyotype.

## Mapping by Chromosome Transfer

Chromosome transfer is a powerful laboratory method that allows entire chromosomes, or segments of chromosomes, to be transferred from a donor cell to a recipient cell in culture. As soon as it became clear that human and other mammalian cells could be maintained in culture, human geneticists began to transfer chromosomes from the cells of one species into cells from another species to separate different genes and their alleles into separate clones of cells. *By correlating which genes are present in a recipient cell when specific chromosomes or chromosome segments have been transferred, the chromosomal location of the transferred genes can be determined.*

### Somatic Cell Hybridization

The most widely used approach for chromosome transfer is to fuse somatic cells from different species to make interspecific **somatic cell hybrids**. When a mixture of human and rodent somatic cells, growing as monolayers or in suspension, is exposed to agents that promote the fusion of plasma membranes of cells, two cells may fuse together into a single hybrid

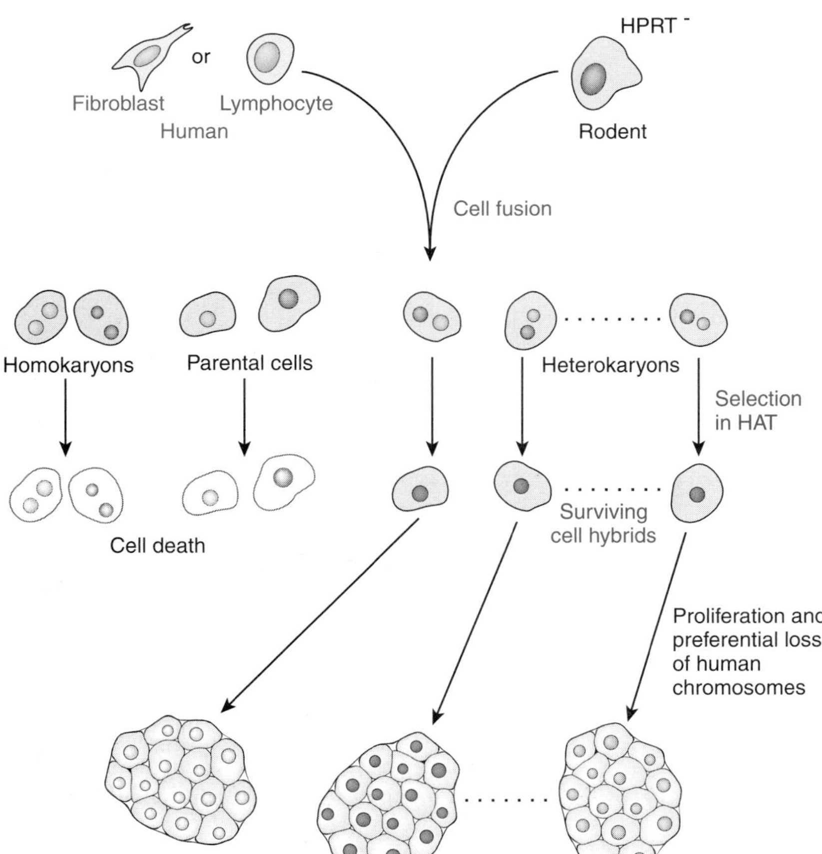


**Figure 8–1.** Interspecific somatic cell hybridization scheme. After cell fusion, human/rodent somatic cell hybrid clones are grown in a selection system, such as hypoxanthine, aminopterin, and thymidine (HAT) medium. These cell hybrids preferentially lose human chromosomes, which makes it possible to isolate hybrid clones containing different combinations of human chromosomes. These clones can then be analyzed for the presence or absence of a particular human gene, thus allowing assignment of the gene to a specific human chromosome.

cell. Immediately after fusion, the two nuclei are maintained separately in the same cytoplasm (Fig. 8–1). If the newly formed hybrids are interspecific hybrids, that is, they contain nuclei from both the rodent and human parental cells, they are known as **heterokaryons**. (**Homokaryons** are hybrids containing nuclei from the same species.) After a heterokaryon undergoes mitosis and cell division, the two nuclear contents unite in a single "hybrid" nucleus and, with further cell division, lose variable numbers of the human chromosomes at random from the human/rodent hybrids; rodent chromosomes are not lost, for reasons that remain unknown.

As a consequence of the random loss of human chromosomes, different daughter hybrid cells contain different numbers and combinations of human chromosomes. Each independent clone of hybrid cells can be isolated and analyzed for its human chromosome content using a number of karyotyping techniques that distinguish between rodent and human chromosomes (see Figs. 8–1 and 8–2).

Somatic cell fusion is not efficient: most cells in culture do not fuse, and, for those that do, there is no method to ensure that a human cell has always fused with a rodent cell and not another human cell (and vice versa for rodent cells). Particular cell culture conditions and techniques are used to render unfused parental cell types, and the hybrids derived from homokaryons, incapable of survival, while allowing hybrids formed from heterokaryons to survive and grow. Although a number of selective schemes have been developed, one of the first and most commonly used involves selection in medium containing hypoxanthine, aminopterin, and thymidine (the so-called HAT medium). Cells can grow in HAT medium only if they possess the enzyme hypoxanthine guanine phosphoribosyltransferase (HPRT), which can salvage the purine base hypoxanthine contained in HAT medium for DNA synthesis (see Fig. 12–3). Cells deficient in HPRT activity ($HPRT^-$) must synthesize purine bases de novo and therefore cannot survive in HAT medium because aminopterin inhibits de novo purine (as well as pyrimidine) biosynthesis.

When $HPRT^-$ rodent cell lines (usually either mouse or hamster) are fused with $HPRT^+$ human cells, only rodent/human somatic cell hybrids are capable of prolonged growth in HAT medium: both the parental $HPRT^-$ rodent line and any homokaryons formed from them die in HAT. Parental human cells and homokaryons derived from them do not survive because they are not transformed and lack long-term growth potential (see Fig. 8–1).

### Somatic Cell Hybrid Mapping Panels

The random loss or retention of human chromosomes in interspecific somatic cell hybrids results in clones containing different subsets of human chromosomes. A set of independent somatic cell hybrid clones, called a **panel**, can be used to map a human gene or DNA segment to a particular human chromosome by simply testing the hybrids in the panel, each of which carries different human chromosomes, for the presence or absence of a particular human gene. The results are matched against the residual human chromosomes present in each hybrid, to determine the concordance between the presence of a particular chromosome and the presence of the gene. In this way, for example, the presence or absence of the gene for hexosaminidase A

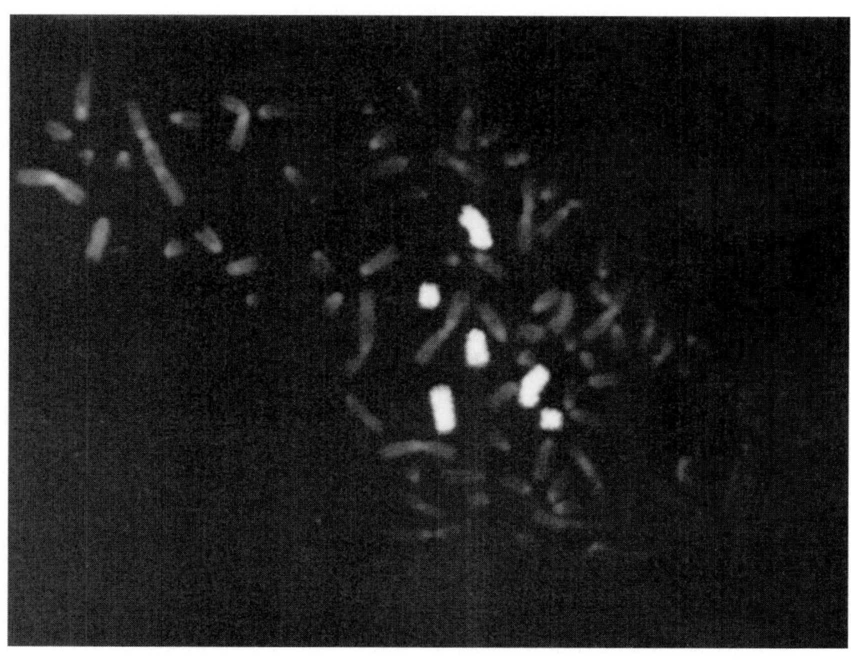

**Figure 8–2.** Metaphase chromosome spread from a mouse/human somatic cell hybrid. Human chromosomes can be identified by a detection method that specifically labels human but not mouse DNA. This hybrid contains six human chromosomes, identified as chromosomes 13, 20 (two copies), and the X (three copies). (Courtesy of V. E. Powers, Stanford University.)

TABLE 8–1

**Mapping a Human Gene by Using Somatic Cell Hybrids**

| | | Human Chromosomes | | | | | | | | | | | | | | | | | | | | | | |
|---|---|---|---|---|---|---|---|---|---|---|---|---|---|---|---|---|---|---|---|---|---|---|---|---|
| *Hybrid* | *HEXA Gene* | *1* | *2* | *3* | *4* | *5* | *6* | *7* | *8* | *9* | *10* | *11* | *12* | *13* | *14* | *15* | *16* | *17* | *18* | *19* | *20* | *21* | *22* | *X* | *Y* |
| I | + | + | − | − | − | − | − | − | − | + | + | − | − | + | − | + | − | − | + | − | + | − | − | + | − |
| II | − | + | + | − | + | − | − | + | + | − | − | − | + | − | + | − | − | − | + | + | − | + | − | + | − |
| III | + | − | − | − | + | − | − | + | + | − | − | + | − | + | + | + | − | − | + | − | − | + | + | + | + |
| IV | − | − | − | − | − | − | − | + | + | − | + | − | + | + | + | − | − | − | + | + | − | + | − | + | − |
| V | − | − | + | + | − | + | − | − | + | − | − | + | − | + | + | − | − | + | − | − | + | + | + | + | + |
| VI | + | + | + | − | − | − | − | − | − | − | − | − | − | − | − | + | − | − | + | + | − | + | − | + | − |
| VII | + | + | − | + | − | − | − | + | + | − | + | + | + | − | + | + | + | − | − | + | + | − | − | + | − |
| VIII | + | − | − | − | − | − | − | − | − | − | − | − | − | − | − | + | − | − | − | − | − | − | − | + | − |

*Note*: A panel of mouse/human somatic cell hybrids, each containing 2 to 13 human chromosomes, was used to test for the presence or absence of the human hexosaminidase A gene (*HEXA*) by means of Southern blotting of DNA prepared from the hybrids (see Fig. 8–3). There is a perfect correlation between the presence or absence of *HEXA* and the presence or absence of human chromosome 15. For all other human chromosomes, there are hybrids that contain *HEXA* but are missing the chromosome, and there are hybrids that contain the chromosome but are missing *HEXA*. Thus these results indicate that the *HEXA* gene must be on human chromosome 15.

(*HEXA*), in which mutations cause Tay-Sachs disease (see Chapter 12), was shown to correlate with the presence of human chromosome 15 in a panel of somatic cell hybrids (Table 8–1). All hybrids that retained a human chromosome 15 contained the human *HEXA* gene; all those without chromosome 15 did not contain human *HEXA*. This perfect concordance was observed only for chromosome 15 and not for any other human chromosome, thus allowing assignment of the *HEXA* gene to chromosome 15. In this type of analysis, the presence of a human gene can be monitored by measuring its biochemical activity if the gene is expressed in somatic cell hybrids and if the human and rodent activities can be distinguished. DNA methods that distinguish the human gene from the rodent gene are now more commonly used (Fig. 8–3). These methods include polymerase chain reaction (PCR) with human versus rodent specific primer pairs and Southern blotting to visualize restriction fragment length differences that distinguish the human and rodent DNA sequences. This type of concordance analysis in a panel of interspecific somatic cell hybrids has allowed thousands of genes to be assigned to individual human chromosomes.

## Mapping a Gene to a Specific Region of a Chromosome

Studies using human/rodent hybrids allow assignment of a gene to a particular chromosome. Additional resolution can be gained by isolating structurally abnormal human chromosomes, such as those described in Chapters 9 and 10, in somatic cell hybrids. If a particular gene is present only in those hybrids with a deleted or translocated chromosome, then the gene can be localized to the portion of the chromosome retained in the hybrids. Alternatively, if a gene is known to map to a particular chromosome but is absent from a hybrid containing a deleted or translocated copy of that chromosome, then the gene can be assigned to the portion of the chromosome that is missing. Figure 8–4 depicts how two structurally abnormal X chromosomes are used in gene mapping to localize X-linked genes and DNA sequences to particular regions of the X chromosome. By examination of different hybrids, each containing one of the translocation chromosomes, the X chromosome can be divided into three intervals and different genes assigned to each. Extension of this

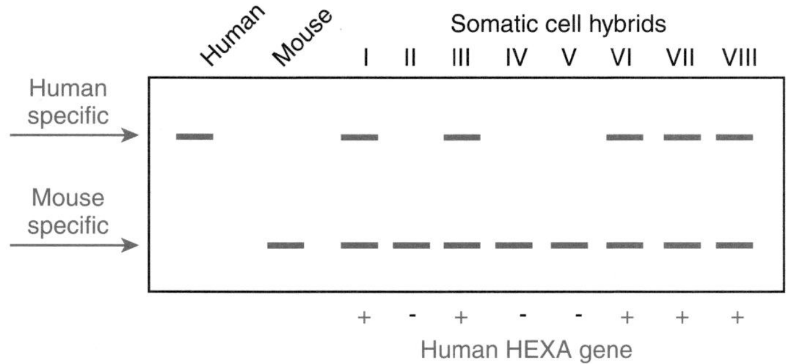


**Figure 8–3.** Gel electrophoresis of a polymerase chain reaction (PCR) experiment to map the human *HEXA* gene to chromosome 15, in a series of mouse/human somatic cell hybrids. Only hybrids I, III, VI, VII, and VIII contain human *HEXA* sequences, which can be distinguished from the mouse gene sequences by the use of different primer pairs for PCR that are specific for the human sequence or the mouse sequence and amplify different sized fragments in the two species. The human and mouse specific fragments are then separated by gel electrophoresis.

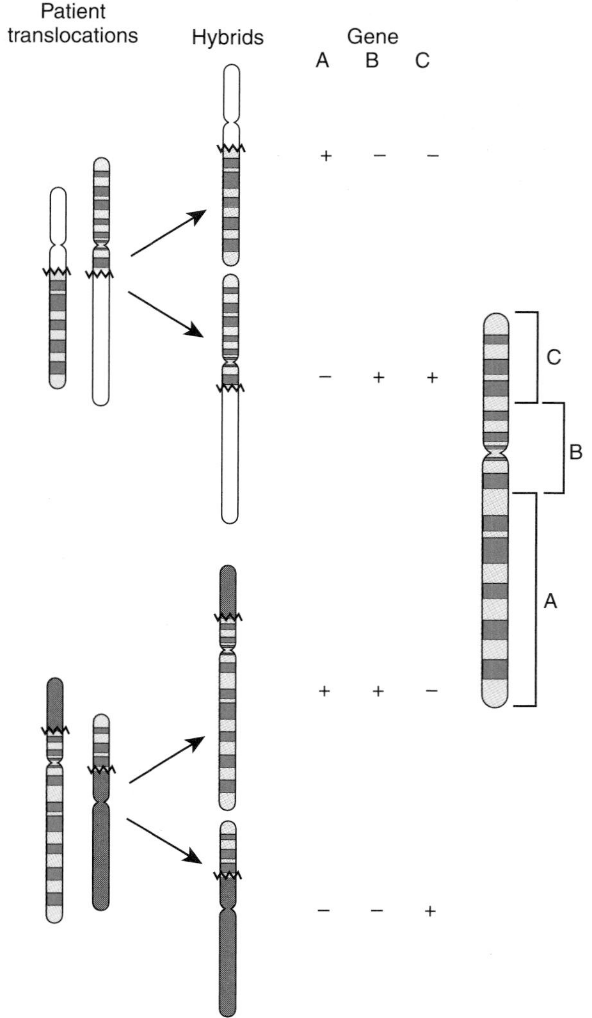


Figure 8–4. Regional mapping of X-linked genes by analysis of X;autosome translocation chromosomes in somatic cell hybrids. The reciprocal products of two different X;autosome translocations are segregated in somatic cell hybrid clones and can be analyzed for the presence or absence of genes from the human X chromosome. The combined results allow regional localization of the three genes to different portions of the X, as indicated at the right.

strategy and examination of increasingly smaller regions of the chromosome of interest in hybrids has made it possible to localize genes to even smaller regions.

### Radiation Hybrid Mapping

Although somatic cell hybridization of structurally abnormal chromosomes can provide regional localization of a gene to a particular portion of a chromosome, the chromosome regions defined are still quite large in comparison with the size of an average gene. Much higher resolution gene mapping can be achieved with **radiation hybrid mapping**, a somatic cell hybridization technique that takes advantage of the ability of x-rays to cause double-strand breaks in DNA. Human cells are x-irradiated to fragment their human chromosomes, and the fragments are separated into a large number of hybrids by somatic cell fusion to $HPRT^-$ rodent cells. Hybrids containing human chromosomal fragments can be isolated by selecting in HAT because hybrids containing the fragment of the X chromosome carrying *HPRT* invariably contain a random assortment of fragments from other human chromosomes as well (Fig. 8–5). Unfused human cells or human homokaryons die from massive chromosome damage, whereas unfused $HPRT^-$ rodent cells or rodent homokaryons die in HAT.

The closer two human genes are on a chromosome, the less likely it is that an x-ray–induced break will occur between them; as a result, two genes in physical proximity are retained in many of the same hybrids, whereas genes that are not close together usually reside on different chromosome fragments and therefore are usually not present in the same hybrids. A statistical analysis of how often two genes are concordant in radiation hybrid clones provides a measure of the distance between the genes. The resolution of radiation hybrid mapping can be adjusted by using smaller or larger doses of x-rays to generate different frequencies of breaks and therefore varying sized fragments.

## Mapping by Gene Dosage Using Patient Cells

Another approach to gene mapping also takes advantage of structurally rearranged chromosomes but does not rely on having to first separate the abnormal chromosomes into somatic cell hybrids. This approach depends on detection of dosage differences in either gene products or the gene sequences themselves between patients' cell lines containing different numbers of copies of a particular gene. The gene dosage strategy was originally used to assign genes to chromosome 21 by detecting levels of enzyme activity in cell lines from patients with Down syndrome (who have three copies or doses of chromosome 21) that were 1.5-fold higher than levels in cell lines from chromosomally normal persons (two doses). At the DNA level, the dosage approach has been used increasingly to assign DNA markers to the X chromosome (by comparing DNA dosage in persons with one [i.e., a normal male karyotype] to five [i.e., a 49,XXXXX karyotype] X chromosomes) (Fig. 8–6) or to small regions of a particular chromosome (by examining collections of patients with partial trisomies [three copies] or monosomies [one copy]; see Chapters 9 and 10).

One of the most direct applications of mapping by gene dosage is the assignment of X-linked disease genes to specific regions of the X chromosome by

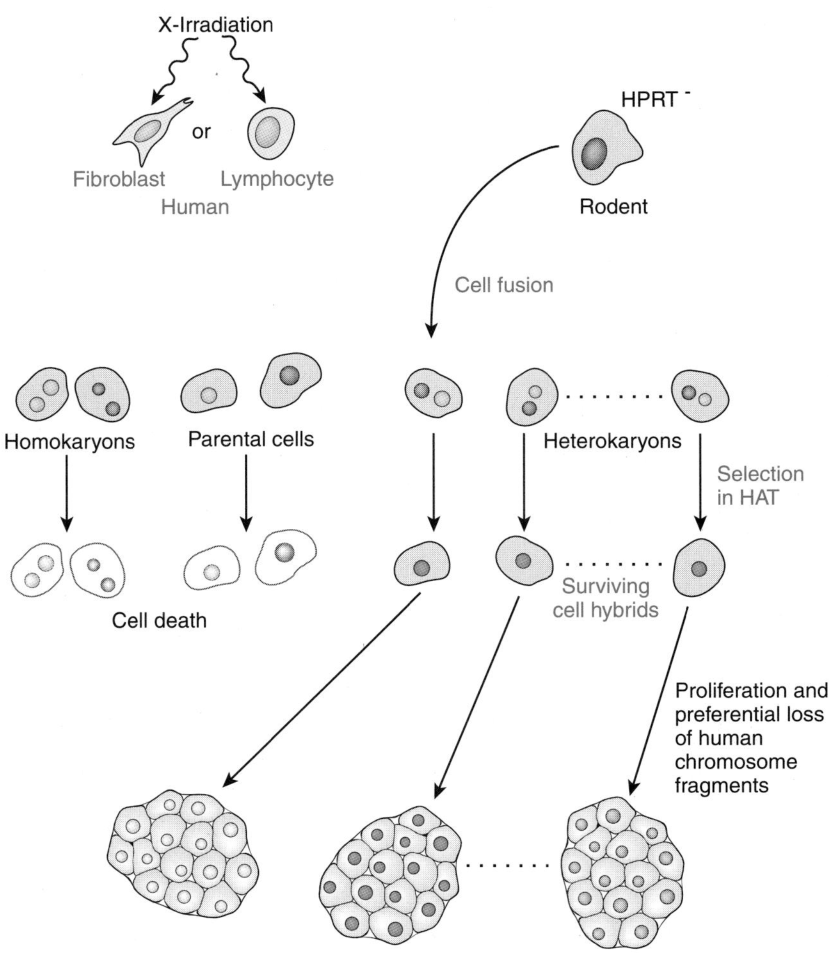


**Figure 8–5.** Radiation hybrid mapping. Human cells are lethally irradiated to fragment the chromosomes and then hybridized to rodent somatic cells. Hybrids containing a human fragment carrying a selectable biochemical marker, such as hypoxanthine guanine phosphoribosyltransferase (HPRT), survive selective media. Each cell hybrid contains a random set of chromosomal fragments (except for the fragment carrying the biochemical marker used to select the interspecific hybrids).

examining males with cytogenetically detectable deletions of part of the X chromosome. In one well-studied example, a boy with no known family history of any genetic disease presented with four ordinarily distinct X-linked conditions: Duchenne muscular dystrophy (DMD), chronic granulomatous disease (CGD), retinitis pigmentosa (RP), and a rare red blood cell phenotype. Careful cytogenetic analysis revealed a small but detectable deletion in band Xp21 (Fig. 8–7). The coexistence of four single-gene disorders with the small chromosome deletion led to the conclusion that the genes for these four X-linked traits mapped to the deleted interval. Extension of this type of analysis to other individuals simultaneously affected with multiple X-linked diseases has allowed the regional assignment of a number of genes in this region of the X chromosome (see Fig. 8–7). The patient with the Xp21 deletion turned out to be even more significant for medical genetics because (as described more fully later in this chapter) his deleted X chromosome was used to identify and isolate the genes for both DMD and CGD. This patient provides yet another example of how recognition of the unusual in medicine—in this case, the occurrence of multiple genetic diseases in a single individual—can provide important new information about normal genes, their organization, and their function.

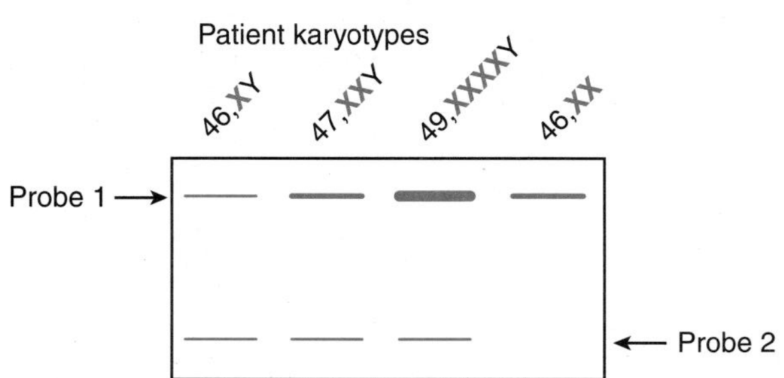


**Figure 8–6.** Examples of mapping by dosage analysis. DNA probe 1 used at the left can be mapped to the X chromosome because the intensity of hybridization appears to be a function of the number of Xs present in each DNA sample. DNA probe 2 shows the same intensity of hybridization in lanes 1 to 3, but is missing from lane 4. This locus maps to the Y chromosome.

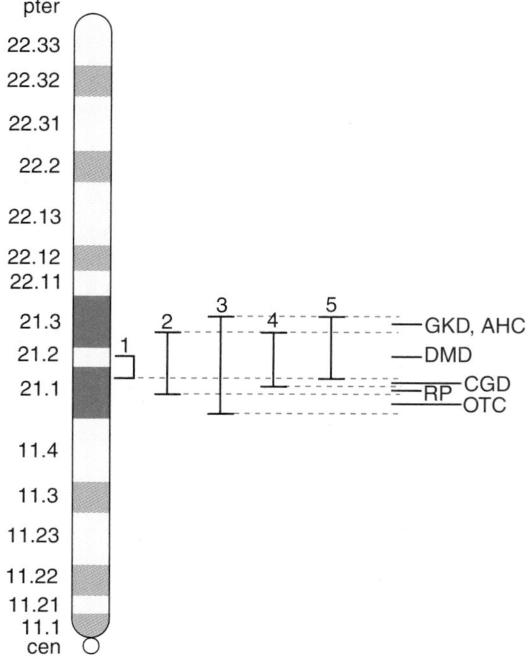


**Figure 8–7.** Regional localization of X-linked genes in patients with X chromosome deletions. Correlation of the extent of the cytogenetic deletion with the particular disorders present in each case allows fine mapping of the individual disease genes to particular regions on the X chromosome. DMD = Duchenne muscular dystrophy, OTC = ornithine transcarbamylase deficiency, CGD = chronic granulomatous disease, RP = retinitis pigmentosa, GKD = glycerol kinase deficiency, AHC = congenital adrenal hypoplasia. (Courtesy of U. Francke, Stanford University.)

## Gene Mapping by Fluorescence In Situ Hybridization

The mapping methods just discussed are indirect in that they provide information on the physical location of a gene on a particular chromosome but do not actually allow the map position of the gene to be visualized. Direct visualization can be achieved using the method of **in situ hybridization**, which involves hybridizing labeled DNA (or RNA) probes directly to metaphase chromosomes (see Chapter 4). The DNA in metaphase chromosomes is denatured in place (hence, in situ) on the slide, to allow hybridization of a labeled probe to proceed. The location of the hybridization signal, and thus the location of the gene to which the probe hybridizes, is then determined under a microscope.

Methods for mapping single-copy gene sequences by in situ hybridization have been developed that enable rapid detection of hybridized probes labeled nonradioactively with compounds that can be visualized by fluorescence microscopy (Fig. 8–8). Even in a single metaphase spread, one can easily see the position of the gene being mapped. In combination with banding methods for chromosome identification (see Chapters 2 and 9), **fluorescence in situ hybridization** (FISH) is used to map genes to a region of 1 million to 2 million base pairs along the highly condensed chromatin of a metaphase or prometaphase chromosome.

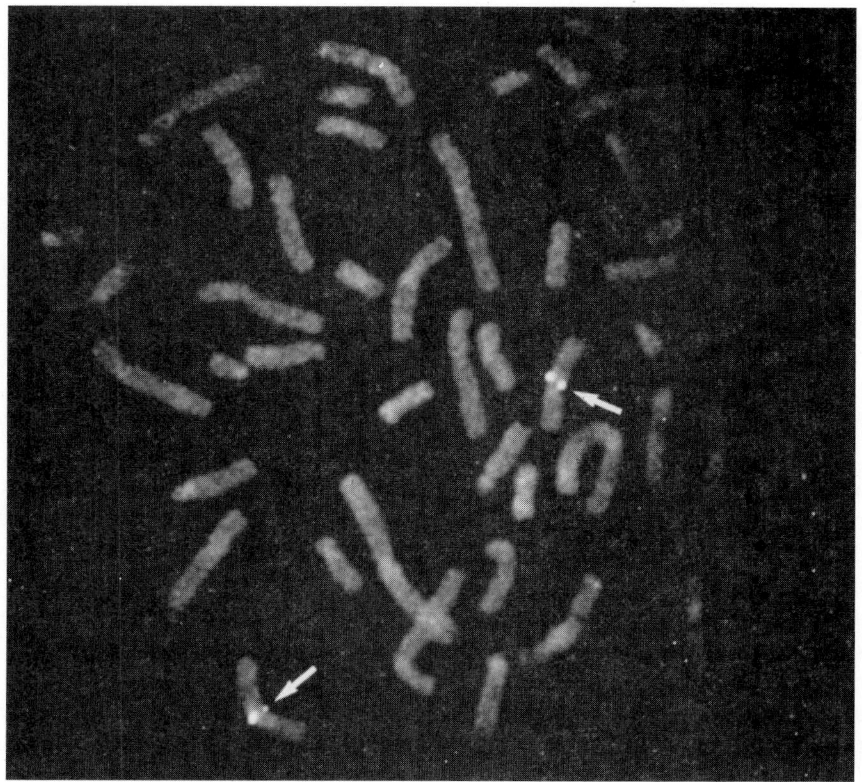

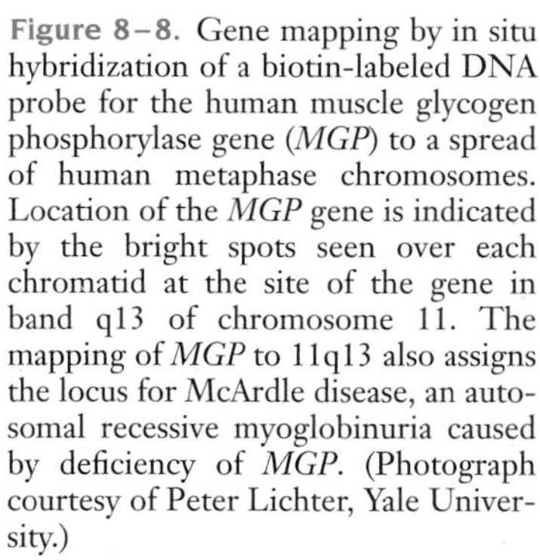

**Figure 8–8.** Gene mapping by in situ hybridization of a biotin-labeled DNA probe for the human muscle glycogen phosphorylase gene (*MGP*) to a spread of human metaphase chromosomes. Location of the *MGP* gene is indicated by the bright spots seen over each chromatid at the site of the gene in band q13 of chromosome 11. The mapping of *MGP* to 11q13 also assigns the locus for McArdle disease, an autosomal recessive myoglobinuria caused by deficiency of *MGP*. (Photograph courtesy of Peter Lichter, Yale University.)

Somewhat higher resolution mapping has been achieved by FISH mapping of DNA fragments using interphase chromatin fibers (fiber-FISH), which are far less condensed than metaphase chromosomes; markers as close as a few hundred kb apart have been resolved when labeled with different colored dyes, allowing their order relative to one another to be determined. Fiber-FISH has been extremely helpful in research aimed at the identification of human disease genes because the technique provides researchers with detailed information on the order and distance between individual genes in the vicinity of a disease gene.

## MAPPING HUMAN GENES BY LINKAGE ANALYSIS

**Linkage** can be defined as the tendency for alleles close together on the same chromosome to be transmitted together, as an intact unit, through meiosis. **Genetic linkage analysis** is a method of mapping genes that uses family studies to determine whether two genes show linkage (are **linked**) when passed on from one generation to the next. Mapping by genetic linkage analysis differs from mapping by physical methods because physical mapping relies on having a laboratory method to localize a gene by FISH or by somatic cell hybridization. In contrast, linkage analysis is a tremendously important and powerful approach in medical genetics because *it is the only method that allows mapping of genes, including disease genes, that are detectable only as phenotypic traits.* The vast majority of genes that underlie genetic disease fall into this category because neither their biochemical nor their molecular basis has yet been elucidated.

### Linkage, Synteny, and Recombination

#### HOMOLOGOUS RECOMBINATION IN MEIOSIS

To understand fully the concepts underlying genetic linkage analysis, it is necessary to review briefly the behavior of chromosomes and genes during meiosis. Homologous chromosomes pair during meiosis I, and the pairs line up along the meiotic spindle. The paternal and maternal homologs exchange homologous segments by crossing over and creating new chromosomes that are a "patchwork," consisting of alternating portions of the grandmother's chromosomes and the grandfather's chromosomes (Fig. 8–9). The creation of such patchwork chromosomes emphasizes the notion of human genetic individuality: *each chromosome inherited by a child from a parent is essentially never exactly the same as either of the two copies of that chromosome in the parent but instead contains some segments derived from the child's grandfather and other segments from the child's grandmother.*

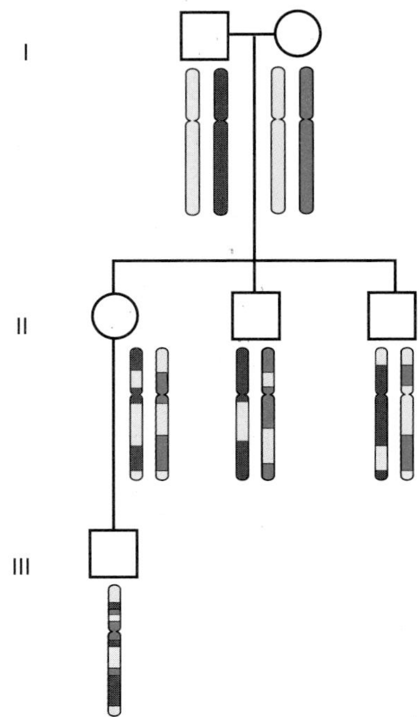


Figure 8–9. The effect of recombination on the origin of various portions of a chromosome. Because of meiotic crossing over, the copy of a chromosome inherited by the boy in generation III is actually a mosaic of parts of all four of the grandparental copies of that chromosome.

If homologous chromosomes generally look identical under the microscope, we must have a way of differentiating the homologs; only in that way can we trace the grandparental origin of each segment of a chromosome inherited by a particular child and thereby determine if and where the recombination events have occurred along the homologous chromosomes. For this purpose, we use **genetic markers**, which are defined as any characteristic located at the same place on a pair of homologous chromosomes that allows us to distinguish one homolog from the other. In the past, genes that encoded electrophoretic enzyme variants or cell surface antigens served as markers; however, in the era of the Human Genome Project, genetic markers are most commonly DNA sequence polymorphisms that can be detected by PCR amplification of the segment of DNA containing the marker (see Chapter 6).

How are genetic markers used for genetic linkage mapping? Suppose there are two genetic marker loci, *1* and *2*, with alleles *D* and *M* on the paternally derived chromosome and alleles *d* and *m* on the maternally derived chromosome in an individual (Fig. 8–10). If the two loci are located on different chromosomes, they will assort independently in meiosis; thus, one observes four types of offspring (i.e., four types of gametes) *in equal proportions*: *DM* and *dm*, which are called **nonre-**

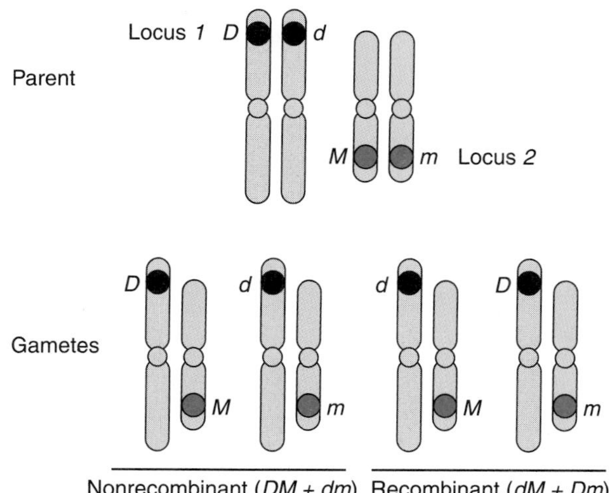


**Figure 8–10.** Meiotic behavior of alleles at two loci, *1* and *2*, when they are located on separate chromosomes.

**combinant** because they match the two original parental chromosomes, and genotypes *Dm* and *dM*, termed **recombinant** because they represent a new combination of alleles that differs from the parental chromosomes. When equal numbers of recombinant and nonrecombinant genotypes are seen (such as when two loci are not located on the same chromosome), the loci are said to be **unlinked**.

## Loci on the Same Chromosome Are Not Necessarily Linked

Suppose, however, that loci *1* and *2* are on the same chromosome? Genes that reside on the same chromosome are said to be **syntenic** (literally, "on the same thread"), regardless of how close together or how far apart they lie on that chromosome. We know that crossing over takes place at the four-strand stage of meiosis, when there are four chromatids per chromosome pair. If no crossover occurs between the loci, only nonrecombinant genotypes *DM* and *dm* are seen in the offspring. If one or more crossovers occur between them, however, the ratio of nonrecombinant genotypes to recombinant genotypes becomes 1:1. In fact, an average of 1 to 3 recombination events occurs somewhere along every chromosome per meiosis. As shown in Figure 8–11, one, two, or more recombinations occurring between two loci result in offspring that are 50 percent recombinant and 50 percent nonrecombinant. Thus, if two syntenic loci are so far apart on the same chromosome that there is going to be at least one crossover between them with every meiosis, recombinant and nonrecombinant genotypes will occur in the offspring in equal proportions, and the two loci will appear to be unlinked, just as if the loci were on separate chromosomes.

**Genetic linkage analysis** takes advantage of these properties of meiosis by using the frequency of recombination to measure how close genetically different loci are to each other. As shown in Figure 8–12*A*, if at least one crossover occurs in the segment of the chromosome between loci *1* and *2*, both the nonrecombinant genotypes *DM* and *dm* and recombinant genotypes *Dm* and *dM* will be seen, on average, in equal proportions in the offspring. On the other hand, if two loci are so close together on

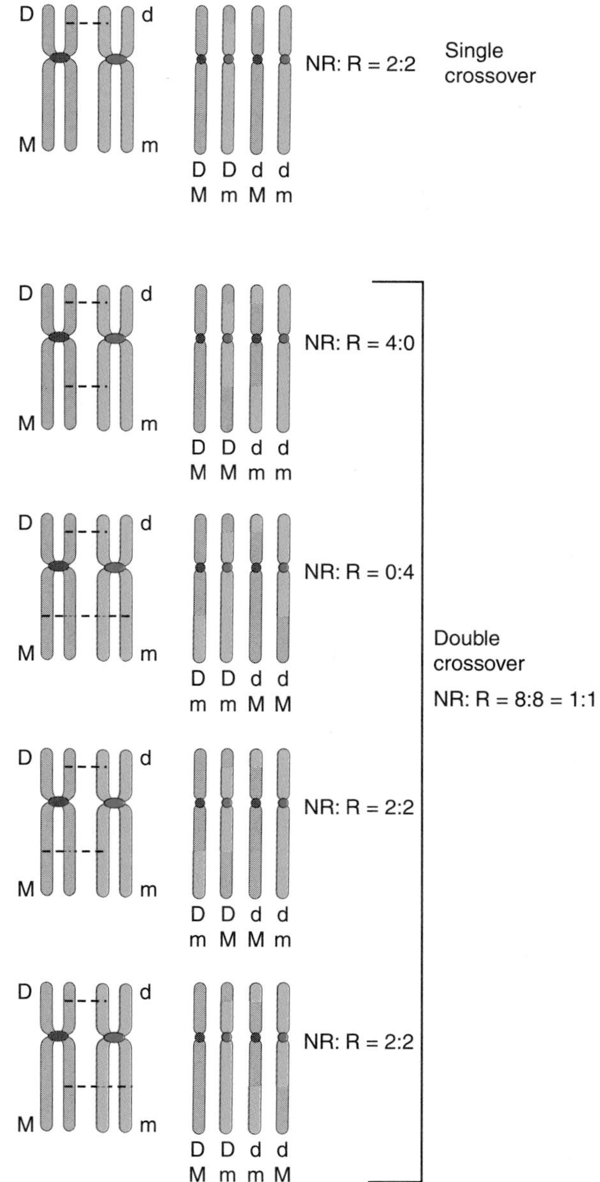


**Figure 8–11.** Crossing over between homologous chromosomes in meiosis, resulting in a new combination of maternally and paternally derived alleles on the recombinant chromosomes. If no crossover occurs in the interval between loci *1* and *2*, only parental (nonrecombinant) genotypes *DM* and *dm* occur in offspring. If one or two crossovers occur in the segment between the loci, half of the offspring will contain a nonrecombinant genotype and half the recombinant genotype. The same is true if > 2 crossovers occur between the loci (not illustrated here).

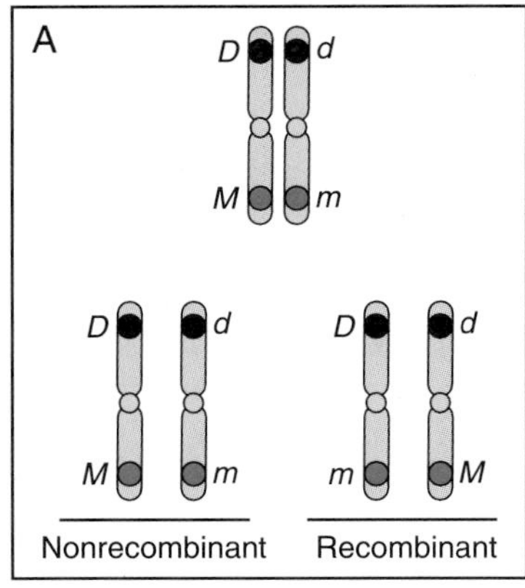


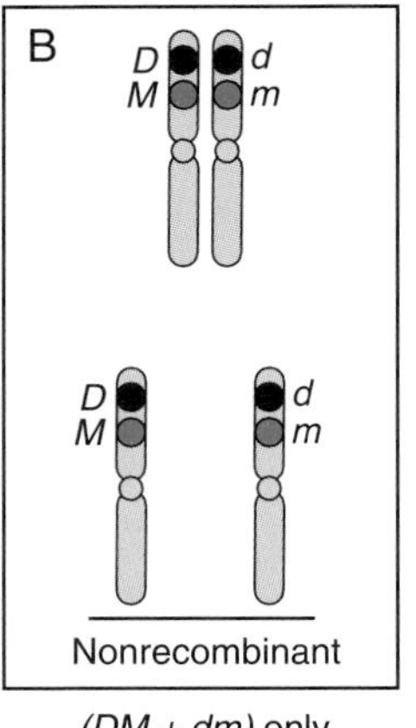


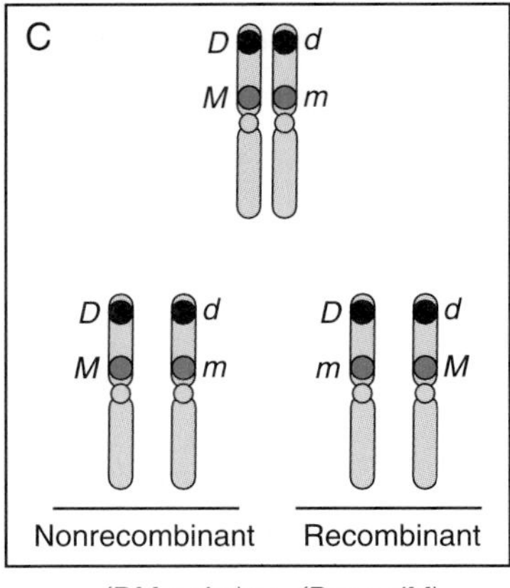


**Figure 8–12.** Meiotic behavior of alleles at two loci, *1* and *2*, when (*A*) they are located very far apart on the same chromosome, (*B*) they are located very close together on the same chromosome, and (*C*) when they are located on the same chromosome but sufficiently far apart for meiotic crossovers to occur.

the same chromosome that crossovers never occur between them, there is complete linkage: the nonrecombinant genotypes (parental chromosomes *DM* and *dm* in Fig. 8–12*B*) are transmitted together all of the time, only the nonrecombinant allele combinations *DM* and *dm* at these two loci will occur, and the frequency of the recombinant genotypes *Dm* and *dM* will be 0. In between these two extremes is the situation in which two loci are far enough apart that a recombination between them occurs in some meioses and not in others (see Fig. 8–12*C*). We will observe nonrecombinant and recombinant combinations of alleles in the offspring, but the frequency of recombinant genotypes at the two loci will fall between 0 percent (completely linked) and 50 percent (completely unlinked): *the smaller the recombination frequency, the closer together two loci are.* A common notation for recombination frequency is the Greek letter $\theta$.

**Figure 8–13.** Linkage of the gene for an autosomal dominant form of retinitis pigmentosa, RP9, to a marker locus. The mother (I-1) is affected with this dominant disease and is heterozygous at the *RP9* locus (*Dd*), as well as at two other loci, *1* and *2*, on chromosome 7. She carries the *A* and *B* alleles on the same chromosome as the mutant *RP9* allele (*D*). The unaffected father is homozygous normal (*dd*) at the *RP9* locus, as well as at the two marker loci (*AA* and *BB*); his contributions are not considered further. All three affected offspring have inherited the *B* allele at locus *2* from their mother, whereas the three unaffected offspring have inherited the *b* allele. Thus all six offspring are nonrecombinant for *RP9* and marker locus *2*. However, individuals II-1, II-3, and II-5 are recombinant for *RP9* and marker locus *1*, indicating that meiotic crossing over has occurred between these two loci.

## Detection of Linkage and Measurement of Genetic Distance

Detecting the recombination events that allow an assessment of linkage between two loci requires that a parent be heterozygous ("informative") at both loci. If the mother (I-1) in the family shown in Figure 8–13 had been homozygous at the marker loci, it would be impossible to determine whether recombination had occurred. The loci most informative for linkage analysis, therefore, are the ones that are highly polymorphic, such as microsatellite markers analyzed by PCR, and are therefore heterozygous in a large proportion of individuals (see Chapter 6).

### Measuring Genetic Distance

With these introductory comments, we can now examine how one measures linkage between two loci. Suppose that one is interested in evaluating possible linkage between two loci in a series of families. Among the offspring of informative meioses (those in which a parent is heterozygous at both loci), 80 percent are nonrecombinant and 20 percent are recombinant. The recombination frequency $\theta$, therefore, is 20 percent.

Genetic distance is measured in units called **centiMorgans** (cM), defined as the genetic length over which, on average, one observes recombination 1 percent of the time. (The cM is 1/100 of a Morgan, named after Thomas Hunt Morgan, who first observed genetic crossing over, in the fruit fly *Drosophila*.) Therefore, translating a recombination fraction of 20 percent into genetic distance, the two can be estimated to lie approximately 20 cM apart genetically. This estimate, however, is valid only if the number of offspring has been sufficient to be confident that the observed 80:20 ratio of nonrecombinants to recombinants is really different from the 50:50 ratio expected for loci that assort independently because they are far apart on the same chromosome or on different chromosomes. In fact, if four of five children were nonrecombinant and one was recombinant, this ratio would not be significantly different from the result expected for completely unlinked, randomly assorting loci (would you consider it significant if you flipped a coin five times and it came up heads four times out of five?). If one observes the same 80:20 ratio after scoring several dozen children from several families, however, it would certainly be considered different from 50:50, just as you would find it very unusual to flip a coin 50 times and have it come up heads 40 times out of 50.

### LOD SCORES: ARE TWO LOCI LINKED?

Suppose we want to determine whether two loci are linked. To do that, we need two pieces of information. First, we must determine the recombination fraction $\theta$ between two loci because determining whether two loci are linked is equivalent to asking whether the recombination fraction between them differs significantly from the 0.5 fraction expected for unlinked loci. Second, we must determine whether a deviation, if any, from 0.5 is truly significant using a statistical tool called the likelihood odds ratio, as follows: One examines a set of actual family data, counts the number of children who show or do not show recombination between the loci, and, finally, calculates the likelihood of observing the data at various possible values of $\theta$ ranging from $\theta = 0.0$ (no recombination) to $\theta = 0.50$ (random assortment). We take the ratio of these two likelihoods to calculate the odds of obtaining the observed data assuming the two loci *are* linked at some recombination fraction $\theta$, in comparison with the situation in which they are *not* linked at all. The odds in favor of a given value of $\theta$ are therefore =

$$\frac{\text{likelihood of data if loci are linked at a particular } \theta}{\text{likelihood of data if loci are unlinked } (\theta = 0.50)}$$

The computed odds ratios are usually expressed as the $\log_{10}$ of this ratio and called a **lod score** ($Z$) for "logarithm of the odds." (The use of logarithms allows data collected from different families to be combined by simple addition.)

The odds ratio is important in two ways. First, it provides a statistically valid method for using the family data to estimate the recombination frequency between the loci: the value of $\theta$ that gives the greatest value for Z is, in fact, the best estimate of the recombination fraction you can make given the data. This value of $\theta$ is called $\theta_{max}$. If $\theta_{max}$ differs from 50 percent, you have evidence of linkage. However, even if $\theta_{max}$ is the best estimate of $\theta$ you can make, how good an estimate is it? The odds ratio also provides you with an answer to this question because *the higher the value of Z, the better an estimate $\theta_{max}$ is.* Positive values of Z (odds >1) suggest that the two loci are linked, whereas negative values (odds <1) suggest that linkage is less likely (at that value of $\theta$) than the possibility that the two loci are unlinked. *By convention, a combined lod score of +3 or greater (equivalent to greater than 1000:1 odds in favor of linkage) is considered definitive evidence that two loci are linked.*

Localization of genes by linkage analysis provides an opportunity to identify medically relevant genes that are not understood in biochemical or molecular terms. Consider the family shown in Figure 8–13. The mother has an autosomal dominant form of RP (RP9). She is also heterozygous for two loci on chromosome 7, one close to the *RP9* gene and one not. One can see that transmission of the *RP9* mutant allele (*D*) invariably "follows" that of allele *B* at marker locus *2* from the first generation to the second generation in this family. All three offspring who inherited their mother's mutant *RP9* allele also inherited the *B* allele at marker locus *2*, whereas all the offspring who inherited their mother's normal allele inherited the *b* allele. The *RP9* gene, however, shows no tendency to follow the allele at marker locus *1*.

Suppose we let $\theta$ be the "true" recombination fraction between *RP9* and locus 2, the fraction we would see if we had unlimited numbers of offspring to test. Viewed in this way, $\theta$ can be considered to be the probability, with each meiosis, that a recombination will occur between the two loci. Because either a recombination occurs or it does not, the probability of a recombination, $\theta$, and the probability of no recombination must add up to 1. Therefore, the probability that no recombination will occur is $1 - \theta$.

In fact, there are only six offspring, all of whom show no recombination. The likelihood of seeing 0 offspring that are recombinant and 6 offspring with no recombination between *RP9* and marker locus *2* is given by $(\theta)^0(1 - \theta)^6$. The lod score between *RP9* and marker 2 is therefore

$$Z = \log_{10} \frac{(\theta)^0(1 - \theta)^6}{(1/2)^0(1/2)^6}$$

The maximum value of Z is 1.81 when $\theta = 0$, which is suggestive but not definite evidence for linkage

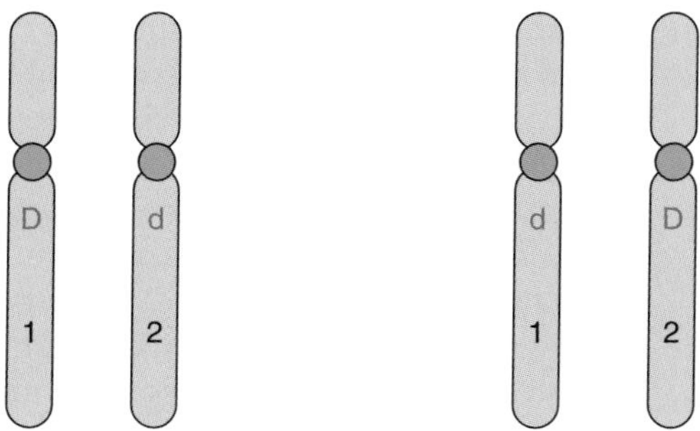


**Figure 8–14.** Possible linkage phases of alleles *1* and *2* at a marker locus with alleles *D* and *d* at a disease locus.

because Z is positive but less than 3. If similar results were obtained from the study of other families, the lod scores could be added together to reach significance ($Z > 3$). In that case, one could definitively say that the *RP9* gene and marker locus *2* are linked, whereas the *RP9* and locus *1* are not (even though they are still syntenic). Because the chromosomal location of locus *2* was known to be at 7p15 by physical mapping methods, the location of the *RP9* locus is now also known to be close to 7p15.

## Phase in Linkage Analysis

Being heterozygous for a linked polymorphic marker and the disease gene (as in Fig. 8–13) is, however, not enough for detecting linkage; we also need to know which of the two polymorphic alleles is located on the same chromosome as the disease allele, that is, the **phase** must be known. Alleles on the same homolog are said to be **in coupling** (or ***cis***), whereas alleles on different homologs are said to be **in repulsion** (or ***trans***) (Fig. 8–14). The alleles in coupling at a set of closely linked markers constitute what is known as the **haplotype** for those loci. To illustrate the concept of phase, we consider two examples that demonstrate the importance of knowing phase information in linkage analysis. Figure 8–15 shows pedigrees of two families with autosomal dominant neurofibromatosis, type 1 (NF1). In the two-generation family, the affected mother is heterozygous at both the *NF1* locus (*D/d*) and a marker locus (*1/2*), but we do not know whether the *NF1* allele is in coupling with allele *1* or allele *2* at the marker locus. The father in this analysis is uninformative because he is homozygous for the normal allele *d* at the *NF1* locus and for allele *1* at the marker locus; he transmits to his offspring a chromosome that has the normal allele (*d*) and the *1* allele, regardless of how far apart the loci are or whether recombination has occurred. By inspection, then, we can infer which alleles in each child have come from the mother. Two children have inherited the *D* and *2* alleles, and one has received *d* and *1*. Depending on the actual phase of these alleles in the mother, either all three offspring are recombinants, or all three are nonrecombinants (see Fig. 8–15, *left*).

Which of these two possibilities is correct? There is no way to know for certain, and thus we must compare the likelihoods of the two possible results. Half of the time, the correct phase is *D2* and *d1*, and all three children have inherited a chromosome in which *no recombination* occurred between *NF1* and the marker locus. If the probability of recombination between *NF1* and the marker is $\theta$, the probability of

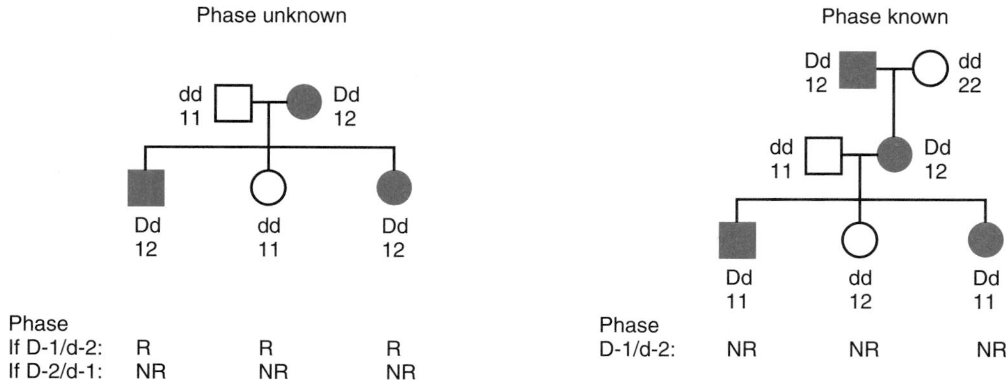


**Figure 8–15.** Comparison of linkage information in phase-unknown and phase-known pedigrees. R = recombinants; NR = nonrecombinants. See text for discussion.

TABLE 8–2

**Maximum Liklihood Analysis for Linkage Between NF1 and Marker Locus in Pedigrees in Figure 8–15**

| | Lod Scores (Z) at Various Values of $\theta$ | | | | | | | | |
|---|---|---|---|---|---|---|---|---|---|
| **Type of Pedigree** | *0.00* | *0.01* | *0.05* | *0.10* | *0.20* | *0.30* | *0.40* | $Z_{max}$ | $\theta_{max}$ |
| Phase unknown | .602 | .589 | .533 | .465 | .318 | .170 | .049 | .602 | .00 |
| Phase known | .903 | .890 | .837 | .765 | .612 | .438 | .237 | .903 | .00 |

no recombination is $(1 - \theta)$, and the likelihood of three nonrecombinant chromosomes is $(1 - \theta)^3$. The overall probability, then, assuming this phase, is $1/2\ (1 - \theta)^3$. The other half of the time, however, the correct phase is *D1* and *d2*, which makes each of these three children *recombinants*; the probability assuming this alternative phase is $1/2\ \theta^3$. To calculate the overall likelihood of the NF1 disease allele *D* being in coupling with marker allele 2 in all three children, we add the likelihood calculated assuming one phase in the mother is correct to the likelihood calculated assuming the other phase is correct. Therefore, the overall likelihood $= 1/2(1 - \theta)^3 + 1/2\ \theta^3$.

On the other hand, if there is no linkage between these loci, one expects independent segregation of the two loci, and the probabilities of a recombinant and a nonrecombinant genotype in the offspring are both equal to 1/2. The probability of having three children with these genotypes, under the assumption of no linkage, is $(1/2)^3$, or 1/8. The relative odds for this pedigree, then, are

$$\frac{1/2(1 - \theta)^3 + 1/2\ \theta^3}{1/8}$$

By evaluating the relative odds for values of $\theta$ from 0 to 0.5, the maximum value of the lod score, $Z_{max}$, is found to be $\log_{10}(4) = 0.602$ when $\theta = 0.0$ (Table 8–2). Because this is far short of a lod score greater than 3, we would need at least five equivalent families to establish linkage (at $\theta = 0.0$) between this marker locus and *NF1*. With slightly more complex calculations (made much easier by computer programs written to facilitate linkage analysis), one can calculate the lod scores for other values of $\theta$ (see Table 8–2).

**Phase Known and Unknown Pedigrees.** The second family in Figure 8–15 is similar, except that the mother's parents are available for analysis. By inspection, it is clear that the maternal grandfather must have transmitted both the *NF1* allele (*D*) and the *1* allele to his daughter. (This finding does not require any assumption about whether a crossover occurred in the grandfather's germline; such an assumption would have been unwarranted.) The phase in the mother must, therefore, be *D1* on one chromosome and *d2* on the other. The availability of a third generation makes this a **phase-known pedigree**. The three children can now be scored definitively as nonrecombinant. Comparing the likelihoods of linkage and nonlinkage is now simplified because we do not have to consider the opposite phase. The probability of having three children with the observed genotypes is now $(1 - \theta)^3$. As in the previous, phase-unknown pedigree, the probability of the observed data if there is no linkage between the loci is $(1/2)^3 = 1/8$. Overall, the relative odds for this pedigree are $(1 - \theta)^3$:1/8 in favor of linkage, and the maximum lod score *Z* at $\theta = 0.0$ is 0.903 (see Table 8–2). Thus, the strength of the evidence supporting linkage is twice as great in the phase-known situation as in the phase-unknown situation.

**Determining Phase in X-Linked Pedigrees.** For linkage analysis in X-linked pedigrees, the mother's father's genotype is particularly important because, as illustrated in Figure 8–16, it provides direct information on linkage phase in the mother. Because there can be no recombination between X-linked genes in a male and because the mother always receives her father's only X, any X-linked marker present in her genotype, but not in her father's, must have been inherited from her mother. Knowledge of phase, so important for genetic counseling, can thus be readily ascertained from the appropriate male members of an X-linked pedigree, if they are available for study.

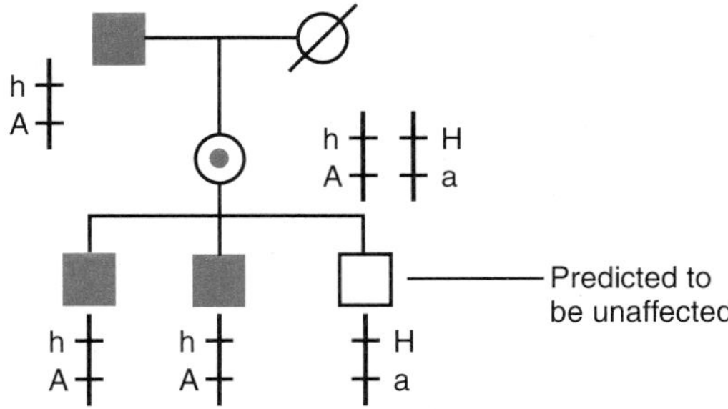


**Figure 8–16.** In X-linkage, the maternal grandfather's phenotype can reveal the linkage phase in his daughter. In this pedigree, the affected maternal grandfather's X chromosome carries allele *A* at a marker locus closely linked to the gene for hemophilia A (*h*). Thus, his daughter carries these alleles on one of her X chromosomes and alleles *a* and *H* on the other, even though there is no direct information on her mother's genotype. Knowledge of genotype phase can be used to predict the genotypes of her male offspring, including a male fetus diagnosed prenatally.

### LINKAGE EQUILIBRIUM

The two families in Figure 8–15 illustrate another very important concept. In one family, the *NF1* mutant allele was associated with the *1* allele at the closely linked marker locus; in the other family, *NF1* was associated with the *2* allele. In general, there is no association between disease alleles and particular alleles at a linked polymorphic locus. The linkage phase has to be established for each family independently of any unrelated families. The allelic frequencies at the two loci are said to be in **linkage equilibrium**; the relative proportions of the possible allelic combinations can be predicted by the product of the population frequencies of the alleles at the individual loci. Thus, if a disease is linked to a polymorphic marker with two alleles of equal frequency, the disease allele will be in coupling with one of the marker alleles in half of affected families and with the other allele in half of the families. Contrast this situation to one in which a disease-producing mutation is found to be in coupling with only one particular allele at a locus linked to the disease gene. This situation, referred to as **linkage disequilibrium**, is infrequent but extremely valuable for genetic analysis, as illustrated later in this chapter with reference to the cystic fibrosis (CF) gene.

## Genetic Linkage Maps

Linkage maps of large numbers of loci, even of entire chromosomes, have been created by combining measurements of genetic distance between closely linked loci taken two at a time. Suppose two loci, *A* and *B*, are linked at a distance of approximately 10 cM. With this information, we can now begin to construct a genetic map for the chromosome on which the *A* and *B* loci map. Additional loci can be added to the linkage map if their distances from the *A* and *B* loci can be measured. For example, consider a third locus *C*, which we find is linked to *A* with a maximum lod score at $\theta = 0.12$ and linked to *B* with a maximum lod score at $\theta = 0.05$. With only these two-point data, the order of the three loci relative to one another can be established by inspection: the likely order would be *A-B-C*, with the following map.

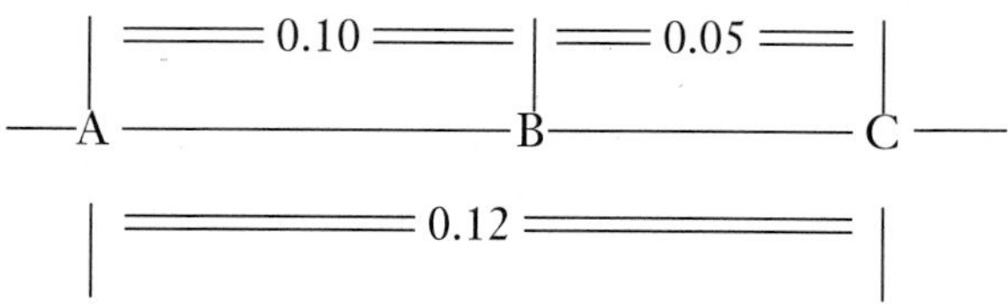


Note that the *A–C* distance as measured by recombination frequency is less than the sum of the *A–B* and *B–C* distances. This discrepancy is due to the fact that double crossovers (one in the *A–B* interval and one in the *B–C* interval) do not result in recombination between *A* and *C* and, therefore, lead to an underestimate of the distance between them.

## Multipoint Linkage Analysis

An alternative method for determining order among three loci is to consider all the data together, a process termed **multipoint analysis**, rather than the individual two-point crosses separately. The principle of multipoint analysis is to establish marker order by minimizing the number of apparent multiple crossovers (Fig. 8–17). Particularly in very complex mapping studies, involving dozens of marker loci, multipoint analysis can provide strong statistical support that a particular order of markers is correct.

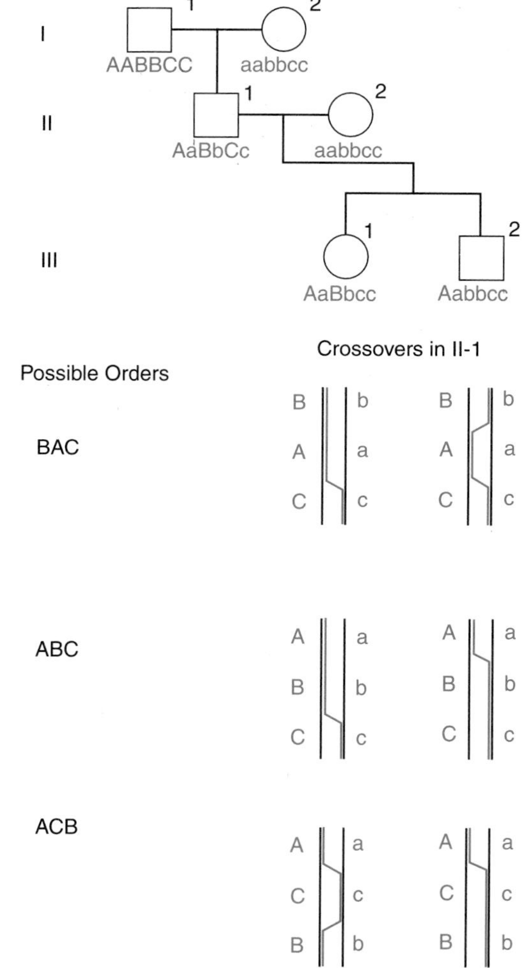


**Figure 8–17.** Determination of marker order by using multipoint crosses. Individuals III-1 and III-2 both received gametes from their father, II-1, in which crossing over must have occurred. There are three possible orders, with either locus *A*, *B*, or *C* located between the other two. Double crossovers are required to explain the genotypes of III-1 and III-2 if either *A* or *C* sits between the other two loci. Only the order that places *B* between *A* and *C* would explain the genotypes of individuals III-1 and III-2 by single crossover events. Other orders are much less likely.

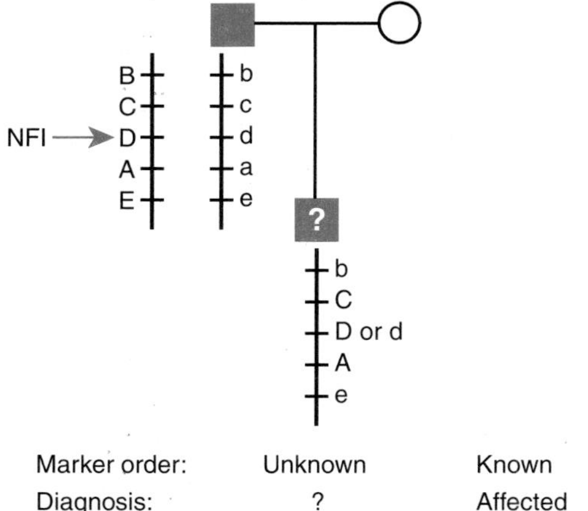


**Figure 8–18.** Normal genetic linkage map of chromosome 17 and its application to genetic counseling for *NF1*. Knowing the order of markers on the chromosome 17 map allows interpretation of linkage data in the family and diagnosis in the male fetus, who is predicted to be affected. Without the normal map for comparison, the family would have been uninformative because the position of the observed crossovers with respect to the *NF1* locus would have been unknown. Thus, no diagnosis would have been possible.

Maps created by multipoint analysis can then be used as frameworks to provide diagnostic information for use in genetic counseling (Fig. 8–18).

With increased attention focused on gene mapping as part of the Human Genome Project (see later discussion), detailed genetic linkage maps of the entire human genome have been constructed using a battery of large three-generation families to measure as accurately and finely as possible the frequency of recombination among thousands of informative microsatellite DNA markers (see, for example, the database of human linkage maps generated by the Cooperative Human Linkage Center). There is no longer any genetically "uncharted territory," and new genes, including many medically relevant ones, are being placed on the human genetic map weekly.

### Relationship between Genetic and Physical Distance

The total genetic length of the 23 chromosomes in the haploid human genome was initially estimated to be approximately 3000 cM, on the basis of the observed number of chiasmata seen in meiosis I in spermatogenesis (see Chapter 2); a recent and more accurate measurement of approximately 4300 cM was generated by adding together all the distances between the thousands of genetic markers that have been placed on the human genetic map by the Cooperative Human Linkage Center. If the genome, with a haploid physical length of approximately $3 \times 10^9$ base pairs, measures approximately 4300 cM in genetic distance, 1 cM translates roughly into 700,000 base pairs. Table 8–3 summarizes the relationships among cytogenetic landmarks, physical distances, and genetic distances and correlates them with approximate gene content. The frequency of recombination is not constant along the length of a chromosome or throughout the genome, however; furthermore, recombination frequency between two loci is also not always identical in male and female meiosis. As a consequence, genetic distance (measured as percentage recombination in meiosis) and physical distance (measured in base pairs or chromosome bands) can only be compared as a rough first approximation and provide very different, although related, measures of the distance between genes.

## APPLICATIONS OF HUMAN GENE MAPPING

The major application of gene mapping to medical genetics is the localization and identification of disease genes. Markers linked to disease genes can then serve as landmarks for the physical maps used for cloning genes responsible for genetic disease. Genetic mapping is aided by the knowledge of the physical map position of polymorphic markers being used in linkage analysis. Physical mapping efforts to finely localize a gene can be guided by the existence of specific meiotic crossovers, detected as part of linkage analyses, which can define the limits within which the disease gene must reside. *Genetic maps and physical maps are interdependent and complementary.*

### Mapping Disease Genes by Linkage Analysis

#### THE IMPORTANCE OF FAMILY STUDIES

Mapping disease genes begins with identifying and enrolling a sufficient number of families to establish linkage. Finding suitable families, however, can be a

TABLE 8–3

**Comparison of Cytogenetic, Physical, and Genetic Parameters in the Genome**

| Cytogenetic | Physical Size | Genetic Distance | Gene Content |
|---|---|---|---|
| Haploid genome of 23 chromosomes | $3 \times 10^9$ base pairs | 4300 cM | ~ 50,000 genes |
| An average chromosome | $1.5 \times 10^8$ base pairs | ~ 200 cM | ~ 2200 genes |
| 1 chromosomal band | $3 \times 10^6$ base pairs | ~ 5 cM | ~ 50 genes |

challenge, particularly for rare disorders or for disorders in which affected persons die at a young age (and DNA samples may be unavailable for analysis). Family members are carefully examined to determine who is affected and who is not affected with the disease. DNA is obtained from all available, relevant family members. Any nucleated cell can serve as a source of DNA: peripheral blood white cells are most frequently used, but buccal cells scraped from inside the cheek, cultured cells, even tissues from fixed specimens embedded in paraffin can provide DNA for analysis. Once the disease status of all family members is known, their DNA samples are used to find their genotypes at a set of polymorphic markers across the genome. The gene responsible for the disease phenotype can then be analyzed for linkage to each of the polymorphic markers.

Two kinds of families have been used to map disease genes (Fig. 8–19). In one, a small number of very large families is ascertained. The advantage of this approach is that all affected members of the pedigree are known to have the same genetic disease, caused by a mutation in the same gene. The alternative approach is to collect a large number of somewhat smaller families. This strategy is easier to do for relatively common diseases, such as CF (see Fig. 8–19), but it carries the risk that not all families may have the genetically identical disorder. **Locus heterogeneity** is the situation in which identical clinical symptoms are caused by defects at two or more genetic loci. The presence of unrecognized locus heterogeneity can confound genetic linkage analysis by giving the impression that a marker is unlinked to a disease locus when in fact it may be linked, but only in a subset of the families analyzed. This situation is illustrated later in the case of linkage in autosomal dominant RP.

## THE 10 CENTIMORGAN LIMIT

In practice in human genetics, one can hope to find linkage only at a distance of approximately 10 cM or less because at longer distances one usually cannot find sufficient family material to establish significant evidence for linkage (a lod score >3). In other words, a polymorphic marker generally has to be within roughly 7.5 million base pairs of the disease gene of interest for linkage to be detected. For an autosomal trait, 7.5 million base pairs is approximately 1/400 of the genome, and so one would predict that, on average, 400 or so well-spaced polymorphic markers would serve as an adequate set of markers to test for linkage in the family collection. It should be clear that the situation is considerably easier for X-linked diseases because one already knows the chromosomal location of the gene. Consequently, an X-linked disease can be mapped to a specific region of the X chromosome using only 15 to 20 X-linked markers.

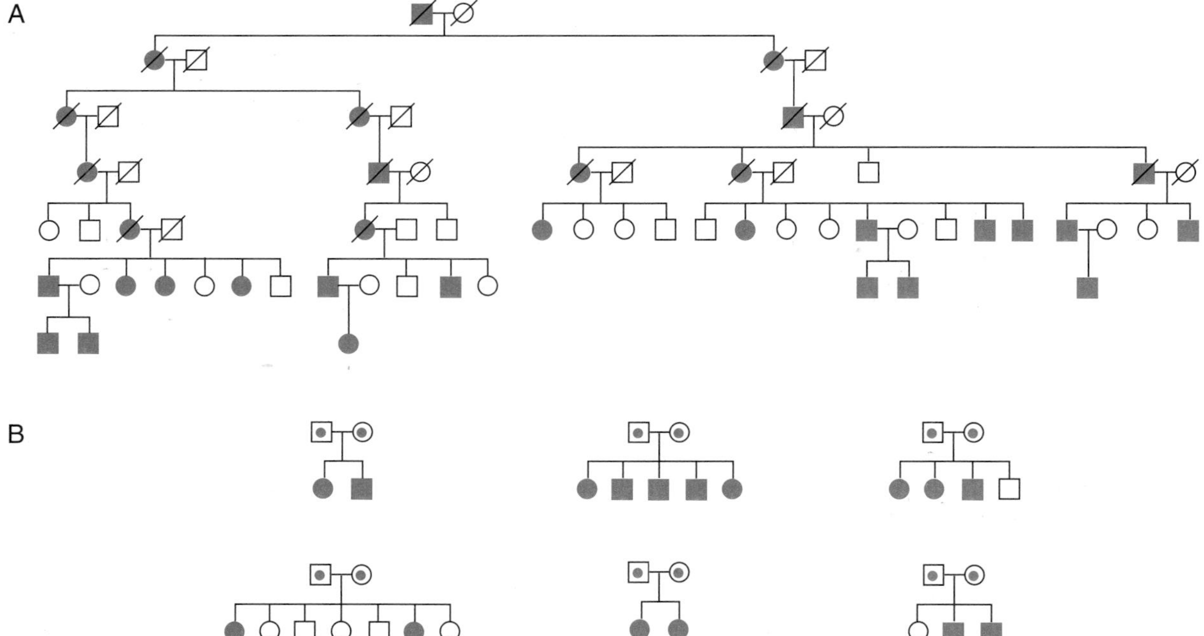


**Figure 8–19.** Two approaches for collecting families for linkage analysis. The successful linkage of Huntington disease to a polymorphic marker on chromosome 4 relied in large part on a single large Venezuelan pedigree, a small part of which is shown in *A*. The successful linkage of cystic fibrosis to a polymorphic marker on chromosome 7, however, relied on a collection of many smaller families, some of which are shown in *B*. (Adapted from Gusella JF, Wexler NS, Conneally PM, et al [1983] A polymorphic DNA marker genetically linked to Huntington's disease. Nature 306:224–238, and Tsui L-C, Zengerling A, Willard HF, Buchwald M [1986] Mapping of the cystic fibrosis locus on chromosome 7. Cold Spring Harbor Symp Quant Biol 51:325–335.)

### Confirming Linkage and Defining the Smallest Interval of Linkage

When one begins a search for linkage, the expectation for any given polymorphic marker is that, by chance, it will *not* be linked to the disease gene (in fact, by chance, any marker is unlikely to be even on the same chromosome as the disease gene). It may therefore take only a few informative meioses to establish that a marker is not close to the gene of interest. When a marker shows suggestive evidence of linkage (a combined maximum lod score of between 2 and 3, for instance), the integration of already extensive physical and genetic maps of each human chromosome becomes extremely valuable. Other markers known to be in the same region as the linked marker can be tested immediately to determine whether the linkage can be confirmed. If, for example, the marker maps to a position on the long arm of chromosome 7, then one can focus attention on other polymorphic markers in that region to confirm or reject the suggested linkage result. After one or more markers are found within about 5 cM of the disease gene, they can be used to track the inheritance of disease genes in families for diagnostic purposes. They can also serve as starting points for fine mapping studies directed toward identifying and isolating the disease gene itself.

Once a suspected linkage result is confirmed, one tests other markers that map near to the known linked markers to find markers that are so tightly linked that they show no recombination with the disease gene ($\theta_{max} = 0$). At this stage, it also becomes extremely important to identify the closest markers on either side of the disease gene that *do* recombine at least once with the disease gene in the families being studied; markers that show at least one recombination event define the boundaries of the interval in which the disease gene must reside.

### High Resolution Mapping

Techniques such as somatic cell hybridization, radiation hybrids, and FISH on metaphase chromosomes can localize genes to regions ranging in size from an entire chromosome down to a segment of a chromosome of approximately 350,000 base pairs, or about 0.1 to 0.7 percent of the linear length of a typical chromosome. The resolution of genetic linkage mapping is even more limited for two reasons. First, the value of $\theta$ always has the imprecision inherent in a statistical estimate and depends on what family material is available for study. Second, after one eventually identifies a set of markers across a region, all of which show no recombination with the disease gene, no further increase in resolution is possible: the disease gene could be anywhere among the markers that do not recombine in the families. Reducing a linkage interval further requires additional families in hopes that additional recombinations will be found in what is already a limited region to allow further narrowing of the interval around a disease gene (although higher resolution is possible if linkage disequilibrium is present; see later discussion). The increase in precision needed to pinpoint the location of genes responsible for genetic disease and to allow their identification and isolation requires high-resolution mapping approaches to map and clone regions of DNA down to the nucleotide sequence (single base pairs), a level of resolution well below the range of cytogenetic and linkage methods.

## Contigs of Artificial Chromosomes

High-resolution mapping relies on the isolation of a set of overlapping large DNA fragments (called a **contig**) that spans the entire contiguous segment of DNA containing both a gene of interest and the genetic markers used to map the gene. Using methods described in Chapter 4, such large fragments are generally isolated from libraries of cloned human DNA prepared in a variety of bacterial or **yeast artificial chromosomes** (YACs). YACs contain fragments up to 1000 kb long; isolating a contig of YACs containing all the markers in the vicinity of a gene of interest is a rapid way to isolate considerable stretches of genomic DNA in a cloned form suitable for further detailed analysis (Fig. 8–20). The DNA segment contained in each YAC can be further subdivided by constructing a contig of overlapping **bacterial artificial chromosomes** (BACs) that spans the segment of DNA contained in the YAC. BACs usually contain 100 to 200 kb of DNA, are smaller than YACs, and are suitable for further subcloning into smaller and smaller fragments and, ultimately, sequencing. In this way, the location and structure of a gene can be determined not only to the resolution of individual exons and introns but even to its actual DNA sequence, including mutations responsible for disease. The techniques used for physical mapping are listed and compared in Table 8–4.

## Human Gene Mapping and Disease Gene Identification

The application of gene mapping to medical genetics has met with many spectacular successes. The overall strategy—mapping the location of a disease gene by linkage analysis to define markers for use in disease diagnosis and genetic counseling, followed by attempts to clone the gene based on its map position—can best be illustrated by specific examples. The examples to be discussed illustrate several approaches; the one that is ultimately successful for a given disease depends on the unique characteristics and circumstances of that disease.

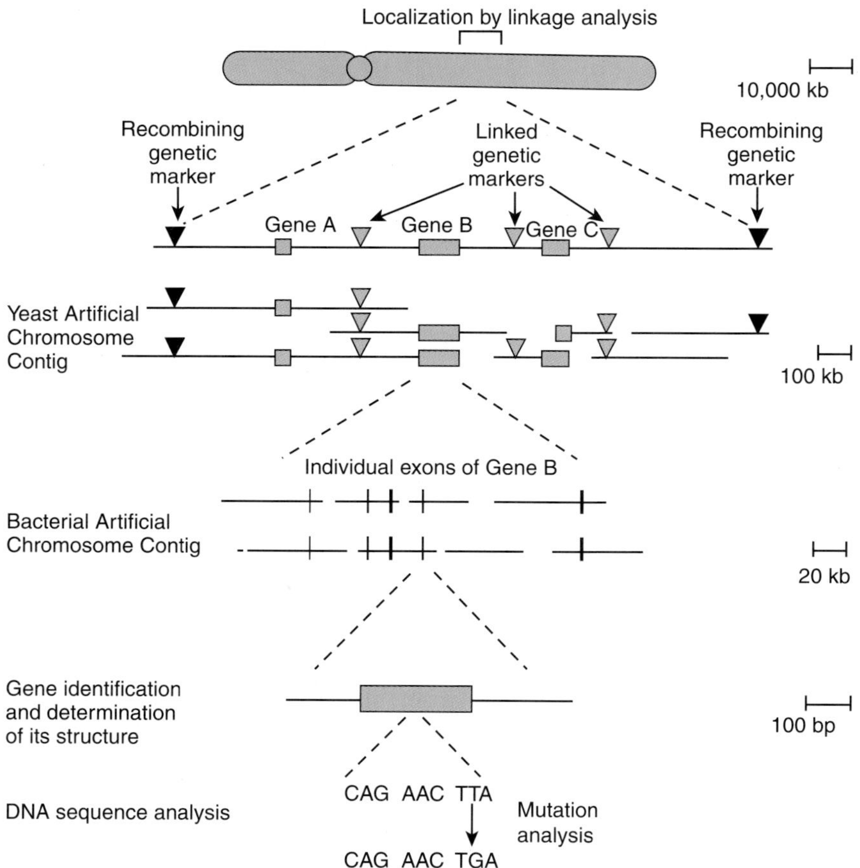


**Figure 8–20.** High-resolution mapping for cloning and analysis of a hypothetical disease gene. Mapping begins with genetic linkage analysis, with tightly linked markers within an interval defined by flanking markers that show recombination with the disease locus. Resolution increases from linkage analysis to cloning in yeast artificial chromosomes and bacterial artificial chromosomes, to gene isolation and characterization, and finally to identification of a molecular defect by DNA sequence determination.

The approach of cloning a gene purely on the basis of its *map position*, without knowing much if anything about what the gene does or what it might look like, is called **positional cloning** to distinguish it from the alternative strategy for gene identification in which one begins with a known protein, determines its amino acid sequence, and uses that information to isolate the gene (see Chapter 4).

### Positional Cloning Using Structural Chromosome Abnormalities: Duchenne Muscular Dystrophy

The X-linked *DMD* gene, in which mutations cause Duchenne muscular dystrophy and the less severe Becker allelic form (BMD), was one of the first disease genes localized by genetic linkage analysis and one of the first cloned by a positional strategy. The molecular genetics of DMD (and BMD) and the nature of the encoded protein, dystrophin, are discussed in Chapter 12. Once the gene was localized by linkage analysis to Xp21, successful cloning of the gene relied on two different approaches, both of which used DNA from unusual patients with DMD whose disease was the result of structural abnormalities involving the X chromosome.

In the first approach, the *DMD* gene was cloned by using DNA from a patient who had DMD plus three other genetic disorders due to the deletion of four genes resulting from a cytogenetically visible deletion of Xp21 (see Fig. 8–7). DNA sequences from Xp21 that were missing from the patient's X chromosome were isolated and tested in a panel of affected boys with *no* apparent cytogenetic deletion; some of these fragments were found to be deleted also in patients with much smaller, submicroscopic deletions. Further analysis of some of these fragments revealed them to be exons of the *DMD* gene.

The second approach took advantage of DNA samples from females with DMD. Females affected with DMD are very rare because the disease is an X-linked recessive disorder, but the etiology of DMD in these females became clear once cytogenetic investigations showed the patients carried balanced X;autosome translocations (see Chapter 10). The autosome involved differed in each case, but the site of the translocation on the X was always the same: Xp21. Researchers hypothesized that the break at Xp21 disrupted the *DMD* gene in these girls. DNA was isolated from the translocation breakpoint of an X;autosome translocation and used to search for and then identify gene sequences in the vicinity of the translocation breakpoint.

TABLE 8–4
**Methods Used in Physical Gene Mapping**

| Method | Goal | Typical Mapping Resolution (in base pairs) |
|---|---|---|
| Rodent/human somatic cell hybrids | Chromosome assignment | $50–250 \times 10^6$ |
| Rodent/human hybrids containing rearranged human chromosomes | Regional localization | $5–20 \times 10^6$ |
| Radiation hybrid mapping | Regional localization | $3.5–5 \times 10^5$ |
| Gene dosage analysis | X-chromosomal and regional localization | $5–20 \times 10^6$ |
| Fluorescence in situ hybridization (FISH) | Chromosome assignment and regional localization within a chromosome band | $1–2 \times 10^6$ |
| Long-range restriction mapping | Fine mapping of gene region | $10^5–10^6$ |
| Chromatin fiber FISH | Fine mapping of gene region and determining marker order | $10^5–10^6$ |
| Cloning in artificial chromosomes | Gene cloning (large fragments) | $10^5–10^6$ |
| Cloning in bacteria | Gene cloning (medium and small fragments) | $10^3–10^5$ |
| Polymerase chain reaction | Gene cloning and mapping | $10^2–10^4$ |
| DNA sequencing | Nucleotide sequence | 1 |

The cloning of the *DMD* gene and its cDNA has allowed intensive study of this disorder and its basic defect. Unlike the situation with CF (see next section), the majority of mutations in *DMD* are due to partial gene deletions.

### Positional Cloning Using Genetic Linkage Mapping: Cystic Fibrosis

Because of its relatively high frequency, particularly in Caucasian populations, and the nearly total lack of understanding of its underlying physiological pathogenesis, CF represented another prime target for positional cloning. Because no structural chromosome abnormalities were known to be involved in CF, genetic linkage mapping was used to localize and clone the gene. DNA samples from nearly 50 CF families were analyzed for linkage between CF and hundreds of DNA markers throughout the genome until linkage of CF to markers on the long arm of chromosome 7 was finally identified. Linkage to additional DNA markers in 7q31 to q32 narrowed the localization of the *CF* gene in this region of chromosome 7. Because of the large number of meioses available for study, it was possible to pinpoint the location of the *CF* locus between the *MET* and *D7S8* loci, two markers approximately 1500 kb apart that were shown to flank the *CF* locus by inspection of crossover events. The location of the gene was then narrowed even further to a region of some 500 kb by using more polymorphic markers between *MET* and *D7S8* to find additional individual crossovers in many hundreds of CF families studied worldwide.

**Linkage Disequilibrium in CF.** At this point, however, an unusual feature of CF genetics emerged: although the closest markers were still some distance from the *CF* gene, it became clear that 90 percent of CF chromosomes had a particular haplotype at loci tightly linked to CF (i.e., the alleles in coupling with the *CF* mutation at these loci), whereas only about 25 percent of normal (non-CF) chromosomes had this haplotype. This result, which is known as **linkage disequilibrium**, is in contradistinction to the linkage equilibrium usually observed between markers linked to a disease, such as with NF1 (discussed earlier) or DMD, in which the alleles at loci linked to the disease gene are different in different families. Linkage disequilibrium is defined as the preferential association of a disease gene with particular alleles at closely linked markers. The usual interpretation of linkage disequilibrium is that it is a founder effect (see Chapter 7) in which most chromosomes carrying the disease mutation are descended from a common ancestor. The ancestral genotype at markers in and around the mutant allele persists at a disproportionately high frequency on chromosomes carrying the disease mutation, as illustrated in Figure 8–21, because the markers are located too close to the gene for recombination to have shuffled different alleles into coupling with the disease allele. This model predicts that the highest degree of disequilibrium should be found closest to the disease mutation. This is because the closer the disease gene and the markers in linkage disequilibrium are, the less likely it is for the disease allele and the alleles at flanking markers that were present on the ancestral chromosome to have been separated through the generations by meiotic crossing over. Therefore, to take advantage of the existence of linkage disequilibrium for positional cloning, one should focus attention on regions with the highest degree of disequilibrium because these will generally be closest to the site of the ancestral mutation.

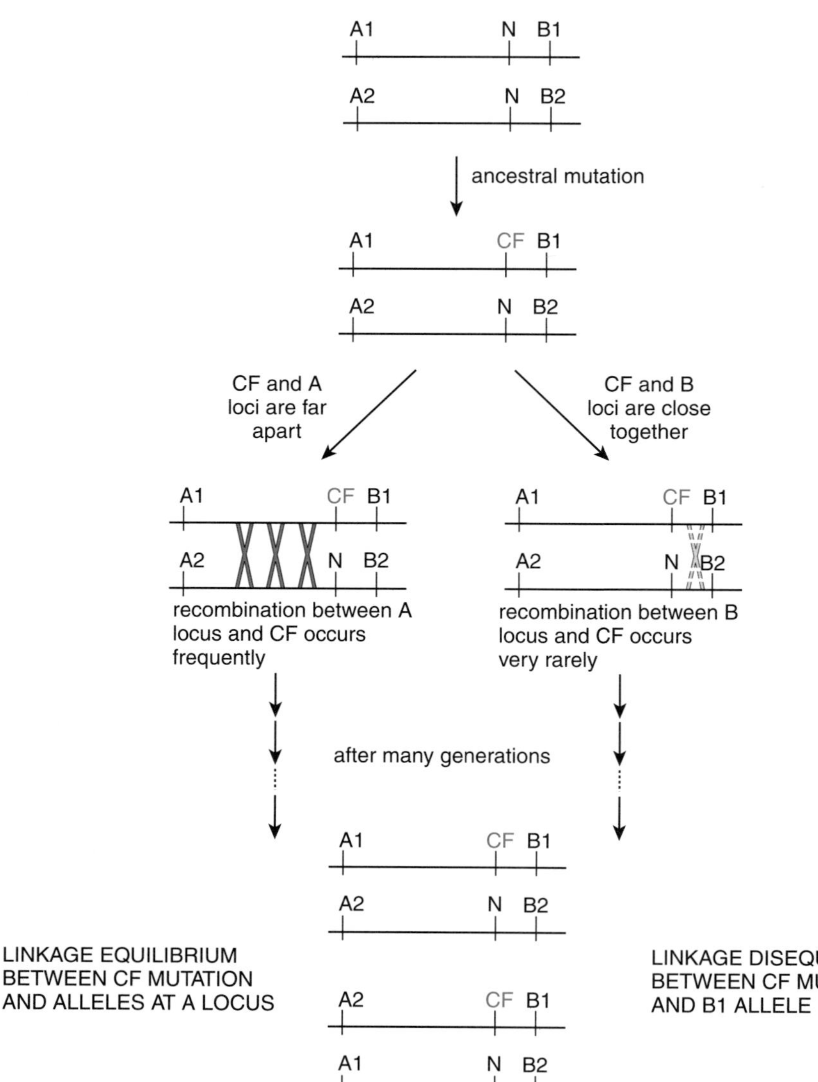


**Figure 8–21.** An explanation for linkage disequilibrium between a disease locus, such as cystic fibrosis, and a closely linked marker locus. Frequencies of haplotypes reach equilibrium if the marker locus is far enough away from the disease locus for many crossovers to have occurred through many generations, since the time of the original "ancestral" mutation. For markers very closely linked to the disease locus, little recombination has occurred, and thus the distribution of alleles observed in chromosomes with the *CF* mutation will resemble those present on the chromosome when the ancestral mutation occurred and not the present day distribution of haplotypes in the population.

The *CF* gene was isolated in 1989 after an intensive series of investigations that illustrate the importance of both physical and genetic mapping. First, all the genes located in the 500-kb interval of DNA believed to contain the *CF* gene needed to be identified. Two gene identification strategies were used: (1) the DNA sequence was examined for regions conserved through evolution, because conserved regions are more likely to represent genes, and (2) DNA fragments from the region were tested to see whether they contained segments that corresponded to mRNA transcripts. Four genes were identified within the interval that was known to contain the *CF* gene by linkage mapping. Only one of the genes showed a molecular defect in patients with CF: a 3 base-pair deletion in the coding sequence was found in approximately 70 percent of all CF chromosomes in Northern European populations but never in normal alleles at this locus. Since 1989, more than 900 different mutations causing CF have been identified in many ethnic groups around the world (see Chapter 12).

### Cloning Disease Genes by Combining Functional and Positional Information: Retinitis Pigmentosa

The hereditary eye disease RP illustrates still another strategy for identifying disease genes. RP is a group of inherited diseases associated with retinal degeneration that, initially, predominantly affects the rod photoreceptors. Clinical features typically include reduced night and peripheral vision in the early stages, but progression to complete blindness is a common outcome. RP is a major cause of blindness in humans, with an estimated prevalence of about 1 in 4000. On the basis of its mode of inheritance alone, RP shows clear locus heterogeneity, because 30 percent of pedigrees can be classified as X-linked, whereas the rest are autosomal (25 percent dominant, 45 percent recessive).

Autosomal dominant RP has been further subclassified clinically on the basis of age of onset and differential patterns of rod and cone degeneration. Because this clinical heterogeneity raised the possibility of multiple responsible loci, linkage studies have concentrated on single large pedigrees, rather than on a collection of smaller ones, and have revealed at least 12 distinct loci for the autosomal dominant forms of RP.

In one large Irish pedigree, very close linkage of RP to a marker locus on the long arm of chromosome 3 was demonstrated. The mapping of autosomal dominant RP to the long arm of chromosome 3 immediately suggested a strong **candidate gene** for the *RP* locus: the gene for rhodopsin, a critical photosensitive rod photoreceptor protein. The gene for rhodopsin had previously also been assigned to the long arm of chromosome 3, and mutations in this gene, therefore, might be responsible for RP in this family. Indeed, a single base mutation was ultimately identified in the rhodopsin gene in this family, and more than 100 other different mutations have subsequently been found in the rhodopsin gene in other RP patients. In other families with autosomal dominant RP, the inherited defect does *not* cosegregate with polymorphisms at the rhodopsin locus. In these families, mutations in other autosomal genes are responsible, and several of these genes have also been identified.

### Cloning Disease Genes by Combining Functional and Positional Information: Hereditary Nonpolyposis Colon Cancer

Another striking example of successful disease gene identification is illustrated by an autosomal dominant familial colon cancer syndrome known as hereditary nonpolyposis colon cancer (HNPCC) (see Chapter 16). The name HNPCC is meant to distinguish this form of autosomal dominant colon cancer from another disorder, familial adenomatous polyposis of the colon (FAP), in which patients develop hundreds to thousands of colonic polyps that undergo malignant transformation (see Chapter 16).

Linkage analysis in families with autosomal dominant HNPCC revealed immediately that there was locus heterogeneity: some families, but not all, showed linkage to the short arm of chromosome 2 (called *HNPCC1*), others showed linkage to chromosome 3p (*HNPCC2*), and a few to neither 2p or 3p. Most surprisingly, however, when the genotypes of patients with the disease were determined both in blood and tumor DNA using microsatellite markers on 2p and elsewhere, the DNA from the cancer was found to contain more than two alleles, many of which had tandem repeat lengths not found in the DNA from the blood of the same patient. These numerous new alleles in tumor tissue suggested that the DNA in the tumor was actually unstable and that short tandem repeat polymorphisms throughout the genome were not being replicated faithfully during mitosis. Such **microsatellite instability**, discussed further in Chapter 16, had been seen before: in yeast defective for a DNA mismatch repair gene called *MSH2* (an obscure acronym for *mutS* homolog, a term derived from the similarity between the yeast gene and a bacterial DNA repair gene called *mutS*). When the human gene most closely related to yeast *MSH2* was mapped to chromosome 2p16, the human gene, also called *MSH2*, quickly became a leading candidate for HNPCC1. Indeed, patients with HNPCC linked to chromosome 2p were found to be heterozygotes for mutations that inactivate the human *MSH2* gene. Carriers of *MSH2* mutations develop colon cancer when their other, normal copy of the gene is lost or mutated in an epithelial cell lining the colon. The DNA in that cell becomes unstable because mismatch repair during cell division is disrupted leading to numerous secondary mutations, some of which inevitably inactivate genes important to the control of cell growth (see Chapter 16).

The discovery of mutations in the *MSH2* gene as a cause of a large fraction of HNPCC (those families with HNPCC1 linked to chromosome 2p) led almost immediately to the elucidation of the genetic cause for HNPCC in other families whose disease was *not* linked to 2p. Chromosome 3p was the known location of another human gene, *MLH1* (standing for *mutL* homolog) that showed strong similarity to the DNA repair proteins *MLH1* in yeast and *mutL* in bacteria. The discovery of the role of *MSH2* in HNPCC1 made *MLH1* a strong candidate for the gene involved in HNPCC2. This hypothesis was quickly confirmed by the discovery of *MLH1* mutations in HNPCC2 (see Chapter 16).

### The Candidate Gene Approach

Identification of rhodopsin as the gene underlying at least one form of autosomal dominant RP or the discovery of *MSH2* and *MLH1* as causes of HNPCC illustrate how genes of known function can become strong candidates for disease loci when (1) the function of the gene relates in some way to what is known about the pathogenesis of the disease, and (2) the candidate gene maps to the same region of the genome as does the disease gene. A variety of methods for finding mutations (see Chapter 4) are then used to screen the candidate gene for defects in a group of patients. Contrast the candidate gene approach to the purely positional methodology used to identify the genes involved in CF and DMD: in those cases, the successful isolation of the responsible genes was not based on any features of the gene other than chromosomal location.

The success of the candidate gene approach illustrates nicely the value of gene mapping. Rhodopsin was originally cloned and mapped for reasons unrelated to RP; *MSH2* and *MLH1* were identified because of their fundamental role in protecting the fidelity of

DNA during replication. If these genes had not been placed on the gene map, however, it is unlikely that the defect in these disorders would have been uncovered so quickly. The candidate gene approach allows the raising and testing of hypotheses about the cause of an inherited disease based on the disease phenotype (at the clinical and cellular level), the map positions of the disease locus and the candidate gene, and the role of candidate proteins in the relevant tissue.

### Expressed Sequence Tags

The positional candidate gene approach to cloning a disease gene requires that the function and position of the gene be known so that an assessment can be made of whether the gene is a reasonable candidate locus for the disease. The more genes that are known and mapped, the more candidates one has once a disease gene is mapped to a location in the genome. In addition to the known, mapped genes listed in public databases, an important supplementary source of candidate genes for disease loci is the growing collection of **expressed sequence tags** (ESTs). ESTs are partial cDNA sequences obtained by sequencing clones, chosen at random, from a wide variety of cDNA libraries made from many different tissues (see Chapter 4). Each EST corresponds to a transcribed gene, and each EST sequence is sufficient to specify (or "tag") the gene to which it corresponds uniquely. Although most ESTs contain sequences that correspond to hitherto unknown and uncharacterized genes, many have sequence homology to known genes in humans or other organisms, or both, which provides some clues as to function. Computerized molecular genetics databases already contain millions of entries of EST sequences. As more and more ESTs are mapped, the genes to which these ESTs correspond are becoming a rich source of additional candidates to consider when a disease gene has been mapped in the neighborhood.

## THE HUMAN GENOME PROJECT

Human and medical geneticists have been identifying and mapping genes for decades. However, a radical departure to the "map-as-map-can" approach was proposed in 1986 by Dulbecco, who suggested that if scientists really wanted to understand the role of genes in cancer—not to mention in genetic disorders in general—all they had to do was sequence the entire 3 billion base pairs and find all the genes! After much discussion and debate, the Human Genome Project, an international effort to first map and eventually sequence all of the estimated 50,000 genes, was born. The initial emphasis of the project was on building both physical and genetic linkage maps of all 22 autosomes and the sex chromosomes and on assembling overlapping collections of clones, or contigs, covering each chromosome from telomere to telomere, in order to facilitate gene identification, isolation, and sequencing of the entire human genome.

The number of mapped loci in the human genome has increased exponentially since the early 1980s. No static description can possibly do justice to the enormous amount of information on human gene discovery and mapping that is accumulating rapidly through the Human Genome Project and other related efforts. At this time, physical and genetic mapping strategies have contributed to the development of a human gene map that now includes more than 6000 mapped genes. For many genes involved in human diseases, mapping methods can be immediately translated into diagnostic assays for presymptomatic or prenatal detection. In addition, as the relevant disease genes are cloned and characterized, many by positional cloning strategies, an enormous increase in the understanding of the molecular basis of human genetic disease is expected to result. In addition to the known disease genes that have been mapped and characterized, there is an even greater number of mapped unique ESTs representing additional genes that we know must be transcribed into mRNA but their full length sequences are unknown and their functions are under investigation. Finally, as the Human Genome Project races to its conclusion, all of the approximately 50,000 genes in the human genome will be uncovered by sequencing of genomic DNA and their precise sequence and map position known. As illustrated by the candidate gene approach, the involvement of many of these genes in an inherited condition is expected to become apparent over time. Much of the progress to date has been made in single-gene disorders, which is not surprising given the emphasis of current approaches on pedigree analysis and linkage detection. In the future, however, it is likely that more progress will be made in unraveling the genetic components involved in conditions such as hypertension, behavioral disorders, and cancer (see Chapters 15 and 16). Gene mapping strategies, together with sophisticated methods for pedigree analysis, are just beginning to be applied to these more complex disorders.

The accelerating pace of gene mapping and disease gene discovery depends on critical technological advances in two areas. One is in the realm of molecular biology. In Chapter 4 and in this chapter, we have discussed the techniques that are the underpinning of the effort to map and sequence the human genome and discover disease genes (see Table 8–3). Hand in hand with the explosive growth of technology for molecular biology has been the equally important development and expansion of electronic databases of genetic information from human and other organisms. These databases, and the software for analyzing and comparing the data, allow the integration of disparate types of data such as genomic and cDNA sequence information, genetic and physical maps, studies of gene structure and function, descriptions of disease phenotypes, and catalogs of mutations responsible for disease. Most of these databases are accessible directly through the National Center for Biotechnology of the National Library of Medicine, including Online Mendelian Inheritance in Man, or through links on the homepage of the National Human Genome Research Institute.

With the Human Genome Project's focus on human gene mapping and sequencing, a map of the estimated 50,000 human genes including the complete sequence of at least one human genome will be available by the year 2001. The combined approach of linkage analysis to assign a particular gene for an inherited disorder to a specific chromosomal region, followed by positional cloning or candidate gene strategies to identify the responsible gene and establish the molecular defect or defects, should continue to reap a bountiful harvest.

## General References

Green ED (2000) The Human Genome Project and its impact on the study of human disease. *In* Scriver CR, Beaudet AL, Sly WS, Valle D, et al (eds) The Metabolic and Molecular Bases of Inherited Disease, 8th ed. McGraw-Hill, New York.

McKusick VA (1998) Mendelian Inheritance in Man: Catalogs of Autosomal Dominant, Autosomal Recessive, and X-Linked Phenotypes, 12th ed. Johns Hopkins University Press, Baltimore.

Terwilliger JD, Ott J (1994) Handbook of Human Genetic Linkage. Johns Hopkins University Press, Baltimore.

White R (1998) Mapping markers and genes in the human genome. *In* Singer M, Berg P (eds) Exploring Genetic Mechanisms. University Science Books, Sausalito, California, pp. 271–300.

## References Specific to Particular Topics

Collins FS (1997) Sequencing the human genome. Hosp Practice 32:35–54.

Dulbecco R (1986) A turning point in cancer research: Sequencing the human genome. Science 231:1055–1056.

Gardiner K, Patterson D (1992) The role of somatic cell hybrids in physical mapping. Cytogenet Cell Genet 59:82–85.

Kerem B, Rommens JM, Buchanan JA, Markiewicz, D, et al (1989). Identification of the cystic fibrosis gene: Genetic analysis. Science 245:1073–1080.

McCarthy LC (1996) Whole genome radiation hybrid mapping. Trends Genet 12:491–493.

The International Human Sequencing Consortium (2001) The human genome: Sequencing and initial analysis. Nature.

White R, Lalouel JM (1988) Chromosome mapping with DNA markers. Sci Am 258:40–48.

Zallen DT, Burian RM (1992) On the beginnings of somatic cell hybridization: Boris Ephrussi and chromosome transplantation. Genetics 132:1–8.

## URLs for Genome Project Databases

NHGRI *http://www.nhgri.nih.gov*. Homepage of National Human Genome Research Institute. Up-to-date information on the status of the Human Genome Project and access to detailed chromosome specific physical maps. Links to many other sites at *http://www.nhgri.nih.gov/Data/*

NCBI *http://www.ncbi.nlm.nih.gov*. National Center for Biotechnology Information, a division of the National Library of Medicine. DNA sequence repository for cloned genes, genomic sequence, and expressed sequence tags.

OMIM *http://www3.ncbi.nlm.nih.gov/Omim*. Online version of Mendelian Inheritance in Man. An online, searchable "knowledge base" of human genetic disorders including clinical description, genetic data, and molecular characterization of known disease genes.

Whitehead Genome Institute *http://www-genome.wi.mit.edu*. Genome Center based at the Whitehead Institute at the Massachusetts Institute of Technology. Physical contig maps of all human chromosomes.

Cooperative Human Linkage Center *http://www.chlc.org*. United States Genetic Mapping Program. Extensive database of polymorphic markers and genetic maps.

Sanger Center *http://www.sanger.ac.uk/* Large-scale sequencing center at Sanger Center in Cambridge, England.

Généthon *http://www.genethon.fr/genethon_en.html*. French Genetic Mapping Program. Extensive database of polymorphic markers and genetic maps.

## Problems

1. The Huntington disease (*HD*) locus was found to be tightly linked to a DNA polymorphism on chromosome 4. In the same study, however, linkage was ruled out between *HD* and the locus for the MNSs blood group polymorphism, which also maps to chromosome 4. What is the explanation?

2. Linkage disequilibrium was an important observation in the positional cloning of the cystic fibrosis gene. Referring to Chapters 5 and 12 as necessary, would you expect to find linkage disequilibrium for an autosomal dominant disease such as HD? Type 1 neurofibromatosis? Why or why not?

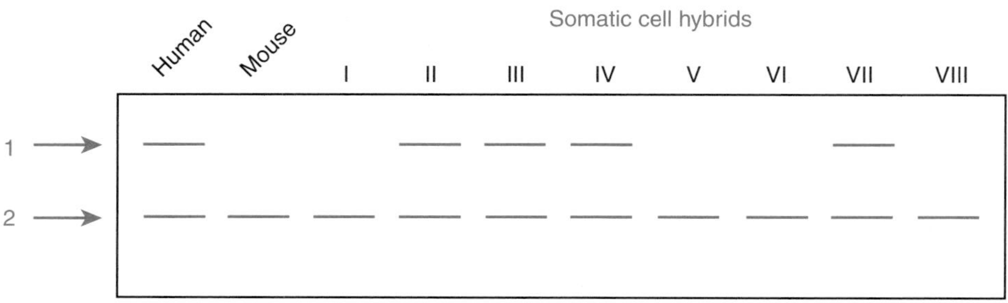


Southern blot data for question 3

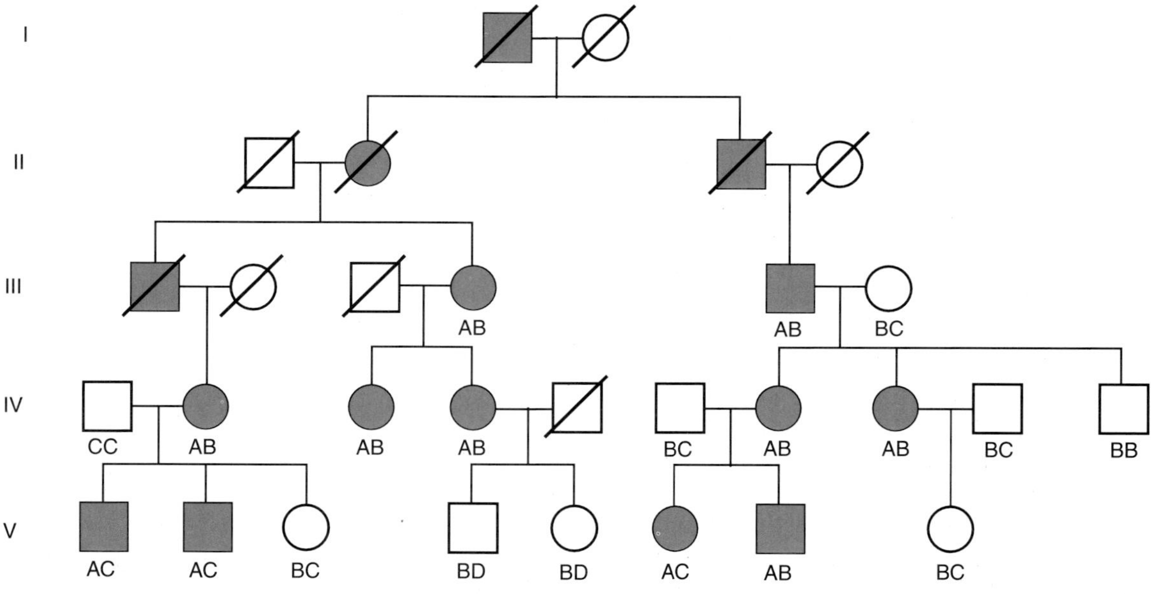


Pedigree for question 5

3. The data shown were obtained with a human cDNA probe for gene *Q* in the same panel of rodent/human somatic cell hybrids analyzed in Figure 8–3 and Table 8–1. What do you conclude about fragment 1 in the Southern blot? Fragment 2? In reference to Table 8–1, where does the *Q* gene map?

4. Linkage between a polymorphism in the α-globin locus on the short arm of chromosome 16 and autosomal dominant polycystic kidney disease, a common and progressive multiorgan condition, was analyzed in a series of British and Dutch families, with the following data:

| $\theta$ | 0.00 | 0.01 | 0.10 | 0.20 | 0.30 | 0.40 |
|---|---|---|---|---|---|---|
| Lod scores (*Z*) | $-\infty$ | 23.4 | 24.6 | 19.5 | 12.85 | 5.5 |

$Z_{max} = 25.85$ at $\theta_{max} = 0.05$

How would you interpret these data?

In a subsequent study, a large family from Sicily with polycystic kidney disease was also investigated for linkage to α-globin, with the following results:

| $\theta$ | 0.00 | 0.10 | 0.20 | 0.30 | 0.40 |
|---|---|---|---|---|---|
| Lod scores (*Z*) | $-\infty$ | −8.34 | −3.34 | −1.05 | −0.02 |

How would you interpret the data in this second study? What implications do these data have for use of linkage information in presymptomatic diagnosis and genetic counseling?

5. The following data were obtained in a study designed to test the hypothesis that a defect in a gene for γ-crystallin, one of the major proteins of the eye lens, may be responsible for the inherited eye defect in Coppock's cataract, an autosomal dominant disorder. The filled-in symbols in the pedigree indicate family members with cataracts. The letters indicate DNA haplotypes at the polymorphic γ-crystallin locus on chromosome 2, detected with a cDNA clone. What would you conclude from this study? What additional studies might be performed to confirm or reject the hypothesis?

6. The following pedigree shows an example of molecular diagnosis in Wiskott-Aldrich syndrome, an X-linked immunodeficiency, by using a linked DNA polymorphism with a map distance of approximately 5 cM between the polymorphic locus and the Wiskott-Aldrich syndrome gene. What is the likely phase in the carrier mother? How did you determine this? What diagnosis would you make regarding the current prenatal diagnosis?

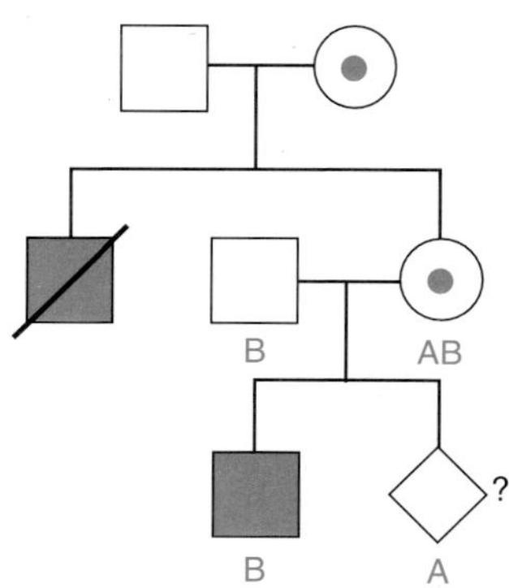


Pedigree for questions 6 and 7

7. In the family described in Question 6, the maternal grandfather becomes available for DNA testing and shows allele *B* at the linked locus. How does this finding affect your determination of phase in the mother? What can you conclude about the affected son? What further studies might be performed to verify this? What diagnosis would you make now in regard to the current prenatal diagnosis?

8. What are some of the implications of knowing the map position of a particular gene for medical genetics? In other words, why map genes?

9. What is the one region of the genome for which radiation hybrid mapping is not possible when performed as described using $HPRT^{-}$ rodent cells? How can that region of the genome be mapped by radiation hybrids?

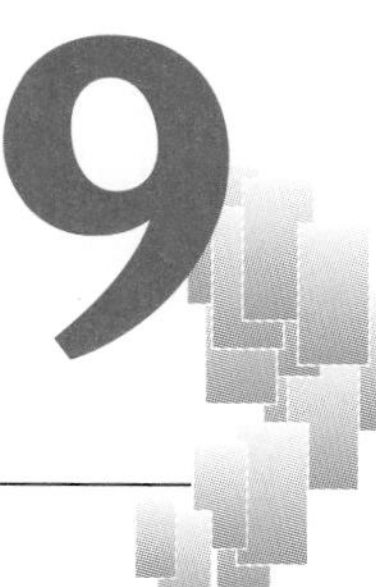

# Principles of Clinical Cytogenetics

Clinical cytogenetics is the study of chromosomes, their structure and their inheritance, as applied to the practice of medical genetics. It has been apparent for more than 40 years that microscopically visible changes in the number or structure of chromosomes could account for a number of clinical conditions. Today, chromosome analysis—now with dramatically improved resolution and precision—is an increasingly important diagnostic procedure in numerous areas of clinical medicine.

Chromosome disorders form a major category of genetic disease. They account for a large proportion of all reproductive wastage, congenital malformations, and mental retardation and play an important role in the pathogenesis of malignancy. Specific chromosome abnormalities are responsible for more than 100 identifiable syndromes that are collectively more common than all the mendelian single-gene disorders together. Cytogenetic disorders are present in nearly 1 percent of live births, in about 2 percent of pregnancies in women older than 35 years who undergo prenatal diagnosis, and in fully half of all spontaneous first-trimester abortions.

In this chapter, we discuss the general principles of clinical cytogenetics and the various types of numerical and structural abnormalities observed in human karyotypes. Some of the most common and best-known abnormalities of the autosomes and the sex chromosomes are described in the next chapter.

## INTRODUCTION TO CYTOGENETICS

The general morphology and organization of human chromosomes, as well as their molecular composition, were introduced in Chapters 2 and 3. To perform a chromosome analysis for routine clinical purposes, cells must be capable of growth and rapid division in culture. The most readily accessible cells that meet this requirement are white blood cells, specifically T lymphocytes. To prepare a short-term culture of these cells suitable for analysis, a sample of peripheral blood is obtained, usually by venipuncture, and mixed with heparin to prevent clotting. The white blood cells are collected, placed in tissue culture medium, and stimulated to divide. After a few days, the dividing cells are arrested in **metaphase** with chemicals that inhibit the mitotic spindle, collected, and treated with a hypotonic solution to release the chromosomes. Chromosomes are then fixed, spread on slides, and stained by one of several techniques, depending on the particular diagnostic procedure being performed. They are then ready for analysis.

### Clinical Indications for Chromosome Analysis

Chromosome analysis is indicated as a routine diagnostic procedure for a number of specific phenotypes encountered in clinical medicine, as described in this chapter and in Chapter 10. In addition, there are also some nonspecific general clinical situations and findings that indicate a need for cytogenetic analysis:

1. **Problems of early growth and development**. Failure to thrive, developmental delay, dysmorphic facies, multiple malformations, short stature, ambiguous genitalia, and mental retardation are frequent findings in children with chromosome abnormalities, although not restricted to that group. Unless there is a definite nonchromosomal diagnosis, chromosome analysis should be performed for patients presenting with a combination of such problems.
2. **Stillbirth and neonatal death**. The incidence of chromosome abnormalities is much higher among stillbirths (up to approximately 10 percent) than

among live births (about 0.7 percent). It is also elevated among infants who die in the neonatal period (about 10 percent). Chromosome analysis should be performed for all stillbirths and neonatal deaths that might have a cytogenetic basis to identify a possible specific cause or, alternatively, to rule out chromosome abnormality as the reason for the loss. In such cases, karyotyping is essential for accurate genetic counseling and may provide important information for prenatal diagnosis in future pregnancies.

3. **Fertility problems**. Chromosome studies are indicated for women presenting with amenorrhea and for couples with a history of infertility or habitual abortion. A chromosome abnormality is seen in one or the other parent in a significant proportion (3 to 6 percent) of cases in which there is infertility or two or more miscarriages.
4. **Family history**. A known or suspected chromosome abnormality in a first-degree relative is an indication for chromosome analysis under some circumstances.
5. **Neoplasia**. Virtually all cancers are associated with one or more chromosome abnormalities (see Chapter 16). Chromosome evaluation in the appropriate tissue sample (the tumor itself or bone marrow in the case of hematologic malignancies) can provide useful diagnostic or prognostic information.
6. **Pregnancy in a woman of advanced age**. There is an increased risk of chromosome abnormality in fetuses conceived by women older than the age of 30 to 35 years (see Chapter 18). Fetal chromosome analysis should be offered as a routine part of prenatal care in such pregnancies.

Although ideal for rapid clinical analysis, cell cultures prepared from peripheral blood have the disadvantage of being short-lived (3 to 4 days). Long-term cultures can be derived from a variety of other tissues (see Chapter 8). Skin biopsy, a minor surgical procedure, can provide samples of tissue that in culture produce **fibroblasts**, which can be used for a variety of biochemical and molecular studies, as well as for chromosome analysis. White blood cells can also be transformed in culture to form **lymphoblastoid** cell lines that are potentially immortal. **Bone marrow** can be obtained only by the relatively invasive procedure of marrow biopsy, but it has the advantage of containing a high proportion of dividing cells, so that little if any culturing is required. Its main use is in the diagnosis of suspected hematological malignancies. Its disadvantage is that the chromosome preparations obtained from marrow are relatively poor, with short, poorly resolved chromosomes that are more difficult to analyze than are those from peripheral blood. **Fetal cells** derived from amniotic fluid (amniocytes) or obtained by chorionic villus biopsy can also be cultured successfully for cytogenetic, biochemical, or molecular analysis. Chorionic villus cells can also be analyzed directly, without the need for culturing (see Chapter 18 for further discussion).

## Chromosome Identification

The 24 types of human chromosome can be readily identified by a number of specific staining procedures. There are three commonly used staining methods that can distinguish among human chromosomes. In Chapter 2, we examined chromosomes stained by Giemsa banding (**G banding**), the most common method used in clinical laboratories. Other procedures used in some laboratories or for specific purposes, or both, include the following:

**Q Banding.** This method requires staining with quinacrine mustard or related compounds and examination by fluorescence microscopy. The chromosomes stain in a specific pattern of bright and dim bands (Q bands), the bright Q bands corresponding almost exactly to the dark G bands. Q banding, as well as C banding (see next section), is particularly useful for detecting occasional variants in chromosome morphology or staining, called **heteromorphisms**. These variants are generally benign and reflect differences in the amount or type of satellite DNA sequences at a particular location along a chromosome.

**R Banding.** If the chromosomes receive special treatment (such as heating) before staining, the resulting dark and light bands (R bands) are the reverse of those produced by G or Q banding. Especially when examining regions that stain poorly by G or Q banding, R banding gives a pattern that is easier to analyze than that given by G or Q banding. It is the standard method in some laboratories, particularly in Europe.

A uniform system of chromosome classification is internationally accepted for identification of human chromosomes stained by any of the three staining procedures mentioned. Figure 9–1 is an ideogram of the banding pattern of a set of normal human chromosomes at metaphase, illustrating the alternating pattern of dark and light bands used for chromosome identification. The pattern of bands on each chromosome is numbered on each arm from the centromere to the telomere, as shown in detail in Figure 9–2 for several chromosomes. Using this numbering system, the location of any particular band, as well as the DNA sequences and genes within it, and its involvement in a chromosomal abnormality can be described unambiguously and precisely.

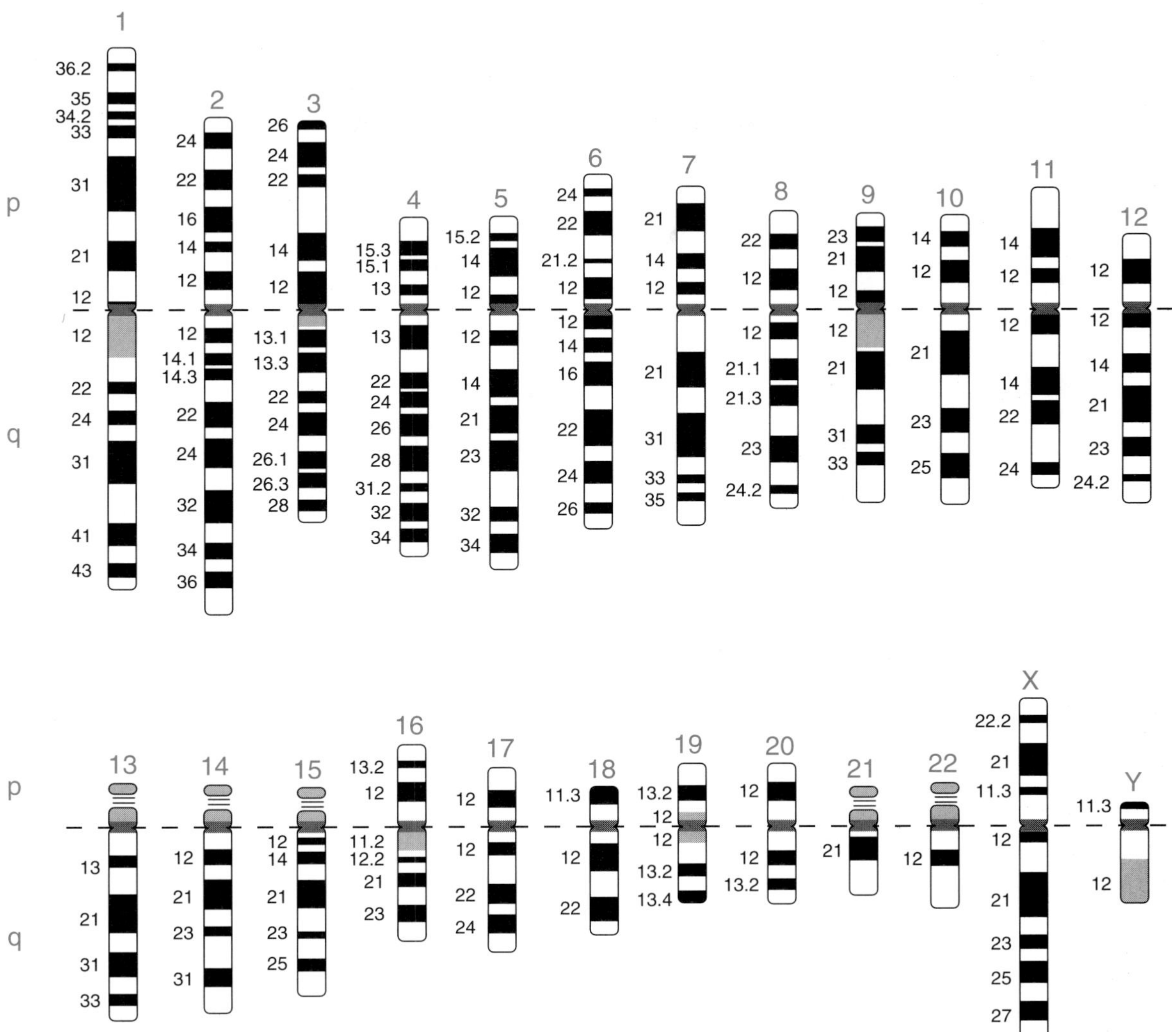


**Figure 9–1.** Ideogram showing G-banding patterns for human chromosomes at metaphase, with about 400 bands per haploid karyotype. As drawn, chromosomes are typically represented with the sister chromatids so closely aligned that they are not recognized as distinct structures. Centromeres are indicated by the narrow dark gray regions separating the p and q arms. For convenience and clarity, only the G-positive bands are numbered. For examples of full numbering scheme, see Figure 9–2. (Redrawn from ISCN, 1995.)

Human chromosomes are often classified by the position of the **centromere** into three types that can be easily distinguished at metaphase (see Fig. 9–1): **metacentric**, with a more or less central centromere and arms of approximately equal length; **submetacentric**, with an off-center centromere and arms of clearly different lengths; and **acrocentric**, with the centromere near one end. A potential fourth type, **telocentric**, with the centromere at one end and only a single arm, does not occur in the normal human karyotype, but it is occasionally observed in chromosome rearrangements and is a common type in some other species. The human acrocentric chromosomes (chromosomes 13, 14, 15, 21, and 22) have small, distinctive masses of chromatin known as **satellites** attached to their short arms by narrow stalks (secondary constrictions). The stalks of these five chromosome pairs contain hundreds of copies of genes encoding ribosomal RNA.

## Special Procedures

For particular situations, a number of specialized techniques can be used:

**C Banding.** This method specifically involves staining the centromeric region of each chromosome and other regions containing **constitutive heterochromatin**: namely, sections of chromosomes 1q, 9q, and 16q adjacent to the centromere and the distal part of Yq. Heterochromatin is the type of chromatin defined by its property of remaining in the condensed state and staining darkly in nondividing (interphase) cells.

**High-Resolution Banding** (also called **prometaphase banding**). This type of banding is achieved through G-banding or R-banding techniques to stain chromosomes that have been obtained at an early

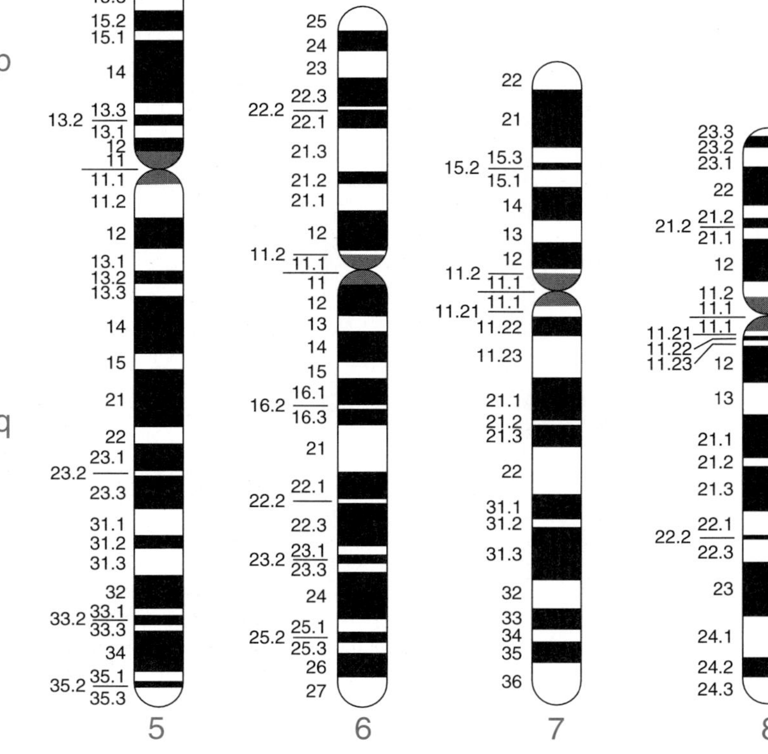


**Figure 9–2.** Examples of G-banding patterns for chromosomes 5, 6, 7, and 8 at the 550-band stage of condensation. Band numbers permit unambiguous identification of each G-positive or G-negative band, e.g., chromosome 5p15.2 or chromosome 8q24.2. (Redrawn from ISCN, 1995.)

stage of mitosis (prophase or prometaphase), when they are still in a relatively uncondensed state (see Chapter 2). High-resolution banding is especially useful when a subtle structural abnormality of a chromosome is suspected; some laboratories, however, routinely use prometaphase banding, as shown in Figures 2–3 and 2–4. Prometaphase chromosomes reveal 550 to 850 bands or even more in a haploid set, whereas standard metaphase preparations show only about 450. A comparison of the banding patterns of the X chromosome at three different stages of resolution is shown in Figure 9–3. The increase in diagnostic precision obtained with these longer chromosomes is evident.

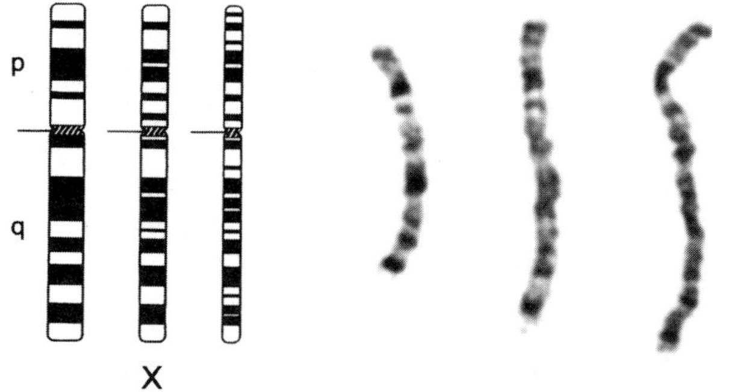


**Figure 9–3.** The X chromosome: ideograms and photomicrographs at metaphase, prometaphase, and prophase (*left* to *right*). (Ideograms redrawn from ISCN, 1995; photomicrographs courtesy of Yim Kwan Ng, The Hospital for Sick Children, Toronto.)

**Fragile Sites.** Fragile sites are nonstaining gaps that are occasionally observed in characteristic sites on several chromosomes. To demonstrate fragile sites, it is usually necessary to expose the cells to growth conditions or chemicals that alter or inhibit DNA synthesis. Many fragile sites are known to be heritable variants. The fragile site most clearly shown to be clinically significant is seen near the end of Xq both in males with a specific and quite common form of X-linked mental retardation and in some female carriers of the same genetic defect (see discussion of the **fragile X syndrome**, Chapter 12). In conjunction with molecular testing to detect expansion of the CGG repeat in the *FMR1* gene characteristic of this disorder, detection of the fragile site on the X chromosome is a diagnostic procedure specific for the fragile X syndrome (see Fig. 12–28).

## Fluorescence In Situ Hybridization

As introduced in Chapter 4, the development of fluorescence in situ hybridization (**FISH**) techniques to examine the presence or absence of a particular DNA sequence or to evaluate the number or organization of a chromosome or chromosomal region has revolutionized both research and clinical cytogenetics. This confluence of molecular and cytogenetic approaches—**molecular cytogenetics**—has dramat-

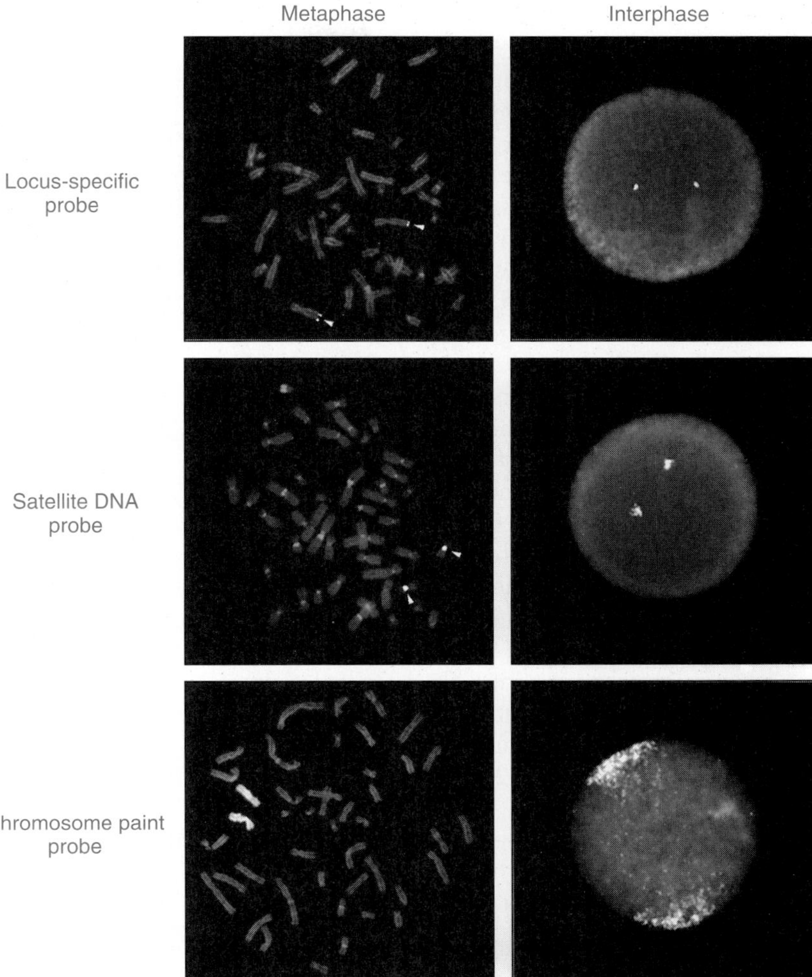


**Figure 9–4.** Fluorescence in situ hybridization to human chromosomes at metaphase and interphase, using three different types of DNA probe. *Top*, A single-copy DNA probe specific for the factor VIII gene on the X chromosome. *Middle*, A repetitive alpha satellite DNA probe specific for the centromere of chromosome 17. *Bottom*, A whole chromosome "paint" probe specific for the X chromosome. (Images courtesy of Karen Gustashaw, Case Western Reserve University.)

ically expanded both the range and precision of routine chromosome analysis.

In FISH, DNA probes specific for individual chromosomes, chromosomal regions, or genes can be used to identify particular chromosomal rearrangements or to rapidly diagnose the existence of an abnormal chromosome number in clinical material (Fig. 9–4). Suitable probes can be prepared by any number of techniques introduced in Chapter 4. Gene-specific or locus-specific probes can be used to detect the presence, absence, or location of a particular gene (see Fig. 8–8), both in metaphase chromosomes and in interphase cells. Repetitive DNA probes allow detection of satellite DNA or other repeated DNA elements (such as the repeated TTAGGG hexamer found at human telomeres) (see Fig 9-5*A*, *color insert*) at specific chromosomal loci including centromeres, telomeres, or regions of heterochromatin; satellite DNA probes, especially those belonging to the alpha satellite family of centromere repeats (see Chapter 3), are extremely useful for determining the number of copies of a particular chromosome (see Fig. 9–4). Last, probes for entire chromosomes or chromosome arms contain a mixture of single-copy DNA sequences that map along the length of the entire chromosome (or arm). These probes "paint" the target chromosome (both in metaphase and in interphase); a comparison of the two images, as in Figure 9–4, visually documents the dynamic nature of chromosome condensation and decondensation throughout the cell cycle, as introduced in Chapter 2 (compare with Fig. 2–5).

One of the more important applications of FISH technology in clinical cytogenetics involves the use of different fluorochromes to detect multiple probes simultaneously. Two-color and three-color applications are routinely used to diagnose specific deletions, duplications, or rearrangements, both in prometaphase or metaphase preparations, as well as in interphase. With highly specialized imaging procedures, it is even possible to detect and distinguish 24 different colors simultaneously by spectral karyotyping (SKY; see Chapter 4), allowing dramatic evaluation of the karyotype in a single experiment (see Figs. 9–5*B* and 9–5*C*, *color insert*).

## CHROMOSOME ABNORMALITIES

Abnormalities of chromosomes may be either numerical or structural and may involve one or more autosomes, sex chromosomes, or both simultaneously. By far the most common type of clinically significant chromosome abnormality is **aneuploidy**, an abnormal chromosome number due to an extra or missing chromosome, which is always associated with physical or mental maldevelopment, or both. **Reciprocal translocations** (an exchange of segments between nonhomologous chromosomes) are also relatively common but usually have no phenotypic effect, although, as explained later, there may be an associated increased risk of abnormal offspring. The clinical and social impact of chromosome abnormalities is enormous. The relative frequencies of numerical and structural abnormalities observed in spontaneous abortions, in fetuses of mothers older than 35 years of age that are analyzed in amniocentesis, and in live births are presented in Table 9–1.

Chromosome abnormalities are described using a standard set of abbreviations and nomenclature. These abbreviations and examples of abnormal karyotypes are listed in Table 9–2.

### Abnormalities of Chromosome Number

A chromosome complement with any chromosome number other than 46 is said to be **heteroploid**. An exact multiple of the haploid chromosome number (n) is called **euploid**, and any other chromosome number is **aneuploid**.

#### TRIPLOIDY AND TETRAPLOIDY

In addition to the diploid (2n) number characteristic of normal somatic cells, two other euploid chromosome complements, **triploid** (3n) and **tetraploid** (4n), are occasionally reported. Both triploidy and tetraploidy have been seen in fetuses, and although triploid infants can be liveborn, they do not survive long. Triploidy most frequently results from fertilization by two sperm (dispermy). Failure of one of the meiotic divisions, resulting in a diploid egg or sperm, can also account for a proportion of cases. The phenotypic expression of a triploid karyotype depends on the source of the extra chromosome set; triploids with an extra set of paternal chromosomes typically have an abnormal placenta and are classified as **partial hydatidiform moles** (see later section), but those with an additional set of maternal chromosomes are spontaneously aborted earlier in pregnancy. Tetraploids are always 92,XXXX or 92,XXYY, suggesting that tetraploidy results from failure of completion of an early cleavage division of the zygote.

#### ANEUPLOIDY

Aneuploidy is the most common and clinically significant type of human chromosome disorder, occurring in at least 3 to 4 percent of all clinically recognized pregnancies. Most aneuploid patients have either **trisomy** (three instead of the normal pair of a particular chromosome) or, less often, **monosomy** (only one representative of a particular chromosome). Either trisomy or monosomy can have severe phenotypic consequences.

Trisomy can exist for any part of the genome, but trisomy for a whole chromosome is rarely compatible with life. By far the most common type of trisomy in liveborn infants is **trisomy 21** (karyotype 47,XX or XY, +21), the chromosome constitution seen in 95 percent of patients with Down syndrome (Fig. 9–6). Monosomy for an entire chromosome is almost always lethal; an important exception is monosomy for the X chromosome, as seen in Turner syndrome. Both Down syndrome and Turner syndrome are described in greater detail in Chapter 10.

Although the causes of aneuploidy are not well understood, it is known that the most common chromosomal mechanism is meiotic **nondisjunction**. This refers to the failure of a pair of chromosomes to disjoin properly during one of the two meiotic divisions,

TABLE 9–1

**Incidence of Chromosome Abnormalities at Different Stages of Fetal or Postnatal Life**

| Abnormal Karyotype | First-Trimester Abortuses | Fetuses of Mothers > 35 Years* | Live Births |
|---|---|---|---|
| Total incidence | 1/2 | 1/50 | 1/160 |
| Percentage of abnormalities | | | |
| *Numerical abnormalities* | 96% | 85% | 60% |
| *Structural abnormalities* | | | |
| Balanced | — | 10% | 30% |
| Unbalanced | 4% | 5% | 10% |

*Studied at amniocentesis; data summarized from Hsu LYF (1998) Prenatal diagnosis of chromosomal abnormalities through amniocentesis. *In* Milunsky A (ed) Genetic Disorders and the Fetus, 4th ed. Johns Hopkins University Press, Baltimore, pp. 179–248.

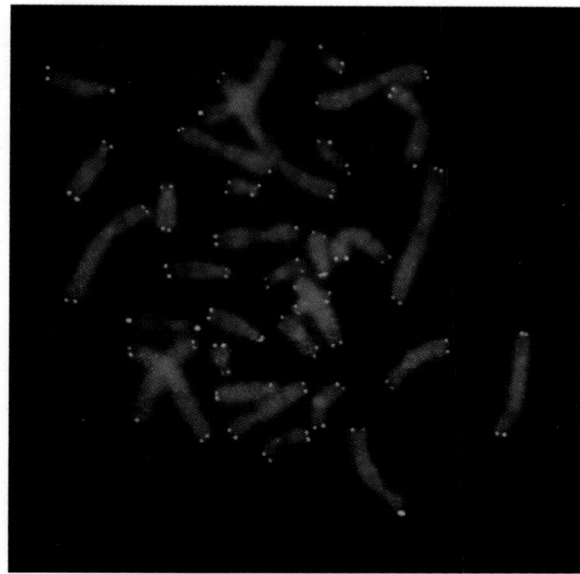

**Figure 9–5.** *A*, Detection of telomeres at the ends of each chromosome by fluorescence in situ hybridization (FISH) using a repeated TTAGGG probe. The two sister chromatids are evident by the double yellow hybridization signal at the end of most chromosome arms. (Courtesy of Stuart Schwartz, Case Western Reserve University and University Hospitals of Cleveland.)

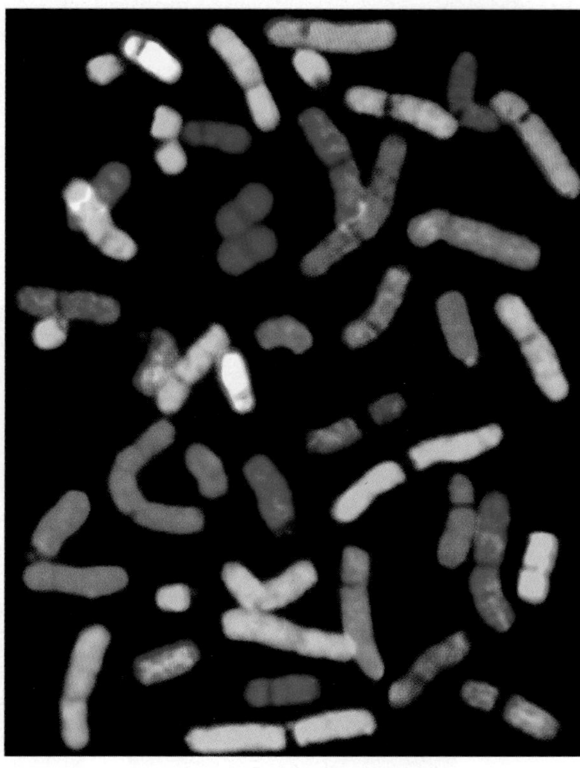

**Figure 9–5.** *B*, Spectral karyotyping (SKY). Twenty-four individual chromosome painting probes are labeled with different fluorescent dyes and used as a total genome chromosome paint. The fluorescent signals are analyzed by sophisticated imaging software and stored in a computer. To generate the photograph, the computer assigns a different color to each of the 24 different fluorescence spectra generated by the individual chromosome painting probes. (Figure courtesy of Dr. Amalia Dutra, National Human Genome Research Institute). In this metaphase from a 46,XX female, only 23 colors are present; the unique color generated by the Y chromosome painting probe is not seen.

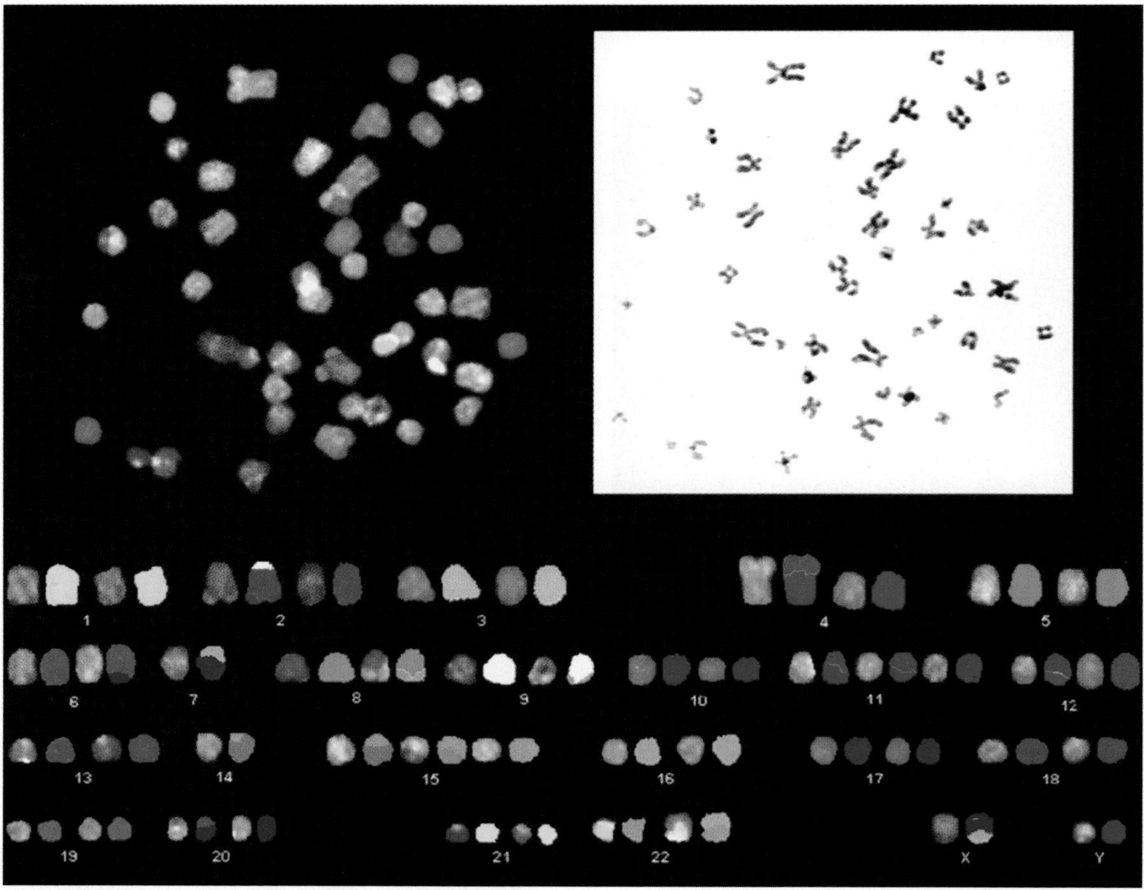


**Figure 9–5.** *C*, Spectral karyotyping analysis of chromosomes from a medulloblastoma cell line. Numerous structural and numerical abnormalities are evident and can be identified by image analysis of the 24 different chromosome painting probes used. Karyotype shows both original image (*left member of each pair*) and false-colored image (*right member of each pair*) in which each of the 24 chromosome types is assigned a different color to aid visual scoring. (Courtesy of Amalia Dutra, National Human Genome Research Institute.)

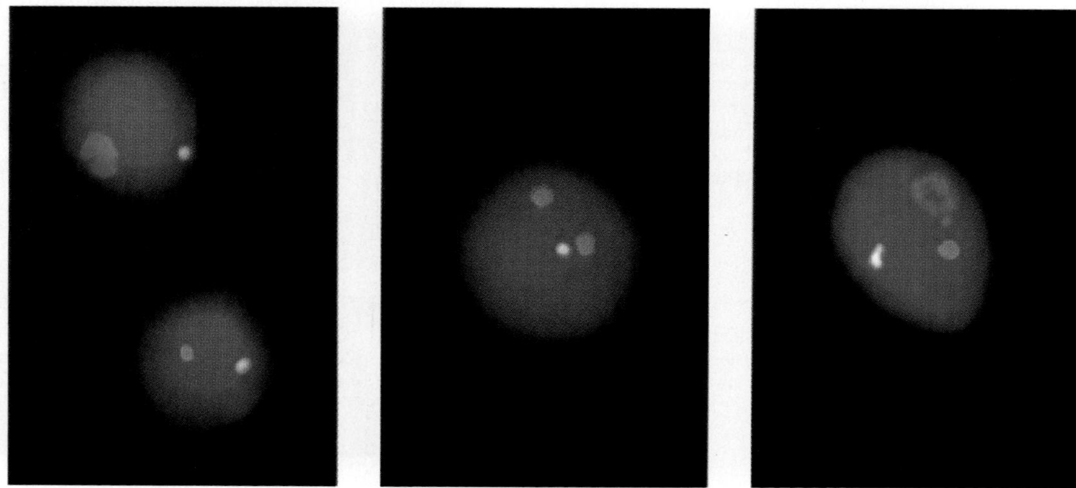

**Figure 9–5.** *D*, Three-color fluorescence in situ hybridization analysis of human sperm, using repetitive probes for chromosome 18 (*yellow*), the Y chromosome (*green*), and the X chromosome (*red*). The two haploid sperm on the left are monosomic for these chromosomes (one 23,X and one 23,Y sperm). The sperm in the middle panel is disomic for the X chromosome (24,XX karyotype), whereas the sperm on the right is disomic for the sex chromosomes (24,XY karyotype). (Courtesy of Terry Hassold, Case Western Reserve University School of Medicine, Cleveland.)

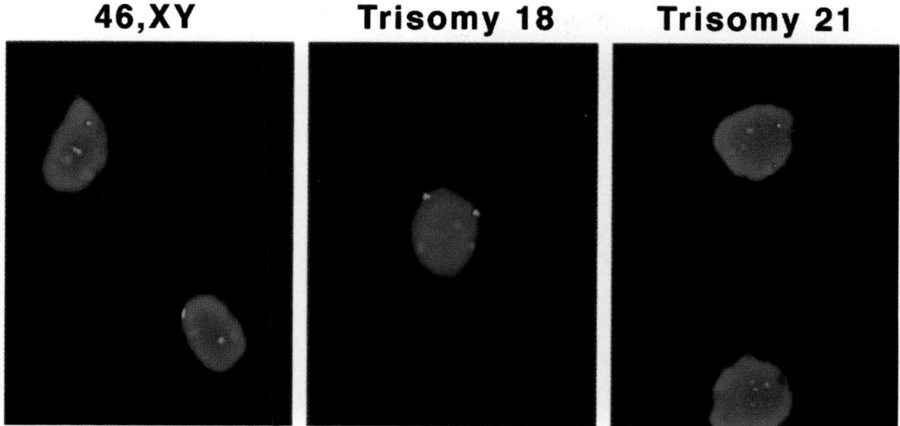


**Figure 9–5.** *E,* Multicolor fluorescence in situ hybridization analysis of interphase amniotic fluid cells. *Left panel,* 46,XY cells (chromosome 18 aqua, X chromosome green, Y chromosome red). *Middle panel,* 47,XX,+18 cell (chromosome 18 aqua, X chromosome green). *Right panel,* trisomy 21 cells (chromosome 13 green, chromosome 21 red). (Courtesy of Stuart Schwartz, Case Western Reserve University and University Hospitals of Cleveland.)

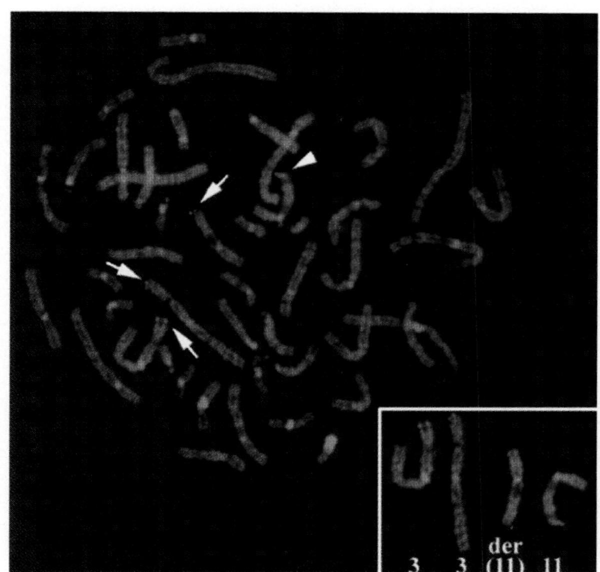


**Figure 9–5.** *F,* Fluorescence in situ hybridization detection of a cryptic translocation in a developmentally delayed proband, using specific probes for the telomere of chromosome 3p (*red*) and chromosome 11q (*green*). An unbalanced translocation between 3p and 11q was not evident by standard G-band analysis, but was revealed by FISH. The arrows show three chromosome 3p hybridization signals, indicative of partial trisomy for 3p, whereas the arrowhead shows only a single hybridization signal for 11q, indicating partial monosomy for 11q. (Courtesy of Christa Lese and David Ledbetter, University of Chicago.)

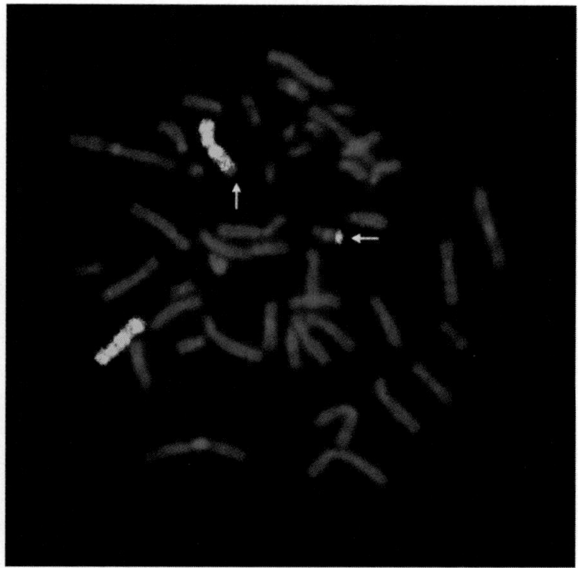

**Figure 9–5.** *G,* Fluorescence in situ hybridization detection of balanced translocation between chromosomes 11 and 16, using a painting probe for chromosome 11 (*yellow*). Karyotype is 46,XY,t(11;16)(q24;q23). Arrows indicate the translocation products. (Courtesy of Stuart Schwartz, Case Western Reserve University and University Hospitals of Cleveland.)

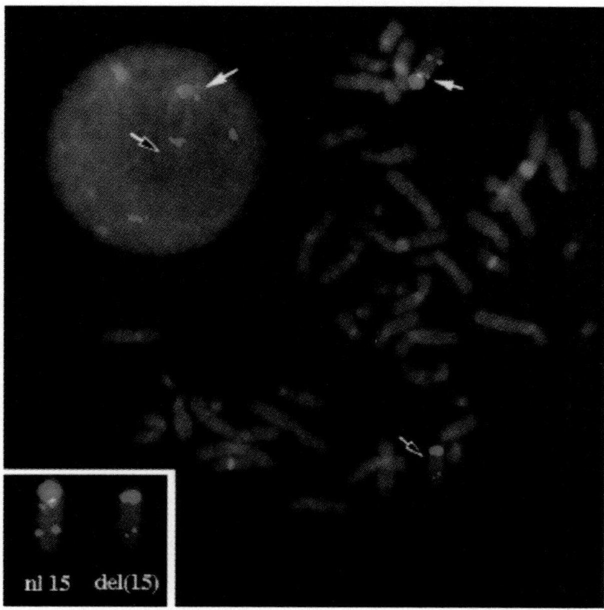


**Figure 9–5.** *H,* Two-color fluorescence in situ hybridization analysis of proband with Prader-Willi syndrome, demonstrating deletion of 15q11-q13 on one homolog. Green signal is hybridization to alpha satellite DNA at the chromosome 15 centromere. Red signal on distal 15q is a control single-copy probe. Red signal on proximal 15q is a probe for the *SNRPN* gene, which is present on one chromosome 15 (*white arrow*), but is deleted from the other (*dark arrow*). (Courtesy of Christa Lese and David Ledbetter, University of Chicago.)

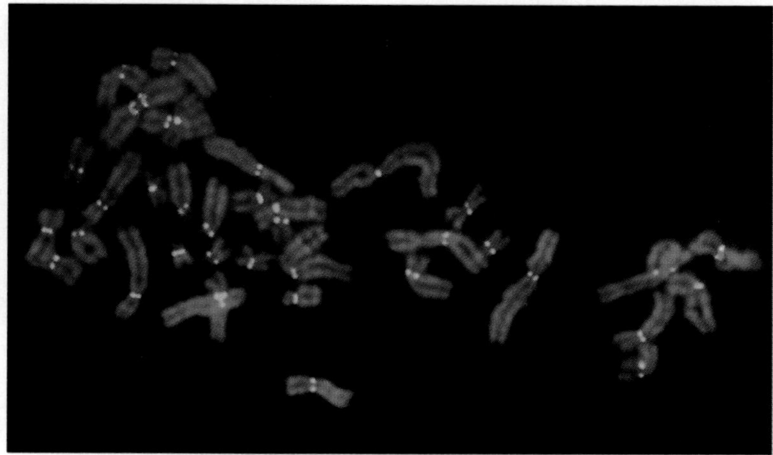

**Figure 9–5.** *I,* Combined fluorescence in situ hybridization and centromere analysis in a 46,X,idic(X) patient, with a dicentric isochromosome of the X chromosome. Chromosomes are stained blue with DAPI, a DNA stain. Paired green signals indicate functional centromeres, as detected with antibodies against a protein specific for active centromeres/kinetochores. X centromeres (*in red*) are detected by FISH using a specific alpha satellite probe from the X. The normal X (with its active centromere) is at the right. The dicentric X is at the left and has two active centromeres, because both centromeres stain with the antibody. (Courtesy of Anne Higgins, Case Western Reserve University School of Medicine, Cleveland.)

TABLE 9–2

**Some Abbreviations Used for Description of Chromosomes and Their Abnormalities and Representative Examples**

| Abbreviation | Meaning | Example | Condition |
|---|---|---|---|
| | | 46,XX | Normal female karyotype |
| | | 46,XY | Normal male karyotype |
| cen | centromere | | |
| del | deletion | 46,XX,del(5p) | Female with cri du chat syndrome due to deletion of part of short arm of one chromosome 5 |
| der | derivative chromosome | der(1) | Translocation chromosome derived from chromosome 1 and containing the centromere of chromosome 1 |
| dic | dicentric chromosome | dic(X;Y) | Translocation chromosome containing centromeres from both the X and the Y chromosomes |
| dup | duplication | | |
| fra | fragile site | 46,Y,fra(X)(q27.3) | Male with fragile X chromosome |
| i | isochromosome | 46,X,i(Xq) | Female with isochromosome for the long arm of the X chromosome |
| ins | insertion | | |
| inv | inversion | inv(3)(p25q21) | Pericentric inversion of chromosome 3 |
| mar | marker chromosome | 47,XX,+mar | Female with an extra, unidentified chromosome |
| mat | maternal origin | 47,XY,+der(1)mat | Male with additional der(1) translocation chromosome inherited from his mother |
| p | short arm of chromosome | | |
| pat | paternal origin | | |
| q | long arm of chromosome | | |
| r | ring chromosome | 46,X,r(X) | Female with ring X chromosome |
| rcp | reciprocal translocation | | |
| rob | Robertsonian translocation | | |
| t | translocation | 46,XX,t(2;8)(q21;p13) | Female with balanced translocation between chromosome 2 and chromosome 8, with breaks in 2q21 and 8p13 |
| ter | terminus | 46,X,Xq$^{-}$(pter→q21:) | Female with partial deletion of the long arm from Xq21 to Xqter (nomenclature shows the portion of the chromosome that is present) |
| + | gain of | 47,XX,+21 | Female with trisomy 21 |
| − | loss of | 45,XX,−14,−21,rob(14q21q) | Normal female carrier of a Robertsonian translocation between the long arms of chromosomes 14 and 21; karyotype is missing a normal 14 and a normal 21 |
| | | 4p$^{-}$ | Chromosome 4 with a portion of the short arm deleted |
| : | break | 5qter→5p15: | Deleted chromosome 5 in a patient with cri du chat syndrome, with a deletion breakpoint in band p15 |
| :: | break and join | 2pter→2q21::8p13→8pter | Description of der(2) portion of t(2;8) |
| / | mosaicism | 46,XX/47,XX,+8 | Female with two populations of cells, one with a normal karyotype and one with trisomy 8 |

Abbreviations from ISCN (1995) Report of the Standing Committee of Human Cytogenetic Nomenclature (1995). Karger, Basel.

usually during meiosis I. The consequences of nondisjunction during meiosis I and meiosis II are different (Fig. 9–7). If the error occurs during meiosis I, the gamete with 24 chromosomes contains both the paternal and the maternal members of the pair. If it occurs during meiosis II, the gamete with the extra chromosome contains both copies of either the paternal or the maternal chromosome. (Strictly speaking, the statements mentioned refer only to the paternal or maternal centromere, because recombination between homologous chromosomes has usually taken place in the preceding meiosis I, resulting in some genetic differences between the chromatids and thus between the corresponding daughter chromosomes; see Chapter 2.) The propensity of a chromosome pair to nondisjoin has been strongly associated with aberrations in the frequency or placement, or both, of recombination events in meiosis I. A chromosome pair

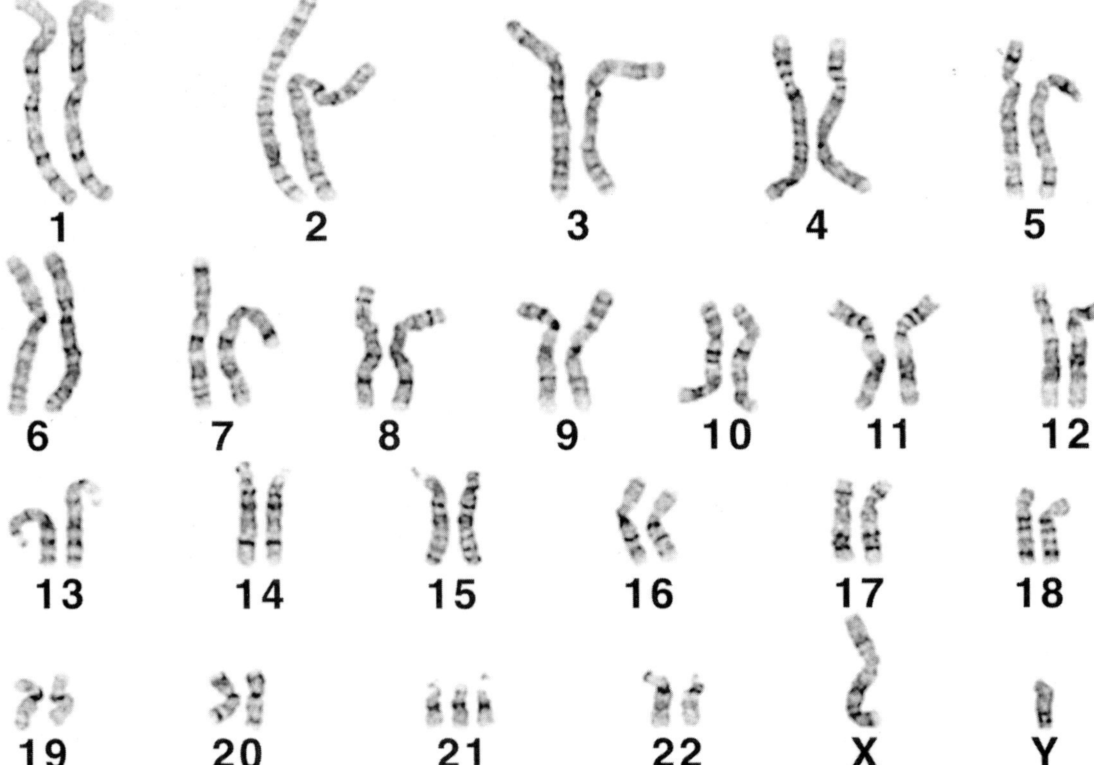


**Figure 9–6.** Karyotype from a male patient with Down syndrome, showing three copies of chromosome 21. (Courtesy of Center for Human Genetics Laboratory, University Hospitals of Cleveland.)

with too few recombinations or with recombination too close to the centromere or telomere may be more susceptible to nondisjunction than a chromosome pair with a more typical number and distribution of recombination events.

In addition to classic nondisjunction, in which improper chromosome segregation is the result of the failure of chromosomes either to pair or to recombine properly, or both, another mechanism involves premature separation of sister chromatids in meiosis I instead of meiosis II. If this happens, the separated chromatids may by chance segregate to the oocyte or to the polar body, leading to an unbalanced gamete.

More complicated forms of multiple aneuploidy have been reported. A gamete occasionally has an extra representative of more than one chromosome.

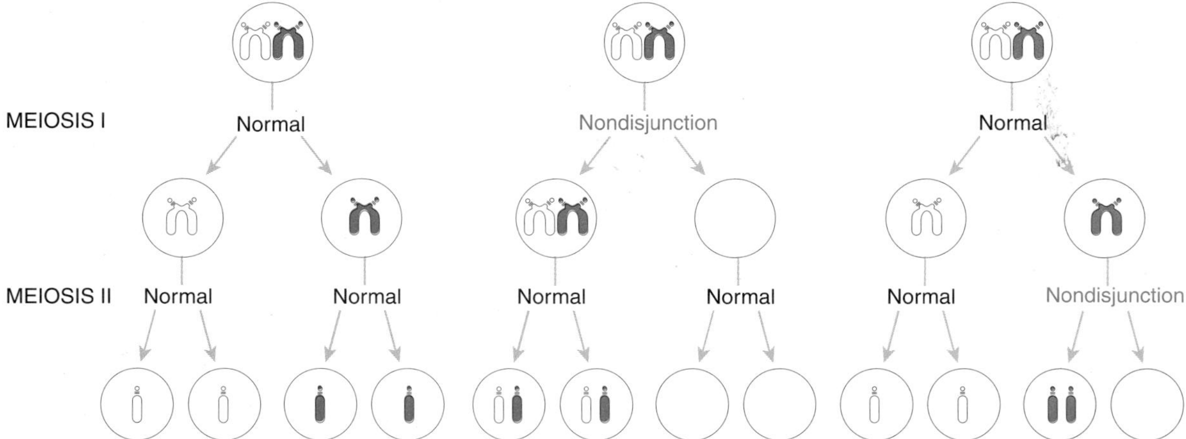


**Figure 9–7.** The different consequences of nondisjunction at meiosis I (*center*) and meiosis II (*right*), compared with normal disjunction (*left*). If the error occurs at meiosis I, the gametes either contain a representative of both members of the chromosome 21 pair or lack a chromosome 21 altogether. If nondisjunction occurs at meiosis II, the abnormal gametes contain two copies of one parental chromosome 21 (and no copy of the other) or lack a chromosome 21.

Nondisjunction can take place at two successive meiotic divisions or by chance in both male and female gametes simultaneously, resulting in zygotes with unusual chromosome numbers, which are extremely rare except for the sex chromosomes (see Fig. 9–5*D*, *color insert*). Nondisjunction can also occur in a mitotic division after formation of the zygote. If this happens at an early cleavage division, clinically significant **mosaicism** may result (see later section). In some malignant cell lines and some cell cultures, mitotic nondisjunction can lead to highly abnormal karyotypes.

An important development in the diagnosis of aneuploidy, especially prenatally, is the application of multicolor FISH to interphase cells (see Fig. 9–5*E*, *color insert*). This approach allows very rapid diagnosis without the need to culture cells. A large number of prenatal cytogenetics laboratories are now performing prenatal interphase analysis to evaluate aneuploidy for chromosomes 13, 18, 21, X, and Y, the five chromosomes that account for the vast majority of aneuploidy in liveborn individuals (see Chapter 18).

## Abnormalities of Chromosome Structure

Structural rearrangements result from chromosome breakage, followed by reconstitution in an abnormal combination. Rearrangement can take place in many ways, which together are less common than aneuploidy; overall, structural abnormalities are present in about 1 in 375 newborns. Chromosome exchange occurs spontaneously at a low frequency and may also be induced by breaking agents (clastogens), such as ionizing radiation, some viral infections, and many chemicals. Like numerical abnormalities, structural rearrangements may be present in all cells of a person or in mosaic form.

Structural rearrangements are defined as **balanced**, if the chromosome set has the normal complement of chromosomal material, or **unbalanced**, if there is additional or missing material. Some rearrangements are stable, capable of passing through mitotic and meiotic cell divisions unaltered, whereas others are unstable. To be stable, a rearranged chromosome must have normal structural elements, including a functional centromere and two telomeres. Some of the types of structural rearrangements observed in human chromosomes are illustrated in Figure 9–8.

### Unbalanced Rearrangements

In unbalanced rearrangements, the phenotype is likely to be abnormal because of deletion, duplication, or (in some cases) both. Duplication of part of a chromosome is comparable with partial trisomy; deletion leads to a partial monosomy. Any change that disturbs the normal balance of functional genes can result in abnormal development.

An important class of unbalanced rearrangement involves submicroscopic changes involving telomeres of many chromosomes in patients with idiopathic mental retardation. Small deletions, duplications, and translocations have been detected in several percent of such patients. Targeted cytogenetic analysis of telomeric regions by FISH may be indicated in unexplained mental retardation because of the profound implications of a positive result for genetic counseling (see Figs. 9–5*F* and *G*, *color insert*).

### Deletions

Deletions involve loss of a chromosome segment, resulting in chromosome imbalance (see Fig. 9–8*A*). A carrier of a chromosomal deletion (with one normal homolog and one deleted homolog) is monosomic for the genetic information on the corresponding segment of the normal homolog. The clinical consequences generally reflect **haploinsufficiency** (literally, the inability of a single copy of the genetic material to carry out the functions normally performed by two copies) and, where examined, appear to depend on the size of the deleted segment and the number and function of the genes that it contains. Cytogenetically visible autosomal deletions have an incidence of approximately 1 in 7000 live births.

A deletion may be terminal or interstitial. Deletions may originate simply by chromosome breakage and loss of the acentric segment. Alternatively, unequal crossing over between misaligned homologous chromosomes or sister chromatids may account for deletion in some cases (see Fig. 9–8*B*). Deletions can also be generated by abnormal segregation from a balanced translocation or inversion, as described later. Numerous deletions have been identified in the investigation of dysmorphic patients and in prenatal diagnosis, but knowledge of the functional genes lost in the deleted segments and their relation to the phenotypic consequences is still limited at present. Specific examples of these syndromes are discussed in Chapter 10.

Both high-resolution banding techniques and FISH can reveal deletions that are too small to be seen in ordinary metaphase spreads. To be identifiable cytogenetically by high-resolution banding, a deletion must span at least 2000 to 3000 kb, but karyotypically undetectable deletions with phenotypic consequences can be detected routinely by FISH using probes specific for the region of interest (see Fig. 9–5*H*, *color insert*).

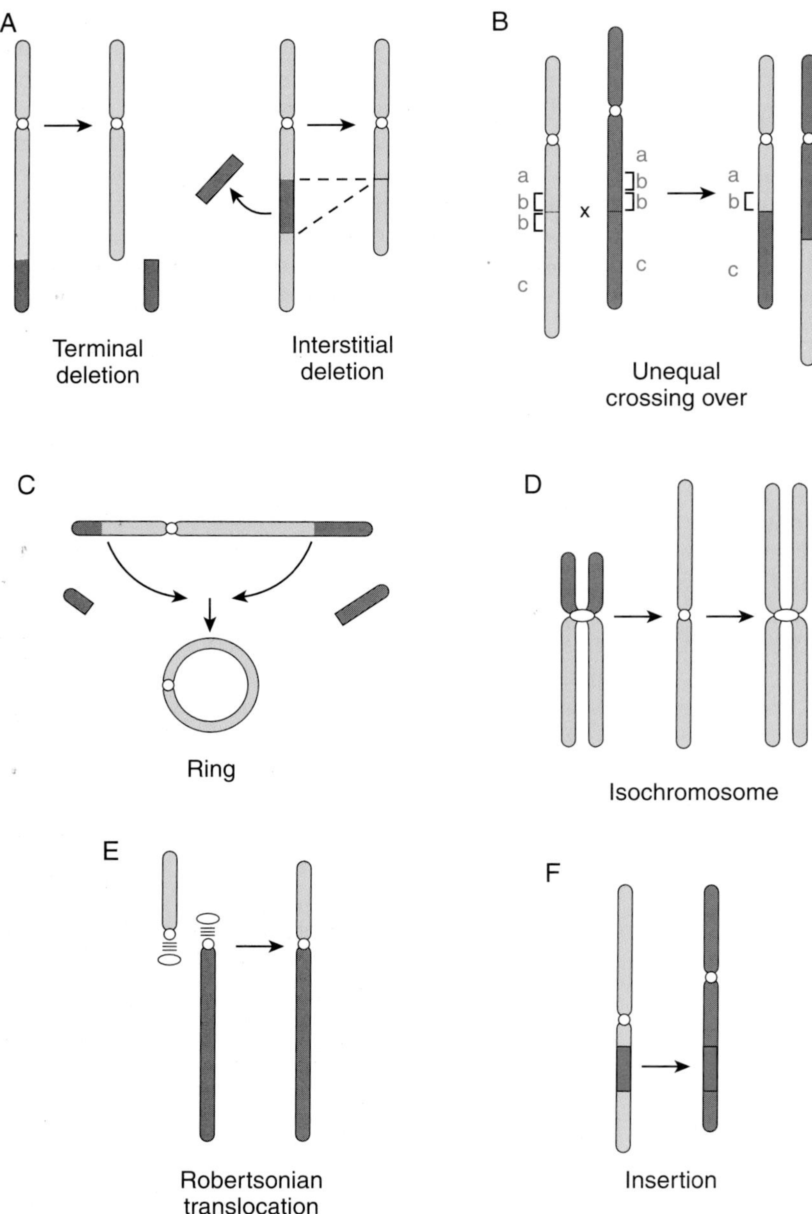


**Figure 9–8.** Structural rearrangements of chromosomes, described in the text. *A*, Terminal and interstitial deletions, each generating an acentric fragment. *B*, Unequal crossing over between segments of homologous chromosomes or between sister chromatids (duplicated or deleted segment indicated by the brackets). *C*, Ring chromosome with two acentric fragments. *D*, Generation of an isochromosome for the long arm of a chromosome. *E*, Robertsonian translocation between two acrocentric chromosomes. *F*, Insertion of a segment of one chromosome into a nonhomologous chromosome.

## Duplications

Duplications, like deletions, can originate by unequal crossing over (see Fig. 9–8*B*) or by abnormal segregation from meiosis in a carrier of a translocation or inversion. In general, duplication appears to be less harmful than deletion. Because duplication in a gamete results in chromosomal imbalance (i.e., partial trisomy), however, and because the chromosome breaks that generate it may disrupt genes, duplication often leads to some phenotypic abnormality.

Although many duplications have been reported, very few of any one kind have been studied thus far. Nonetheless, certain phenotypes appear to be associated with duplications of particular chromosomal regions.

## Marker and Ring Chromosomes

Very small, unidentified chromosomes, called "marker" chromosomes, are occasionally seen in chromosome preparations, frequently in a mosaic state. They are usually in addition to the normal chromosome complement and are thus also referred to as **supernumerary chromosomes** or **extra structurally abnormal chromosomes (ESACs)**. Cytogeneticists find markers very hard to characterize specifically by banding, even by high-resolution techniques, because they are usually so small that the banding pattern is ambiguous or not apparent. FISH with various probes is usually required for precise identification. Tiny marker chromosomes often consist of little more than centric heterochromatin that can be identified using a variety of chromosome-specific satellite or "paint" FISH probes. Spectral karyotyping may be particularly well suited to this purpose.

Larger marker chromosomes certainly contain some material from one or both chromosome arms, creating an imbalance for whatever genes are present. The prenatal frequency of de novo supernumerary marker chromosomes has been estimated to be approximately 1 in 2500. Because of the problem of identification, the clinical significance of a marker is difficult to assess, and the finding of a marker in a fetal karyotype can present a serious problem in assessment and genetic counseling. Depending on the origin of the marker, the risk of a fetal abnormality can range from very low to as high as 100 percent. A relatively high proportion of such markers derives from chromosome 15 and from the sex chromosomes. Specific syndromes are associated with bisatellited chromosome 15–derived markers and with markers derived from the centric portion of the X chromosome (see Chapter 10).

An intriguing subclass of marker chromosomes lack identifiable centromeric DNA sequences, including alpha satellite, despite being mitotically stable. These markers represent small fragments of chromosome arms (often some distance from the normal centromere) that have somehow acquired centromere activity. Such markers are said to contain **neocentromeres.**

Many marker chromosomes lack identifiable telomeric sequences and are thus likely to be small rings. Ring chromosomes are formed when a chromosome undergoes two breaks and the broken ends of the chromosome reunite in a ring structure (see Fig. 9–8*C*). Ring chromosomes are quite rare but have been detected for every human chromosome. If the centromere is within the ring, a ring chromosome would be expected to be mitotically stable. Many rings experience difficulties at mitosis, however, when the two sister chromatids of the ring chromosome become tangled in their attempt to disjoin at anaphase. There may be breakage of the ring followed by fusion, and larger and smaller rings may thus be generated. Because of this mitotic instability, it is not uncommon for ring chromosomes to be found in only a proportion of cells.

### Isochromosomes

An isochromosome (see Fig. 9–8*D*) is a chromosome in which one arm is missing and the other duplicated in a mirror-image fashion. A person with 46 chromosomes carrying an isochromosome, therefore, has a single copy of the genetic material of one arm (partial monosomy) and three copies of the genetic material of the other arm (partial trisomy). A person with two normal homologs in addition to the isochromosome is tetrasomic for the chromosome arm involved in the isochromosome (Fig. 9–9). Although the basis for isochromosome formation is not precisely known, at least two mechanisms have been documented: (1) misdivision through the centromere in meiosis II and, more commonly, (2) exchange involving one arm of a chromosome and its homolog (or sister chromatid) at the proximal edge of the arm, adjacent to the centromere. (Formally, these latter isochromosomes are isodicentric chromosomes, although the two centromeres are usually not distinguishable cytogenetically because they are so close together.)

The most common isochromosome is an isochromosome of the long arm of the X chromosome, i(Xq), in some individuals with Turner syndrome (see Chapter 10). Isochromosomes for a number of autosomes have also been described, however, including isochromosomes for the short arm of chromosome 18, i(18p) (see Fig. 9–9), and for the short arm of chromosome 12, i(12p). Isochromosomes are also frequently seen in kary-

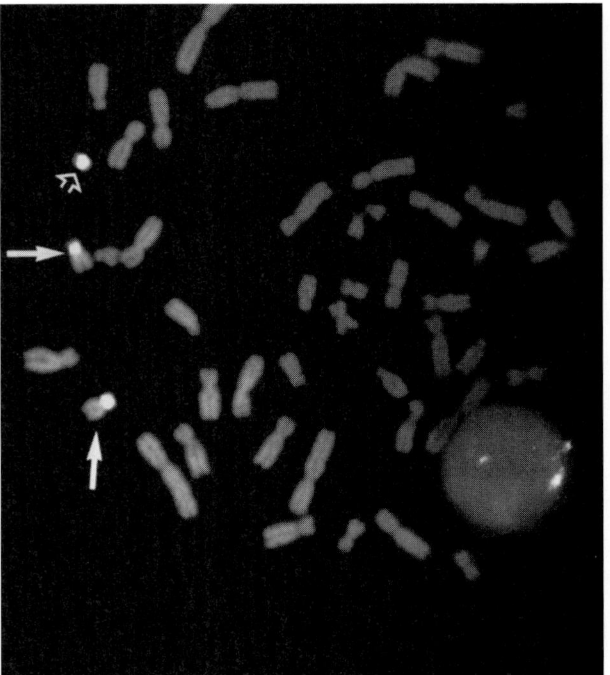

**Figure 9–9.** Identification of a supernumerary marker chromosome as i(18p), an isochromosome for the short arm of chromosome 18, by fluorescence in situ hybridization, using a specific DNA probe for the centromere of chromosome 18. *Open arrow* indicates the i(18p). *White arrows* indicate the two normal chromosome 18s. (Photograph courtesy of VE Powers, Case Western Reserve University School of Medicine.)

otypes of both solid tumors and hematological malignancies (see Chapter 16).

### Dicentric Chromosomes

A dicentric is a rare type of abnormal chromosome in which two chromosome segments (from different chromosomes or from the two chromatids of a single one), each with a centromere, fuse end to end, with loss of their acentric fragments. Dicentrics, despite their two centromeres, may be mitotically stable if one of the two centromeres is inactivated or if the two centromeres always coordinate their movement to one or the other pole during anaphase. Such chromosomes are formally called **pseudodicentric**. The most common pseudodicentrics involve the sex chromosomes or the acrocentric chromosomes (Robertsonian translocations; see later). Evaluation of centromere function by FISH combined with immunofluorescence analysis of centromere and kinetochore proteins is a specialized procedure in some clinical cytogenetics laboratories (see Fig. 9–5*I*, *color insert*).

## BALANCED REARRANGEMENTS

Chromosomal rearrangements do not usually have a phenotypic effect if they are balanced, because all the chromosomal material is present even though it is packaged differently. (It is important to distinguish here between truly balanced rearrangements and those that, although appearing balanced cytogenetically, are really unbalanced at the molecular level.) Even when structural rearrangements are truly balanced, they can pose a threat to the subsequent generation, because carriers are likely to produce a high frequency of unbalanced gametes and therefore have an increased risk of having abnormal offspring with unbalanced karyotypes; depending on the specific rearrangement, the risk can range from 1 percent to as high as 20 percent. There is also a possibility that one of the chromosome breaks will disrupt a gene, leading to mutation. This is a well-documented cause of X-linked diseases in female carriers of balanced X; autosome translocations (see Chapter 10), and such translocations can be a useful clue to the location of the gene responsible for a genetic disease, as discussed in Chapter 8 with the example of Duchenne muscular dystrophy.

### Inversions

An inversion occurs when a single chromosome undergoes two breaks and is reconstituted with the segment between the breaks inverted. Inversions are of two types: **paracentric** (not including the centromere), in which both breaks occur in one arm, and **pericentric** (including the centromere), in which there is a break in each arm. Because paracentric inversions do not change the arm ratio of the chromosome, they can be identified only by banding or FISH with locus-specific probes, if at all. Pericentric inversions are easier to identify cytogenetically because they may change the proportion of the chromosome arms as well as the banding pattern.

An inversion does not usually cause an abnormal phenotype in carriers, because it is a balanced rearrangement. Its medical significance is for the progeny; a carrier of either type of inversion is at risk of producing abnormal gametes that may lead to unbalanced offspring (Fig. 9–10). When an inversion is present, a loop is formed when the chromosomes pair in meiosis I. Although recombination is somewhat suppressed within inversion loops, when it occurs it can lead to the production of unbalanced gametes. Both gametes with balanced chromosome complements (either normal or possessing the inversion) and gametes with unbalanced complements are formed, depending on the location of recombination events. When the inversion is paracentric, the unbalanced recombinant chromosomes are typically acentric or dicentric and may not lead to viable offspring (see Fig. 9–10*A*), although there have been rare exceptions. Thus, the risk that a carrier of a paracentric inversion will have a liveborn child with an abnormal karyotype is very low indeed.

A pericentric inversion, on the other hand, can lead to the production of unbalanced gametes with both **duplication** and **deficiency** of chromosome segments (see Fig. 9–10*B*). The duplicated and deficient segments are the segments that are distal to the inversion. *Overall, the apparent risk of a carrier of a pericentric inversion producing a child with an unbalanced karyotype is estimated to be 5 to 10 percent.* Each pericentric inversion, however, is associated with a particular risk, and large pericentric inversions are more likely than are smaller ones to lead to viable recombinant offspring because the unbalanced segments in the recombinant progeny are smaller in the case of large inversions. Three well-described inversions illustrate this point.

A pericentric inversion of chromosome 3, originating in a couple from Newfoundland married in the early 1800s, is one of the few for which sufficient data have been obtained to allow an estimate of the segregation of the inversion chromosome in the offspring of carriers. The inv(3)(p25q21) has since been reported from a number of North American centers, in families whose ancestors have been traced to the maritime provinces of Canada. Carriers of the inv(3) chromosome are normal, but some of their offspring have a characteristic abnormal phenotype (Fig. 9–11) associated with a recombinant chromosome 3, in which there is duplication of the segment distal to 3q21 and deficiency of the segment distal to 3p25 (see Fig. 9–10). Nine individuals who were carriers of the in-

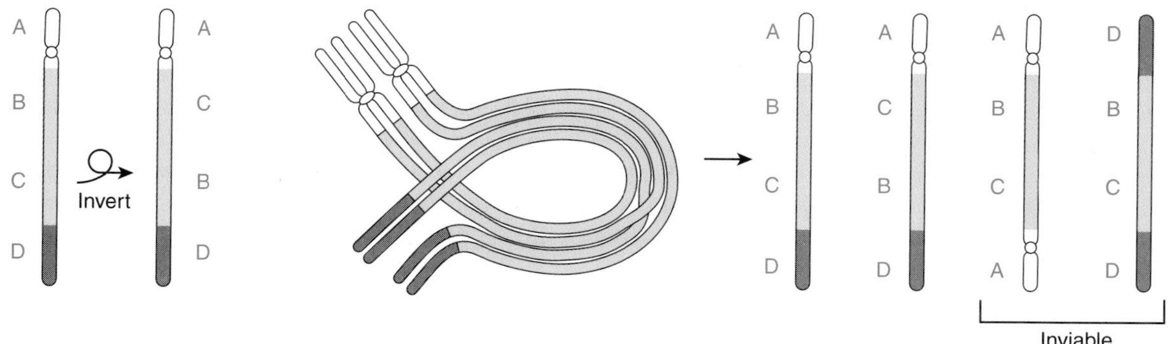


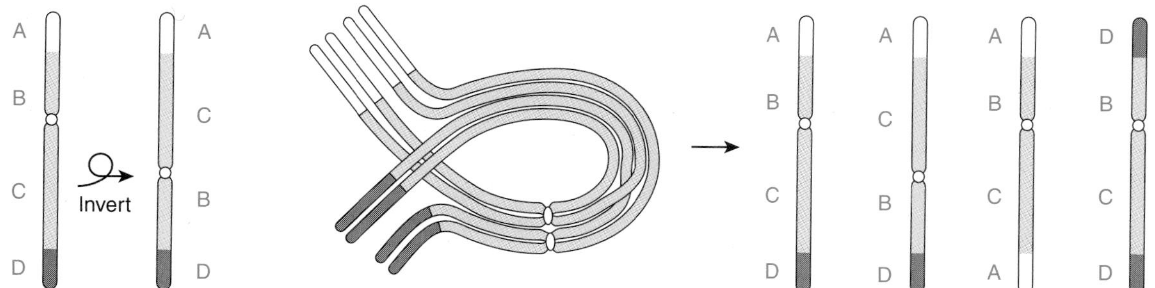


Figure 9–10. Crossing over within inversion loops formed at meiosis I in carriers of a chromosome with segment B-C inverted (order A-C-B-D, instead of A-B-C-D). *A*, Paracentric inversion. Gametes formed after the second meiosis usually contain either a normal (A-B-C-D) or a balanced (A-C-B-D) copy of the chromosome, because the acentric and dicentric products of the crossover are inviable. *B*, Pericentric inversion. Gametes formed after the second meiosis may be normal, balanced, or unbalanced. Unbalanced gametes contain a copy of the chromosome with a duplication or a deficiency of the material flanking the inverted segment (A-B-C-A or D-B-C-D).

version have had 53 recorded pregnancies. The high empiric risk of an abnormal pregnancy outcome in this group (22/53, or >40 percent) indicates the importance of family chromosome studies to identify carriers and to offer genetic counseling and prenatal diagnosis.

Another pericentric inversion associated with a severe duplication/deficiency syndrome in recombinant offspring involves chromosome 8, inv(8)(p23.1q22.1), and is found primarily among Hispanics from the southwestern United States. Empiric studies have shown that carriers of the inv(8) have a 6 percent chance of having a child with the recombinant 8 syndrome, a lethal disorder with severe cardiac abnormalities and mental retardation. The recombinant chromosome is duplicated for sequences distal to 8q22.1 and deleted for sequences distal to 8p23.1.

The most common inversion seen in human chromosomes is a small pericentric inversion of chromosome 9, which is present in up to 1 percent of all individuals tested by cytogenetics laboratories. The inv(9)(p11q12) has no known deleterious effect on carriers and does not appear to be associated with a significant risk of miscarriage or unbalanced offspring; it is, therefore, generally considered a normal variant.

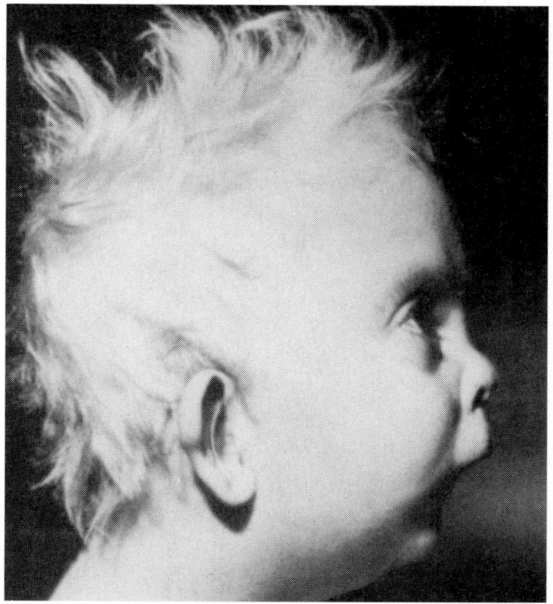

Figure 9–11. A child with an abnormal karyotype, offspring of a carrier of a pericentric inversion. See text for discussion. (From Allderdice PW, Browne N, Murphy DP [1975] Chromosome 3 duplication q21-qter, deletion p25-pter syndrome in children of carriers of a pericentric inversion inv(3) (p25q21). Am J Hum Genet 27: 699–718.)

Translocations

Translocation involves the exchange of chromosome segments between two, usually nonhomologous, chromosomes. There are two main types: reciprocal and Robertsonian.

**Reciprocal Translocations.** This type of rearrangement results from breakage of nonhomologous chromosomes, with reciprocal exchange of the broken-off segments. Usually only two chromosomes are involved, and because the exchange is reciprocal, the total chromosome number is unchanged (Fig. 9–12*A*). (Complex translocations involving three or more chromosomes are rare.) Reciprocal translocations are relatively common and are found in approximately 1 in 600 newborns. Such translocations are usually harmless, although they are more common in institutionalized mentally retarded individuals than in the general population. Like other balanced struc-

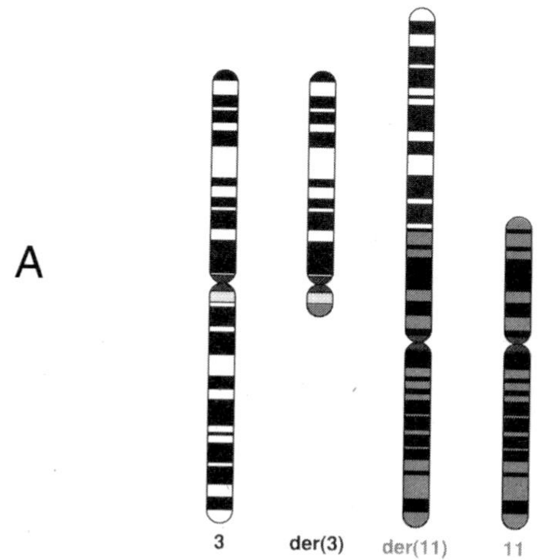


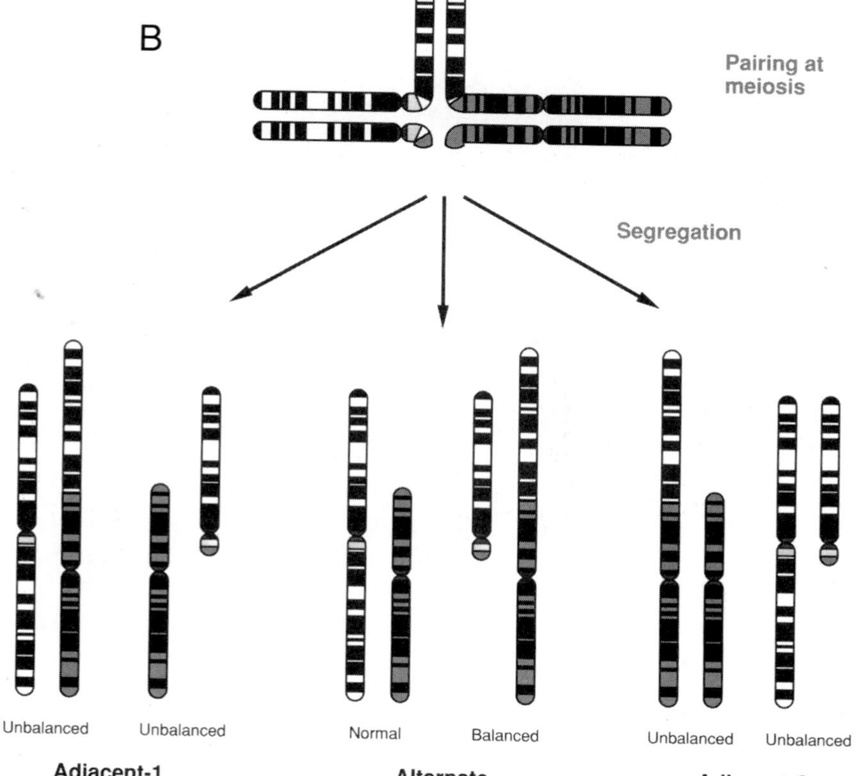


**Figure 9–12.** *A*, Diagram of a balanced translocation between chromosome 3 and chromosome 11, t(3;11)(q12;p15.5). *B*, Quadrivalent formation in meiosis and 2:2 segregation in a carrier of the t(3; 11), leading to either balanced or unbalanced gametes. See text for discussion.

tural rearrangements, they are associated with a high risk of unbalanced gametes and abnormal progeny. They come to attention either during prenatal diagnosis or when the parents of an abnormal child with an unbalanced translocation are karyotyped. Balanced translocations are more commonly found in couples who have had two or more spontaneous abortions and in infertile males than in the general population.

When the chromosomes of a carrier of a balanced reciprocal translocation pair at meiosis, a **quadrivalent** (cross-shaped) figure is formed, as shown in Figure 9–12*B*. At anaphase, the chromosomes usually segregate from this configuration in one of three ways, described as **alternate, adjacent-1**, and **adjacent-2 segregation**. Alternate segregation, the usual type of meiotic segregation, produces gametes that have either a normal chromosome complement or the two reciprocal chromosomes; both types of gamete are balanced. In adjacent-1 segregation, homologous centromeres go to separate daughter cells, whereas in adjacent-2 segregation (which is rare), homologous centromeres pass to the same daughter cell. Both adjacent-1 and adjacent-2 segregation yield unbalanced gametes (see Fig. 9–12*B*).

In addition to the examples mentioned of 2:2 segregation (i.e., two chromosomes to each pole), balanced translocation chromosomes can also segregate 3:1, leading to gametes with 22 or 24 chromosomes. Although monosomy in a resulting fetus is rare, trisomy can result. Such 3:1 segregation is observed in 5 to 20 percent of sperm from balanced translocation carriers, depending on the specific translocation.

**Robertsonian Translocations.** This type of rearrangement involves two acrocentric chromosomes that fuse near the centromere region with loss of the short arms (see Fig. 9–8*E*). The resulting balanced karyotype has only 45 chromosomes, including the translocation chromosome, which, in effect, is made up of the long arms of two chromosomes. Because the short arms of all five pairs of acrocentric chromosomes have multiple copies of genes for ribosomal RNA, loss of the short arms of two acrocentric chromosomes is not deleterious. Robertsonian translocations can be either monocentric or pseudodicentric, depending on the location of the breakpoint on each acrocentric chromosome.

Although Robertsonian translocations involving all combinations of the acrocentric chromosomes have been detected, two (13q14q and 14q21q) are relatively common. The translocation involving 13q and 14q is found in about 1 person in 1300 and is thus by far the single most common chromosome rearrangement in our species.

Although a carrier of a Robertsonian translocation is phenotypically normal, there is a risk of unbalanced gametes and therefore of unbalanced offspring. The chief clinical importance of this type of translocation is that carriers of a Robertsonian translocation involving chromosome 21 are at risk of producing a child with translocation Down syndrome (see Chapter 10).

**Insertions.** An insertion is a nonreciprocal type of translocation that occurs when a segment removed from one chromosome is inserted into a different chromosome, either in its usual orientation or inverted (see Fig. 9–8*F*). Because they require three chromosome breaks, insertions are relatively rare. Abnormal segregation in an insertion carrier can produce offspring with duplication or deletion of the inserted segment, as well as normal offspring and balanced carriers. The average risk of producing an abnormal child is quite high, up to 50 percent, and prenatal diagnosis is indicated.

## Mosaicism

When a person has a chromosome abnormality, the abnormality is usually present in all of his or her cells. Sometimes, however, two or more different chromosome complements are present in an individual. This situation is called **mosaicism**. Mosaicism may be either numerical (the most common type) or structural.

A common cause of mosaicism is nondisjunction in an early postzygotic mitotic division. For example, a zygote with an additional chromosome 21 might lose the extra chromosome in a mitotic division and continue to develop as a 46/47,+21 mosaic. The significance of a finding of mosaicism is often difficult to assess, especially if it is identified prenatally. The effects of mosaicism on development vary with the timing of the nondisjunctional event, the nature of the chromosome abnormality, the proportions of the different chromosome complements present, and the tissues affected. An additional problem is that the proportions of the different chromosome complements seen in the tissue being analyzed (for example, cultured amniocytes or lymphocytes) may not necessarily reflect the proportions present in other tissues or in the embryo during its early developmental stages. In laboratory studies, cytogeneticists attempt to differentiate between true mosaicism, present in individuals, and **pseudomosaicism**, in which the mosaicism probably arose in cell culture. The distinction is not always easy or certain. Mosaicism is relatively common in cytogenetic studies of chorionic villus cultures and can lead to major interpretive difficulties in prenatal diagnosis (see Chapter 18).

Clinical studies of the phenotypic effects of mosaicism have two main weaknesses. First, because people are hardly ever karyotyped without some clinical indications, clinically normal mosaic persons are rarely ascertained; second, there have been few follow-up studies of prenatally diagnosed mosaic fetuses.

Nonetheless, it is often believed that individuals who are mosaic for a given trisomy, such as mosaic Down syndrome or mosaic Turner syndrome, are less severely affected than nonmosaic individuals.

## Population Incidence of Chromosome Anomalies

The incidence of different types of chromosomal aberration has been measured in a number of large population surveys (Tables 9–3 and 9–4). The major numerical disorders of chromosomes are three autosomal trisomies (trisomy 21, trisomy 18, and trisomy 13) and four types of sex chromosomal aneuploidy: Turner syndrome (usually 45,X); Klinefelter syndrome (47,XXY); 47,XYY; and 47,XXX (see Chapter 10). Triploidy and tetraploidy account for a small percentage of cases, particularly in spontaneous abortions. The classification and incidence of chromosomal defects measured in these surveys can be used to summarize the fate of 10,000 conceptuses, as presented in Table 9–5.

### Live Births

The overall incidence of chromosome abnormalities in newborns has been found to be about 1 in 160 births (0.7 percent). The findings are summarized in Table 9–3, classified separately for specific numerical abnormalities of sex chromosomes and autosomes and for balanced and unbalanced structural rearrangements. Most of the autosomal abnormalities can be diagnosed at birth, but most sex chromosome abnormalities, with the exception of Turner syndrome, are not recognized clinically until puberty (see Chapter 10). Balanced rearrangements are rarely identified clinically unless a carrier of a rearrangement gives birth to a child with an unbalanced chromosome complement and family studies are initiated; unbalanced rearrangements are likely to come to clinical attention because of dysmorphism and delayed physical and mental development in the chromosomally abnormal individual.

### Spontaneous Abortions

The overall frequency of chromosome abnormalities in spontaneous abortions is at least 40 to 50 percent, and the kinds of abnormalities differ in a number of ways from those seen in liveborns (see Table 9–4). The single most common abnormality in abortuses is 45,X (Turner syndrome), which accounts for nearly 20 percent of chromosomally abnormal spontaneous abortuses but less than 1 percent of chromosomally abnormal live births. The other sex chromosome abnormalities, which are quite common in live births, are rare in abor-

TABLE 9–3

**Incidence of Chromosomal Abnormalities in Newborn Surveys**

| Type of Abnormality | Number | Approximate Incidence |
|---|---|---|
| **Sex Chromosome Aneuploidy** | | |
| Males (43,612 newborns) | | |
| 47,XXY | 45 | 1/1000 |
| 47,XYY | 45 | 1/1000 |
| Other X or Y aneuploidy | 32 | 1/1350 |
| **Total** | **122** | **1/360 male births** |
| Females (24,547 newborns) | | |
| 45,X | 6 | 1/4000 |
| 47,XXX | 27 | 1/900 |
| Other X aneuploidy | 9 | 1/2700 |
| **Total** | **42** | **1/580 female births** |
| **Autosomal Aneuploidy** (68,159 newborns) | | |
| Trisomy 21 | 82 | 1/830 |
| Trisomy 18 | 9 | 1/7500 |
| Trisomy 13 | 3 | 1/22,700 |
| Other aneuploidy | 2 | 1/34,000 |
| **Total** | **96** | **1/700 live births** |
| **Structural Abnormalities** (68,159 newborns) | | |
| (Sex chromosomes and autosomes) | | |
| Balanced rearrangements | | |
| Robertsonian | 62 | 1/1100 |
| Other | 77 | 1/885 |
| Unbalanced rearrangements | | |
| Robertsonian | 5 | 1/13,600 |
| Other | 38 | 1/1800 |
| **Total** | **182** | **1/375 live births** |
| **All Chromosome Abnormalities** | **442** | **1/154 live births** |

Data from Hsu LYF (1998) Prenatal diagnosis of chromosomal abnormalities through amniocentesis. *In* Milunsky A (ed) Genetic Disorders and the Fetus, 4th ed. Johns Hopkins University Press, Baltimore, pp. 179–248.

TABLE 9–4

**Frequency of Chromosome Abnormalities in Spontaneous Abortions with Abnormal Karyotypes**

| Type | Approximate Proportion of Abnormal Karyotypes |
|---|---|
| **Aneuploidy** | |
| Autosomal trisomy | 0.52 |
| Autosomal monosomy | <0.01 |
| 45,X | 0.19 |
| **Triploidy** | 0.16 |
| **Tetraploidy** | 0.06 |
| **Other** | 0.07 |

Based on analysis of 8,841 unselected spontaneous abortions, as summarized by Hsu LYF (1998) Prenatal diagnosis of chromosomal abnormalities through amniocentesis. *In* Milunsky A (ed) Genetic Disorders and the Fetus, 4th ed. Johns Hopkins University Press, Baltimore, pp. 179–248.

tuses. Another difference is the distribution of kinds of trisomy; for example, trisomy 16 accounts for about one third of trisomies in abortuses but is not seen at all in live births.

Because the overall spontaneous abortion rate (about 15 percent) is known, as is the overall incidence of specific chromosome defects in both abortuses and live births, one can estimate the proportion of all conceptuses of a given karyotype that are lost by spontaneous abortion (see Table 9–5).

## PARENT-OF-ORIGIN EFFECTS

### Genomic Imprinting

As introduced in Chapter 5, **genomic imprinting** reflects the differential expression of the maternally and paternally inherited alleles at one or more loci. A number of such parent-of-origin effects come to light because of cytogenetic abnormalities and are thus included in this chapter. Evidence of genomic imprinting has been obtained for a number of chromosomes or chromosomal regions throughout the genome, as revealed by comparing phenotypes of individuals carrying the same cytogenetic abnormality affecting either the maternal or paternal homolog (Fig. 9–13). For example, deletion of the maternal or paternal chromosome 15q11-q13 (see Fig. 9–5, *color insert*) leads to either Angelman or Prader-Willi syndrome, respectively, as discussed in Chapter 5.

### Cytogenetics of Hydatidiform Moles and Ovarian Teratomas

Occasionally in an abnormal pregnancy, the placenta is converted into a mass of tissue resembling a bunch of grapes, called a hydatid cyst. This is due to abnormal growth of the chorionic villi, in which the epithelium proliferates and the stroma undergoes cystic cavitation. Such an abnormality is called a **mole**. A mole may be complete, with no fetus or normal placenta present, or partial, with remnants of placenta and perhaps a small atrophic fetus.

Most **complete moles** are diploid, with a 46,XX karyotype. The chromosomes are all paternal in origin, however, and, with rare exceptions, all genetic markers are homozygous. Such moles originate when a single 23,X sperm fertilizes an ovum that lacks a nucleus, and its chromosomes then double. The absence of any maternal contribution is thought to be responsible for the very abnormal development, with hyperplasia of the trophoblast and grossly disorganized or absent fetal tissue. About half of all cases of choriocarcinoma (a malignancy of fetal, not maternal, tissue) develop from hydatidiform moles. The reciprocal genetic condition is apparent in **ovarian teratomas**, benign tumors that arise from 46,XX cells containing only maternal chromosomes; no paternal contribution is evident. *Thus, normal fetal development*

TABLE 9–5

**Outcome of 10,000 Conceptions**

| Outcome | Conceptions | Spontaneous Abortions: *No.* | Spontaneous Abortions: *Percent* | Live Births |
|---|---|---|---|---|
| *Total* | 10,000 | 1500 | 15 | 8500 |
| *Normal Chromosomes* | 9200 | 750 | 8 | 8450 |
| *Abnormal Chromosomes* | | | | |
| Total | 800 | 750 | 94 | 50 |
| Triploid/tetraploid | 170 | 170 | 100 | — |
| 45,X | 140 | 139 | 99 | 1 |
| Trisomy 16 | 112 | 112 | 100 | — |
| Trisomy 18 | 20 | 19 | 95 | 1 |
| Trisomy 21 | 45 | 35 | 78 | 10 |
| Trisomy, other | 209 | 208 | 99.5 | 1 |
| 47,XXY, 47,XXX, 47,XYY | 19 | 4 | 21 | 15 |
| Unbalanced rearrangements | 27 | 23 | 85 | 4 |
| Balanced rearrangements | 19 | 3 | 16 | 16 |
| Other | 39 | 37 | 95 | 2 |

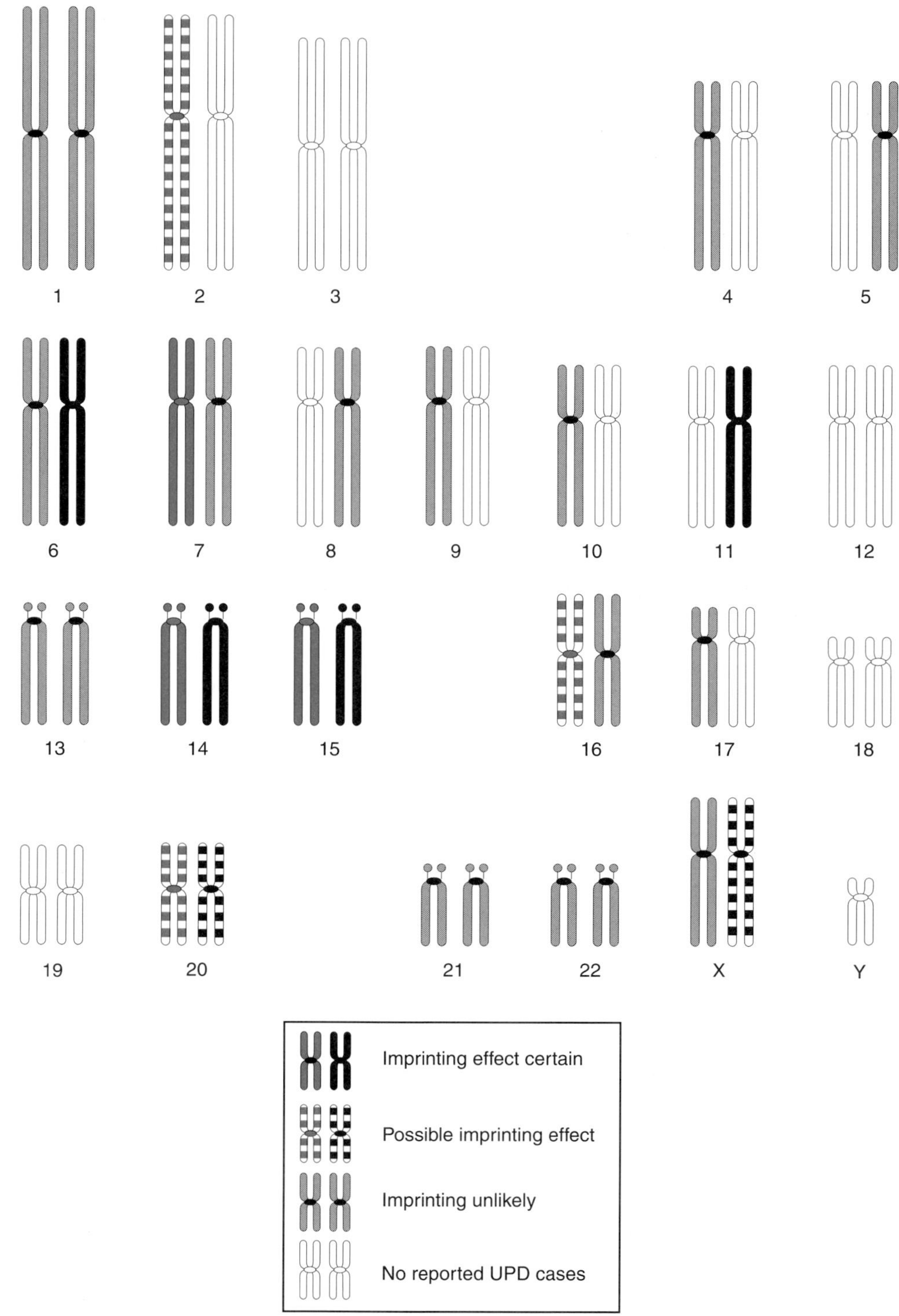


**Figure 9–13.** Map of imprinted regions in the human genome, based on phenotypes detected in cases of uniparental disomy involving the maternally inherited homolog (*left chromosome in each pair*) or the paternally inherited homolog (*right chromosome in each pair*). (Revised from Ledbetter DH, Engel E [1995] Uniparental disomy in humans: Development of an imprinting map and its implications for prenatal diagnosis. Hum Mol Genet 4:1757–1764.) (An updated electronic version of the map, with references, is available from *http://www.genes.uchicago.edu*)

*requires both maternal and paternal genetic contributions.* It appears that the paternal genome is especially important for extraembryonic development, whereas the maternal genome is critical for fetal development.

In contrast to complete moles, **partial moles** are triploid; in about two thirds of cases, the extra chromosome set is of paternal origin. Comparing cases of maternal or paternal origin, fetal development is severely abnormal in both, but the defects are different. An extra paternal set results in abundant trophoblast but poor embryonic development, whereas an extra maternal set results in severe retardation of embryonic growth with a small, fibrotic placenta. The specificity of the effect is a further example of genomic imprinting.

### Confined Placental Mosaicism

One specific type of chromosomal mosaicism occurs when the karyotype of the placenta is mosaic for an abnormality, usually a trisomy, that is not apparent in the fetus. For example, the placenta may be 46,XX/47,XX,+15, whereas the fetus may be 46,XX. This situation, called **confined placental mosaicism**, may lead to a phenotypically abnormal fetus or liveborn, despite the apparently euploid karyotype. In one mechanism, both copies of the relevant chromosome (for example, chromosome 15) in the fetus may originate from the same parent. The interpretation is that a trisomic state, not normally consistent with survival, may be "rescued" by loss of one of the copies of the chromosome involved in the trisomy. By chance, the chromosome lost may be the only copy that originated from one of the parents, leading to **uniparental disomy** in the remaining cells.

The abnormal phenotype seen in the fetus or liveborn can in many cases be explained by the presence of imprinted genes on the chromosome involved in the trisomy rescue (see Fig. 9–13). For example, Prader-Willi syndrome will result in the case of maternal uniparental disomy 15, whereas Angelman syndrome reflects paternal uniparental disomy 15 (see Chapter 5). This mechanism accounts for about 30 percent of Prader-Willi syndrome cases but less than 5 percent of cases of Angelman syndrome.

The possibility of confined placental mosaicism is a frequent diagnostic dilemma in prenatal cytogenetics laboratories (see Chapter 18).

## STUDIES OF CHROMOSOMES IN HUMAN MEIOSIS

Two general approaches have been used to study the chromosome constitution of sperm or ova in human males and females, respectively. In the first approach, one can analyze abnormal meioses retrospectively, using DNA polymorphisms or cytogenetic heteromorphisms to study the parental origin of aneuploid fetuses or liveborns. Extensive analysis of more than 1000 conceptuses has indicated a significantly different contribution of either maternal or paternal nondisjunction to different cytogenetic abnormalities; for example, maternal nondisjunction accounts for more than 90 percent of cases of trisomy 21 and fully 100 percent of trisomy 16 but only about half of cases of Klinefelter syndrome (47,XXY) and only 20 to 30 percent of Turner syndrome (45,X).

A second approach involves direct analysis of chromosomes in human germ cells. Using FISH with chromosome-specific probes, a large number of sperm can be scored quickly to evaluate aneuploidy levels for individual human chromosomes (see Fig. 9–5, *color insert*). A number of very large studies have indicated chromosome-specific rates of disomy of about 1 in 1000 to 2000 sperm, with some variation between chromosomes. Nondisjunction of the sex chromosomes appears to be several-fold more frequent than nondisjunction of the autosomes.

A number of studies have suggested that the frequency of chromosomally abnormal sperm is elevated in males who exhibit infertility. This is an important area of investigation, because of the increasing use of intracytoplasmic sperm injection (ICSI) in human in vitro fertilization (IVF) procedures; in many IVF centers, ICSI is the procedure of choice in male infertility cases. There are a number of indications that suggest a sharp increase in chromosomal abnormalities (particularly involving the sex chromosomes) in ICSI pregnancies.

Sperm FISH can also be used to evaluate the proportion of normal, balanced, or unbalanced sperm in male carriers of reciprocal translocations or inversions. Results of such studies can be useful for genetic counseling, although comparison of the findings in sperm, fetuses, and liveborns must be made with caution. For example, half the sperm in carriers of reciprocal translocations have unbalanced karyotypes; this is in contrast to the observations in liveborn offspring of male translocation carriers, very few of whom have unbalanced chromosome sets.

Direct visualization of chromosomes during oogenesis is more difficult than during spermatogenesis. As a result of improvements in IVF technology, however, oocytes can be obtained at the time of ovulation, matured in vitro, and examined by FISH during the first meiotic division. Such studies are providing insights into mechanisms of maternal nondisjunction and into the relationship between advancing maternal age and the increasing incidence of aneuploidy.

## MENDELIAN DISORDERS WITH CYTOGENETIC EFFECTS

There are several rare single-gene syndromes, in addition to the relatively common fragile X syndrome (see Chapter 12), in which there is a characteristic cytogenetic abnormality (Table 9–6). Collectively, these autosomal recessive disorders are referred to as **chromosome instability syndromes**. In each disorder, a detailed chromosome study can be an important element of diagnosis. The nature of the chromosome defect and presumably the underlying molecular defect in chromosome replication or re-

TABLE 9–6

**Mendelian Disorders with Cytogenetic Effects**

| Disorder | Inheritance | Clinical Features | Cytogenetic Effects |
|---|---|---|---|
| Ataxia telangiectasia | AR | Cerebellar ataxia, telangiectasia, growth retardation, immunoglobin deficiencies, predisposition to malignancy | DNA repair defects, chromatid damage |
| Bloom syndrome | AR | Dwarfism, sun-sensitive butterfly rash of face, predisposition to malignancy | High frequency of SCE (see Fig. 9–14) |
| Fanconi anemia | AR | Short stature, radial hypoplasia, anemia, pancytopenia, bronzing of skin, predisposition to leukemia | Chromosome breakage and nonhomologous interchange |
| Fragile X syndrome | X-linked | Mental retardation, macro-orchidism, large ears, and prominent jaw (see Fig. 12–27) | Fragile site at Xq27.3 (see Fig. 12–28) |
| ICF syndrome | AR | Immunodeficiency, centromere instability, facial anomalies | Hypomethylation of specific DNA sequences, association of centromeres of chromosomes 1, 9, and 16 |
| Roberts syndrome | AR | Growth retardation, developmental delay, limb anomalies, craniofacial deformaties | Separation of heterochromatic regions, "railroad track" sister chromatids |
| Xeroderma pigmentosum | AR | Sensitivity to sunlight, skin changes, predisposition to malignancy | Excision repair defects; increased SCE rate after exposure to UV light or chemical carcinogens |

AR = autosomal recessive; SCE = sister chromatid exchange.
Several of the disorders are genetically heterogeneous.

pair is different in each of these disorders. For example, Bloom syndrome is caused by a defect in a DNA helicase that leads to a striking increase in somatic recombination and **sister chromatid exchange** (Fig. 9–14). ICF syndrome (characterized by **i**mmunodeficiency, **c**entromeric instability, and **f**acial anomalies) is caused by a deficiency in one of the DNA methyltransferases that are required for establishing and maintaining normal patterns of DNA methylation (at 5-methylcytosine residues; see Chapter 10) in the genome. Chromosomes from patients with ICF show a characteristic abnormal association of pericentromeric heterochromatin involving chromosomes 1, 9, and 16.

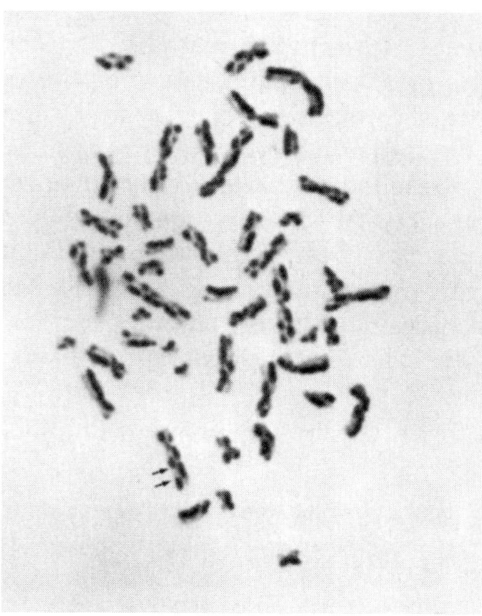

Figure 9–14. Characteristic high frequency of sister chromatid exchanges in chromosomes from a patient with Bloom syndrome. Two exchanges are indicated by the arrows. (Photomicrograph courtesy of Chin Ho, Cytogenetics Laboratory, The Hospital for Sick Children, Toronto.)

Several of the chromosome breakage syndromes listed in Table 9–6 are associated with an increased risk of malignancy. Further analysis of the correlation between decreased ability to replicate or repair DNA and increased risk of malignancies might be expected to provide insight into the relationship between mutagenesis and carcinogenesis (see Chapter 16).

## CYTOGENETIC ANALYSIS IN CANCER

An important field of cancer research is the delineation of cytogenetic changes in specific forms of cancer and the relation of the breakpoints of the various structural rearrangements to oncogenes. The cytogenetic changes seen in cancer cells are numerous and diverse. Many are repeatedly seen in the same type of tumor. Several hundred nonrandom chromosome changes involving all chromosomes except the Y chromosome have been identified in various neoplasias. In the future, the association of cytogenetic analysis with tumor type and with the effectiveness of therapy will be an important part of the management of patients with cancer. The types of chromosome changes seen in cancer and the role of chromosome abnormalities in the etiology or progression, or both, of different malignancies are discussed further in Chapter 16. Their detection in clinical cytogenetics laboratories, using FISH, can have important diagnostic or prognostic value, or both, for oncologists (see Fig. 9–5, *color insert*).

## General References


Epstein CJ (1986) The Consequences of Chromosome Imbalance: Principles, Mechanisms, and Models. Cambridge University Press, New York.

Gardner RJM, Sutherland GR (1996) Chromosome Abnormalities and Genetic Counseling, 2nd ed. Oxford University Press, Oxford, England, 478 pp.

Hsu LYF (1998) Prenatal diagnosis of chromosomal abnormalities through amniocentesis. *In* Milunsky A (ed) Genetic Disorders and the Fetus, 4th ed. Johns Hopkins University Press, Baltimore, pp. 179–248.

Mittleman F (ed) (1995) ISCN 1995: An International System for Human Cytogenetic Nomenclature. Karger, Basel, 114 pp.

Sapienza C, Hall JG (2000) Genome imprinting in human disease. *In* Scriver CR, Beaudet AL, Sly WS, Valle D (eds) The Metabolic and Molecular Basis of Inherited Disease, 8th ed. McGraw-Hill, New York.

Schwartz S (1998) Molecular cytogenetics and prenatal diagnosis. *In* Milunsky A (ed) Genetic Disorders and the Fetus, 4th ed. Johns Hopkins University Press, Baltimore, pp. 286–313.

Shaffer LG, Ledbetter DH, Lupski JR (2000) Molecular cytogenetics of contiguous gene syndromes: Mechanisms and consequences of gene dosage imbalance. *In* Scriver CR, Beaudet AL, Sly WS, Valle D (eds) The Metabolic and Molecular Bases of Inherited Disease, 8th ed. McGraw-Hill, New York.

Therman E, Susman M (1993) Human Chromosomes: Structure, Behavior, Effects, 3rd ed. Springer-Verlag, New York, 376 pp.


## References Specific to Particular Topics


Allderdice PW, Browne N, Murphy DP (1975) Chromosome 3 duplication q21-qter, deletion p25-pter syndrome in children of carriers of a pericentric inversion inv(3)(p25q21). Am J Hum Genet 27:699–718.

American College of Medical Genetics (1993) Prenatal interphase fluorescence in situ hybridization (FISH) policy statement. Am J Hum Genet 53:526–527.

Flint J, Wilke AO, Buckle VJ, et al (1995) The detection of subtelomeric chromosomal rearrangements in idiopathic mental retardation. Nature Genet 9:132–140.

Hassold TJ (1998) Nondisjunction in the human male. Curr Top Dev Biol 37:383–406.

Jacobs PA, Browne C, Gregson N, et al (1992) Estimates of the frequency of chromosome abnormalities detectable in unselected newborns using moderate levels of banding. J Med Genet 29:103–108.

Ledbetter DH, Engel E (1995) Uniparental disomy in humans: Development of an imprinting map and its implications for prenatal diagnosis. Hum Mol Genet 4:1757–1764.

Lengauer C, Kinzler KW, Vogelstein B (1998) Genetic instabilities in human cancers. Nature 396:643–649.

Schrock E, du Manoir S, Veldman T, et al (1996) Multicolor spectral karyotyping of human chromosomes. Science 273: 494–497.

Sutherland GR, Baker E, Richards RI (1998) Fragile sites still breaking. Trends Genet 14:501–506.

Warburton D (1991) De novo balanced chromosome rearrangements and extra marker chromosomes identified at prenatal diagnosis: Clinical significance and distribution of breakpoints. Am J Hum Genet 49:995–1013.

Ward BE, Gersen SL, Carelli MP, et al (1993) Rapid prenatal diagnosis of chromosomal aneuploidies by fluorescence in situ hybridization: Clinical experience with 4500 specimens. Am J Hum Genet 52:854–865.


## Problems

1. You send a blood sample from a dysmorphic infant to the chromosome laboratory for analysis. The laboratory's report states that the child's karyotype is 46,XY, 18q−.
   (a) What does this karyotype mean?
   (b) The laboratory asks for blood samples from the clinically normal parents for analysis. Why?
   (c) The laboratory reports the mother's karyotype as 46,XX and the father's karyotype as 46,XY,−7,−18, +t(7;18)(q35;q12). What does the latter karyotype mean? Referring to the normal chromosome idiograms in Figure 9–1, sketch the translocation chromosome or chromosomes in the father and in his son. Sketch these chromosomes in meiosis in the father. What kinds of gametes can he produce?
   (d) In light of this new information, what does the child's karyotype mean now? What regions are monosomic? Trisomic? Given information from Chapter 3, estimate the number of genes present in the trisomic or monosomic regions.

2. A spontaneously aborted fetus is found to have trisomy 18.
   (a) What proportion of fetuses with trisomy 18 are lost by spontaneous abortion?
   (b) What is the risk that the parents will have a liveborn child with trisomy 18 in a future pregnancy?

3. A newborn child with Down syndrome, when karyotyped, is found to have two cell lines: 70 percent of her cells have the typical 47,XX,+21 karyotype, and 30 percent are normal 46,XX. When did the nondisjunctional event probably occur? What is the prognosis for this child?

4. Which of the following persons is or are expected to be phenotypically normal?
   (a) A female with 47 chromosomes, including a small supernumerary chromosome derived from the centromeric region of chromosome 15.
   (b) A female with the karyotype 47,XX,+13.
   (c) A male with deletion of a band on chromosome 4.
   (d) A person with a balanced reciprocal translocation.
   (e) A person with a pericentric inversion of chromosome 6.

   What kinds of gametes can each of these individuals produce? What kinds of offspring might result, assuming that the other parent is chromosomally normal?

5. For each of the following, state whether chromosome analysis is indicated or not. For which family members, if any? For what kind of chromosome abnormality might the family in each case be at risk?
   (a) A pregnant 29-year-old woman and her 41-year-old husband, with no history of genetic defects.
   (b) A pregnant 41-year-old woman and her 29-year-old husband, with no history of genetic defects.
   (c) A couple whose only child has Down syndrome.
   (d) A couple whose only child has Duchenne muscular dystrophy.
   (e) A couple who have two severely retarded boys.

10

# Clinical Cytogenetics: Disorders of the Autosomes and the Sex Chromosomes

In Chapter 9, we introduced general principles of clinical cytogenetics and the different types of abnormalities detected in clinical practice. In this chapter we present more detailed accounts of several specific chromosomal disorders and their causes and consequences. We first discuss the most common autosomal abnormalities, including Down syndrome, followed by consideration of the X and Y chromosomes, their unique biology, and their abnormalities. Because sex determination is chromosomally determined, we include in this discussion disorders of gonadal development and sexual differentiation. Even though many such disorders are determined by single genes, a clinical approach to evaluating ambiguous genitalia usually includes a detailed cytogenetic analysis.

## AUTOSOMAL DISORDERS

In this section, the major autosomal disorders of clinical significance are described. Although there are numerous rare chromosome disorders in which gain or loss of an entire chromosome or a chromosome segment has been reported, many of these either have been seen only in fetuses that were aborted spontaneously or involve relatively short chromosome segments. There are only three well-defined nonmosaic chromosome disorders compatible with postnatal survival in which there is trisomy for an entire autosome: **trisomy 21** (Down syndrome), **trisomy 18**, and **trisomy 13**.

Each of these autosomal trisomies is associated with growth retardation, mental retardation, and multiple congenital anomalies. Nevertheless, each has a fairly distinctive phenotype. The developmental abnormalities characteristic of any one trisomic state are determined by the extra dosage of the particular genes on the additional chromosome. Knowledge of the specific relationship between the extra chromosome and the consequent developmental abnormality has been limited to date. Current research, however, is beginning to show that specific genes on the extra chromosome are responsible, through direct and indirect modulation of developmental pathways, for specific aspects of the abnormal phenotype. More generally, any chromosomal imbalance, whether it involves addition or loss of genes, is expected to have a specific phenotypic effect determined by the dosage of the specific genes on the extra or missing chromosome segment.

### Down Syndrome

Down syndrome, or trisomy 21, is by far the most common and best known of the chromosome disorders and is the single most common genetic cause of moderate mental retardation. About 1 child in 800 is born with Down syndrome (see Table 9–3), and among liveborn children or fetuses of mothers 35 years of age or older, the incidence rate is far higher (Table 10–1).

The syndrome was first described clinically by Langdon Down in 1866, but its cause remained a deep mystery for almost a century. Two noteworthy features of its population distribution drew attention:

TABLE 10–1

**Incidence of Down Syndrome in Liveborns and Fetuses in Relation to Maternal Age**

| | Incidence | | |
|---|---|---|---|
| **Maternal Age (Years)** | *At Birth* | *At Amniocentesis (16 weeks)* | *At Chorionic Villus Sampling (9–11 weeks)* |
| 15–19 | 1/1250 | — | — |
| 20–24 | 1/1400 | — | — |
| 25–29 | 1/1100 | — | — |
| 30 | 1/900 | — | — |
| 31 | 1/900 | — | — |
| 32 | 1/750 | — | — |
| 33 | 1/625 | 1/420 | 1/370 |
| 34 | 1/500 | 1/333 | 1/250 |
| 35 | 1/385 | 1/250 | 1/250 |
| 36 | 1/300 | 1/200 | 1/175 |
| 37 | 1/225 | 1/150 | 1/175 |
| 38 | 1/175 | 1/115 | 1/115 |
| 39 | 1/140 | 1/90 | 1/90 |
| 40 | 1/100 | 1/70 | 1/80 |
| 41 | 1/80 | 1/50 | 1/50 |
| 42 | 1/65 | 1/40 | 1/30 |
| 43 | 1/50 | 1/30 | 1/25 |
| 44 | 1/40 | 1/25 | 1/25 |
| 45 and over | 1/25 | 1/20 | 1/15 |

Data from Hsu (1998) and Gardner and Sutherland (1996). Figures have been rounded and are approximate.

increased maternal age and a peculiar distribution within families—concordance in monozygotic twins but almost complete discordance in dizygotic twins and other family members. Although it was recognized as early as the 1930s that a chromosome abnormality could explain these observations, at that time no one was prepared to believe that humans were really likely to have chromosome abnormalities. However, when techniques for detailed analysis of human chromosomes became available, Down syndrome was one of the first conditions to be examined chromosomally. In 1959 it was established that most children with Down syndrome have 47 chromosomes, the extra member being a small acrocentric chromosome that has since been designated chromosome 21 (see Fig. 9–6).

## PHENOTYPE

Down syndrome can usually be diagnosed at birth or shortly thereafter by its dysmorphic features, which vary among patients but nevertheless produce a distinctive phenotype (Fig. 10–1). Hypotonia may be the first abnormality noticed in the newborn. In addition to characteristic dysmorphic facial features evident to even the untrained observer, the patients are short in stature and have brachycephaly with a flat occiput. The neck is short, with loose skin on the nape. The nasal bridge is flat, the ears are low-set and have a characteristic folded appearance, the eyes have Brushfield spots around the margin of the iris, and the mouth is open, often showing the furrowed, protruding tongue. Characteristic epicanthal folds and upslanting palpebral fissures gave rise to the term "mongolism," once used to refer to this condition (the term is now considered inappropriate and should not be used). The hands are short and broad, often with a single transverse palmar crease ("simian crease") and incurved fifth digits, or clinodactyly (Fig. 10–2). The dermatoglyphics (patterns of the ridged skin) are highly characteristic. The feet show a wide gap between the first and second toes, with a furrow extending proximally on the plantar surface.

The major cause for concern in Down syndrome is mental retardation. Even though in early infancy the child may not seem delayed in development, the delay is usually obvious by the end of the first year. The intelligence quotient (IQ) is usually 30 to 60 when the child is old enough to be tested. Nevertheless, many children with Down syndrome develop into happy, responsive, and even self-reliant persons in spite of these limitations (see Fig. 10–1).

Congenital heart disease is present in at least one third of all liveborn Down syndrome infants and in a somewhat higher proportion of abortuses with the syndrome. Certain malformations, such as duodenal atresia and tracheoesophageal fistula, are more common in Down syndrome than in other disorders. There is a 15-fold increase in the risk of leukemia.

## PRENATAL AND POSTNATAL SURVIVAL

Because trisomy 21 accounts for about half of all abnormalities identified prenatally, the incidence of Down syndrome seen in live births, in amniocentesis, and in chorionic villus sampling at different maternal ages can provide a basis for estimating the amount of fetal loss between the 11th and 16th weeks and between the 16th week and birth (see Table 10–1). At all the maternal ages shown, there is some loss between the 11th and 16th weeks (as would be expected from the high rate of chromosome abnormality seen in spontaneous abortions) and an additional loss later in pregnancy. In fact, probably only 20 to 25 percent of trisomy 21 conceptuses survive to birth (see Table 9–5).

Among Down syndrome conceptuses, those least likely to survive are those with congenital heart disease; about one fourth of the liveborn infants with heart defects die before their first birthday. Premature senility, associated with the neuropathological findings characteristic of Alzheimer disease (cortical

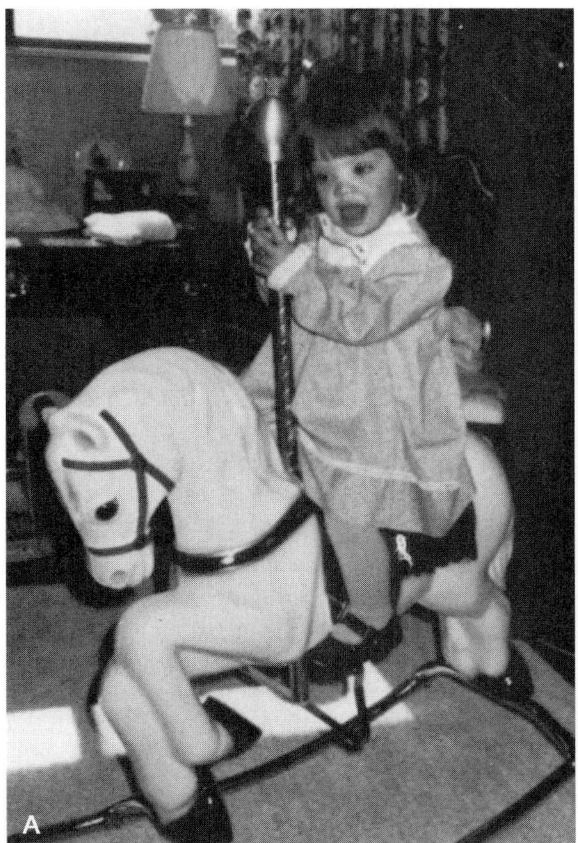


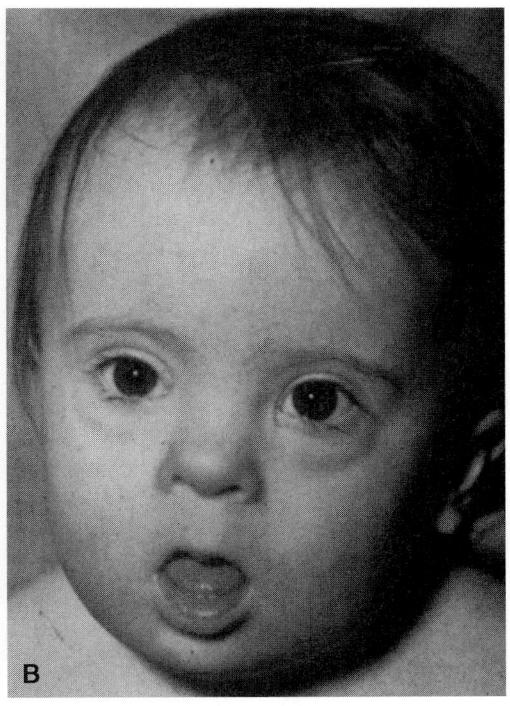


**Figure 10–1.** Two children with Down syndrome. (*A*, Courtesy of David Patterson, Eleanor Roosevelt Institute, Denver. *B*, From Jones KL [1988] Smith's Recognizable Patterns of Human Malformation, 4th ed. WB Saunders, Philadelphia.)

atrophy, ventricular dilatation, and neurofibrillar tangles), affects Down syndrome patients at an age several decades earlier than the typical age of onset of Alzheimer disease in the general population.

### The Chromosomes in Down Syndrome

The clinical diagnosis of Down syndrome usually presents no particular difficulty. Nevertheless, karyotyping is necessary for confirmation and to provide a basis for genetic counseling. Although the particular karyotype responsible for Down syndrome usually has little effect on the phenotype of the patient, it is essential for determining the recurrence risk.

**Trisomy 21.** In about 95 percent of all patients, Down syndrome involves trisomy for chromosome 21 (see Fig. 9–6), resulting from meiotic nondisjunction of the chromosome 21 pair, as discussed in the previous chapter. As noted earlier, the risk of having a child with trisomy 21 increases with maternal age, especially after the age of 30 years (see Table 10–1). The meiotic error responsible for the trisomy usually occurs during maternal meiosis (about 90 percent of cases), predominantly in meiosis I, but can occur in paternal meiosis (about 10 percent of cases), usually in meiosis II.

**Robertsonian Translocation.** About 4 percent of Down syndrome patients have 46 chromosomes, one of which is a Robertsonian translocation between chromosome 21q and the long arm of one of the other acrocentric chromosomes (usually chromosome 14 or 22). The translocation chromosome replaces one of the normal acrocentrics, and the karyotype of a Down syndrome patient with a Robertsonian translocation between chromosomes 14 and 21 is therefore 46,XX or XY,rob(14;21),+21. The standard nomenclature is written rob(14;21), not t(14;21), to denote this special type of translocation. In effect, the patient is trisomic for 21q.

Unlike standard trisomy 21, translocation Down syndrome shows no relation to maternal age but has a relatively high recurrence risk in families when a parent, especially the mother, is a carrier of the translocation. For this reason, karyotyping of the parents and possibly other relatives is necessary before accurate genetic counseling can be provided.

A carrier of a Robertsonian translocation involving chromosomes 14 and 21 has only 45 chromosomes; one chromosome 14 and one chromosome 21 are missing and are replaced by the translocation chromosome; the karyotype, therefore, is 45,XX or XY,rob(14;21). The gametes that can be formed by

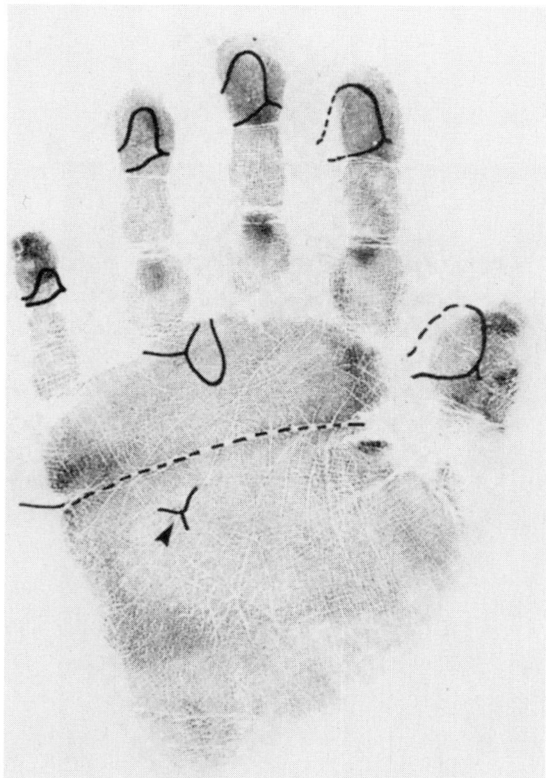

**Figure 10–2.** Characteristic dermal patterns of the palm of a child with Down syndrome: a single flexion crease (simian crease), axial triradius (*arrow*) in distal position, a pattern area on the palm between the third and fourth digits, and ulnar loops on all ten digits.

such a carrier are shown in Figure 10–3. Theoretically, there are six possible types of gamete, but three of these appear unable to lead to viable offspring. Of the three viable types, one is normal, one is balanced, and one is unbalanced, having both the translocation chromosome and the normal chromosome 21. In combination with a normal gamete, this could produce a child with translocation Down syndrome (Fig. 10–4). Theoretically, the three types of gametes are produced in equal numbers, and thus the theoretical risk of a Down syndrome child should be 1 in 3. However, extensive population studies have shown that unbalanced chromosome complements appear in only about 10 to 15 percent of the progeny of carrier mothers and in only a few percent of the progeny of carrier fathers who have translocations involving chromosome 21.

**21q21q Translocation.** A 21q21q translocation chromosome is a chromosome comprising two chromosome 21 long arms; it is seen in a small proportion of Down syndrome patients. It is thought to originate as an isochromosome rather than by Robertsonian translocation. Although this is a rare abnormality, it is particularly important because all gametes of a carrier of such a chromosome must either contain the 21q21q chromosome, with its double dose of chromosome 21 genetic material, or lack it and have no chromosome 21 representative at all. The potential progeny, therefore, inevitably have either Down syndrome or monosomy 21, which is rarely viable. In other words, an individual unfortunate enough to carry a 21q21q chromosome is unable to have normal children and will probably have only children with Down syndrome.

**Mosaic Down Syndrome.** A small percentage of Down syndrome patients are mosaic, usually for cell populations with either a normal or a trisomy 21 karyotype. The phenotype may be milder than that of typical trisomy 21, but there is wide variability in phenotypes among mosaic patients, possibly reflecting the variable proportion of trisomy 21 cells in the embryo during early development. The ascertained patients with mosaic Down syndrome probably

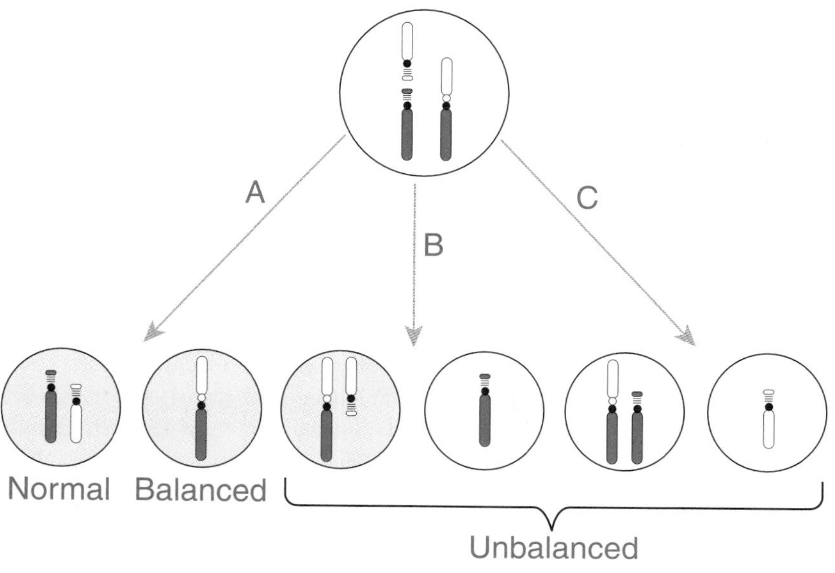


**Figure 10–3.** Chromosomes of gametes that theoretically can be produced by a carrier of a Robertsonian translocation, rob(14;21). *A*, Normal and balanced complements. *B*, Unbalanced, one product with both the translocation chromosome and the normal chromosome 21, the reciprocal product with chromosome 14 only. *C*, Unbalanced, one product with both the translocation chromosome and chromosome 14, the reciprocal product with chromosome 21 only. Only the three shaded gametes at the left can lead to viable offspring; see text for a description of the eventual fate of these gametes.

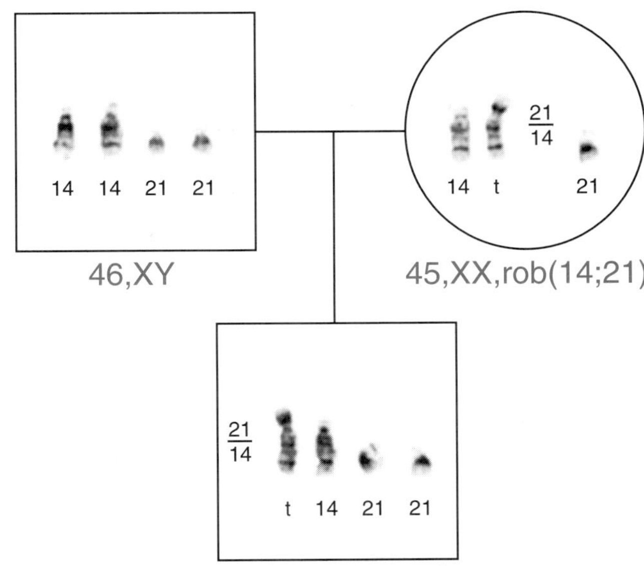


**Figure 10–4.** Translocation 14q21q transmitted by a carrier mother to her child, who has Down syndrome. The father's chromosomes are normal. Only chromosomes 14, 21, and rob(14;21) are shown. t = rob(14;21) (Original karyotype courtesy of R. G. Worton, The Hospital for Sick Children, Toronto.)

represent the more clinically severe cases, because very mildly affected persons are less likely to be karyotyped.

**Partial Trisomy 21.** Very rarely is Down syndrome diagnosed in a patient in whom only a part of the long arm of chromosome 21 is present in triplicate, and a Down syndrome patient with no cytogenetically visible chromosome abnormality is even more rarely identified. These patients are of particular interest because they can show what region of chromosome 21 is likely to be responsible for specific components of the Down syndrome phenotype, and what regions can be triplicated without causing that aspect of the phenotype.

Although sequence information from the Human Genome Project (see Chapter 8) has demonstrated that chromosome 21 contains only a few hundred genes, attempts to correlate triple dosage of specific genes with specific aspects of the Down syndrome phenotype have been largely unsuccessful so far. Sorting out the genes crucial to the expression of Down syndrome from those that merely happen to be syntenic with them on chromosome 21 is a focus of current investigation, especially using the mouse as a surrogate model. Mice engineered to contain extra dosage of genes from human chromosome 21 can show phenotypic abnormalities.

## Etiology of Trisomy 21

Although the chromosomal basis of Down syndrome is clear, the reason for the chromosome abnormality is still poorly understood. The high percentage of all cases of trisomy 21 in which the abnormal gamete originated during maternal meiosis I suggests that something about maternal meiosis I, related to increased maternal age, is the underlying cause. One obvious possibility is the "older egg" model: it has been suggested that the older the oocyte, the greater the chance that the chromosomes will fail to disjoin correctly. As mentioned previously, analyses of trisomy 21 (as well as of other autosomal trisomies) have implicated the number and/or placement of recombination events as a determinant of whether the chromosome pair will disjoin properly during the two meiotic divisions. Older eggs may be less able to overcome a susceptibility to nondisjunction established by the recombination machinery. A remarkable feature of this model (and one that greatly complicates its investigation) is that the etiologic event leading to the birth of a Down syndrome infant today may have been put in place 35 to 40 years ago, when the child's mother was herself a fetus whose primary oocytes were in prophase of the first meiotic division. Despite recognition of the important association between recombination patterns and chromosome segregation, a full understanding of chromosome 21 nondisjunction and the maternal age effect continues to be elusive.

## Risk of Down Syndrome

A frequent problem in genetic counseling, especially in prenatal genetics, is how to assess the risk of the birth of a Down syndrome child. Down syndrome can be detected prenatally by cytogenetic analysis of chorionic villus or amniotic fluid cells, and in fact about 80 percent of prenatal diagnoses are performed because increased maternal age or prenatal biochemical screening gives rise to concern about the risk of Down syndrome in the fetus. A commonly accepted guideline is that a woman is eligible for prenatal diagnosis if the risk that her fetus has Down syndrome outweighs the risk that the procedure of amniocentesis or chorionic villus sampling used to obtain fetal tissue for chromosome analysis will lead to fetal loss (see Chapter 18). The risk depends chiefly on the mother's age but also on both parents' karyotypes.

The population incidence of Down syndrome in live births is currently estimated to be about 1 in 800, reflecting the maternal age distribution for all births and the proportion of older mothers who make use of prenatal diagnosis and selective termination. At about age 30 years the risk begins to rise sharply, reaching 1 in 25 births in the oldest maternal age group (see Table 10–1). Even though younger mothers have a much lower risk, their birth rate is so much higher that more than half of the mothers of all Down syndrome babies are younger than 35 years. The risk of Down syndrome due to translocation or partial trisomy is unrelated to maternal age. The paternal age appears to have no influence on the risk.

In the United States and Canada, 50 percent or more of pregnant women 35 years old and older undergo prenatal diagnosis for fetal chromosome analysis, but only about 1 percent of the fetuses tested is found to have trisomy 21. Current approaches to more precise or efficient identification of fetuses at risk, by means of biochemical screening assays and ultrasonography, are discussed in Chapter 18. Methods to examine rare fetal cells found in the maternal circulation are also being developed.

### Recurrence Risk

The recurrence risk of trisomy 21 or some other autosomal trisomy, after one such child has been born in a family, is about 1 percent overall. For mothers younger than 30 years, the risk is about 1.4 percent, and for older mothers it is the same as the age-related risk; that is, there is an increase in risk for the younger mothers but only the age-related risk for the older mothers. The reason for the increased risk for the younger mothers is not known. One possibility is that unrecognized germline mosaicism in one parent, with a trisomic cell line as well as a normal cell line, may be a factor. A history of trisomy 21 elsewhere in the family, although often a cause of maternal anxiety, does not appear to significantly increase the risk of having a Down syndrome child.

The recurrence risk for Down syndrome due to a translocation is much higher, as described previously.

## Trisomy 18

The phenotype of an infant with trisomy 18 is shown in Figure 10–5. The features of trisomy 18 always include mental retardation and failure to thrive and often include severe malformation of the heart. Hypertonia is a typical finding. The head has a prominent occiput, and the jaw recedes. The ears are low-set and malformed. The sternum is short. The fists clench in a characteristic way, the second and fifth digits overlapping the third and fourth (see Fig. 10–5). The feet have a "rocker-bottom" appearance, with prominent

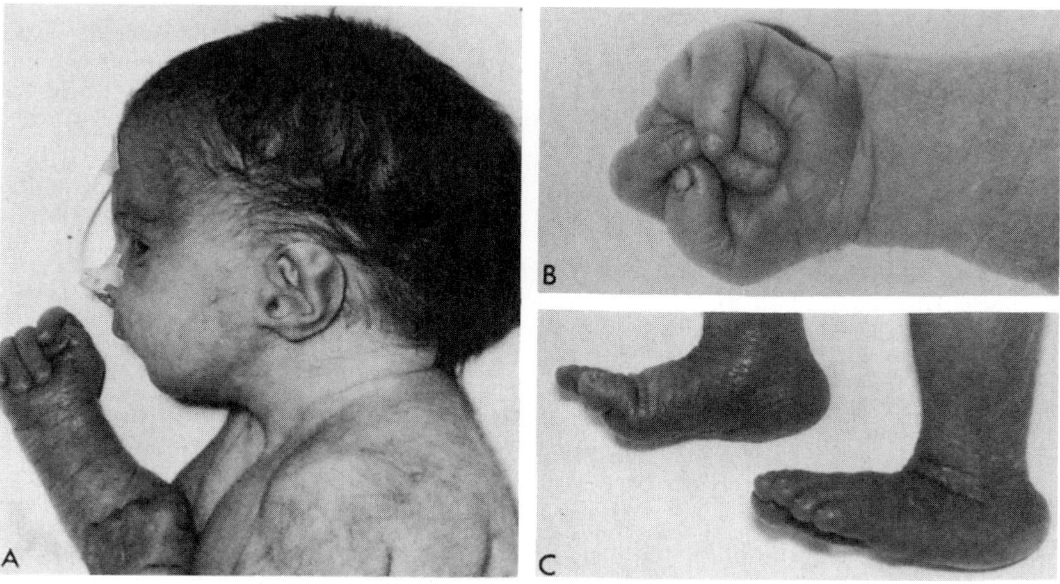


**Figure 10–5.** An infant with trisomy 18. Note the clenched fist with the second and fifth digits overlapping the third and fourth; rocker-bottom feet with prominent calcanei; and large, malformed, and low-set ears. (Courtesy of Dr. H. Medovy, Children's Centre, Winnipeg, Canada.)

calcanei. The dermal patterns are distinctive, with single creases on the palms and arch patterns on most or all digits. The nails are usually hypoplastic.

The incidence of this condition in liveborn infants is about 1 in 7500 births (see Table 9–3). The incidence at conception is much higher, but about 95 percent of trisomy 18 conceptuses are aborted spontaneously. Postnatal survival is also poor, and survival for more than a few months is rare. About 80 percent of the patients are female, perhaps because of their preferential survival. As in most other trisomies, increased maternal age is a factor, and the risk of a trisomy 18 infant is substantially greater for women older than 35 years.

The trisomy 18 phenotype, like that of trisomy 21, can result from a variety of rare karyotypes other than complete trisomy, and karyotyping of affected infants or fetuses is essential. In about 20 percent of cases, there is a translocation involving all or most of chromosome 18, which may be either de novo or inherited from a balanced carrier parent. The trisomy may also be present in mosaic form, with variable but usually somewhat milder expression.

## Trisomy 13

The striking phenotype of trisomy 13 is shown in Figure 10–6. Growth retardation and severe mental retardation are present, accompanied by severe central nervous system malformations such as arhinencephaly and holoprosencephaly. The forehead is sloping, there is microcephaly and wide open sutures, and there may be microphthalmia, iris coloboma, or even absence of the eyes. The ears are malformed. Cleft lip and cleft palate are often present. The hands and feet may show postaxial polydactyly, and the hands clench with the second and fifth digits overlapping the third and fourth, as in trisomy 18. The feet, again as in trisomy 18, have a rocker-bottom appearance. The palms often have simian creases. Internally there are usually congenital heart defects of specific types and urogenital defects, including cryptorchidism in males, bicornuate uterus and hypoplastic ovaries in females, and polycystic kidneys. Of this constellation of defects, the most distinctive are the general facial appearance with cleft lip and palate and ocular abnormalities, polydactyly, the clenched fists, and rocker-bottom feet.

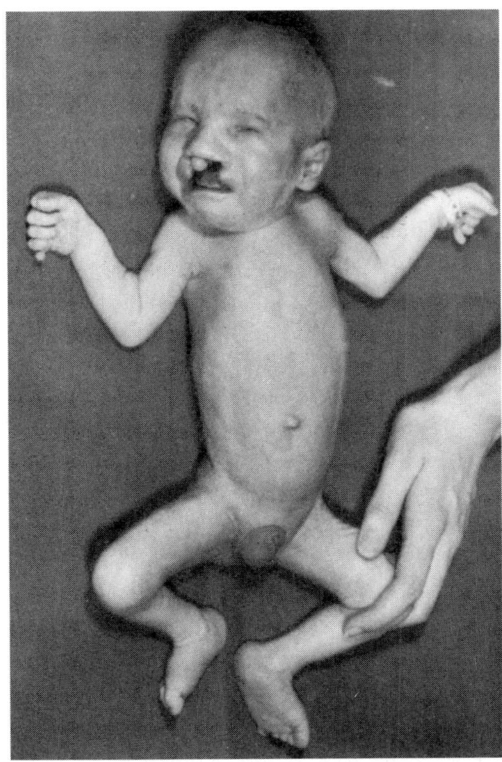

**Figure 10–6.** An infant with trisomy 13. Note particularly the bilateral cleft lip and polydactyly. (Courtesy of P. E. Conen, The Hospital for Sick Children, Toronto.)

The incidence of trisomy 13 is about 1 in 20,000 to 25,000 births. Trisomy 13 is clinically very severe, and about half of such individuals die within the first month. Like most other trisomies, it is associated with increased maternal age, and the extra chromosome usually arises from nondisjunction in maternal meiosis I. Karyotyping of affected infants or fetuses is indicated to confirm the clinical diagnosis; about 20 percent of the cases are caused by an unbalanced translocation. The recurrence risk is low; even when one parent of a translocation patient is a carrier of the translocation, the empiric risk that a subsequent liveborn child will have the syndrome is less than 2 percent.

## Autosomal Deletion Syndromes

There are many reports of cytogenetically detectable deletions in dysmorphic patients, but most of these deletions have been seen in only a few patients and are not associated with recognized syndromes. However, there are a number of well-delineated autosomal deletion syndromes in which a series of patients have the same or similar deletion, resulting in a clearly recognizable syndrome. Overall, cytogenetically visible autosomal deletions occur with an estimated incidence of 1 in 7000 live births.

### Cri du Chat Syndrome

One such syndrome is the cri du chat syndrome, in which there is a large deletion of the short arm of chromosome 5. This deletion syndrome was given its common name because crying infants with this disorder sound like a mewing cat. The syndrome accounts for about 1 percent of all institutionalized mentally retarded patients. The facial appearance, shown in Figure 10–7, is distinctive, with microcephaly,

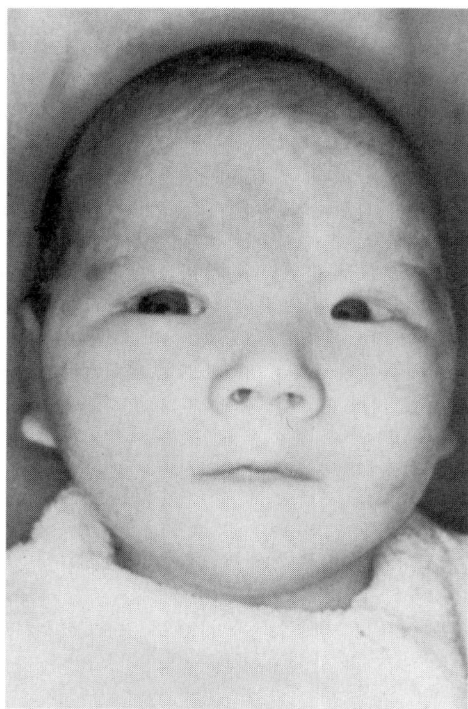

**Figure 10–7.** An infant with cri du chat syndrome, which results from deletion of part of chromosome 5p. Note characteristic facies with hypertelorism, epicanthus, and retrognathia.

hypertelorism, epicanthal folds, low-set ears sometimes with preauricular tags, and micrognathia. Other features include severe mental retardation and heart defects.

Most cases of cri du chat syndrome are sporadic, and 10 to 15 percent of the patients are the offspring of translocation carriers. The breakpoints and extent of the deleted segment of chromosome 5p vary in different patients, but the critical region, missing in all patients with the phenotype, has been identified as band 5p15. A number of genes have been demonstrated to be deleted from $5p^-$ chromosomes, and the basis for the relationship between monosomy for such genes and the clinical phenotype is beginning to be elucidated. Many of the clinical findings appear to be due to haploinsufficiency of a gene or genes within band 5p15.2, and the distinctive cat cry appears to result from deletion of 5p15.3.

## Microdeletion Syndromes

Several dysmorphic syndromes are associated with small, but sometimes cytogenetically visible, deletions, leading to a form of genetic imbalance referred to as **segmental aneusomy** (Table 10–2). These deletions produce syndromes that are usually clinically recognizable and that can be detected either by high-resolution chromosome analysis or by fluorescence in situ hybridization (FISH) (see Fig. 9–5, *color insert*). The term **contiguous gene syndrome** has been applied to many of these conditions, as the phenotype is attributable to haploinsufficiency of multiple, contiguous genes within the deleted region. For other deletion disorders, the phenotype is apparently due to deletion of only a single gene, despite the typical association of a large deletion with the condition.

For each syndrome, the extent of the deletions in different patients is similar. Indeed, for the syndromes listed in Table 10–2, molecular and FISH studies have demonstrated that the location of centromeric and telomeric breakpoints cluster among different patients, suggesting the existence of deletion-prone sequences. Fine mapping in a number of these disorders has suggested that the breakpoints localize to low-copy repeated sequences and that aberrant recombination between nearby copies of the repeats

TABLE 10–2

**Microdeletion or Contiguous Gene Syndromes Involving Recombination Between Repeated Sequences**

| Disorder | Location | Rearrangement *Type* | Rearrangement *Size (kb)* | Repeat Length (kb) |
|---|---|---|---|---|
| Smith-Magenis syndrome | 17p11.2 | Deletion | 5000 | 200 |
| dup(17)(p11.2) | | Duplication | | |
| Prader-Willi/Angelman syndromes | 15q11-q13 | Deletion | 4000 | ~50–400 |
| Williams syndrome | 7q11.23 | Deletion | 2000 | >30 |
| Ichthyosis | Xp22.3 | Deletion | 1900 | 20 |
| Neurofibromatosis | 17q11.2 | Deletion | 1500 | ~15–100 |
| Charcot-Marie-Tooth (*CMT1A*)/HNLPP | 17p12 | Duplication / Deletion | 1500 | 24 |
| DiGeorge syndrome/ velocardiofacial syndrome | 22q11 | Deletion | 3000 | 200 |
| Cat-eye syndrome | | Duplication | | |

HNLPP = hereditary neuropathy with liability to pressure palsies.

Data updated from Lupski JR (1998) Genomic disorders: Structural features of the genome can lead to DNA rearrangements and human disease traits. Trends Genet 14:417–422.

causes the deletions, which span several hundred to several thousand kb. This general mechanism has been implicated in several syndromes involving contiguous gene rearrangements (see Table 10–2). Deletions and duplications mediated by unequal recombination have been documented (Fig. 10–8). For example, unequal recombination between flanking repeats that are nearly 99 percent identical in sequence during meiosis I can result in either duplication or deletion of a 1500-kb region of chromosome 17p11.2. Duplication of the intervening genes leads to a form of Charcot-Marie-Tooth disease, whereas deletion leads to hereditary neuropathy with liability to pressure palsies (see Table 10–2).

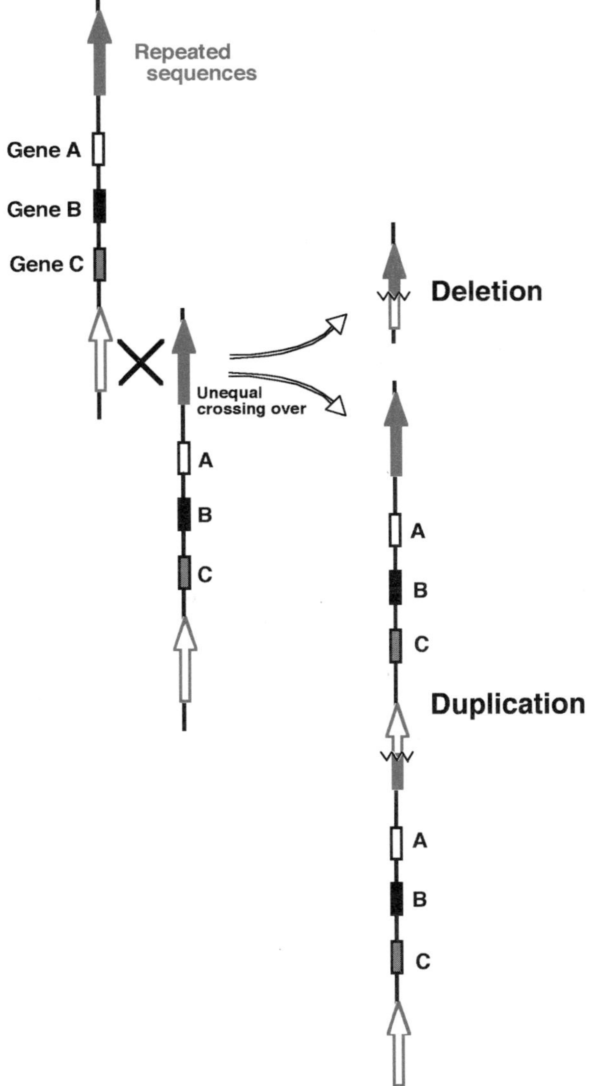


**Figure 10–8.** Unequal crossing over between misaligned sister chromatids or homologous chromosomes containing highly homologous copies of a repeated DNA sequence can lead to two products differing in the number of copies of the sequence. The copy number of any gene(s) (such as *A*, *B*, *C*) that lie between the copies of the repeat will change as a result of this genome rearrangement.

A particularly common microdeletion that is frequently evaluated in clinical cytogenetics laboratories involves chromosome 22q11.2 and is associated with **DiGeorge syndrome** or **velocardiofacial syndrome**. DiGeorge syndrome/velocardiofacial syndrome is an autosomal dominant condition with variable expressivity, caused by a deletion within 22q11, spanning 3000 kb. This microdeletion, also mediated by homologous recombination between low-copy repeated sequences, is one of the most common cytogenetic deletions associated with an important clinical phenotype and is detected in 1 in 2000 to 4000 live births. Patients show characteristic craniofacial anomalies, mental retardation, and heart defects. DiGeorge syndrome/velocardiofacial syndrome deletion is thought to play a role in as many as 5 percent of all congenital heart defects and is a particularly frequent cause of certain defects. For example, more than 40 percent of patients with tetralogy of Fallot and pulmonary atresia and more than 60 percent of patients with tetralogy of Fallot and absent pulmonary valve have this microdeletion. In contrast to the relatively common deletion of 22q11.2, duplication of 22q11.2 is much rarer and leads to the dysmorphic **cat-eye syndrome**, in which patients have a triple or quadruple complement of this segment of chromosome 22.

## THE SEX CHROMOSOMES AND THEIR ABNORMALITIES

The X and Y chromosomes have long attracted interest because they differ between the sexes, because they have their own specific patterns of inheritance, and because they are involved in primary sex determination. They are structurally quite distinct and are subject to different forms of genetic regulation, yet they pair in male meiosis. For all these reasons, they require special attention. In this section, we review the common sex chromosome abnormalities and their clinical consequences, the current state of knowledge concerning the control of sex determination, and other mendelian abnormalities of sexual differentiation.

### The Chromosomal Basis of Sex Determination

The different sex chromosome constitution of normal human male and female cells has been appreciated for more than 50 years. Soon after cytogenetic analysis became feasible, the fundamental basis of the XX/XY system of sex determination became apparent. Males with Klinefelter syndrome were found to have 47 chromosomes with two X chromosomes as well as a Y chromosome (karyotype 47,XXY), whereas most Turner syndrome females were found to have only 45 chromosomes with a single X chromosome (karyotype 45,X). *These findings promptly and firmly established the crucial role of the Y chromosome in normal male development. Furthermore, compared with the dramatic consequences of autosomal aneuploidy, these karyotypes underscored the relatively modest effect of varying the number of X chromosomes in either males or females.* The basis for both observations in terms of the unique biology of the Y and X chromosomes is now understood.

## The Y Chromosome

The structure of the Y chromosome and its role in sexual development have been determined at both the molecular and genomic levels (Fig. 10–9). In male meiosis, the X and Y chromosomes normally pair by segments at the ends of their short arms (see Fig. 2–8) and undergo recombination in that region. The pairing segment includes the **pseudoautosomal region** of the X and Y chromosomes, so called because the X- and Y-linked copies of this region are homologous to one another and undergo homologous recombination in meiosis I, like pairs of autosomes (see Chapter 5). (A second, less well-characterized pseudoautosomal segment is located at the distal ends of Xq and Yq.) By comparison with autosomes and the X chromosome, the Y chromosome is relatively gene-poor and is estimated to contain fewer than 50 genes. However, the functions of a high proportion of these genes are related to gonadal and genital development.

### Embryology of the Reproductive System

The effect of the Y chromosome on the embryology of the male and female reproductive systems is summarized in Figure 10–10. By the sixth week of development in both sexes, the primordial germ cells have migrated from their earlier extraembryonic location to the gonadal ridges, where they are surrounded by the sex cords to form a pair of primitive gonads. Up to this time, the developing gonad, whether chromosomally XX or XY, is bipotential and is often referred to as "indifferent."

The current concept is that development into an ovary or a testis is determined by the coordinated action of a sequence of genes that leads normally to ovarian development when no Y chromosome is present or to testicular development when a Y is present. The ovarian pathway is followed unless a Y-linked gene, designated testis-determining factor (*TDF*), acts as a switch, diverting development into the male pathway.

In the presence of a Y chromosome, the medullary tissue forms typical testes with seminiferous tubules and Leydig cells that, under the stimulation of human chorionic gonadotropin from the placenta, become capable of androgen secretion (see Fig. 10–10). The spermatogonia, derived from the

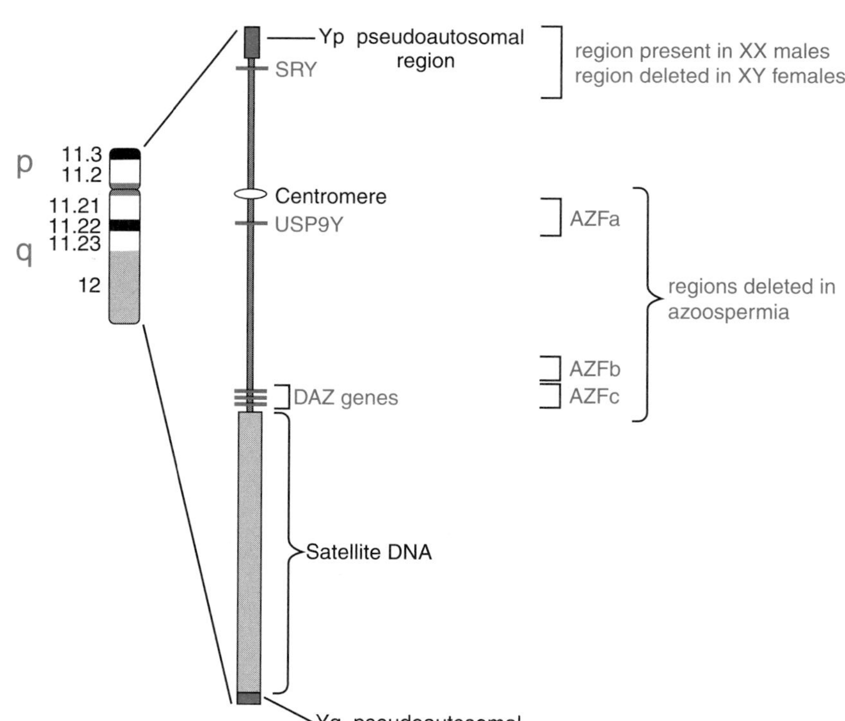


**Figure 10–9.** The Y chromosome in sex determination and in disorders of sexual differentiation. Individual genes and regions implicated in sex determination, sex reversal, and defects of spermatogenesis are indicated.

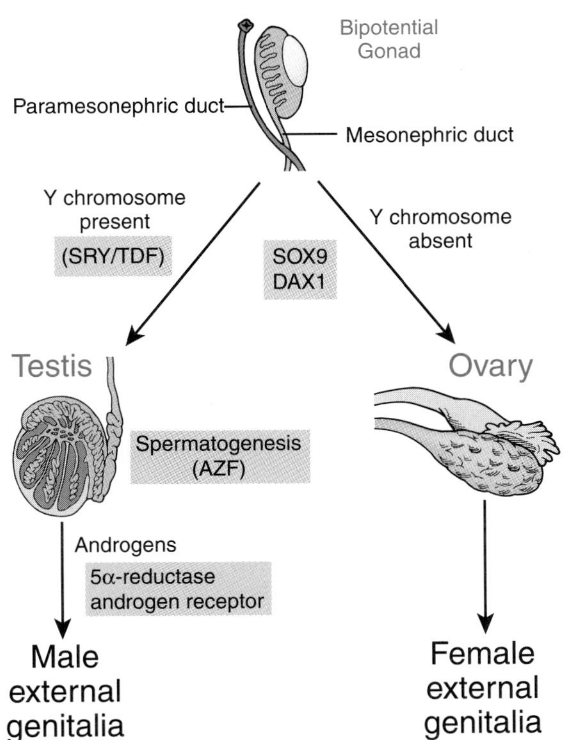


**Figure 10–10.** Scheme of developmental events in sex determination and differentiation of the male and female gonads. Involvement of individual genes in key developmental steps and/or in genetic disorders is indicated in red boxes. See text for discussion.

primordial germ cells by 200 or more successive mitoses, line the walls of the seminiferous tubules, where they reside together with supporting Sertoli cells.

If no Y chromosome is present, the gonad forms an ovary, beginning about the 12th week of gestation; the cortex develops, the medulla regresses, and oogonia begin to develop within follicles (see Fig. 10–10). Beginning at about the end of the third month, the oogonia enter meiosis I, but (as described in Chapter 2) this process is arrested at dictyotene until ovulation occurs many years later.

While the primordial germ cells are migrating to the genital ridges, thickenings in the ridges indicate the developing genital ducts, the **mesonephric** (formerly called wolffian) and **paramesonephric** (formerly called müllerian) ducts. In the male, the Leydig cells of the fetal testes produce androgen, which stimulates the mesonephric ducts to form the male genital ducts. The Sertoli cells produce a hormone (müllerian inhibitory substance) that suppresses formation of the paramesonephric ducts. In the female (or in an embryo with no gonads), the mesonephric ducts regress, and the paramesonephric ducts develop into the female duct system. Duct formation is usually completed by the third month.

In the early embryo, the external genitalia consist of a genital tubercle, paired labioscrotal swellings, and paired urethral folds. From this undifferentiated state, male external genitalia develop under the influence of androgens. In the absence of a testis, female external genitalia are formed regardless of whether an ovary is present.

## The Testis-Determining Gene

The earliest cytogenetic studies established the testis-determining function of the Y chromosome. More recently, different deletions of the pseudoautosomal region and of the sex-specific region of the Y chromosome in sex-reversed individuals have been used to map the precise location of the primary testis-determining region on Yp.

Whereas the X and Y chromosomes normally exchange in meiosis I within the Xp/Yp pseudoautosomal region, in rare instances genetic recombination occurs outside of the pseudoautosomal region (Fig. 10–11), leading to two rare, but highly informative, abnormalities: **XX males** and **XY females**. Each of these sex-reversal disorders occurs with an incidence of approximately 1 in 20,000 births. XX males are phenotypic males with a 46,XX karyotype who usually possess some Y chromosomal sequences translocated to the short arm of the X. Similarly, a proportion of phenotypic females with a 46,XY karyotype have lost the testis-determining region of the Y chromosome.

The *SRY* gene (**s**ex-determining **r**egion on the **Y**) lies near the pseudoautosomal boundary on the Y chromosome, is present in many 46,XX males, and is deleted or mutated in a proportion of female 46,XY patients, thus strongly implicating *SRY* in male sex determination. *SRY* is expressed only briefly early in development in cells of the germinal ridge just before differentiation of the testis. *SRY* encodes a DNA-binding protein that is likely to be a transcription factor, although the specific genes that it regulates are unknown. Importantly, the mouse *Sry* gene, when introduced into an XX mouse, can by itself cause testis formation. Thus, by all available genetic and developmental criteria, *SRY* is equivalent to the *TDF* gene on the Y chromosome.

Other genes in the sex-determination pathway are located on the X chromosome and on the autosomes and are discussed in later sections.

## Y-Linked Genes in Spermatogenesis

Interstitial deletions in Yq have been associated with at least 10 percent of cases of nonobstructive azoospermia (no sperm detectable in semen) and with a smaller number of cases of severe oligospermia (low sperm count). These findings suggest that one or more genes, termed the azoospermia

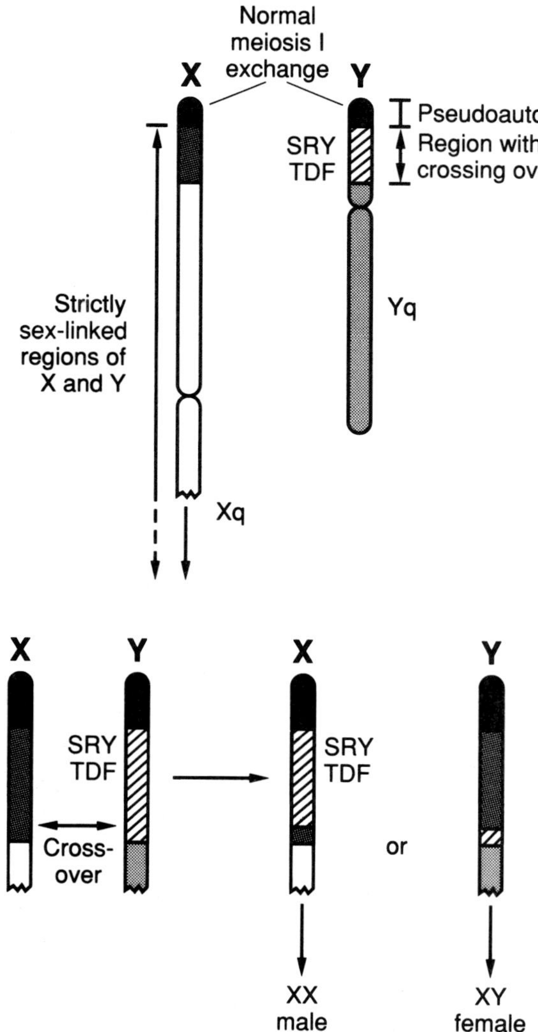


**Figure 10–11.** Etiological factors of XX male or XY female phenotypes by aberrant exchange between X- and Y-linked sequences. X and Y chromosomes normally recombine within the Xp/Yp pseudoautosomal segment in male meiosis. If recombination occurs below the pseudoautosomal boundary, between the X-specific and Y-specific portions of the chromosomes, sequences responsible for male sexual differentiation (including the *SRY* gene) may be translocated from the Y to the X. Fertilization by a sperm containing such an X chromosome leads to an XX male. In contrast, fertilization by a sperm containing a Y chromosome that has lost *SRY* will lead to an XY female.

factor(s) (AZF), are located on the Y chromosome, and three nonoverlapping regions on Yq (AZFa, AZFb, and AZFc) have been defined (see Fig. 10–9). Molecular analysis of these deletions has led to identification of a series of genes that may be important in spermatogenesis. For example, the *DAZ* genes (**d**eleted in **az**oospermia), located within the AZFc deletion region, encode RNA-binding proteins expressed only in the premeiotic germ cells of the testis. Consistent with their causal role in male infertility, deletions in Yq that include *DAZ* have been found to occur de novo and, when tested, are not present in the fertile fathers or brothers of these infertile males.

The prevalence of AZF mutations or deletions in the general male population is unknown. Approximately 2 percent of otherwise healthy males are infertile because of severe defects in sperm production, and de novo deletions or mutations may account for a significant proportion of these. Thus, men with idiopathic infertility should be karyotyped, and Y chromosome molecular testing and genetic counseling may be appropriate prior to initiating assisted reproduction for such couples.

Not all cases of male infertility are due to *DAZ* deletions, as there are at least two other deletion regions on Yq proximal to the *DAZ* genes (see Fig. 10–9). Within one of these regions, a de novo point mutation has been described in one gene, *USP9Y*, the function of which has yet to be explained but which must be required for normal spermatogenesis.

## The X Chromosome

As pointed out in Chapter 9, aneuploidy for the X chromosome is among the most common of cytogenetic abnormalities. The relative tolerance of the human karyotype for X chromosome abnormalities can be explained in terms of **X chromosome inactivation**. X inactivation and its consequences were discussed in relation to X-linked disorders in Chapter 5. Here, we discuss the chromosomal and molecular mechanisms of X inactivation.

## X Chromosome Inactivation

As introduced in Chapter 5, the theory of X inactivation is that in somatic cells in normal females (but not in normal males), one X chromosome is inactivated, thus equalizing the expression of X-linked genes in the two sexes. The inactive X chromosome adopts a unique conformation in the nucleus and is represented in interphase cells by the **Barr body** (Fig. 10–12). In patients with extra X chromosomes, any X chromosome in excess of one is inactivated and forms a Barr body (see Box).

Thus, all diploid somatic cells in both males and females have a single active X chromosome, regardless of the total number of X or Y chromosomes present.

Although the inactive X chromosome was first identified cytologically by the presence of the Barr body, there are many features that distinguish the active and inactive X chromosomes. As well as providing insight into the mechanisms of X inactivation, these features can be useful diagnostically for identifying the inactive X. For example, the inactive X replicates its DNA later in the S phase of the cell cycle than does the active X; this replication asynchrony between early- and late-replicating X chromosomes can be recognized cytogenetically by a specialized banding procedure called "replication banding" (Fig. 10–13).

The promoter region of many genes on the inactive X is extensively modified by addition of a methyl group to cytosine (see Fig. 3–1) by the enzyme DNA methyltransferase. Such **DNA methylation** is restricted to CpG dinucleotides (see Chapter 3) and contributes to formation of an inactive chromatin state. This and other chromatin modifications involving histones appear to be an essential part of the X inactivation mechanism.

As initially mentioned in Chapter 5, the chromosome-wide basis for X inactivation is well established, but not all genes on the X are subject to inactivation. Extensive analysis of expression of over 250 X-linked genes has demonstrated that about 10 to 15 percent of the genes escape inactivation and are expressed from active and inactive X chromosomes (Fig. 10–14). Notably, these genes are not distributed randomly along X; many more genes on Xp escape inactivation than on Xq. Although the evolutionary or genomic basis for this finding is not clear, it has important implications for genetic counseling in cases of partial X chromosome aneuploidy, as imbalance for genes on Xp may have greater clinical significance than imbalance of Xq.

**Sex Chromosomes and the Barr Body**

| Sexual phenotype | Karyotype | Barr bodies |
|---|---|---|
| Male | 46,XY; 47,XYY | 0 |
| | 47,XXY; 48,XXYY | 1 |
| | 48,XXXY; 49,XXXYY | 2 |
| | 49,XXXXY | 3 |
| Female | 45,X | 0 |
| | 46,XX | 1 |
| | 47,XXX | 2 |
| | 48,XXXX | 3 |
| | 49,XXXXX | 4 |

### The X Inactivation Center and the XIST Gene

From the study of structurally abnormal, inactivated X chromosomes, the **X inactivation center** has been mapped to proximal Xq, in band Xq13 (see Fig. 10–14). The X inactivation center contains an unusual gene, ***XIST***, that appears to be a key master regulatory locus for X inactivation. *XIST* (an acronym for inactive X (**Xi**)–**s**pecific **t**ranscripts) has the novel feature that it is expressed only from the allele on the inactive X; it is transcriptionally silent on the active X in both male and female cells. Although the exact mode of action of *XIST* is unknown, X inactivation cannot occur in its absence. The product of *XIST* is a noncoding RNA that stays in the nucleus in close association with the inactive X as part of an *XIST* RNA/Barr body complex (Fig. 10–15).

### Nonrandom X Inactivation

As described in Chapter 5, X inactivation is normally random in female somatic cells and leads to mosaicism for two cell populations expressing

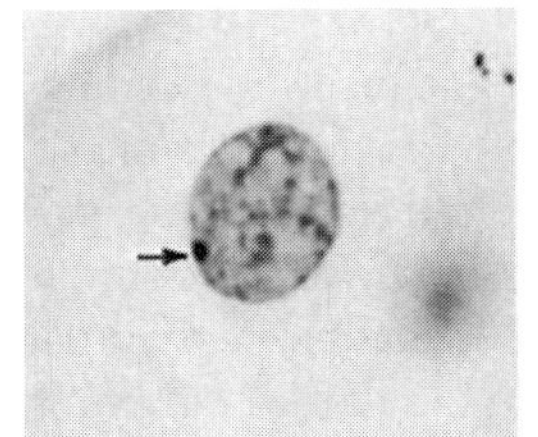
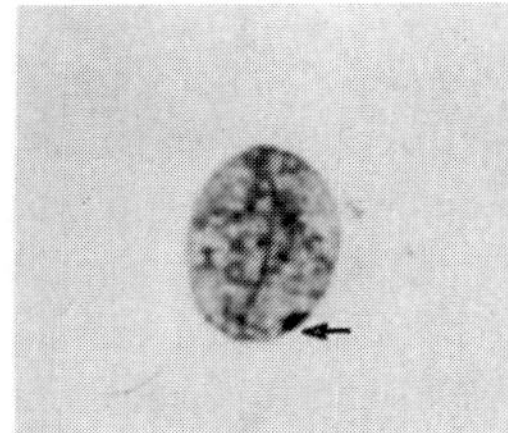
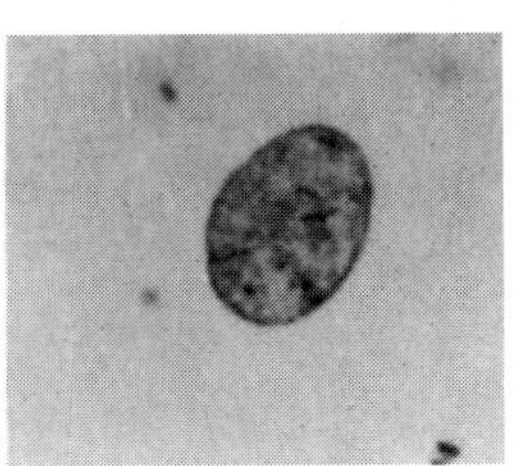

**Figure 10–12.** Barr bodies (sex chromatin) in epithelial cells of human buccal mucosa. Arrows indicate the Barr body close to the nuclear membrane in 46,XX female cells. A male cell (*right*) has no Barr body. (From Moore KL, Barr ML [1955] Smears from the oral mucosa in the determination of chromosomal sex. Lancet 2:57–58.)

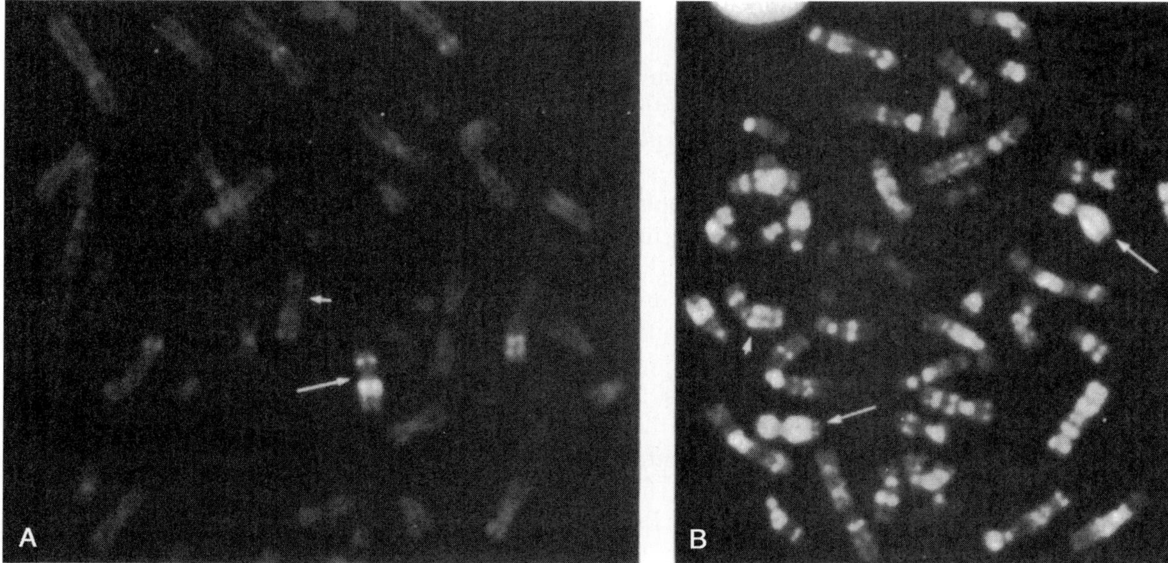


**Figure 10–13.** Replication banding and late replication of the inactive X chromosome in peripheral lymphocytes from a normal 46,XX female (*A*) and a 47,XXX female (*B*). Brightly staining chromosomal regions are those that replicate late in the S phase. Active X chromosomes (*small arrows*) replicate synchronously with the rest of the karyotype. Inactive X chromosomes (*long arrows*) replicate late. (*B* originally courtesy of Samuel A. Latt [deceased], Children's Hospital, Boston.)

alleles from one or the other X (see Fig. 5–16). However, there are exceptions to this when the karyotype involves a structurally abnormal X. For example, in almost all patients with unbalanced structural abnormalities of an X chromosome (including deletions, duplications, and isochromosomes), the structurally abnormal chromosome is always the inactive X, probably reflecting secondary selection against genetically unbalanced cells that could lead to significant clinical abnormalities (Fig. 10–16). Because of this preferential inactivation of the abnormal X, such X chromosome anomalies are tolerated better than similar abnormalities of autosomes and consequently are more frequently observed.

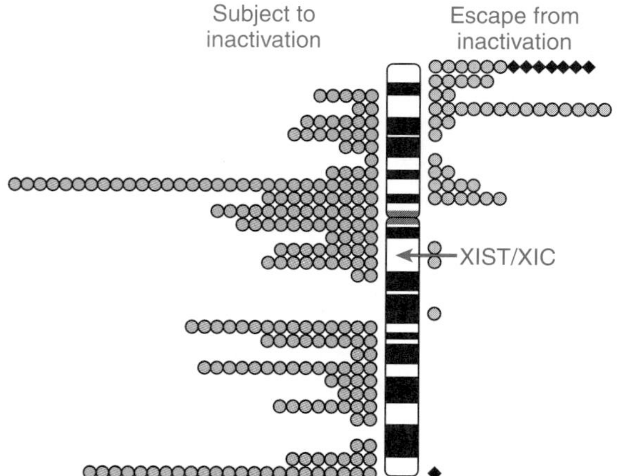


**Figure 10–14.** Profile of gene expression of the X chromosome. Each symbol indicates X inactivation status of an X-linked gene. Location of each symbol indicates its approximate map position on the X chromosome. Genes not expressed from the inactive X (subject to inactivation) are on the left. Genes expressed from the inactive X (escape from inactivation) are on the right. Pseudoautosomal genes are indicated by diamonds. The location of the *XIST* gene and the X inactivation center (XIC) are indicated in Xq13. (Data based on Carrel L, Cottle A, Goglin KC, Willard HF [1999] A first-generation X inactivation profile of the human X chromosome. Proc Natl Acad Sci U S A 96:14440–14444.)

Nonrandom inactivation is also observed in most cases of X;autosome translocations (see Fig. 10–16). If such a translocation is balanced, the normal X chromosome is preferentially inactivated, and the two parts of the translocated chromosome remain active, again probably reflecting selection against cells in which autosomal genes have been inactivated. In the unbalanced offspring of a balanced carrier, however, only the translocation product carrying the X inactivation center is present, and this chromosome is invariably inactivated; the normal X is always active. These nonrandom patterns of inactivation have the general effect of minimizing, but by no means eliminating, the clinical consequences of the particular chromosomal defect. Because patterns of inactivation are strongly correlated with clinical outcome, determination of an individual's X inactivation pattern by cytogenetic (replication studies) or molecular (DNA methylation) analysis is indicated in all cases involving X;autosome translocations.

One consequence sometimes observed in balanced carriers of X;autosome translocations is that the break itself may cause a mutation by disrupting a gene on the X chromosome at the site of the translocation. The only normal copy of the particular gene is inactivated in most or all cells because of nonran-

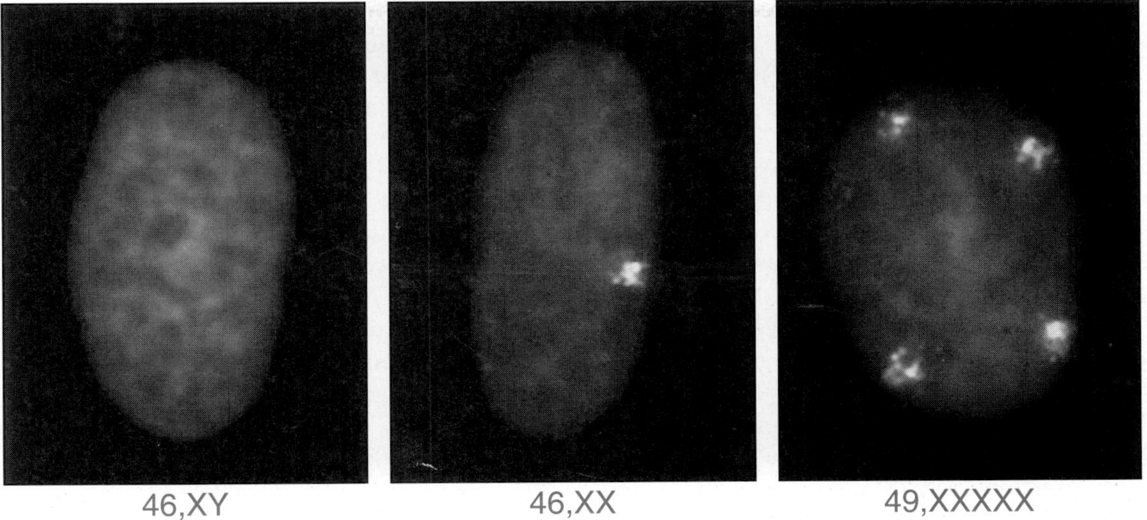


**Figure 10–15.** Detection of XIST RNA in interphase nuclei from a 46,XY male, a 46,XX female, and a 49,XXXXX female. Regions of bright fluorescence indicate presence of XIST RNA/Barr body complexes associated with inactive X chromosomes. (Courtesy of Laura Carrel, Case Western Reserve University School of Medicine, Cleveland.)

dom X inactivation of the normal X, thus allowing expression in a female of an X-linked trait normally observed only in hemizygous males. Several X-linked genes have been mapped to specific regions of the X chromosome when a typical X-linked phenotype has been found in a female who then proved to have an X;autosome translocation (see Chapter 8). The general clinical message of these findings is that if a female patient manifests an X-linked phenotype normally seen only in males, high-resolution chromosome analysis is indicated. The finding of a balanced translocation can explain the phenotypic expression and show the gene's probable map position on the X chromosome.

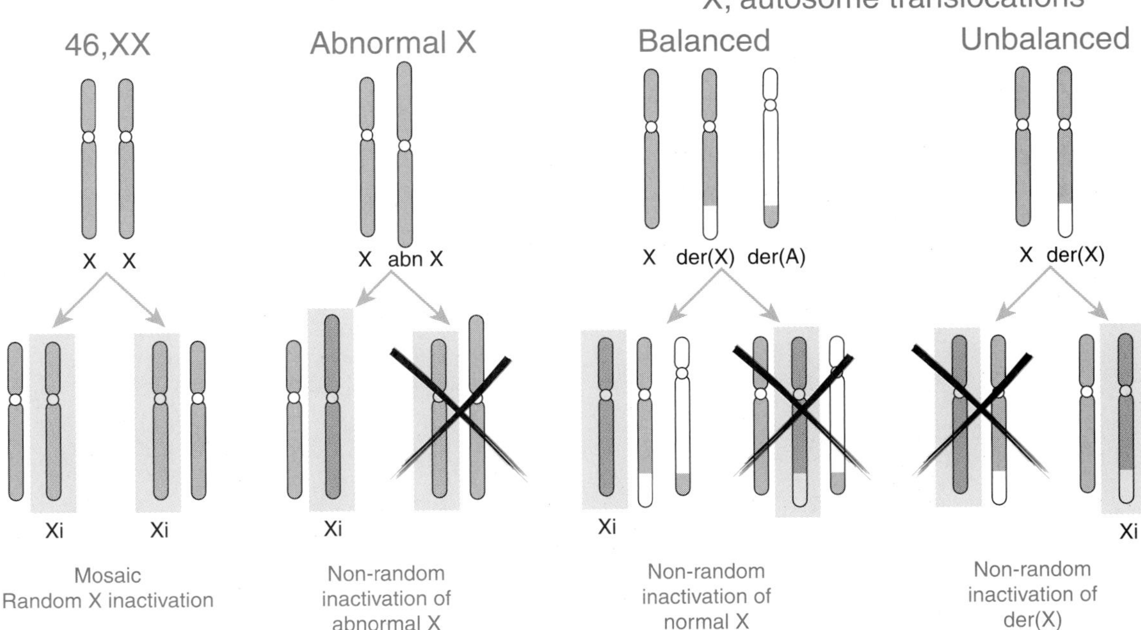


**Figure 10–16.** Nonrandom X chromosome inactivation in karyotypes with abnormal X chromosomes or X;autosome translocations. Normal female cells (46,XX) undergo random X inactivation; resulting tissues are a mosaic of two cell populations in which either the paternal or maternal X is the inactive X (Xi, indicated by red box). Individuals carrying a structurally abnormal X (abn X) or X;autosome translocation in a balanced or unbalanced state show nonrandom X inactivation in which virtually all cells have the same X inactive. The other cell population is inviable and/or at a growth disadvantage because of genetic imbalance and is thus underrepresented or absent. See text for further discussion. der(X) and der(A) represent the two derivatives of the X;autosome translocation.

### X-Linked Mental Retardation

An additional feature of the X chromosome is the high frequency of mutations or microdeletions that cause X-linked mental retardation. The collective incidence of X-linked mental retardation has been estimated to be 1 in 500 to 1000 live births. In many instances, mental retardation is but one of several abnormal phenotypic features that together define an X-linked syndrome. However, there are at least several dozen other genes at which mutations lead to isolated or nonsyndromic X-linked mental retardation, often of the severe to profound kind. The number of such genes is consistent with the finding in many large-scale surveys that there is a 20 to 40 percent excess of males among persons with mental retardation. Detailed chromosome analysis is indicated as an initial evaluation to rule out an obvious cytogenetic abnormality such as a deletion; in addition, molecular testing of the *FMR1* gene in Xq27.3 may be indicated to rule out fragile X syndrome (see Chapter 12).

## Cytogenetic Abnormalities of the Sex Chromosomes

Sex chromosome abnormalities, like abnormalities of the autosomes, can be either numerical or structural and can be present in all cells or in mosaic form. Their incidence rate in liveborn children, in fetuses examined prenatally, and in spontaneous abortions was compared in Chapter 9 with the incidence rate of similar abnormalities of the autosomes and is summarized in Table 10–3. There are a number of clinical indications that would raise the possibility of a sex chromosome abnormality and thus the need for cytogenetic and/or molecular studies. These especially include delay in onset of puberty, amenorrhea, infertility or ambiguous genitalia.

X and Y chromosome aneuploidy is relatively common, and sex chromosome abnormalities are among the most common of all human genetic disorders, with an overall incidence of about 1 in 400 to 500 births. The phenotypes associated with these chromosomal defects are, in general, less severe than those associated with comparable autosomal disorders because X inactivation, and the apparent low gene content of the Y, minimizes the clinical consequences of sex chromosome imbalance. By far the most common sex chromosome defects in liveborn infants and in fetuses are the trisomic types (XXY, XXX, and XYY), but all three are rare in spontaneous abortions. In contrast, monosomy for the X (Turner syndrome) is less frequent in liveborn infants but is the most common chromosome anomaly reported in spontaneous abortions (see Table 9–4).

Structural abnormalities of the sex chromosomes are less common; the defect most frequently observed is an isochromosome of the long arm of the X, i(Xq), seen in complete or mosaic form in at least 15 percent of females with Turner syndrome. Mosaicism is more common for sex chromosome abnormalities than for autosomal abnormalities, and in some patients it is associated with relatively mild expression of the associated phenotype.

As a group, disorders of the sex chromosomes tend to occur as isolated events without apparent predis-

TABLE 10–3

**Incidence of Sex Chromosome Abnormalities**

| Sex | Disorder | Karyotype | Approximate Incidence |
|---|---|---|---|
| Male | Klinefelter syndrome | 47,XXY | 1/1000 males |
| | | 48,XXXY | 1/25,000 males |
| | | Others (48,XXYY; 49,XXXXY; mosaics) | 1/10,000 males |
| | 47,XYY syndrome | 47,XYY | 1/1000 males |
| | Other X or Y chromosome abnormalities | | 1/1500 males |
| | XX males | 46,XX | 1/20,000 males |
| | | | *Overall incidence: 1/400 males* |
| Female | Turner syndrome | 45,X | 1/5000 females |
| | | 46,X,i(Xq) | 1/50,000 females |
| | | Others (deletions, mosaics) | 1/15,000 females |
| | Trisomy X | 47,XXX | 1/1000 females |
| | Other X chromosome abnormalities | | 1/3000 females |
| | XY females | 46,XY | 1/20,000 females |
| | Androgen insensitivity | 46,XY | 1/20,000 females |
| | | | *Overall incidence: 1/650 females* |

Data adapted from Table 9–3 and Robinson A, Linden MG, Bender BG (1998) Prenatal diagnosis of sex chromosome abnormalities. *In* Milunsky A (ed) Genetic Disorders of the Fetus, 4th ed. Johns Hopkins University Press, Baltimore, pp. 249–285.

TABLE 10–4

**Follow-Up Observations on Patients with Sex Chromosome Aneuploidy**

| Disorder | Karyotype | Phenotype | Sexual Development | Intelligence | Behavioral Problem |
|---|---|---|---|---|---|
| Klinefelter syndrome | 47,XXY | Tall male (see text) | Infertile; hypogonadism | Learning difficulties (some patients) | May have poor psychosocial adjustment |
| XYY syndrome | 47,XYY | Tall male | Normal | Normal | Frequent |
| Trisomy X | 47,XXX | Female, usually tall | Usually normal | Learning difficulties (some patients) | Occasional |
| Turner syndrome | 45,X | Short female, distinctive features (see text) | Infertile; streak gonads | Normal (but see text) | Rare |

Data from Ratcliffe SG, Paul N (eds) (1986) Prospective studies on children with sex chromosome aneuploidy. March of Dimes Birth Defects Foundation, Birth Defects Original Article Series 22(3). Alan R. Liss, New York; and from Rovert J, Netley C, Bailey J, et al (1995) Intelligence and achievement in children with extra X aneuploidy: A longitudinal perspective. Am J Med Genet 60:356–363.

posing factors, except for an effect of late maternal age in the cases that originate from errors of maternal meiosis I. Because almost all patients with sex chromosome abnormalities have only mild developmental abnormalities, a parental decision regarding potential termination of a pregnancy in which the fetus is found to have this type of defect can be a difficult one.

The four well-defined syndromes associated with sex chromosome aneuploidy are important causes of infertility or abnormal development or both, and thus warrant a more detailed description. The effects of these chromosome abnormalities on development have been studied in a long-term multicenter study of over 300 affected individuals, some of whom have been monitored for more than 30 years. To avoid the bias inherent in studying cases unusual enough to be referred to a medical center for assessment, only cases ascertained by screening of newborns or by prenatal diagnosis have been used. The major conclusions of this important clinical study are summarized in Table 10–4.

## KLINEFELTER SYNDROME (47,XXY)

The phenotype of Klinefelter syndrome, the first human sex chromosome abnormality to be reported, is shown in Figure 10–17. The patients are tall and thin and have relatively long legs. They appear physically normal until puberty, when signs of hypogonadism become obvious. Puberty occurs at a normal age, but the testes remain small, and secondary sexual characteristics remain underdeveloped. Klinefelter patients are almost always infertile because of the failure of germ cell development, and patients are often identified clinically for the first time because of infertility. Gynecomastia is a feature of some patients.

The incidence is at least 1 in 1000 male live births (1 in 2000 total births). As predicted by the finding that 47,XXY Klinefelter patients have a Barr body, one of the two X chromosomes is inactivated. Because of the relatively mild yet variable phenotype, many cases are presumed to go undetected.

About half the cases of Klinefelter syndrome result from errors in paternal meiosis I because of a failure of normal Xp/Yp recombination in the pseudoautosomal region. Among cases of maternal origin, most result from errors in maternal meiosis I and the remainder from errors in meiosis II or from a postzygotic mitotic error leading to mosaicism. Maternal age is increased in the cases associated with maternal meiosis I errors.

About 15 percent of Klinefelter patients have mosaic karyotypes. As a group, such mosaic patients have

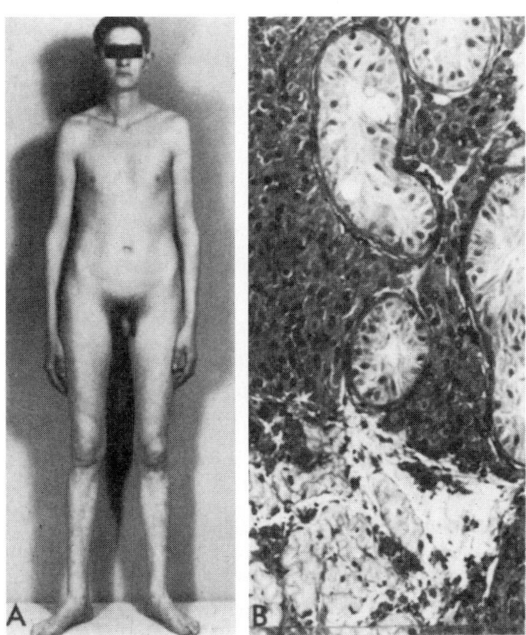


**Figure 10–17.** *A*, Phenotype of an adult male with 47,XXY Klinefelter syndrome. Note long limbs and relatively small genitalia. Gynecomastia, not present in this patient, is a feature of some Klinefelter males. *B*, Section of a testicular biopsy showing seminiferous tubules without germ cells. (From Ferguson-Smith MA [1966]. *In* Moore KL [ed] The Sex Chromatin. WB Saunders, Philadelphia.)

variable phenotypes; some may have normal testicular development. The most common mosaic karyotype is 46,XY/47,XXY, probably as a consequence of loss of one X chromosome in an XXY conceptus during an early postzygotic division.

There are several variants of Klinefelter syndrome, with karyotypes other than 47,XXY, including 48,XXYY, 48,XXXY, and 49,XXXXY. As a rule, the additional X chromosomes (even though they are inactive) cause a correspondingly more abnormal phenotype, with a greater degree of dysmorphism, more defective sexual development, and more severe mental impairment.

Although there is wide phenotypic variation among patients with this and other sex chromosome aneuploidies, some consistent phenotypic differences have been identified between patients with Klinefelter syndrome and chromosomally normal males. Verbal comprehension and ability are below that of normal males, and 47,XXY males score slightly less well on certain intelligence performance tests (IQ tests). Patients with Klinefelter syndrome have a several-fold increased risk of learning difficulties, especially in reading, that may require educational intervention. Many of the affected boys have relatively poor psychosocial adjustment, in part related to poor body image. Language difficulties may lead to shyness, unassertiveness, and immaturity.

### 47,XYY Syndrome

Among all male live births, the incidence of the 47,XYY karyotype is about 1 in 1000. The 47,XYY chromosome constitution is not associated with an obviously abnormal phenotype, and males with this karyotype cannot be distinguished from normal 46,XY males by any marked physical or behavioral features.

The origin of the error that leads to the XYY karyotype must be paternal nondisjunction at meiosis II, producing YY sperm. The less common XXYY and XXXYY variants, which share the features of the XYY and Klinefelter syndromes, probably also originate in the father as a result of sequential nondisjunction in meiosis I and meiosis II.

XYY males identified in newborn screening programs without ascertainment bias are tall and have an increased risk of educational or behavioral problems in comparison with chromosomally normal males. They have normal intelligence and are not dysmorphic. Fertility is usually normal, and there appears to be no particularly increased risk that a 47,XYY male will have a chromosomally abnormal child. About half of 47,XYY boys require educational intervention as a result of language delays and reading and spelling difficulties. Their IQ scores are about 10 to 15 points below average.

Parents whose child is found, prenatally or postnatally, to be XYY are often extremely concerned about the behavioral implications. Attention deficits, hyperactivity, and impulsiveness have been well documented in XYY males, but marked aggression or psychopathology is not a common feature of the syndrome. This is an important point to emphasize because of reports in the 1960s and 1970s that the proportion of XYY males was elevated in prisons and mental hospitals, especially among the tallest inmates. This stereotypic impression is now known to be incorrect.

Nonetheless, inability to predict the outcome in individual cases makes identification of an XYY fetus one of the more difficult genetic counseling problems in prenatal diagnosis programs.

### Trisomy X (47,XXX)

Trisomy X occurs with an incidence of 1 in 1000 female births. Trisomy X females, although somewhat above average in stature, are not abnormal phenotypically. Some are first identified in infertility clinics, but probably most remain undiagnosed. Follow-up studies have shown that XXX females develop pubertal changes at an appropriate age, and they are usually fertile although with a somewhat increased risk of chromosomally abnormal offspring. There is a significant deficit in performance on IQ tests, and about 70 percent of the patients have some learning problems. Severe psychopathology and antisocial behavior appear to be rare; however, abnormal behavior is apparent, especially during the transition from adolescence to early adulthood.

In 47,XXX cells, two of the X chromosomes are inactivated and late-replicating (see Fig. 10–13), as suggested originally by the finding of two Barr bodies. Almost all cases result from errors in maternal meiosis, and of these the majority are in meiosis I. There is an effect of increased maternal age, restricted to those patients in whom the error was in maternal meiosis I.

The tetrasomy X syndrome (48,XXXX) is associated with more serious retardation in both physical and mental development, and the pentasomy X syndrome (49,XXXXX), despite the presence of four inactive X chromosomes (see Fig. 10–15), usually includes severe developmental retardation with multiple physical defects.

### Turner Syndrome (45,X and Variants)

Unlike patients with other sex chromosome aneuploidies, females with Turner syndrome can often be identified at birth or before puberty by their distinctive phenotypic features (Fig. 10–18). Turner syndrome is much less common than other sex chromosome aneuploidies. The incidence of the Turner

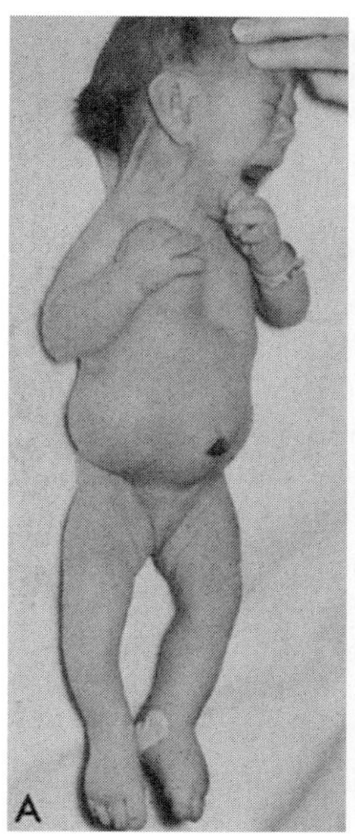


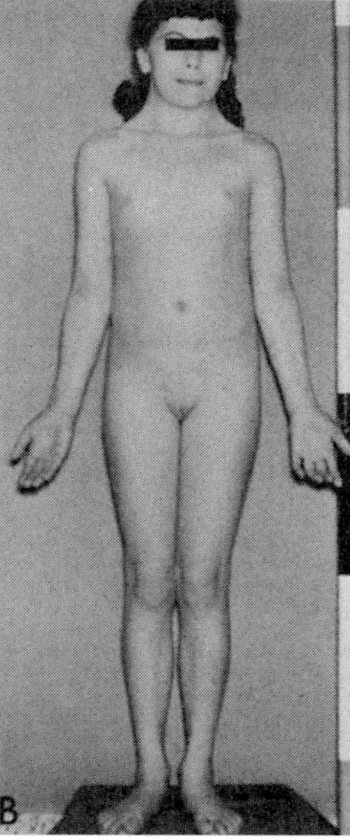


**Figure 10–18.** Phenotype of females with 45,X Turner syndrome. *A*, Newborn infant. Note the webbed neck and lymphedema of the hands and feet. *B*, A 13-year-old girl showing classic Turner features, including short stature, webbed neck, delayed sexual maturation, and broad, shieldlike chest with widely spaced nipples. (From Moore KL [1966] The Sex Chromactin. WB Saunders, Philadelphia.)

syndrome phenotype is approximately 1 in 4000 female live births, although much higher numbers have been reported in some surveys.

The most frequent chromosome constitution in Turner syndrome is 45,X (sometimes written incorrectly as 45,XO) with no second sex chromosome. However, about 50 percent of cases have other karyotypes. About one quarter of Turner syndrome cases involve mosaic karyotypes, in which only a proportion of cells are 45,X. The most common karyotypes and their approximate relative prevalences are as follows:

| | |
|---|---|
| 45,X | 50% |
| 46,X,i(Xq) | 15% |
| 45,X/46,XX mosaics | 15% |
| 45,X/46,X,i(Xq) mosaics | about 5% |
| 45,X, other X abnormality | about 5% |
| Other 45,X/? mosaics | about 5% |

The chromosome constitution is clinically significant; for example, patients with i(Xq) are similar to classic 45,X patients, whereas patients with a deletion of Xp have short stature and congenital malformations, and those with a deletion of Xq often have only gonadal dysfunction.

Typical abnormalities in Turner syndrome include short stature, gonadal dysgenesis (usually streak gonads reflecting a failure of ovarian maintenance), characteristic unusual facies, webbed neck, low posterior hairline, broad chest with widely spaced nipples, and an elevated frequency of renal and cardiovascular anomalies. At birth, infants with this syndrome often have edema of the dorsum of the foot, a useful diagnostic sign (see Fig. 10–18). Many patients have coarctation of the aorta, and Turner syndrome females are at particular risk for cardiovascular abnormalities. Lymphedema may be present in fetal life, causing cystic hygroma (visible by ultrasonography), which is the cause of the neck webbing seen postnatally. Growth hormone therapy is now standard in Turner syndrome and can result in gains of 6 to 10 cm to the final height.

Intelligence in Turner syndrome females is usually average or above average. However, patients often display a deficiency in spatial perception, perceptual motor organization, or fine motor execution. As a consequence, the nonverbal IQ is significantly lower than the verbal IQ, and many patients require educational intervention, especially in mathematics. Turner syndrome females have an elevated risk of impaired social adjustment. A comparison of 45,X girls with a maternal X and those with a paternal X provided evidence of significantly worse social cognition skills in those with a maternally derived X. Because imprinting could explain this parent-of-origin effect, the possibility of an X-linked imprinted gene that increases visuospatial memory is under investigation.

The high incidence rate of 45,X in spontaneous abortions has already been mentioned. This single abnormality is present in an estimated 1 to 2 percent of all conceptuses; survival to term is a rare outcome, and more than 99 percent of such fetuses abort spontaneously. The single X is maternal in origin in about 70 percent of cases; in other words, the chromosome error is usually paternal. The basis for the unusually high frequency of X or Y chromosome loss is unknown. Furthermore, it is not clear why the 45,X karyotype is usually lethal in utero but is apparently fully compatible with postnatal survival. The "missing" genes responsible for the Turner syndrome phenotype must reside on the X and Y chromosomes. It has been suggested that the responsible genes are among those that escape X inactivation (see Fig. 10–14).

Small ring X chromosomes are occasionally observed in patients with short stature, gonadal dysgenesis, and mental retardation. Because mental retardation is not a feature of Turner syndrome, the presence of mental retardation with or without other associated physical anomalies in individuals with a 46,X,r(X) karyotype has been attributed to the fact that small ring X chromosomes lack the X inactivation center and do not express the *XIST* gene. The failure to inactivate the ring X in these patients leads to overexpression of X-linked genes that are normally subject to inactivation. The discovery of a ring X in a prenatal diagnosis can lead to great uncertainty, and studies of *XIST* expression are indicated. Large rings containing the X inactivation center and expressing *XIST* would predict a Turner syndrome phenotype; a small ring lacking or not expressing *XIST* would predict a much more severe phenotype.

## Disorders of Gonadal and Sexual Development

The genetic sex of an embryo is established at the time of fertilization. Earlier in this chapter, we discussed the primary sex-determining role of the Y chromosome. Here we examine the role of various X-linked and autosomal genes in ovarian and testicular development and in the development of male and female external genitalia.

For some newborn infants, determination of sex is difficult or impossible because the genitalia are ambiguous, with anomalies that tend to make them resemble those of the opposite chromosomal sex. Such anomalies may vary from mild hypospadias in males (a developmental anomaly in which the urethra opens on the underside of the penis or on the perineum) to an enlarged clitoris in females. In some patients, both ovarian and testicular tissue is present, a condition known as **hermaphroditism**. Such problems do not necessarily indicate a cytogenetic abnormality of the sex chromosomes but may be due to single-gene defects or to nongenetic causes. Nonetheless, determination of the child's karyotype is an essential part of the investigation of such patients.

### Gonadal Maldevelopment

A number of autosomal and X-linked genes have been implicated in conversion of the bipotential (indifferent) gonad to either a testis or ovary (see Fig. 10–10). Detailed analysis of a subset of **sex-reversed 46,XY females** in whom the *SRY* gene was not deleted or mutated revealed a duplication of a portion of the short arm of the X chromosome. The *DAX1* gene in Xp21 encodes a transcription factor that plays a dosage-sensitive role in determination of gonadal sex, implying a tightly regulated interaction between *DAX1* and *SRY*. An excess of *SRY* at a critical point in development leads to testis formation; an excess of *DAX1*, resulting from duplication of the gene, can suppress the normal male-determining function of *SRY*, and ovarian development results.

**Camptomelic dysplasia**, due to mutations in the *SOX9* gene on chromosome 17q, is an autosomal dominant disorder with usually lethal bone and cartilage malformations. However, about two thirds of 46,XY patients with this disorder are sex-reversed and are phenotypic females. *SOX9* is normally expressed early in development in the genital ridge and thus appears to be required for normal testis formation (in addition to its role in other aspects of development). In its absence, testes fail to form, and the default ovarian pathway is followed. Interestingly, duplication of *SOX9* can lead to XX sex reversal, suggesting that overproduction of *SOX9*, even in the absence of *SRY*, can initiate testis formation.

Other autosomal loci have also been implicated in gonadal development. Chromosomally male patients with **Denys-Drash syndrome** may have female or ambiguous external genitalia. The *WT1* gene in 11p13 (also implicated in Wilms' tumor, a childhood kidney neoplasia) encodes a transcription factor that is involved in interactions between Sertoli and Leydig cells in the developing gonad. Dominant *WT1* mutations apparently disrupt normal testicular development.

A well-characterized cytogenetic defect sometimes associated with 46,XY sex reversal is the **9p deletion syndrome**. By comparing patients with different deletions, the region required for normal male sexual development has been narrowed to 9p24. This region contains the *DMRT1* gene, which encodes another transcription factor expressed exclusively in the developing gonad.

### Female Pseudohermaphroditism

Pseudohermaphrodites are "pseudo" because, unlike true hermaphrodites, they have gonadal tissue of only one sex. Female pseudohermaphrodites have 46,XX karyotypes with normal ovarian tissue but with ambiguous or male external genitalia.

Female pseudohermaphroditism is usually due to **congenital adrenal hyperplasia**, an autosomal recessive disorder arising from specific defects in enzymes of the adrenal cortex required for cortisol biosynthesis and resulting in virilization of female infants. Ovarian development is normal, but excessive production of androgens causes masculinization of the external genitalia, with clitoral enlargement and labial fusion to form a scrotum-like structure (Fig. 10–19).

Although any one of several enzymatic steps may be defective in congenital adrenal hyperplasia, by far the most common defect is deficiency of 21-hydroxylase, which has an incidence of about 1 in 12,500 births. Deficiency of 21-hydroxylase blocks the normal biosynthetic pathway, causing overproduction of the precursors, which are then shunted into the pathway of androgen biosynthesis, causing abnormally high androgen levels. Whereas female infants with 21-hydroxylase deficiency are born with ambiguous genitalia, affected male infants have normal external genitalia and may go unrecognized in early infancy. Of patients with classic 21-hydroxylase deficiency, 25 percent have the simple virilizing type, and 75 per-

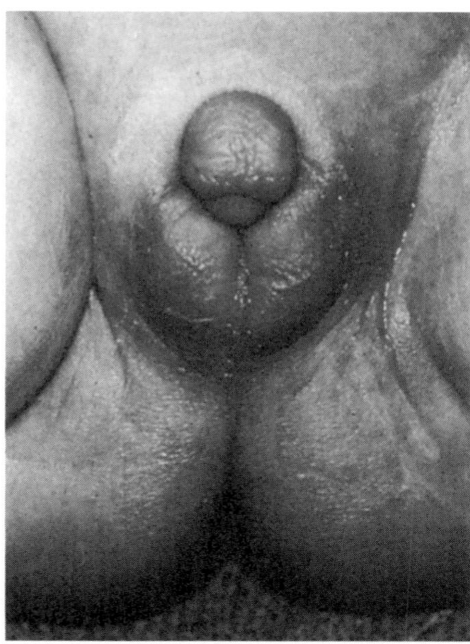

**Figure 10–19.** Masculinized external genitalia of a 46,XX infant caused by congenital adrenal hyperplasia (virilizing form). See text for discussion. (From Moore KL, Persaud TVN [1993] The Developing Human: Clinically Oriented Embryology, 5th ed. WB Saunders, Philadelphia.)

cent have a salt-losing type that is clinically more severe and may lead to neonatal death. A screening test developed to identify the condition in newborns, in which heel-prick blood specimens are blotted onto filter paper, is now in use in many countries. It is valuable in preventing the serious consequences of the salt-losing defect in early infancy and in prompt diagnosis of affected males and females.

### Male Pseudohermaphroditism

In addition to disorders of testis formation during embryological development, causes of pseudohermaphroditism in 46,XY individuals include abnormalities of gonadotropins, inborn errors of testosterone biosynthesis and metabolism, and abnormalities of androgen target cells. These disorders are heterogeneous both genetically and clinically and, in some cases, they may correspond to milder manifestations of the same cause underlying true hermaphroditism.

There are several forms of androgen insensitivity resulting in male pseudohermaphroditism. One example is deficiency of the steroid **5α-reductase**, the enzyme responsible for converting the male hormone testosterone to its active form dihydrotestosterone. This autosomal recessive condition results in feminization of external genitalia in affected males. Although testicular development is normal, the penis is small, and there is a blind vaginal pouch. Gender assignment can be difficult.

Another well-studied disorder is an X-linked syndrome known as **androgen insensitivity syndrome** (formerly known as **testicular feminization**). In this disorder, affected persons are chromosomal males (karyotype 46,XY), with apparently normal female external genitalia, who have a blind vagina and no uterus or uterine tubes (Fig. 10–20). The incidence of androgen insensitivity is about 1 in 20,000 live births. Axillary and pubic hair is sparse. As the alternative name "testicular feminization" indicates, testes are present either within the abdomen or in the inguinal canal, where they are sometimes mistaken for hernias in infants who otherwise appear to be normal females. Although the testes secrete androgen normally, there is end-organ unresponsiveness to androgens, resulting from absence of androgen receptors in the cytosol of the appropriate target cells. The receptor protein, specified by the normal allele at the X-linked androgen receptor locus, has the role of

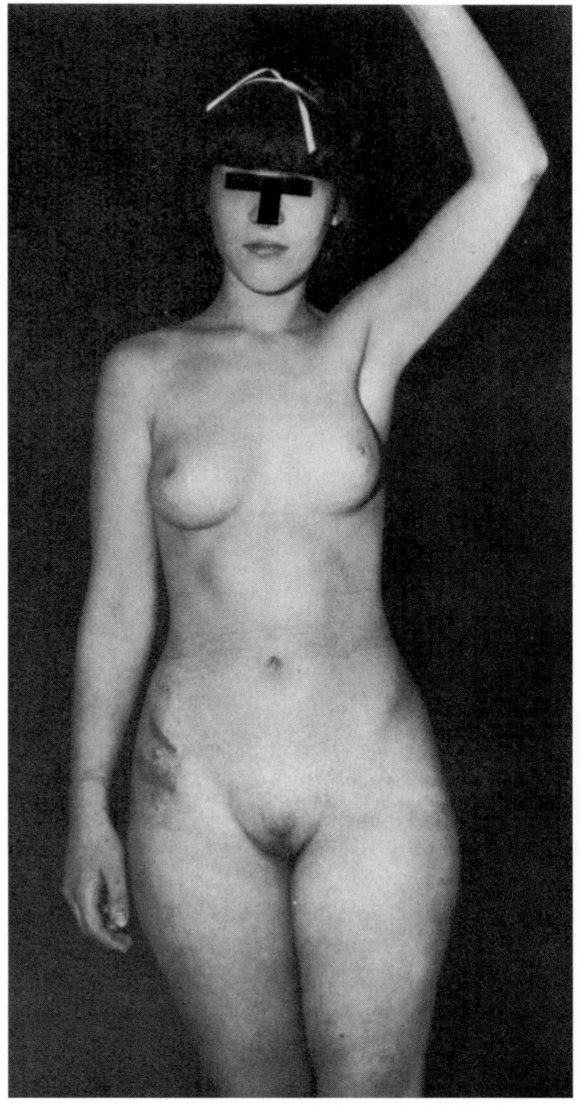

**Figure 10–20.** Complete androgen insensitivity syndrome (testicular feminization) in a 46,XY individual. Note female body contours, absence of axillary hair, sparse pubic hair, and breast development. (Courtesy of L. Pinsky, McGill University, Montreal.)

forming a complex with testosterone and dihydrotestosterone. If the complex fails to form, the hormone fails to enter the nucleus, become attached to chromatin, and stimulate the transcription of target genes required for differentiation in the male direction. The molecular defect has been determined in hundreds of cases and ranges from a complete deletion of the androgen receptor gene on the X chromosome (see Fig. 4–8) to point mutations in the androgen-binding or DNA-binding domains of the androgen receptor protein.

## General References


Gardner RJM, Sutherland GR (1996) Chromosome Abnormalities and Genetic Counseling. 2nd ed. Oxford University Press, Oxford, England.

Grumbach MM, Conte FA (1998) Disorders of sex differentiation. *In* Williams Textbook of Endocrinology, 9th ed. JD Wilson, DW Foster, HM Kronenberg, PR Larson (eds). WB Saunders, Philadelphia.

Hassold TJ, Patterson D (eds) (1999) Down Syndrome: A Promising Future Together. Wiley-Liss, New York.

Hsu LYF (1998) Prenatal diagnosis of chromosomal abnormalities through amniocentesis. *In* Milunsky A (ed) Genetic Disorders and the Fetus, 4th ed. Johns Hopkins University Press, Baltimore, pp. 179–248.

Moore KL, Persaud TVN (1993) The Developing Human: Clinically Oriented Embryology, 5th ed. WB Saunders, Philadelphia.

Pinsky L, Erickson RP, Schimke RN (1999) Genetic Disorders of Human Sexual Development. Oxford University Press, Oxford, England.

Robinson A, Linden MG, Bender BG (1998) Prenatal diagnosis of sex chromosome abnormalities. *In* Milunsky A (ed) Genetic Disorders of the Fetus, 4th ed. Johns Hopkins University Press, Baltimore, pp. 249–285.

Shaffer LG, Ledbetter DH, Lupski JR (2000) Molecular cytogenetics of contiguous gene syndromes: Mechanisms and consequences of gene dosage imbalance. *In* Scriver CR, Beaudet AL, Sly WS, Valle D (eds) The Molecular and Metabolic Bases of Inherited Disease, 8th ed. McGraw-Hill, New York.

Stevenson RE, Schwartz CE, Schroer RJ (2000) X-Linked Mental Retardation. Oxford University Press, Oxford, England.

Willard HF (2000) The sex chromosomes and X chromosome inactivation. *In* Scriver CR, Beaudet AL, Sly WS, Valle D (eds) The Molecular and Metabolic Bases of Inherited Disease, 8th ed. McGraw-Hill, New York.


## References Specific to Particular Topics


Brewer C, Holloway S, Zawalnyski P, et al (1998) A chromosomal deletion map of human malformations. Am J Hum Genet 63:1153–1159.

Budarf ML, Emanuel BS (1997) Progress in the autosomal segmental aneusomy syndromes: Single or multi-locus disorders? Hum Mol Genet 6:1657–1665.

Carrel L, Cottle A, Goglin KC, Willard HF (1999) A first-generation X inactivation profile of the human X chromosome. Proc Natl Acad Sci U S A 96:14440–14444.

Kola I, Hertzog PJ (1997) Animal models in the study of the biological function of genes on human chromosome 21 and their role in the pathophysiology of Down syndrome. Hum Mol Genet 6:1713–1727.

Lamb NE, Freeman SB, Savage-Austin A, et al (1996) Susceptible chiasmate configurations of chromosome 21 predispose to nondisjunction in both maternal meiosis I and meiosis II. Nat Genet 14:400–405.

Lindsay EA, Baldini A (1998) Congenital heart defects and 22q11 deletions: Which genes count? Mol Med Today 4:350–357.

Lupski JR (1998) Genomic disorders: Structural features of the genome can lead to DNA rearrangements and human disease traits. Trends Genet 14:417–422.

Overhauser J, Huang X, Gersh M, et al (1994) Molecular and phenotypic mapping of the short arm of chromosome 5: Sublocalization of the critical region for the cri du chat syndrome. Hum Mol Genet 3:247–252.

Pryor JL, Kent-First M, Muallem A, et al (1997) Microdeletions of the Y chromosome of infertile men. N Engl J Med 336:534–539.

Ratcliffe SG, Paul N (eds) (1986) Prospective studies on children with sex chromosome aneuploidy. March of Dimes Birth Defects Foundation, Birth Defects Original Article Series 22(3). Alan R. Liss, New York.

Reijo R, Lee TY, Salo P, et al (1995) Diverse spermatogenic defects in humans caused by Y chromosome deletions encompassing a novel RNA-binding protein gene. Nat Genet 10:383–393.

Rovert J, Netley C, Bailey J, et al (1995) Intelligence and achievement in children with extra X aneuploidy: A longitudinal perspective. Am J Med Genet 60:356–363.

Skuse DH (1999) Genomic imprinting of the X chromosome: A novel mechanism for the evolution of sexual dimorphism. J Lab Clin Med 133:23–32.

Sun C, Skaletsky H, Birren B, et al (1999) An azoospermic man with a de novo point mutation in the Y chromosomal gene USP9Y. Nat Genet 23:429–432.

The Chromosome 21 Mapping and Sequencing Consortium (2000) The DNA sequence of human chromosome 21. Nature 405:311–319.


## Problems

1. In a woman with a 47,XXX karyotype, what types of gametes would theoretically be formed and in what proportions? What are the theoretical karyotypes and phenotypes of her progeny? (Actually, a triple-X woman almost always has children with normal karyotypes only.)

2. One of your patients is a girl with severe hemophilia A, an X-linked recessive disorder.
   (a) You are advised to arrange for chromosome analysis of this child. Why? What mechanisms can allow the occurrence of an X-linked recessive phenotype in a female?
   (b) The laboratory reports that the child has an X;autosome translocation, with a breakpoint in the X chromosome at Xq28. How could this explain her phenotype?

3. The birth incidence rates of 47,XXY and 47,XYY males are approximately equal. Is this what you would expect on the basis of the possible origins of the two abnormal karyotypes? Explain.

4. How can a person with an XX karyotype differentiate as a phenotypic male?

5. A baby girl presents with bilateral inguinal masses that are thought to be hernias but are found to be testes in the inguinal canals. What karyotype would you expect to find in the child? What is her disorder? What genetic counseling would you offer to the parents?

6. A baby girl with ambiguous genitalia is found to have 21-hydroxylase deficiency of the salt-wasting type. What karyotype would you expect to find? What is the disorder? What genetic counseling would you offer to the parents?

7. What are the expected clinical consequences of the following deletions? If the same amount of DNA is deleted in each case, why might the severity of each be different?
   (a) $46,XX,13p^-$
   (b) $46,XYq^-$
   (c) $46,XX,5p^-$
   (d) $46,XXq^-$

8. Discuss the clinical consequences of X chromosome inactivation. Provide possible explanations for the fact that persons with X chromosome aneuploidy are clinically not completely normal.

9. In genetics clinic, you are counseling five pregnant women who inquire about their risk of having a Down syndrome fetus. What are their risks and why?
   (a) a 23-year-old mother of a previous trisomy 21 child
   (b) a 41-year-old mother of a previous trisomy 21 child
   (c) a 27-year-old woman whose niece has Down syndrome
   (d) a carrier of a 14;21 Robertsonian translocation
   (e) a woman whose husband is a carrier of a 14;21 Robertsonian translocation

# Clinical Case Studies Illustrating Genetic Principles

These 29 clinical vignettes illustrate genetic principles in the practice of medicine. Each vignette is followed by a brief explanation or description of the disease, its etiology, pathophysiology, phenotype, management, and inheritance risk. These explanations and descriptions are based on current knowledge and understanding; therefore, like most things in medicine and science, they are subject to refinement and change as our knowledge and understanding evolve. The description of each case uses standard medical terminology; student readers, therefore, may need to consult a standard medical dictionary for explanations. Each vignette is also followed by a few questions that are intended to initiate discussion of some basic genetic or clinical principles, or both, illustrated by the case. Neither the vignettes nor the ensuing explanations or descriptions are intended to be definitive or comprehensive treatments of a topic.

The cases are not intended to direct medical care or set a standard of care; they are simply illustrations of the application of genetic principles to the practice of medicine. Although loosely based on clinical experience, all individuals and medical details presented are ficticious.

Cornelius F. Boerkoel III, M.D., Ph.D.
Roderick R. McInnes, M.D., Ph.D.
Robert L. Nussbaum, M.D.
Huntington F. Willard, Ph.D.

## Case Presentations

1. Achondroplasia
2. Alzheimer Disease
3. Hereditary Breast and Ovarian Cancer
4. Charcot-Marie-Tooth Disease Type 1A
5. Chronic Myelogenous Leukemia
6. Cystic Fibrosis
7. Duchenne Muscular Dystrophy
8. Familial Adenomatous Polyposis
9. Familial Hypercholesterolemia
10. Fragile X Syndrome
11. Glucose-6-Phosphate Dehydrogenase
12. Hemophilia
13. Hereditary Nonpolyposis Colon Cancer
14. Holoprosencephaly (Nonsyndromic Form)
15. Huntington Disease
16. Insulin-Dependent Diabetes Mellitus
17. Marfan Syndrome
18. Miller-Dieker Syndrome
19. Myoclonic Epilepsy with Ragged-Red Fibers
20. Non–Insulin-Dependent Diabetes Mellitus
21. Polycystic Kidney Disease
22. Prader-Willi Syndrome
23. Retinoblastoma
24. Sex Reversal
25. Sickle Cell Anemia
26. Tay-Sachs Disease
27. Thalassemia
28. Turner Syndrome
29. Xeroderma pigmentosum

# Achondroplasia

## (FGFR3 mutation)

### Autosomal Dominant

## Principles

- Gain-of-function mutations
- Advanced paternal age
- *De novo* mutation

## Major Phenotypic Features

- Age of onset: Prenatal
- Rhizomelic short stature
- Megalencephaly
- Spinal cord compression

## History and Physical Findings

P.S., a 30-year-old healthy woman, was 27 weeks pregnant with her first child. A fetal ultrasound at 26 weeks' gestation identified a female fetus with macrocephaly and rhizomelia (shortening of proximal segments of extremities) of all extremities. P.S.'s spouse was 45 years of age and healthy; he had three healthy children from a previous relationship. Neither parent had a family history of skeletal dysplasia, birth defects, or genetic disorders. The obstetrician explained to the parents that their fetus had the features of achondroplasia. The infant girl was delivered at 38 weeks' gestation by cesarean section. She had the physical and radiographic features of achondroplasia including frontal bossing, megalencephaly, midface hypoplasia, lumbar kyphosis, limited elbow extension, rhizomelia, trident hands, brachydactyly, and hypotonia. Consistent with her physical features, DNA testing identified a G1138A mutation in the fibroblast growth factor receptor 3 gene *(FGFR3)*.

## Background

### Disease Etiology

Achondroplasia, the most common cause of human dwarfism, is an autosomal dominant disorder caused by specific mutations in *FGFR3;* two mutations, G1138A (~98 percent) and G1138C (1 to 2 percent), account for more than 99 percent of cases of achondroplasia. Achondroplasia has an incidence of 1 in 15,000 to 1 in 40,000 live births and affects all races.

### Pathogenesis

FGFR3 is a transmembrane tyrosine kinase receptor that binds fibroblast growth factors (FGF). Binding of FGF to the extracellular domain of FGFR3 activates the intracellular tyrosine kinase domain of the receptor and initiates a signaling cascade. In endochondral bone, FGFR3 activation inhibits proliferation of chondrocytes within the growth plate and thus helps coordinate the growth and differentiation of chondrocytes with the growth and differentiation of bone progenitor cells.

The *FGFR3* mutations associated with achondroplasia are "gain-of-function" mutations that cause ligand-independent activation of FGFR3. Such constitutive activation of FGFR3 inappropriately inhibits chondrocyte proliferation within the growth plate and consequently leads to shortening of the long bones as well as to abnormal differentiation of other bones.

Guanine 1138 in the *FGFR3* gene is one of the most mutable nucleotides identified in any human gene. Mutation of this nucleotide accounts for nearly 100 percent of achondroplasia; more than 80 to 90 percent of patients have a *de novo* mutation. *De novo* mutations of *FGFR3* guanine 1138 occur exclusively in the father's germline and increase in frequency with advanced paternal age (>35 years).

### Phenotype and Natural History

Patients with achondroplasia present at birth with rhizomelic shortening of the arms and legs, a relatively long and narrow trunk, a trident configuration of the hands, and macrocephaly with midface hypoplasia and a prominent forehead. Usually they have a birth length that is slightly less than normal although occasionally within the low normal range; their length or height falls progressively further from the normal range as they grow.

Generally, patients have normal intelligence, although most have delayed motor development. Their delayed motor development arises from a combination of hypotonia, hyperextensible joints (although the elbows have limited extension and rotation), mechanical difficulty balancing their large heads, and, less commonly, spinal canal stenosis with spinal cord compression.

Abnormal growth of the skull and facial bones results in midface hypoplasia, a small cranial base, and small cranial foramina. The midface hypoplasia causes dental crowding, obstructive apnea, and otitis media. Narrowing of the jugular foramina is believed to increase intracranial venous pressure and to thereby cause hydrocephalus. In approximately 10 percent of patients, narrowing of the foramen magnum often causes compression of the brain stem at the craniocervical junction and thereby an increased frequency of hypotonia, quadriparesis, failure to thrive, central apnea, and sudden death. Three to 7 percent of patients die unexpectedly during their first year of life because of brain stem compression (central apnea) or obstructive apnea. Other medical complications include obesity, lumbar spinal stenosis, and genu varum.

### Management

Suspected on the basis of clinical features, the diagnosis of achondroplasia is usually confirmed by radiographic findings. DNA testing for *FGFR3* mutations can be helpful in ambiguous cases but is usually not necessary to make the diagnosis.

Throughout life, management should focus on the anticipation and treatment of the complications of achondroplasia. During infancy and early childhood, patients must be monitored for chronic otitis media, hydrocephalus, brain-stem compression, and obstructive apnea, and treated as necessary. Treatment of patients with brain-stem compression by decompression of their craniocervical junction usually results in marked improvement of neurological function. During later childhood and through early adulthood, patients must be monitored for symptomatic spinal stenosis, symptomatic genu varum, obesity, dental complications, and chronic otitis media and treated as necessary. Treatment of the spinal stenosis usually requires surgical decompression and stabilization of the spine. Obesity is difficult to prevent and control and often complicates the management of obstructive apnea and joint and spine problems.

Both growth hormone therapy and surgical lengthening of the lower legs have been promoted as treatments for the short stature. Both therapies remain controversial.

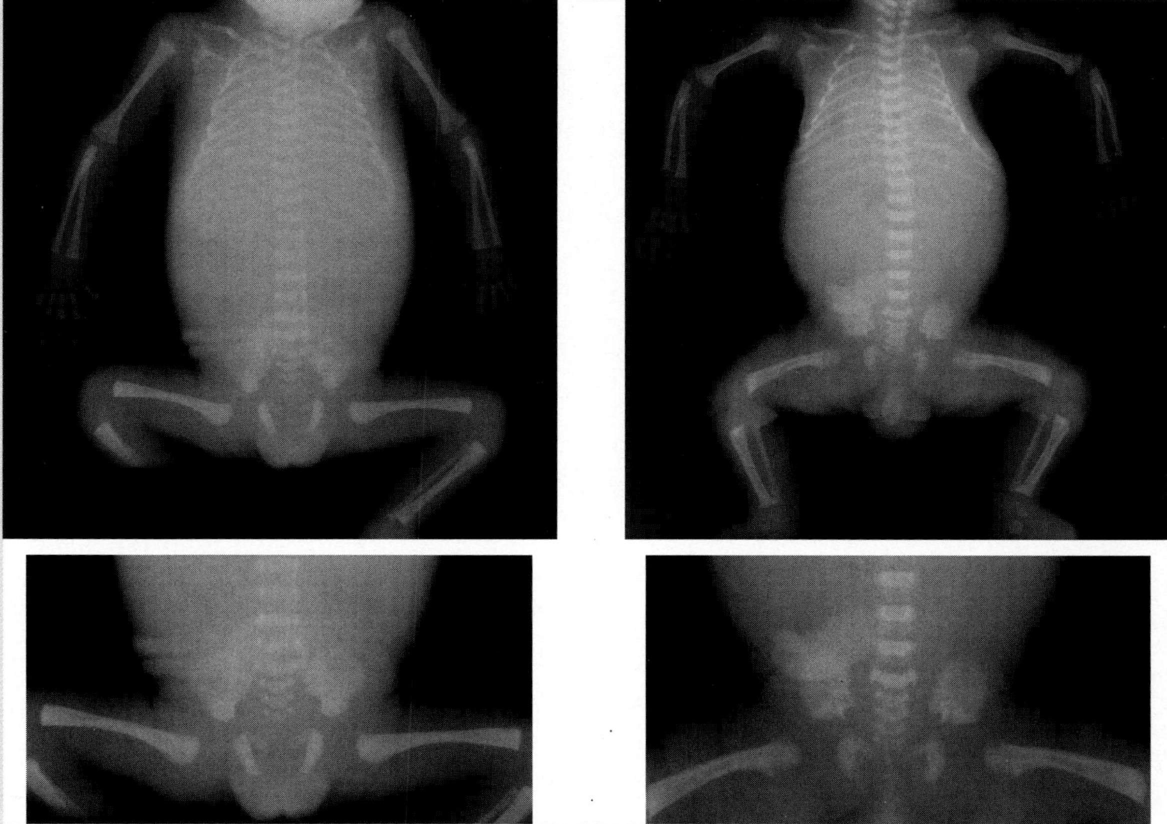

**Figure C–1.** Radiographs of a normal 34-week fetus *(left)* and a 34-week fetus with achondroplasia *(right)*. Comparison of the upper frames shows rhizomelia and trident positioning of the fingers in the fetus with achondroplasia. Comparison of the lower frames illustrates the caudal narrowing of the interpedicular distance in the fetus with achondroplasia versus the interpedicular widening in the normal fetus. Also, the fetus with achondroplasia has small iliac wings shaped like an elephant's ear and narrowing of the sacrosciatic notch. (Courtesy of S. Unger, R. S. Lachman, and D. L. Rimoin, Cedars-Sinai Medical Center, Los Angeles.)

In addition to management of their medical problems, patients often need help with social adjustment both because of the psychological aspects of their appearance and short stature and because of their physical handicaps. Support groups often assist by providing interaction with similarly affected peers and social awareness programs.

## Inheritance Risk

For normal parents with a child affected with achondroplasia, the risk of recurrence in their future children is very low, although it is higher than the general population risk because of possible germline mosaicism. For relationships in which one partner is affected with achondroplasia, the risk of recurrence in each child is 50 percent because achondroplasia is an autosomal dominant disorder with full penetrance. For relationships in which both partners are affected, each child has a 50 percent risk of having achondroplasia, a 25 percent risk of having lethal homozygous achondroplasia, and a 25 percent chance of being of normal stature.

Prenatal diagnosis before 20 weeks of gestation is available only by molecular testing of fetal DNA, although the diagnosis can be made late in pregnancy by analysis of a fetal skeletal radiograph. The features of achondroplasia cannot be detected by prenatal ultrasound before 24 weeks' gestation, whereas the more severe thanatophoric dysplasia can be detected earlier (Fig. C–1).

## *Questions for Small Group Discussion*

1. Name other disorders that increase in frequency with increasing paternal age. What types of mutations are associated with these disorders?

2. Discuss possible reasons why the *FGFR3* mutations G1138A and G1138C arise exclusively during spermatogenesis.

3. Marfan syndrome, Huntington disease, and achondroplasia all arise as a result of dominant gain-of-function mutations. Compare and contrast the pathological mechanisms of these gain-of-function mutations.

4. In addition to achondroplasia, *FGFR3* gain-of-function mutations are associated with hypochondrodysplasia and thanatophoric dysplasia. Explain how phenotypic severity of these three disorders correlates with the level of constitutive FGFR3 tyrosine kinase activity.

## *Reference*

GeneClinics
*http://www.geneclinics.org/*

# Alzheimer Disease

## (Cerebral Neuronal Dysfunction and Death)

### Autosomal Dominant or Multifactorial

## Principles

- Variable expressivity
- Genetic heterogeneity
- Gene dosage
- Toxic gain of function
- Risk modifier

## Major Phenotypic Features

- Age of onset: Middle to late adulthood
- Dementia
- $\beta$-amyloid plaques
- Neurofibrillary tangles
- Amyloid angiopathy

## History and Physical Findings

L.W. was an elderly woman with dementia. Eight years before her death, she and her family noticed a deficit in her short-term memory. Initially, they ascribed this to the forgetfulness of "old age"; her cognitive decline continued, however, and progressively interfered with her ability to drive, shop, and keep house. L.W. did not have findings suggestive of thyroid disease, vitamin deficiency, a brain tumor, drug intoxication, chronic infection, depression, or strokes; magnetic resonance imaging of her brain showed diffuse cortical atrophy. L.W.'s brother, father, and two other paternal relatives had died of dementia in their seventies. A neurologist explained to L.W. and her family that normal aging is not associated with dramatic declines in memory or judgment and that declining cognition with behavioral disturbance and impaired daily functioning suggested a clinical diagnosis of familial dementia, possibly Alzheimer disease (AD). The suspicion of AD was supported by her apolipoprotein E genotype: $\epsilon$4/4. L.W.'s condition deteriorated rapidly during the next year, and she died of malnutrition at 75 years of age. Her autopsy confirmed the diagnosis of AD.

## Background

### Disease Etiology

Approximately 10 percent of persons older than 70 years have dementia, and about half of them have AD. AD is a panethnic genetically heterogeneous disease; less than 5 percent of patients have early-onset familial disease, 15 to 25 percent have late-onset familial disease, and 75 percent have sporadic disease. Approximately 10 percent of familial AD exhibits autosomal dominant inheritance; the remainder exhibits multifactorial inheritance. Less than 1 percent of patients with AD have Down syndrome (see Chapters 12 and 15).

Current evidence suggests that defects of $\beta$-amyloid precursor protein metabolism cause the neuronal dysfunction and death observed with AD. Consistent with this hypothesis, mutations associated with early-onset autosomal dominant AD have been identified in the $\beta$-amyloid precursor protein gene (*APP*), the presenilin 1 gene *(PSEN1)*, and the presenilin 2 gene *(PSEN2)* (see Chapter 12). The prevalence of mutations in these genes varies widely depending on the inclusion criteria of the study; 20 to 70 percent of patients with early-onset autosomal dominant AD have mutations in *PSEN1*, 10 to 15 percent have mutations in *APP*, and less than 5 percent have mutations in *PSEN2*.

No mendelian causes of late-onset AD have been identified; however, both familial and sporadic late-onset AD are strongly associated with allele $\epsilon$4 at the apolipoprotein E gene *(APOE)*. The frequency of $\epsilon$4 is 12 to 15 percent in normal controls compared with 35 percent in all patients with AD and 45 percent in patients with a family history of dementia.

### Pathogenesis

A$\beta$-amyloid precursor protein (APP) undergoes endoproteolytic cleavage to produce peptides with neurotrophic and neuroprotective activities. Cleavage of APP within the endosomal-lysosomal compartment produces a carboxyl-terminal peptide of 40 amino acids ($A\beta_{40}$); the function of $A\beta_{40}$ is unknown. In contrast, cleavage of APP within the endoplasmic reticulum or cis-Golgi produces a carboxyl-terminal peptide of 42 or 43 amino acids ($A\beta_{42/43}$). $A\beta_{42/43}$ readily aggregates and is neurotoxic in vitro and possibly in vivo. Patients with AD have a significant increase in $A\beta_{42/43}$ aggregates within their brains. Mutations in *APP*, *PSEN1*, and *PSEN2* increase the relative or absolute production of $A\beta_{42/43}$. Patients with Down syndrome overexpress APP (the gene for which is on chromosome 21) and thus $A\beta_{42/43}$. The role of *APOE* $\epsilon$4 is uncertain.

AD is a central neurodegenerative disorder, especially of cholinergic neurons of the hippocampus, neocortical association area, and other limbic structures. Neuropathology includes cortical atrophy, extracellular neuritic plaques, intraneuronal neurofibrillary tangles (Fig. C–2), and amyloid deposits in the walls of cerebral arteries. The neuritic plaques (see Fig. C–2) contain many different proteins including $A\beta_{42/43}$ and ApoE. The neurofibrillary tangles are composed predominantly of hyperphosphorylated tau protein; tau helps maintain neuronal integrity, axonal transport, and axonal polarity by promoting the assembly and stability of microtubules.

### Phenotype and Natural History

AD is characterized by a progressive loss of cognitive function including recent memory, abstract reasoning, concentration, language, visual perception, and visual-spatial function. Beginning with a subtle failure of memory, AD is often attributed initially to benign "forgetfulness." Some patients perceive their cognitive decline and become frustrated and anxious, whereas others are unaware. Eventually, patients are unable to work, and they require supervision. Social etiquette and superficial conversation are often retained surprisingly well. Ultimately, most patients develop rigidity, mutism, and incontinence and are bedridden. Other symptoms associated with AD include agitation, social withdrawal, hallucinations, seizures, myoclonus, and parkinsonian features. Death usually results from malnutrition, infection, or heart disease.

Aside from the age of onset, early- and late-onset AD are clinically indistinguishable. Mutations in *PSEN1* are fully penetrant and usually cause rapidly progressive disease with a mean onset at 45 years. Mutations in *APP* are fully penetrant and cause a rate of AD progression similar to that of late-onset AD; the age of onset ranges from 40s to early 60s. Mutations in *PSEN2* may not be fully penetrant and

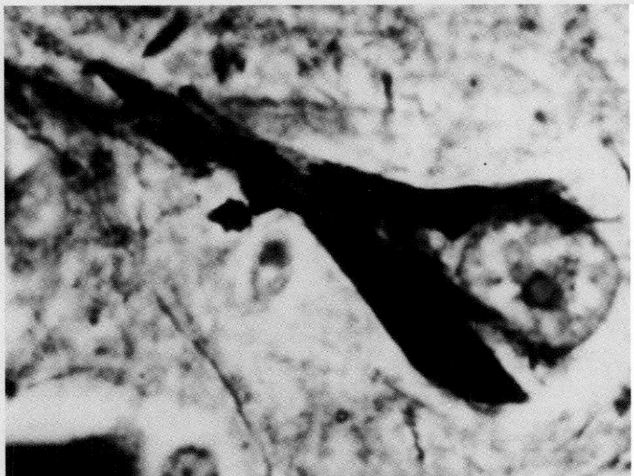
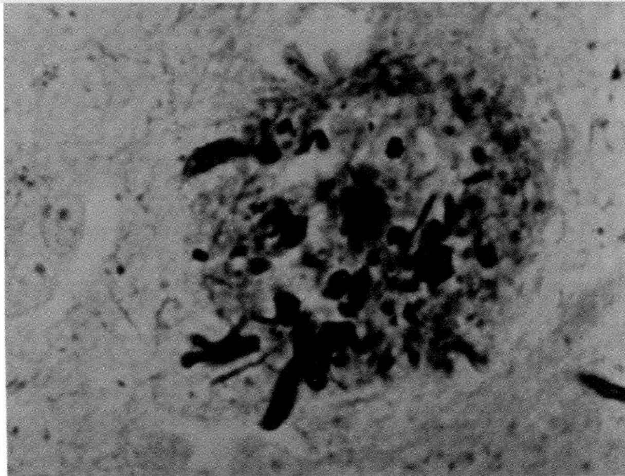

**Figure C–2.** Photograph of a neurofibrillary tangle *(left)* and a neuritic plaque *(right)* observed on brain histopathology from an individual with Alzheimer disease. (Courtesy of D. Armstrong, Baylor College of Medicine and Texas Children's Hospital, Houston.)

usually cause slowly progressive disease with onset ranging from 40 to 75 years. In contrast to early-onset AD, late-onset AD develops after 60 to 65 years of age; the duration of disease is usually 8 to 10 years, although the range is 2 to 25 years. For both late-onset AD and AD secondary to *APP* mutations, the *APOE* allele ϵ4 is a dose-dependent modifier of onset; that is, the age of onset varies inversely with the number of copies of the ϵ4 allele.

## Management

Except for patients in families segregating an AD-associated mutation, patients with dementia can be definitively diagnosed with AD only by autopsy; however, with rigorous adherence to diagnostic criteria, a clinical suspicion of AD is confirmed by neuropathology 80 to 90 percent of the time. The accuracy of the clinical suspicion increases to 97 percent if the patient is homozygous for allele ϵ4 of *APOE*.

Because no curative therapies are available for AD, treatment is focused on the amelioration of associated behavioral and neurological problems. Approximately 10 to 20 percent of patients have a modest decrease in the rate of cognitive decline if treated early in the disease course with agents that increase cholinergic activity.

## Inheritance Risk

Old age, family history, female gender, and Down syndrome are the most important risk factors for AD. In Western populations, the empiric lifetime risk for AD is 5 percent. If patients have a first-degree relative in whom AD developed after 65 years, they have a three- to sixfold relative risk of AD. If patients have a sibling in whom AD developed before 70 years and an affected parent, their relative risk is seven- to ninefold. *APOE* testing is an adjunct diagnostic test and should not be used for predictive testing for AD in asymptomatic patients.

Patients with Down syndrome have an increased risk for AD. After age 40, patients with Down syndrome consistently have neuropathological findings of AD, and approximately 50 percent experience cognitive decline.

For families segregating autosomal dominant AD, each person has a 50 percent risk of inheriting an AD-causing mutation. With the exception of some *PSEN2* mutations, full penetrance and relatively consistent age of onset within a family allow genetic counseling. Currently, clinical DNA testing is available for *APP*, *PSEN1*, and *PSEN2*; DNA testing should be done only in the context of genetic counseling.

## Questions for Small Group Discussion

1. Why is the *APOE* genotype not useful for predicting AD in asymptomatic individuals?
2. Why is AD usually a neuropathological diagnosis? What is the differential diagnosis for AD?
3. Mutation of *MAPT*, the gene encoding tau protein, causes frontotemporal dementia; however, *MAPT* mutations have not been detected in AD. Compare and contrast the proposed mechanisms by which abnormalities of tau cause dementia in AD and frontotemporal dementia.
4. Approximately 30 to 50 percent of the population risk for AD is attributed to genetic factors. What environmental factors are proposed for the remaining risk? What are the difficulties with conclusively identifying environmental factors as risks?

## Reference

GeneClinics
*http://www.geneclinics.org/*

# Hereditary Breast and Ovarian Cancer

## (BRCA1 or BRCA2 Mutation)

### Autosomal Dominant

## Principles

- Tumor suppressor gene
- Multistep carcinogenesis
- Somatic mutation
- Incomplete penetrance
- Variable expressivity
- Founder effect

## Major Phenotypic Features

- Age of onset: Adulthood
- Breast cancer
- Ovarian cancer
- Prostate cancer
- Multiple primary cancers

## History and Physical Findings

S.M., a 27-year-old previously healthy woman, was referred to the cancer genetics clinic by her gynecologist after being diagnosed with breast cancer. She was concerned about her children's risk for developing cancer and about her risk for developing ovarian cancer. Her mother, two maternal aunts, and maternal grandfather had breast cancer; her mother had also had ovarian cancer (Fig. C–3). The findings from S.M.'s physical examination were remarkable only for a scar on her right breast. The genetic counselor explained that the family history of breast cancer was indicative of an inherited predisposition. Based on the ensuing discussion of prognosis and recurrence risks, S.M. chose to pursue DNA sequencing of the breast cancer susceptibility genes *BRCA1* and *BRCA2*. This testing showed that she had a germline mutation in one *BRCA2* allele. During the discussion of the results, S.M. requested that her 6- and 7-year-old girls be tested. The genetic counselor explained that the decision to have genetic testing was better left until the children were mature enough to decide on the utility of such testing. Five adult relatives elected to have predictive testing, and four were found to be carriers of the mutation; one of these four pursued prophylactic bilateral mastectomy, and another underwent prophylactic bilateral salpingo-oophorectomy.

## Background

### Disease Etiology

Mutations of major cancer predisposition genes account for 3 to 10 percent of cases of breast cancer and have an estimated overall prevalence of 1 in 300 to 1 in 800. Two of these genes are *BRCA1* and *BRCA2*. In the general North American population, the prevalence of *BRCA1* mutations is between 1 in 500 and 1 in 1000; the prevalence of *BRCA2* mutations is undefined. Mutations of *BRCA1* or *BRCA2* account for approximately 70 to 80 percent of **familial** breast cancer.

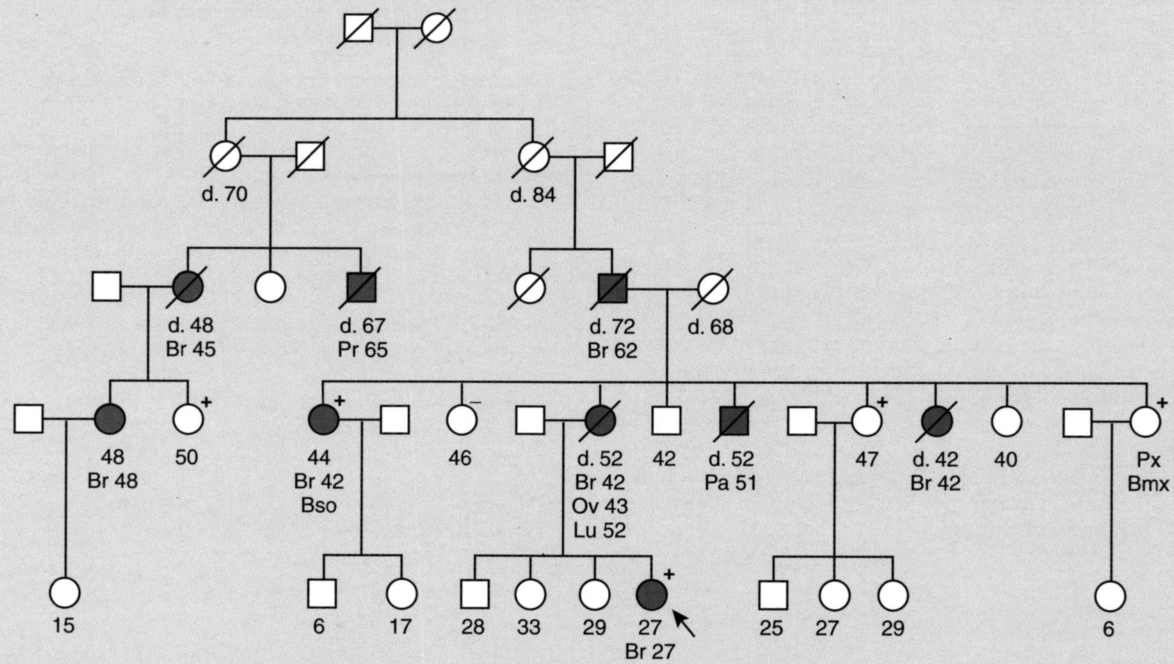


**Figure C–3.** Family segregating a *BRCA2* C3590G mutation. Note the frequent occurrence of breast cancer, including male breast cancer. Also, note the incomplete penetrance in generations I and II. The proband, S.M., is indicated by an arrow. Red symbols indicate a diagnosis of cancer. Ages are shown directly below the symbol. A "+" identifies carriers of the *BRCA2* mutation and a "−" noncarriers as determined by DNA sequencing. Cancer diagnoses are followed by the age at diagnosis. Cancer abbreviations: Br = breast; Ov = ovarian; Lu = lung; Pa = pancreatic; Pr = prostate. Other abbreviations: Bso = bilateral salpingo-oophorectomy; d. = age at death; Px Bmx = prophylactic bilateral mastectomy. (Courtesy of A. Liede and S. Narod, Women's College Hospital and University of Toronto.)

| Population | Cumulative Risk at Age 70 Years (%) *Female* | | *Male* | |
|---|---|---|---|---|
| | Breast Cancer | Ovarian Cancer | Breast Cancer | Prostate Cancer |
| *BRCA1* mutation carriers | 40–87 | 16–63 | ? | 25 |
| *BRCA2* mutation carriers | 28–84 | 27 | 6–14 | 20 |
| General population | 8–10 | 1.5 | <0.1 | 10 |

## Pathogenesis

*BRCA1* and *BRCA2* encode ubiquitously expressed nuclear proteins that are believed to maintain genomic integrity by regulating DNA repair, transcriptional transactivation, and the cell cycle. Many experimental observations suggest that *BRCA1* and *BRCA2* act in the same pathway.

Despite the ubiquitous expression of *BRCA1* and *BRCA2*, mutation of these genes predisposes predominantly to breast and ovarian neoplasias. Loss of *BRCA1* or *BRCA2* function probably permits the accumulation of other mutations that are directly responsible for neoplasia. Consistent with this hypothesis, breast and ovarian carcinomas from patients with mutations of *BRCA1* or *BRCA2* have chromosomal instability and frequent mutations in other tumor suppressor genes.

Tumor formation in carriers of *BRCA1* or *BRCA2* germline mutations follows the "two-hit" hypothesis; that is, both alleles of either *BRCA1* or *BRCA2* lose function in tumor cells (see Chapter 16). Somatic loss of function by the second allele occurs by loss of heterozygosity, intragenic mutation, or promoter hypermethylation. Because of the high frequency with which the second allele of *BRCA1* or *BRCA2* loses function, families segregating a germline *BRCA1* or *BRCA2* mutation exhibit autosomal dominant inheritance of neoplasia.

The population prevalence of *BRCA1* or *BRCA2* germline mutations varies widely and often suggests a founder effect. In Iceland, the *BRCA2* 999del5 mutation occurs on a specific haplotype and has a prevalence of 0.6 percent. Among Ashkenazic Jews, the *BRCA1* 185delAG and 5382inC mutations and the *BRCA2* 6174delT mutation also occur on specific haplotypes and have prevalences of 1, 0.4, and 1.2 percent, respectively.

## Phenotype and Natural History

Patients with *BRCA1* or *BRCA2* germline mutations have an increased risk for several cancers. In addition to the increased risk of ovarian and female breast cancer, *BRCA1* mutations confer an increased risk for prostate cancer and, possibly, for colon cancer. Similarly, in addition to ovarian and female breast cancer, germline *BRCA2* mutations increase the risk of prostate, pancreatic, bile duct, gall bladder, and male breast cancers.

Among female carriers of a *BRCA1* or *BRCA2* germline mutation, the overall penetrance of breast or ovarian cancer, or both, is estimated to be approximately 50 to 80 percent. Approximately two thirds of families with a history of breast and ovarian cancer segregate a *BRCA1* mutation, whereas approximately two thirds of families with a history of male and female breast cancer segregate a *BRCA2* mutation.

Patients with *BRCA1* or *BRCA2* mutations and breast or ovarian cancer, or both, have outcomes and prognoses similar to those of patients with sporadic breast and ovarian cancer; prognosis is determined largely by the tumor stage. In contrast to patients with sporadic breast carcinomas, however, patients with *BRCA1* or *BRCA2* mutations usually have breast carcinomas that are of a higher grade and that are estrogen-receptor negative.

## Management

Current recommendations for women with a germline *BRCA1* or *BRCA2* mutation include frequent breast and ovarian examinations as well as imaging studies; unfortunately, current screening methods for ovarian cancer have not increased survival. Management of at-risk males includes frequent prostate and breast examinations and laboratory tests for evidence of prostate cancer. In families with known germline mutations, molecular analysis can focus surveillance or prophylaxis on members carrying a mutation. Total bilateral mastectomy may reduce the risk of breast cancer by more than 90 percent, although the risk is not abolished because some breast tissue often remains. Similarly, bilateral salpingo-oophorectomy may reduce the risk of ovarian cancer by more than 90 percent. Studies of chemoprevention of breast cancer using estrogen antagonists and oral contraceptives are ongoing.

## Inheritance Risk

Female gender, age, and family history are the most important risk factors for breast cancer. In Western populations, the cumulative female breast cancer incidence is 1 in 200 at 40 years, 1 in 50 at 50 years, and 1 in 10 by 70 years. If patients have a first-degree relative in whom breast cancer developed after 55 years, they have a 1.6 relative risk for breast cancer, whereas the relative risk increases to 2.3 if the breast cancer developed in the family member before 55 years and to 3.8 if it developed before 45 years. If the first-degree relative had bilateral breast cancer, the relative risk is 6.4.

Children of a patient with a *BRCA1* or *BRCA2* germline mutation have a 50 percent risk of inheriting that mutation. Because of incomplete penetrance and variable expressivity, the development and onset of cancer cannot be precisely predicted.

## Questions for Small Group Discussion

1. At what age and under what conditions might testing of an at-risk child be appropriate?
2. What is the risk for a son developing prostate cancer if a parent carries a *BRCA1* germline mutation? A *BRCA2* germline mutation?
3. Currently, sequencing of the coding region of *BRCA1* detects only 60 to 70 percent of mutations in families with linkage to the gene. What mutations would sequencing miss? How should a report of "no mutation detected by sequencing" be interpreted and counseled? How would testing of an affected family member clarify the testing results?

## Reference

GeneClinics
*http://www.geneclinics.org/*

# Charcot-Marie-Tooth Disease Type 1A

## (PMP22 Mutation or Duplication)

### Autosomal Dominant

## Principles

- Genetic heterogeneity
- Gene dosage
- Recombination between repeated DNA sequences

## Major Phenotypic Features

- Age of onset: Childhood to adulthood
- Progressive distal weakness
- Distal muscle wasting
- Hyporeflexia

## History and Physical Findings

During the past few years, J.T., an 18-year-old woman, had noticed a progressive decline in her strength, endurance, and ability to run and walk. She also complained of frequent leg cramps exacerbated by cold and recent difficulty stepping over objects and climbing stairs. She did not recollect a precedent illness or give a history suggestive of an inflammatory process. No other family members had similar problems or a neuromuscular disorder. On examination, J.T. was thin and had atrophy of her lower legs, mild weakness of ankle extension and flexion, absent ankle reflexes, reduced patellar reflexes, an equine gait, and enlarged peroneal nerves. She had difficulty walking on her toes and could not walk on her heels. The findings from her examination were otherwise normal. As part of her evaluation, the neurologist requested several studies, including nerve conduction velocities (NCV). J.T.'s NCVs were abnormal; her median NCV was 25 m/sec (normal >43 m/sec). Results of a subsequent nerve biopsy showed segmental demyelination, myelin sheath hypertrophy (redundant wrappings of Schwann cells around nerve fibers), and no evidence of inflammation. The neurologist explained that these results were strongly suggestive of a demyelinating neuropathy such as type 1 Charcot-Marie-Tooth disease (CMT1), also known as hereditary motor and sensory neuropathy type 1. Explaining that the most common cause of CMT1 is a duplication of the peripheral myelin protein 22 gene (*PMP22*), the neurologist requested testing for this duplication. This test confirmed that J.T. had a duplicated *PMP22* allele and the disease CMT1A.

## Background

### *Disease Etiology*

CMT is a genetically heterogeneous group of hereditary neuropathies characterized by chronic motor and sensory polyneuropathy. CMT has been subdivided according to patterns of inheritance, neuropathology, and clinical features. By definition, CMT1 is an autosomal dominant demyelinating neuropathy; it has a prevalence of approximately 15 in 100,000 and is also genetically heterogeneous. CMT1 is most commonly caused by increased dosage of PMP22 secondary to duplication of the *PMP22* gene on chromosome 17. This duplication accounts for 70 percent of CMT1 overall and 90 percent of sporadic CMT1 cases. More than 90 percent of *de novo* duplications arise during male meiosis.

### *Pathogenesis*

PMP22 is an integral membrane glycoprotein. Within the peripheral nervous system, PMP22 is found in compact but not noncompact myelin. The function of PMP22 has not been fully elucidated, but evidence suggests that it plays a key role in myelin compaction.

Dominant negative mutations within *PMP22* or increased dosage of PMP22 cause a demyelinating peripheral polyneuropathy. Increased dosage of PMP22 arises by tandem duplication of band p11.2 on chromosome 17. This 1.5 megabase (Mb) region is flanked by repeated DNA sequences that are approximately 98 percent identical. Misalignment of these flanking repeat elements during meiosis can lead to unequal crossing over and formation of one chromatid with a duplication of the 1.5 Mb region and another with the reciprocal deletion. (The reciprocal deletion causes the disease hereditary neuropathy with pressure palsies [HNPP]). An individual inheriting a chromatid with the duplication will have three copies of a normal *PMP22* gene and, thus, overexpress PMP22.

Overexpression of PMP22 or expression of dominant negative forms of PMP22 results in an inability to form and maintain compact myelin. Nerve biopsy specimens from severely affected infants show a diffuse paucity of myelin, and nerve biopsy specimens from more mildly affected patients show segmental demyelination and myelin sheath hypertrophy. The mechanism by which PMP22 overexpression causes this pathology remains unclear.

The muscular weakness and atrophy observed in CMT1 result from muscular denervation secondary to axonal degeneration. Longitudinal patient studies have shown an age-dependent reduction in the nerve fiber density that correlates with the development of disease symptoms. In addition, evidence in murine models suggests that myelin is necessary for maintenance of the axonal cytoskeleton. The mechanism by which demyelination alters the axonal cytoskeleton and effects axonal degeneration has not been elucidated completely.

### *Phenotype and Natural History*

CMT1A has nearly full penetrance, although the severity, onset, and progression of CMT1 vary markedly within and among families. Many affected individuals do not seek medical attention, either because their symptoms are not noticeable or because their symptoms are accommodated easily. On the other hand, others have severe disease that manifests in infancy or in childhood.

Symptoms of CMT1A usually develop in the first 2 decades of life; onset after 30 years of age is rare. Typically, symptoms begin with an insidious onset of slowly progressive weakness and atrophy of the distal leg muscles and mild sensory impairment (Fig. C–4). The weakness of the feet and legs leads to abnormalities of gait, a dropped foot, and, eventually, to foot deformities (pes cavus and hammer toes) and loss of balance; it rarely causes patients to lose their ability to walk. Weakness of the intrinsic hand muscles usually occurs late in the disease course and, in severe cases, causes claw hand deformities. Other associated findings include decreased or absent reflexes, upper-extremity ataxia and tremor, scoliosis, and palpably enlarged superficial nerves. Occasionally, the phrenic and autonomic nerves are also involved.

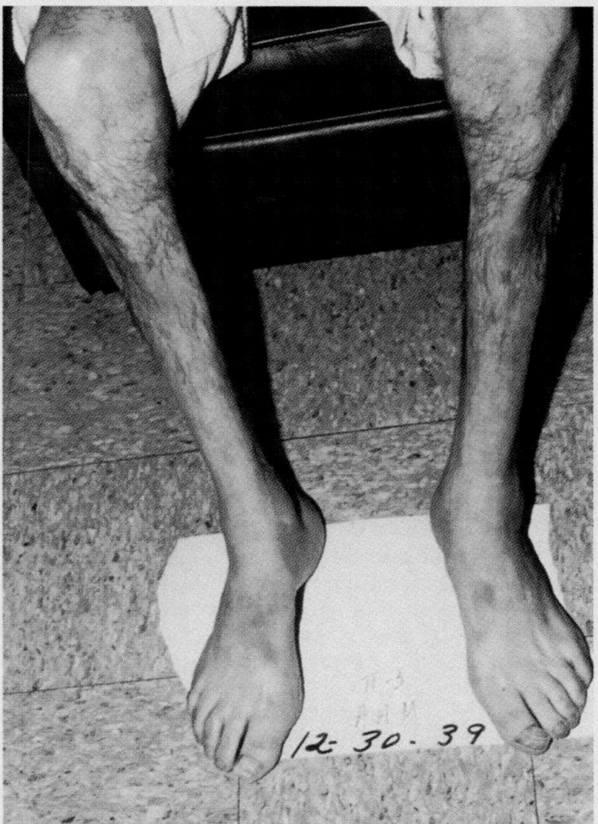


**Figure C–4.** Distal leg muscle wasting in an elderly gentleman with the *PMP22* duplication. (Courtesy of J. R. Lupski, Baylor College of Medicine, Houston, and C. Garcia, Tulane University, New Orleans.)

In electrophysiological studies, the hallmark of CMT1A is uniform slowing of NCVs in all nerves and nerve segments as a result of demyelination. The full reduction in NCVs is usually present by 2 to 5 years of age, although clinically apparent symptoms may not manifest for many years.

### *Management*

Although the diagnosis of CMT1 is suspected because of clinical, electrophysiological, and pathological features, a definitive diagnosis often depends on detection of a mutation. Inflammatory peripheral neuropathies are frequently difficult to distinguish from CMT1 and HNPP, and before the advent of molecular testing, many patients with inherited neuropathies were treated with immunosuppressants and experienced the associated morbidity without improvement of their neuropathy.

Treatment focuses on symptomatic management because curative therapies are currently unavailable for CMT1. Paralleling disease progression, therapy generally follows three stages: strengthening and stretching exercises to maintain gait and function, use of orthoses and special adaptive splints, and orthopedic surgery. Further deterioration may require use of ambulatory supports such as canes or walkers or, in rare, severely affected patients, the use of a wheelchair. All patients should be counseled to avoid exposure to neurotoxic medications and chemicals.

## Inheritance Risk

Because the *PMP22* duplication and most *PMP22* point mutations are autosomal dominant and fully penetrant, each child of an affected parent has a 50 percent chance of developing CMT1A. The variable expressivity of the *PMP22* duplication and *PMP22* mutations, however, makes prediction of disease severity impossible.

## *Questions for Small Group Discussion*

1. Genomic deletions and duplications frequently arise by recombination between repetitive sequences within the human genome (see Chapter 10). Name three disorders caused by deletion following presumed recombination between repetitive sequences. Which of these deletions are associated with a reciprocal duplication? What does the identification of a reciprocal duplication suggest about the mechanism of recombination? What does the absence of a reciprocal duplication suggest?
2. At least two different mechanisms cause human chromosomal deletions. Contrast the molecular mechanism leading to the HNPP deletion with that leading to the Jacobsen syndrome deletion.
3. Generally, genomic duplications are associated with less severe disease than are genomic deletions. Duplication of a *PMP22* allele, however, usually causes more severe disease than deletion of a *PMP22* allele. Discuss possible reasons for this.
4. Name two other diseases that are caused by a gene dosage effect.

## *Reference*


GeneClinics
*http://www.geneclinics.org/*

# Chronic Myelogenous Leukemia

## (BCR-ABL Oncogene Activation)

### Somatic Mutation

## Principles

- Chromosomal reciprocal translocation
- Oncogene activation
- Fusion protein
- Multi-hit hypothesis

## Major Phenotypic Features

- Age of onset: Middle to late adulthood
- Leukocytosis
- Splenomegaly
- Fatigue and malaise

## History and Physical Findings

E.S., a 45-year-old woman, presented to her family physician for her annual checkup. She had been in good health and had no specific complaints. On examination, she had a palpable spleen tip but no other abnormal findings. Results of her complete blood count unexpectedly showed a white blood cell count of $31 \times 10^9$/L and a platelet count of $650 \times 10^9$/L. The peripheral smear revealed basophilia and immature granulocytes. Her physician referred her to the oncology department for further evaluation. Her bone marrow was found to be hypercellular with an increased number of myeloid and megakaryocytic cells and an increased ratio of myeloid to erythroid cells. Cytogenetic analysis of her marrow identified several myeloid cells with a Philadelphia chromosome, der(22)t(9;22)(q34;q11.2). Her oncologist explained that she had chronic myelogenous leukemia (CML) and that the only potentially curative therapy currently available was allogenic bone marrow transplantation.

## Background

### *Disease Etiology*

CML is a clonal expansion of transformed hematopoietic progenitor cells that increases circulating myeloid and erythroid cells and platelets. Transformation of progenitor cells occurs by expression of the *BCR-ABL* oncogene. CML accounts for 15 percent of adult leukemia and has an incidence of 1 to 2 per 100,000; the age-adjusted incidence is higher in men than in women (1.3 to 1.7 versus 1.0) (see Chapter 16).

### *Pathogenesis*

Approximately 95 percent of patients with CML have a Philadelphia chromosome, and the remainder have complex or variant translocations (see Chapter 16). The Abelson proto-oncogene *(ABL)*, which encodes a nonreceptor tyrosine kinase, resides on 9q34, and the breakpoint cluster region gene *(BCR)*, which encodes a phosphoprotein, resides on 22q11. During the formation of the Philadelphia chromosome, the *ABL* gene is disrupted in intron 1 and the *BCR* gene in one of three breakpoint cluster regions; the *BCR* and *ABL* gene fragments are joined head to tail on the derivative chromosome 22 (Fig. C–5). The *BCR-ABL* fusion gene on the derivative chromosome 22 generates a fusion protein that varies in size depending on the length of the Bcr peptide attached to the amino terminus.

To date, the normal functions of Abl and Bcr have not been clearly defined. Abl has been conserved fairly well throughout metazoan evolution. It is found in both the nucleus and cytoplasm and as a myristolated product associated with the inner cytoplasmic membrane. The relative abundance of Abl in these compartments varies among cell types and in response to stimuli. Abl participates in the cell-cycle, stress responses, integrin signaling, and neural development. The functional domains of Bcr include a coiled-coil motif for polymerization with other proteins, a serine-threonine kinase domain, a GDP-GTP exchange domain involved in regulation of ras family members, and a guanosine triphosphatase-activating domain for regulating Rac and Rho GTPases.

Expression of Abl does not result in cellular transformation, whereas expression of the Bcr-Abl fusion protein does. Transgenic mice expressing Bcr-Abl develop acute leukemia at birth, and infection of normal mice with a retrovirus expressing Bcr-Abl causes a variety of acute and chronic leukemias depending on the genetic background. In contrast to Abl, Bcr-Abl has constitutive tyrosine kinase activity and is confined to the cytoplasm where it avidly binds actin microfilaments. Bcr-Abl phosphorylates several cytoplasmic substrates and thereby activates signaling cascades that control growth and differentiation and, possibly, adhesion of hematopoietic cells. Unregulated activation of these signaling pathways results in unregulated proliferation of the hematopoietic stem cell, release of immature cells from the marrow, and, ultimately, CML.

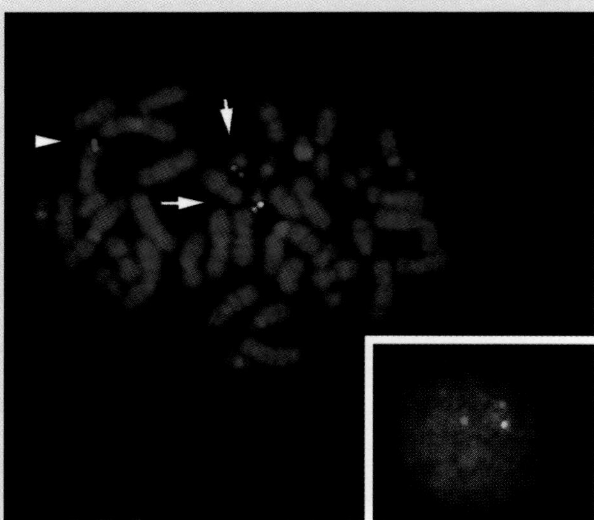

**Figure C–5.** Fluorescence in situ hybridization of a locus-specific probe to metaphase and interphase *(inset)* cells for the detection of the t(9;22)(q34;q11.2) in chronic myelogeneous leukemia. The DNA is counterstained with DAPI. The probe is a mixture of DNA probes for the *BCR* gene *(red)* at 22q11.2 and for the *ABL* gene *(green)* at 9q34. In normal cells, the green signal is observed on both chromosome 9 homologs, and the red signal is observed on both chromosome 22 homologs. In cells with the t(9;22), a green signal is observed on the normal chromosome 9 *(arrowhead)*, a red signal on the normal chromosome 22 *(short arrow)*, and a yellow fusion signal *(long arrow)*, resulting from the presence of both green and red signals together on the Philadelphia chromosome as a result of the translocation of *ABL* to the derivative 22 chromosome. (Courtesy of M. M. LeBeau and H. T. Abelson, University of Chicago.)

As CML progresses, it becomes increasingly aggressive. During this evolution, tumor cells of 50 to 80 percent of patients acquire other chromosomal changes as (trisomy 8, i(17q), or trisomy 19) or another Philadelphia chromosome, or both. In addition to the cytogenetic changes, tumor suppressor genes and proto-oncogenes are also frequently mutated in the progression of CML.

### Phenotype and Natural History

CML is a biphasic or triphasic disease. The initial or chronic stage is characterized by an insidious onset with subsequent development of fatigue, malaise, weight loss, and minimal-to-moderate splenic enlargement. Over time, CML typically evolves to an accelerated phase and then to a blast crisis, although some patients progress directly from the chronic phase to the blast crisis. CML progression includes development of additional chromosomal abnormalities within tumor cells, progressive leukocytosis, anemia, thrombocytosis or thrombocytopenia, increasing splenomegaly, fever, and bone lesions. Blast crisis is an acute leukemia in which the blasts can be myeloid, lymphoid, erythroid, or undifferentiated. The accelerated phase is intermediate between the chronic phase and blast crisis.

Approximately 85 percent of patients are diagnosed in the chronic phase. Depending on the study, the median age of diagnosis ranges from 45 to 65 years, although all ages can be affected. The rate of progression from the chronic phase to blast crisis is approximately 5 to 10 percent during the first 2 years and then 20 percent per year subsequently. Because blast crisis is rapidly fatal, demise parallels progression to blast crisis.

### Management

Allogeneic bone marrow transplantation (BMT) is the only known curative therapy. The success of BMT depends on the stage of CML, the age and health of the patient, the bone marrow donor (related versus unrelated), the preparative regimen, development of graft-versus-host disease, and post-transplantation treatment. Much of the long-term success of BMT depends on a graft-versus-leukemia effect, that is, a graft-versus-host response directed against the leukemic cells. After BMT, patients are monitored frequently for relapse and treated as necessary.

Unfortunately, only 30 percent of patients have a related or unrelated HLA-matched donor. Patients ineligible for BMT are usually treated with interferon-$\alpha$ because it can induce hematological and cytogenetic remissions in some patients with chronic phase CML. The durability of these remissions has not been fully defined. The mechanism of action of interferon in CML is poorly understood but is possibly mediated through the immune system. As with acute leukemia, patients in blast crisis are usually treated with cytotoxic agents and, if possible, BMT. Unfortunately, the outcome of these therapies is poor.

## Inheritance Risk

Because CML arises from a somatic mutation that is not found in the germline, the risk of a patient passing the disease to his or her children is zero.

---

### Questions for Small Group Discussion

1. What is the multi-hit hypothesis? How does it apply to neoplasia?
2. Discuss two additional mechanisms of proto-oncogene activation in human cancer, for example, n-*myc* in neuroblastoma and the *ras* oncogenes in carcinomas.
3. Neoplasias graphically illustrate the effects of the accumulation of somatic mutations; however, other less dramatic diseases arise, at least in part, through the accumulation of somatic mutations. Discuss the effect of somatic mutations on aging.
4. Many somatic mutations and cytogenetic rearrangements are never detected because the cells containing them do not have a selective advantage. What advantage does the Philadelphia chromosome confer?

### Reference

Faderl S, Talpaz M, Estrov Z, et al (1999) The biology of chronic myeloid leukemia. N Engl J Med 341:164–172.

# Cystic Fibrosis

## (CFTR Mutation)

### Autosomal Recessive

## Principles

- Ethnic variation in mutation frequency
- Variable expressivity
- Tissue-specific expression of mutations
- Genetic modifiers
- Environmental modifiers

## Major Phenotypic Features

- Age of onset: Neonatal to adulthood
- Progressive pulmonary disease
- Exocrine pancreatic insufficiency
- Obstructive azoospermia
- Elevated sweat chloride
- Growth failure
- Meconium ileus

## History and Physical Findings

J.B., a 2-year-old girl, was referred to the pediatric clinic for evaluation of poor growth. During infancy, J.B. had had diarrhea and colic that had resolved when an elemental formula was substituted for her standard formula. She developed malodorous stools containing food particles as table foods were added to her diet. During her second year, J.B. grew poorly, developed a chronic cough, and had frequent upper respiratory infections. No one else in the family had poor growth, feeding disorders, or pulmonary illnesses. On physical examination, J.B.'s weight and height plotted less than the 3rd percentile and her head circumference at the 10th percentile. She had a severe diaper rash, diffuse rhonchi, and mild clubbing of her digits. The findings from her examination were otherwise normal. After briefly discussing a few possible causes of J.B.'s illness, the pediatrician requested several tests, including a test for sweat chloride level; the sweat chloride level was 75 mmol/L, a level consistent with cystic fibrosis (CF) (normal, 40 mmol/L; indeterminate, 40 to 60 mmol/L). Based on this result and the clinical course, the pediatrician diagnosed J.B's condition as CF. The parents and J.B. were referred to the CF clinic for further counseling and treatment.

## Background

### *Disease Etiology*

CF is an autosomal recessive disorder of epithelial ion transport caused by mutations in the CF transmembrane conductance regulator gene *(CFTR)*. Although CF has been observed in all races, it is predominantly a disease of northern Europeans. The live birth incidence of CF ranges from 1 in 313 among the Hutterites of southern Alberta, Canada, to 1 in 90,000 among the Asian population of Hawaii.

### *Pathogenesis*

CFTR is a cAMP-regulated chloride channel that regulates other ion channels. CFTR maintains the hydration of secretions within airways and ducts through the excretion of chloride and inhibition of sodium uptake (see Chapter 12).

Dysfunction of CFTR can affect many different organs, particularly those that secrete mucus including the upper and lower respiratory tracts, pancreas, biliary system, male genitalia, intestine, and sweat glands.

The dehydrated and viscous secretions in the lungs of patients with CF interfere with mucociliary clearance, inhibit the function of naturally occurring antimicrobial peptides, provide a medium for growth of pathogenic organisms, and obstruct air flow. Within the first months of life, these secretions and the bacteria colonizing them initiate an inflammatory reaction. The release of inflammatory cytokines, host antibacterial enzymes, and bacterial enzymes damages the bronchioles. Recurrent cycles of infection, inflammation, and tissue destruction decrease the amount of functional lung tissue and eventually lead to respiratory failure (Fig. C–6).

Loss of the CFTR chloride transport into the pancreatic duct impairs the hydration of secretions and leads to the retention of exocrine enzymes in the pancreas. Damage from these retained enzymes eventually causes fibrosis of the pancreas.

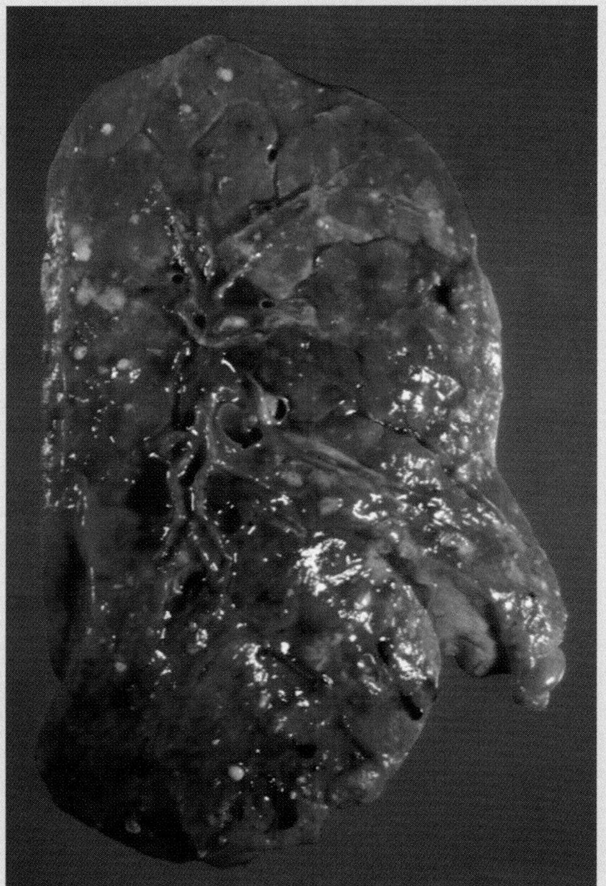

**Figure C–6.** Photograph of a median cross section of a lung from a patient with cystic fibrosis. Note the mucus plugs and purulent secretions within the airways. (Courtesy of J. Rutledge, University of Washington and Children's Hospital and Medical Center, Seattle.)

CFTR also regulates the uptake of sodium and chloride from sweat as it moves through the sweat duct. In the absence of functional CFTR, the sweat has an increased sodium chloride content, and this is the basis of the historical "salty-baby syndrome" and the diagnostic sweat chloride test.

### Phenotype and Natural History

CF classically manifests in early childhood, although approximately 4 percent of patients are diagnosed in adulthood. Ten to 20 percent of patients present at birth with meconium ileus, and the remainder present with chronic respiratory complaints (rhinitis, sinusitis or obstructive lung disease, or both) or poor growth, or both, later in life. The poor growth results from a combination of increased caloric expenditure because of chronic lung infections, and malnutrition from pancreatic exocrine insufficiency. Five to 15 percent of patients with CF with pulmonary disease do not develop pancreatic insufficiency. More than 95 percent of male patients with CF are azoospermic because of obliteration of or failure to develop wolffian duct structures. The progression of lung disease is the chief determinant of morbidity and mortality; most patients die of respiratory failure and cor pulmonale between 30 and 40 years of age.

In addition to CF, mutations within *CFTR* have been associated with a spectrum of diseases including obstructive azoospermia, idiopathic pancreatitis, disseminated bronchiectasis, allergic bronchopulmonary aspergillosis, atypical sinopulmonary disease, and asthma. Some of these disorders are associated with mutations within a single *CFTR* allele, whereas others, like CF, are observed with mutations in both *CFTR* alleles. A direct causative role for mutant *CFTR* alleles has been established for some, but not all, of these disorders.

A correlation between particular *CFTR* mutant alleles and disease severity exists only for pancreatic insufficiency. Secondary mutations or polymorphisms within a *CFTR* allele may alter the efficiency of splicing or protein maturation and thereby extend the spectrum of disease associated with some mutations. In addition, some mutations are predominantly expressed in certain tissues; for example, some mutations affecting the efficiency of splicing have a greater effect on CFTR expression in wolffian duct derivatives than in other tissues. Environmental factors, such as exposure to cigarette smoke, markedly worsen the severity of lung disease among patients with CF.

### Management

Because nearly 900 different mutations and variants have been described across the *CFTR* gene, the diagnosis of CF in North America is usually based on clinical criteria and sweat chloride concentration. One to 2 percent of patients with CF have normal sweat chloride concentrations; in these patients, however, the nasal transepithelial potential difference is usually diagnostic of CF.

Currently, there are no curative treatments for CF, although improved symptomatic management has increased the average longevity from early childhood to between 30 and 40 years. The objectives of medical therapy for CF are clearance of pulmonary secretions, control of pulmonary infection, adequate nutrition, and prevention of intestinal obstruction. Although medical therapy ameliorates the progression of pulmonary disease, the only effective treatment for respiratory failure in CF is lung transplantation. Pancreatic enzyme replacement and supplementation of fat soluble vitamins treat the malabsorption effectively; because of increased caloric needs and anorexia, however, many patients also require caloric supplements. Most patients also require extensive counseling to deal with the psychological effects of having a chronic fatal disease.

## Inheritance Risk

A couple's empiric risk for having a child affected with CF varies greatly depending on the frequency of CF in their ethnic groups. For North Americans who do not have a family history of CF and are of northern European ancestry, their empiric risk for each being a carrier is approximately 1 in 25, and such a couple's risk of having an affected child is therefore 1 in 2500. For couples who already have a child affected with CF, the risk of future children having CF is 1 in 4.

Prenatal diagnosis is based on identification of the *CFTR* mutations in DNA from fetal tissue such as chorionic villi or amniocytes. Effective identification of affected fetuses usually requires that the mutations responsible for CF in a family have already been identified.

### Questions for Small Group Discussion

1. Because some studies suggest that nutritional and possibly medical intervention before the development of symptoms improves the quality of life, screening tests for affected infants or carrier parents, or both, are currently being considered and tested. What criteria must a newborn screening test for CF meet to be implemented?

2. The most common CF mutation is ΔF508; it accounts for approximately 70 percent of all mutant *CFTR* alleles. For a couple of northern European extraction, what is their risk of having an affected child if each tests negative for ΔF508? If one tests positive and the other tests negative for ΔF508?

3. What constitutes disease, a mutation in a gene or the phenotype caused by that mutation? Does detection of a mutation in the *CFTR* gene of patients with congenital bilateral absence of the vas deferens mean they have CF?

### References


Cystic Fibrosis Mutation Data Base *http://www.genet.sickkids. on.ca/cftr/*

Welsh MJ, Ramsey BW, Accurso F, Cutting GR (2001) Cystic fibrosis. *In* Scriver CR, Beaudet AL, Sly WS, et al (eds) The Metabolic and Molecular Bases of Inherited Disease, 8th ed, McGraw-Hill, New York, pp. 5121–5188.

# Duchenne Muscular Dystrophy

## (DMD Mutation)

### X-Linked

## Principles

- High frequency of new mutations
- Allelic heterogeneity
- Manifesting carriers
- Phenotypic variability

## Major Phenotypic Features

- Age of onset: Childhood
- Muscular weakness
- Calf hypertrophy
- Moderate intellectual compromise
- Elevated serum creatine kinase level

## History and Physical Findings

A.Y. was a 6-year-old boy referred for mild developmental delay. He had difficulty climbing stairs, running, and participating in vigorous physical activities; he had both decreased strength and endurance. His parents, two brothers, and one sister were all healthy; no other family members were similarly affected. On examination, he had difficulty jumping onto the examination table, a Gowers sign (a sequence of maneuvers for rising from the floor, Fig. C–7), proximal weakness, a waddling gait, tight heel cords, and enlarged calf muscles. His serum creatine kinase (CK) level was 50-fold higher than normal. Because the history, physical examination findings, and elevated CK level strongly suggested a myopathy, A.Y. was referred to the neurogenetics clinic for further evaluation. Results of his muscle biopsy showed marked variation of muscle fiber size, fiber necrosis, fat and connective tissue proliferation, and no staining for dystrophin. Based on these results, A.Y.'s condition was given a provisional diagnosis as Duchenne muscular dystrophy (DMD), and he was tested for deletions of the dystrophin gene; he was found to have a deletion of exons 45 through 48. Subsequent testing showed that his mother was a carrier. The family was counseled, therefore, that the risk for affected sons was 50 percent, the risk for affected daughters was low but dependent on skewing of X-inactivation, and the risk of carrier daughters was 50 percent. Because her carrier status placed her at a high risk for cardiac complications, the mother was referred for a cardiac evaluation.

## Background

### Disease Etiology

DMD is an X-linked panethnic progressive myopathy caused by mutations within the *DMD* gene. It has an incidence of approximately 1 in 3500 male births.

### Pathogenesis

*DMD* encodes dystrophin, an intracellular protein that is expressed predominantly in smooth, skeletal, and cardiac muscle, as well as in some brain neurons (see Chapter 12). In skeletal muscle, dystrophin is part of a large complex of sarcolemma-associated proteins that confers stability to the sarcolemma.

*DMD* mutations associated with DMD include large deletions (50 to 70 percent); large duplications (5 to 10 percent); and small deletions, insertions, or nucleotide changes (25 to 30 percent). Most large deletions occur in one of two hotspots. Nucleotide changes occur throughout the gene, predominantly at CpG dinucleotides. *De novo* mutations arise with comparable frequency during oogenesis and spermatogenesis; most *de novo* large deletions arise during oogenesis, whereas most *de novo* nucleotide changes arise during spermatogenesis.

Mutations causing a dystrophin null phenotype effect more severe muscular disease than mutant *DMD* alleles ex-

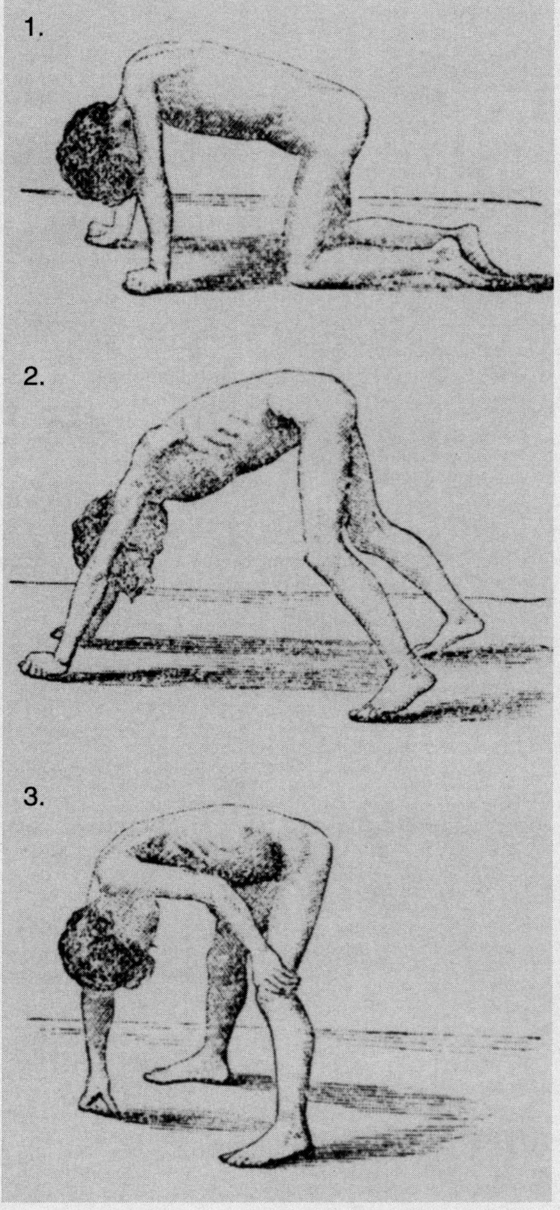


**Figure C–7.** Drawing of a boy with Duchenne muscular dystrophy rising from the ground (the Gowers maneuver). (From Gowers WR [1879] Pseudohypertrophic Muscular Paralysis. A Clinical Lecture. J. and A. Churchill, London.)

pressing partially functional dystrophin. A consistent genotype-phenotype correlation has not been defined for the intellectual impairment.

## Phenotype and Natural History

**Males.** DMD is a progressive myopathy resulting in muscle degeneration and weakness. Beginning with the hip girdle muscles and neck flexors, the muscular weakness progressively involves the shoulder girdle and distal limb and trunk muscles. Although occasionally manifesting in the newborn period with hypotonia or failure to thrive, male patients usually present between ages 3 and 5 years with gait abnormalities. By age 5, most patients use a Gowers maneuver and have calf pseudohypertrophy, that is, enlargement of the calf through replacement of muscle by fat and connective tissue. By age 12, most patients are confined to a wheelchair and have or are developing contractures and scoliosis. Most patients die of impaired pulmonary function and pneumonia; the median age at death is 18 years.

Nearly 95 percent of patients with DMD have some cardiac compromise (dilated cardiomyopathy or electrocardiographic abnormalities, or both), and 84 percent have demonstrable cardiac involvement at autopsy. Chronic heart failure develops in nearly 50 percent of patients. Rarely, cardiac failure is the presenting complaint for patients with DMD.

Although dystrophin is also present in smooth muscle, smooth muscle complications are rare. These complications include gastric dilatation and ileus and bladder paralysis.

Patients with DMD have an average intelligence quotient approximately 1 standard deviation below the mean, and nearly a third have some degree of mental retardation. The basis of this impairment has not been established.

**Females.** The age of onset and severity of DMD in females depends on the degree of skewing of X-inactivation (see Chapter 5). If the X chromosome carrying the mutant *DMD* allele is active in most cells, females develop DMD, whereas if the X chromosome carrying the normal *DMD* allele is predominantly active, females have few or no symptoms of DMD. Regardless of whether they develop clinical symptoms of skeletal muscle weakness, most carrier females develop cardiac abnormalities such as dilated cardiomyopathy, left ventricle dilatation, or electrocardiographic changes.

## Management

The diagnosis of DMD is based on family history and either DNA analysis or muscle biopsy to test for immunoreactivity for dystrophin.

Currently, there are no curative treatments for DMD, although improved symptomatic management has increased the average longevity from late childhood to early adulthood. The objectives of therapy are slowing disease progression, maintenance of mobility, prevention and correction of contractures and scoliosis, weight control, and optimization of pulmonary and cardiac function. Glucocorticoid therapy can slow the progression of DMD for several years. Most patients also require extensive counseling to deal with the psychological effects of having a chronic fatal disease.

## Inheritance Risk

Approximately a third of mothers who have a single affected son will not themselves be carriers of a mutation in the *DMD* gene. Determination of carrier status remains quite difficult, however, because currently available molecular methods do not detect small alterations such as nucleotide changes. Determination of carrier risk in families without identifiable deletions or duplications must rely on linkage analysis, serial serum CK levels, and mosaic expression of dystrophin in muscle biopsy specimens (due to random X-chromosome inactivation). Counseling of recurrence risk must take into account the high rate of germline mosaicism (approximately 14 percent).

If a mother is a carrier, each son has a 50 percent risk of DMD and each daughter has a 50 percent risk of inheriting the *DMD* mutation. Reflecting the random nature of X-chromosome inactivation, daughters inheriting the *DMD* mutation have a low risk of DMD; however, for reasons not fully understood, their risk of cardiac abnormalities may be as high as 50 to 60 percent. If a mother is apparently not a carrier by DNA testing she still has an approximately 7 percent risk of having a boy with DMD. This elevated risk is due to germline mosaicism (see Chapter 5). Counseling and, possibly, prenatal diagnosis is indicated for these mothers.

## Questions for Small Group Discussion

1. Why is DMD considered a genetic lethal condition? What features define a condition as being genetically lethal?
2. Discuss what mechanisms may cause a gender bias in origin of mutation types. Name two or three diseases other than DMD in which this occurs. In particular, discuss the mechanism and high frequency of mutations at CpG dinucleotides during spermatogenesis.
3. How is the rate of germline mosaicism determined for a disease? Name two or three other diseases with a high rate of germline mosaicism.
4. Contrast the phenotype of Becker muscular dystrophy with DMD. What is the postulated mechanism for the milder phenotype of Becker muscular dystrophy?

## References


Gene Clinics
*http://www.geneclinics.org/*

Worton RG, Molnar MJ, Brais B, Karpati G (2001) The muscular dystrophies. *In* Scriver CR, Beaudet AL, Sly WS, et al (eds) The Metabolic and Molecular Bases of Inherited Disease, 8th ed, McGraw-Hill, New York, pp. 5493–5524.

# Familial Adenomatous Polyposis

## (APC Mutation)

### Autosomal Dominant

## Principles

- Tumor suppressor gene
- Multistep carcinogenesis
- Somatic mutation
- Cytogenetic instability
- Variable expressivity

## Major Phenotypic Features

- Age of onset: Adolescence through mid-adulthood
- Colorectal adenomatous polyps
- Colorectal cancer
- Multiple primary cancers

## History and Physical Findings

R.P. was a 35-year-old man who was referred to the cancer genetics clinic by his oncologist. He had just undergone a total colectomy; the colonic mucosa had more than 2000 polyps and pathology consistent with adenomatous polyposis coli. In addition to his abdominal scars and colostomy, he had retinal pigment abnormalities consistent with congenital hypertrophy of the retinal pigment epithelium. Several of his relatives had died of cancer. He did not have a medical or family history of other health problems. Based on the medical history and suggestive family history, the geneticist counseled R.P. that he most likely had familial adenomatous polyposis (FAP). The geneticist explained the surveillance protocol for R.P.'s children and the possibility of using molecular testing to identify those children at risk for FAP. Because R.P. did not have contact with his family, linkage analysis was not possible, and R.P. elected to proceed with screening of the adenomatous polyposis coli gene (*APC*); he had a nonsense mutation in exon 15 of one APC allele.

## Background

### Disease Etiology

At least 50 percent of individuals in western populations develop a colorectal tumor by age 70, and approximately 10 percent of these individuals eventually develop colorectal carcinoma. Approximately 15 percent of colorectal cancer is familial, including FAP and hereditary nonpolyposis colorectal cancer (HNPCC). FAP is an autosomal dominant cancer predisposition syndrome caused by mutations in the *APC* gene. It has a prevalence of 2 to 3 per 100,000 and accounts for less than 1 percent of colon cancer. *APC* mutations also occur in more than 80 percent of sporadic colorectal tumors (see Chapter 16).

### Pathogenesis

Apc directly or indirectly regulates transcription, cell adhesion, the microtubular cytoskeleton, cell migration, crypt fission, apoptosis, and cell proliferation. It forms complexes with several different proteins including β-catenin.

In both humans and mice, both alleles of *APC* must be inactivated for adenoma formation. The high frequency of somatic loss of function in the second *APC* allele defines FAP as an autosomal dominant condition. This somatic loss of function occurs by loss of heterozygosity, intragenic mutation, transcriptional inactivation, and, rarely, by dominant negative effects of the inherited mutant allele. More than 95 percent of intragenic *APC* mutations cause truncation of the Apc protein. Loss of functional Apc usually results in high levels of free cytosolic β-catenin; free β-catenin migrates to the nucleus, binds to T cell factor 4, and inappropriately activates gene expression. Consistent with this mechanism, mutations of the β-catenin gene have been identified in some colorectal carcinomas without *APC* mutations.

Although loss of functional Apc causes affected cells to form dysplastic groups of cells within intestinal crypts, these cells are not cancerous and must acquire other somatic mutations to progress to cancer (see Chapter 16). This progression is characterized by cytogenetic instability resulting in the loss of large chromosomal segments and, consequently, loss of heterozygosity. Specific genetic alterations implicated in this progression include activation of the Ki-*ras* or N-*ras* oncogenes, inactivation of a tumor suppressor gene on 18q, inactivation of the *TP53* gene, and alterations in methylation leading to transcriptional silencing of tumor suppressor genes. As cells accumulate mutations, they become increasingly neoplastic and eventually form invasive and metastatic carcinomas.

### Phenotype and Natural History

FAP is characterized by hundreds to thousands of colonic adenomatous polyps (Fig. C–8). It is diagnosed clinically either by the presence of more than 100 colorectal adenomatous polyps or between 10 and 100 polyps in an individual with a relative with FAP. Adenomatous polyps usually appear between 7 and 40 years of age and rapidly increase in number. Untreated, 7 percent of patients develop colorectal cancer by 21 years, 87 percent by 45 years, and 93 percent by 50 years.

Although nonpenetrance is very rare, patients with germline mutations of *APC* do not necessarily develop adenomas or colorectal cancer; they are only predisposed. The rate-limiting step in adenoma formation is somatic mutation of the wild-type *APC* allele. Progression of an adenoma to carcinoma requires the accumulation of other genetic alterations. Patients with FAP are at much greater risk than is the general population for developing colorectal carcinoma for two reasons. First, although the average time to progress from adenoma to carcinoma is approximately 23 years, these patients develop adenomas earlier in life and are less likely to die of other causes before the development of carcinoma. Second, although less than 1 percent of adenomas progress to carcinoma, patients have tens to thousands of adenomas, each with the potential to transform to carcinoma.

The penetrance and expressivity of *APC* mutations depend on the particular *APC* mutation, genetic background, and environment. Mutations in different regions of the gene are variously associated with Gardner syndrome (an association of colonic adenomatous polyposis, osteomas, and soft tissue tumors), with congenital hypertrophy of the retinal pigment epithelium, or with attenuated adenomatous polyposis coli. Among mice strains with an *APC* mutation, alleles of a secreted phospholipase A2 modify the number of adenomas; similar modifiers may cause patients with identical germline mutations to have dissimilar clinical features. Many studies of sporadic colo-

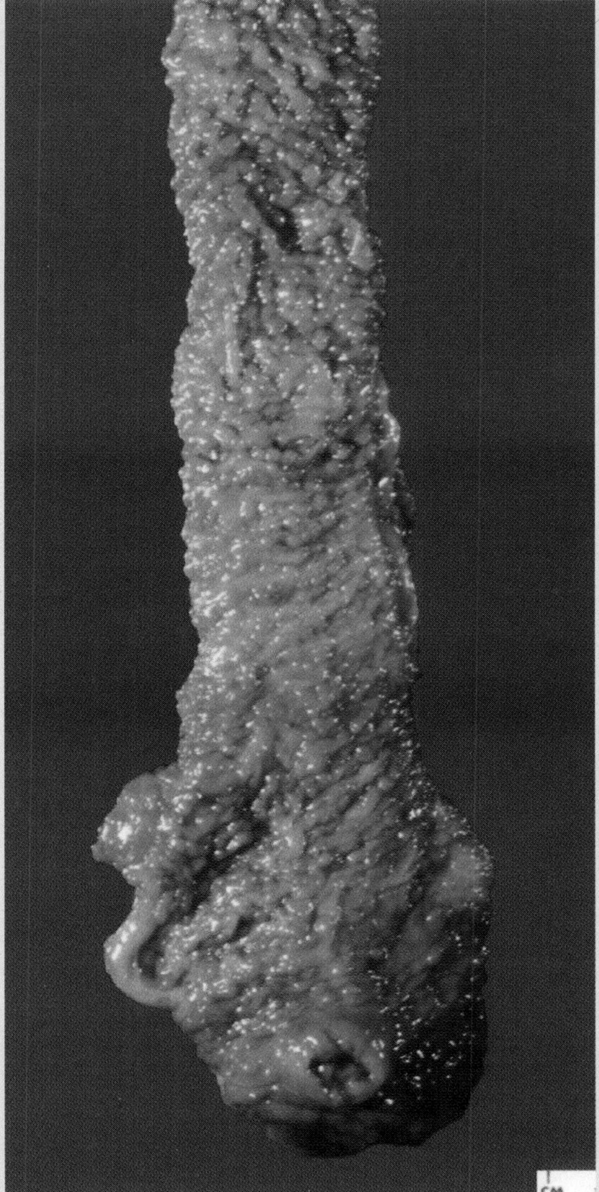


**Figure C–8.** Photograph of the mucosa of an ascending colon resected from a patient with familial adenomatous polyposis. Note the enormous number of polyps. (Courtesy of J. Rutledge, University of Washington and Children's Hospital and Medical Center, Seattle.)

rectal tumorigenesis identify an enhanced risk for individuals consuming diets high in animal fat; therefore, given the common mechanism of tumorigenesis, diet likely plays a role in FAP, as well.

### *Management*

Early recognition of FAP is necessary for effective intervention, that is, prevention of colorectal cancer. After the development of polyps, definitive treatment is total colectomy with ileo-anal pull through. Recommended surveillance for patients at risk for FAP is sigmoidoscopy every 1 to 2 years beginning at age 10 to 12 years. To focus this surveillance, molecular testing is recommended to identify at-risk family members.

## Recurrence Risk

The empiric lifetime risk for colorectal cancer among western populations is 5 to 6 percent. This risk is markedly modified by family history. Patients who have a sibling with adenomatous polyps but no family history of colorectal cancer have a 1.78 relative risk; the relative risk increases to 2.59 if a sibling developed adenomas before age 60 years. Patients with a first-degree relative with colorectal cancer have a 1.72 relative risk; this relative risk increases to 2.75 if two or more first-degree relatives had colorectal cancer. If an affected first-degree relative developed colorectal cancer before 44 years of age, the relative risk increases to more than 5.

In contrast, a patient with FAP or an *APC* germline mutation has a 50 percent risk of having a child affected with FAP in each pregnancy. The absence of a family history of FAP does not preclude the diagnosis of FAP in a parent because approximately 20 to 30 percent of patients have a new germline *APC* mutation. Prenatal diagnosis is available using linkage analysis or by testing for the mutation if the mutation in the parent has been defined. Because of intrafamilial variation in expressivity, the severity, time of onset, and associated features unfortunately cannot be predicted.

### *Questions for Small Group Discussion*

1. Name additional disorders that demonstrate autosomal dominant inheritance but are recessive at the cellular level. Why do these diseases exhibit autosomal dominant inheritance if two mutations are required for expression of the disease? What does the observation that two mutations are required for expression of the disease suggest about disease prevention?

2. Discuss some other rare genetic disorders that have modeled or provided insights into more common diseases, including at least one for cancer and one for dementia.

3. What does the association of attenuated adenomatous polyposis coli with early truncations of Apc suggest about the biochemical basis of attenuated adenomatous polyposis coli compared with classic FAP?

### *Reference*

GeneClinics
*http://www.geneclinics.org/*

# Familial Hypercholesterolemia

## (Low-Density-Lipoprotein–Receptor Mutation)

### Autosomal Dominant

## Principles

- Environmental modifiers
- Founder effects
- Gene dosage
- Genetic modifiers

## Major Phenotypic Features

- Age of onset:
  Heterozygote: Early to middle adulthood
  Homozygote: Childhood
- Hypercholesterolemia
- Atherosclerosis
- Xanthomas
- Arcus cornea

## History and Physical Findings

L.L. was a previously healthy 45-year-old French Canadian poet admitted for a myocardial infarction. He had a small xanthoma on his right Achilles tendon. His brother also had coronary heart disease (CHD); his mother, maternal grandmother, and two maternal uncles had died of CHD. In addition to his family history and gender, his risk factors for CHD and atherosclerosis included an elevated level of low-density-lipoprotein (LDL) cholesterol, mild obesity, physical inactivity, and cigarette smoking. Based on the family history, L.L. was believed to have an autosomal dominant form of hypercholesterolemia. Confirming this suspicion, molecular analysis revealed that he was heterozygous for a deletion of the 5′ end of the LDL-receptor gene (*LDLR*), a mutation found in 59 percent of French Canadians with familial hypercholesterolemia (FH). Screening of his children revealed that two of the three children had elevated LDL-cholesterol levels. The cardiologist explained to L.L. that, in addition to drug therapy, effective treatment of his CHD required dietary and lifestyle changes, such as a low saturated fat and low-cholesterol diet, increased physical activity, weight loss, and smoking cessation. L.L. was not compliant with treatment and died a year later of a myocardial infarction.

## Background

### Disease Etiology

FH is an autosomal dominant disorder of cholesterol and lipid metabolism caused by mutations in *LDLR*. FH occurs among all races and has a prevalence of 1 in 200 to 1 in 1000 in most Caucasian populations. It accounts for somewhat less than 5 percent of patients with hypercholesterolemia (see Chapter 12).

### Pathogenesis

The LDL receptor, a transmembrane glycoprotein predominantly expressed in the liver and adrenal cortex, plays a key role in cholesterol homeostasis. It binds apo B-100, the sole protein of LDL, and apo E, a protein found on very-low-density lipoproteins, intermediate-density lipoproteins (IDL), chylomicron remnants, and some high-density lipoproteins. Hepatic LDL receptors clear approximately 50 percent of IDL and 66 to 80 percent of LDL from the circulation by endocytosis; poorly understood LDL-receptor independent pathways clear the remainder of the LDL.

Mutations associated with FH occur throughout *LDLR*; 2 to 10 percent are large insertions, deletions, or rearrangements mediated by recombination between *Alu* repeats within *LDLR*. Some mutations appear to be dominant negative. Most mutations are private mutations, although some populations—such as Lebanese, French Canadians, South African Indians, South African Ashkenazic Jews, and Afrikaners—have common mutations and a high prevalence of disease because of founder effects.

Homozygous or heterozygous mutations of *LDLR* decrease the efficiency of IDL and LDL endocytosis and cause accumulation of plasma LDL by increasing production of LDL from IDL and decreasing hepatic clearance of LDL. The elevated plasma LDL levels cause atherosclerosis by increasing the clearance of LDL through LDL-receptor independent pathways such as endocytosis of oxidized LDL by macrophages and histiocytes. Monocytes, which infiltrate the arterial intima and endocytose oxidized LDL, form foam cells and release cytokines that cause proliferation of smooth muscle cells of the arterial media. Initially, the smooth muscle cells produce sufficient collagen and matrix proteins to form a fibrous cap over the foam cells; because foam cells continue to endocytose oxidized LDL, however, the foam cells eventually rupture through the fibrous cap into the arterial lumen and trigger thrombus formation. Such thrombus formation is a common cause of strokes and myocardial infarction.

Environment, gender, and genetic background modify the effect of LDL-receptor mutations on LDL plasma levels and thereby the occurrence of atherosclerosis. Diet is the major environmental modifier of LDL plasma levels. Most Tunisian FH heterozygotes have "normal North American" LDL levels and rarely develop cardiovascular disease and xanthomas. Similarly, Chinese FH heterozygotes living in China rarely have xanthomas and cardiovascular disease, whereas Chinese FH heterozygotes living in western societies have clinical manifestations similar to those of Caucasian FH heterozygotes. Dietary cholesterol suppresses the synthesis of LDL receptors and thereby raises plasma LDL levels; this effect of dietary cholesterol is potentiated by saturated fatty acids such as palmitate from dairy products and ameliorated by unsaturated fatty acids such as oleate and linoleate. Because a similar diet does not elevate LDL levels equally among patients, other environmental and genetic factors must also influence LDL metabolism. Supporting a genetic modifier, a few families with FH segregate an autosomal dominant locus that reduces plasma LDL.

### Phenotype and Natural History

Hypercholesterolemia, the earliest finding in FH, usually manifests at birth and is the only clinical finding through the first decade; at all ages, the plasma cholesterol concentration is greater than the 95th percentile in more than 95 percent of patients. Arcus corneae and tendon xanthomas begin to appear by the end of the second decade, and by death, 80 percent of FH heterozygotes have xanthomas (Fig. C–9). Nearly 40 percent of adult patients have recurrent nonprogressive polyarthritis and tenosynovitis. As tabulated above, the development of CHD among FH heterozygotes depends on age and gender.

| Age | Percent Affected FH Males | | Percent Affected FH Females | |
|---|---|---|---|---|
| | *CHD* | *Death* | *CHD* | *Death* |
| 30 | 5 | – | 0 | – |
| 40 | 20–24 | – | 0–3 | 0 |
| 50 | 45–51 | 25 | 12–20 | 2 |
| 60 | 75–85 | 50 | 45–57 | 15 |
| 70 | 100 | 80 | 75 | 30 |

## *Management*

Elevated plasma LDL cholesterol and a family history of hypercholesterolemia, xanthomas, or premature CHD, strongly suggest a diagnosis of FH. Confirmation of the diagnosis is difficult, however, because it requires quantification of LDL-receptor function in the patient's skin fibroblasts or identification of the *LDLR* mutation. In most populations, the plethora of *LDLR* mutations precludes direct DNA analysis unless a particular mutation is strongly suspected. Fortunately, a definitive molecular diagnosis of FH does not provide prognostic or therapeutic information beyond that derived from the family history and determination of plasma LDL cholesterol.

Regardless of whether they have FH, all patients with elevated LDL-cholesterol levels require aggressive normalization of their LDL cholesterol to reduce their risk of CHD; rigorous normalization of LDL cholesterol can prevent and reverse atherosclerosis. Among FH heterozygotes, rigorous adherence to a low-fat, high-carbohydrate diet usually produces a 10 to 20 percent reduction in LDL cholesterol. Because this reduction is usually insufficient, patients are often also treated with one or a combination of three classes of drugs: bile-acid sequestrants, 3-hydroxy-3-methylglutaryl coenzyme A reductase inhibitors, and nicotinic acid (see Chapter 13). In addition, treatment of postmenopausal women with estrogen reduces LDL cholesterol. Current recommendations are initiation of drug therapy at age 10 years for patients with an LDL-cholesterol level of more than 190 mg/dl and a negative family history for premature CHD, and at age 10 years for patients with an LDL-cholesterol level of more than 160 mg/dl and a positive family history for premature CHD.

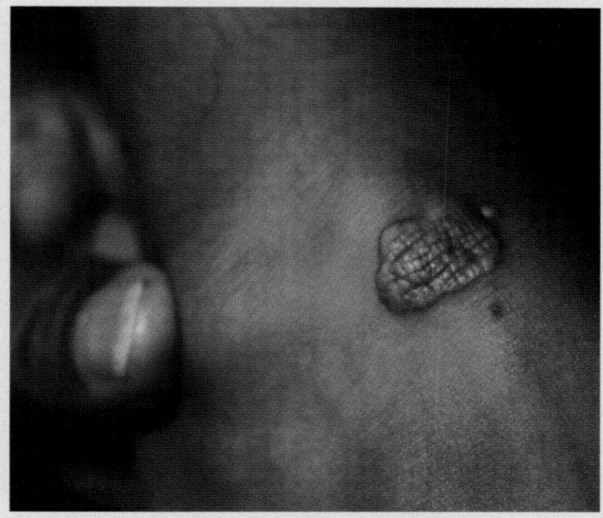

**Figure C–9.** Photograph of an Achilles tendon xanthoma from a patient with familial hypercholesterolemia. (Courtesy of M. L. Levy, Baylor College of Medicine and Texas Children's Hospital, Houston.)

## Inheritance Risk

Because FH is an autosomal dominant disorder, each child of an affected parent has a 50 percent chance of inheriting the mutant *LDLR* allele. Untreated FH heterozygotes have a 100 percent risk of developing CHD by age 70 if male and a 75 percent risk if female. Current medical therapy markedly reduces this risk by normalizing plasma cholesterol.

## *Questions for Small Group Discussion*

1. What insights does FH provide into the more common polygenic causes of atherosclerosis and CHD?
2. Familial defective apo B-100 is a phenocopy of FH. Why?
3. Vegetable oils are hydrogenated to make margarine. What effect would margarine consumption have on LDL-receptor expression as compared with vegetable oil consumption?
4. Discuss genetic susceptibility to infection and potential heterozygote advantage in the context of the role of the LDL receptor in hepatitis C infection.

## *Reference*

Goldstein JL, Hobbs HH, Brown MS (2001) Familial hypercholesterolemia. *In* Scriver CR, Beaudet AL, Sly WS, et al (eds) The Metabolic and Molecular Bases of Inherited Disease, 8th ed. McGraw-Hill, New York, pp. 2863–2914.

# Fragile X Syndrome

## (FMR1 Mutation)

### X-Linked

## Principles

- Triplet repeat expansion
- Somatic mosaicism
- Gender-specific anticipation
- Methylation
- Haplotype effect

## Major Phenotypic Features

- Age of onset: Childhood
- Mental deficiency
- Dysmorphic facies
- Male macro-orchidism

## History and Physical Findings

R.L., a 6-year-old boy, was referred to the developmental pediatrics clinic for evaluation of mental retardation and hyperactivity. He had failed kindergarten because he was disruptive, unable to attend to tasks, and had poor speech and motor skills. His development was delayed, but he had not lost developmental milestones: he sat by 10 to 11 months, walked by 20 months, and spoke two to three clear words by 24 months. He had otherwise been in good health. His mother and maternal aunt had mild childhood learning disabilities, and a maternal uncle was mentally retarded. The findings from his physical examination were normal except for hyperactivity. The physician recommended several tests, including a karyotype, thyroid-function studies, and DNA analysis for fragile X syndrome. The Southern blot analysis of the *FMR1* gene was consistent with fragile X syndrome.

## Background

### Disease Etiology

Fragile X syndrome is an X-linked mental retardation disorder that is caused by mutations in the *FMR1* gene on Xq27.3 (see Chapter 12). Fragile X syndrome has an estimated prevalence of 16 to 25 per 100,000 in the general male population and half that in the general female population. Fragile X syndrome accounts for 3 to 6 percent of mental retardation among boys with a positive family history of mental retardation and no birth defects.

### Pathogenesis

The *FMR1* gene product, Fmrp, is expressed in many cell types but most abundantly in neurons. Fmrp may chaperone a subclass of mRNA from the nucleus to the translational machinery.

More than 99 percent of *FMR1* mutations are expansions of a $(CGG)_n$ repeat sequence in the 5′ untranslated region of the gene (see Chapter 12). In normal alleles of *FMR1*, the number of CGG repeats ranges from 6 to approximately 50. In disease-causing alleles or full mutations, the number of repeats is more than 230. Alleles with more than 230 CGG repeats usually have hypermethylation of the CGG repeat sequence and the adjacent *FMR1* promoter (Fig. C–10). Hypermethylation inactivates the *FMR1* promoter, causing a loss of Fmrp expression.

Full mutations arise from premutation alleles (approximately 55 to 230 CGG repeats) with maternal transmission of a mutant *FMR1* allele but not with paternal transmission; in fact, premutations often shorten with paternal transmission. Full mutations do not arise from normal alleles. Because the length of an unstable CGG repeat increases each generation if transmitted by a female, increasing numbers of affected offspring are usually observed in later generations of an affected family; this phenomenon is genetic anticipation.

The risk of premutation expansion to a full mutation increases as the repeat length of the premutation increases (see Fig. C–10). Not all premutations, however, are equally predisposed to expand because, although premutations are relatively common, progression to a full mutation has been observed only on a limited number of haplotypes, that is, there is a haplotype predisposition to expansion. This haplotype predisposition may relate partly to the presence of a few AGG triplets embedded within the string of CGG repeats; these AGG triplets appear to inhibit expansion of the string of CGG repeats.

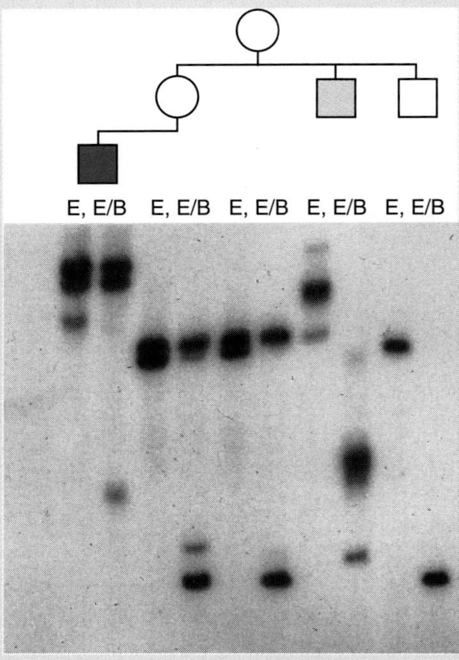


**Figure C–10.** Southern blot showing a family segregating *FMR1* premutations and expansion of a premutation into a full mutation in the third generation. Note that the unaffected grandmother carries a very small amount of premutation, the unaffected mother carries a larger amount of a slightly larger premutation, and the affected boy carries a full mutation. The grandmother also has a mildly affected son with a full mutation that is not methylated and a son with a normal allele.

Genomic DNA was digested with either endonuclease *Eco*RI (E) alone or in combination with *Bss*H2(EB). Expansion of the CGG repeat was detected using a probe from the 5′ end of the *FMR1* gene; the normal *Eco*RI band is 5.2 kb and the normal *Eco*RI/*Bss*H2 band is 2.8 kb. Because *Bss*H2 digestion is inhibited by DNA methylation, it does not cut within the methylated CGG repeats of the *FMR1* allele on the inactive X or of a methylated *FMR1* full mutation. (Courtesy of P. Ray, The Hospital for Sick Children and University of Toronto.)

### *Phenotype and Natural History*

Fragile X syndrome causes moderate mental retardation in affected males and mild mental retardation in affected females. Most affected individuals also have behavioral abnormalities, including hyperactivity, hand flapping or biting, temper tantrums, poor eye contact, and autistic features. The physical features of males vary in relation to puberty such that before puberty they have somewhat large heads but few other distinctive features, whereas after puberty they frequently have more distinctive features (long face with prominent jaw and forehead, large ears, and macro-orchidism). Because these clinical findings are not unique to fragile X syndrome, the diagnosis depends on molecular detection of mutations. Patients with fragile X syndrome have a normal life span.

Nearly all males and 40 to 50 percent of females who inherit a full mutation will have fragile X syndrome. The severity of the phenotype depends on repeat length mosaicism and repeat methylation. Because full mutations are mitotically unstable, some patients have a mixture of cells with repeat lengths ranging from premutation to full mutation (repeat length mosaicism). All males with repeat length mosaicism are affected but often have higher mental function than do those with a full mutation in every cell; females with repeat length mosaicism are normal to fully affected. Similarly, some patients have a mixture of cells with and without methylation of the CGG repeat (repeat methylation mosaicism). All males with methylation mosaicism are affected but often have higher mental function than do those with a hypermethylation in every cell; females with methylation mosaicism are normal to fully affected. Very rarely, patients have a full mutation that is unmethylated in all cells; whether male or female, these patients vary from normal to fully affected. Additionally, in females, the phenotype is dependent on the degree of skewing of X-chromosome inactivation (see Chapter 5).

### *Management*

No curative treatments are currently available for fragile X syndrome. Therapy focuses on educational intervention and pharmacological management of the behavioral problems.

## Inheritance Risk

The risk that a woman with a premutation will have an affected child is determined by the size of the premutation, the gender of the fetus, and the family history. Empirically, the recurrence risk can be as high as 50 percent for each male child and 25 percent for each female child. Based on the analysis of a relatively small number of carrier mothers, however, the recurrence risk appears to decline from this empiric risk as the premutation decreases from 100 to 56 repeats. For a premutation of 56 to 59 repeats, therefore, the recurrence risk is approximately 7 percent for an affected son and 3.5 percent for an affected daughter. Prenatal testing is available using fetal DNA derived from chorionic villi or amniocytes.

---

### *Questions for Small Group Discussion*

1. Discuss haplotype bias in disease, that is, the effect of haplotype on mutation development (fragile X syndrome), disease severity (sickle cell disease), or predisposition to disease (autoimmune diseases).
2. Fragile X syndrome, myotonic dystrophy, Friedreich ataxia, Huntington disease, and several other disorders are caused by expansion of repeat sequences. Contrast the mechanisms or proposed mechanisms by which expansion of the repeat causes disease for each of these disorders. Why do some of these disorders show anticipation whereas others do not?
3. The gender bias in transmission of *FMR1* mutations is believed to arise because Fmrp expression is necessary for production of viable sperm. Compare the bias in transmitting gender for fragile X syndrome and Huntington disease. Discuss mechanisms that could explain biases in the transmitting gender for various diseases.
4. What family history and diagnostic information are necessary before undertaking prenatal diagnosis for fragile X syndrome?
5. How would you counsel a pregnant woman carrying a 46,XY fetus with 60 repeats? A 46,XX fetus with 60 repeats? A 46,XX fetus with more than 300 repeats?

### *References*


GeneClinics
*http://www.geneclinics.org/*

Warren ST, Sherman SL (2001) The fragile X syndrome. *In* Scriver CR, Beaudet AL, Sly WS, et al (eds) The Metabolic and Molecular Bases of Inherited Disease, 8th ed, McGraw-Hill, New York, pp. 1257–1280.

# Glucose-6-Phosphate Dehydrogenase Deficiency

## (G6PD Mutation)

### X-Linked

## Principles

- Heterozygote advantage
- Pharmacogenetics

## Major Phenotypic Features

- Age of onset: Neonatal
- Hemolytic anemia
- Neonatal jaundice

## History and Physical Findings

On a quiet summer evening, L.M., a previously healthy 5-year-old boy, presented to the emergency department febrile, pale, tachycardic, tachypneic, and minimally responsive; findings of his physical examination were otherwise normal. The morning before presentation, he had been in good health, but during the afternoon, he developed abdominal pain, headache, and fever; by late evening, he was tachypneic and incoherent. He had not ingested any medications or known toxins, and results of a urine toxicology screen were negative. Results of other laboratory tests showed massive nonimmune intravascular hemolysis and hemoglobinuria. After resuscitation, L.M. was admitted to the hospital; the hemolysis resolved without further intervention. L.M. was of Greek ethnicity; his parents were unaware of a family history of hemolysis, although his mother had some cousins in Europe with a "blood problem." Further inquiry revealed that the morning before admission, L.M. had been eating fava beans in the garden while his mother was working in the yard. The physician explained to the parents that L.M. probably was deficient for glucose-6-phosphate dehydrogenase (G6PD) and that because of this he had become ill after eating fava beans. Subsequent measurement of L.M.'s erythrocyte G6PD activity confirmed that he had G6PD deficiency. The parents were counseled concerning L.M.'s risk of acute hemolysis after exposure to certain drugs and toxins and given a list of compounds that L.M. should avoid.

## Background

### Disease Etiology

G6PD deficiency, a hereditary predisposition to hemolysis, is an X-linked disorder of antioxidant homeostasis that is caused by mutations in the *G6PD* gene. In areas in which malaria is endemic, G6PD deficiency has a prevalence of 5 to 25 percent, whereas in nonendemic areas, it has a prevalence of less than 0.5 percent (Fig. C–11). Like sickle cell disease, G6PD deficiency appears to have reached a substantial frequency in some areas because it confers to individuals heterozygous for G6PD deficiency some resistance to malaria and, thus, a survival advantage (see Chapter 12).

### Pathogenesis

G6PD is the first enzyme in the hexose monophosphate shunt, a pathway critical for generating nicotinamide adenine dinucleotide phosphate (NADPH). NADPH is required for the regeneration of the reduced glutathione. Within erythrocytes, reduced glutathione is used for the detoxification of oxidants produced by the interaction of hemoglobin and oxygen and by exogenous factors such as drugs, infection, and metabolic acidosis.

Most G6PD deficiency arises because mutations in the X-linked *G6PD* gene decrease the catalytic activity or the stability of G6PD, or both. When G6PD activity is sufficiently depleted or deficient, insufficient NADPH is available to regenerate reduced glutathione during times of oxidative stress; this results in the oxidation and aggregation of intracellular proteins (Heinz bodies) and the formation of rigid erythrocytes that readily hemolyze.

With the more common *G6PD* alleles, which cause the protein to be unstable, deficiency of G6PD within erythrocytes worsens as erythrocytes age. Because erythrocytes do not have nuclei, new G6PD mRNA cannot be transcribed; thus, erythrocytes are unable to replace G6PD as it is degraded. During exposure to an oxidative stress episode, therefore, hemolysis begins with the oldest erythrocytes and progressively involves younger erythrocytes, depending on the severity of the oxidative stress.

### Phenotype and Natural History

As an X-linked disorder, G6PD deficiency predominantly and most severely affects males. Rare symptomatic females have a skewing of X-chromosome inactivation such that the X chromosome carrying the *G6PD* disease allele is the active X chromosome in erythrocyte precursors.

Besides gender, the severity of G6PD deficiency depends on the specific *G6PD* mutation. In general, the mutation common in the Mediterranean basin (i.e., G6PD $B^-$ or Mediterranean) tends to be more severe than those mutations common in Africa (i.e., G6PD $A^-$ variants) (see Fig. C–11). In erythrocytes of patients with the Mediterranean variant, G6PD activity decreases to insufficient levels 5 to 10 days after erythrocytes appear in the circulation, whereas in the erythrocytes of patients with the G6PD $A^-$ variants, G6PD activity decreases to insufficient levels 50 to 60 days after erythrocytes appear in the circulation. Therefore, most erythrocytes are susceptible to hemolysis in patients with severe forms of G6PD deficiency, such as G6PD Mediterranean, but only 20 to 30 percent are susceptible in patients with G6PD $A^-$ variants.

G6PD deficiency most commonly manifests as either neonatal jaundice or acute hemolytic anemia. The peak incidence of neonatal jaundice occurs during days 2 and 3 of life. The severity of the jaundice ranges from subclinical to levels compatible with kernicterus; the associated anemia is rarely severe. Episodes of acute hemolytic anemia usually begin within hours of an oxidative stress and end when G6PD-deficient erythrocytes have hemolyzed; therefore, the severity of the anemia associated with these acute hemolytic episodes is proportionate to the deficiency of G6PD and the oxidative stress. Viral and bacterial infections are the most common triggers, but many drugs and toxins can also precipitate hemolysis. The disorder favism results from hemolysis secondary to the ingestion of fava beans by patients with more severe forms of G6PD deficiency, such as G6PD Mediterranean; fava beans contain $\beta$-glycosides, naturally occurring oxidants.

In addition to neonatal jaundice and acute hemolytic anemia, G6PD deficiency rarely causes congenital or chronic nonspherocytic hemolytic anemia. Patients with

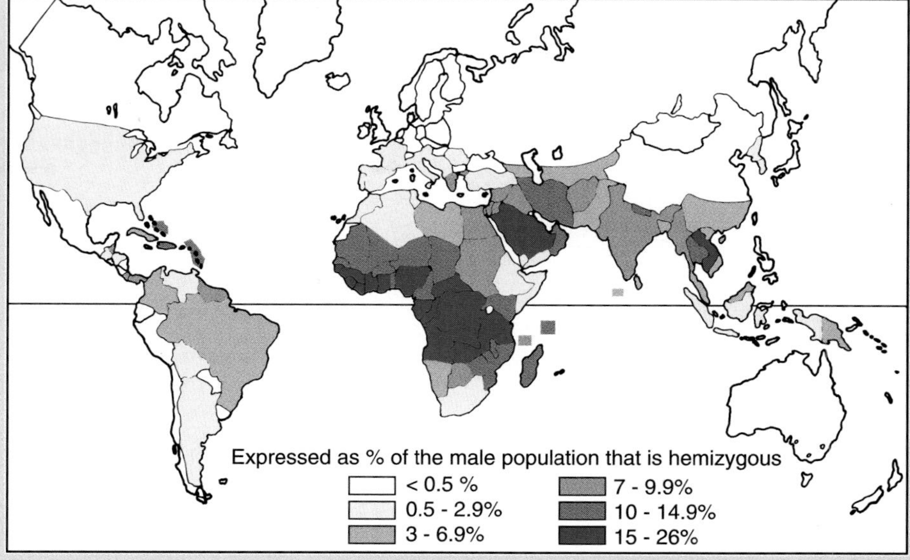


**Figure C–11.** World distribution of G6PD deficiency. The frequencies of G6PD-deficient males in the various countries are also the allele frequencies because the gene is X-linked. (Redrawn from WHO Working Group [1989] Glucose-6-phosphate dehydrogenase deficiency. Bull WHO 67:601, by permission.)

chronic nonspherocytic hemolytic anemia generally have a profound deficiency of G6PD that causes severe anemia and an increased susceptibility to infection. The susceptibility to infection arises because the NADPH supply within granulocytes is inadequate to sustain the oxidative burst necessary for killing of phagocytosed bacteria.

### *Management*

G6PD deficiency should be suspected in patients of African, Mediterranean, or Asian ancestry who present with either an acute hemolytic episode or neonatal jaundice. G6PD deficiency is diagnosed by measurement of G6PD activity in erythrocytes; this activity should be measured when the patient has had neither a recent transfusion nor a recent hemolytic episode. (Because G6PD deficiency occurs primarily in older erythrocytes, measurement of G6PD activity in the predominantly young erythrocytes present during or immediately following a hemolytic episode often gives a false-negative result.)

The key to management of G6PD deficiency is prevention of hemolysis by prompt treatment of infections and avoidance of oxidant drugs (e.g., sulfonamides, sulfones, nitrofurans) and toxins (e.g., naphthalene). Although most patients with a hemolytic episode will not require medical intervention, those with severe anemia and hemolysis may require resuscitation and erythrocyte transfusions. Patients presenting with neonatal jaundice respond well to the same therapies as other infants with neonatal jaundice (hydration, light therapy, and exchange transfusions).

## Inheritance Risk

Each son of a mother carrying a *G6PD* mutation has a 50 percent chance of being affected, and each daughter has a 50 percent chance of being a carrier. Each daughter of an affected father will be a carrier, but each son will be unaffected because an affected father does not contribute an X chromosome to his sons. The risk that carrier daughters will have clinically significant symptoms is low because sufficient skewing of X-chromosome inactivation is relatively uncommon.

### *Questions for Small Group Discussion*

1. The consumption of fava beans and the occurrence of G6PD deficiency are coincident in many areas. What evolutionary advantage might the consumption of fava beans give populations with G6PD deficiency?

2. Several hundred different mutations have been described that cause G6PD deficiency. Presumably, all of these mutations have persisted because of selection. Discuss heterozygote advantage in the context of G6PD deficiency.

3. What is pharmacogenetics? How does G6PD deficiency illustrate the principles of pharmacogenetics?

### *Reference*

Luzzatto L, Melta A, Vulliamy T (2001) Glucose-6-phosphate dehydrogenase deficiency. *In* Scriver CR, Beadet AL, Sly WS, et al (eds) The Metabolic and Molecular Bases of Inherited Disease, 8th ed, McGraw-Hill, New York, pp. 4517–4553.

# Hemophilia

## (F8C or F9 mutation)

### X-Linked

## Principles

- Replacement therapy
- Intrachromosomal recombination
- Transposable element insertion
- Variable expressivity

## Major Phenotypic Features

- Age of onset: Infancy to adulthood
- Bleeding diathesis
- Hemarthroses
- Hematomas

## History and Physical Findings

S.T., a healthy 38-year-old woman, scheduled an appointment for counseling regarding her risk of having a child with hemophilia. She had a maternal uncle who had died in childhood from hemophilia and a brother who had had bleeding problems as a child. Her brother's bleeding problems had resolved during adolescence. No other family members had bleeding disorders. The geneticist explained to S.T. that her family history was suggestive of an X-linked abnormality of coagulation such as hemophilia A or B and that her brother's improvement was particularly suggestive of the hemophilia B variant factor IX Leyden. To confirm the diagnosis of hemophilia, the geneticist told S.T. that her brother should be evaluated first because identification of an isolated carrier is difficult. S.T. talked to her brother, and he agreed to an evaluation. Review of his records showed that he indeed had been diagnosed with factor IX deficiency as a child but now had nearly normal plasma levels of factor IX. DNA mutation analysis confirmed that he had a mutation in the *F9* gene promoter, consistent with factor IX Leyden. Subsequent testing of S.T. showed that she did not carry the mutation identified in her brother.

## Background

### Disease Etiology

Hemophilia A and B are X-linked disorders of coagulation caused by mutations in the *F8C* and *F9* genes, respectively. Mutations of *F8C* cause deficiency or dysfunction of clotting factor VIII; mutations of *F9* cause deficiency or dysfunction of clotting factor IX.

Hemophilia is a panethnic disorder without racial predilection. Hemophilia A has an incidence of 1 in 5000 to 10,000 newborn males; hemophilia B is far rarer, with an incidence of 1 in 100,000.

### Pathogenesis

The coagulation system maintains the integrity of the vasculature through a delicate balance of clot formation and inhibition. The proteases and protein cofactors composing the clotting cascade are present in the circulation as inactive precursors and must be sequentially activated at the site of injury to form a fibrin clot. Timely and efficient formation of a clot requires exponential activation or amplification of the protease cascade. Clotting factors IX and VIII, which complex together, are key to this amplification; they activate clotting factor X, and active factor X, in turn, activates more factor IX and factor VIII. Factor IX functions as a protease and factor VIII as a cofactor. Deficiency or dysfunction of either factor IX or factor VIII causes hemophilia.

Mutations of *F8C* include deletions, insertions, inversions, and point mutations. The most common mutation is an inversion deleting the carboxyl terminus of factor VIII; it accounts for 25 percent of all hemophilia A and for 40 to 50 percent of severe hemophilia A. This inversion results from an intrachromosomal recombination between sequences located in intron 22 of *F8C* and homologous sequences telomeric to *F8C*. An intriguing class of mutation involves retrotransposition of L1 repeats into the gene. For all *F8C* mutations, the residual enzymatic activity of the factor VIII-factor IX complex correlates with the severity of clinical disease.

Many different *F9* mutations have been identified in patients with hemophilia B, but in contrast to the frequent partial inversion of *F8C* in hemophilia A, a common *F9* mutation has not been identified for hemophilia B. Factor IX Leyden is an unusual *F9* variant caused by point mutations in the *F9* promoter; it is associated with very low levels of factor IX and severe hemophilia during childhood but spontaneous resolution of hemophilia occurs at puberty, as factor IX levels nearly normalize. For each *F9* mutation, the residual enzymatic activity of the factor VIII-factor IX complex correlates with the severity of clinical disease.

### Phenotype and Natural History

Hemophilia is classically a male disease, although rare females are affected because of skewed X-chromosome inactivation. Clinically, hemophilia A and B are indistinguishable. Both are characterized by bleeding into soft tissues, muscles, and weight bearing joints (Fig. C–12). Bleeding occurs within hours to days following trauma and often continues for days or weeks. Those with severe disease are usually diagnosed as newborns because of excessive cephalohematomas or prolonged bleeding from umbilical or circumcision wounds. Patients with moderate disease often do not develop hematomas or hemarthroses until they begin to crawl or walk and, therefore, escape diagnosis until that time. Patients with mild disease frequently present in adolescence or adulthood with hemarthroses or prolonged bleeding after surgery or trauma.

Hemophilia A and B are diagnosed and distinguished by measuring factor VIII and IX activity levels. For both hemophilia A and B, the level of factor VIII or IX activity predicts the clinical severity.

| Classification | % Activity (Factor VIII or IX) |
|---|---|
| Severe | <5% |
| Moderate | 1%–5% |
| Mild | 5%–25% |

### Management

Although current gene therapy trials show great promise, no curative treatments are available for hemophilia A and B except for liver transplantation. Currently, the standard of care is intravenous replacement of the deficient factor. Factor-replacement therapy has increased life expectancy from an average of 1.4 years in the early 1900s to approximately 65 years today.

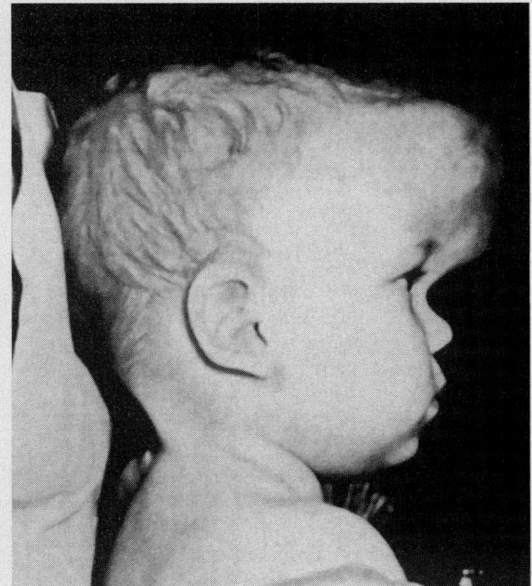

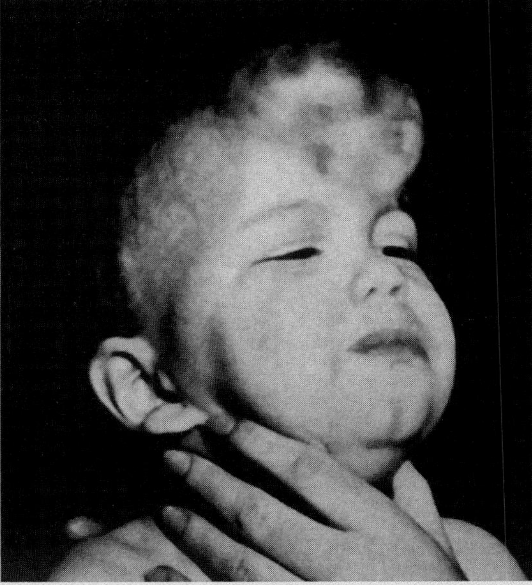

**Figure C–12.** Subcutaneous hematoma of the forehead in a young boy with hemophilia. The photograph was taken 4 days after a minor contusion. The appearance of the forehead returned to normal in 6 months. (Adapted from Stefanini M, Dameshek W [1962] The Hemorrhagic Disorders: A Clinical and Therapeutic Approach, Grune & Stratton, New York, p. 252, by permission. Photographic restoration courtesy of B. Moseley-Fernandini.)

## Inheritance Risk

If a woman has a family history of hemophilia, her carrier status can be determined by linkage analysis or by identification of the *F8C* or *F9* mutation segregating in the family. Routine mutation identification is available only for the common *F8C* inversion, however. Carrier detection by enzyme assay is difficult and not widely available.

If a mother is a carrier, each son has a 50 percent risk of hemophilia and each daughter a 50 percent risk of inheriting the *F8C* or *F9* mutation. Reflecting the frequency of skewing of X-chromosome inactivation, daughters inheriting an *F8C* or *F9* mutation have a low risk of hemophilia.

If a mother has a son with hemophilia but no other affected relatives, her a priori risk of being a carrier is 2 in 3 because approximately a third of patients have a new mutation in *F8C* or *F9*. Through the application of Bayes' theorem, this risk can be modified by considering the number of unaffected sons in the family (see Chapter 19).

### Questions for Small Group Discussion

1. What other diseases are caused by recombination between repeated nucleotide sequences? Compare and contrast the recombination mechanism observed with hemophilia A with that observed with Smith-Magenis syndrome and with familial hypercholesterolemia (low-density-lipoprotein–receptor mutations).
2. One of the more unusual mutations in *F8C* is insertion of an L1 element into exon 14. What are transposable elements? How do transposable elements move within a genome? Name another disease effected by movement of transposable elements?
3. What is Haldane's hypothesis? Name two other diseases that are consistent with this hypothesis.
4. In patients with factor IX Leyden, why does the deficiency of factor IX resolve during puberty?
5. Compare and contrast enzyme replacement for hemophilia to that for Gaucher disease. Approximately 10 percent of patients with hemophilia develop a clinically significant antibody titer against factor VIII or IX. Why? Is there a genetic predisposition to developing antibodies against the replacement factors? How could this immune reaction be circumvented? Would gene therapy be helpful for patients with antibodies?
6. Discuss current approaches to gene therapy in hemophilia B.

### References


GeneClinics
*http://www.geneclinics.org/*

Kay MA, Manno CS, Ragni MV (2000) Evidence for gene transfer and expression of factor IX in haemophilia B patients treated with an AAV vector. Nat Genet 24:257–261.

# Hereditary Nonpolyposis Colon Cancer

## (DNA Mismatch Repair Gene Mutations)

### Autosomal Dominant

## Principles

- Tumor susceptibility genes
- Multistep carcinogenesis
- Somatic mutation
- Microsatellite instability
- Variable expressivity
- Incomplete penetrance

## Major Phenotypic Features

- Age of onset: Middle adulthood
- Colorectal cancer
- Multiple primary cancers

## History and Physical Findings

P.P. was a 38-year-old banker and mother of three children who was referred to the cancer genetics clinic by her physician for counseling regarding her family history of cancer. Her father, brother, nephew, niece, paternal uncle, and paternal grandmother developed colorectal cancer at ages 47, 46, 40, 35, 80, and 40 years, respectively. In addition, a sister had colorectal cancer at 26 years and endometrial cancer at 43 years; a paternal aunt developed endometrial cancer at 38 years, and another paternal aunt developed ovarian cancer at 44 years. P.P. did not have a history of medical or surgical problems. The findings from her physical examination were normal. The geneticist explained to P.P. that her family history was suggestive of hereditary nonpolyposis colon cancer (HNPCC) and that the most efficient and effective way to determine the genetic cause of HNPCC in her family was through molecular testing of a living affected family member. After some discussion with her niece, the only surviving affected family member, P.P. and her niece returned to the clinic for testing. Testing of an archived tumor sample from the niece's resected colon identified microsatellite instability and, subsequently, a germline mutation in *MLH1*. P.P. did not carry the mutation; therefore, the geneticist counseled that her and her children's risk of developing cancer was similar to that of the general population. Her unaffected brother was found to carry the mutation and continued to have an annual colonoscopy. Her paternal uncle who developed colorectal cancer at age 80 did not carry the mutation.

## Background

### Disease Etiology

At least 50 percent of individuals in western populations develop a colorectal tumor by age 70, and approximately 10 percent of these individuals eventually develop colorectal cancer. HNPCC is a genetically heterogeneous autosomal dominant cancer predisposition syndrome that is often caused by mutations in DNA mismatch repair genes. HNPCC has a prevalence of 2 to 5 per 1000 and accounts for approximately 3 to 8 percent of colorectal cancer.

### Pathogenesis

In most colorectal cancers, including familial adenomatous polyposis, the karyotype becomes progressively more aneuploid (see Chapter 16). Approximately 13 to 15 percent of colorectal cancers do not have such chromosomal instability but have insertion or deletion mutations in repetitive sequences (microsatellite instability). Microsatellite instability occurs in 85 to 90 percent of HNPCC tumors. Consistent with this observation, approximately 70 percent of HNPCC families with carcinomas exhibiting microsatellite instability have germline mutations in one of six DNA mismatch repair genes: *MSH2*, *MSH6*, *MLH1*, *MLH3*, *PMS1*, or *PMS2*.

DNA mismatch repair reduces DNA replication errors by 1000-fold. Errors of DNA synthesis cause mispairing and deform the DNA double helix. MutS$\alpha$, a heterodimer of MSH2 and MSH6, binds these deformations, and MutL$\alpha$, a heterodimer of MLH1 and PMS2, binds to MutS$\alpha$ and identifies the newly synthesized DNA strand. This protein complex then recruits other enzymes to effect repair. Using the process of long patch excision, this complex excises the errant fragment of the newly synthesized DNA strand and then resynthesizes it.

Both alleles of a DNA mismatch repair gene must lose function to cause microsatellite instability. The high frequency of somatic loss of function in the second allele defines HNPCC as an autosomal dominant disease with approximately 80 percent penetrance. This somatic loss of function can occur by loss of heterozygosity, intragenic mutation, or hypermethylation.

In HNPCC, an increasing number of microsatellite loci mutate during the progression from adenoma to carcinoma. Inactivation of genes containing microsatellite sequences could play key roles in tumor progression. For example, microsatellite instability induces frameshift mutations in the transforming growth factor receptor II gene (*TGFBR2*). Mutations within *TGFBR2* cause the loss of TGF$\beta$RII expression, and because the TGF$\beta$ system inhibits the growth of colonic epithelial cells, its loss allows escape from growth control. In support of the role of *TGFBR2* in HNPCC, one affected family without mutations in a DNA mismatch repair gene has a germline mutation in *TGFBR2*. *TGFBR2* mutations occur in early HNPCC lesions and might be responsible for the growth of adenomas.

### Phenotype and Natural History

Although patients with HNPCC develop polyps similar in number to those of the general population, they develop them at younger ages. Their median age at diagnosis with a colorectal adenocarcinoma is younger than 50 years, that is, 10 to 15 years younger than the general population (Fig. C–13). Patients with HNPCC and a defined germline mutation have an 80 percent lifetime risk of developing colorectal cancer. Sixty to 70 percent of the colonic adenomas and carcinomas occur proximal to the splenic flexure.

In addition to colorectal cancer, HNPCC-associated cancers include cancer of the stomach, small bowel, pancreas, kidney, endometrium, and ovaries; cancers of the lung and breast are not associated with HNPCC (see Fig. C–13). Patients with HNPCC and a defined germline mutation have a more than 90 percent lifetime risk of developing colorectal cancer or one of these associated cancers, or both. The variable penetrance and expressivity of HNPCC likely depends on both genetic background and environment.

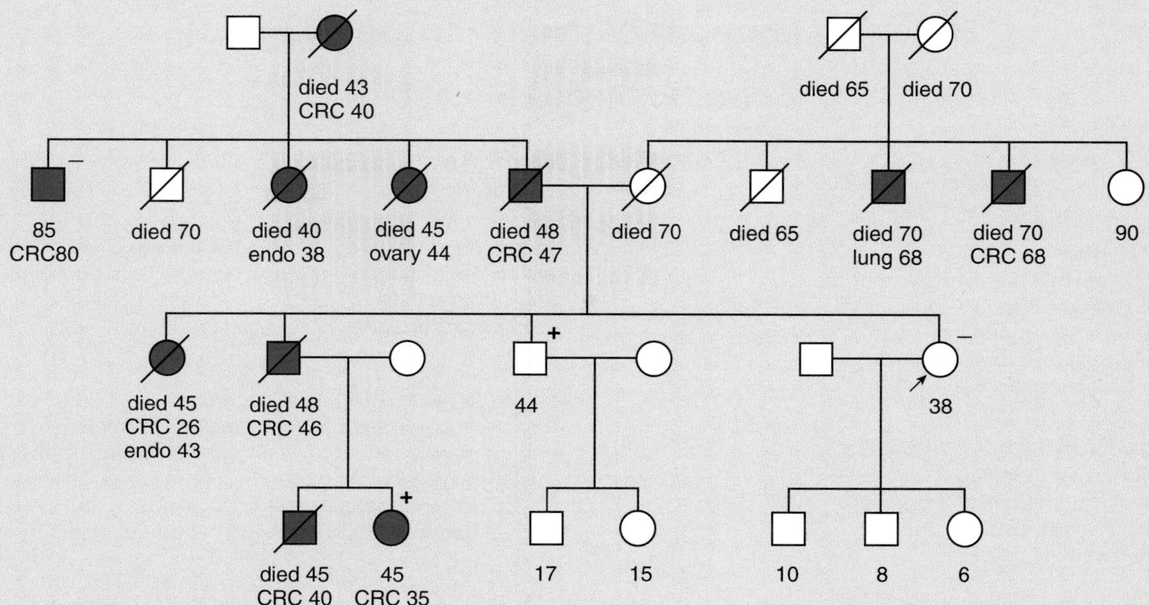


**Figure C–13.** Family segregating an *MLH1* mutation. Note the frequent occurrence of colon cancer as well as other HNPCC-associated cancers such as endometrial cancer, pancreatic cancer, and ovarian cancer. Note that one family member had cancers of the colorectum and endometrium and that another had sporadic colon cancer (tested negative for the family mutation). The proband is indicated by an *arrow*. Shaded symbols indicate a diagnosis of cancer. Ages are shown directly below the symbol. A "+" sign identifies carriers of the *MLH1* mutation, and "−" sign identifies noncarriers. Cancer diagnoses are followed by the age at diagnosis. Cancer abbreviations: CRC = colorectal cancer; endo = endometrial cancer; ovary = ovarian cancer; lung = lung cancer. (Courtesy of T. Pal and S. Narod, Women's College Hospital and University of Toronto.)

Compared with patients with familial adenomatous polyposis or colorectal tumors with chromosome instability, patients with HNPCC have a better prognosis when adjusted for stage and age. The mechanism underlying this observation is not understood.

### Management

Family history defines HNPCC; patients do not have distinguishing physical features. The criteria necessary to identify patients are evolving as the diagnosis of HNPCC moves from the research to the clinical arena. Early recognition of HNPCC is necessary for effective intervention; surveillance colonoscopy of the proximal colon beginning at age 25 years increases life-span expectancy by 13.5 years, and proctocolectomy at age 25 years increases life-span expectancy by 15.6 years. Surveillance endometrial biopsies and abdominal ultrasound scans for at-risk women have not proved to be effective preventive measures. In families with known germline mutations, identification of the DNA mismatch repair gene mutation can focus surveillance on those patients carrying the mutation, but in HNPCC families without an identified germline mutation, the absence of a mutation does not negate the need for frequent surveillance.

## Inheritance Risk

The empiric western general population risk for the development of colorectal cancer is 5 to 6 percent. This risk is markedly modified by family history. Patients with a first-degree relative with colorectal cancer have a 1.7 relative risk; this relative risk increases to 2.75 if two or more first-degree relatives had colorectal cancer. If an affected first-degree relative developed colorectal cancer before 44 years of age, the relative risk increases to more than 5.

In contrast, a patient with a DNA mismatch repair gene germline mutation has a 50 percent risk of having a child carrying a germline mutation, and each child has a cancer risk of approximately 45 percent. Prenatal diagnosis is not routine but is theoretically possible if the germline mutation has been identified in the parent. Because of incomplete penetrance and variation in expressivity, the severity and onset of HNPCC and the occurrence of associated cancers cannot be predicted.

### Questions for Small Group Discussion

1. Compare the mechanisms of tumorigenesis in disorders of nucleotide excision repair, chromosomal instability, and microsatellite instability.
2. How should a patient with a family history of HNPCC be counseled if testing for DNA mismatch repair gene mutations is positive? If negative?
3. Discuss the ethics of testing of minors for HNPCC.

### References


Boland CR (2001) Hereditary nonpolyposis colorectal cancer (HNPCC). *In* Scriver CR, Beaudet AL, Sly WS, et al (eds) The Metabolic and Molecular Bases of Inherited Disease, 8th ed. McGraw-Hill, New York, pp. 769–783.

Kinzler KW, Vogelstein B (1996) Lessons from hereditary colorectal cancer. Cell 87:159–170.

Lengauer C, Kinzler KW, Vogelstein B (1998) Genetic instabilities in human cancers. Nature 396:643–649.

# Holoprosencephaly (Nonsyndromic Form)

## (Sonic Hedgehog Mutation)

### Autosomal Dominant

## Principles

- Developmental regulatory gene
- Genetic heterogeneity
- Position-effect mutations
- Variable expressivity
- Variable penetrance

## Major Phenotypic Features

- Age of onset: Prenatal
- Ventral forebrain maldevelopment
- Facial dysmorphism
- Developmental delay

## History and Physical Findings

Dr. D., a 37-year-old physicist, presented to the genetics clinic with his wife because their first child died at birth of holoprosencephaly (HPE). The pregnancy had been uncomplicated, and the child had a normal karyotype. Neither he nor his wife reported any major medical problems. Dr. D. had been adopted as a child and did not know the history of his biological family; his wife's family history was not suggestive of any genetic disorders. Careful examination of Dr. D. and his wife showed that he had an absent superior labial frenulum and slight hypotelorism but no other dysmorphic findings. His physician explained to him that the HPE in his child and his absent superior labial frenulum and slight hypotelorism were suggestive of autosomal dominant HPE. Subsequent molecular testing confirmed that Dr. D. had a mutation in the sonic hedgehog gene (*SHH*).

## Background

### *Disease Etiology*

HPE, which has a birth incidence of 1 in 10,000 to 1 in 20,000, is the most common human congenital brain defect. It affects twice as many girls as boys.

HPE results from a variety of causes, including chromosomal and single-gene disorders and environmental factors such as maternal diabetes. The disorder occurs both in isolation and as a feature of various syndromes such as Smith-Lemli-Opitz syndrome. Nonsyndromic familial HPE exhibits autosomal dominant, autosomal recessive, or X-linked inheritance. Approximately 25 to 50 percent of all HPE is associated with a chromosomal abnormality; the nonrandom distribution of chromosomal abnormalities predicts at least 12 different HPE loci including 7q36, 13q32, 2p21, 18p11.3, and 21q22.3.

*SHH*, the first gene identified with mutations causing HPE, maps to 7q36. *SHH* mutations account for approximately 30 to 40 percent of familial nonsyndromic autosomal dominant HPE but for less than 5 percent of nonsyndromic HPE overall.

### *Pathogenesis*

Shh is a secreted signaling protein required for developmental patterning in both mammals and insects (see Chapter 17).

Human *SHH* mutations are loss-of-function mutations. Some of the cytogenetic abnormalities affecting *SHH* expression are translocations that occur 15 to 256 kb 5′ to the coding region of *SHH*. These translocations are referred to as "position-effect" mutations because they do not mutate the coding sequence but disrupt distant regulatory elements or chromatin structure, or both, and thereby alter *SHH* expression.

### *Phenotype and Natural History*

The prosencephalic malformations of HPE follow a continuum of severity but are usually subdivided into alobar HPE (no evidence of an interhemispheric fissure), semilobar HPE (posterior interhemispheric fissure only), and lobar HPE (ventricular separation and almost complete cortical separation) (Fig. C–14). Among HPE patients with a normal karyotype, 63 percent have alobar HPE, 28 percent have semilobar HPE, and 9 percent have lobar HPE. Other commonly associated central nervous system (CNS) malformations include undivided thalami, dysgenesis of the corpus callosum, hypoplastic olfactory bulbs, hypoplastic optic bulbs and tracts, and pituitary dysgenesis.

The spectrum of facial dysmorphism in HPE extends from cyclopia to normal and usually reflects the severity of the CNS malformations. Dysmorphic features associated with but not diagnostic of HPE include micro- or macrocephaly, an- or microphthalmia, hypo- or hypertelorism, dysmorphic nose, palatal anomalies, bifid uvula, a single central incisor, and absence of a superior labial frenulum.

Delayed development occurs in nearly all patients with HPE; the severity of delay correlates with the severity of CNS malformation, that is, patients with normal brain imaging usually have normal intelligence. In addition to delayed development, patients frequently have seizures, brainstem dysfunction, and sleep dysregulation.

Among HPE patients without chromosomal abnormalities, survival varies inversely with the severity of the facial phenotype. Patients with cyclopia or ethmocephaly usually do not survive a week; approximately 50 percent of patients with alobar HPE die before 4 to 5 months of age and 80 percent before a year. Approximately 50 percent of patients with isolated semilobar or lobar HPE survive the first year.

### *Management*

Patients with HPE require an expeditious evaluation within the first few days of life. Treatment is symptomatic and supportive. Aside from the medical concerns of the patient, a major part of the management includes counseling and supporting the parents as well as defining the cause of HPE.

## Inheritance Risk

Etiologically, HPE is extremely heterogeneous, and the recurrence risk in a family is dependent on identification of the underlying cause. Diabetic mothers have a 1 percent risk of having a child with HPE. For parents of a patient with a cytogenetic anomaly, the recurrence risk depends on whether one of them has a cytogenetic abnormality that gave rise to the abnormality in the patient. For parents of patients with syndromic HPE, the recurrence risk depends on the recurrence risk for that syndrome. In the absence of a family history of HPE or a cytogenetic or syndromic cause of HPE, parents and siblings must be examined closely for microforms, subtle features associated with HPE such as an absent frenulum or a single upper incisor. For parents with a negative family history, no identifiable

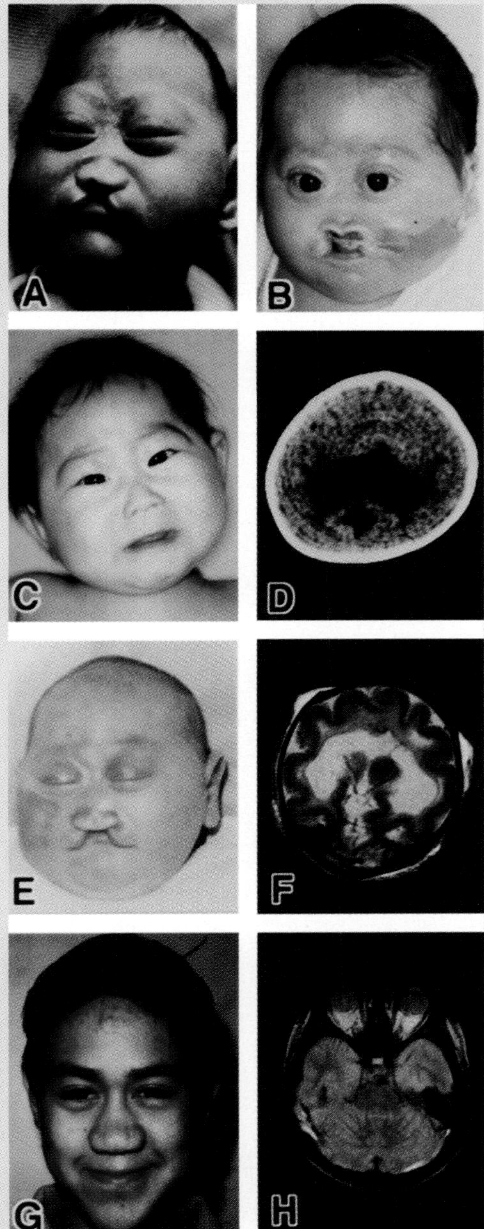


**Figure C–14.** Holoprosencephaly (HPE) in patients with *SHH* mutations. *A*, Microcephaly, absence of nasal bones, midline cleft palate, and semilobar HPP. *B*, Semilobar HPE, premaxillary agenesis and midline cleft lip. *C*, *D*, Mild facial findings with severe semilobar HPE on magnetic resonance imaging (MRI). *E*, *F*, Microcephaly, prominent optic globes, premaxillary agenesis and cleft lip, with semilobar HPE on MRI. *G*, *H*, Microcephaly, ocular hypotelorism, flat nose without palpable cartilage, midface and philtrum hypoplasia, normal intelligence, and normal brain MRI. All patients have *SHH* mutations. Patients *A* and *B* also have mutations of *TGIF*, and patient *C* also has a mutation in *ZIC2*. *TGIF* mutations indirectly decrease Shh expression. (Courtesy of M. Muenke, National Human Genome Research Institute, National Institutes of Health, Bethesda, Maryland. Adapted by permission from Nanni, L, Ming JE, Bocian M, et al [1999] The mutational spectrum of the *Sonic Hedgehog* gene in holoprosencephaly: *SHH* mutations cause a significant portion of autosomal dominant holoprosencephaly. Hum Mol Genet 8:2479.)

causes of HPE, and no microforms suggestive of autosomal dominant HPE, the empiric recurrence risk is approximately 4 to 5 percent.

Although autosomal recessive and X-linked HPE have been reported, most families with an established mode of inheritance exhibit autosomal dominant inheritance. The penetrance of autosomal dominant HPE is approximately 70 percent. Among obligate carriers of autosomal dominant HPE, the risk of having a child affected with severe HPE is 16 to 21 percent and with a microform, 13 to 14 percent. The phenotype of the carrier does not affect the risk of having an affected child.

Molecular testing for HPE mutations is not currently available as a clinical service. Severe HPE can be detected by prenatal ultrasound at 16 to 18 weeks of gestation.

## Questions for Small Group Discussion

1. What factors might explain the variable expressivity and penetrance of *SHH* mutations among siblings?

2. Discuss genetic disorders with a sex bias and the mechanisms underlying the sex bias. As examples, consider Rett syndrome to illustrate embryonic sex-biased lethality, pyloric stenosis to illustrate a sex bias in disease frequency, and coronary heart disease in familial hypercholesterolemia to illustrate a sex bias in disease severity.

3. Considering the many loci associated with HPE, discuss why mutations in different genes give rise to identical phenotypes?

4. Considering that *GLI3* is in the signal transduction cascade of Shh, discuss why *GLI3* loss-of-function mutations do not give rise to the same phenotype as *SHH* loss-of-function mutations.

## References

Ming JE, Roessler E, Muenke M (1998) Human developmental disorders and the sonic hedgehog pathway. Mol Med Today 4:343–349.

Muenke M, Beachy PA (2001) Holoprosencephaly. *In* Scriver CR, Beaudet AL, Sly WS, et al (eds) The Metabolic and Molecular Bases of Inherited Disease, 8th ed. McGraw-Hill, New York, pp. 6203–6230.

# Huntington Disease

## (HD Mutation)

### Autosomal Dominant

## Principles

- Triplet repeat expansion
- Gain-of-function mutation
- Gender-specific anticipation
- Variable expressivity
- Reduced penetrance
- Presymptomatic counseling

## Major Phenotypic Features

- Age of onset: Late childhood to late adulthood
- Movement abnormalities
- Cognitive abnormalities
- Psychiatric abnormalities

## History and Physical Findings

M.P., a 45-year-old man, presented initially with declining memory and concentration. As his intellectual function deteriorated during the ensuing year, he developed involuntary movements of his fingers and toes as well as facial grimacing and pouting. He was aware of his condition and became depressed. He had been previously healthy and did not have a history of any similarly affected relatives; his parents had died in their 40s in an automobile accident. M.P. had one healthy daughter. After an extensive evaluation, the neurologist diagnosed M.P.'s condition as Huntington disease (HD). The diagnosis of HD was confirmed by a DNA analysis showing 43 CAG repeats in one of his *HD* alleles (normal, <26). Subsequent presymptomatic testing of M.P.'s daughter showed that she had also inherited the mutant *HD* allele (Fig. C–15). Both received extensive counseling.

## Background

### Disease Etiology

HD is a panethnic autosomal dominant progressive neurodegenerative disorder that is caused by mutations in the *HD* gene (see Chapter 12). The prevalence of HD ranges from 3 to 7 per 100,000 among western Europeans to 0.1 to 0.38 per 100,000 among Japanese. This variation in prevalence reflects the variation in distribution of *HD* alleles and haplotypes that are predisposed to mutation.

### Pathogenesis

The *HD* gene product, huntingtin, is ubiquitously expressed. The function of huntingtin remains unknown.

Disease-causing mutations in *HD* usually result from an expansion of a polyglutamine-encoding CAG repeat sequence in exon 1; normal *HD* alleles have 10 to 26 CAG repeats, whereas mutant alleles have more than 36 repeats (see Chapter 12). Approximately 3 percent of patients develop HD as the result of a new CAG repeat expansion, whereas 97 percent inherit a mutant *HD* allele from an affected parent. New mutant *HD* genes arise from expansion of a premutation (27 to 35 CAG repeats) to a full mutation. To date, all patients reported have inherited the new full mutation from their father.

Expansion of the HD polyglutamine tract appears to confer a deleterious gain of function. In addition to the diffuse, severe atrophy of the neostriatum that is the hallmark of HD, expression of mutant huntingtin causes neuronal dysfunction, generalized brain atrophy, changes in neuroreceptor levels, and accumulation of neuronal nuclear and cytoplasmic aggregates. Ultimately, expression of mutant huntingtin leads to neuronal death; however, studies of murine models suggest that clinical symptoms and neuronal

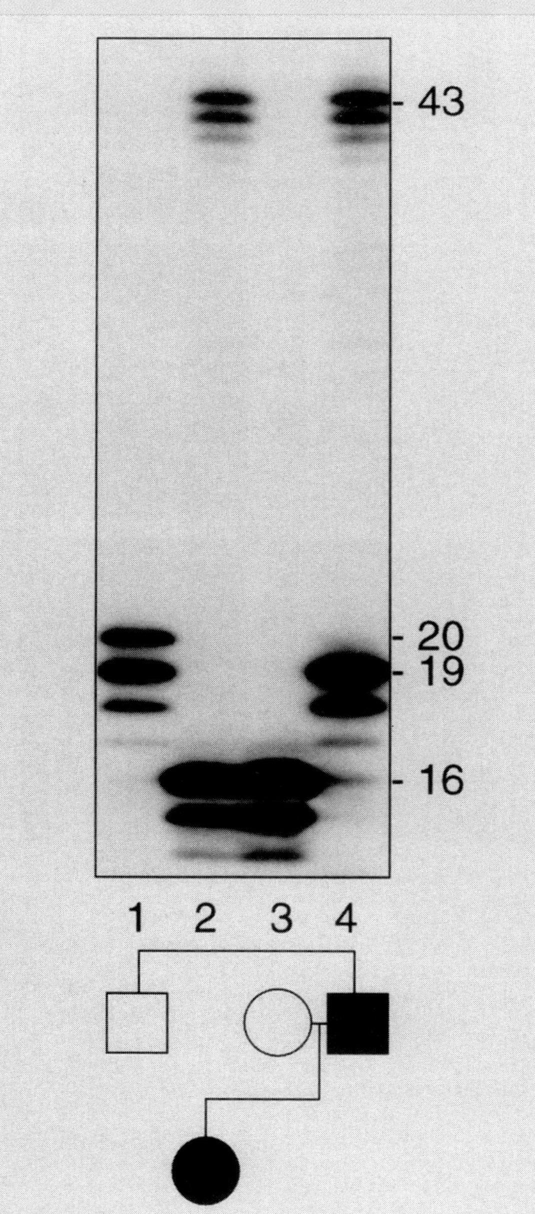


**Figure C–15.** Segregation of an *HD* gene mutation in a family with HD. Photograph of a Southern blot of polymerase chain reaction products derived from amplification of the CAG repeats in exon 1 of the *HD* gene. Notice that the affected father and daughter both have an allele with a full mutation (43 CAG repeats) and a normal allele (19 and 16 repeats, respectively). The daughter's unaffected mother and her unaffected paternal uncle have *HD* alleles with a normal number of CAG repeats. (Courtesy of M. R. Hayden, University of British Columbia, Vancouver, Canada.)

dysfunction precede the development of intracellular aggregates and neuronal death. Furthermore, studies in mice suggest that expression of the expanded polyglutamine tract alone is necessary and sufficient for the induction of an HD-like phenotype. Consistent with this observation, shutting off expression of the expanded polyglutamine tract in mice displaying an HD-like phenotype results in resolution of many features of HD. The mechanism by which expression of this expanded polyglutamine tract causes HD remains unclear.

### Phenotype and Natural History

Patient age at disease onset is inversely proportional to the number of *HD* CAG repeats; patients with adult-onset disease usually have 40 to 55 repeats, whereas those with juvenile-onset disease usually have more than 60 repeats. Patients with 36 to 41 *HD* CAG repeats exhibit reduced penetrance; that is, they may or may not develop HD in their lifetime. Apart from the relationship to the age of onset, the number of repeats does not correlate with other features of HD.

Instability in the number of CAG repeats within mutant *HD* alleles often results in anticipation, that is, progressively earlier ages of onset with succeeding generations. Once the number of CAG repeats is 36 or more, the CAG repeat length generally expands during paternal transmission; expansions during maternal transmission are less frequent and shorter than are expansions during paternal transmission. Because the CAG repeat length is inversely correlated with the age of onset, individuals inheriting a mutation from their father have an increased risk of developing early-onset disease; approximately 80 percent of juvenile patients inherit the mutant *HD* gene from their father.

Approximately one-third of patients present with psychiatric abnormalities; two-thirds present with a combination of cognitive and motor disturbances. Patients' mean age at presentation is 35 to 44 years; approximately one quarter of patients develop HD after age 50 years, however, and one tenth before age 20 years (see Chapter 12). The median survival after diagnosis is 15 to 18 years, and the mean age at death is 54 to 55 years.

HD is characterized by progressive motor, cognitive, and psychiatric abnormalities. The motor disturbances involve both voluntary and involuntary movement. Initially, these movements interfere little with daily activities but generally become incapacitating as HD progresses. Chorea, which is present in more than 90 percent of patients, is the most common involuntary movement; it is characterized by nonrepetitive, nonperiodic jerks that cannot be suppressed voluntarily. Cognitive abnormalities begin early in the disease course and affect all aspects of cognition; language is usually affected later than are other cognitive functions. Behavioral disturbances, which usually develop later in the disease course, include social disinhibition, aggression, outbursts, apathy, sexual deviation, and increased appetite. The psychiatric manifestations, which can develop anytime in the disease course, include personality changes, affective psychosis, and schizophrenia.

In the end stages of HD, patients usually develop such severe motor impairments that they are fully dependent on others. They also experience weight loss, sleep disturbances, incontinence, and mutism. Their behavioral disturbances decrease as the disease advances.

### Management

Currently, no curative treatments are available for HD. Therapy focuses on supportive care as well as pharmacological management of the behavioral and neurological problems.

## Inheritance Risk

Each child of a parent with HD has a 50 percent risk of inheriting a mutant *HD* allele. Except for those alleles with incomplete penetrance (36 to 41 CAG repeats), all children inheriting a mutant *HD* allele will develop HD if they have a normal life span.

Children of fathers carrying a premutation have an empiric risk of approximately 3 percent of inheriting an *HD* allele in which the premutation has expanded to a full mutation. Not all males carrying a premutation, however, are equally likely to transmit a full mutation.

Presymptomatic and prenatal testing are available through analysis of the number of CAG repeats within exon 1 of the *HD* gene. Presymptomatic and prenatal testing are a form of predictive testing and are interpreted best after confirmation of a CAG expansion in an affected family member.

---

### Questions for Small Group Discussion

1. Patients with heterozygous and homozygous mutations of *HD* have similar clinical expression of HD, whereas individuals with deletion of one *HD* allele on chromosome 4p have a normal phenotype. How can this be explained?

2. Some studies suggest that a father with a premutation and an affected child has a higher risk of transmitting a full mutation than does a father with a premutation and no affected children. Discuss possible mechanisms for this predisposition to transmit *HD* mutations.

3. Expansion of *HD* premutations to full mutations occurs through the male germline, whereas expansion of *FMR1* (fragile X syndrome) premutations to full mutations occurs through the female germline. Discuss possible mechanisms for gender biases in disease transmission.

4. By international consensus, asymptomatic at-risk children are not tested for *HD* mutations because testing removes the child's choice to know or not know, testing results open the child to familial and social stigmatization, and testing results could affect educational and career decisions. When would it be appropriate to test asymptomatic at-risk children? What advances in medicine are necessary to make testing of all asymptomatic at-risk children acceptable? (Consider the reasoning underlying newborn screening.)

### Reference

GeneClinics
*http://www.geneclinics.org/*

# Insulin-Dependent Diabetes Mellitus

## (Autoimmune Destruction of Islet Beta Cells)

### Multifactorial

## Principles

- Polygenic disease
- Environmental trigger
- Susceptibility allele
- Protective allele

## Major Phenotypic Features

- Age of onset: Childhood through adulthood
- Polyuria, polydipsia, polyphagia
- Hyperglycemia
- Ketosis
- Wasting

## History and Physical Findings

F.C. was a 45-year-old father with late-onset diabetes mellitus who was referred to the endocrinology clinic for counseling regarding his children's risk for diabetes. F.C. developed glucose intolerance (inability to maintain normal blood glucose levels after ingestion of sugar) at age 39 and fasting hyperglycemia at age 45. He did not have a history of other medical or surgical problems. The findings from his physical examination were normal except for moderate abdominal obesity. He had five children by two different partners; a child from each relationship had developed insulin-dependent diabetes mellitus (IDDM) before age 10. His sister developed IDDM as a child and died during adolescence from diabetic ketoacidosis. The geneticist explained that, given his family history, F.C. might have a late-onset form of IDDM and that his current non–insulin-dependent diabetes mellitus was likely an antecedent to developing IDDM. After discussing the possible causes of and prognostic factors for the development of IDDM, F.C. elected to enroll himself and his children in a research protocol studying the prevention of IDDM. As part of that study, he and his children were tested for anti-islet antibodies. Both he and an unaffected daughter had a high titer of anti-islet antibodies; the daughter also had an abnormal glucose tolerance test but not fasting hyperglycemia. As part of the study protocol, F.C. and his daughter were prescribed low-dose insulin injections.

## Background

### *Disease Etiology*

IDDM (sometimes called type 1 diabetes) is usually caused by autoimmune destruction of islet $\beta$ cells in the pancreas; this autoimmune reaction is triggered by an unknown mechanism. The destruction of islet $\beta$ cells causes insulin deficiency and thereby dysregulation of anabolism and catabolism, resulting in metabolic changes similar to those observed in starvation (Fig. C–16). Among North American Caucasians, IDDM is the second most common chronic disease of childhood, increasing in prevalence from 1 in 2500 at 5 years of age to 1 in 300 at age 18.

### *Pathogenesis*

**Genetics.** IDDM usually results from a genetic susceptibility and subsequent environmental insult (see Chapter 15); it is believed rarely to result only from an environmental insult or only from a genetic mutation. Although approximately 90 percent of IDDM occurs in patients without a family history of diabetes, observations supporting a genetic predisposition include differences in concordance between monozygotic (33 to 50 percent) and dizygotic twins (1 to 14 percent), familial clustering, and differences in prevalence among different populations. More than 13 different genetic susceptibility loci have been reported in humans, although few have been identified consistently and reproducibly. One of the few is the HLA locus that may account for as much as 30 to 60 percent of the genetic susceptibility. Approximately 95 percent of Caucasian patients express a DR3 or a DR4 allele, or both, compared with 50 percent of controls; this association apparently arises not because DR3 and DR4 are susceptibility alleles but because of linkage disequilibrium between DR and DQ. The DQ$\beta_1$*0201 allele, which segregates with DR3, and DQ$\beta_1$*0302, which segregates with DR4, appear to be the primary susceptibility alleles. In contrast, DQ$\beta_1$*602, which segregates with DR2, appears to be a protective allele; that is, it negates the effect of a susceptibility allele when both are present. Both of the DQ$\beta_1$ susceptibility alleles have a neutral amino acid at position 57, a site within the putative antigen binding cleft, whereas protective or neutral DQ$\beta_1$ alleles have an aspartic acid at position 57. This substitution of an uncharged amino acid for aspartic acid is predicted to change the specificity of antigen binding to the DQ molecule.

**Environment.** Evidence supporting an environmental component to the induction of IDDM in genetically susceptible individuals includes a concordance of less than 50 percent among monozygotic twins, seasonal variation in incidence, and an increased incidence of diabetes among children with congenital rubella. Proposed environmental triggers include viral infections and early exposure to bovine albumin. Exposure to viruses and bovine albumin could cause autoimmune destruction of $\beta$ cells by molecular mimicry, that is, sharing of antigenic determinants between $\beta$-cell proteins and the virus or bovine albumin. Approximately 80 to 90 percent of newly diagnosed patients with IDDM have islet-cell antibodies. These autoantibodies recognize cytoplasmic and cell surface determinants such as glutamic acid decarboxylase (GAD), carboxy peptidase H, ganglioside antigens, islet-cell antigen 69 (ICA69), and a protein tyrosine phosphatase. GAD and ICA69, respectively, share epitopes with coxsackievirus B4 and bovine serum albumin.

In sum, IDDM appears to be an autoimmune disease, although the precise role of islet-cell autoantibodies remains uncertain. Additional evidence for an autoimmune mechanism in IDDM includes an increased prevalence of other autoimmune diseases, mononuclear cell infiltrates of islets, and recurrent $\beta$ cell destruction after transplantation from a monozygotic twin. But two lines of evidence suggest that progression to IDDM involves more than the development of autoantibodies. First, less than 1 percent of the general population develops diabetes although 10 percent have islet autoantibodies; and second, first-degree relatives and school children have remission rates of 10 to 78 percent for islet-cell antibodies.

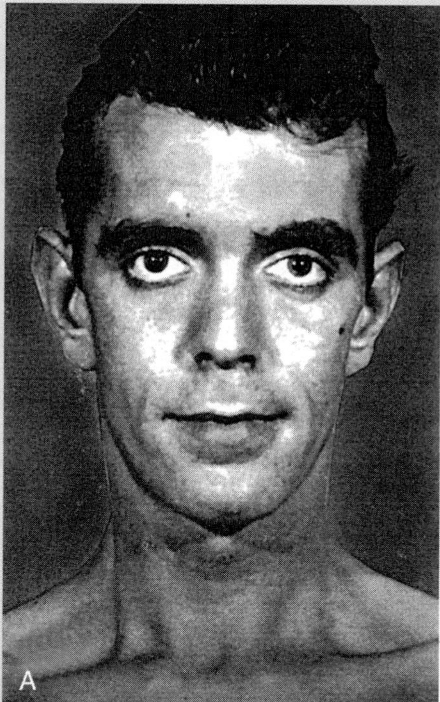


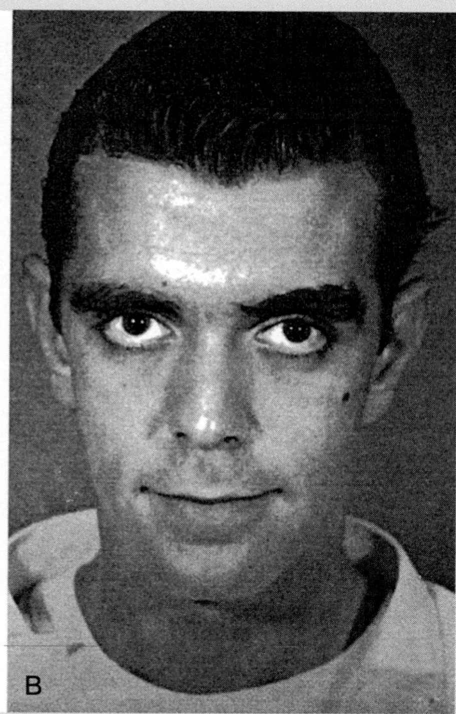


**Figure C–16.** A 28-year-old man with insulin-dependent diabetes mellitis. Panel *A*, Photograph after 3 weeks of polydipsia and polyuria. Panel *B*, Photograph after gaining 5 kg after 10 days of insulin replacement. (Adapted from Oakley WG, Pyke DA, Taylor KW [1968] Clinical Diabetes and Its Biochemical Basis. Blackwell Scientific Publications, Oxford, p. 258, by permission. Photographic restoration courtesy of B. Moseley-Fernandini.)

## Phenotype and Natural History

Loss of insulin reserve occurs over a few to many years. The earliest sign of abnormality is the development of islet autoantibodies when blood glucose, glucose tolerance (ability to maintain normal blood glucose levels after ingestion of sugar), and insulin responses to glucose are normal. This period is followed by a phase of decreased glucose tolerance but normal fasting blood glucose. With continued loss of $\beta$ cells, fasting hyperglycemia eventually develops but sufficient insulin is still produced to prevent ketosis; during this period, patients have non–insulin-dependent diabetes mellitus (NIDDM). Eventually, insulin production falls below a critical threshold, and patients become dependent on exogenous insulin supplements and have a propensity to ketoacidosis. Younger patients generally progress through these phases more rapidly than do older patients.

Although the acute complications of diabetes can be controlled by administration of exogenous insulin, the loss of endogenous insulin production causes many problems, including atherosclerosis, peripheral neuropathy, renal disease, cataracts, and retinopathy. Approximately 50 percent of patients eventually die of renal failure. The development and severity of these complications is related to the genetic background and degree of metabolic control. Rigorous control of blood glucose levels reduces the risk of complications by 35 to 75 percent.

## Management

Although pancreatic or islet transplantation can cure IDDM, the paucity of tissue for transplantation and complications of immunosuppression limit this therapy. Management of most patients emphasizes intensive control of blood glucose levels by injection of exogenous insulin.

The development of islet autoantibodies several years before the onset of IDDM has led to the development of studies to predict and prevent IDDM. The administration of insulin or nicotinamide appears to delay the development of IDDM in some patients.

## Inheritance Risk

The risk of IDDM in the general population is approximately 1 in 300. With one affected sibling, the risk increases to 1 in 14 (1 in 6 if HLA-identical, 1 in 20 if HLA-haplotype identical). With a second affected first-degree relative in addition to an affected sibling, the risk increases to 1 in 6 and with an affected monozygotic twin to 1 in 3. Children of an affected mother have a 1 in 50 to 1 in 33 risk of developing IDDM, whereas children of an affected father have a 1 in 25 to 1 in 16 risk. This paternity-related increased risk appears to be limited to fathers with an HLA DR4 allele.

## Questions for Small Group Discussion

1. Discuss the difficulties of identifying the genetic components of polygenic diseases.
2. How might HLA susceptibility alleles effect susceptibility and protective alleles effect protection?
3. Discuss the underlying mechanism(s) for prevention of IDDM by exogenous insulin injections.
4. Compare risk counseling for fathers and mothers with IDDM. Discuss the teratogenic risks and mechanisms of maternal diabetes.

## Reference

Sperling MA (1999) Diabetes Mellitus. *In* Behrman RE, Kliegman RM, Jenson HB (eds) Nelson Textbook of Pediatrics, 16th ed. WB Saunders, Philadelphia, pp. 1767–1786.

# Marfan Syndrome

## (FBN1 Mutation)

### Autosomal Dominant

### Principles
- Dominant negative mutations
- Variable expressivity
- Genocopy

### Major Phenotypic Features
- Age of onset: Early childhood
- Disproportionate tall stature
- Skeletal anomalies
- Ectopia lentis
- Mitral valve prolapse
- Aortic dilatation and rupture
- Spontaneous pneumothorax
- Lumbosacral ectasia

### History and Physical Findings
J.L., a healthy 16-year old high school basketball star, was referred to the genetics clinic for evaluation for Marfan syndrome. Her physique was similar to that of her father. Her father, a tall thin man, had died during a morning jog; no other family members had a history of skeletal abnormalities, sudden death, vision loss, or congenital anomalies. On physical examination, J.L. had an asthenic habitus with a high arched palate, mild pectus carinatum, arachnodactyly, an arm span to height ratio of 1.1, a diastolic murmur, and stretch marks on her shoulders and thighs. She was referred for echocardiography; this showed dilatation of the ascending aorta with aortic regurgitation. An ophthalmologic examination showed bilateral iridodonesis and slight displacement of the lens superiorly. Based on her physical examination and testing results, the geneticist explained to J.L. that she had Marfan syndrome. Eventually, J.L. married and adopted children but declined to become pregnant herself.

## Background

### Disease Etiology
Marfan syndrome is a panethnic autosomal dominant connective tissue disorder that results from mutations in the fibrillin-1 gene (*FBN1*). Marfan syndrome has an incidence of 1 in 10,000 to 1 in 20,000. Approximately 25 to 35 percent of patients have *de novo* mutations.

### Pathogenesis
*FBN1* encodes fibrillin-1, an extracellular glycoprotein with ubiquitous distribution. Fibrillin-1 polymerizes to form microfibrils, structural molecules in load-bearing tissues such as the aortic adventitia, ciliary zonules, and skin.

Mutations leading to Marfan syndrome are scattered across the gene, and each mutation is usually unique to a family. These mutations affect fibrillin-1 synthesis, processing, secretion, polymerization, or stability. Studies of fibrillin-1 deposition and cell culture expression assays have generally suggested a dominant negative pathogenesis; that is, production of mutant fibrillin-1 inhibits formation of normal microfibrils by normal fibrillin-1 or stimulates inappropriate proteolysis of extracellular microfibrils.

In addition to Marfan syndrome, mutations in *FBN1* cause neonatal Marfan syndrome, familial arachnodactyly, autosomal dominant ectopia lentis, MASS phenotype (Marfanoid signs involving *m*itral valve, *a*orta *s*keleton, and *s*kin), and isolated marfanoid skeletal features. Generally, the phenotypes are fairly consistent within a family, although the severity of the phenotype may vary considerably. Occasionally, however, an *FBN1* mutation within a family causes more than one of these phenotypes. To date, clear genotype-phenotype correlations have not emerged. The intra- and interfamilial variability suggests that environmental and epigenetic factors play a significant role in determining the phenotype.

### Phenotype and Natural History
Marfan syndrome is a multisystem disorder with skeletal, ocular, cardiovascular, pulmonary, skin, and dural abnormalities. The skeletal abnormalities include disproportionate tall stature (arm span:height $>1.05$, normal $<1.05$), arachnodactyly, pectus deformities, scoliosis, joint laxity, and a narrow palate. The ocular abnormalities include ectopia lentis (Fig. C–17), flat corneas, increased globe length, and hypoplastic irides. The cardiovascular abnormalities include mitral valve prolapse, aortic regurgitation, and dilatation and dissection of the ascending aorta. The pulmonary abnormalities include spontaneous pneumothorax and apical blebs. The skin abnormalities include striae atrophicae and recurrent herniae. The dural abnormalities include lumbosacral ectasia.

Many features of Marfan syndrome develop with age. Skeletal anomalies such as anterior chest deformities and scoliosis worsen with bone growth. Subluxation of the lens tends to progress during early childhood or adolescence. Secondary glaucoma usually develops several years after lens subluxation and after displacement of the lens into the

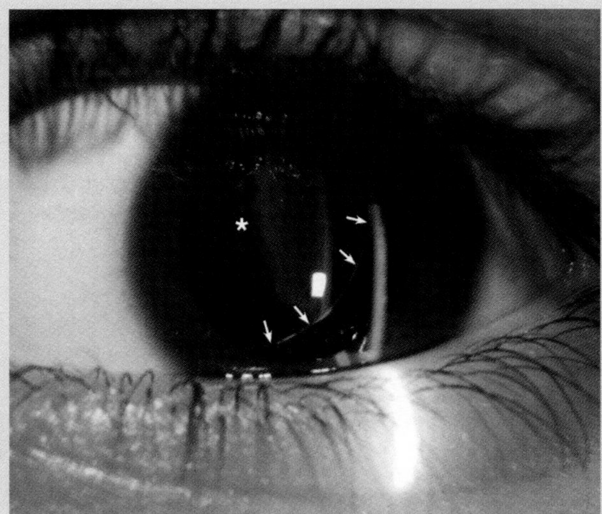

**Figure C–17.** Ectopia lentis. Slit lamp view of the left eye of a patient with Marfan syndrome. *Asterisk* indicates the center of the lens that is displaced superior nasally; normally, the lens is in the center of the pupil. The *arrows* indicate the edge of the lens that is abnormally visible in the pupil. (Courtesy of A. V. Levin, The Hospital for Sick Children and University of Toronto.)

anterior chamber. Cardiovascular complications manifest at any age and progress throughout life.

The major causes of premature death in patients with Marfan syndrome are heart failure from aortic regurgitation and aortic dissection and rupture. As surgical and medical management of the aortic dilatation have improved, however, so has survival. Between 1972 and 1993, the age at which 50 percent of patients are predicted to be alive rose from 49 to 74 years for women and from 41 to 70 years for men.

### *Management*

Marfan syndrome is a clinical diagnosis defined by the presence of particular features. Confirmation of Marfan syndrome by identification of mutations in *FBN1* is not currently practical because extreme allelic heterogeneity makes identifying the causative mutation in each family prohibitively labor intensive and because of the lack of reliable genotype-phenotype correlation. In families segregating Marfan syndrome, at-risk individuals can be identified by linkage analysis if an informative marker segregates with the disease.

No curative treatments are available for Marfan syndrome; therefore, treatment focuses on prevention and symptomatic management. Ophthalmological management includes frequent examinations, correction of the myopia, and, often, lens replacement. Orthopedic management includes bracing or surgery for scoliosis, or both, chest-wall reconstruction for pulmonary compromise, and physical therapy and orthotics for joint instability. Cardiovascular management is a combination of medical and surgical therapy. Medical therapy attempts to prevent or slow progression, or both, of aortic dilatation by reducing ventricular ejection force with beta-adrenergic blockers and through restriction of participation in stressful activities and exposure to emotional stress. Prophylactic replacement of the proximal aorta and aortic root is recommended when aortic dilatation becomes sufficiently severe.

The hemodynamic changes associated with pregnancy are particularly difficult to manage. Although most women with Marfan syndrome do not have major complications during pregnancy and delivery, most aortic dissections in young patients occur in pregnant women. The aortic dissections are believed to be secondary to the hormonal, blood volume, and cardiac output changes associated with pregnancy and parturition.

## Inheritance Risk

Patients with Marfan syndrome have a 50 percent risk of having a child affected with Marfan syndrome. Prenatal diagnosis is available only for those families in which linkage studies are possible or in which the *FBN1* mutation has been identified.

---

## *Questions for Small Group Discussion*

1. Homocystinuria was long considered a genocopy of Marfan syndrome. Why? How can these two disorders be distinguished by medical history? By physical examination? By biochemical testing?

2. Discuss the difference between a prenatal diagnosis made by linkage analysis and one made by identification of a "disease-causing" mutation. What factors influence the accuracy of each diagnosis? How should the results of such testing be presented to parents?

3. What are dominant negative mutations? What are novel property mutations? Contrast the two. Why are dominant negative mutations common in connective tissue disorders?

4. If one wished to design a curative treatment for a disorder caused by dominant negative mutations, what must the therapy accomplish at a molecular level? How is this different than treatment of a disease caused by loss-of-function mutations?

## *Reference*

Dietz HC, Pyeritz RE (2001) Marfan syndrome and related disorders. *In* Scriver CR, Beaudet AL, Sly WS, et al (eds) The Metabolic and Molecular Bases of Inherited Disease, 8th ed. McGraw-Hill, New York, pp. 5287–5311.

# Miller-Dieker Syndrome

## (17p13.3 Hemizygous Deletion)

### Chromosomal

## Principles
- Microdeletion syndrome
- Contiguous gene disorder
- Haploinsufficiency

## Major Phenotypic Features
- Age of onset: Prenatal
- Lissencephaly type 1 or 2
- Facial dysmorphism
- Severe global mental deficiency
- Seizures
- Early death

## History and Physical Findings
B.B., a 5-day-old boy born at 38 weeks of gestation, was admitted to the neonatal intensive care unit because of marked hypotonia and feeding difficulties. He was the product of an uncomplicated pregnancy; a fetal ultrasound at 14 weeks of gestation and a maternal triple screen at 16 weeks of gestation had been normal. B.B. was born by spontaneous vertex vaginal delivery; his Apgar scores were 8 at 1 minute and 9 at 5 minutes. He did not have a family history of genetic, neurological, or congenital disorders. On physical examination, B.B. had hypotonia and mild dysmorphic facial features including bitemporal narrowing, a depressed nasal bridge, a small nose with anteverted nares, and micrognathia. The findings from the examination were otherwise normal. His evaluation had included normal serum electrolytes, a normal metabolic screen, normal studies for congenital infections, and an abnormal brain ultrasound scan. The ultrasound had shown a hypoplastic corpus callosum, mild ventricular dilatation, and a smooth cortex. In addition to those studies, the genetics consultation team recommended a chromosome analysis, fluorescence in situ hybridization (FISH) for *LIS1* (17p13.3), and magnetic resonance imaging (MRI) of the brain. The MRI showed a thickened cerebral cortex, complete cerebral agyria, multiple cerebral heterotopias, a hypoplastic corpus callosum, a normal cerebellum, and a normal brain stem. The chromosome analysis was normal (46,XY), but FISH showed a deletion of *LIS1* on one chromosome 17. Based on these results, the geneticist explained to the parents that B.B. had Miller-Dieker syndrome (MDS). The parents declined further measures other than those to keep the baby comfortable, and B.B. died at 2 months of age.

## Background

### Disease Etiology
MDS is a contiguous gene syndrome caused by hemizygous deletion of 17p13.3; the mechanism underlying recurrent deletion of 17p13.3 has not yet been elucidated, but may (like other microdeletion syndromes; see Chapter 10) involve repetitive DNA sequences. MDS is a rare disorder of undefined incidence that occurs in all populations.

### Pathogenesis
More than 50 genes have been mapped within the MDS deletion region in 17p13.3, but only the *LIS1* gene has been associated with a specific phenotypic feature of MDS; hemizygosity for *LIS1* causes lissencephaly. *LIS1* encodes the brain isoform of the noncatalytic $\beta$ subunit of platelet-activating factor acetylhydrolase (PAFAH). PAFAH hydrolyzes platelet activating factor, an inhibitor of neuronal migration. PAFAH also binds to and stabilizes microtubules; preliminary observations suggest PAFAH may play a role in the microtubule reorganization required for neuronal migration.

Haploinsufficiency of *LIS1* does not cause the other dysmorphic features associated with MDS. Point mutations within or isolated deletions of *LIS1* cause isolated lissencephaly sequence (ILS), that is, lissencephaly without other dysmorphism. Because all patients with MDS have facial dysmorphology, this dysmorphism must be caused by haploinsufficiency of a different gene(s) in the common MDS deletion interval.

### Phenotype and Natural History
The features of MDS include brain dysgenesis, hypotonia, failure to thrive, and facial dysmorphism. The brain dysgenesis is characterized by lissencephaly type 1 (complete agyria) or type 2 (widespread agyria with a few sulci at the frontal or occipital poles), a cerebral cortex with four instead of six layers, gray matter heterotopias, and attenuated white matter. Some patients also have heart malformations and omphaloceles.

Patients with MDS feed and grow poorly. Smiling, brief visual fixation, and nonspecific motor responses are the only developmental skills most patients acquire. In addition to mental deficiency, patients usually suffer from opisthotonos, spasticity, and seizures. Nearly all patients die by 2 years of age.

### Management
A patient's facial features and an MRI finding of lissencephaly often suggest a diagnosis of MDS (Fig. C–18). Confirmation of the diagnosis, however, requires detection of a 17p13.3 deletion by chromosome analysis or by FISH with a *LIS1*-specific probe. Approximately 60 percent of patients have a visible deletion of the MDS critical region.

MDS is incurable; therefore, treatment focuses on the management of symptoms and palliative care. Nearly all patients require pharmacological management of their seizures. Also, many patients receive nasogastric or gastrostomy tube feedings because of poor feeding and repeated aspiration.

## Inheritance Risk
Eighty percent of patients have a *de novo* microdeletion of 17p13.3, and 20 percent inherit the deletion from a parent who carries a balanced chromosomal rearrangement. Because of the frequency with which the deletion is inherited from a parent with a balanced translocation, karyotypes and FISH for *LIS1* should be checked in both parents. A parent with a balanced translocation involving 17p13.3 has approximately a 26 percent risk of having an abnormal liveborn child (MDS or dup17p) and approximately a 22 percent risk of pregnancy loss. In contrast, if a patient has MDS as a result of a *de novo* deletion, the parents have a low risk for recurrence of MDS in future children.

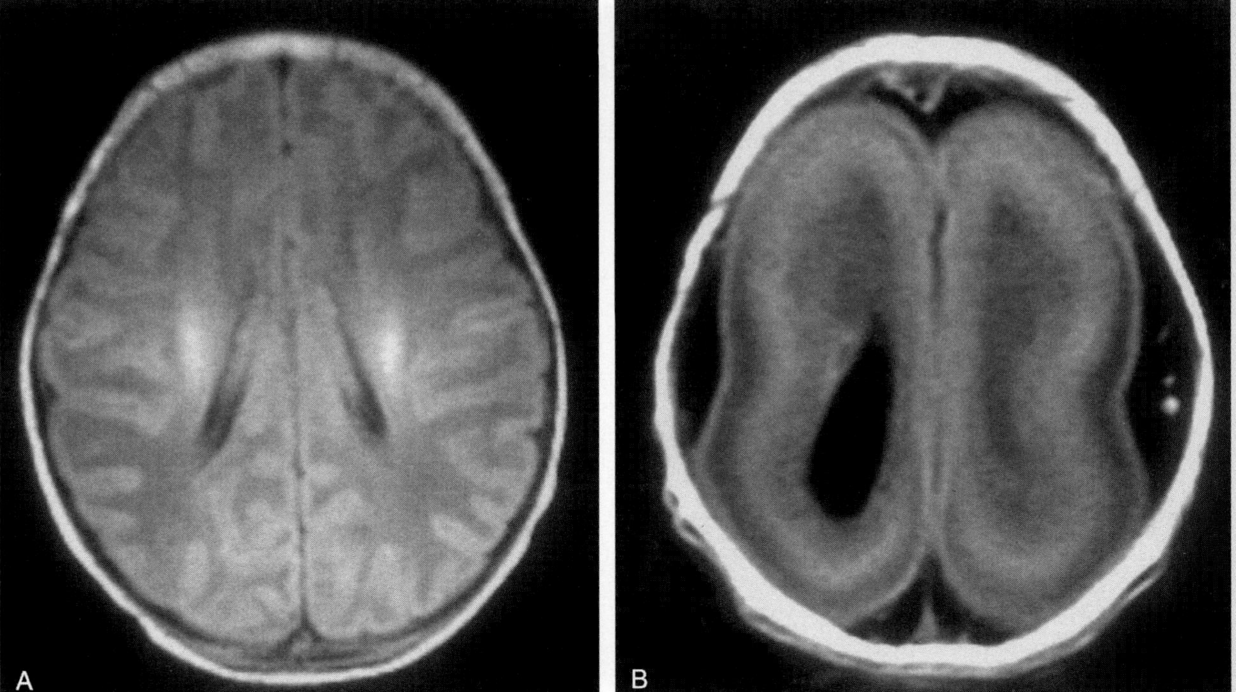


**Figure C–18.** Brain magnetic resonance images of an infant without lissencephaly (*A*) and an infant with Miller-Dieker syndrome (MDS) (*B*). Note the smooth cerebral surface, the thickened cerebral cortex, and the classic "figure-8" appearance of the brain of the patient with MDS. (Courtesy of D. Chitayat, The Hospital for Sick Children and University of Toronto.)

Although the brain malformations of MDS result from incomplete migration of neurons to the cerebral cortex during the third and fourth months of gestation, lissencephaly is not detected by fetal MRI or ultrasound until late in gestation. Prenatal diagnosis of MDS requires detection of a 17p13.3 deletion in fetal chorionic villi or amniocytes.

## Questions for Small Group Discussion

1. Rubenstein-Taybi syndrome is caused either by deletion of 16p13.3 or by mutation of the *CREBBP* transcription factor. Compare and contrast the relationship of *CREBBP* and Rubenstein-Taybi syndrome with the relationship of *LIS1* and MDS. Why is MDS a contiguous gene deletion syndrome, whereas Rubenstein-Taybi syndrome is not?

2. Mutations of either *LIS1* on chromosome 17 or *DCX* on the X chromosome account for approximately 75 percent of isolated lissencephaly sequence. What features of the family history and brain MRI can be used to focus testing on *DCX* as opposed to on *LIS1*?

3. At 30 weeks of gestation, a woman had a fetal ultrasound showing fetal lissencephaly. The pregnancy was otherwise uncomplicated, and fetal ultrasound findings earlier in gestation had been normal. What counseling and evaluation are indicated? Discuss your counseling approach if she and her spouse wish to terminate the pregnancy at 32 weeks of gestation.

## Reference

GeneClinics
*http://www.geneclinics.org/*

# Myoclonic Epilepsy with Ragged-Red Fibers

## (Mitochondrial *t*RNA$^{lys}$ Mutation)

### Matrilineal, Mitochondrial

## Principles

- Mitochondrial DNA mutations
- Replicative segregation
- Expression threshold
- High mutation rate
- Accumulation of mutations with age

## Major Phenotypic Features

- Age of onset: Childhood through adulthood
- Myopathy
- Dementia
- Myoclonic seizures
- Ataxia
- Deafness

## History and Physical Findings

R.S., a 15-year-old boy, was referred to the neurogenetics clinic for myoclonic epilepsy; his electroencephalogram was characterized by bursts of slow wave and spike complexes. Before the seizures developed, he had been well and developing normally. His family history was remarkable for a maternal uncle who had died of an undiagnosed myopathic disorder at 53 years; a maternal aunt with progressive dementia who had presented with ataxia at 37 years; and an 80-year-old maternal grandmother with deafness, diabetes, and renal dysfunction. On examination, R.S. had generalized muscle wasting and weakness, myoclonus, and ataxia. Initial evaluation detected neurosensory hearing loss, slowed nerve conduction velocities, and mildly elevated blood and cerebrospinal fluid lactate levels. Results of a subsequent muscle biopsy identified abnormal mitochondria, deficient staining for cytochrome oxidase, and ragged-red fibers—muscle fibers with subsarcolemmal mitochondria that stained red with Gomori trichrome stain. Molecular testing for mutations within the mitochondrial genome (mtDNA) identified a mutation (G8344A, *tRNA$^{lys}$* gene) that is associated with myoclonic epilepsy with ragged-red fibers (MERRF). Subsequent testing of blood samples from R.S.'s mother, aunt, and grandmother confirmed that they also carried this mutation. A review of the autopsy of the deceased uncle identified ragged-red fibers in some muscle groups. The physician counseled the family members that they each were either manifesting or nonmanifesting carriers of a deleterious mtDNA mutation compromising oxidative phosphorylation (OXPHOS). No other family members chose to be tested for the mutation.

## Background

### Disease Etiology

MERRF is a rare panethnic disorder that is caused by mutations within mtDNA. More than 90 percent of patients have a mutation (G8344A or T8356C) within the mitochondrial *tRNA$^{lys}$* gene. The disease is inherited maternally, because mitochondria are inherited only from the mother (see Chapter 5).

### Pathogenesis

Mitochondria generate energy for cellular processes by producing adenosine triphosphate through OXPHOS. Five enzyme complexes, I to V, comprise the OXPHOS pathway. Except for complex II, each complex has some components encoded within the mtDNA and some in the nuclear genome. The mtDNA encodes 13 of the polypeptides in the OXPHOS complexes as well as 2 rRNAs and 22 tRNAs (see Chapter 12).

In MERRF, the activities of complexes I and IV are usually most severely reduced. The *tRNA$^{lys}$* mutations associated with MERRF reduce the amount of charged tRNA$^{lys}$ in the mitochondria by 50 to 60 percent and thereby decrease the efficiency of translation such that at each lysine codon there is a 26 percent chance of termination. Because complexes I and IV have the most components synthesized within the mitochondria, they are most severely affected.

Because each mitochondrion contains multiple mtDNAs and each cell contains multiple mitochondria, a cell can contain mtDNAs of either one genotype (homoplasmy) or multiple genotypes (heteroplasmy); therefore, expression of the MERRF phenotype in any cell, organ, or individual ultimately depends on the overall reduction in OXPHOS capacity. The threshold for expression of a deleterious phenotype depends on the balance between oxidative supply and demand. This threshold varies with age and among individuals, organ systems, and tissues.

The threshold for expression of the MERRF phenotype can be met by either decreasing the efficiency of expression from the normal mtDNA or increasing the proportion of mutant mtDNA. In contrast to nuclear DNA, mtDNA has a 10-fold higher mutation rate; this may result from exposure to a high concentration of oxygen free radicals from OXPHOS, a lack of protective histones, and ineffective DNA repair. Because mtDNA has no introns, random mutations usually affect coding sequences. Consistent with this increased mutation rate, mitochondrial efficiency declines gradually throughout adulthood, and as reserve OXPHOS activity declines, expression of defects in the OXPHOS pathway becomes increasingly likely.

Increases in the proportion of mutant mtDNA can occur by a combination of inheritance, preferential replication of mutant mtDNA, and selection. First, the children of heteroplasmic mothers have widely varying proportions of mtDNA genotypes because of replicative segregation, that is, random partitioning of mitochondria during expansion of the oogonial population. Second, as heteroplasmic cells within an individual undergo mitosis, the proportion of mtDNA genotypes in daughter cells changes from that of the parent cell by replicative segregation. Third, because changes in the proportion of mtDNA genotypes affect the cellular phenotype, the mtDNA is subject to strong selective pressures; the selective pressures vary among tissues and result in different mtDNA populations in different tissues of the same person. Thus, both intercellular and intergenerational mtDNA transmission follow the principles of population genetics.

### Phenotype and Natural History

The classic MERRF phenotype includes myoclonic epilepsy and mitochondrial myopathy with ragged-red fibers (Fig. C–19). Other associated findings include abnormal brain stem evoked responses, sensory neural hearing loss, ataxia, renal dysfunction, diabetes, cardiomyopathy, and dementia. Onset of symptoms can be in childhood

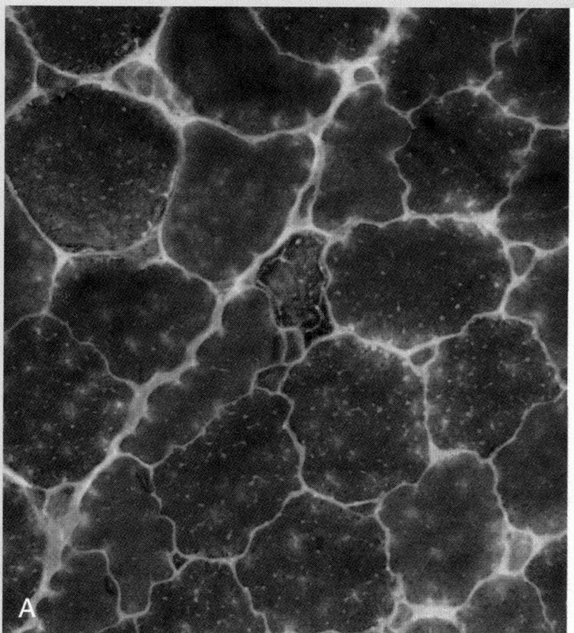

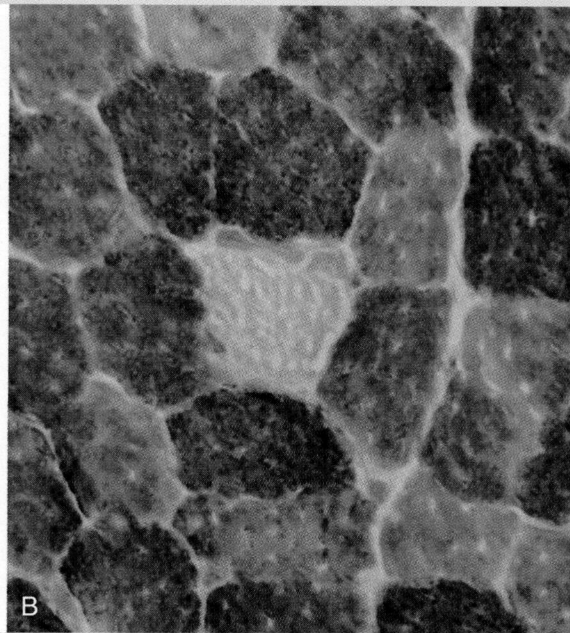


**Figure C–19.** Quadriceps muscle histology. *A*, Modified Gomori trichrome stain illustrating a ragged-red fiber. Magnification, X525. *B*, Cytochrome oxidase stain illustrating absence of cytochrome oxidase in an affected muscle fiber, consistent with a mitochondrial DNA defect. Magnification, X525. (Courtesy of Annette Feigenbaum, The Hospital for Sick Children and University of Toronto.)

or adult life, and the course can be slowly progressive or rapidly downhill.

Because mtDNA genetics follows quantitative and stochastic principles, clinical features of affected relatives vary in pattern and severity and do not have an easily defined clinical course. The absence of ragged-red fibers in a muscle biopsy specimen does not exclude MERRF. Within pedigrees, phenotypes generally correlate well with the severity of the OXPHOS deficit, but correlation with the percentage of mutant mtDNA in skeletal muscle requires adjustment for age. In one pedigree, a young adult with 5 percent normal mtDNA in skeletal muscle had a severe clinical and biochemical phenotype; other young adults with 15 percent normal mtDNA had normal phenotypes; and an elderly adult with 16 percent normal mtDNA had a severe phenotype. This expression pattern demonstrates that symptoms accumulate progressively as OXPHOS capacity drops below organ expression thresholds and that age-related declines in OXPHOS play a critical role in the appearance and progression of symptoms.

### *Management*

Treatment is symptomatic and palliative. No specific therapies are currently available. Most patients are given vitamin supplements to optimize the activity of the OXPHOS complexes.

## Inheritance Risk

The risk to children of affected males is zero because children do not inherit paternal mtDNA. The risk to children of affected or unaffected females with a MERRF mutation cannot be estimated accurately by prenatal testing because the critical parameters defining disease in the child (replicative segregation, tissue selection, and somatic mtDNA mutations) cannot be predicted in advance.

Similarly, molecular testing of blood samples from at-risk family members is complicated by two general problems. First, because of replicative segregation and tissue selection, the mutation may not be detectable in blood; therefore, a negative result does not exclude a family member as a mtDNA mutation carrier. Second, because of replicative segregation, a positive result predicts neither the proportion of mutant mtDNA in other tissues nor the expected severity of disease.

## *Questions for Small Group Discussion*

1. How does a mutant mtDNA molecule, arising in a cell with hundreds of normal molecules, become such a significant fraction of the total that energy-generating capacity is compromised and symptoms develop?
2. How could mitochondrial mutations affecting oxidative phosphorylation accelerate the mutation rate of mtDNA?
3. How would mitochondrial mutations affecting oxidative phosphorylation accelerate aging?
4. In the fetus, oxygen tension is low and most energy is derived from glycolysis. How could this observation affect the prenatal expression of deleterious OXPHOS mutations?

## *References*


Nyhan WL, Ozand PT (1998) Myoclonic epilepsy and ragged red fiber (MERRF) disease. *In* Atlas of Metabolic Diseases. Chapman & Hall Medical, New York, pp. 292–296.

Wallace DC (1999) Mitochondrial diseases in man and mouse. Science 283:1482–1488.

# Non–Insulin-Dependent Diabetes Mellitus

## (Insulin Deficiency and Resistance)

### Multifactorial

## Principles

- Polygenic disease
- Environmental modifiers

## Major Phenotypic Features

- Age of onset: Childhood through adulthood
- Hyperglycemia
- Relative insulin deficiency
- Insulin resistance
- Obesity
- Acanthosis nigricans

## History and Physical Findings

M.P. was a 38-year-old healthy Pima Indian who requested information on his risk of developing non–insulin-dependent diabetes mellitus (NIDDM), a disease that affects nearly 50 percent of Pima people by the age of 35 years. Both of his parents had had NIDDM; his father died at 60 years from a myocardial infarction and his mother at 55 years from renal failure. His paternal grandparents and one older sister also had NIDDM, but he and his four younger siblings did not have the disease. The findings from M.P.'s physical examination were normal except for mild obesity; he had a normal fasting blood glucose level but an elevated blood insulin level and abnormally high blood glucose levels after an oral glucose challenge. These results were consistent with an antecedent to NIDDM. His physician advised M.P. to change his lifestyle so that he would lose weight and increase his physical activity. M.P. sharply reduced his dietary fat consumption, began commuting to work by bicycle, and jogging three times per week; his weight decreased 10 kg, and his glucose tolerance and blood insulin level normalized.

## Background

### *Disease Etiology*

NIDDM accounts for 80 to 90 percent of all diabetes mellitus and has a prevalence of 6 to 7 percent in the United States. It is a heterogeneous disease composed of type 1 (autoimmune) and type 2 (nonautoimmune) diabetes mellitus. Approximately 5 to 10 percent of patients with NIDDM have type 1 diabetes (see the case describing patient F.C., insulin-dependent diabetes mellitus [IDDM]), 5 to 10 percent have maturity-onset diabetes of youth, 5 to 10 percent have a rare genetic disorder, and the remaining 70 to 85 percent have "typical NIDDM," a form of type 2 diabetes mellitus characterized by relative insulin deficiency and resistance. The molecular and genetic bases of "typical NIDDM" remain poorly defined.

### *Pathogenesis*

"Typical NIDDM," hereafter referred to as NIDDM, results from a combination of genetic susceptibility and environmental factors. Observations supporting a genetic predisposition include differences in concordance between monozygotic and dizygotic twins, familial clustering, and differences in prevalence among populations. Human inheritance patterns and rat models of NIDDM suggest polygenic inheritance, but identification of the relevant genes in humans is confounded by the effects of age, gender, ethnicity, physical fitness, diet, smoking, obesity, and fat distribution on insulin sensitivity and secretion. Genome-wide screens and analyses of more than 250 candidate genes have not identified common major genetic loci, although screens of Finnish and Mexican-American groups have identified predisposition loci apparently specific to those populations. Evidence for an environmental component includes a concordance of less than 100 percent in monozygotic twins, differences in prevalence in genetically similar populations, and associations with lifestyle, diet, obesity, pregnancy, and stress. The body of experimental evidence suggests that, although genetic susceptibility is a prerequisite for NIDDM, clinical expression of NIDDM is possibly largely determined by environmental factors.

NIDDM results from a derangement of insulin secretion and resistance to insulin action. Normally, basal insulin secretion follows a rhythmic pattern interrupted by responses to glucose loads. In patients with NIDDM, the rhythmic basal release of insulin is markedly deranged, responses to glucose loads are inadequate, and basal insulin levels are elevated although low relative to the hyperglycemia of these patients.

Persistent hyperglycemia and hyperinsulinemia develop before NIDDM and initiate a cycle leading to NIDDM. The persistent hyperglycemia desensitizes the islet $\beta$ cell such that less insulin is released for a given blood glucose level. Similarly, the chronic elevated basal levels of insulin downregulate insulin receptors and thereby increase insulin resistance. Furthermore, as sensitivity to insulin declines, glucagon is unopposed and oversecreted; consequently, glucose release by the liver increases, worsening the hyperglycemia. Ultimately, this cycle leads to NIDDM and to progression of NIDDM.

### *Phenotype and Natural History*

NIDDM usually affects obese individuals in middle age or beyond, although an increasing number of children and younger individuals are affected as more and more become obese and sedentary.

NIDDM has an insidious onset and is diagnosed usually by an elevated glucose level on routine examination. In contrast to patients with IDDM, patients with NIDDM usually do not develop ketoacidosis. Generally, the development of NIDDM is divided into three clinical phases. First, the plasma glucose remains normal despite insulin resistance. Second, postprandial hyperglycemia develops despite elevated insulin concentrations. Third, declining insulin secretion causes fasting hyperglycemia and overt diabetes.

In addition to hyperglycemia, the metabolic dysregulation resulting from islet $\beta$-cell dysfunction and insulin resistance causes atherosclerosis, peripheral neuropathy, renal disease, cataracts, and retinopathy (Fig. C–20). The development of these complications is related to the genetic background and degree of metabolic control. Rigorous control of blood glucose levels reduces the risk of complications by 35 to 75 percent.

### *Management*

Weight loss, increased physical activity, and dietary changes help many patients with NIDDM by markedly improving insulin sensitivity and control. Unfortunately, many patients

**Comparison of Type 1 and Type 2 Diabetes Mellitus**

| Characteristic | Type 1 | Type 2 |
|---|---|---|
| Gender | Female = Male | Female > Male |
| Age of onset | Childhood and adolescence | Adolescence through adulthood |
| Ethnic predominance | Caucasians | African Americans, Mexican Americans, Native Americans |
| Concordance | | |
| Monozygotic twins | 33%–50% | 69%–90% |
| Dizygotic twins | 1%–14% | 24%–40% |
| Family history | Uncommon | Common |
| Autoimmunity | Common | Uncommon |
| Body habitus | Normal to wasted | Obese |
| Acanthosis nigricans | Uncommon | Common |
| Plasma insulin | Low to absent | Normal to high |
| Plasma glucagon | High, suppressible | High, resistant |
| Acute complication | Ketoacidosis | Hyperosmolar coma |
| Insulin therapy | Responsive | Responsive to resistant |
| Sulfonylurea therapy | Unresponsive | Responsive |

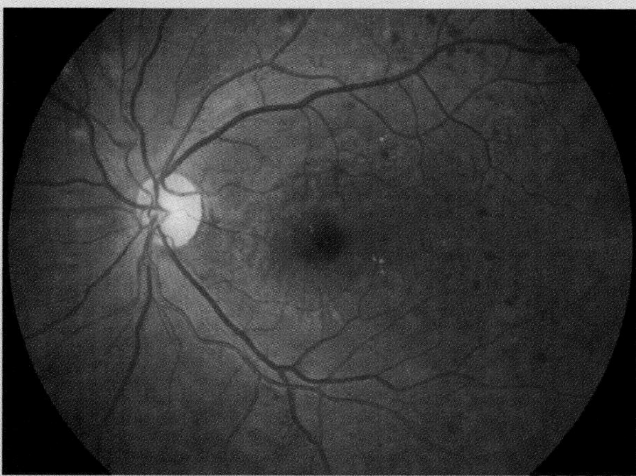

**Figure C–20.** Photograph of nonproliferative diabetic retinopathy in a patient with non–insulin-dependent diabetes mellitus. Note the multiple "dot-and-blot" hemorrhages, the scattered "bread crumb" patches of intraretinal exudate, and, superonasally, a few cotton-wool patches. (Courtesy of R. A. Lewis, Baylor College of Medicine, Houston.)

are unable or unwilling to change their lifestyle sufficiently to accomplish this control and require treatment with oral hypoglycemic agents, such as sulfonylureas and biguanides. Oral hypoglycemics are not as effective as weight loss, increased physical activity, and dietary changes for achieving glycemic control. To achieve glycemic control and, possibly, reduce the risk of diabetic complications, some patients require treatment with exogenous insulin; however, insulin therapy accentuates insulin resistance by increasing hyperinsulinemia and obesity.

## Inheritance Risk

The risk of NIDDM in the general population is highly dependent on the population under consideration; in most populations, this risk is from 1 to 5 percent, although it is 6 to 7 percent in the United States. If a patient has one affected sibling, the risk increases to 1 in 10; if an affected sibling and another first-degree relative, the risk is 1 in 5; and if an affected monozygotic twin, the risk is 1 in 2 to 1 in 1.1. In addition, because some forms of NIDDM are antecedents to IDDM (see case describing F.C.), children of parents with NIDDM have an empiric risk of 1 in 10 for developing IDDM.

### *Questions for Small Group Discussion*

1. How could civil engineering have a major impact on the treatment of patients with NIDDM?
2. What counseling should members, including children, of NIDDM families be given?
3. What factors are contributing to the rising prevalence of NIDDM?

### *Reference*

Foster DW (1998) Diabetes mellitus. *In* Fauci AS, Braunwald E, Isselbacher KJ, et al (eds) Harrison's Principles of Internal Medicine, 14th ed. McGraw-Hill, Philadelphia, pp. 2060–2081.

# Polycystic Kidney Disease

## (PKD1 and PKD2 Mutations)

### Autosomal Dominant

## Principles

- Variable expressivity
- Genetic heterogeneity
- Two-hit hypothesis

## Major Phenotypic Features

- Age of onset: Childhood through adulthood
- Progressive renal failure
- Hepatic cysts
- Intracranial saccular aneurysms
- Mitral valve prolapse
- Colonic diverticula

## History and Physical Findings

Four months ago, P.J., a 35-year-old woman with a history of mitral valve prolapse, developed intermittent flank pain. She eventually presented to her local emergency department with severe pain and hematuria. A renal ultrasound scan showed nephrolithiasis and polycystic kidneys consistent with polycystic kidney disease. The findings from her physical examination were normal except for a systolic murmur consistent with mitral valve prolapse, mild hypertension, and a slight elevation of her serum creatinine. Her father and his sister had died of ruptured intracranial aneurysms, and P.J.'s son had died at 1 year of age from polycystic kidney disease. At the time of her son's death, the physicians had discussed that P.J. and her husband should be evaluated to see whether either of them had polycystic kidney disease; however, the parents elected not to pursue this evaluation because of guilt and grief about their son's death. P.J. was admitted for management of her nephrolithiasis. During this admission, the nephrologists told P.J. that she had autosomal dominant polycystic kidney disease (ADPKD).

## Background

### Disease Etiology

ADPKD is genetically heterogeneous. Approximately 85 percent of patients have mutations in the *PKD1* gene (ADPKD-1), whereas most of the remainder have mutations of *PKD2* (ADPKD-2). A few families have not shown linkage to either of these loci, suggesting that there is at least one additional, as yet unidentified, locus.

ADPKD is one of the most common genetic disorders and has a prevalence of 1 in 300 to 1 in 1000 among all races studied. In the United States, it accounts for 8 to 10 percent of end-stage renal disease.

### Pathogenesis

*PKD1* encodes polycystin-1, a transmembrane receptor–like protein of unknown function. *PKD2* encodes polycystin-2, an integral membrane protein with homology to the voltage-activated sodium and calcium $\alpha 1$ channels. Polycystin-1 and polycystin-2 may interact as part of a heteromultimeric complex.

Cyst formation in ADPKD appears to follow a "two-hit" mechanism such as that observed with tumor suppressor genes and neoplasia (see Chapter 16); that is, both alleles of either *PDK1* or *PDK2* must lose function for cysts to form. The mechanism by which loss of either polycystin-1 or polycystin-2 function causes cyst formation has not been defined.

### Phenotype and Natural History

ADPKD may manifest at any age, but most frequently causes symptoms in the third or fourth decades. Patients present with urinary tract infections, hematuria, urinary tract obstruction (clots or nephrolithiasis), nocturia, hemorrhage into a renal cyst, or complaints of flank pain from the mass effect of the enlarged kidneys (Fig. C–21). Hypertension affects 20 to 30 percent of children with ADPKD and nearly 75 percent of adults with ADPKD. The hypertension is a secondary effect of intrarenal ischemia and activation of the renin-angiotensin system. Nearly half of patients develop end-stage renal disease by 60 years of age. Hypertension, recurrent urinary tract infections, male sex, and early age of symptoms are most predictive of early renal failure. Approximately 43 percent of patients presenting with ADPKD before or shortly after birth die of renal failure within the first year of life; the survivors develop end-stage renal disease or hypertension, or both, by 30 years of age.

ADPKD exhibits both inter- and intrafamilial variation in the age of onset and severity. Part of the interfamilial variation is secondary to genetic heterogeneity because patients with ADPKD-2 have milder disease than do patients with ADPKD-1. Intrafamilial variation appears to result from a combination of environment and genetic background because the variability is more marked between generations than among siblings.

In addition to renal cysts, patients with ADPKD develop hepatic, pancreatic, ovarian, and splenic cysts as well as intracranial aneurysms, mitral valve prolapse, and colonic diverticula. Hepatic cysts are common in both ADPKD-1 and ADPKD-2 whereas pancreatic cysts are generally observed

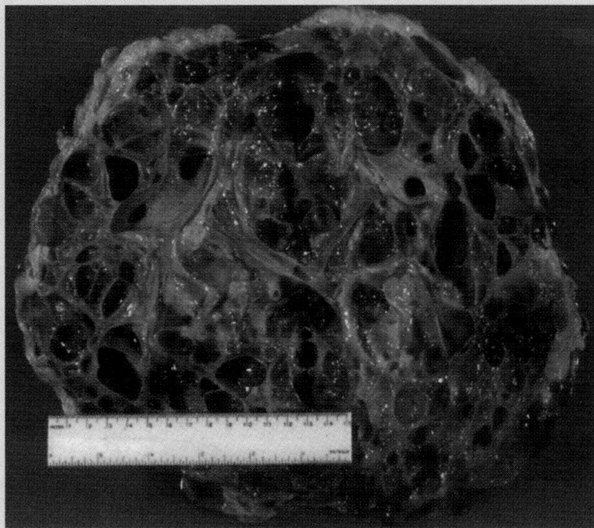

**Figure C–21.** Photograph of a cross section of a kidney from a patient with autosomal dominant polycystic kidney disease. (Courtesy of J. Rutledge, Department of Pathology, University of Washington, Seattle.)

with ADPKD-1. Five to 10 percent of patients with ADPKD develop intracranial saccular aneurysms; however, not all patients have an equal risk for developing these because aneurysms exhibit familial clustering. Patients with ADPKD have an increased risk of aortic and tricuspid valve insufficiency, and approximately 25 percent develop mitral valve prolapse. Colonic diverticula are the most common extrarenal abnormality; the diverticula associated with ADPKD are more likely to perforate than are those observed in the general population.

### *Management*

Generally, ADPKD is diagnosed by family history and renal ultrasound. The detection of renal cysts by ultrasound increases with age such that by age 20 years 80 to 90 percent of patients have detectable cysts and by 30 years nearly 100 percent have them. If necessary for prenatal diagnosis or identification of a related kidney donor, the diagnosis can be confirmed by linkage or mutation detection, or both, in some families.

The management and treatment of patients with ADPKD focuses on slowing the progression of renal disease and minimizing its symptoms. Hypertension and urinary tract infections are treated aggressively to preserve renal function. Pain from the mass effect of the enlarged kidneys is managed often by drainage and sclerosis of the cysts.

## Inheritance Risk

Ninety percent of patients have a family history of ADPKD. Parents with ADPKD have a 50 percent risk of having an affected child in each pregnancy. If the parents have had a child with in utero onset disease, the risk of having another severely affected child is approximately 25 percent. In general, however, the severity of disease cannot be predicted because of variable expressivity. For families in which the mutation is known or in which linkage analysis is possible, the recurrence risk can be modified by analysis of fetal DNA.

Siblings and parents of patients with ADPKD also have an increased risk of disease. Only 10 percent of ADPKD results from *de novo* mutations of either *PDK1* or *PDK2*. Renal ultrasound is the recommended method for the screening of family members.

---

### *Questions for Small Group Discussion*

1. Compare the molecular mechanism of cyst development in ADPKD to the development of neurofibromas in neurofibromatosis type 1.
2. Many mendelian diseases have variable expressivity that might be accounted for by modifier loci. How would one identify such loci?
3. Why is ADPKD frequently associated with tuberous sclerosis? How might this illustrate a contiguous gene deletion syndrome?
4. How can ADPKD be distinguished from autosomal recessive polycystic kidney disease?
5. Linkage analysis of families segregating ADPKD requires the participation of family members in addition to the patient. What should be done if individuals crucial to the study do not want to participate?

### *Reference*

Wu G, Somlo S (2000) Molecular genetics and mechanism of autosomal dominant polycystic kidney disease. Mol Genet Metab 69:1–15.

# Prader-Willi Syndrome

## (Absence of Paternally Derived 15q11-q13)

### Uniparental Disomy, Chromosomal

## Principles

- Imprinting
- Uniparental disomy
- Microdeletion
- Recombination between repeated DNA sequences

## Major Phenotypic Features

- Age of onset: Infancy
- Infantile feeding difficulties
- Childhood hyperphagia and obesity
- Hypotonia
- Cognitive impairment
- Sterility
- Dysmorphism

## History and Physical Findings

J.T. was born at 38 weeks' gestation after an uncomplicated pregnancy and delivery. He was the second child of nonconsanguineous parents. Shortly after birth, his parents and the nurses noticed that J.T. was hypotonic and feeding poorly. His parents and older sister were in good health; J.T. did not have a family history of neuromuscular, developmental, genetic, or feeding disorders. Review of the patient record did not reveal a history of overt seizures, hypoxic insults, infection, cardiac abnormalities, or blood glucose or electrolyte abnormalities. On examination, J.T. did not have respiratory distress or dysmorphic features except for a hypoplastic scrotum and cryptorchidism; his weight and length were appropriate for gestational age; he was severely hypotonic with lethargy, weak cry, decreased reflexes, and poor suck. Subsequent evaluation included testing for congenital infections, brain magnetic resonance imaging, a blood ammonium level, an evaluation of urine organic acids, an amino acid screen, an evaluation for hypothyroidism, and a karyotype with fluorescence in situ hybridization (FISH) for deletion of the Prader-Willi syndrome (PWS) locus (chromosome 15q11-q13) (see Chapter 9). The results of the tests were normal except for the FISH assay, which showed a deletion of chromosome 15q11-q13. The geneticist explained to the parents that J.T. had Prader-Willi syndrome (PWS). After much discussion and thought, J.T.'s parents decided that they were unable to care for a disabled child and gave J.T. up for adoption.

## Background

### *Disease Etiology*

PWS is a panethnic developmental disorder caused by loss of expression of genes on paternally derived 15q11-q13. Loss of paternally expressed genes arises by several mechanisms; approximately 70 percent of patients have a deletion of 15q11-q13, 25 percent have maternal uniparental disomy, less than 5 percent have mutations within the imprinting control element, and less than 1 percent have a chromosomal abnormality (see Chapter 5). PWS has an incidence of 1 in 10,000 to 1 in 15,000 live births.

### *Pathogenesis*

Many genes within the region 15q11-q13 are differentially expressed depending on whether the region is inherited from the father or the mother. In other words, many genes expressed by paternal 15q11-q13 are not expressed by maternal 15q11-q13, and many genes expressed by maternal 15q11-q13 are not expressed by paternal 15q11-q13. This phenomenon of differential expression of a gene depending on whether it is inherited from the father or mother is known as imprinting (see Chapter 5). Maintenance of correct expression of imprinted genes requires switching of the imprint on passage through the germline; that is, paternal imprints are switched to maternal on passage through the maternal germline, and maternal imprints are switched to paternal on passage through the paternal germline. Switching of imprinting on passage through the germline is regulated by the imprinting control element and reflected by changes in the DNA methylation regulating gene expression.

Deletion of 15q11–q13 during male meiosis gives rise to children with PWS because children inheriting a sperm carrying the deletion will not be able to express genes active only on the paternally derived 15q11–q13. The mechanism underlying this recurrent deletion is illegitimate recombination between repeat sequences flanking the deletion interval. Less commonly, inheritance of a deletion spanning this region occurs if a patient inherits an unbalanced karyotype from a parent who has a balanced translocation.

Failure to switch the maternal imprints during male meiosis to paternal imprints gives rise to children with PWS because children inheriting a sperm with a maternally imprinted 15q11–q13 will not be able to express genes active only on the paternally imprinted 15q11–q13. Imprinting failure arises from mutations within the imprinting control element.

Maternal uniparental disomy also gives rise to PWS because the child has two maternal chromosomes 15 and no paternal chromosome 15. Maternal uniparental disomy is thought to develop secondary to trisomy rescue, that is, loss of the paternal chromosome 15 from a conceptus with chromosome 15 trisomy secondary to maternal nondisjunction.

Despite the observations that loss of a paternally imprinted 15q11–q13 gives rise to PWS and despite the identification of many imprinted genes within this region, the precise cause of PWS is still unknown. No abnormal gene product associated with PWS has been identified.

### *Phenotype and Natural History*

In early infancy, PWS is characterized by severe hypotonia, feeding difficulties, and hypogonadism with cryptorchidism. The hypotonia improves over time, although adults remain mildly hypotonic. The hypogonadism, which is of hypothalamic origin, does not improve with time and usually causes delayed and incomplete pubertal development as well as infertility. The feeding difficulties usually resolve within the first year of life, and between 1 and 6 years, the patients develop extreme hyperphagia and food-seeking behavior (hoarding, foraging, and stealing). This behavior and a low metabolic rate cause marked obesity. The obesity is a major cause of morbidity including cardiopulmonary disease and type 2 diabetes mellitus. Longevity can be nearly normal if obesity is avoided.

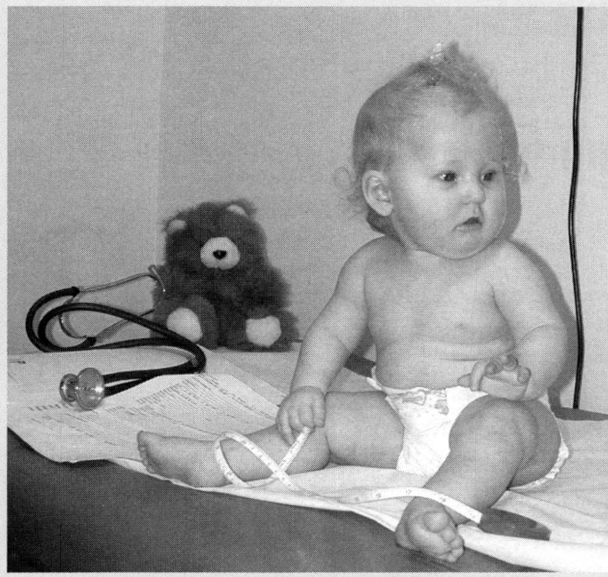

**Figure C–22.** A 12-month-old girl with Prader-Willi syndrome. Note her fair coloring, narrow bifrontal diameter, almond-shaped eyes, and downturned mouth. The hyperphagia, with resulting central obesity, generally does not begin until ages 2 to 6 years. (Photograph courtesy of S. Heeger, University Hospitals of Cleveland.)

Most children with PWS have delayed motor and language development as well as mild mental retardation (mean IQ, 60 to 80) and severe learning disabilities. They also have behavioral problems including temper tantrums, obsessive-compulsive disorders, and poor adaptation to changes in routine. These behavioral problems continue into adulthood and remain very disabling. Approximately 5 to 10 percent of patients also develop psychoses during early adulthood.

Other anomalies associated with PWS include short stature, scoliosis, osteoporosis, and dysmorphism. Dysmorphic features include a narrow bifrontal diameter, almond-shaped eyes, a triangular mouth, and small hands and feet (Fig. C–22). Also, many patients have hypopigmentation of their hair, eyes, and skin.

## *Management*

Although often suspected on the basis of history and physical features, a diagnosis of PWS is defined by absence of a paternally imprinted 15q11–q13. Loss of the paternal imprint is detected by DNA analyses showing that the imprinted genes have only a maternal methylation pattern. If the DNA studies confirm PWS, genetic counseling requires a subsequent karyotype and FISH for 15q11–q13 to determine whether PWS arose from inheritance of a chromosomal translocation.

No medications are currently available to treat the hyperphagia; diet and exercise remain the mainstays for controlling the obesity. Sex hormone replacement promotes secondary sexual features but frequently worsens behavioral problems in males and increases the risk of stroke in females. Behavioral management and serotonin reuptake inhibitors are the most effective therapies currently available for the behavioral disorder. Adult patients usually perform best in sheltered living (group homes) and employment environments.

## Inheritance Risk

The risk for recurrence of PWS in future children of parents is related to the molecular cause. For imprinting defects, the risk can be as high as 50 percent, whereas for either deletion of 15q11–q13 or maternal uniparental disomy, the recurrence risk is less than 1 percent. The risk for recurrence if a parent carries a balanced translocation depends on the translocation but could be as high as 25 percent; to date, however, all reported PWS patients with an unbalanced translocation have had a *de novo* chromosomal rearrangement.

## *Questions for Small Group Discussion*

1. Angelman syndrome also arises from imprinting defects of 15q11–q13. Compare and contrast the phenotypes and causative molecular mechanisms of Prader-Willi syndrome and Angelman syndrome.
2. How might imprinting explain the phenotypes associated with triploidy?
3. Beckwith-Wiedemann syndrome and Russell-Silver syndrome also appear to be caused by abnormal expression of imprinted genes. Explain.
4. J.T.'s parents gave up J.T. for adoption. Should the genetic counseling have been done differently? What is nondirective genetic counseling?

## *Reference*

GeneClinics
*http://www.geneclinics.org/*

# Retinoblastoma

## (RB1 Mutation)

### Autosomal Dominant

## Principles

- Tumor suppressor gene
- Two-hit hypothesis
- Somatic mutation
- Tumor predisposition
- Cell cycle regulation
- Variable expressivity

## Major Phenotypic Features

- Age of onset: Childhood
- Leukocoria
- Strabismus
- Visual deterioration
- Conjunctivitis

## History and Physical Findings

B.B. was a 2-year-old boy who was referred by his pediatrician for evaluation of right strabismus and leukocoria, a reflection from a white mass within the eye giving the appearance of a white pupil (for an example, see Fig. 16–7). His mother reported that he had developed progressive right esotropia during the month before seeing his pediatrician. He had not complained of pain, swelling, or redness of his right eye. He was otherwise healthy. He had healthy parents and a 4-month-old sister; no other family members had had ocular disease. Except for the leukocoria and strabismus, the findings from his physical examination were normal. His ophthalmologic examination defined a solitary retinal tumor of 8 disk diameters arising near the macula. Magnetic resonance imaging of the head did not show extension of the tumor outside the globe. He received chemotherapy combined with focal irradiation (brachytherapy). DNA analysis showed that he had a germline mutation (C to T transition) in one allele of his retinoblastoma (*RB1*) gene.

## Background

### Disease Etiology

Retinoblastoma is a rare embryonic neoplasm of retinal origin (Fig. C–23) that results from germline or somatic mutations, or both, in both alleles of *RB1*. It occurs in all races with an incidence of 1 in 18,000 to 30,000.

### Pathogenesis

The retinoblastoma protein (Rb) is a tumor suppressor that plays an important role in regulating the progression of proliferating cells through the cell cycle and the exit of differentiating cells from the cell cycle. Rb effects these two functions by sequestration of other transcription factors and by promoting deacetylation of histones, a chromatin modification associated with gene silencing.

Retinoblastoma-associated *RB1* mutations occur throughout the coding region and promoter of the gene. Mutations within the coding region of the gene either destabilize Rb or compromise its association with enzymes necessary for histone deacetylation. Mutations within the promoter region reduce expression of normal Rb. Both types of mutations result in a loss of functional Rb.

Forty percent of patients with retinoblastoma have an *RB1* germline mutation, but only 10 percent of all patients have a history of other affected family members. *RB1* mutations include cytogenetic abnormalities of 13q14, single-base substitutions, and small insertions or deletions. Some evidence suggests that the majority of new germline mutations arise on the paternal allele, whereas somatic mutations arise with equal frequency on the maternal and paternal alleles. Nearly half of the mutations occur at CpG dinucleotides. After either the inheritance of a mutated allele or the generation of a somatic mutation on one allele, the other *RB1* allele must also lose function for a cell to proliferate unchecked and develop into a retinoblastoma (see Chapter 16). Loss of a functional second allele occurs by occurrence of a novel mutation, loss of heterozygosity, or promoter CpG island hypermethylation; deletion or the development of isodisomy occurs most frequently, and promoter hypermethylation occurs least frequently.

Retinoblastoma usually segregates as an autosomal dominant disorder with full penetrance; a few families have been described with reduced penetrance, however. The *RB1* mutations identified within these families include missense mutations, in-frame deletions, and promoter mutations. In contrast to the more common null *RB1* alleles, these mutations are believed to represent alleles with some residual function.

### Phenotype and Natural History

Patients with bilateral retinoblastoma generally present during the first year of life, whereas those with unilateral disease present somewhat later with a peak between 24 and 30 months. Seventy percent of patients have unilateral retinoblastoma, and 30 percent have bilateral retinoblastoma. All patients with bilateral disease have germline *RB1* mutations, but not all patients with germline mutations develop bilateral disease. The disease in approximately 80 to

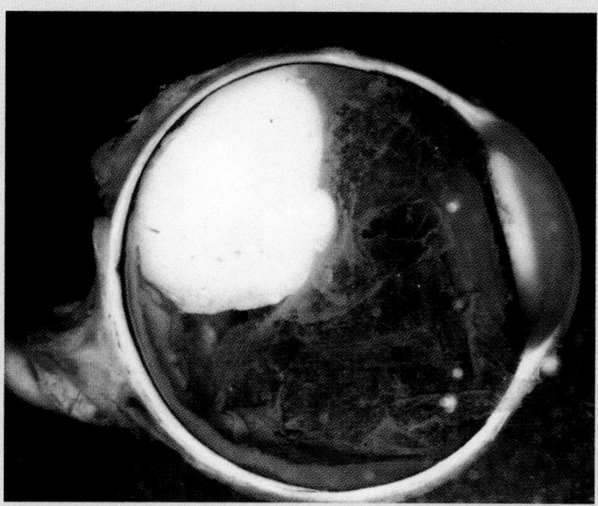

**Figure C–23.** Midline cross section of an enucleated eye from a patient with retinoblastoma. Notice the large primary tumor in the posterior third of the globe and a few white vitreous seeds. (The brown discoloration of the vitreous is a fixation artifact.) (Courtesy of R. A. Lewis, Baylor College of Medicine, Houston.)

95 percent of patients is diagnosed before 5 years. The disease is almost uniformly fatal if not treated, but with appropriate therapy, more than 80 to 90 percent of patients are free of disease 5 years after diagnosis.

As might be expected with mutation of a key cell cycle regulator, patients with germline *RB1* mutations have a markedly increased risk of secondary neoplasms; this risk is increased by environmental factors such as treatment of the initial retinoblastoma with radiotherapy. The most common secondary neoplasms are osteosarcomas, soft-tissue sarcomas, and melanomas. There is no increase in second malignancies in patients with nonhereditary retinoblastoma.

### *Management*

Early detection and treatment are essential for optimal outcome. The goals of therapy are to cure the disease and to preserve as much vision as possible. Treatment is tailored according to the tumor size and involvement of adjacent tissues. Treatment options for intraocular retinoblastoma include enucleation, various modes of radiotherapy, cryotherapy, light coagulation, and chemotherapy.

If the disease is unilateral at the time of patient presentation, the patient needs frequent examinations for the development of new retinoblastomas in the unaffected eye because 30 percent of apparently sporadic cases are caused by the inheritance of a new germline mutation. Such frequent examinations are usually continued until at least 7 years of age.

To direct follow-up more efficiently, patients should receive molecular testing to identify the mutations in the *RB1* gene. Ideally, a tumor sample is tested first, and then another patient tissue such as blood is examined to determine whether one of those mutations is a germline mutation. If neither mutation is a germline mutation, then the patient does not require such frequent follow-up.

## Inheritance Risk

If a parent had bilateral retinoblastoma and thus likely carries a germline mutation, the empiric risk of an affected child is 45 percent; this reflects the high likelihood of a second, somatic mutation (or "hit") occurring in the second *RB1* allele of the child. On the other hand, if the parent had unilateral disease, the empiric risk of an affected child is 7 to 15 percent; this reflects the relative proportion of germline mutations versus somatic mutations in patients with unilateral disease. Ninety percent of children who develop retinoblastoma are the first individual affected within the family. Approximately 1 percent of parents without a clinical history of retinoblastoma have evidence of a spontaneously resolved retinoblastoma on retinal examination; therefore, for these families, the risk of an affected child is 45 percent. Except for the rare situation in which one parent is a nonpenetrant carrier of an *RB1* mutation, families in which neither parent had retinoblastoma have a risk of recurrence equivalent to that of the general population (1 in 18,000 to 30,000).

---

## *Questions for Small Group Discussion*

1. What other diseases develop as a result of a high frequency of mutations in CpG dinucleotides? What is the mechanism of mutation at CpG dinucleotides? What could explain the increased frequency of CpG dinucleotide mutations with increasing paternal age?

2. Compare and contrast the type and frequency of tumors observed in Li-Fraumeni syndrome with those observed in retinoblastoma. Both Rb and p53 are tumor suppressors; why are *TP53* mutations associated with a different phenotype than are *RB1* mutations?

3. Discuss four diseases that arise as a result of somatic mutations. Examples should illustrate chromosomal recombination, loss of heterozygosity, gene amplification, and accumulation of point mutations.

4. Both Sry (see Chapter 10) and Rb regulate development by modulating gene expression through the modification of chromatin structure. Compare and contrast the two different mechanisms that each uses to modify chromatin structure.

## *Reference*

GeneClinics
*http://www.geneclinics.org/*

# Sex Reversal

## (SRY Mutation or Translocation)

### Y-Linked or Chromosomal

## Principles

- Sex reversal
- Developmental regulatory gene
- Illegitimate recombination
- Incomplete penetrance
- Fertility loci

## Major Phenotypic Features

- Age of onset: Prenatal
- Sterility
- Reduced secondary sexual features
- Unambiguous genitalia

## History and Physical Findings

Ms. R., a 37-year-old executive, was pregnant with her first child. Because of her age-related risk of having a child with a chromosomal abnormality, she had elected to have an amniocentesis to assess the fetal karyotype; the karyotype result was normal 46,XX. At 18 weeks' gestation, a fetal ultrasound scan revealed a normal male fetus; a subsequent detailed ultrasound scan confirmed a male fetus. Ms. R had been in good health before and during the pregnancy; she did not have any exposures during the pregnancy. Neither she nor her partner had a family history of ambiguous genitalia, sterility, or congenital anomalies. Re-evaluation of the chromosome analysis confirmed a normal 46,XX karyotype, but fluorescence in situ hybridization identified a sex determining region-Y gene (*SRY*) signal on one X chromosome (Fig. C–24). At 38 weeks of gestation, Ms. R. had an uncomplicated spontaneous vaginal delivery of a phenotypically normal male child.

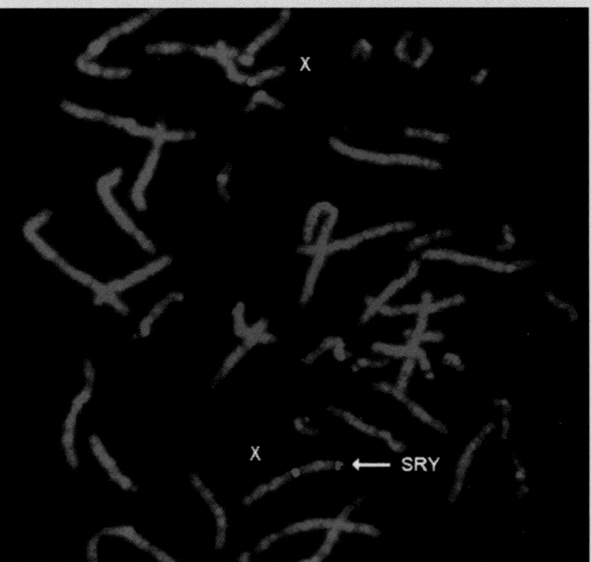


**Figure C–24.** Fluorescence in situ hybridization of a locus-specific probe to metaphase chromosomes for the detection of the t(X;Y)(p22.3; p11.2) in an $SRY^+$ XX male. The chromosomes are counterstained with DAPI. The probe for *SRY* is a mixture of locus-specific sequences *(red)*. The centromere of chromosome X is probed with sequences that map to the alpha satellite DNA *(green)*. In normal cells, the red signal is observed only on the Y chromosome. In cells with t(X;Y)(p22.3; p11.2), a red signal is observed on the abnormal chromosome X and a green signal on both X chromosomes. (Courtesy of B. Bejjani and L. Shaffer, Baylor College of Medicine, Houston.)

## Background

### Disease Etiology

Sex reversal is panethnic and genetically heterogeneous. In patients with complete gonadal dysgenesis, point mutations, deletions, or translocations of *SRY* are the most common cause of sex reversal (see Chapter 10). Approximately 80 percent of 46,XX males with complete gonadal dysgenesis have a translocation of *SRY* onto an X chromosome, and 20 to 30 percent of 46,XY females with complete gonadal dysgenesis have a mutation or deletion involving *SRY*. The incidence of 46,XX males and 46,XY females is about 1 in 20,000.

### Pathogenesis

Sry is a DNA-binding protein that alters chromatin structure by bending DNA. These DNA-binding and DNA-bending properties suggest that Sry regulates gene expression.

During normal human development, Sry is necessary for formation of male genitalia, and its absence is permissive for formation of female genitalia. The precise mechanism through which Sry effects development of male genitalia is undefined, although some observations suggest that Sry represses a negative regulator of testicular development.

*SRY* mutations identified in XY females cause a loss of Sry function. Ten to 15 percent of XY females have a deletion of *SRY* ($SRY^-$ XY females), and 10 to 15 percent have point mutations within *SRY*. The point mutations within *SRY* impair either DNA binding or DNA bending.

The *SRY* alteration observed in XX males is a translocation of *SRY* from Yp to Xp ($SRY^+$ XX males; see Fig. C–24). During male meiosis, an obligatory crossing over occurs between the pseudoautosomal regions of Xp and Yp; this crossing over ensures proper segregation of the chromosomes and maintains sequence identity between the X and Y pseudoautosomal regions. Occasionally, however, recombination occurs centromeric to the pseudoautosomal region and results in the transfer of Yp-specific sequences including *SRY* to Xp (see Chapter 10).

In addition to *SRY*, the Y chromosome contains at least three loci (azoospermic-factor loci AZFa, AZFb, and AZFc) required for normal sperm development. The absence of these loci at least partially explains the infertility of $SRY^+$ XX males.

The X chromosome also contains several loci necessary for ovarian maintenance and female fertility. Oocyte development requires a single X chromosome, but maintenance of those oocytes requires two X chromosomes. Consistent with these observations, XY female fetuses develop oocytes, but their ovarian follicles degenerate by or shortly after birth. The absence of a second X chromosome therefore explains the infertility of XY females.

### Phenotype and Natural History

$SRY^+$ XX males have many features of Klinefelter syndrome (47,XXY), including hypogonadism, azoospermia, hyalinization of seminiferous tubules, and gynecomastia.

Despite decreased testosterone production, most patients enter puberty spontaneously, although they may require testosterone supplementation to attain full virilization. In contrast to patients with Klinefelter syndrome, most 46,XX male patients have normal to short stature, normal skeletal proportions, normal intelligence, and fewer psychosocial problems. Patients with an extensive portion of Yp on an X chromosome resemble patients with Klinefelter syndrome more closely.

*SRY*⁻ XY females have complete gonadal dysgenesis and are usually taller than average for normal women. These patients have physical features of Turner syndrome only when the deletion of *SRY* is associated with an extensive deletion of Yp. Because these patients have only streak gonads, they do not enter puberty spontaneously.

In contrast to the complete penetrance and relatively uniform expressivity observed with translocation or deletion of *SRY*, point mutations of *SRY* exhibit both incomplete penetrance and variable expressivity. Usually patients with *SRY* point mutations have complete gonadal dysgenesis, are taller than average for normal women, and do not spontaneously develop secondary sexual characteristics. A few *SRY* point mutations, however, have been associated with an infertile (complete gonadal dysgenesis) female phenotype and a fertile male phenotype within the same family.

## *Management*

In patients with complete gonadal dysgenesis, the diagnosis of sex reversal usually arises either because of discordance between the fetal ultrasound and fetal karyotype or because of absent or incomplete secondary sexual development and infertility. Confirmation that the sex reversal is secondary to an abnormality of *SRY* expression requires demonstration of the appropriate *SRY* alteration.

For *SRY*⁺ XX males, androgen supplementation is usually effective for virilization, but treatment of the azoospermia is not currently possible. Administration of supplemental androgens does not prevent gynecomastia. Patients need surgical treatment if the gynecomastia becomes sufficiently disconcerting or severe.

For *SRY*⁻ XY females and XY females with point mutations of *SRY*, estrogen therapy is usually initiated at about 14 to 15 years of age to promote development of secondary sexual characteristics. Progesterone therapy is added to the regimen to induce menses either at the time of the first vaginal breakthrough bleeding or in the second year of estrogen therapy. In addition, because of the risk of developing gonadoblastoma, it is recommended that dysgenic gonads be removed once skeletal growth is complete.

As with all disorders of genital ambiguity or of discord between genetic and phenotypic sex, the psychosocial management and counseling of the family and patient are extremely important. Many families and patients have difficulty understanding the medical data and making appropriate psychosocial adjustments.

## Inheritance Risk

*De novo* illegitimate recombination is the most common cause of *SRY*⁺ XX males and *SRY*⁻ XY females; therefore, most couples with an affected child have a low risk of recurrence in future children. Rarely, however, *SRY*⁺ XX males and *SRY*⁻ XY females arise as a result of inheriting a *SRY* deletion or translocation from a father with a balanced translocation between Xp and Yp. If the father is a translocation carrier, all children will be either an *SRY*⁺ XX boy or an *SRY*⁻ XY girl. Because *SRY*⁺ XX males and *SRY*⁻ XY females are invariably sterile, they are at no risk of passing on the disorder.

Most XY females with point mutations in *SRY* have *de novo* mutations. Parents of an affected child, therefore, usually have a low risk of recurrence in future children; however, because some *SRY* mutations have incomplete penetrance, normal fertile fathers can carry *SRY* mutations that may or may not cause sex reversal among their XY children.

---

## *Questions for Small Group Discussion*

1. Mutations of other genes, such as *WT1*, *SOX9*, *SF-1*, and *DAX-1*, can also result in sex reversal. Compare and contrast the phenotypes observed with these mutations with those observed with *SRY* mutations.

2. The association of *SRY* point mutations with an infertile female phenotype and a fertile male phenotype within the same family suggests either stochastic variation dependent on the reduced Sry activity or segregation of another locus that interacts with *SRY*. Why? How could this be resolved?

3. Mutations affecting steroid synthesis or steroid responsiveness are usually associated with ambiguous genitalia, whereas *SRY* mutations are generally associated with reversed but unambiguous genitalia. Discuss the reasons for this generalization.

4. Discuss genetic, gonadal, phenotypic, and psychological gender and the importance of each to genetic counseling.

## *Reference*

Grumbach MM, Conte FA (1998) Disorders of sex differentiation. *In* Wilson JD, Foster DW, Kronenberg HM, Larsen PR (eds) Williams Textbook of Endocrinology, 9th ed. WB Saunders, Philadelphia, pp. 1303–1425.

# Sickle Cell Anemia

## (Beta-Globin Val6Glu Mutation)

### Autosomal Recessive

## Principles

- Heterozygote advantage
- Novel property mutation
- Genetic compound
- Ethnic variation in allele frequencies

## Major Phenotypic Features

- Age of onset: Childhood
- Anemia
- Infarction
- Asplenia

## History and Physical Findings

For the second time in 6 months, a Caribbean couple brought their 24-month-old daughter, C.W., to the emergency department for refusing to bear weight on her feet. There was no history of fever, infection, or trauma, and her medical history was otherwise unremarkable; findings from the previous visit were normal except for a low hemoglobin level and a mildly enlarged spleen. Findings from the physical examination were normal except for a palpable spleen tip and swollen feet. Her feet were very tender to palpation, and she refused to bear weight. Both parents had siblings who died in childhood of infection and others who may have had sickle cell disease. In view of this history and the recurrent painful swelling of her feet, her physician tested C.W. for sickle cell disease by hemoglobin electrophoresis. This test result documented sickle cell hemoglobin in C.W.

## Background

### *Disease Etiology*

Sickle cell disease is an autosomal recessive disorder of hemoglobin in which the $\beta$ subunit genes have a missense mutation causing the substitution of valine for glutamine at amino acid 6. The disease is most commonly due to homozygosity for the sickle cell mutation, although genetic compound between the sickle allele and a hemoglobin C or a $\beta$-thalassemia allele can also have the disease. The prevalence of sickle cell disease varies widely among populations in proportion to past and present exposure to malaria (Table). The sickle mutation appears to have evolved because it confers some resistance to malaria and thus a survival advantage to individuals heterozygous for the mutation.

**Frequencies of the Sickle Cell Mutation among California Newborns**

| Ethnicity | Hb SS | Hb AS |
|---|---|---|
| African American | 1/700 | 1/14 |
| Asian Indian | 0/1600 | 1/700 |
| Hispanic | 1/46,000 | 1/180 |
| Middle Eastern | 0/22,000 | 1/360 |
| Native American | 1/17,000 | 1/180 |
| Caucasian | 1/160,000 | 1/600 |
| Asian | 0/200,000 | 1/1300 |

### *Pathogenesis*

Hemoglobin is composed of four subunits, two $\alpha$ and two $\beta$ subunits (see Chapter 11). The Val6Glu mutation in $\beta$ globin decreases the solubility of deoxygenated hemoglobin and causes it to form a gelatinous network of fibrous polymers that stiffen and distort the cell, that is, sickle-shaped cells (Fig. C–25). These rigid sickled erythrocytes occlude capillaries and cause infarctions. Initially, oxygenation causes the hemoglobin polymer to dissolve and the erythrocyte to regain its normal shape and plasticity; however, repeated sickling and unsickling produce irreversibly sickled cells that are removed from the circulation. The removal of erythrocytes from the circulation exceeds the production capacity of the marrow and causes a hemolytic anemia.

### *Phenotype and Natural History*

Patients with sickle cell disease generally present in the first 2 years of life with anemia, failure to thrive, splenomegaly, repeated infections, and dactylitis (painful swelling of the hands or feet from the occlusion of the capillaries in small bones). Vaso-occlusive infarctions occur in many tissues causing strokes, "acute chest syndrome," renal papillary necrosis, "autosplenectomy," leg ulcers, priapism, bone aseptic necrosis, and visual loss. Bony vaso-occlusion causes painful "crises," and if untreated, these "crises" can persist for days or weeks. The functional asplenia, from infarction and other poorly understood factors, increases susceptibility to bacterial infections such as pneumococcal sepsis and *Salmonella* osteomyelitis. Infection is a major cause of death at all ages, although progressive renal and pulmonary failure are also common causes of death in the fourth and fifth decades. Patients also have a high risk of developing life-threatening aplastic anemia after parvovirus infection because parvovirus infection causes a temporary cessation of erythrocyte production.

In contrast to sickle cell disease, sickle cell trait, seen in heterozygotes for the mutation, is unaccompanied by anemia and is usually clinically silent. Under conditions of severe anoxia such as ascent to high altitudes, however, erythrocytes of patients with sickle cell trait may sickle and cause symptoms similar to those observed with sickle cell disease.

### *Management*

In a given patient with sickle cell disease, there are no accurate predictors for the severity of the disease course. Although the molecular basis of this disease has been known longer than that of any other single gene defect, current treatment is only supportive. No specific therapy that prevents or reverses the sickling process in vivo has been identified. Although gene therapy has the potential to ameliorate and cure this disease (see Chapter 13), effective gene transfer has not been achieved. Allogenic bone marrow transplantation is the only treatment currently available that can cure sickle cell disease.

## Inheritance Risk

Because sickle cell disease is an autosomal recessive disorder, future siblings of an affected child have a 25 percent risk of sickle cell disease and a 50 percent risk of sickle cell trait. Using fetal DNA derived from chorionic villi or amniocytes, prenatal diagnosis is available by molecular analysis for the sickle mutation.

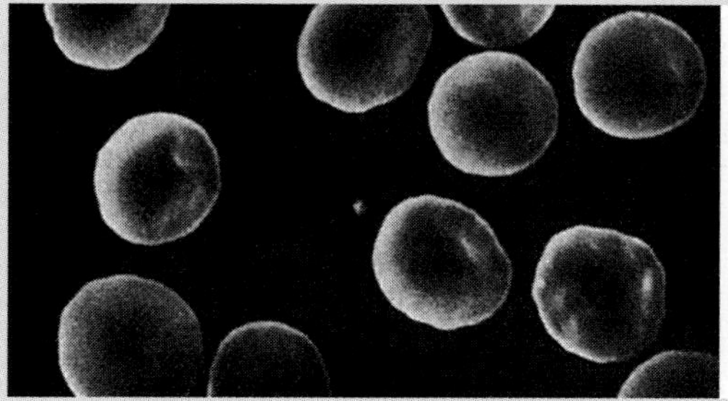
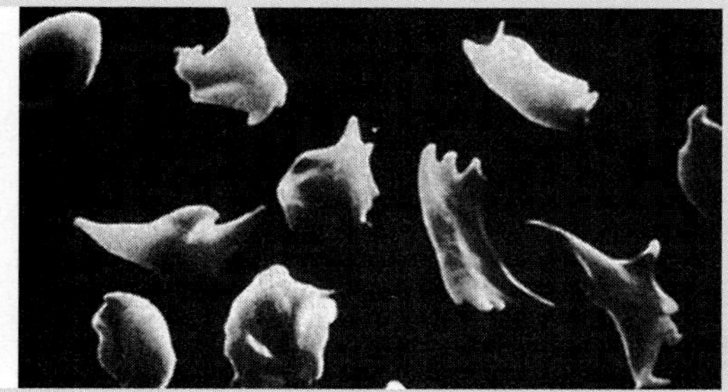

**Figure C–25.** A scanning electron micrograph of red cells from a patient with sickle cell disease. The classic sickle shape is produced only when the cells are in the deoxygenated state *(right)*. Oxygenated cells are on the *left*. (From Kaul DK, Fabry ME, Windisch P, et al [1983] J Clin Invest 72:22, by permission.)

## Questions for Small Group Discussion

1. What are the difficulties with gene therapy for this disorder?
2. Name two other diseases that may have become prevalent because of a heterozygote survival advantage. What is the rationale for hypothesizing a heterozygote advantage for those diseases?
3. Although always a severe disease, the severity of sickle cell disease is determined partially by the haplotype on which the mutation occurs. How could the haplotype affect disease severity?
4. Using the incidence figures in the table, what is the risk that an unrelated African-American woman and man will have a child affected with sickle cell disease? With sickle cell trait?

## References


Reed W, Vichinsky EP (1998) New considerations in the treatment of sickle cell disease. Annu Rev Med 49:461–474.

Weatherall DJ, Clegg JB, Higgs DR, Wood WG (2001) The hemoglobinopathies. *In* Scriver CR, Beaudet AL, Sly WS, et al (eds) The Metabolic and Molecular Bases of Inherited Disease, 8th ed. McGraw-Hill, New York, pp. 4571–4636.

# Tay-Sachs Disease

## (HEXA Mutation)

### Autosomal Recessive

## Principles

- Lysosomal storage disease
- Ethnic variation in allele frequencies
- Genetic drift
- Pseudodeficiency
- Population screening

## Major Phenotypic Features

- Age of onset: Infancy through adulthood
- Neurodegeneration
- Retinal cherry-red spot
- Psychosis

## History and Physical Findings

R.T. and S.T., an Ashkenazic Jewish couple, were referred to the genetics clinic for evaluation of their risk of having a child with Tay-Sachs disease. S.T. had a sister who died of Tay-Sachs disease as a child. R.T. had a paternal uncle living in a psychiatric home, but he did not know what disease his uncle had. The family history was otherwise unremarkable. Both R.T. and S.T. had declined screening for Tay-Sachs carrier status as teenagers. Enzymatic carrier testing showed that both R.T. and S.T. had extremely reduced hexosaminidase A activity. Subsequent molecular analysis for *HEXA* mutations predominant in Ashkenazic Jews confirmed that S.T. carried a disease-causing mutation, whereas R.T. had a pseudodeficiency allele but no disease-causing mutation.

## Background

### Disease Etiology

Tay-Sachs disease, infantile $G_{M2}$ gangliosidosis, is a panethnic autosomal recessive disorder of ganglioside catabolism that is caused by a deficiency of hexosaminidase A (see Chapter 12). In addition to severe infantile-onset disease, hexosaminidase A deficiency causes milder disease with juvenile or adult onset.

The incidence of hexosaminidase A deficiency varies widely among different populations; the incidence of Tay-Sachs disease ranges from 1 in 3600 Ashkenazic Jewish births to 1 in 360,000 non–Ashkenazic Jewish North American births. French Canadians, Louisiana Cajuns, and Pennsylvania Amish have an incidence of Tay-Sachs comparable to that of Ashkenazic Jews. The increased carrier frequency in these four populations appears to be secondary to genetic drift.

### Pathogenesis

Gangliosides, a type of sphingoglycolipid, are a group of ceramide oligosaccharides that have at least one sialic acid residue. Gangliosides reside in all cell surface membranes but are most abundant in the brain. Ganglioside content and distribution vary widely among brain regions, cell types, and cell surface domains. Gangliosides are concentrated in neuronal surface membranes, particularly in the dendrites and axonal termini. They function as receptors for various glycoprotein hormones and bacterial toxins and are involved in cell differentiation and cell-cell interaction.

Hexosaminidase A is a lysosomal enzyme that is composed of two subunits. The $\alpha$ subunit is encoded by the *HEXA* gene on chromosome 15 and the $\beta$ subunit by the *HEXB* gene on chromosome 5. In the presence of activator protein, hexosaminidase A removes the terminal *N*-acetylgalactosamine from the ganglioside $G_{M2}$. Mutations of the $\alpha$ subunit or the activator protein cause the accumulation of $G_{M2}$ in the lysosome and thereby Tay-Sachs disease or a variant thereof. (Mutation of the $\beta$ subunit causes Sandoff disease). The mechanism by which the accumulation of $G_{M2}$ ganglioside causes neuronal death has not been fully defined, although by analogy with Gaucher and Krabbe diseases, toxic byproducts of $G_{M2}$ ganglioside (e.g., lysoganglioside $G_{M2}$) could effect the neuropathology.

The level of residual hexosaminidase A activity correlates inversely with the severity of the disease. Patients with infantile-onset $G_{M2}$ gangliosidosis have two null alleles, that is, no hexosaminidase A enzymatic activity. Patients with juvenile- or adult-onset forms of $G_{M2}$ gangliosidosis are usually compound heterozygotes for a null *HEXA* allele and an allele with low residual hexosaminidase A activity.

### Phenotype and Natural History

Infantile-onset $G_{M2}$ gangliosidosis is characterized by neurological deterioration beginning between ages 3 and 6 months and progressing to death by 2 to 4 years. Motor development usually plateaus or begins to regress by 8 to 10 months and progresses to loss of voluntary movement within the second year of life. Visual loss begins within the first year and progresses rapidly; almost uniformly it is associated with a "cherry-red" spot on fundoscopic examination (Fig. C–26). Seizures usually begin near the end of the first year and progressively worsen. Further deterioration in the second year of life results in decerebrate posturing, difficulties in swallowing, worsening seizures, and, finally, an unresponsive, vegetative state.

Manifesting between 2 and 4 years and progressing to death usually in the second decade, juvenile-onset $G_{M2}$ gangliosidosis is characterized by neurological deterioration beginning with ataxia and incoordination. By the end of the first decade, most patients experience spasticity and seizures; by 10 to 15 years, most develop decerebrate rigidity and enter a vegetative state. Loss of vision is not consistently associated with a cherry-red spot; optic atrophy and retinitis pigmentosa often occur late in the disease course.

Adult-onset $G_{M2}$ gangliosidosis exhibits marked clinical variability (progressive dystonia, spinocerebellar degeneration, motor neuron disease, or psychiatric abnormalities). As many as 40 percent of patients have progressive psychiatric manifestations without dementia. Vision is rarely affected, and the ophthalmological examination is generally normal.

### Management

The diagnosis of a $G_{M2}$ gangliosidosis relies on the demonstration of both absent to nearly absent hexosaminidase A activity in the serum or white blood cells and normal to elevated activity of hexosaminidase B. Mutation analysis of the *HEXA* gene can also be used for diagnosis but is more typically reserved to clarify carrier status and for prenatal testing.

Tay-Sachs disease is currently an incurable disorder; therefore, treatment focuses on management of symptoms and palliative care. Nearly all patients require pharmacological management of their seizures. The psychiatric mani-

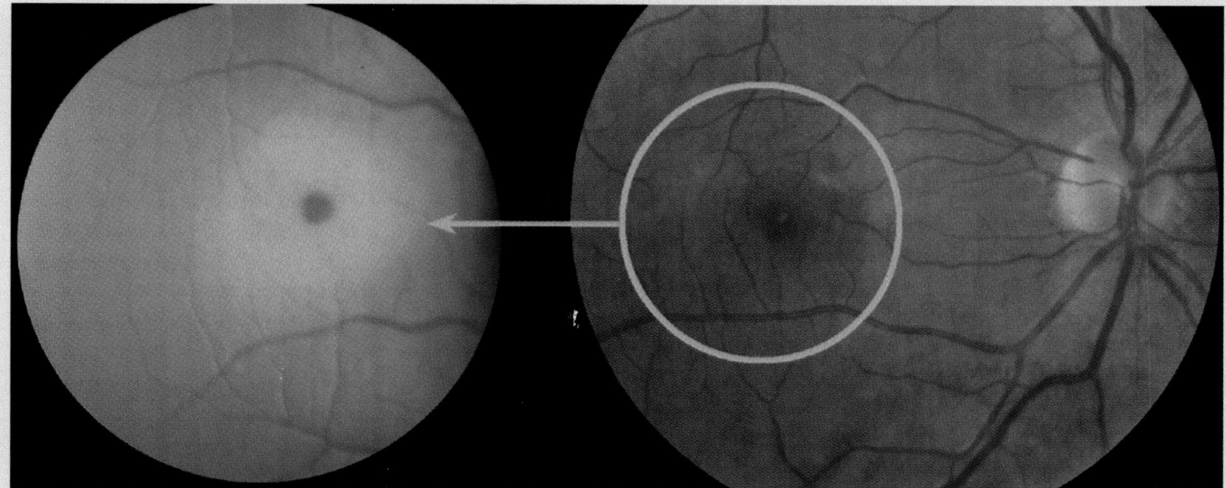

**Figure C–26.** Cherry-red spot in Tay-Sachs disease. *Right* frame shows normal retina. The *circle* surrounds the macula, lateral to the optic nerve. *Left* frame shows the macula of a child with Tay-Sachs disease. The "cherry-red" center is the normal retina of the fovea at the center of the macula that is surrounded by macular retina made white by abnormal storage of $G_{M2}$ in retinal neurons. (Courtesy of A. V. Levin, Hospital for Sick Children and University of Toronto.)

festations of patients with adult-onset $G_{M2}$ gangliosidosis are not usually responsive to conventional antipsychotic or antidepressant medications; lithium and electroconvulsive therapy are most effective.

## Inheritance Risk

For potential parents without a family history of $G_{M2}$ gangliosidosis, their empiric risk for having a child affected with $G_{M2}$ gangliosidosis depends on the frequency of $G_{M2}$ gangliosidosis in their ethnic groups. For most North Americans, their empiric risk of being a carrier is approximately 1 in 250 to 1 in 300, whereas for Ashkenazic Jewish individuals, the empiric risk of being a carrier is approximately 1 in 30. For couples who are each carriers, the risk of having a child with $G_{M2}$ gangliosidosis is 1 in 4.

Prenatal diagnosis relies on identification of the *HEXA* mutations or hexosaminidase A deficiency in fetal tissue such as chorionic villi or amniocytes. Effective identification of affected fetuses by *HEXA* mutation analysis usually requires that the mutations responsible for $G_{M2}$ gangliosidosis in a family have already been identified.

Screening of high-risk populations for carriers and subsequent prevention has reduced the incidence of Tay-Sachs disease among Ashkenazic Jews by nearly 90 percent. Traditionally, such screening is performed by determining the serum activity of hexosaminidase A using an artificial substrate. This sensitive assay, however, cannot distinguish between pathological mutations and pseudodeficiency (reduced catabolism of the artificial substrate but normal catabolism of the natural substrate); therefore, carrier status is usually confirmed by molecular analysis of *HEXA*. Two pseudodeficiency alleles and more than 70 pathological mutations have been identified in *HEXA*. Among Ashkenazic Jews who are positive by enzymatic carrier screening, 2 percent are heterozygous for a pseudodeficiency allele and 95 to 98 percent are heterozygous for one of three pathological mutations, two causing infantile- and one causing adult-onset $G_{M2}$ gangliosidosis. In contrast, among non-Jewish North Americans who are positive by enzymatic carrier screening, 35 percent are heterozygous for a pseudodeficiency allele.

## Questions for Small Group Discussion

1. Screening for what other diseases is complicated by "pseudodeficiency"?
2. Name two other diseases that exhibit genetic drift. What is genetic drift? What are causes of genetic drift?
3. Should population screening be instituted to identify carriers of other diseases?
4. What diseases are genocopies of adult-onset hexosaminidase A deficiency? Consider psychiatric disorders and adult-onset neuronal ceroid lipofuscinosis. Of infantile-onset hexosaminidase A deficiency? Consider $G_{M2}$ activator mutations. How would you distinguish between a genocopy and hexosaminidase A deficiency?

## Reference

GeneClinics
*http://www.geneclinics.org/*

# Thalassemia

## (Alpha- or Beta-Globin Deficiency)

### Autosomal Recessive

## Principles
- Heterozygote advantage
- Ethnic variation in allele frequencies
- Gene dosage

## Major Phenotypic Features
- Age of onset: Childhood
- Hypochromic microcytic anemia
- Hepatosplenomegaly
- Extramedullary hematopoiesis

## History and Physical Findings
J.Z., a 25-year-old healthy Canadian woman, presented to her obstetrician for routine prenatal care. Results of her complete blood count showed a mild microcytic anemia (hemoglobin [Hb], 98 g/L; mean corpuscular volume, 75 $\mu m^3$). She was of Vietnamese origin, and her spouse, T.Z., was of Greek origin. J.Z. was unaware of any blood disorders in her or T.Z's family. Nonetheless, Hb electrophoresis showed a mildly elevated Hb $A_2$ ($\alpha_2\delta_2$) and Hb F ($\alpha_2\gamma_2$), which suggested that J.Z. had $\beta$-thalassemia trait. Molecular testing detected a nonsense mutation in one $\beta$-globin allele and no $\alpha$-globin deletions. The results of T.Z.'s testing showed that he also had a nonsense mutation of one $\beta$-globin allele and no $\alpha$-globin deletions. After referral to the genetics clinic, the geneticist explained to J.Z. and T.Z. that their risk for a child with $\beta$-thalassemia major was 25 percent. After discussing prenatal diagnosis, J.Z. and T.Z. chose to carry the pregnancy to term without further investigation.

## Background
### Disease Etiology
Thalassemias are autosomal recessive anemias caused by deficient synthesis of either $\alpha$ or $\beta$ globin relative to the other chain. A relative deficiency of $\alpha$ globin causes $\alpha$-thalassemia and a relative deficiency of $\beta$ globin causes $\beta$-thalassemia (see Chapter 11).

Thalassemia predominates among persons of Mediterranean, African, Middle Eastern, Indian, Chinese, and Southeast Asian descent. Thalassemias appear to have evolved because they confer some resistance to malaria (see Chapter 7); therefore, the prevalence of thalassemia in an ethnic group reflects past and present exposure of a population to malaria. The prevalence of $\alpha$-thalassemia trait ranges from less than 0.01 percent in natives from nonmalarial areas such as the United Kingdom, Iceland, and Japan to approximately 49 percent among natives of some Southwest Pacific islands; Hb H disease and hydrops fetalis (Table) are restricted to the Mediterranean and Southeast Asia. The incidence of $\beta$-thalassemia trait ranges from approximately 1.5 percent among Africans and African Americans to 30 percent in some villages of Sardinia.

### Pathogenesis
Thalassemia arises from inadequate Hb production and unbalanced accumulation of globin subunits. Inadequate Hb production causes hypochromia and microcytosis. Unbalanced accumulation of globin causes ineffective erythropoiesis and hemolytic anemia. The severity of thalassemia is proportionate to the severity of the imbalance between $\alpha$ globin and $\beta$ globin.

Nearly 200 different mutations have been associated with thalassemia; only a few mutations account for most thalassemia, however. Deletion of $\alpha$-globin genes accounts for 80 to 85 percent of $\alpha$-thalassemia, and approximately 15 mutations account for more than 90 percent of $\beta$-thalassemia. Molecular studies of both $\alpha$-globin and $\beta$-globin mutations strongly suggest that the various mutations have arisen independently in different populations and then achieved their high frequency by selection.

### Phenotype and Natural History
The $\alpha$-globin mutations are separated into four clinical groups that reflect the impairment of $\alpha$-globin production (see Table).

The phenotypes observed in a population reflect the types of $\alpha$-globin mutations in that population. Chromosomes with deletion of both $\alpha$-globin genes are observed in Southeast Asia and the Mediterranean basin; therefore, Hb H disease and hydrops fetalis usually occur in these populations and not in Africans who usually have chromosomes with deletion of one $\alpha$-globin gene.

| Phenotype | No. of Functional $\alpha$-Globin Genes | $\alpha$:$\beta$-Globin Ratio | $\alpha$-Globin Genotypes | Hb H Inclusions | Complications |
|---|---|---|---|---|---|
| Normal | 4 | 1 | $\alpha\alpha/\alpha\alpha$ | None | None |
| Silent carrier | 3 | 0.8 | $-\alpha/\alpha\alpha$<br>$--/\alpha\alpha\alpha$ | Rare | None |
| $\alpha$-thalassemia trait | 2 | 0.6 | $-\alpha/-\alpha$<br>$--/\alpha\alpha$ | Occasional | Mild anemia |
| Hb H disease | 1 | 0.3 | $--/-\alpha$ | Many | Moderate anemia, jaundice, hepatosplenomegaly, gallstones, increased susceptibility to infection, folic acid deficiency. |
| Hydrops fetalis | 0 | 0.0 | $--/--$ | Present | Severe anemia, congestive heart failure, fatal *in utero* or shortly after birth. |

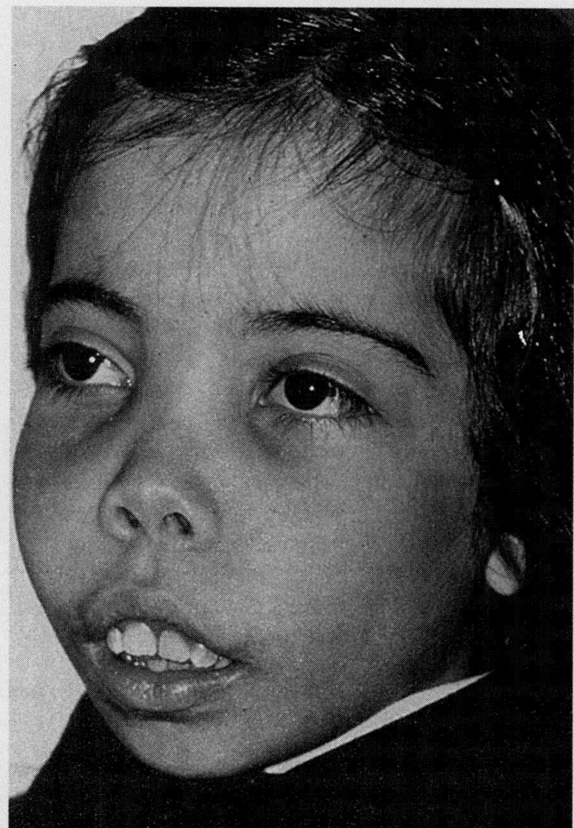

**Figure C–27.** The typical facial appearance of a child with untreated $\beta$-thalassemia. Note the prominent cheek bones and the protrusion of the upper jaw that results from the expansion of the marrow cavity in the bones of the skull and face. (Courtesy of N. Olivieri, The Hospital for Sick Children and University of Toronto.)

The $\beta$-globin mutations are also divided into clinical groups reflecting the impairment of $\beta$-globin production (see Table). Beta-thalassemia trait is associated with a mutation in one $\beta$-globin allele and $\beta$-thalassemia major with mutations in both $\beta$-globin alleles. Generally, patients with $\beta$-thalassemia trait have a mild hypochromic microcytic anemia, mild bone marrow erythroid hyperplasia, and, occasionally, hepatosplenomegaly; they are usually asymptomatic. Patients with $\beta$-thalassemia major present with anemia when the postnatal production of Hb F decreases. The severe hemolytic anemia and ineffective erythropoiesis cause growth retardation, jaundice, hepatosplenomegaly (extramedullary hematopoiesis), and bone marrow expansion (Fig. C–27). Approximately 80 percent of untreated patients die by 5 years; patients receiving transfusion therapy alone die before 30 years of infection or hemachromatosis; patients receiving transfusion therapy with iron chelation therapy usually survive beyond the third decade. Iron overload from repeated transfusions and increased intestinal absorption causes cardiac, hepatic, and endocrine complications.

## Management

Initial screening for $\alpha$- or $\beta$-thalassemia trait is usually done by determination of erythrocyte indices. For patients without iron deficiency anemia, the diagnosis of $\beta$-thalassemia trait is usually confirmed by quantitative determination of Hb $A_2$ and Hb F or DNA mutation analysis, or both. Unassociated with Hb $A_2$ or Hb F, $\alpha$-thalassemia trait is confirmed by DNA mutation analysis or demonstration of a high $\beta/\alpha$-globin ratio.

Treatment of Hb H disease is primarily supportive. Therapy includes folate supplementation, avoidance of oxidant drugs and iron, prompt treatment of infection, and judicious transfusion. Splenectomy is rarely required.

Treatment of $\beta$-thalassemia includes blood transfusions, iron chelation, prompt treatment of infection, and, frequently, splenectomy. Bone marrow transplantation is the only currently available cure.

## Inheritance Risk

If each parent has $\beta$-thalassemia trait, the couple has a 25 percent risk of having a child with $\beta$-thalassemia major and a 50 percent risk of having a child with $\beta$-thalassemia trait. If one parent has $\beta$-thalassemia trait and the other parent a triplication of the $\alpha$-globin gene, this couple could also have a 25 percent risk of having a child with $\beta$-thalassemia major.

For parents with $\alpha$-thalassemia trait, their risk for a child with Hb H disease or hydrops fetalis depends on the nature of their $\alpha$-globin mutations. Parents with $\alpha$-thalassemia trait can have either a $-\alpha/-\alpha$ or $--/\alpha\alpha$ genotype; therefore, depending on their genotypes, they have a 25 percent risk of having a child with Hb H disease or hydrops fetalis.

For both $\alpha$- and $\beta$-thalassemia, prenatal diagnosis is possible by molecular analysis of fetal DNA from either chorionic villi or amniocytes. Molecular prenatal diagnosis of thalassemia is most efficient if the mutations have already been identified in the carrier parents.

## Questions for Small Group Discussion

1. A father has the genotype $\alpha\alpha\alpha/\alpha-$, $\beta/\beta$ and a mother $\alpha\alpha/\alpha\alpha$, $\beta/-$. If their child has the genotype $\alpha-/\alpha\alpha$, $\beta/-$, what is the most likely phenotype? Why? If the child's genotype is $\alpha\alpha\alpha/\alpha\alpha$, $\beta/-$, what is the most likely phenotype? Why?
2. What are the molecular mechanisms of $\alpha$-globin gene deletion? Of $\alpha$-globin gene triplication?
3. How does expression of $\gamma$ globin protect against $\beta$-thalassemia?
4. Describe carrier screening for thalassemia. To what ethnic groups should carrier screening be applied? Should individuals from classically low-risk ethnic groups be screened if their partner has $\alpha$- or $\beta$-thalassemia trait? Consider population admixture.
5. $\alpha$-Thalassemia is the most common single gene disorder in the world. Three mechanisms can increase the frequency of a mutation in a population: selection, genetic drift, and founder effects. Describe each mechanism and the reason(s) selection likely accounts for the high frequency of $\alpha$-thalassemia.

## Reference

Orkin S, Nathan D (1998) The thalassemias. *In* Orkin S, Nathan D (eds) Nathan and Oski's Hematology of Infancy and Childhood. WB Saunders, Philadelphia, pp. 811–886.

# Turner Syndrome

## (Female Monosomy X)

### Chromosomal

## Principles

- Nondisjunction
- Prenatal selection
- Haploinsufficiency

## Major Phenotypic Features

- Age of onset: Prenatal
- Short stature
- Ovarian dysgenesis
- Sexual immaturity

## History and Physical Findings

L.W., a 14-year-old girl, was referred to the endocrinology clinic for evaluation of absent secondary sexual characteristics (menses and breast development). Although born small for gestational age, she had been in good health and had normal intellect. No other family members had similar problems. The findings from her examination were normal except for short stature, Tanner stage I sexual development, and a broad chest with widely spaced breasts. After briefly discussing some causes of short stature and delayed or absent sexual development, her physician requested a follicle stimulating hormone (FSH) level, growth hormone (GH) level, bone age analysis, and chromosome analysis. These tests showed a normal growth hormone level, an elevated FSH level, and an abnormal karyotype (45,X). The physician explained that L.W. had Turner syndrome (TS). L.W. was treated with growth hormone supplements to maximize her linear growth; a year later, she started estrogen and progesterone therapy to induce the development of secondary sexual characteristics.

## Background

### *Disease Etiology*

TS is a panethnic disorder caused by complete or partial absence of a second X chromosome in females. It has an incidence of between 1 in 2000 to 1 in 5000 among liveborn girls. Fifty percent of TS is associated with a 45,X karyotype, 25 percent with a structural abnormality of the second X chromosome, and 25 percent with 45,X mosaicism (see Chapter 10).

Monosomy for the X chromosome can arise either by failure to include a sex chromosome in one of the gametes or by loss of a sex chromosome from the zygote or early embryo. Failure to include a sex chromosome in a gamete is the most common cause of a 45,X karyotype; 70 to 80 percent of patients with a 45,X karyotype are conceived from a sperm lacking a sex chromosome. Loss of a sex chromosome by a cell in the early embryo is likely the cause of 45,X mosaicism.

### *Pathogenesis*

The mechanism by which X chromosome monosomy causes TS in girls is poorly understood. The X chromosome contains several loci necessary for ovarian maintenance and female fertility. Although oocyte development requires only a single X chromosome, maintenance of those oocytes requires two X chromosomes. In the absence of a second X chromosome, therefore, oocytes in fetuses and neonates with TS degenerate, and their ovaries atrophy into streaks of fibrous tissue. The genetic bases for the other features of TS such as the cystic hygroma, lymphedema, broad chest, cardiac anomalies, renal anomalies, and sensorineural hearing deficit have not been defined, but presumably reflect to some degree haploinsufficiency for one or more X-linked gene(s).

### *Phenotype and Natural History*

Although 45,X conceptuses account for between 1 and 2 percent of all pregnancies, less than 1 percent of 45,X conceptions result in a liveborn infant. In view of the mild phenotype observed in patients with TS, this high rate of miscarriage is remarkable and suggests that a second sex chromosome is required for intrauterine survival.

All patients with TS have short stature, and more than 90 percent have ovarian dysgenesis. The ovarian dysgenesis is sufficiently severe that only 10 to 20 percent of patients have spontaneous pubertal development (breast budding and pubic hair growth) and only 2 to 5 percent develop spontaneous menses. Many individuals also have physical anomalies, such as a webbed neck, low nuchal hairline, broad chest, cardiac anomalies, renal anomalies, sensorineural hearing deficit, edema of the hands and feet, and dysplastic nails. Nearly 50 percent of patients have a bicuspid aortic valve and, therefore, an increased risk of aortic root dilatation; nearly 60 percent have renal anomalies and, therefore, an increased risk of renal dysfunction.

Most patients have normal intellectual development. Those with intellectual impairment usually have an X-chromosome structural abnormality. Socially, individuals with TS tend to be shy and withdrawn (see Chapter 10).

In addition to the complications resulting from their congenital anomalies, women with TS have an increased incidence of osteoporotic fractures, thyroiditis, diabetes mellitus type 1 and type 2, inflammatory bowel disease, and cardiovascular disease. The causes of the diabetes mellitus, thyroid disorders, and inflammatory bowel disease are unclear. Estrogen deficiency, however, is probably largely responsible for the osteoporosis and for the increased incidence of atherosclerosis, ischemic heart disease, and stroke, although diabetes mellitus likely accentuates the cardiovascular effects of estrogen deficiency.

### *Management*

When a TS patient's stature falls below the fifth percentile, she is usually treated with growth hormone supplements until her bone age reaches 15 years (Fig. C–28). On average, this treatment results in a gain of 10 cm in predicted height; the improvement in final height decreases the later growth hormone therapy is started, however. Concurrent estrogen therapy decreases the effectiveness of growth hormone.

Estrogen therapy is usually initiated at about 14 to 15 years of age to promote development of secondary sexual characteristics. Progesterone therapy is added to the regimen to induce menses either at the time of the first vaginal breakthrough bleeding or in the second year of estrogen therapy.

In addition, medical management usually includes echocardiography for evaluation of aortic root dilatation and valvular heart disease, a renal ultrasound for evaluation

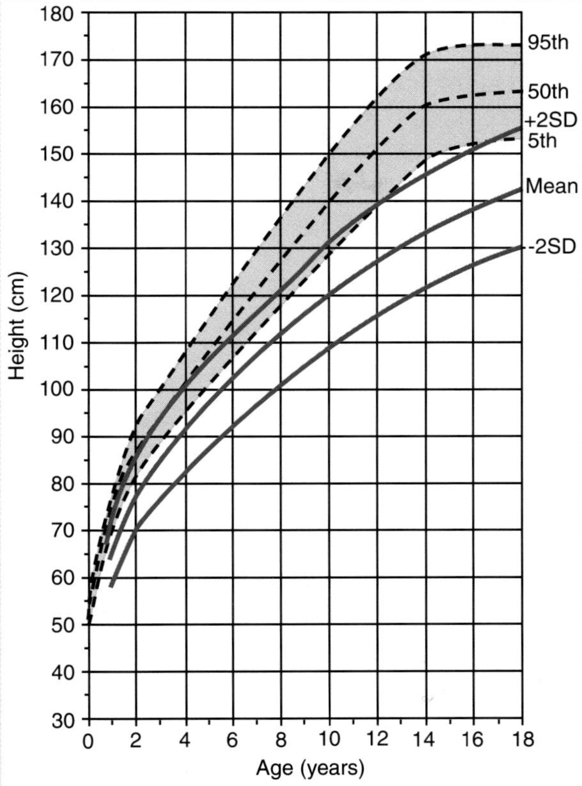


**Figure C–28.** Growth curves for normal girls *(shaded)* and girls with Turner syndrome. None of the girls received hormone treatment. (Adapted from Lyon AJ, Preece MA, Grant DB [1985] Arch Dis Child 60:932, by permission from the BMJ Publishing Group.)

of congenital renal anomalies, and a glucose tolerance test for detection of diabetes.

Patients who have complete ovarian dysgenesis do not ovulate spontaneously or conceive children. If they have adequate cardiovascular and renal function, however, women with TS can have children using in vitro fertilization and ovum donation.

## Inheritance Risk

TS is not associated with advanced maternal or paternal age. Although there have been a few familial recurrences, TS is usually sporadic, and the empiric recurrence risk for future pregnancies is not increased over that of the general population. If TS is suspected based on fetal ultrasound findings such as a cystic hygroma, the diagnosis should be confirmed by karyotyping of chorionic villi or amniocytes.

Only a few pregnancies have been reported among spontaneously menstruating patients with TS. Among the resulting offspring, one in three has had congenital anomalies such as congenital heart disease, Down syndrome, and spina bifida. The cause or causes of this increased risk for congenital anomalies has not been defined.

## *Questions for Small Group Discussion*

1. Some observations have suggested that patients with TS who inherit a paternal X chromosome are more outgoing and have better social adaptation than those who inherit a maternal X chromosome. What molecular mechanisms could explain this?
2. X-chromosome monosomy is the only viable human monosomy. Discuss possible reasons.
3. Discuss possible reasons for the high rate of birth defects among the children of women with TS.
4. Maternal meiotic nondisjunction gives rise more frequently to Down syndrome and paternal meiotic nondisjunction to Turner syndrome. Discuss possible reasons.
5. Discuss the psychosocial support and counseling that are appropriate and necessary for patients with TS.

## *References*


Saenger P (1996) Turner's syndrome. N Engl J Med 335:1749–1754.

Zinn AR, Ross JL (1998) Turner syndrome and haploinsufficiency. Curr Opin Genet Dev 8:322–327.

# Xeroderma Pigmentosum

## (Defect of Nucleotide Excision Repair)

### Autosomal Recessive

## Principles

- Variable expressivity
- Genetic heterogeneity
- Genetic complementation

## Major Phenotypic Features

- Age of onset: Childhood
- Ultraviolet light sensitivity
- Skin cancer
- Neurological dysfunction

## History and Physical Findings

W.S., a 3-year-old girl, was referred to the dermatology clinic for evaluation of severe sun sensitivity and freckling. On physical examination, she was photophobic and had conjunctivitis and prominent freckled hyperpigmentation in sun-exposed areas; her development and findings from the physical examination were otherwise normal. W.S. was the child of nonconsanguineous Japanese parents; no one else in the family was similarly affected. The dermatologist explained that W.S. had classic features of xeroderma pigmentosum (XP), that is, "parchment-like pigmented skin." To confirm the diagnosis, W.S. had a skin biopsy to evaluate DNA repair and ultraviolet (UV) radiation sensitivity in her skin fibroblasts. The results of this testing confirmed the diagnosis of XP. Despite appropriate preventive measures, W.S. developed metastatic melanoma at 15 years of age and died 2 years later. Her parents had two more children; neither was affected with XP.

## Background

### *Disease Etiology*

XP is a genetically heterogeneous panethnic autosomal recessive disorder of DNA repair that causes marked sensitivity to UV irradiation. In the United States and Europe, the prevalence is approximately 1 in 1 million, but in Japan, the prevalence is 1 in 100,000 (see Chapter 9).

### *Pathogenesis*

Repair of DNA damaged by UV irradiation occurs by three mechanisms: excision repair, postreplication repair, and photoreactivation. Excision repair mends DNA damage by nucleotide excision repair or base excision repair. Postreplication repair is a damage tolerance mechanism that allows replication of DNA across a damaged template. Photoreactivation reverts damaged DNA to the normal chemical state without removing or exchanging any genetic material.

Nucleotide excision repair is a complex but versatile process involving at least 30 proteins. The basic principle is the removal of a small single-stranded DNA segment containing a lesion by dual incision of the damaged strand and subsequent gap-filling repair synthesis using the intact complementary strand as a template. Within transcribed genes, DNA damage blocks RNA polymerase II progression; the stalled RNA polymerase II initiates nucleotide excision repair (transcription coupled repair). In the rest of the genome and on nontranscribed strands of genes, a nucleotide excision repair complex identifies DNA damage by detection of helical distortions within the DNA (global genome repair).

Occasionally, nucleotide excision repair will not have repaired a lesion before DNA replication. Because such lesions inhibit the progression of DNA replication, postreplication repair bypasses the lesion, allowing DNA synthesis to continue. DNA polymerase $\eta$ mediates translesional DNA synthesis; it efficiently and accurately catalyzes synthesis past dithymidine lesions.

XP is caused by mutations affecting the global genome repair subpathway of nucleotide excision repair or by mutations affecting postreplication repair. In contrast, Cockayne syndrome, a related disorder, is caused by mutations affecting the transcription coupled repair subpathway of nucleotide excision repair. XP and Cockayne syndrome have been separated into 10 biochemical complementation groups; each group reflects a mutation of a different component of nucleotide excision repair or postreplication repair (Table).

The reduced or absent capacity for global genome repair or postreplication repair results in the accumulation of mutations within cells. Cutaneous neoplasms from patients with XP have a higher level of oncogene and tumor-suppressor gene mutations than have tumors from the normal population, and those mutations appear to be highly UV-specific.

### *Phenotype and Natural History*

Patients with XP develop symptoms at a median age of 1 to 2 years, although in approximately 5 percent of patients, onset occurs after 14 years. Initial symptoms commonly include easy sunburning, acute photosensitivity, freckling, and photophobia. Continued cutaneous damage causes premature skin aging (thinning, wrinkling, solar lentigines,

| Complementation Group | Gene | Process Affected | Phenotype |
|---|---|---|---|
| XPA | *XPA* | DNA damage recognition | XP |
| XPB | *ERCC3* | DNA unwinding | XP-CS, TTD |
| XPC | *XPC* | DNA damage recognition | XP |
| XPD | *ERCC2* | DNA unwinding | XP, TTD, XP-CS |
| XPE | *DDB2* | DNA damage recognition | XP |
| XPF | *ERCC4* | Endonuclease | XP |
| XPG | *ERCC5* | Endonuclease | XP, XP-CS |
| XPV | *POLH* | Translesional DNA synthesis | XP |
| CSA | *CKN1* | Transcription coupled repair | CS |
| CSB | *ERCC6* | Transcription coupled repair | CS |

CS = Cockayne syndrome; TTD = trichothiodystrophy; XP-CS = combined XP and Cockayne syndrome phenotype.

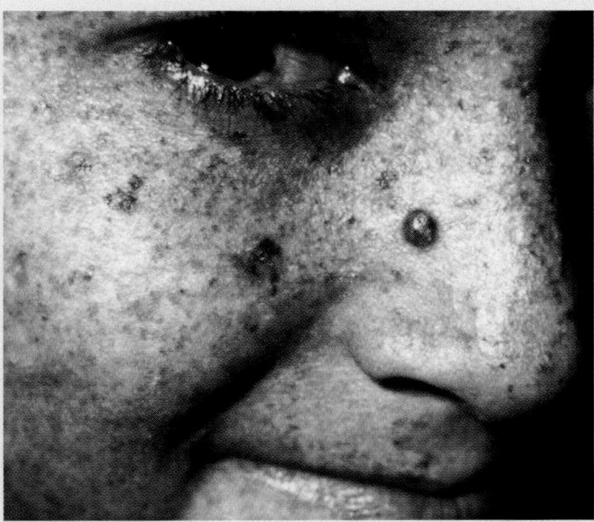

**Figure C–29.** Cutaneous and ocular findings of xeroderma pigmentosum. Note the freckled hyperpigmentation and the papillomatous and verrucous lesions on the skin and the conjunctivitis. (Courtesy of M. L. Levy, Baylor College of Medicine and Texas Children's Hospital, Houston.)

telangiectasis), premalignant actinic keratoses, and benign and malignant neoplasms (Fig. C–29). Nearly 45 percent of patients develop basal cell or squamous cell carcinomas, or both, and approximately 5 percent develop melanomas. Ninety percent of the carcinomas occur at the sites of greatest UV exposure—the face, neck, head, and tip of the tongue. Before the introduction of preventive measures, the median age for developing cutaneous neoplasms was 8 years, 50 years younger than the general population, and the frequency of such neoplasms was more than 1000-fold greater than that of the general population.

In addition to cutaneous symptoms, 60 to 90 percent of patients experience ocular abnormalities. Symptoms include photophobia, conjunctivitis, blepharitis, ectropion, and neoplasia. Again, the distribution of ocular damage and neoplasms corresponds to the sites of greatest UV exposure.

Approximately 18 percent of patients experience progressive neuronal degeneration. Symptoms include sensorineural deafness, mental retardation, spasticity, hyporeflexia or areflexia, segmental demyelination, ataxia, choreoathetosis, and supranuclear ophthalmoplegia. The severity of neurological symptoms is usually proportionate to the severity of the nucleotide excision repair deficit. The neurodegeneration may result from an inability to repair DNA damaged by endogenously generated oxygen free radicals.

Nucleotide excision repair also corrects DNA damage from many chemical carcinogens, such as cigarette smoke, charred food, and cisplatin. Consequently, patients have a 10- to 20-fold increase in the incidence of internal neoplasms, such as brain tumors, leukemia, lung tumors, and gastric carcinomas.

Patients with XP have a shortened life span; without preventive protection, their life span is about 30 years shorter than that of individuals without XP. Metastatic melanoma and squamous cell skin carcinoma are the most common causes of death.

### Management

Confirmation of the diagnosis of XP relies on functional tests of DNA repair and UV sensitivity; such tests are usually performed on cultured skin fibroblasts. Diagnostic confirmation by identification of mutations in an XP-associated gene is not currently clinically available.

The management of patients with XP includes avoiding exposure to sunlight, protective clothing, physical and chemical sunscreens, and careful surveillance for and excision of cutaneous malignancies. No curative treatments are currently available.

## Inheritance Risk

Because XP is an autosomal recessive disease, many patients do not have a family history of the disease. For parents who already have a child affected with XP, the risk for future children having XP is 1 in 4. Prenatal diagnosis is possible by functional testing of DNA repair and UV sensitivity in cultured amniocytes or chorionic villi.

---

### Questions for Small Group Discussion

1. Define complementation groups and explain their use for defining the biochemical bases of diseases.
2. Compare and contrast XP and Cockayne syndrome. Why is Cockayne syndrome not associated with an increased risk of neoplasia?
3. Patients with XP have a defect of cutaneous cellular immunity. How could the sensitivity of patients with XP to UV radiation explain this immunodeficiency? How could this immunodeficiency contribute to cancer susceptibility?
4. Werner syndrome, Bloom syndrome, XP, ataxia telangiectasia, and Fanconi anemia are inherited diseases of genomic instability. What are the molecular mechanisms underlying each of these disorders? What types of genomic instability are associated with each disorder?

### Reference

de Boer J, Hoeijmakers JHJ (2000) Nucleotide excision repair and human syndromes. Carcinogenesis 21:453–460.

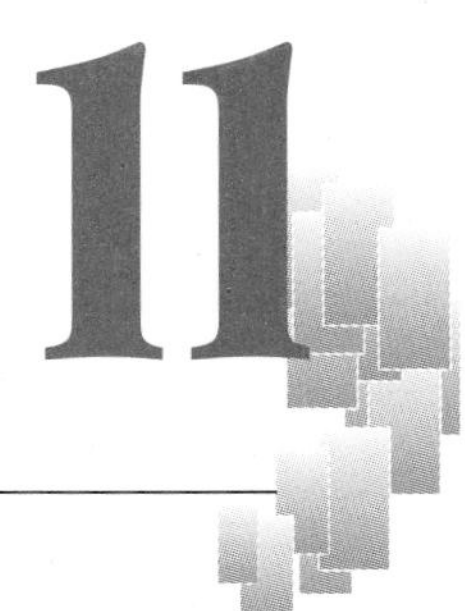

# 11 Principles of Molecular Disease: Lessons from the Hemoglobinopathies

A molecular disease is one in which the primary disease-causing event is a mutation, either inherited or acquired. This chapter outlines the basic genetic and biochemical mechanisms underlying genetic disease, using disorders of hemoglobin—the **hemoglobinopathies**—as examples. This overview of mechanisms is expanded in Chapter 12 to include other genetic diseases that are important because they illustrate additional principles of genetics in medicine.

Knowledge of molecular pathology is the foundation of rational therapy and management for genetic diseases. Moreover, such knowledge is also often instructive about normal function. The study of phenotype at the level of proteins, biochemistry, and metabolism constitutes the discipline of **biochemical genetics**. A genetic disease occurs when an alteration in the DNA of an essential gene changes the amount or function, or both, of the gene products (messenger RNA [mRNA] and protein). Single-gene disorders almost always result from mutations that alter the function of a protein. The only known exceptions to this generalization are mutations found in several genes of the mitochondrial DNA that encode transfer RNAs (tRNAs); these mutations lead to serious neurological conditions affecting muscle or brain (see Chapter 12).

Understanding the pathogenesis of a genetic disease is not possible without knowledge of the primary biochemical abnormalities that result from the alteration in gene function. Disease-causing mutations have been identified in more than 1000 of the approximately 4500 single-gene diseases (both autosomal and X-linked) currently recognized. Although it is impressive that the basic molecular defect has been found in so many disorders, it is sobering to realize that the pathophysiology is not entirely understood for *any* genetic disease. **Sickle cell disease,** discussed later, is among the best characterized of inherited disorders, and, even here, knowledge is incomplete—although it was the first molecular disease to be recognized (by Linus Pauling in 1949). Nevertheless, the study of genetic disease at its various phenotypic levels (gene, protein, cell, tissue, whole body) has informed medicine greatly, not only about specific disorders, but also about the normal biology of the human body.

## THE EFFECT OF MUTATION ON PROTEIN FUNCTION

The four possible effects of disease-causing mutations on protein function are outlined in Figure 11–1. A **loss of function** of the protein is the most common consequence of mutation. Many important conditions arise, however, from one of three other mechanisms: (1) a **gain of function**; (2) the acquisition of a **novel property** by the mutant protein; or (3) the expression of a gene at the wrong time (**heterochronic expression**), or in the wrong place (**ectopic expression**), or both.

### Loss-of-Function Mutations

Loss of function of a gene may result from mutations in either its coding or its regulatory elements or from the disruption by insertions or deletions of critical sequences. The loss of function due to a reduction in gene dosage is exemplified by the **α-thalassemias,** which are due most commonly to deletions of α-globin genes (see later discussion); by chromosome-loss

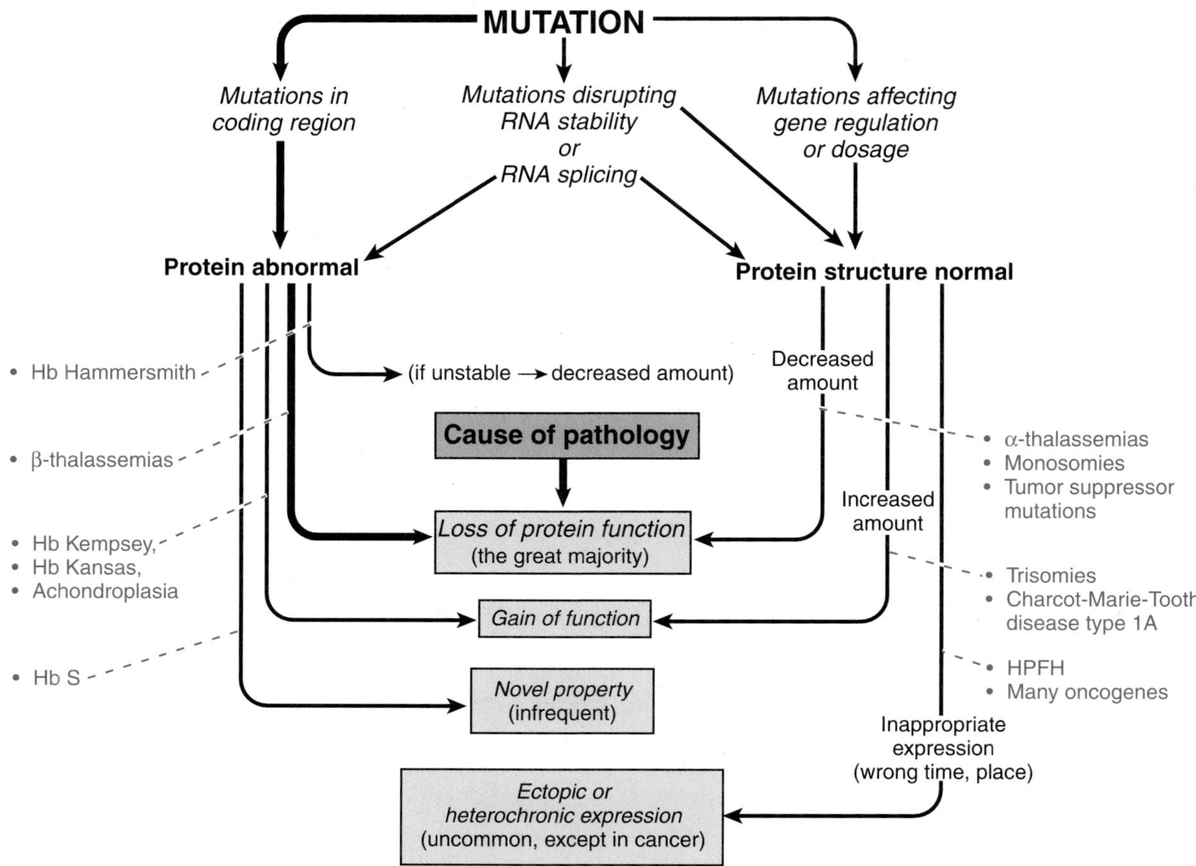


**Figure 11–1.** A general outline of the mechanisms by which disease-causing mutations produce pathology. Mutations in the coding region result in structurally abnormal proteins that have a loss or gain of function or a novel property that causes disease. Mutations in noncoding sequences are of two general types: (1) those that alter the stability or splicing of the mRNA, or (2) those that disrupt regulatory elements or that change gene dosage. Mutations in regulatory elements alter the abundance of the mRNA or the time or cell type in which the gene is expressed. Mutations in either the coding region or regulatory domains can decrease the amount of the protein produced.

diseases such as monosomies like Turner syndrome (see Chapters 9 and 10); and by acquired somatic mutations—often deletions—that occur in tumor suppressor genes in many cancers (such as **retinoblastoma,** see Chapter 16). In addition to reduction in gene dosage, a complete loss of function may also result from the introduction of a premature stop codon, due either to a nonsense mutation that converts a codon to a stop or a frameshift mutation that alters the reading frame and introduces a stop codon. Missense and other mutations in the coding sequence may also abolish or impair function or make the protein unstable, thereby reducing its abundance. All of these classes of mutation are illustrated by the ***β*-thalassemias** (see later discussion), a group of hemoglobinopathies that result from a reduction in the abundance of $\beta$ globin, one of the major adult hemoglobin proteins in red blood cells. As might be expected, the severity of the disease that results from loss-of-function mutations is generally related to the amount of function lost. In many instances, the retention of very small amounts of residual function by the mutant protein can greatly reduce the severity of the disease, a situation well illustrated by enzyme defects leading to various degrees of hyperphenylalaninemia, the most severe form of which is termed **phenylketonuria (PKU)** (see Chapter 12).

## Gain-of-Function Mutations

Mutations can also alter the biochemical phenotype by enhancing the function of a protein. More is not necessarily better, however, and disease may result. This effect is due to either (1) an increase in the level of the protein's expression or (2) an increase in the ability of each protein molecule to perform one or more normal functions. It is critical to recognize when a disease is due to a gain-of-function mutation because treatment of the resulting disease must necessarily differ from disorders that arise from other mechanisms, such as diseases due to loss-of-function mutations. In addition, gain-of-function mutations often provide insight into the regulation of the expression of the affected gene or into the molecular basis of a protein's function.

**Mutations That Enhance One Normal Function of a Protein.** Rarely, mutations in the coding region may increase the ability of each protein molecule to perform a normal function but are detrimental to the overall physiological activity of the protein. Once again, mutations in globin genes are among the best understood of mutations of this type and include missense mutations such as hemoglobin Kempsey, which locks hemoglobin in its high oxygen-affinity state, thereby reducing oxygen delivery to tissues. Another example of this phenomenon occurs in the form of short stature called **achondroplasia,** in which a single amino acid substitution in fibroblast growth factor receptor 3 (FGFR3) leads to activation of this receptor even in the absence of its ligand, FGF. Mutations of this type, which lead to the increase of a *normal* function, are conceptually and physiologically quite different from those that lead to the acquisition of a totally *new* functional property by the mutant protein—novel property mutations (see later).

**Mutations That Increase Production of a Normal Protein.** Some mutations cause disease by increasing the synthesis of a normal protein in cells in which the protein is normally present. The most common mutations of this type are due to increased gene dosage—the presence of three or more copies of a gene—which is generally the result of the duplication of part or all of a chromosome, as occurs in trisomy 21 (Down syndrome). Another important example is the peripheral nerve degeneration Charcot-Marie-Tooth disease type 1A, which results from duplication of only one gene, the gene for peripheral myelin protein 22 (*PMP22*). Increases in gene dosage are also prevalent as somatic mutations in cancer cells and can result from increased copies of part or all of a chromosome; mutations of this type more often contribute to tumor progression rather than to initiation (discussed in Chapter 16).

### Novel Property Mutations

In a few important diseases, a change in the amino acid sequence causes pathology by conferring a novel property on the protein, without necessarily altering its normal functions. The classic example is **sickle cell disease** (see later discussion), which is due to an amino acid substitution that has *no* effect on the ability of sickle hemoglobin to transport oxygen. Rather, unlike normal hemoglobin, sickle hemoglobin chains aggregate when deoxygenated, to form polymeric fibers that deform red blood cells. This behavior has not been observed with any other hemoglobin mutant. That novel property mutations are infrequent is not surprising, because most amino acid substitutions are either neutral or detrimental to the function or stability of a protein that has been finely tuned by evolution. Only rarely does a mutation introduce a new property of pathological significance.

### Mutations Associated with Heterochronic or Ectopic Gene Expression

An interesting and important class of mutations are those that alter the regulatory regions of a gene and cause inappropriate expression of the gene at an abnormal time or place. One of the most common genetic diseases, cancer, is frequently due to the abnormal expression of a gene that normally promotes cell proliferation—an **oncogene**—in cells in which the gene is not normally expressed, resulting in malignancy (see Chapter 16). Comparably, some mutations in hemoglobin regulatory elements lead to the continued expression in the adult of the $\gamma$-globin gene, which is normally expressed at high levels only in fetal and not postnatal life. Such mutations lead to a phenotype called the **hereditary persistence of fetal hemoglobin** (see later discussion).

## HOW MUTATIONS DISRUPT THE FORMATION OF BIOLOGICALLY NORMAL PROTEINS

To develop a biologically active protein, information must be transcribed from the nucleotide sequence of the gene to the mRNA and then translated into the polypeptide, which then undergoes progressive stages of maturation. Changes in any of these steps (Table 11–1, second column) due to alterations of the structural gene are termed **primary abnormalities.** Abnormalities in seven of the eight different steps are illustrated by various hemoglobinopathies (see Table 11–1, first column).

In some instances, the formation of a mature protein may depend on modifying events that are mediated by *other* proteins or on the association of a protein with other proteins (see Table 11–1, third column). When these modifying events fail to occur, the alteration of function is due to a **secondary abnormality** in the protein, as illustrated by the examples shown in the last column of Table 11–1 (Most of these examples are discussed in Chapter 12). Of course, when a secondary abnormality alters a protein in a genetic disease, the primary defect lies in the structural gene of some other protein necessary for the modification.

TABLE 11–1

**Steps at which Mutation Can Disrupt Formation of Normal Protein**

| **Primary Abnormalities (Changes in Steps Directly Dependent on the DNA Sequence of the Structural Gene)** | | **Secondary Abnormalities (Changes in Modifying Events or in the Synthesis of Associated Molecules Required for Function)** | |
|---|---|---|---|
| *Disease Example (Largely Hemoglobinopathies)* | *Step Affected* | *Event Modified* | *Disease Example (Various Diseases, See Chapter 12)* |
| | NUCLEOTIDE SEQUENCE | | |
| Thalassemias in which decreased mRNA is due to deletions or defects in regulatory or splice sites. HPFH: Increased postnatal transcription. | Transcription | Regulation of transcription | Acute intermittent porphyria: Drugs that induce cytochrome P450 decrease free heme → induction of ALA synthetase → symptoms. |
| | MESSENGER RNA | | |
| Thalassemias due to nonfunctional mRNAs with nonsense or frameshift mutations. | Translation | Regulation of protein synthesis | Acute intermittent porphyria: Decreased heme increases both transcription and translation of ALA synthetase. |
| | ABNORMAL POLYPEPTIDE FOLDING | | |
| Thirteen different Hb mutants in which an amino acid in an $\alpha$ helix is replaced by proline, introducing kinks that disrupt the helix and, thus, the tertiary structure. | Polypeptide folding (secondary and tertiary structure) | Post-translational modifications e.g., glycosylation, hydroxylation | Ehlers-Danlos syndrome type VI: Lysyl hydroxylase deficiency → poorly cross-linked collagen |
| | THREE-DIMENSIONAL CONFORMATION | | |
| *Methylmalonic aciduria: A defect in the leader sequence in one allele of methylmalonyl CoA acid mutase. | Subcellular localization directed by information in the amino acid sequence | Subcellular localization directed by post-translational modifications of the polypeptide | I-cell disease: failure to add a recognition marker to lysosomal enzymes |
| Hb Philly: A substitution at the $\alpha1{:}\beta1$ interface increases the dissociation constant of Hb tetramers to monomers. | For multimeric proteins: –subunit association –subunit interaction | Formation of multiprotein complexes and organelles | Zellweger syndrome, a defect in peroxisome biogenesis |
| | LOCALIZATION & ASSEMBLY† | | |
| Hb Hammersmith: The heme pocket is deformed by the $\beta42$ Phe → Ser substitution → a change in the tilt of the heme → low $O_2$ affinity → cyanosis. | Cofactor or prosthetic group binding (noncovalent or covalent) | Cofactor or prosthetic group binding (covalent) or removal | Holocarboxylase synthase deficiency; biotinidase deficiency |
| | BIOLOGICAL FUNCTION | | |
| Hb Kempsey: Impaired subunit interaction locks Hb in its high $O_2$-affinity state. Hb Kansas: Locks Hb in its low $O_2$-affinity state. | The mutant protein is normal in virtually every way, except that one or more of its biological activities is altered by an amino acid substitution. | Cofactor or prosthetic group synthesis or transport | Mutations in vitamin $B_{12}$ metabolism → methylmalonic aciduria and/or homocystinuria |
| | PROTEOLYTIC DEGRADATION | | |
| Over 70 abnormal hemoglobins have unstable structure due to amino acid substitutions or deletions (e.g., the proline substitutions cited above) → degradation. | Changes in primary amino acid sequence that impair folding and destabilize the protein | Regulation of protein degradation | No examples yet known |

*Methylmalonic aciduria and most of the diseases in column 4 are discussed in Chapter 12. †Which of these two steps occurs first varies with the type of protein. HPFH = hereditary persistance of fetal hemoglobin.

## HEMOGLOBINS AND THEIR DISEASES

Disorders of human hemoglobins, called the hemoglobinopathies, occupy a unique position in medical genetics for several reasons. They are easily the most common single-gene diseases in the world, and they cause substantial morbidity. The World Health Organization has estimated that more than 5 percent of the world's population are carriers of genes for clinically important disorders of hemoglobin. Moreover, because hemoglobin was one of the first protein structures to be deduced and because the human globin genes were the first disease-related genes to be cloned, their molecular and biochemical pathology is better understood than perhaps any other group of genetic diseases. The globins also cast light on the process of evolution at both the molecular and the population levels and provide a model of gene action during development.

## Structure and Function of Hemoglobin

Hemoglobin is the oxygen carrier in vertebrate red blood cells. The molecule contains four subunits: two $\alpha$ chains and two $\beta$ chains. Each subunit is composed of a polypeptide chain, globin, and a prosthetic group, heme, which is an iron-containing pigment that combines with oxygen to give the molecule its oxygen-transporting ability.

**Human Hemoglobins and Their Genes.** The hemoglobin molecule consists of two each of two different types of polypeptide chains. In normal adult hemoglobin (hemoglobin A, or Hb A), these globin chains are designated $\alpha$ and $\beta$ (the structure of the $\beta$-globin gene is described in Chapter 3). The four chains are folded and fitted together to form a globular tetramer with a molecular weight of approximately 64,500, a structure that, for Hb A, is abbreviated as $\alpha_2\beta_2$. The two types of chains are almost equal in length, the $\alpha$-globin chain having 141 amino acids and the $\beta$ chain 146. The chains resemble one another markedly both in amino acid sequence (primary structure) and in three-dimensional configuration (tertiary structure). Because the $\alpha$- and $\beta$-globin chains are encoded by genes at separate loci, a point mutation affects one chain or the other but not both.

In addition to Hb A, there are five other normal human hemoglobins, each of which has a tetrameric structure comparable to that of Hb A in consisting of two $\alpha$ or $\alpha$-like chains and two non-$\alpha$ chains (Fig. 11–2). The genes for the $\alpha$ and $\alpha$-like chains are clustered in a tandem arrangement on chromosome 16, and those for the $\beta$ and $\beta$-like chains are on chromosome 11. There are two identical $\alpha$-globin genes, designated $\alpha_1$ and $\alpha_2$, on each copy of chromosome 16. Within the $\beta$-globin gene complex, a close homology exists between the different genes. For example, the $\beta$ and $\delta$ globins differ in only 10 of their 146 amino acids. All of the globin genes undoubtedly arose from a common ancestral gene.

**Features of Globin Structure Relevant to the Hemoglobinopathies.** The major features of globin structure have been highly conserved during evolution and are central to an understanding of the hemoglobinopathies. Above all, the tertiary structure of the globin polypeptide has been preserved, so that virtually all globins examined have seven or eight helical regions (depending on the chain) designated A through H in Figure 11–3. Only two amino acid residues have been conserved in all globins throughout nature and mutations in either of these residues are associated with disease (see Fig. 11–3).

The study of the structure of hemoglobin allows one to predict which types of mutations are likely to

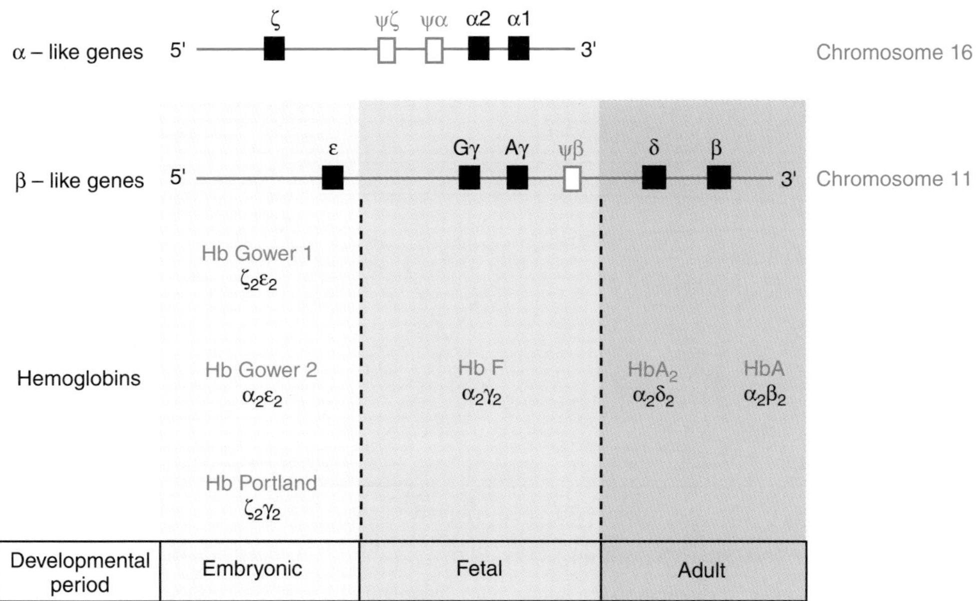


Figure 11–2. Organization of the human globin genes and hemoglobins produced in each stage of human development. (Redrawn from Stamatoyannopoulos G, Nienhuis AW [1987] Hemoglobin switching. *In* Stamatoyannopoulos G, Nienhuis AW, Leder P, Majerus PW (eds) The Molecular Basis of Blood Diseases. WB Saunders, Philadelphia, pp. 66–105.)

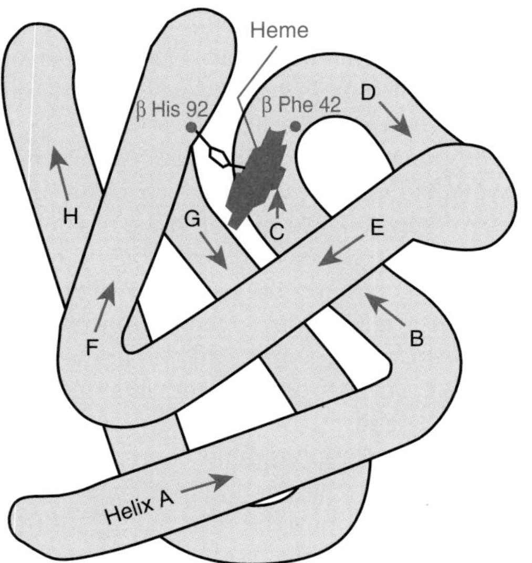


Figure 11–3. The tertiary structure of a hemoglobin molecule. The molecule has eight helical regions, designated A to H. The two most conserved amino acids are shown: at His 92, the histidine to which the iron of heme is covalently linked, and at Phe 42, the phenylalanine that wedges the porphyrin ring of heme into the heme "pocket" of the folded protein. See discussion of Hb Hammersmith and Hb Hyde Park, which have substitutions for Phe 42 and His 92, respectively.

be pathogenic. Thus, a mutation that alters globin conformation, substitutes highly conserved amino acids, or disrupts the hydrophobic shell—that excludes water from the interior of the molecule—by replacing one of the nonpolar residues, is likely to cause a hemoglobinopathy. Like all proteins, globin has "sensitive areas," in which mutations cannot occur without affecting function, and "insensitive areas," in which variation is tolerated more freely.

## Developmental Expression of Globin Genes and Globin Switching

The change in the expression during development of the various globin genes (Fig. 11–4) (also referred to as **globin switching**) is a classic example of the ordered regulation of developmental gene expression (see Chapter 17). Note that the genes in the $\alpha$ and $\beta$ clusters are arranged in the same transcriptional orientation and, remarkably, that the genes in each cluster are situated in the same sequential order in which they are expressed during development. There is equimolar production of the $\alpha$-like and $\beta$-like globin chains.

Interestingly, the temporal switches of globin synthesis are accompanied by changes in the major site of erythropoiesis (see Fig. 11–4). Embryonic globin synthesis occurs in the yolk sac from the third to eighth weeks of gestation, but at about the fifth week of gestation, the major site of hematopoiesis begins to move from the yolk sac to the fetal liver. Hb F ($\alpha_2\gamma_2$) is the predominant hemoglobin throughout fetal life and constitutes approximately 70 percent of total hemoglobin at birth, but in adult life, Hb F represents less than 1 percent of the total hemoglobin.

Although $\beta$ chains can be detected in early gestation, their synthesis becomes significant only near the time of birth; by 3 months of age, almost all the hemoglobin present is of the adult type, Hb A. Synthesis of the $\delta$ chain also continues after birth, but Hb $A_2$ ($\alpha_2\delta_2$) never accounts for more than about 2 percent of adult hemoglobin. Some of the transcription factors that control the developmental expression of the globin genes are known. The mechanism of regulation of globin-chain production is of potential therapeutic importance in the thalassemias (see Chapter 13).

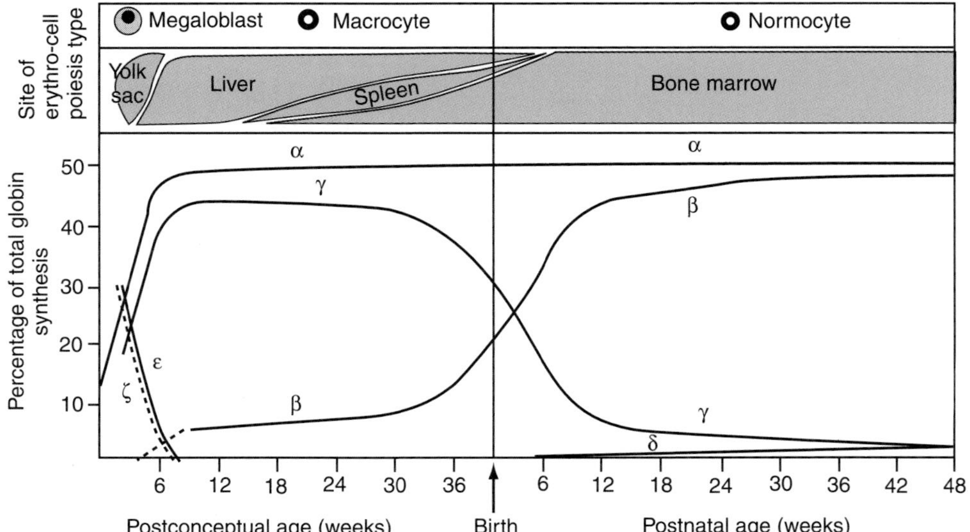


Figure 11–4. Development of erythropoiesis in the human fetus and infant. Types of cells responsible for hemoglobin synthesis, organ(s) involved, and types of globin chain synthesized at successive stages are shown. (Redrawn from Wood WG [1976] Haemoglobin synthesis during fetal development. Br Med Bull 32:282–287, by permission.)

**The Beta-Globin Locus Control Region.** The expression of the $\beta$-globin gene is only partly controlled by the promoter and two enhancers in the immediate flanking DNA (see Chapter 3). The existence of additional regulatory elements was first suggested by the identification of a unique group of patients who had no gene expression from *any* of the genes in the $\beta$-globin cluster, even though the genes themselves (including their individual regulatory elements) were intact. These patients were found to have large deletions upstream of the $\beta$-globin complex, deletions that removed an approximately 20 kb domain called the **locus control region** (LCR), situated 20 kb upstream of the $\varepsilon$-globin gene. The resulting disease, $\varepsilon\gamma\delta\beta$-thalassemia (Fig. 11–5), is described later. The LCR is required for the expression of all the $\beta$-globin genes.

The LCR is responsible both for appropriate high-level expression of the genes within the cluster and for the correct developmental timing of expression of each gene. The control of gene expression in the $\beta$-globin cluster by the LCR is achieved by two mechanisms. First, the LCR provides an open chromatin domain that gives transcription factors access to the regulatory elements within the cluster. Second, it acts as a "super-enhancer" of transcription of the genes in the cluster. An LCR has also been identified for the $\alpha$-globin locus; this LCR is located about 40 kb upstream of the $\zeta$-globin gene.

The clinical significance of the LCR is threefold. First, as mentioned, patients who have deletions of the LCR fail to express the genes of the $\beta$-globin cluster. Second, and of wider significance, components of the LCR are likely to be essential for gene therapy of disorders of the $\beta$-globin cluster (see Chapter 13). Third, knowledge of the molecular mechanisms that underlie globin switching may make it feasible, for example, to upregulate the expression of the $\gamma$-globin gene in patients with $\beta$-thalassemia, who have severely impaired $\beta$-globin expression. Such upregulation would be an effective treatment for $\beta$-thalassemia, because Hb F ($\alpha_2\gamma_2$) is an effective oxygen carrier in the adult (see Chapter 13).

**Gene Dosage, Ontogeny, and Clinical Disease.** The differences in gene dosage (four $\alpha$- and two $\beta$-globin genes per diploid genome) and ontogeny of the $\alpha$ and $\beta$ globins are important to an understanding of the pathogenesis of many hemoglobinopathies. Mutations in the $\beta$-globin gene are more likely to cause disease because a single mutation affects 50 percent of the $\beta$ chains, whereas a single $\alpha$-chain mutation affects only 25 percent of the $\alpha$ chains. On the other hand, $\beta$-globin mutations have no prenatal consequences, because $\gamma$ globin is the major $\beta$-like globin before birth, and Hb F constitutes three quarters of the total hemoglobin at term. Because $\alpha$ chains are the only $\alpha$-like components of all hemoglobins 6 weeks after conception (see Fig. 11–4), $\alpha$-globin mutations cause severe disease in both fetal and postnatal life.

## GENETIC DISORDERS OF HEMOGLOBIN

The hereditary disorders of hemoglobin can be separated into three broad groups, depending on whether the mutation alters the globin protein, its synthesis, or globin developmental switching:

1. **Structural variants** that alter the globin polypeptide without affecting its rate of synthesis.
2. **Thalassemias**, in which there is decreased synthesis (or, rarely, extreme instability) of one or more of the globin chains, resulting in an imbalance in the relative amounts of the $\alpha$ and $\beta$ chains.
3. **Hereditary persistence of fetal hemoglobin**, a group of clinically benign conditions that are of interest because they impair the perinatal switch from $\gamma$- to $\beta$-globin synthesis.

### Hemoglobin Structural Variants

Most of the variant hemoglobins result from point mutations in one of the globin structural genes, but a few are formed by other, more complex, molecular mechanisms. More than 400 abnormal hemoglobins have been described, and approximately half of these are clinically significant. The hemoglobin structural variants can be separated into three classes (Table 11–2), depending on the clinical phenotype:

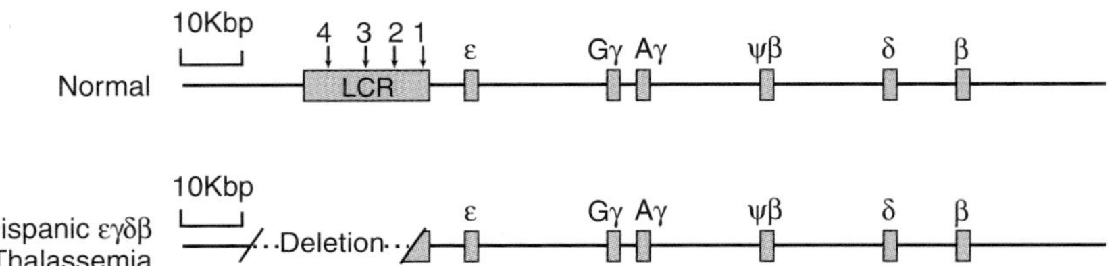


Figure 11–5. The $\beta$-globin locus control region (LCR). Each of the four regions of open chromatin (*arrows*) contains several consensus binding sites for both erythroid-specific and ubiquitous transcription factors. The precise mechanisms by which the LCR regulates gene expression is unclear. Also shown is a deletion of the LCR that has led to $\varepsilon\gamma\delta\beta$-thalassemia, which is discussed in the text. (Redrawn from Kazazian HH Jr, Antonarakis S [1997] Molecular genetics of the globin genes. *In* Singer M, Berg P [eds] Exploring Genetic Mechanisms. University Science Books, Sausalito, California, pp. 301–336.)

TABLE 11–2

**The Major Classes of Hemoglobin Structural Variants***

| Variant Class | Molecular Basis of Mutation | Change in Polypeptide | Pathophysiological Effect of Mutation | Inheritance |
|---|---|---|---|---|
| ***Variants causing hemolytic anemia*** **(1) Hemoglobins with novel physical properties** | | | | |
| Hb S | Single nucleotide substitution | β chain: Glu6Val | Deoxygenated Hb S polymerizes → sickle cells → vascular occlusion and hemolysis | AR |
| Hb C | Single nucleotide substitution | β chain: Glu6Lys | Oxygenated Hb C tends to crystallize → less deformable cells → mild hemolysis. The disease in Hb S/Hb C compounds is like mild sickle cell disease. | AR |
| ***Variants causing hemolytic anemia*** **(2) Unstable hemoglobins** | | | | |
| Hb Hammersmith | Single nucleotide substitution | β chain: Phe42Ser | An unstable Hb → Hb precipitation → hemolysis; also low $O_2$ affinity. | AD |
| Hb Gun Hill | Mispairing of homologous sequences and unequal crossing over within *same* gene (vs. Hb Lepore and Hb Miyada, below) | β chain: a 5 amino acid deletion | An unstable Hb, with increased oxygen affinity | AD |
| ***Hemoglobins with altered $O_2$ transport*** | | | | |
| Hb Hyde Park (a Hb M) | Single nucleotide substitution | β chain: His92Tyr | The substitution makes oxidized heme iron resistant to methemoglobin reductase → Hb M, which can't carry $O_2$ → cyanosis (asymptomatic) | AD |
| Hb Kempsey | Single nucleotide substitution | β chain: Asp99Asn | The substitution keeps the Hb in its high $O_2$-affinity structure → less $O_2$ to tissues → polycythemia | AD |
| Hb Kansas | Single nucleotide substitution | β chain: Asn102Thr | The substitution keeps the Hb in its low $O_2$-affinity structure → asymptomatic cyanosis | AD |
| Hb Tak | Frameshift near end of chain allows readthrough to a downstream stop in new frame | β chain: An additional 11 residues | Greatly increased oxygen affinity, due to the "new" C-terminal hydrophobic tail preventing formation of a stable "deoxy" structure | AR |
| ***Variants with thalassemia phenotypes*†** | | | | |
| Hb E | Single nucleotide substitution | β chain: Glu26Lys | The mutation → an abnormal Hb *and* to decreased synthesis (abnormal RNA splicing) → mild thalassemia (see Fig. 11–14) | AR |
| Hb Lepore and Hb Miyada (an anti-Lepore Hb) | Mispairing of homologous sequences and unequal crossing over between *different* genes → 7 kb deletion (Lepore) → 7 kb insertion (Miyada) (see Fig. 11–10) | Hb Lepore: A δβ fusion chain Hb Miyada: A βδ fusion chain | Both: Ineffective synthesis of the fusion chain → severe δβ-thalassemia in homozygotes, or in genetic compounds with β-thalassemia alleles | Both: AR |

TABLE 11–2 *Continued*

**The Major Classes of Hemoglobin Structural Variants***

| Variant Class | Molecular Basis of Mutation | Change in Polypeptide | Pathophysiological Effect of Mutation | Inheritance |
|---|---|---|---|---|
| Hb Constant Spring | Substitution in the stop codon: UAA or UAG to CAA or CAG → readthrough to next stop codon in the reading frame | $\alpha$ chain: An additional 31 amino acids | Impaired synthesis and instability of the elongated $\alpha$ chain → hemolysis. $\alpha$-thalassemia in genetic compounds with $\alpha$-thalassemia mutations ($- \; -/\alpha^{CS}\alpha$) | AR |

*Hemoglobin variants are named after the hometown of the first reported patient. †Additional $\beta$ chain structural variants that cause $\beta$-thalassemia are depicted in Table 11–4.

1. Variants that cause **hemolytic anemia**. The great majority of mutant hemoglobins that cause hemolytic anemia make the hemoglobin tetramer unstable. However, two of the best-known variants associated with hemolysis, sickle cell globin and Hb C, are not unstable but cause the mutant globin proteins to assume unusual rigid structures.
2. Mutants with **altered oxygen transport**, due either to increased or decreased oxygen affinity or to the formation of methemoglobin, a form of globin incapable of reversible oxygenation.
3. Variants due to mutations in the coding region that cause **thalassemia** because they reduce the abundance of the globin polypeptide. Most of these mutations impair the rate of synthesis of the mRNA or the protein. Some rare variants cause gross instability of the hemoglobin monomer, greater instability than do those variants associated with hemolytic anemia.

The structural mutants described in this chapter (see Table 11–2) are presented either because they are common and representative of one of the three groups described above or because they illustrate the dramatic and variable biochemical and clinical consequences of mutations, both single nucleotide substitutions as well as other types of changes in the DNA.

## Hemolytic Anemias

### Hemoglobins with Novel Physical Properties: Sickle Cell Disease

Sickle cell hemoglobin (Hb S) was the first abnormal hemoglobin to be detected and is of great clinical importance. It is due to a single nucleotide substitution that changes the codon of the sixth amino acid of $\beta$ globin from glutamic acid to valine (GAG → GTG: Glu6Val) (see Table 11–2). Homozygosity for this mutation is the cause of **sickle cell disease**, a serious disorder that is common in some parts of the world. The disease has a characteristic geographic distribution, occurring most frequently in equatorial Africa and less commonly in the Mediterranean area and India and in countries to which people from these regions have migrated. About 1 in 600 African Americans is born with this disease, which may be fatal in early childhood although longer survival is becoming more common.

**Clinical Features.** Sickle cell disease is a severe autosomal recessive hemolytic condition characterized by a tendency of the red blood cells to become grossly abnormal in shape (i.e., sickled) under conditions of low oxygen tension (see Fig. 11–6). Heterozygotes, who are said to have **sickle cell trait,** are clinically normal, but their red blood cells sickle when subjected to very low oxygen pressure in vitro. Occasions when this might happen in vivo are very unusual, although heterozygotes appear to be at risk for splenic infarction, especially when flying at high altitudes in airplanes with reduced cabin pressure. The heterozygous state is present in approximately 8 percent of African Americans, but in areas where the gene frequency is high (e.g., West Central Africa), up to 25 percent of the newborn population are heterozygotes.

**The Molecular Pathology of Hb S.** In 1956, Ingram discovered that the abnormality in sickle cell hemoglobin was a replacement of one of the 146 amino acids in the $\beta$ chain of the hemoglobin molecule. All the clinical manifestations of sickle cell hemoglobin are consequences of this single change in the $\beta$-globin gene. This was the first demonstration *in any organism* that a mutation in a structural gene could cause an amino acid substitution in the corresponding protein.

Because the abnormality of Hb S is localized in the $\beta$ chain, the formula for sickle cell hemoglobin may be written as $\alpha_2\beta_2^S$, or, more precisely, as $\alpha_2^A\beta_2^S$. A heterozygote has a mixture of the two types of hemoglobin, A and S. The relationship of clinical status, hemoglobin types, and genes can be summarized as follows:

| Clinical Status | Hemoglobin | Hemoglobin Composition | Genotype |
|---|---|---|---|
| Normal | Hb A | $\alpha_2^A\beta_2^A$ | $\alpha\alpha/\alpha\alpha$<br>$\beta/\beta$ |
| Sickle cell trait | Hb A, Hb S | $\alpha_2^A\beta_2^A$<br>$\alpha_2^A\beta_2^S$ | $\alpha\alpha/\alpha\alpha$<br>$\beta/\beta^S$ |
| Sickle cell disease | Hb S | $\alpha_2^A\beta_2^S$ | $\alpha\alpha/\alpha\alpha$<br>$\beta^S/\beta^S$ |

**Sickling and Its Consequences.** The molecular and cellular pathology of sickle cell disease is summarized in Figure 11–6. Hemoglobin molecules containing the mutant $\beta$-globin subunits are normal in their ability to perform their principal function of binding oxygen (provided they have not polymerized, as described next), but, in deoxygenated blood, they are only one fifth as soluble as normal hemoglobin. The relative insolubility of deoxyhemoglobin S is the physical basis of the sickling phenomenon. Under conditions of low oxygen tension, the sickle hemoglobin molecules aggregate in the form of rod-shaped polymers or fibers, which distort the shape of the erythrocyte to a sickle shape. These misshapen erythrocytes are less deformable than normal and, unlike normal red blood cells, cannot squeeze in single file through capillaries, thereby blocking blood flow and causing local ischemia.

**Multiple Origins of the Hb S Mutation.** In one of the seminal uses of a polymorphic DNA marker to study the genetics of patients and populations, Kan and Dozy showed in 1978 that the normal $\beta$-globin gene is contained within a 7.6 kb restriction fragment of DNA in most individuals of African origin (Fig. 11–7). In contrast, they discovered that the sickle globin allele is frequently found in a fragment of 13 kb in certain parts of Africa, such as Ghana (see Fig. 11–7), and in nearly 70 percent of African Americans. This high carrier frequency allowed the 13-kb fragment to be used as a marker of sickle cell disease in these groups. In other parts of Africa (e.g., Kenya), the sickle cell mutation is typically associated with the 7.6 kb fragment (see Fig. 11–7). These findings imply that the sickle mutation arose in West Africa on a chromosome that contained the $\beta$-globin gene on the 13 kb fragment and that it occurred independently at least once elsewhere. The protection that the sickle cell gene confers against malaria in heterozygotes accounts for the high frequency that the gene has reached in malarial areas of the world (see Chapter 7).

### Hemoglobins with Novel Physical Properties: Hemoglobin C

Hb C was the second hemoglobin variant to be identified, and coincidentally, like Hb S, it is also due to a substitution at the sixth position of the $\beta$ chain, the glutamic acid being replaced by lysine (Glu6Lys) (see Table 11–2). Hb C is less soluble than Hb A and thus tends to crystallize in red blood cells, reducing their deformability in capillaries and causing a mild hemolytic disorder.

The $\beta^C$ allele is frequent in West Africa and in descendants of people of this region (about 1 percent of African Americans are carriers). Thus, it is not uncommon to find individuals with Hb C who have a $\beta^S$ allele or a thalassemia allele at the other $\beta$-globin locus. Persons who are **genetic compounds** for the $\beta^C$ and $\beta^S$ mutations (Hb SC disease) have a hemolytic disorder that is milder than

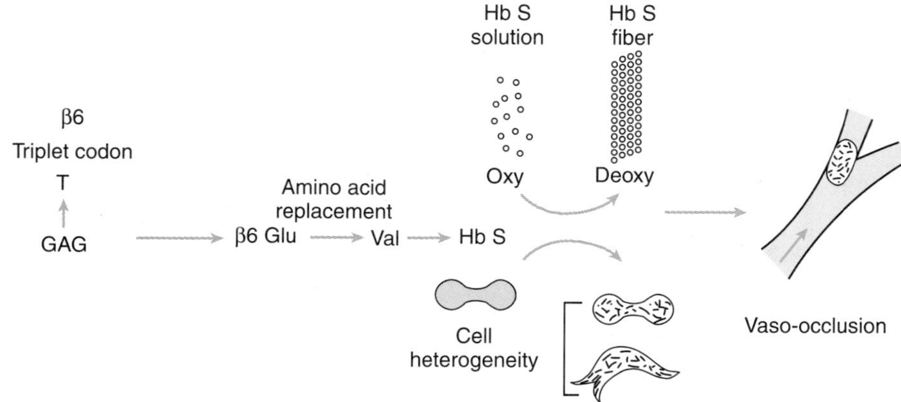


**Figure 11–6.** Scheme of the pathogenesis of sickle cell disease. (Redrawn from Ingram V [1986] Sickle cell disease: molecular and cellular pathogenesis. *In* Bunn HF, Forget BG [eds] Hemoglobin: Molecular, Genetic and Clinical Aspects. WB Saunders, Philadelphia, pp. 453–501.)

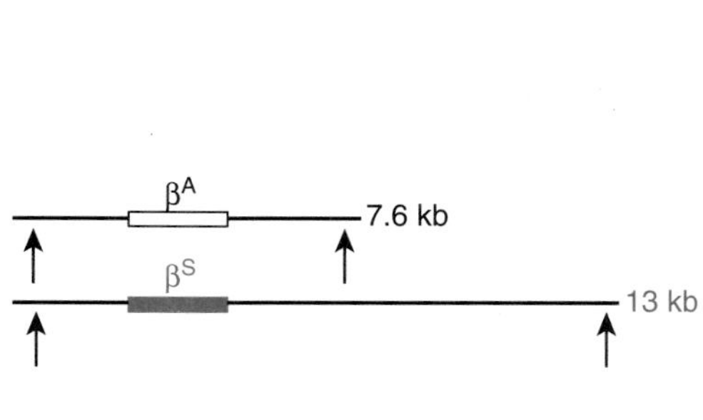


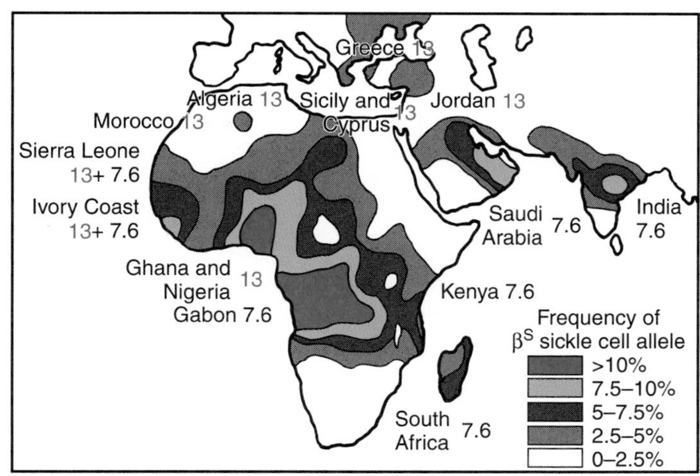


Figure 11–7. The *HpaI* restriction fragment length polymorphism adjacent to the $\beta^S$ gene and the geographic distribution of the sickle cell gene in relation to *HpaI* fragments 7.6 kb and 13 kb in length. The mutation associated with the 13 kb fragment originated in West Africa and spread from there. The mutation associated with the 7.6 kb fragment arose separately and probably had multiple origins. (From Kan YW [1978] *In* The Harvey Lectures, Series 76, Academic Press, New York, pp. 75–93, by permission.)

sickle cell anemia and may have no clinical problems until, unexpectedly, a serious complication develops as a result of vascular occlusion, particularly in the retina.

### Unstable Hemoglobins

**Hb Hammersmith.** The unstable hemoglobins are generally due to point mutations that cause denaturation of the hemoglobin *tetramer*. (Note that the instability is much less pronounced than in the rare variants that so destabilize the globin *monomer* that they cause chain imbalance and thalassemia.) The denatured globin tetramers are insoluble and precipitate to form inclusions (Heinz bodies) that contribute to damage of the red cell membrane and cause hemolysis. The amino acid substitution in Hb Hammersmith ($\beta$ chain: Phe42Ser) (see Table 11–2) is particularly noteworthy because the substituted phenylalanine residue (see Fig. 11–3) is one of the two amino acids that are conserved in all globins. It is therefore not surprising that substitutions at this position produce serious disease. The role of the bulky phenylalanine is to wedge the heme into its pocket in $\beta$ globin. Its replacement with serine, a smaller residue that leaves a gap, allows the heme to drop out of its pocket. In addition to its instability, Hb Hammersmith has a low oxygen affinity, which causes cyanosis.

**Hb Gun Hill.** Most hemoglobin variants are caused by single nucleotide substitutions, but other types of molecular abnormalities, such as small deletions, have been recognized. The mechanism believed to underlie most small deletions, called **slipped mispairing**, is illustrated by Hb Gun Hill. The Hb Gun Hill allele has a 15 base-pair deletion in the $\beta$-globin gene. The $\beta$-globin open reading frame is maintained, but five amino acids are removed from the polypeptide. The mutant $\beta$ chain is able to fold, but the Hb Gun Hill tetramer is unstable (see Table 11–2), leading to hemolysis. It has been noted that small deletions most commonly occur at sites at which direct repeat sequences are present in the DNA. The slipped mispairing mechanism by which the presence of such repeats is thought to cause a deletion is outlined in Figure 11–8 (top). The 15 base-pair region deleted from Hb Gun Hill is flanked by two nearly identical repeat sequences that are in the region of codons 90 to 98 of the $\beta$-globin gene (see Fig. 11–8 bottom).

## Variants with Altered Oxygen Transport

Mutations that alter the ability of hemoglobin to transport oxygen, although rare, are of general interest because they illustrate how a mutation can impair one set of functions of a protein (in this case, oxygen binding and release) that is the responsibility of one domain and yet leave relatively intact the other properties of the molecule; for example, the mutations to be described generally have little or no effect on hemoglobin stability.

### Methemoglobins

Oxyhemoglobin is the form of hemoglobin that is capable of reversible oxygenation; its heme iron is in the reduced (or ferrous) state. The heme iron tends

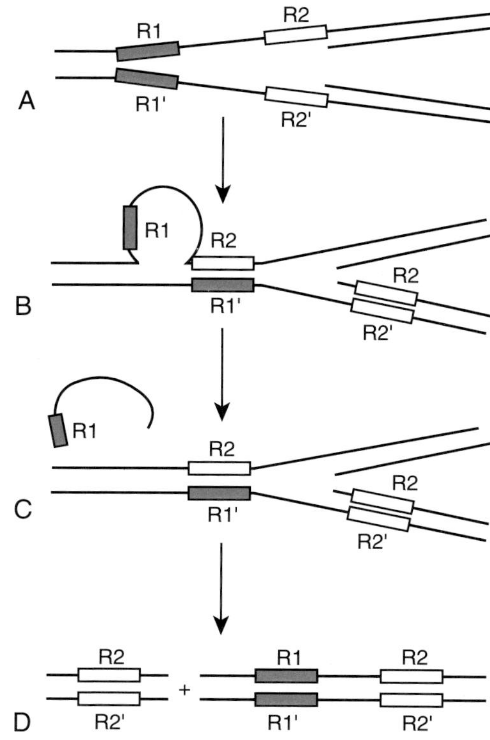


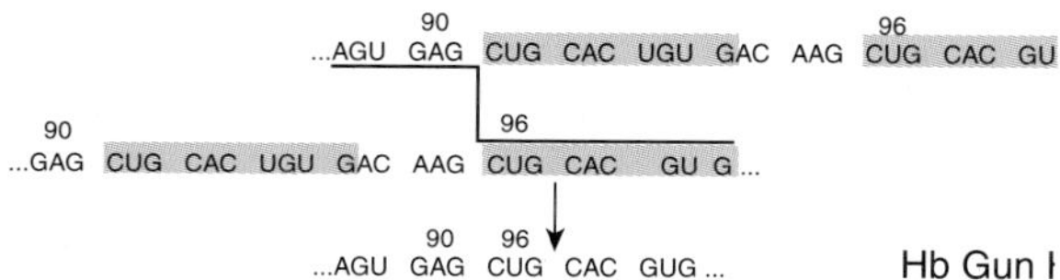


Figure 11–8. (*Top*) The slipped mispairing mechanism thought to underlie most small deletions, such as Hb Gun Hill. (A) A duplex DNA, containing the two direct repeat sequences R1 and R2, becomes single-stranded at the replication fork. (B) The R2 repeat mispairs with the complementary R1′ repeat, looping out the R1 repeat and its adjacent sequence. (C) After the single-stranded loop is excised, the DNA strand is repaired. (D) The daughter duplexes, one of which has only one repeat and lacks the sequence between the repeats. (Redrawn from Cooper DN, Krawczak M [1993] Human Gene Mutation, BIOS Scientific Publishers, Oxford.) (*Bottom*) Hb Gun Hill is a $\beta$-chain structural variant with a deletion of codons 91–95. This deletion probably arose by the slipped mispairing mechanism shown above. The two flanking repeats and their misalignment are shown, together with the sequence of the Hb Gun Hill allele.

to oxidize spontaneously to the ferric form, and the resulting molecule, referred to as methemoglobin, is incapable of reversible oxygenation. If significant amounts of methemoglobin accumulate in the blood, cyanosis results. Maintenance of the heme iron in the reduced state is the role of the enzyme methemoglobin reductase. In several mutant globins (either $\alpha$ or $\beta$), substitutions in the region of the heme pocket affect the heme-globin bond in a way that makes the iron resistant to the reductase. Although heterozygotes for these mutant hemoglobins are cyanotic, they are asymptomatic. The homozygous state is presumably lethal. One example of a $\beta$-chain methemoglobin is Hb Hyde Park, in which the conserved histidine (see His92 in Fig. 11–3) to which heme is covalently bound has been replaced by tyrosine (His92Tyr).

### Hemoglobins with Altered Oxygen Affinity

**Hemoglobins Kempsey and Kansas.** Mutations that alter oxygen affinity are of significance because they demonstrate the importance of subunit interaction for the normal function of a multimeric protein such as hemoglobin. In the Hb A tetramer, the chains are arranged as shown in Figure 11–9.

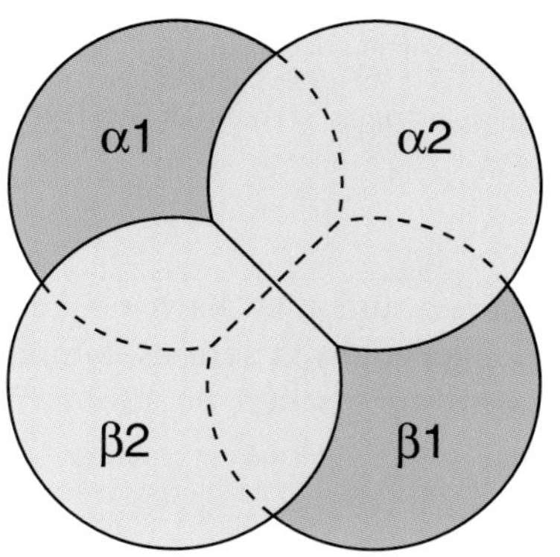


Figure 11–9. Representation of a molecule of normal adult hemoglobin (Hb A). There are two $\alpha$ and two $\beta$ chains, each associated with a heme moiety. As hemoglobin shifts from the oxygenated to the deoxygenated state, critical movement of the chains occurs at the $\alpha1{:}\beta2$ contacts. Substitutions at the subunit interfaces can alter oxygen affinity (e.g., Hb Kempsey and Hb Kansas—see text) or the stability of the molecule.

The $\alpha_1{:}\beta_2$ interface has been very highly conserved throughout evolution because it is subject to significant movement between the chains when the hemoglobin shifts from the oxygenated (relaxed) to the deoxygenated (tense) form of the molecule. Predictably, substitutions in residues at this interface, exemplified by the $\beta$-globin mutants Hb Kempsey and Hb Kansas, have serious pathological effects because they prevent the oxygen-related movement between the chains. These two mutant proteins have structural and clinical abnormalities, however, that are the inverse of each other. In Hb Kempsey ($\beta$-chain Asp99Asn), the mutation "locks" the hemoglobin into the relaxed structure, which has high oxygen affinity, and causes polycythemia. Carriers of Hb Kansas ($\beta$-chain Asn102Thr), on the other hand, have cyanosis, because the mutation inhibits the formation of the relaxed (oxygenated) structure, so that the hemoglobin has a lowered oxygen affinity. Nevertheless, at least one carrier of Hb Kansas is healthy enough to be an excellent tennis player, suggesting that he can extract a larger-than-normal fraction of oxygen from blood.

**Hb Tak.** The increased oxygen affinity of Hb Tak (see Table 11–2) is the result of a small (two base-pair) insertion between codons 146 and 147 of the $\beta$ chain. This mutation illustrates a different principle—that insertions or deletions in the reading frame of a gene that are not a multiple of 3 will change the reading frame to alter the length of the polypeptide. Because codon 146 is the last amino acid codon before the termination codon of $\beta$ globin (see Fig. 3–10), the effect of the two base-pair insertion is to increase the length of the $\beta$ chain by 11 residues, an alteration that increases the oxygen affinity of the protein (see Table 11–2).

### Variant Hemoglobins with Thalassemia Phenotypes

#### Hemoglobin E: An Abnormal Beta-Globin Polypeptide with Reduced mRNA Synthesis

Hb E is a $\beta$-globin structural variant (Glu26Lys) that causes thalassemia because it is synthesized at a reduced rate. It is probably the most common structurally abnormal hemoglobin in the world, occurring at high frequency in Southeast Asia, where there are at least 1 million homozygotes and 30 million heterozygotes. This allele is noteworthy for several reasons: its frequency, its allelic interaction with other $\beta$-globin mutants, and its effect on RNA splicing (see Table 11–2). Although Hb E homozygotes are asymptomatic and only mildly anemic, genetic compounds with the Hb E mutation and different $\beta$-thalassemia alleles have abnormal phenotypes that are largely determined by the severity of the other allele. Hb E is also notable because its mutation, although located in the coding region, reduces normal splicing of the $\beta^E$-globin RNA, producing a mild thalassemia phenotype. The mechanism by which this mutation impairs splicing is reviewed in the discussion of $\beta$-thalassemia, later.

#### Lepore and Anti-Lepore Hemoglobins: Fusion Genes

Some patients with moderate to severe $\beta$-thalassemia have an unusual non-$\alpha$ chain that consists of the N-terminal half (50 to 80 residues) of a normal $\delta$ chain fused to the C-terminal half (60 to 90 residues) of a normal $\beta$ chain, to form a new $\delta\beta$ fusion chain, termed Hb Lepore (see Table 11–2). This variant has arisen by homologous but unequal crossing over between the very similar $\delta$-globin and $\beta$-globin genes (Fig. 11–10). During meiosis, misalignment based on the sequence homology between the $\delta$ gene of one chromatid and the $\beta$ gene of the corresponding chromatid could happen as a relatively rare accident. Crossing over between the chromatids would then be possible, forming two abnormal products, a deleted fusion gene such as Hb Lepore and an "anti-Lepore" fusion gene with an insertion, one example being Hb Miyada (see Fig. 11–10 and Table 11–2). Note that this mechanism of deletion differs from the slipped mispairing mechanism that is believed to be responsible for small deletions, such as the deletion in Hb Gun Hill (see Fig. 11–8).

## Thalassemia: An Imbalance of Globin-Chain Synthesis

The thalassemias, collectively the most common human single-gene disorders, are a heterogeneous group of diseases of hemoglobin synthesis in which mutations reduce the synthesis or stability of either the $\alpha$- or $\beta$-globin chain, to cause **$\alpha$- or $\beta$-thalassemia**, respectively. The resulting imbalance in the ratio of the $\alpha$:$\beta$ chains underlies the pathophysiology. The chain that is produced at the normal rate is in relative excess; in the absence of a complementary chain with which to form a tetramer, the excess normal chains eventually precipitate in the cell, damaging the membrane and leading to premature red

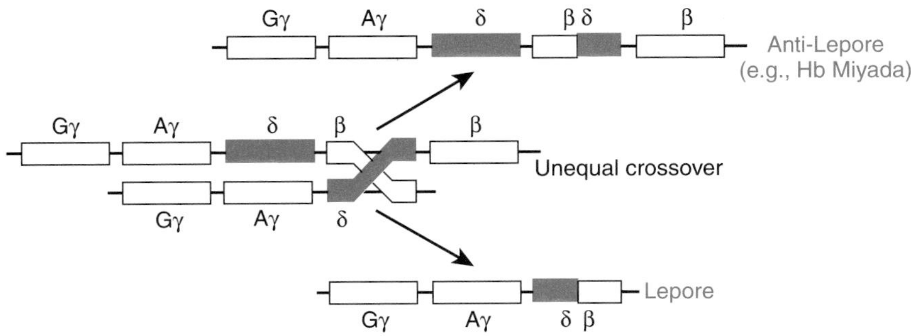


**Figure 11–10.** Model for the origin of a Lepore gene and of an anti-Lepore gene, such as Hb Miyada, by unequal crossing over. The adjacent $\gamma$ and $\beta$ genes differ at only 10 of their 146 residues. If mispairing occurs, followed by intragenic crossing over, two hybrid genes result: one with a deletion of part of each locus (a Lepore gene), the other with a corresponding duplication (an anti-Lepore gene such as that encoding Hb Miyada). (Redrawn from Weatherall DJ, Clegg JB [1981] The Thalassemia Syndromes, 3rd ed. Blackwell Scientific Publications, Oxford.)

blood cell destruction. In addition, the defect in hemoglobin synthesis produces a hypochromic, microcytic anemia.

The name "thalassemia" is derived from the Greek word for sea, *thalassa*, and signifies that the disease was first discovered in persons of Mediterranean origin. Both $\alpha$- and $\beta$-thalassemia, however, have a high frequency in many populations, although $\alpha$-thalassemia is more prevalent and widely distributed. The frequency of thalassemia is due to the protective advantage against malaria that it confers on carriers, analogous to the heterozygote advantage (see Chapter 7) of sickle hemoglobin carriers. There is a characteristic distribution of the thalassemias in a band around the Old World: in the Mediterranean, the Middle East, and parts of Africa, India, and Asia. In most countries, thalassemia carriers are sufficiently numerous to pose the important problem of differential diagnosis from iron deficiency anemia and to be a relatively common source of referral for homozygote detection in prenatal diagnosis.

An important clinical consideration is that it is not unusual for alleles for both types of thalassemia, as well as for structural hemoglobin abnormalities, to coexist in an individual. As a result, clinically important interactions may occur among different alleles of the same gene or among mutant alleles of different globin genes. These interactions are outlined in the Box at the end of this chapter.

### THE ALPHA-THALASSEMIAS

Genetic disorders of $\alpha$-globin production affect the formation of *both* fetal and adult hemoglobins (see Figs. 11–2 and 11–4) and therefore cause intrauterine as well as postnatal disease. In the absence of $\alpha$-globin chains with which to associate, the chains from the $\beta$-globin cluster are free to form a homotetrameric hemoglobin. Hemoglobin with a $\gamma_4$ composition is known as Hb Bart's, and the $\beta_4$ tetramer is called Hb H. Because neither of these hemoglobins is capable of releasing oxygen to tissues in normal conditions, they are completely ineffective oxygen carriers. Consequently, infants with severe $\alpha$-thalassemia and high levels of Hb Bart's suffer severe intrauterine hypoxia and are born with massive generalized fluid accumulation, a condition called **hydrops fetalis**. In milder $\alpha$-thalassemias, an anemia develops because of the gradual precipitation of the Hb H in the erythrocyte. This leads to the formation of inclusions in the mature red blood cell, and the removal of these inclusions by the spleen damages the cells, leading to their premature destruction.

**Deletions of the Alpha-Globin Genes.** The most common forms of $\alpha$-thalassemia are the result of deletions. The reason for the frequency of this type of abnormality in mutants of the $\alpha$ and not the $\beta$ chain is revealed by comparison of these genes and their local chromosomal contexts (see Fig. 11–2). Not only are there two identical $\alpha$ genes on each chromosome 16, but the intron sequences around the two $\alpha$ genes are also very similar.

The arrangement of tandem regions of homology in and around the $\alpha$ genes facilitates misalignment due to homologous pairing and subsequent recombination between the $\alpha 1$ gene domain on one chromosome and the corresponding $\alpha 2$ gene region on the other (Fig. 11–11). Evidence that this explanation for the deletions is correct is provided by reports of rare normal individuals with a triplicated $\alpha$ gene complex (see Fig. 11–11). Deletions or other alterations of one, two, three, or all four of these genes cause a correspondingly severe hematological abnormality, as summarized in Table 11–3.

Although the $\alpha$-thalassemias are distributed throughout the world, the homozygous deletion type of $\alpha$-thalassemia leading to hydrops fetalis is largely restricted to Southeast Asia. The high gene frequency

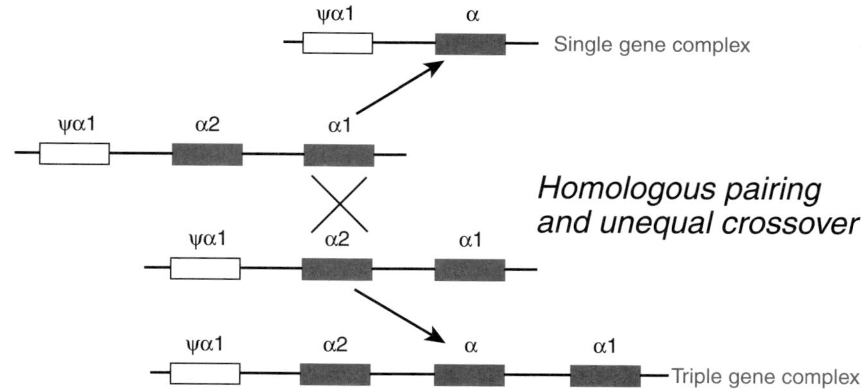


**Figure 11–11.** The probable mechanism of the most common form of $\alpha$-thalassemia, which is due to deletions of one of the two $\alpha$-globin genes on a chromosome. Misalignment, homologous pairing, and recombination between the $\alpha 1$ gene on one chromosome and the $\alpha 2$ gene on the homologous chromosome results in the deletion of one $\alpha$ gene. (Redrawn from Orkin SH [1987] Disorders of hemoglobin synthesis: The thalassemias. *In* Stamatoyannopoulos G, Nienhuis AW, Leder P, Majerus PW [eds] The Molecular Basis of Blood Diseases. WB Saunders, Philadelphia, pp. 106–126.)

TABLE 11–3

**Clinical States of Alpha-Thalassemia Genotypes**

| Clinical Condition | Number of Functional $\alpha$ Genes | Genotype | $\alpha$ Chain Production |
|---|---|---|---|
| Normal | 4 | $\alpha\alpha/\alpha\alpha$ | 100% |
| Silent carrier | 3 | $\alpha\alpha/\alpha-$ | 75% |
| $\alpha$-thalassemia trait (mild anemia, microcytosis) | 2 | $\alpha-/\alpha-$ or $\alpha\alpha/--$ | 50% |
| Hb H ($\beta$4) disease (moderately severe hemolytic anemia) | 1 | $\alpha-/--$ | 25% |
| Hydrops fetalis or homozygous $\alpha$-thalassemia (Hb Bart's: $\gamma$4) | 0 | $--/--$ | 0% |

in this population (up to 15 percent in some regions) can be explained by the nature of the deletion. The heterozygous state, called $\alpha$-thalassemia trait (two normal and two mutant $\alpha$ genes), can result from either of two genotypes ($-\alpha/-\alpha$ or $--/\alpha\alpha$). The latter is relatively common among Southeast Asians, and offspring may consequently receive two ($--/--$) chromosomes. In other groups, however, heterozygosity is usually the result of the ($-\alpha/-\alpha$) genotype, from which there is virtually no possibility of transmitting the hydrops fetalis phenotype.

In addition to $\alpha$-thalassemia mutations that result in deletion of the $\alpha$ genes per se, mutations that delete only the LCR of the $\alpha$-globin complex (see Fig. 11–2) have also been found to cause $\alpha$-thalassemia. In fact, such mutations first indicated the existence of this regulatory element.

**Nondeletion Forms of Alpha-Thalassemia.** These occur less commonly than do the deletion genotypes just described. Four $\alpha$-chain termination mutations, including the structural variant Hb Constant Spring (see Table 11–2), cause $\alpha$-thalassemia, apparently because of a pronounced instability of the mutant $\alpha$-globin chain.

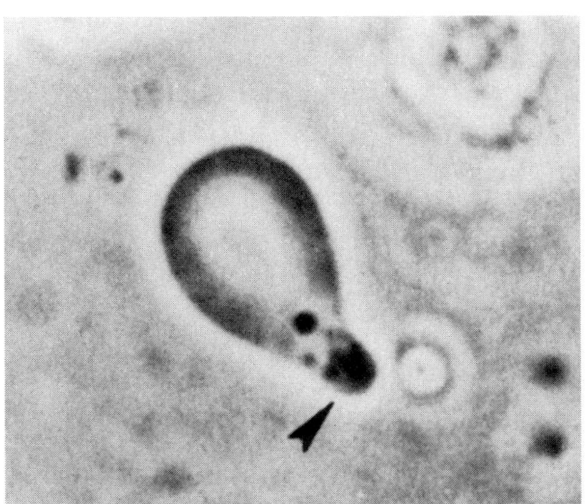

Figure 11–12. Visualization of one pathological effect of the deficiency of $\beta$ chains in $\beta$ thalassemia: The precipitation of the excess normal $\alpha$ chains to form a Heinz body in the red blood cell. Phase microscopy of a wet preparation of scrapings from the spleen of a patient with homozygous $\beta$-thalassemia, showing an $\alpha$-chain inclusion body (*arrow*) within a teardrop-shaped red blood cell. Such inclusions are removed from the erythrocyte by reticuloendothelial cells, damaging the cell membrane and causing premature destruction of the cell. (From Nathan DG [1972] Thalassemia. N Engl J Med 286:586–594, by permission.)

## THE BETA-THALASSEMIAS

The $\beta$-thalassemias share many features with $\alpha$-thalassemia. Decreased $\beta$-globin production causes a hypochromic, microcytic anemia, and the imbalance in globin synthesis leads to precipitation of the excess $\alpha$ chains, which in turn leads to damage of the red cell membrane. In contrast to $\alpha$ globin, however, the $\beta$ chain is important only in the postnatal period (see Fig. 11–4). Consequently, the onset of $\beta$-thalassemia is not apparent until a few months after birth, when $\beta$ globin normally replaces $\gamma$ globin as the major non-$\alpha$ chain, and only the synthesis of the major adult hemoglobin, Hb A, is reduced. The excess $\alpha$ chains are insoluble, so that they precipitate in red cell precursors and are destroyed in the bone marrow; this process causes ineffective erythropoiesis (Fig. 11–12). Because the $\delta$ gene is intact, Hb $A_2$ production continues, and, in fact, elevation of the Hb $A_2$ level is unique to $\beta$-thalassemia heterozygotes. The level of Hb F is also increased, not because of a reactivation of the $\gamma$-globin gene expression that was switched off at birth, but because of selective survival and perhaps also increased production of the minor population of adult red blood cells that contain Hb F.

In contrast to $\alpha$-thalassemia, the $\beta$-thalassemias are usually due to single base-pair substitutions rather than to deletions. There are so many different $\beta$-thalassemia mutations that persons carrying two $\beta$-thalassemia alleles are more likely to be genetic compounds than to be true homozygotes for one allele. Most individuals with two $\beta$-thalassemia alleles have **thalassemia major**, a condition characterized by severe anemia and the need for lifelong medical management. When the $\beta$-thalassemia alleles allow so little production of $\beta$ globin that no Hb A is present, the condition is designated **$\beta^0$-thalassemia**. If some Hb A is detectable, the patient is said to have **$\beta^+$-thalassemia**. Although the severity of the clinical disease depends on the combined effect of the two alleles present, survival into adult life was, until recently, unusual.

Infants affected with homozygous $\beta$-thalassemia present with anemia once the postnatal production of Hb F decreases, generally before 2 years of age. The red cells in peripheral blood are all markedly hypochromic and variable in size and shape. At present, treatment of the thalassemias is based on correction of the anemia and the increased marrow expansion by blood transfusion and on control of the consequent iron accumulation by the administration of chelating agents. Bone marrow transplantation is effective, but this is an option only if an HLA-matched family member can be found. Experimental therapies offer promise and are discussed in Chapter 13.

Carriers of one $\beta$-thalassemia allele are clinically well and are said to have **thalassemia minor**. Such individuals have hypochromic, microcytic red blood cells and may have a slight anemia that can be misdiagnosed initially as iron deficiency. The diagnosis of thalassemia minor can be supported by hemoglobin electrophoresis, which generally reveals an increase in the level of Hb $A_2$ ($\alpha_2\delta_2$).

### Beta-Thalassemia, Complex Thalassemias, and Hereditary Persistence of Fetal Hemoglobin

Almost every type of mutation known to reduce the synthesis of an mRNA or protein has been identified as a cause of $\beta$-thalassemia. The following overview of these genetic defects is, therefore, instructive about mutational mechanisms in general, while describing in particular the molecular basis of one of the most common and severe genetic diseases in the world. Mutations of the $\beta$-globin complex are separated into two broad groups with different clinical phenotypes. One group of defects, which accounts for the great majority of patients, impairs the production of $\beta$ globin alone and causes **simple $\beta$-thalassemia**. The second group of mutations is one in which large deletions cause the **complex thalassemias**, in which the $\beta$-globin gene *as well as* one or more of the other genes—or the LCR—in the $\beta$-globin cluster is removed. Some deletions within the $\beta$-globin cluster do not cause thalassemia, but rather a fascinating phenotype termed the **hereditary persistence of fetal hemoglobin** (i.e., the persistence of $\gamma$-globin gene expression throughout adult life).

#### *The Molecular Basis of Simple Beta-Thalassemia*

Simple $\beta$-thalassemia results from many different types of molecular abnormalities, mostly point mutations, in the $\beta$-globin gene (Table 11–4 and Fig. 11–13). The only common $\beta$-globin deletion in any racial group is a 619 base-pair partial deletion of the 3′ end of the gene in patients of Asian Indian origin (see Table 11–4). Hb Lepore, an Hb structural variant discussed earlier, is due to unequal crossing over that produces an approximately 7-kb deletion involving the $\delta$ and $\beta$ genes.

Most $\beta$-thalassemia mutations decrease the abundance of the $\beta$-globin mRNA, and they are of three types: promoter mutants, RNA splicing mutants (the most common), and mRNA capping or tailing mutants (see Fig. 11–13). A smaller number of patients with $\beta$-thalassemia have nonsense or frameshift mutations in the coding region of the gene, which lead to the synthesis of short, unstable $\beta$-globin polypeptides. A few hemoglobin structural variants also impair processing of the $\beta$-globin mRNA, as exemplified by Hb E, described earlier.

**Defective mRNA Synthesis.** The majority of $\beta$-thalassemia patients with defective mRNA synthesis have abnormalities in RNA splicing. More than 24 defects of this type have been described, and their combined clinical burden is substantial. These mutations have also acquired high visibility because their effects on splicing are often unexpectedly complex, and analysis of the mutant mRNAs has contributed extensively to knowledge of the sequences critical to normal RNA processing (introduced in Chapter 3). The splice defects are separated into three groups (Fig. 11–14), depending on the region of the unprocessed RNA in which the mutation is located.

**Group 1. Splice Junction Mutations.** This group includes mutations at the 5′ donor or 3′ acceptor splice junctions of the introns or in the consensus sequences surrounding the junctions. The critical nature of the conserved GT dinucleotide at the 5′ intron donor site and of the AG at the 3′ intron receptor site (see Chapter 3) is apparent from the complete loss of normal splicing that results from mutations in these dinucleotides (see Fig. 11–14*B*). The inactivation of the normal acceptor site elicits the use of other acceptor-like sequences elsewhere in the RNA precursor. These alternative sites are termed **cryptic splice sites** because they are normally not used by the splicing apparatus when the correct site is available. Cryptic donor or acceptor slice sites can be found in either exons or introns and may be used alone or in competition with other cryptic sites or the normal splice site.

The importance of the consensus sequences adjacent to the donor or acceptor dinucleotides is also illustrated by the effect of mutations. Thus, substitution of the fifth or sixth nucleotide of the donor sequence of intron 1 reduces the effectiveness of the normal splice event, but because some normal splicing still occurs, phenotypes are those of $\beta^+$-thalassemia.

TABLE 11–4
**The Molecular Basis of Simple Beta-Thalassemia**

| Type | Example | Phenotype | Affected Population |
|---|---|---|---|
| ***Deletions**** | | | |
| β-globin gene deletions | 619 base-pair deletion | $\beta^0$ | Indian |
| ***Defective mRNA synthesis*** | | | |
| RNA splicing defects (see Fig. 11–14) | Abnormal acceptor site of intron 1: **A**G → **G**G | $\beta^0$ | African American |
| Promoter mutants | Mutation in the ATA box<br>−31 −30 −29 −28 → −31 −30 −29 −28<br>**A** T A A → **G** T A A | $\beta^+$ | Japanese |
| Abnormal RNA cap site | A → C transversion at the mRNA cap site | $\beta^+$ | Asian |
| Polyadenylation signal defects | AATAAA → AA**C**AAA | $\beta^+$ | African American |
| ***Nonfunctional mRNAs*** (Note: early premature stop codons such as the two shown below also reduce the abundance of the mRNA—see text) | | | |
| Nonsense mutations | codon 39<br>gln → stop<br>**C**AG → **U**AG | $\beta^0$ | Mediterranean (especially Sardinia) |
| Frameshift mutations | codon 16 (1 base-pair deletion)<br>*normal* trp 15 UGG; gly 16 G**G**C; lys 17 AAG; val 18 GUG; asn 19 AAC<br>UGG GCA AGG UGA<br>*mutant* trp ala arg stop | $\beta^0$ | Indian |
| ***Coding region mutations that also alter splicing**** | | | |
| Synonymous mutations | codon 24<br>gly → gly<br>GG**U** → GG**A** | $\beta^+$ | African American |

* Two other hemoglobin structural variants that cause β-thalassemia are shown in Table 11–2.
Derived in part from Weatherall DJ, Clegg JB, Higgs DR, Wood WG (1995) The hemoglobinopathies. *In* Scriver CR, Beaudet AL, Sly WS, Valle D (eds) The Metabolic and Molecular Bases of Inherited Disease, 7th ed. McGraw-Hill, New York, pp. 3417–3484 and Orkin SH (1987) Disorders of hemoglobin synthesis: The thalassemias. *In* Stamatoyannopoulos G, Nienhuis AW, Leder P, Majerus PW (eds) The Molecular Basis of Blood Diseases. WB Saunders, Philadelphia, pp. 106–126.

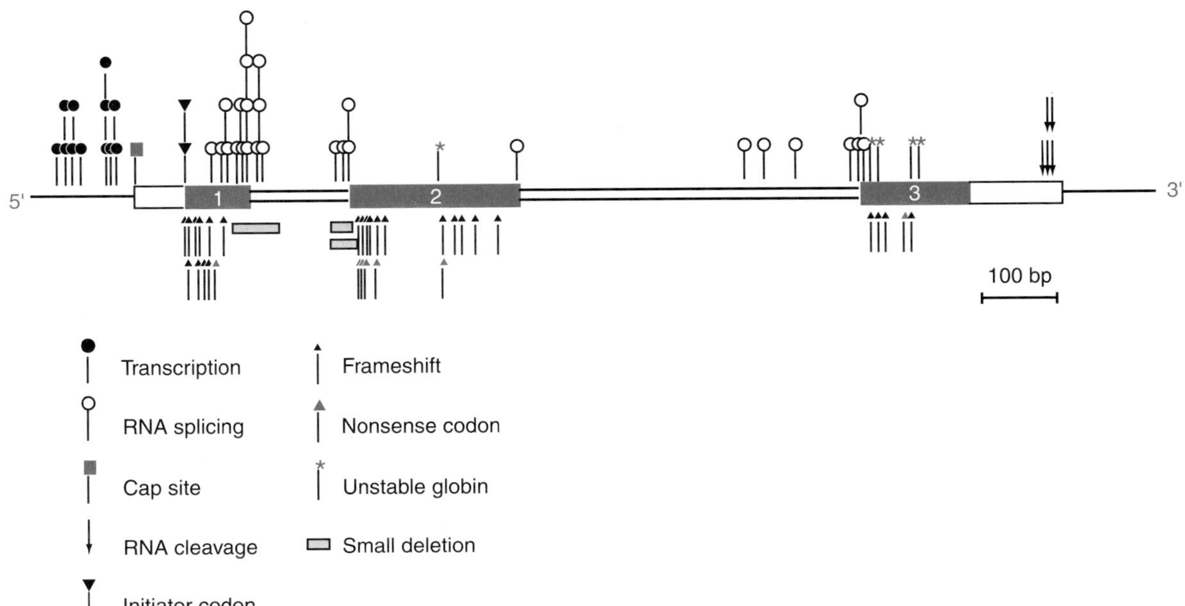


**Figure 11–13.** Representative point mutations that cause β-thalassemia. Note the distribution of mutations throughout the gene and that the mutations affect virtually every process required for the production of normal β globin. More than 100 different β-globin point mutations are associated with simple β-thalassemia. (Redrawn from Kazazian HH [1990] The thalassemia syndromes: Molecular basis and prenatal diagnosis in 1990. *In* Miescher LA, Jaffé ER [eds] Seminars in Hematology 27. WB Saunders, Philadelphia, pp. 209–228.)

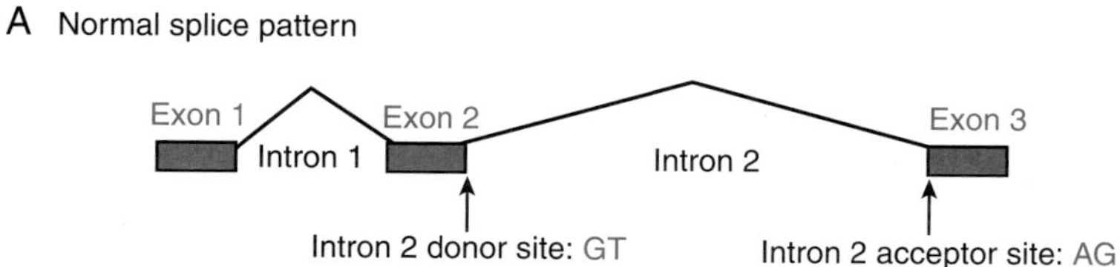


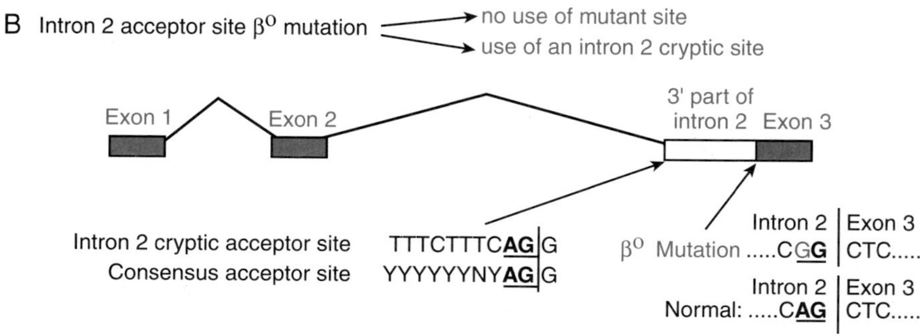


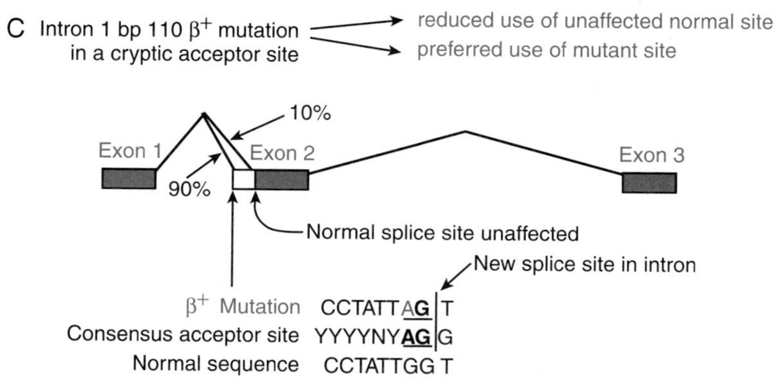


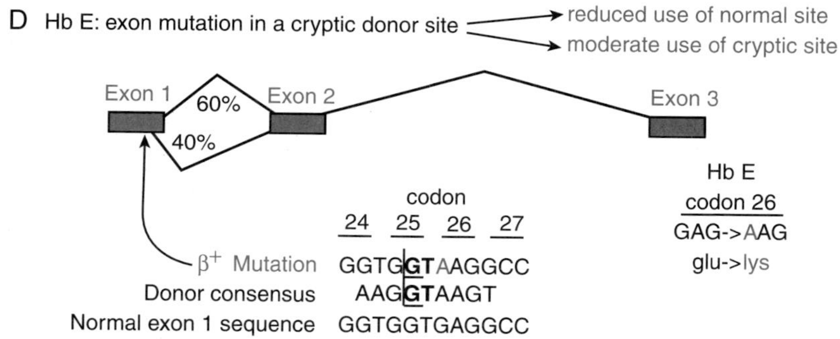


**Figure 11-14.** Examples of mutations that disrupt normal splicing (*A*) of the β-globin gene to cause β-thalassemia. *B*, An *intron 2 mutation* (A → G) in the normal splice acceptor site aborts normal splicing. This mutation results in the use of a cryptic acceptor site in intron 2. The cryptic site conforms perfectly to the consensus acceptor splice sequence (where Y = either pyrimidine, T or C). mRNA made from this mutant gene cannot encode β globin because exon 3 has been enlarged at the 5′ end by inclusion of intron 2 sequences in the alternatively spliced mRNA. *C*, An *intron 1 mutation* (G → A in base pair 110 of intron 1) activates a cryptic acceptor site by creating an AG dinucleotide and increasing the resemblance of the site to the consensus acceptor sequence. The globin mRNA thus formed is elongated (19 extra nucleotides) at the 5′ side of exon 2; a premature stop codon is introduced into the transcript. A $\beta^+$-thalassemia phenotype results because the correct acceptor site is still used, although at only 10% of the wild type level. *D*, In the *Hb E defect*, the missense mutation (Glu26Lys) in codon 26 in exon 1 activates a cryptic donor splice site that competes quite effectively with the normal donor site. Moderate use is made of this alternative splicing pathway, but the majority of RNA is still processed from the correct site, and mild $\beta^+$-thalassemia results.

**Group 2. Intron Mutations.** A mutation within an intron cryptic splice site may enhance its use by making it more similar or identical to the normal splice site. An activated cryptic site then competes with the normal site, with variable effectiveness, thereby reducing the abundance of the normal mRNA by decreasing splicing from the correct site, which remains perfectly intact (see Fig. 11–14*C*). Cryptic splice site mutations are often "leaky," which means that some use of the normal site occurs, producing a $\beta^+$-thalassemia phenotype.

**Group 3. Exon Mutations That Affect Splicing.** Disease-causing mutations in the coding region generally alter the amino acid sequence of the protein, whereas mutations outside the coding region cause disease by altering the abundance of the specific mRNA. The structural variant Hb E illustrates that both problems may result from a single mutation (see Fig. 11–14*D*). This dual effect is possible because mutations in exons can also activate cryptic splice sites. A comparable defect causing mild $\beta^+$-thalassemia has been found in codon 24 (see Table 11–4), but notably, this mutation does not change the encoded amino acid (both GGT and GGA code for glycine); this is an example of a **synonymous mutation** that is not neutral in its effect.

**Nonfunctional mRNAs.** Some mRNAs are nonfunctional and cannot direct the synthesis of a complete polypeptide because the mutation generates a premature stop codon, which prematurely terminates translation. Two $\beta$-thalassemia mutations near the amino terminus exemplify this effect and are shown in Table 11–4. In one (Gln39Stop), the failure in translation is due to a single nucleotide substitution that creates a nonsense mutation. In the other, a frameshift mutation results from a single base-pair deletion early in the coding sequence (Gly16[$\Delta$1 bp]); in the new reading frame, a premature stop codon is quickly encountered downstream, well before the normal termination signal (see Table 11–4). Because no $\beta$ globin is made, both of these types of nonfunctional mRNA mutations cause $\beta^0$-thalassemia. In contrast, frameshifts near the carboxyl terminus of the protein allow most of the mRNA to be translated normally, or to produce elongated globin chains such as Hb Tak (see Table 11–2), resulting in a variant hemoglobin rather than thalassemia.

In addition to ablating the production of the $\beta$-globin polypeptide, nonsense codons, including the two described, often lead to a reduction in the abundance of the mutant mRNA. The mechanisms underlying this phenomenon, called **nonsense-mediated mRNA decay**, are incompletely understood, but the effect appears to be restricted to nonsense codons located more than 50 base pairs 5′ to the final exon: exon junction.

**Defects in Capping and Tailing of Beta-Globin mRNA.** Two $\beta^+$-thalassemia mutations highlight the critical nature of the post-transcriptional modifications of all mRNAs, the capping of the RNA at its extreme 5′ end (at the cap site) and the polyadenylation of the 3′ end of the mRNA (see Table 11–4). An Asian patient was discovered to have an A → C transversion in the first nucleotide of the message (the cap site is a purine in 90 percent of eukaryotic mRNAs). This mutation may impair the addition of the cap, a 7-methylguanosine, thus exposing the RNA to degradation. The polyadenylation of mRNA occurs after its enzymatic cleavage, and the signal for the cleavage site, AAUAAA, is found near the 3′ end of most eukaryotic mRNAs. A patient with a substitution that changed the signal sequence to AACAAA produced only a minor fraction of $\beta$-globin mRNA that was polyadenylated at the normal position.

## The Molecular Basis of Complex Thalassemias and the Hereditary Persistence of Fetal Hemoglobin

The large deletions that cause the **complex thalassemias** remove both the $\beta$-globin gene plus one or more other genes—or the LCR—from the $\beta$-globin cluster. Thus, affected individuals have reduced expression of $\beta$ globin and one or more of the other $\beta$-like chains. These conditions are named according to the genes deleted—that is, $\delta\beta^0$-thalassemia or $\gamma\delta\beta^0$-thalassemia, and so on. Deletions that remove the $\beta$-globin LCR start approximately 50 to 100 kb upstream of the $\beta$-globin gene cluster and extend 3′ to varying degrees (Fig. 11–15). Although some of these deletions—such as the Hispanic deletion—leave all or some of the genes at the $\beta$-globin locus completely intact, they ablate expression from the entire cluster, to cause $\varepsilon\gamma\delta\beta$-thalassemia. Such mutations demonstrate the total dependence on the LCR of gene expression from the $\beta$-globin gene cluster (see Fig. 11–5).

A second group of large $\beta$-globin gene cluster deletions of medical significance are those that leave at least one of the $\gamma$ genes intact (see Fig. 11–15). Patients carrying such mutations have one of two clinical manifestations, depending on the deletion: $\delta\beta^0$ thalassemia, or hereditary persistence of fetal hemoglobin (HPFH), a benign condition due to disruption of the perinatal switch from $\gamma$- to $\beta$-globin synthesis. Homozygotes with either of these conditions are viable because the remaining $\gamma$ gene or genes are still active after birth, instead of switching off as would normally occur. As a result, Hb F ($\alpha_2\gamma_2$) synthesis continues postnatally at a high level, compensating for the absence of Hb A.

The clinically innocuous nature of HPFH is due to a substantial production of $\gamma$ chains, producing a

## Clinical Heterogeneity Due to Genetic Heterogeneity: Examples from the Hemoglobinopathies

Clinical heterogeneity in genetic disease can often be explained by genetic heterogeneity, which is of three general types exemplified by the hemoglobinopathies:

1. **Different alleles and allelic interactions in genetic compounds**. Different alleles of a single gene can be associated with phenotypes of variable severity (e.g., $\beta$-thalassemia alleles associated with either $\beta^0$- or $\beta^+$-thalassemia). If a patient with a recessive disease carries two different disease-causing alleles at a locus (i.e., is a genetic compound—see Chapter 5), the phenotype may vary if there are interactions between the alleles.
2. **Different genes**. Mutations in different genes may produce similar but often distinguishable phenotypes (e.g., $\alpha$- versus $\beta$-thalassemia).
3. **Modifier genes (locus interactions)**. Specific wild-type or disease alleles of one or more genes (modifier genes) can sometimes dramatically modify the clinical severity of the phenotype due to mutations in a disease-causing gene. This source of clinical heterogeneity is undoubtedly the most common and is vaguely encompassed by the term "**genetic background**," but, to date, few modifier genes have been identified, and the vast majority of clinical heterogeneity in genetic disease remains unexplained. One known modifier gene affecting the severity of $\beta$-thalassemia is described later.

### Allelic Interactions at the Beta-Globin Locus

One mechanism by which different mutations in a single gene can produce phenotypic variation is demonstrated by genetic compounds at the $\beta$-globin locus. Two or more of the most common $\beta$-globin mutations, such as those leading to Hb C, Hb S, and Hb E, and some of the thalassemia alleles, are sometimes present at relatively high frequencies in the same population. Consequently, it is not uncommon to find people in certain parts of the world (e.g., Africa) who are genetic compounds (an alternative term is "compound heterozygotes") for different mutations at the $\beta$-globin locus and who have clinical phenotypes that result from the interaction of the two different mutant alleles. For example, patients who carry both sickle cell and $\beta$-thalassemia alleles ($\beta^{thal}\beta^S$) have a disease that varies in severity depending on the particular $\beta$-thalassemia mutation they inherited: those with a severe ($\beta^0$) thalassemia allele have a severe disorder that resembles sickle cell disease, whereas those with a mild $\beta^+$ allele are clinically well, as are patients with sickle cell trait. This allelic interaction results from the fact that $\beta^0$ carriers produce less Hb A and therefore have a higher fraction of Hb S than do the mild $\beta^+$ carriers.

### Modifier Genes (Locus Interactions) in Beta-Thalassemia

The geographic distributions of many of the common $\alpha$- and $\beta$-globin mutant alleles frequently overlap (e.g., in the Mediterranean). As a result, occasional patients who have coinherited mutations at both the $\alpha$- and $\beta$-globin loci are recognized. The study of such patients has indicated that significant modification of the biochemical and clinical phenotype of mutations at one locus can occur when the other locus also has a mutant allele. For example, $\beta$-thalassemia homozygotes who also inherit an $\alpha$-thalassemia allele sometimes have less severe $\beta$-thalassemia. The imbalance of globin-chain synthesis that occurs in $\beta$-thalassemia, reflecting the relative excess of $\alpha$ chains, is ameliorated by the decrease in $\alpha$-chain production that results from the $\alpha$-thalassemia mutation. This example of gene interaction illustrates, at a molecular level, why the same mutant gene may have variable phenotypic effects in different individuals, even different affected members of a single family. Variable expressivity and penetrance in other disorders may sometimes be due to comparable interactions between gene products.

higher level of Hb F in heterozygotes (17 to 35 percent Hb F) than is generally seen in heterozygotes for $\delta\beta^0$-thalassemia (5 to 18 percent Hb F). The deletions that cause $\delta\beta^0$-thalassemia overlap with those that cause HPFH (see Fig. 11–15), and it is not clear why patients with HPFH have higher levels of $\gamma$-gene expression. One possibility is that some HPFH deletions bring enhancers closer to the $\gamma$-globin genes (see Fig. 11–15). Insight into the mechanism leading to the high postnatal $\gamma$-gene expression in patients with HPFH may make it possible to express Hb F at high levels in patients with $\beta$-

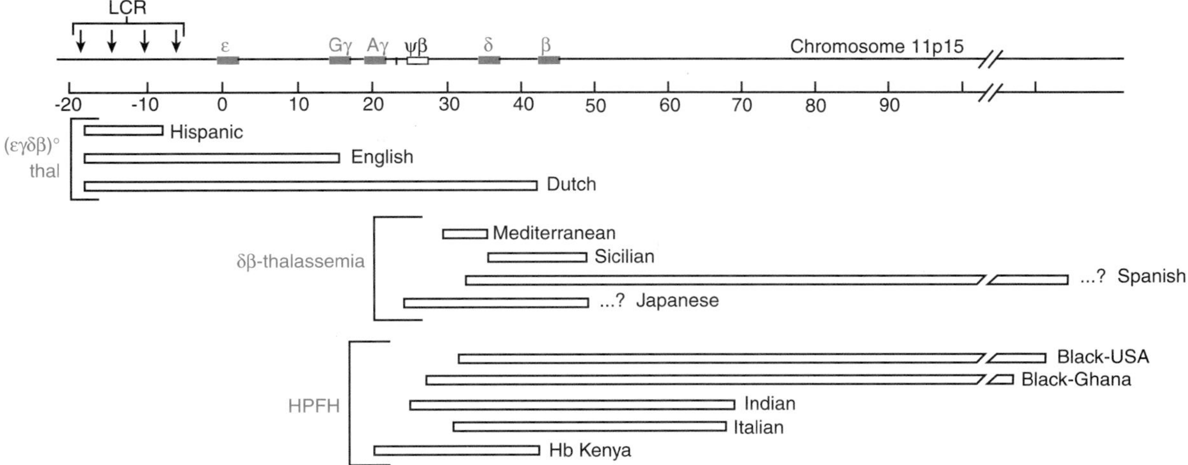


**Figure 11–15.** Location and size of deletions of various $\varepsilon\gamma\delta\beta$-thalassemia, $\delta\beta$ thalassemia and HPFH mutants. Note that deletions of the locus control region (LCR) abrogate the expression of all genes in the $\beta$-globin cluster. The deletions responsible for HPFH and $\delta\beta$-thalassemia overlap (see text). (HPFH = hereditary persistance of fetal hemoglobin; Redrawn from Stamatoyannopoulos G, Nienhuis AW [1994] Hemoglobin switching. *In* Stamatoyannopoulos G, Nienhuis AW, Leder P, Varmus H [eds] The Molecular Basis of Blood Diseases. WB Saunders, Philadelphia, pp. 107–155.)

thalassemia, a switch that would treat the disorder (see Chapter 13).

A few patients with HPFH have single base-pair substitutions in the upstream regulatory region of either the $^{A}\gamma$ or $^{G}\gamma$ genes. In Greek $^{A}\gamma$ HPFH, for example, there is a G → A change a few bases 5′ to a CCAAT box (a promoter element; see Chapter 3) of the $^{A}\gamma$ gene. These mutations are presumed to alter the affinity of regulatory (DNA-binding) proteins required for the postnatal repression of $\gamma$-gene expression. Individuals with nondeletion HPFH are clinically normal; their genetic condition is recognized incidentally during hematological studies undertaken for other reasons.

## CONCLUSION

In retrospect, it is fortunate that the hemoglobinopathies were the first group of genetic diseases to be examined at a molecular level because they exhibit such a diversity of molecular pathology. Most other genetic conditions have been found to result from mechanisms of altered gene function that had been initially recognized, in some form, in a hemoglobin disorder. Thus, although the hemoglobinopathies are paradigms for the genetic and mutational basis of "molecular disease," the biochemical pathology of each disease reflects different and often unique aspects of the structure and function of the protein altered by the mutation. The next chapter extends the concepts learned from the hemoglobinopathies, and, by describing some of the most important genetic diseases that are understood at a biochemical and molecular level, provides an overview of the pathophysiology that results from mutations in various classes of proteins.

## General References


Bunn HF, Forget BG (1986) Hemoglobin: Molecular, Genetic, and Clinical Aspects. WB Saunders, Philadelphia.

Kazazian HH Jr, Antonarakis S (1997) Molecular genetics of the globin genes. *In* Singer M, Berg P (eds) Exploring Genetic Mechanisms. University Science Books, Sausalito, California, pp. 301–336.

McKusick VA (1998) Mendelian Inheritance in Man, Catalogs of Human Genes and Genetic Disorders, 12th ed. Johns Hopkins University Press, Baltimore. See online version at *http://www.ncbi.nlm.nih.gov/omim/*

Perutz MF (1987) Molecular anatomy, physiology, and pathology of hemoglobin. *In* Stamatoyannopoulos G, Nienhuis AW, Leder P, Majerus PW (eds) The Molecular Basis of Blood Diseases. WB Saunders, Philadelphia, pp. 127–178.

Stamatoyannopoulos G, Nienhuis AW (1994) Hemoglobin switching. *In* Stamatoyannopoulos G, Nienhuis AW, Majerus PW, Varmus H (eds) The Molecular Basis of Blood Diseases, 2nd ed. WB Saunders, Philadelphia, pp. 107–155.

Weatherall DJ, Clegg JB, Higgs DR, Wood WG (1995) The hemoglobinopathies. *In* Scriver CR, Beaudet AL, Sly WS, Valle D (eds) The Metabolic and Molecular Bases of Inherited Disease, 7th ed. McGraw-Hill, New York, pp. 3417–3484.

Wood WG (1996) The complexities of $\beta$-globin gene regulation. Trends Genet 12:204–206.


## References Specific to Particular Topics


Ingram VM (1956) Specific chemical difference between the globins of normal human and sickle-cell anemia hemoglobin. Nature 178:792–794.

Kan YW, Dozy AM (1978) Polymorphism of DNA sequence adjacent to human-globin structural gene: Relationship to sickle mutation. Proc Natl Acad Sci U S A 75:5631–5635.

Lucarelli G, Galimberti M, Polchi P, et al (1990) Bone marrow transplantation in patients with thalassemia. N Engl J Med 322: 417–421.

Pauling L, Itano HA, Singer SJ, Wells IG (1949) Sickle cell anemia, a molecular disease. Science 110:543–548.

## Problems

1. A child dies of hydrops fetalis. Draw a pedigree with genotypes that illustrates to the carrier parents the genetic basis of the infant's thalassemia. Explain why a Melanesian couple whom they met in the hematology clinic, who also have the $\alpha$-thalassemia trait, are unlikely to have a similarly affected infant.

2. Why are most patients with $\beta$-thalassemia likely to be genetic compounds? In what situations might you anticipate that a patient with $\beta$-thalassemia would have two identical $\beta$-globin alleles?

3. Tony, a young Italian boy, is found to have moderate $\beta$-thalassemia, with a Hb of 7 g/dl (normal amounts are 10 to 13 g/dl). When you perform a Northern blot of his reticulocyte RNA, you unexpectedly find three $\beta$-globin mRNA bands, one of normal size, one larger than normal, and one smaller than normal.

   What mutational mechanisms could account for the presence of three bands like this in a patient with $\beta$-thalassemia? In *this* patient, the fact that the anemia is mild suggests that a significant fraction of normal $\beta$-globin mRNA is being made. What types of mutation would allow this to occur?

4. A man is heterozygous for Hb M Saskatoon, a hemoglobinopathy in which the normal amino acid His is replaced by Tyr at position 63 of the $\beta$ chain. His mate is heterozygous for Hb M Boston, in which His is replaced by Tyr at position 58 of the $\alpha$ chain. Heterozygosity for either of these mutant alleles produces methemoglobinemia. Outline the possible genotypes and phenotypes of their offspring.

5. A child has a paternal uncle and a maternal aunt with sickle cell disease; both of her parents do not. What is the probability that the child has sickle cell disease?

6. A woman has sickle cell trait, and her mate is heterozygous for Hb C. What is the probability that their child has no abnormal hemoglobin?

7. Match the following:

| | | |
|---|---|---|
| _______ | complex $\beta$-thalassemia | 1. Detectable Hb A |
| _______ | $\beta^+$-thalassemia | 2. Three |
| _______ | number of $\alpha$-globin genes missing in Hb H disease | 3. $\beta$-thalassemia |
| _______ | two different mutant alleles at a locus | 4. $\alpha$-thalassemia |
| _______ | prenatal diagnosis of sickle cell disease | 5. High-level $\beta$-chain expression |
| _______ | insoluble $\beta$-chains | 6. $\alpha$-thalassemia trait |
| _______ | number of $\alpha$-globin genes missing in hydrops fetalis with Hb Bart's | 7. Genetic compound |
| _______ | locus control region | 8. $\delta\beta$ genes deleted |
| _______ | $\alpha-/\alpha-$ genotype | 9. Four |
| _______ | increased Hb $A_2$ | 10. Restriction enzyme HpaI |

8. Mutations in noncoding sequences change the number of protein molecules produced, but, generally, each protein molecule made will have a normal amino acid sequence. Give examples of some exceptions to this rule, and describe how the alterations in the amino acid sequence are generated.

9. In Hb Tak, the insertion of two base pairs (either AC or CA—it is not possible to know which insertion occurred, and the effect on the reading frame of either one is the same) between codons 146 and 147 of the $\beta$-globin chain leads to the addition of 11 amino acids to the end of the polypeptide. Using the nucleotide sequence of the coding region of the $\beta$-globin gene shown in Fig. 3–10, determine the sequence of the novel C-terminal peptide responsible for the increased oxygen affinity of this globin variant.

12

# The Molecular and Biochemical Basis of Genetic Disease

The examination of the molecular and biochemical basis of genetic disease that began in the previous chapter with the hemoglobinopathies is extended in this chapter to other proteins and their corresponding diseases. In Chapter 11, we presented an outline of the general mechanisms by which disease-causing mutations cause pathology (see Fig. 11–1) and reviewed the steps at which mutations can disrupt the synthesis or function of a protein (see Table 11–1). These outlines provide a framework for understanding the pathogenesis of all genetic disease. Although the hemoglobinopathies have taught geneticists much about the mechanisms that underlie genetic disease, there are many other molecular and biochemical disease processes that require consideration. Mutations in other classes of proteins often disrupt cell and organ function by processes that differ from those illustrated by the hemoglobinopathies.

In this chapter, we extend the description of the general mechanisms by which mutations impair the synthesis, processing, or molecular associations of proteins, and the consequent effects on protein function. The relationships between a molecular defect and the location and nature of its clinical pathology are also examined. To illustrate disease mechanisms, in most instances we use well-known diseases such as **phenylketonuria (PKU)**, **cystic fibrosis (CF)**, **familial hypercholesterolemia**, **Duchenne muscular dystrophy (DMD)**, and **Alzheimer disease (AD)**. In some instances, less common disorders such as **acute intermittent porphyria** and **I-cell disease** are included because they best demonstrate a specific principle.

The importance of teaching medical genetics from general principles is illustrated by the fact that more than 1000 genes associated with single-gene disorders have now been identified. It would be impossible to remember the molecular pathology and pathophysiology of each condition or even of every biochemical category of disease. Moreover, there are at least 3000 other single-gene diseases in which the biochemical defect remains to be identified and, overall, 30,000 to 50,000 genes in the genome, many of which will be shown in the coming decades to be implicated in genetically determined conditions.

## DISEASES DUE TO MUTATIONS IN DIFFERENT CLASSES OF PROTEINS

Proteins carry out an astounding number of different functions, a few of which are presented in Table 12–1 with their associated genetic diseases. As the list suggests, mutations in virtually every functional class of protein can lead to a genetic disorder. The recognition that a disease results from abnormality in a protein of a particular class is often useful in understanding its pathogenesis and inheritance, and in devising therapy. In this section, we describe important genetic diseases that affect representative proteins from many of the groups listed. Not every disease listed in Table 12–1 is reviewed here. The interested reader can find a wealth of information on genetic diseases that are understood at the biochemical level in the comprehensive references listed at the

TABLE 12–1

**Some Examples of the Classes of Proteins Associated with Monogenic Diseases**

| Function | | Examples of Proteins Affected by Mutations (Disease)* | Inheritance |
|---|---|---|---|
| Enzymes | Literally hundreds, in all areas of metabolism, including | | |
| | *Amino acids* | • phenylalanine hydroxylase (PKU) | AR |
| | *Carbohydrates* | • galactose-1-phosphate uridyl transferase (galactosemia) | AR |
| | *Organic acids* | • methylmalonyl-CoA mutase (methylmalonic aciduria) | AR |
| | *Fatty acids* | • medium chain acyl CoA dehydrogenase (MCAD deficiency) | AR |
| | *Complex lipids* | • hexosaminidase A (Tay-Sachs disease) | AR |
| | *Purines* | • adenosine deaminase (severe combined immunodeficiency) | AR |
| | *Porphyrins* | • porphobilinogen deaminase (acute intermittent porphyria) | AD |
| Transport and storage | *Interorgan* | • hemoglobin (the thalassemias, hemoglobin variants) | AR |
| | *Organelle membrane* | • a lysosomal cystine transport protein (cystinosis) | AR |
| | *Intracellular transport* | • a copper transport protein (Menkes syndrome) | XR |
| | *Epithelial membrane* | • Cftr, a $Cl^-$ channel in the epithelia of tissues affected in cystic fibrosis (e.g., lung, pancreas) | AR |
| Structure of cells and organs | *Extracellular* | • types I and II collagen (osteogenesis imperfecta) | AR, AD |
| | *Cell membrane and cytoskeleton* | • the red cell membrane skeleton protein, spectrin (hereditary spherocytosis) | AD |
| | | • dystrophin (Duchenne and Becker muscular dystrophy) | XR |
| | *Organelle biogenesis* | • PEX1, an ATPase required for peroxisome membrane biogenesis (Zellweger syndrome) | AR |
| Extracellular homeostasis | *Immune protection* | • proteins of the complement system (e.g., complement C3 deficiency → recurrent bacterial infections) | AD, AR |
| | *Hemostasis* | • Factor VIII (hemophilia A) | XR |
| | *Protease inhibition* | • $\alpha_1$-antitrypsin (deficiency → lung and liver disease) | AR |
| Developmental gene expression | *Transcription factors* | • PAX6, a homeodomain transcription factor (aniridia) | AD |
| | | • WT1, a zinc finger transcription factor (Wilms' tumor) | AD |
| | *Signaling molecules* | • sonic hedgehog (holoprosencephaly) | AD |
| | *Signaling receptors* | • FGFR3 receptor (achondroplasia) | AD |
| | *Ribosomal proteins* | • S19 ribosomal protein (Diamond-Blackfan anemia) | AD |
| Control of growth and differentiation | *Tumor suppressors* | • Rb gene product (retinoblastoma and osteosarcoma) | AR |
| | *Oncogenes* | • the Ret receptor tyrosine kinase (multiple endocrine neoplasia or MEN2) | AD |
| Intercellular metabolism and communication | *Cell-cell channels* | • connexin 43 gap junction protein (cardiac malformations, defects in laterality) | AR |
| | | • connexin 26 gap junction protein (nonsyndromic hearing loss) | AR |
| | *Metabolite receptors* | • low-density-lipoprotein receptor (familial hypercholesterolemia) | AD |
| | *Light receptors* | • rhodopsin (one form of AD retinitis pigmentosa) | AD |
| | | • green and red light opsins (X-linked color blindness) | XR |
| | *Hormones* | • growth hormone (dwarfism) | AR |
| | | • insulin (rare forms of type 2 diabetes mellitus) | AD |
| | *Hormone receptors* | • vasopressin V2 receptor (diabetes insipidus) | XR |
| | | • androgen receptor (androgen insensitivity) | XR |
| | | • insulin receptor (Donohue syndrome) | AR |
| | *Signal transducers* | • the stimulatory guanine nucleotide-binding protein of adenylate cyclase (pseudohypoparathyroidism) | AD |

*The protein classification has been adapted and modified from Stryer L (1981) Biochemistry, 2nd ed. WH Freeman, San Francisco.
AD = autosomal dominant pattern of inheritance; AR = autosomal recessive pattern of inheritance; XR = X-linked recessive pattern of inheritance.

end of the chapter. The treatment of genetic disease, including that of many of the conditions described in this chapter, is presented in Chapter 13.

## Housekeeping Proteins, Specialty Proteins, and Genetic Disease

Proteins can be separated into two general classes based on their pattern of expression: **housekeeping proteins** that are present in virtually every cell and have fundamental roles in the maintenance of cell structure and function, and tissue-specific **specialty proteins** that are produced in only one or a limited number of cell types; they have unique functions that contribute to the individuality of the cells in which they are expressed. This class distinction is not necessarily absolute, however. A protein with a housekeeping role in most cells may be present at a higher level in a few tissues in which it has a more specialized function. Most tissues of higher eukaryotes, such as humans, express 10,000 to 15,000 genes. As many as 90 percent of the messenger RNA (mRNA) species found in a tissue are also present in many other tissues and encode shared housekeeping proteins. The remaining 10 percent or so encode the specialty proteins of the tissue.

Knowledge of the tissues in which a protein is expressed, and of the tissues in which it is expressed at high levels, is often useful in understanding the pathogenesis of a disease. Several generalizations can be made about the relationship between the site of a protein's expression and the site of pathology.

First, mutation in a tissue-specific protein most often produces a disease restricted to that tissue, although there may be secondary effects on other tissues. However, the relationship between the site at which a protein is expressed and the site of pathology in a genetic disease may, at times, be unpredictable. For example, mutation in a tissue-specific protein may produce its primary clinical abnormalities in cells and organs other than those in which the protein is expressed; ironically, the tissue that lacks the mutant protein may even be left unaffected by pathology. Consequently, one cannot necessarily infer that pathology in an organ results from a mutation in a gene expressed principally or only in that organ, or in that organ at all.

Second, although housekeeping proteins are by definition expressed in most or all tissues, genetic diseases that affect these proteins rarely cause pathology in every tissue. (Mutations in genes that are essential to every tissue, such as actin, are likely, in most instances, to be incompatible with live birth.) Rather, the clinical effects of mutations in a housekeeping protein are frequently limited to one or a few tissues, often tissues in which the protein is abundant and serves a specialty function.

## The Relationship Between Genotype and Phenotype in Genetic Disease

Variation in the clinical phenotype observed in an inherited disease may be due to one of three types of genetic variation: allelic heterogeneity, locus heterogeneity, or the effect of modifier genes.

**Allelic Heterogeneity.** As discussed in Chapter 5, genetic heterogeneity is most commonly due to the presence of multiple alleles at a locus, a situation referred to as **allelic heterogeneity** (Table 12–2). In many instances, there is a clear **genotype-phenotype** correlation between a specific allele and a specific phenotype. The most common explanation for the effect of allelic heterogeneity on the clinical phenotype is that alleles that confer more *residual function* are often associated with a milder phenotype (e.g., see later discussion of phenylalanine hydroxylase alleles). In other instances, alleles that confer some residual function on a protein are associated with a partial phenotype of the whole clinical spectrum associated with a null allele. This situation prevails with certain variants of the *CFTR* gene associated with congenital absence of the vas deferens but no other manifestations of CF (see later).

A second explanation for allele-based variation in phenotype is that the phenotypic variation may reflect the *specific subfunction* of the protein most perturbed by the mutation. In this situation, some alleles may be associated with remarkably distinct clinical phenotypes. These points are well illustrated by some of the $\beta$-globin disease–causing alleles described in Chapter 11 (see Table 11–1). Thus, $\beta$-globin alleles that alter the oxygen affinity of hemoglobin produce polycythemia or cyanosis. These specific phenotypes are often so different from the phenotypes associated with severe loss-of-function alleles (e.g., thalassemia in the case of the globin chains) that it is not at all obvious, from a clinical perspective, that these diseases result from mutations affecting the same protein.

Finally, it should be noted that the biochemical and clinical consequences of a specific mutation in a protein are often unpredictable and may be unique to that allele. For example, no one would have foreseen that the allele most commonly associated with $\alpha_1$-antitrypsin ($\alpha_1$-AT) deficiency (the *Z* allele) would cause liver disease because the mutation leads the protein to form intracellular aggregates in hepatocytes (see later).

**Locus Heterogeneity.** Genetic heterogeneity also arises from the association of more than one locus with a specific clinical condition, a situation termed **locus heterogeneity** (Table 12–2). This phenomenon is illustrated by the discovery that mutations in any one of five genes can lead to hyperphenylalaninemia (Table 12–3). Once locus heterogeneity has been documented, careful comparison of the phenotype associated with each gene commonly reveals that the phenotype is not as homogeneous as initially believed.

**Modifier Genes.** Sometimes even the most robust genotype-phenotype relationships are found not to hold for a specific patient. For example, CF patients homozygous for the most common CF mutation have highly variable lung disease, as discussed later. Such phenotypic variation can, in principle, be ascribed to environmental factors or to the action of other genes, termed **modifier genes**. To date, few modifier genes for human monogenic disorders have been identified. One example is cited at the end of Chapter 11: the amelioration of disease in $\beta$-thalassemia homozygotes who also inherit an $\alpha$-thalassemia allele. Modifier genes will only infrequently be disease-causing alleles at other loci, however. More often, they will be polymorphisms or rare benign variants that in some way

TABLE 12–2

**The Various Types of Heterogeneity Associated with Genetic Disease**

| Type of Heterogeneity | Definition | Example |
|---|---|---|
| **Genetic heterogeneity** | | |
| Allelic heterogeneity | The occurrence of more than one allele at a locus | • $\beta$-thalassemia alleles<br>• Phenylalanine hydroxylase mutations |
| Locus heterogeneity | The association of more than one locus with a specific clinical phenotype | • Biopterin defects causing hyperphenylalaninemia<br>• Sanfilippo syndrome |
| **Clinical or phenotypic heterogeneity** | The association of more than one phenotype with mutations at a single locus | • Phenylalanine hydroxylase mutations causing PKU, variant PKU, or non-PKU hyperphenylalaninemia<br>• $\alpha$-iduronidase mutations causing Hurler syndrome or Scheie syndrome |

PKU = Phenylketonuria.

modulate the severity of disease due to pathogenic mutations at another locus. The modifier effect of alleles of the apolipoprotein E gene (*APOE*) on the age of onset of AD, reviewed later, is a prominent example.

## ENZYME DEFECTS

Enzymes are the biological catalysts that mediate, with great efficiency, the conversion of a substrate to a product. Apart from the few catalytic ribonucleic acids (RNAs) involved in RNA processing, enzymes are proteins. The diversity of substrates on which enzymes act is barely suggested in Table 12–1; the list includes only a few important enzymopathies, which at present number in the hundreds. We first discuss one of the best-known groups of inborn errors of metabolism, the hyperphenylalaninemias, which arise from deficient activity of phenylalanine hydroxylase. Several additional enzyme defects of significance are then briefly examined. In a summary section, general features of the pathophysiology of enzymopathies are presented.

### Aminoacidopathies

#### THE HYPERPHENYLALANINEMIAS

The abnormalities that lead to an increase in the blood level of phenylalanine, most notably PKU, illustrate almost every principle of biochemical genetics of relevance to enzyme defects. The biochemical causes of hyperphenylalaninemia are illustrated in Figure 12–1, and the principal features of the disease associated with mutations at the five hyperphenylala-

TABLE 12–3

**The Locus Heterogeneity of the Hyperphenylalaninemias**

| Biochemical Defect | Incidence/ $10^6$ Births | Enzyme Affected | Gene Location | Inheritance | Treatment |
|---|---|---|---|---|---|
| ***Mutations in the phenylalanine hydroxylase apoenzyme*** | | | | | |
| Classic PKU | 5–350 | PAH | 12q24.1 | AR | Low phenylalanine diet |
| Variant PKU | Less than classic PKU | PAH | 12q24.1 | AR | Low phenylalanine diet (less restrictive than that required to treat PKU) |
| Non-PKU hyperphenylalaninemia | 15–75 | PAH | 12q24.1 | AR | None, or less restrictive low phenylalanine diet |
| ***Mutations in genes encoding enzymes of tetrahydrobiopterin metabolism*** | | | | | |
| Impaired $BH_4$ recycling | 1–2 | PCD | 10q22 | AR | Low phenylalanine diet + L-dopa, 5-HT, carbidopa |
| | | DHPR | 4p15.31 | AR | Low phenylalanine diet + L-dopa, 5-HT, carbidopa + folinic acid |
| Impaired $BH_4$ synthesis | Rare | GTP-CH | 14q22 | AR | Low phenylalanine diet + L-dopa, 5-HT, carbidopa + folinic acid + pharmacologic doses of $BH_4$ |
| | | 6-PTS | 11q22.3–23.3 | AR | As above |

5-HT = 5-hydroxytryptophan; 6-PTS = 6-pyruvoyltetrahydropterin synthase; $BH_4$ = tetrahydrobiopterin; DHPR = dihydropteridine reductase; GTP-CH = guanosine triphosphate cyclohydrolase; PAH = phenylalanine hydroxylase; PCD = pterin 4-$\alpha$-carbinolamine dehydratase; PKU = phenylketonuria.

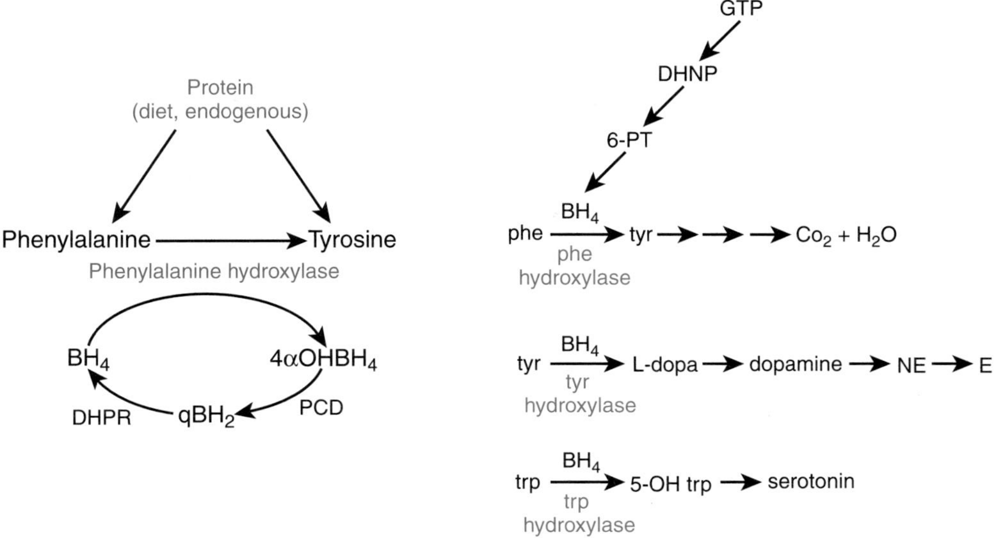


**Figure 12–1.** The biochemical pathways affected in the hyperphenylalaninemias. $BH_4$ = tetrahydrobiopterin; $qBH_2$ = quininoid dihydrobiopterin, the oxidized product of the hydroxylation reactions, which is reduced to $BH_4$ by dihydropteridine reductase (DHPR); phe = phenylalanine; tyr = tyrosine; trp = tryptophan; L-dopa = L-dihydroxyphenylalanine; NE = norepinephrine; E = epinephrine; 5-OH trp = 5-hydroxytryptophan; GTP = guanosine triphosphate; DHNP = dihydroneopterin triphosphate; 6-PT = 6-pyruvoyltetrahydropterin; PCD = pterin 4-$\alpha$-carbinolamine dehydratase.

ninemia loci are presented in Table 12–2. All of the genetic abnormalities of phenylalanine metabolism are due to loss-of-function mutations in the gene encoding phenylalanine hydroxylase (*PAH*) (Fig. 12–1) or in genes required for the synthesis or reutilization of its cofactor, tetrahydrobiopterin ($BH_4$). Thus, in the latter conditions, the loss of PAH function is a *secondary abnormality* (as described in Table 11–1) of a mutation in a gene encoding a component of the biopterin pathway.

**Phenylketonuria.** Classic PKU has been justifiably termed the epitome of inborn errors of metabolism. It is an autosomal recessive disorder of phenylalanine catabolism, resulting from mutations in the gene encoding PAH, the enzyme that converts phenylalanine to tyrosine (see Fig. 12–1 and Table 12–3). The discovery of PKU by Følling in 1934 marked the first demonstration of a genetic defect as a cause of mental retardation. Because of their inability to degrade phenylalanine, patients with PKU accumulate this amino acid in body fluids. The hyperphenylalaninemia damages the developing central nervous system in early childhood and interferes with the function of the mature brain. A small fraction of total phenylalanine is metabolized by alternative pathways, producing increased amounts of phenylpyruvic acid (a keto acid and the compound responsible for the name of the disease) and other minor metabolites, which are excreted in the urine. Ironically, although the enzymatic defect has been known for decades, the exact neuropathological mechanism by which the increase in phenylalanine damages the brain is still unknown. The neurological damage due to the metabolic block in classic PKU may be largely avoided by dietary modifications that prevent phenylalanine accumulation. The management of PKU is a paradigm of the treatment of many metabolic diseases whose outcome can be improved by preventing accumulation of an enzyme substrate and its derivatives; this concept is described further in Chapter 13.

**Newborn Screening.** Population screening of newborns for PKU is done widely. It is the prototype of genetic diseases for which mass newborn screening is justified (see Chapter 20); the disorder is relatively common in some populations (up to about 1/2,900 live births). Treatment, if begun early in life, is effective; without treatment, severe retardation is inevitable. The screening test is performed a few days after birth. A droplet of blood is obtained from a heel prick, dried on filter paper, and sent to a central laboratory for assay of blood phenylalanine levels. In the past, samples were collected before an infant left the hospital. The trend toward very short postdelivery hospitalizations for mothers and newborns has modified that practice, however. The test is preferably not done before 3 to 4 days of age because the phenylalanine level in PKU increases in relation to time after birth in the first week of life. Positive tests must be confirmed quickly because delays beyond 4 weeks postnatally in the initiation of treatment have profound effects on the intellectual outcome of patients with PKU.

**Variant Phenylketonuria and Non-Phenylketonuria Hyperphenylalaninemia.** Whereas PKU results from a virtual absence of PAH activity (less than 1 percent of controls), less severe phenotypes, designated non-PKU hyperphenylalaninemia and variant PKU (see Table 12–3), result when the mutant PAH enzyme has some residual activity. **Non-PKU hyperphenylalaninemia** is defined by plasma phenylalanine concentrations below 1 mM when the patient is receiving a normal diet. This degree of hyperphenylalaninemia is only about 10-fold above normal, lower than the concentrations found in classic PKU (>1 mM). The moderate increase in phenylalanine in non-PKU hyperphenylalaninemia is less damaging to the brain or may even be benign if the increase is small (<0.4 mM), and affected individuals come to clinical attention only because they are identified by newborn screening. Their normal phenotype has been the best indication of the "safe" level of plasma phenylalanine that must not be exceeded in the treatment of patients with classic PKU. **Variant PKU** is a category that includes patients with phenylalanine tolerance intermediate between that of classic PKU and non-PKU hyperphenylalaninemia; such patients require some phenylalanine restriction in their diet but less than that required by patients with classic PKU. The association of these three clinical phenotypes with mutations in the *PAH* gene is a clear example of clinical heterogeneity (see Table 12–2).

### The Hyperphenylalaninemias: Allelic and Locus Heterogeneity

**The Molecular Defects in Phenylalanine Hydroxylase.** The gene for PAH was isolated in 1986, and, subsequently, a striking degree of allelic heterogeneity (see Table 12–3) has been demonstrated in the PAH-deficient population. More than 400 different alleles have been recognized. The great majority are rare mutations that impair PAH enzymatic activity and lead to hyperphenylalaninemia, although benign polymorphisms or less common benign variants have also been identified. Six different mutations account for about two thirds of known mutant chromosomes in populations of European descent (Fig. 12–2). Notably, six other mutations are responsible for slightly more than 80 percent of *PAH* mutations in Asian populations (Fig. 12–2). The remaining disease-causing mutations are individually rare. To record and make this information publicly available, a *PAH* database has been developed by an international consortium.

In all populations, there is substantial genetic heterogeneity in the *PAH* mutant population. Owing to the high degree of allelic heterogeneity at the locus, most PKU patients in most populations are **genetic compounds** (i.e., have two different disease-causing alleles), a finding entirely in agreement with enzymatic and clinical observations of phenotypic heterogeneity in PAH defects. Although it first seemed that knowledge of the *PAH* genotype would reliably predict details of the phenotype, this expectation has not been borne out. For example, two of the common European mutations are associated with phenotypes ranging from classic PKU to variant PKU to non-PKU hyperphenylalaninemia (Table 12–4). Thus, it is now clear that other unidentified biological variables—including modifier genes—generate phenotypic inconsistency in PKU, even in the presence of genotypic identity at the *PAH* locus. Consequently, it has been recognized that even monogenic traits like PKU are not simple.

In Northern Europe, three of the principal mutant alleles are largely restricted to specific haplotypes (Table 12–4), although more than 80 restriction

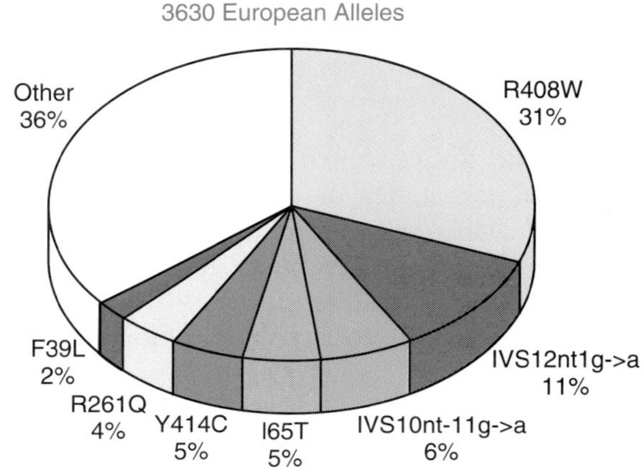


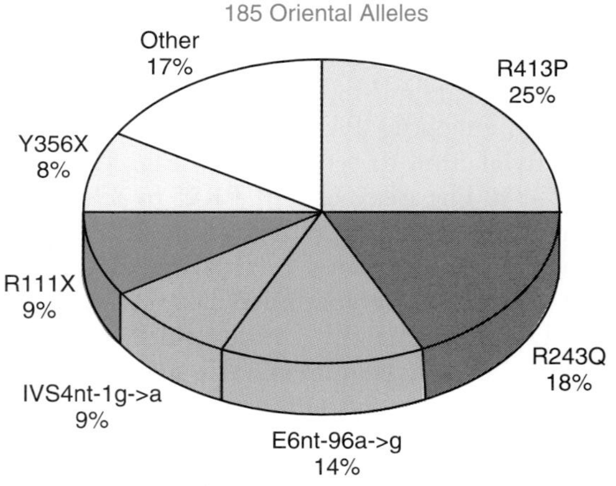


Figure 12–2. The nature and identity of *PAH* mutations in populations of European and Asian descent (the latter from China, Korea, and Japan). (Derived from Nowacki PM, Byck S, Prevost L, and Scriver CR [1998] PAH mutation analysis consortium database: 1997. Prototype for relational locus-specific mutation databases. Nucl Acids Res 26:220–225, by permission of Oxford University Press). The one-letter amino acid code is used (see Table 3–1) and mutation nomenclature is as described in Chapter 6.

TABLE 12–4

**Phenylalanine Hydroxylase Gene: Mutations, Haplotypes, and Clinical Phenotypes in Populations of European Descent**

| Mutation | % Activity | Representation among Mutations* | Associated Haplotype† | Associated Phenotype in Homozygotes‡ |
|---|---|---|---|---|
| Arg 408 Trp | <1% | 31% | 1, 2, 5, 44 | Classic PKU |
| IVS12nt1g → a§ | <1% | 11% | 3 | Classic PKU |
| IVS10nt − 11g → a | unknown | 6% | 6, 10, 34, 36 | Classic PKU |
| Ile 65 Thr | ~25% | 5% | 9 | Classic PKU, Variant PKU, Non-PKU HPA |
| Tyr 414 Cys | 30–50%‖ | 5% | 4 | Variant PKU, Non-PKU HPA |
| Arg 261 Gln | 30%‖ | 4% | 1, 2, 4, others | PKU or variant PKU |

*From Nowacki P et al (1998) PAH mutation analysis consortium database: 1997. Prototype for relational locus-specific mutation databases. Nucl Acids Res 26:220–225.

†From the PAH database (*www.mcgill.ca/pahdb*).

‡From Kayaalp E, et al (1997) Human phenylalanine hydroxylase mutations and hyperphenylalaninemia phenotypes: A metanalysis of genotype-phenotype correlations. Am J Hum Genet 61:1309–1317.

§IVS 12nt1g → a means that the first nucleotide of the 12th intron is "a" substituted for "g."

‖Whether these activities, obtained by in vitro assays, reflect in vivo function is unclear.

fragment length polymorphism (RFLP) haplotypes centered around the *PAH* gene have now been identified. As discussed in Chapter 8, a particular haplotype is often associated with a particular mutation *in a specific population*. The association of a specific mutation with a particular chromosomal haplotype in different population subgroups suggests that the mutation originated on a chromosome with that haplotype. In the case of PKU, the data suggest single origins for several alleles in Northern Europe. The most common *PAH* mutation (Arg408Trp) appears to have arisen independently on several different chromosomes, because it is found on several different haplotypes; it involves a hypermutable CpG site. For this reason, one cannot assume that a particular haplotype is associated with a specific mutation in PKU, except in well-defined populations.

### Defects in Tetrahydrobiopterin Metabolism

It was initially believed that all children with hereditary hyperphenylalaninemia had a primary deficiency of PAH. It is now clear, however, that in about 1 to 3 percent of these patients the *PAH* gene is normal, and their hyperphenylalaninemia is the result of a genetic defect in the formation or recycling of the cofactor of PAH, tetrahydrobiopterin ($BH_4$) (see Fig. 12–1 and Table 12–3). The association of a single phenotype, such as hyperphenylalaninemia, with mutations in different genes is an example of locus heterogeneity (see Table 12–2). As illustrated by mutations in the genes encoding the PAH apoenzyme and the biopterin cofactor pathways (see Fig. 12–1), the proteins encoded by genes that manifest locus heterogeneity generally act at different steps in a single biochemical pathway. $BH_4$-deficient patients were first recognized because, despite the successful administration of a low-phenylalanine diet, they developed profound neurological problems in early life. This poor outcome is due in part to the requirement for the $BH_4$ cofactor of two other enzymes, tyrosine hydroxylase and tryptophan hydroxylase. Both of these hydroxylases are critical for the synthesis of monoamine neurotransmitters such as dopa, norepinephrine, epinephrine, and serotonin (see Fig. 12–1).

$BH_4$-deficient patients have defects either in one of the steps in the biosynthesis of $BH_4$ from guanosine triphosphate (GTP) or in the regeneration of $BH_4$ (see Fig. 12–1). It is critical to recognize these conditions because their treatment differs markedly from that for classic PKU. For this reason, all hyperphenylalaninemic infants should also be tested for $BH_4$ deficiency. Apart from controlling blood phenylalanine levels, the object of treatment for these patients is to try to normalize the neurotransmitters in the brain by administering the products of tyrosine hydroxylase and tryptophan hydroxylase, L-dopa and 5-hydroxytryptophan, respectively (see Fig. 12–1 and Table 12–3). Like classic PKU, these disorders are inherited as autosomal recessive traits.

**Maternal Phenylketonuria.** The generally successful treatment of PKU allows affected homozygotes to lead an independent life and have near-normal prospects for parenthood. In the past, most patients with PKU were taken off a low phenylalanine diet in mid-childhood on the assumption (now shown to be incorrect) that function of the mature nervous system would not be impaired by the return of hyperphenylalaninemia. Subsequently, it was discovered that almost all the offspring of women with PKU who were not receiving treatment were abnormal. Most are mentally retarded and many have microcephaly, growth impairment, and malformations, particularly of the heart. As predicted by principles of mendelian inheritance, most of these children are heterozygotes. Thus, their retardation is not due to their own genetic constitution but to the highly teratogenic effect of elevated levels of phenylalanine in the maternal circulation. Accordingly, it is imperative that women with PKU who are planning pregnancies commence a low-phenylalanine diet before conceiving.

## Defects in Purine Metabolism

### LESCH-NYHAN SYNDROME

A good example of a genotype-phenotype relationship due to allelic heterogeneity is provided by mutations at the *HPRT* locus encoding the X-linked enzyme hypoxanthine guanine phosphoribosyltransferase (Hprt) (Fig. 12–3). Patients with no residual Hprt activity have a remarkable phenotype called the Lesch-Nyhan syndrome, characterized by choreoathetosis (a movement disorder), spasticity, variable mental retardation, uric acid overproduction that causes gout and renal stones, and, most striking, self-mutilation. The neurological abnormalities may result from changes in brain purine levels produced by the disease, consistent with the theory that some purines are putative neurotransmitters. Finally, patients with Hprt deficiency also illustrate how loss of normal feedback inhibition on the regulation of a metabolic pathway can have pathophysiological consequences, an important principle of biochemical genetic disease (Fig. 12–3).

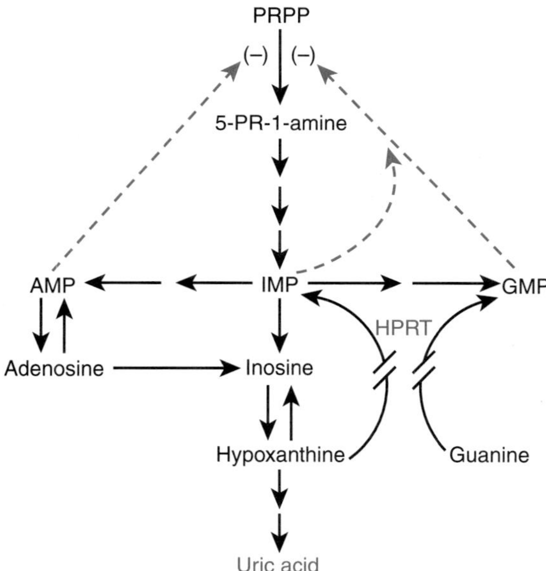


**Figure 12–3.** An outline of the purine synthetic pathway. In the absence of HPRT, the ability to reutilize hypoxanthine and guanine to make IMP and GMP is lost. As a consequence, the normal feedback inhibition by IMP and GMP (*broken arrows*) on an early step in purine synthesis is greatly reduced, and the de novo synthesis of purines, and ultimately uric acid, is increased (*heavy central arrows*). PRPP = phosphoribosylpyrophosphate; 5-PR-1-amine = 5-phosphoribosyl-1-amine; AMP = adenosine monophosphate; IMP = inosine monophosphate; GMP = guanosine monophosphate; HPRT = hypoxanthine guanine phosphoribosyltransferase.

Some subjects with mutations in the *HPRT* gene manifest only a partial phenotype of the Lesch-Nyhan syndrome, hyperuricemia, with gout. In contrast to patients with Lesch-Nyhan syndrome, these individuals carry alleles associated with levels of Hprt activity ranging from approximately 1 to 30 percent of normal. None of the dramatic neurological findings are present. Partial Hprt deficiency of this type, however, accounts for less than 2 percent of all adult male patients with gout.

## Lysosomal Storage Diseases

Lysosomes are membrane-bound organelles containing an array of hydrolytic enzymes involved in the degradation of a variety of biological macromolecules. Genetic defects of these hydrolases lead to the accumulation of their substrates inside the lysosome, resulting in cellular dysfunction and, eventually, cell death. The gradual accumulation of the substrate is responsible for the one uniform clinical feature of these diseases: their unrelenting progression. In most of these conditions, substrate storage is manifested clinically as an increase in the mass of the affected tissues and organs. When the brain is affected, however, as is often the case, the picture is one of neurodegeneration. The clinical phenotypes often make the diagnosis of a storage disease straightforward and usually suggest the class of storage disease, if not the specific disorder. More than 48 lysosomal hydrolase or lysosomal membrane transport deficiencies have been described. Almost all are autosomal recessive in inheritance. Finally, as shown by several examples discussed later, the lysosomal storage diseases provide dramatic examples of both allelic and locus heterogeneity.

### TAY-SACHS DISEASE

Tay-Sachs disease is one of a group of heterogeneous lysosomal storage diseases, the $G_{M2}$ gangliosidoses, that result from the inability to degrade a sphingolipid, $G_{M2}$ ganglioside (Fig. 12–4). The biochemical lesion is a marked deficiency of hexosaminidase A (hex A). Although the enzyme is ubiquitous, the disease has its clinical impact almost solely on the brain, the predominant site of $G_{M2}$ ganglioside synthesis. Catalytically active hex A is the product of a three-gene system (Fig. 12–4). These genes encode the $\alpha$ and $\beta$ subunits of the enzyme (the *HEXA* and *HEXB* genes, respectively) and an activator protein that must associate with the substrate and the enzyme before the latter can cleave the terminal *N*-acetyl-$\beta$-galactosamine residue from the ganglioside.

The clinical manifestations of defects in the three genes are indistinguishable, but they can be differentiated by enzymatic analysis. Mutations in the *HEXA*

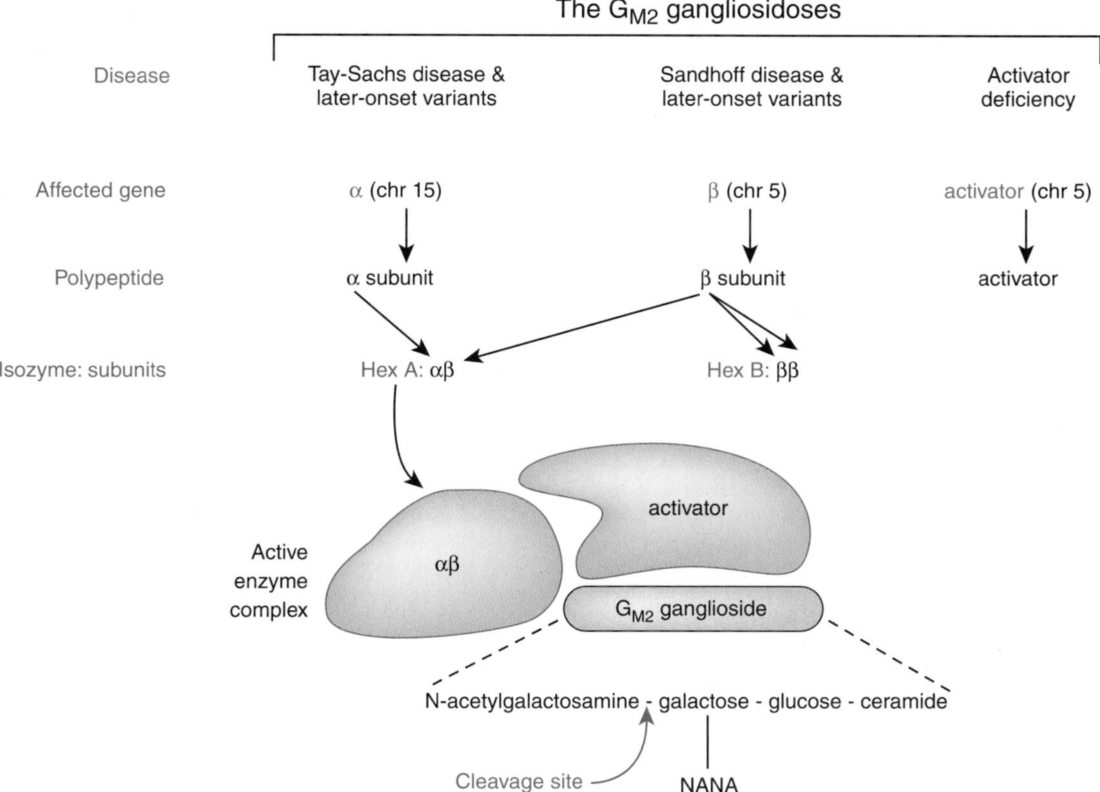


**Figure 12–4.** The three-gene system required for hexosaminidase A activity, and the diseases that result from defects in each of the genes. The function of the activator protein is to bind the ganglioside substrate and present it to the enzyme. (Modified from Sandhoff K, Conzelmann E, Neufeld EF, et al [1989] The $G_{M2}$ gangliosidoses. *In* Scriver CR, Beaudet AL, Sly WS, Valle D [eds] The Metabolic Bases of Inherited Disease, 6th ed. McGraw-Hill, New York, pp. 1807–1839.)

gene affect the $\alpha$ subunit and disrupt hex A activity to cause Tay-Sachs disease (or less severe variants of hex A deficiency). Most Tay-Sachs alleles lead to a profound deficiency of the $\alpha$ subunit mRNA and of hex A activity (Table 12–5). The most common mutation responsible for Tay-Sachs disease in both Ashkenazic Jewish and other populations is the null allele shown in Figure 12–5. Defects in the *HEXB* gene, or in the gene encoding the activator protein, impair the activity of both hex A and hex B (see Fig. 12–4) to produce Sandhoff disease and activator protein deficiency (which is very rare), respectively.

The clinical course of Tay-Sachs disease is particularly tragic. Affected infants appear normal until about 3 to 6 months of age but then gradually undergo progressive neurological deterioration until

TABLE 12–5

**Nature and Frequency of Hexosaminidase A Alleles in Ashkenazic Jewish and Other Populations***

| Mutation | Effect on Gene Product | Estimated Frequency in Ashkenazic Jews | Frequency in Non-Ashkenazic Populations | Homozygous Phenotype |
|---|---|---|---|---|
| 4 bp insertion (exon 11) | Premature stop codon | 80% | 32% | Tay-Sachs disease |
| Exon 12 splice junction: G→C | Defective mRNA splicing | 10–15% | <1% | Tay-Sachs disease |
| Gly269Ser plus abnormal splicing | <3% Residual activity | 2–3% | <1% | Adult-onset $G_{M2}$ gangliosidosis |
| Other alleles | Variable | <1% | >80% | Variable |

*Derived from Triggs-Raine BL, Feigenbaum ASJ, Natowicz M, et al (1990) Screening for carriers of Tay-Sachs disease among Ashkenazi Jews. N Engl J Med 323:6–12; and Gravel RA, Clarke JTR, Kaback MM, et al (1995) The $G_{M2}$ gangliosidoses. *In* Scriver CR, Beaudet AL, Sly WS, Valle D [eds] The Metabolic and Molecular Bases of Inherited Disease, 7th ed. McGraw-Hill, New York, pp. 2839–2879.

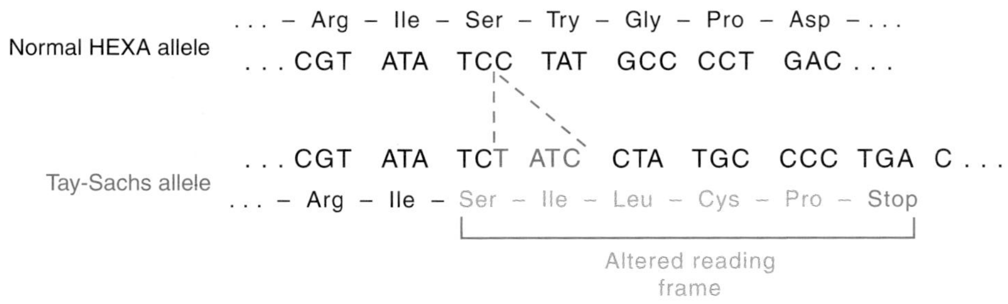

Normal HEXA allele

. . . – Arg – Ile – Ser – Try – Gly – Pro – Asp – . . .
. . . CGT ATA TCC TAT GCC CCT GAC . . .

. . . CGT ATA TCT ATC CTA TGC CCC TGA C . . .
. . . – Arg – Ile – Ser – Ile – Leu – Cys – Pro – Stop

Tay-Sachs allele

Altered reading frame

**Figure 12–5.** Four-base insertion in the hexosaminidase A gene in Tay-Sachs disease, leading to a frameshift mutation. This mutation is the major cause of Tay-Sachs disease in Ashkenazic Jews (see Table 12–5). No detectable hex A protein is made, accounting for the complete enzyme deficiency observed in these infantile-onset patients.

death at 2 to 4 years. The effects of neuronal cell death can be seen directly in the form of the so-called cherry-red spot in the retina, which is the prominent red fovea centralis surrounded by a pale macula. Multiple alleles have been identified at the *HEXA* locus and are responsible for remarkable clinical heterogeneity in hex A deficiency (see Table 12–5). In later-onset variants of the disease, there are small but definite amounts of functioning residual enzyme, and the age of onset of symptoms is very roughly proportional to the residual activity. In the chronic form, which can even be of adult onset, the manifestations commonly include lower motor neuron dysfunction and ataxia due to spinocerebellar degeneration, but in contrast to the infantile disease, vision and intelligence usually remain normal, although psychosis develops in one third of these patients.

**Population Genetics.** About 1 in 27 Ashkenazic Jews is a carrier of a Tay-Sachs allele, and the incidence of affected infants is 100 times higher than in other populations, as discussed in Chapter 7. Either founder effect or heterozygote advantage has been considered to be the most likely explanation. Although one predominant allele is often associated with a high carrier frequency of a disease gene in a single population, molecular analysis has shown, unexpectedly, that three alleles account for 99 percent of the mutations in all Ashkenazic Jewish patients and carriers (see Table 12–5). Thus, the reason for the high frequency of hex A deficiency in the Ashkenazic Jewish population is not apparent. The presence of three alleles does not necessarily confirm the heterozygote advantage hypothesis, because they may each owe their frequency to a founder effect. A practical benefit of the molecular characterization of the disease in this population is the degree to which it has facilitated carrier screening (because most carriers will have one of the three common alleles).

**Hex A Pseudodeficiency Alleles.** An unexpected consequence of screening for Tay-Sachs carriers in the Ashkenazic Jewish population was the discovery of a unique class of hex A alleles, the pseudodeficiency alleles. As their name implies, the two pseudodeficiency alleles are clinically benign. Individuals identified as pseudodeficient in screening tests are genetic compounds with pseudodeficiency alleles on one chromosome and a common Tay-Sachs mutation on the other chromosome. These individuals have a low level of hex A activity (about 20 percent of controls in leukocytes) that is still adequate to prevent the accumulation of the substrate, $G_{M2}$ ganglioside. The importance of hex A pseudodeficiency alleles is twofold. First, they complicate prenatal diagnosis, because a pseudodeficient fetus may be incorrectly diagnosed as affected. More generally, the existence of the hex A pseudodeficiency alleles indicates that screening programs for other genetic diseases must recognize that comparable alleles are likely to exist at other loci and may confound the correct characterization of individuals in screening or diagnostic tests.

## THE MUCOPOLYSACCHARIDOSES

Mucopolysaccharides, or glycosaminoglycans (GAGs), are polysaccharide chains synthesized by connective tissue cells as normal constituents of many tissues. They are made up of long disaccharide repeating units; the nature of the two sugar molecules is the distinguishing feature of a specific GAG. The degradation of these macromolecules occurs in the lysosome and requires the stepwise removal of the monosaccharide unit at the end of the chain by an enzyme specific to the monosaccharide and the bond involved. A series of enzymes is thus required for the degradation of any one GAG, and a single enzyme often participates in the catabolism of more than one GAG.

The mucopolysaccharidoses are a heterogeneous group of storage diseases in which mucopolysaccharides accumulate in lysosomes as a result of a deficiency of one of the enzymes required for their degradation (Table 12–6). In a specific mucopolysaccharidosis, one or more GAGs may accumulate if the defective enzyme is required for their catabolism. The nondegraded GAGs appear in the urine, in which they can be detected by screening tests.

TABLE 12–6

## Examples of Mucopolysaccharidoses

| Syndrome | Clinical Features | Enzyme Defect; Stored/Excreted Mucopolysaccharide | Genetics | Comment |
|---|---|---|---|---|
| Hurler | Diagnosed at 6–18 months, corneal clouding, skeletal changes on radiograph called dysostosis multiplex, hepatosplenomegaly, coarse facies, stiff joints, nasal discharge, hydrocephalus, death <10 years | α-L-Iduronidase; dermatan sulfate, heparan sulfate | AR | Probably due to any allele that abolishes the activity of the enzyme. Most patients are likely to be genetic compounds |
| Scheie | Onset after age 5 years, normal intelligence and life span, corneal clouding, stiff joints, valvular heart disease, visual impairment | α-L-Iduronidase; dermatan sulfate, heparan sulfate | AR | Complementation tests show that this milder phenotype affects the same gene as does Hurler syndrome |
| Hurler/Scheie | Intermediate phenotype between Hurler and Scheie syndrome | α-L-Iduronidase; dermatan sulfate, heparan sulfate | AR | Some cases are probably genetic compounds of Hurler and Scheie alleles |
| Hunter | Similar to Hurler syndrome, but with slower progression, no corneal clouding, and a unique pebbly skin lesion | Iduronate sulfatase; dermatan sulfate, heparan sulfate | XR | A milder phenotype without central nervous system disease also occurs, with a much less aggressive somatic course |
| Sanfilippo A | Hyperactivity and retardation, progressive neurodegeneration; mild somatic features → underdiagnosis | Heparan *N*-sulfatase; heparan sulfate | AR | Predominantly neurological, with little to distinguish the phenotypes associated with the four Sanfilippo genes |
| Sanfilippo B | Similar to Sanfilippo A syndrome | α-*N*-acetylglucosaminidase; heparan sulfate | AR | As above |

Modified from Neufeld EF, Muenzer J (1995) The mucopolysaccharidoses. *In* Scriver CR, Beaudet AL, Sly WS, Valle D (eds) The Metabolic and Molecular Bases of Inherited Disease, 7th ed. McGraw-Hill, New York, pp. 2465–2494.

The first two mucopolysaccharidoses to be recognized were X-linked recessive **Hunter syndrome** in 1917 and the more severe autosomal recessive **Hurler syndrome** in 1919. Each of these conditions was originally called "gargoylism" because of the coarseness of the facial features of affected individuals (Fig. 12–6). Affected children are mentally retarded, have skeletal abnormalities and short stature, and manifest other abnormalities listed in Table 12–6.

Hurler syndrome is due to a severe deficiency of $\alpha$-L-iduronidase. A clinically distinct disorder, **Scheie syndrome**, was originally thought to involve a different locus, principally because of its much milder phenotype. However, the Scheie and Hurler syndromes are allelic, but the $\alpha$-L-iduronidase mutations that cause Scheie syndrome appear to be associated with higher residual activity. An intermediate phenotype, Hurler/Scheie syndrome, in at least some cases, is a genetic compound of Hurler and Scheie alleles. It could also result from two alleles with activity intermediate between Hurler and Scheie alleles.

The difference in the pattern of inheritance of the autosomal Hurler and X-linked Hunter syndromes indicated that they were due to mutations in different genes. This difference was also demonstrated in cell culture. Although fibroblasts from patients of either type accumulated mucopolysaccharides in the culture medium, the accumulation could be corrected by cocultivation of both cell types in the same culture dish. The interpretation, which proved correct, was that the lysosomal enzyme deficient in one mutant cell type was taken up from the medium, into which it had been released by the other cell type. This simple experiment was a powerful demonstration that the two diseases affected different proteins. The demonstration that the genome of one mutant can correct the biochemical defect in another mutant is termed **complementation**; this phenomenon is discussed in the next section. In contrast, cocultivation of Scheie and Hurler cells failed to induce any biochemical correction, indicating, as enzyme assays later showed, that they were due to defects in the same protein.

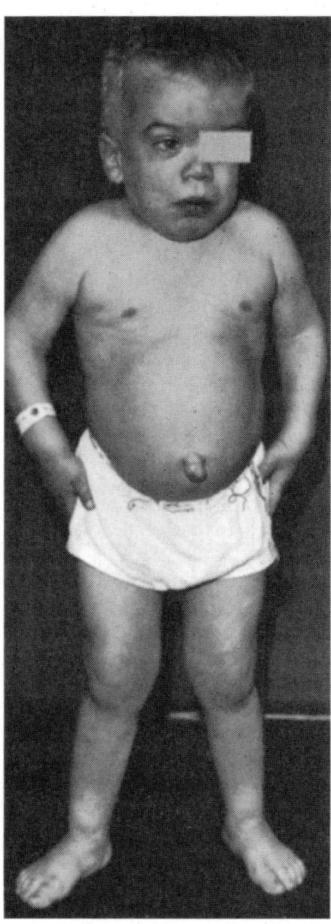

Figure 12–6. A child with Hurler syndrome, showing the typical coarse facial features. At 5 years of age, he is only as tall as a typical 3-year-old. (From Smith DW [1982] Recognizable Patterns of Human Malformation, 3rd ed. WB Saunders, Philadelphia.)

The ability of a cell to take up the lysosomal enzyme that it lacks, from the extracellular fluid, is one mechanism by which the transplantation of normal cells (that would secrete the enzyme) into patients with storage diseases may allow correction of the biochemical defect in the rest of the body. Dramatic therapeutic benefits have been obtained by treatment of some patients with mucopolysaccharidoses, including Hurler syndrome, with bone marrow transplantation (see Chapter 13).

Another mucopolysaccharidosis, **Sanfilippo syndrome**, illustrates the extensive locus heterogeneity that can underlie a relatively homogeneous clinical phenotype. An important clinical feature of patients with Sanfilippo syndrome is that intellectual and behavioral abnormalities are evident well before physical changes, which tend to be mild. Initially regarded as a single entity, this syndrome can result from one of four enzyme deficiencies, two of which are outlined in Table 12–6. The clinical phenotypes of individual patients provide little basis for suggesting which enzyme (and, therefore, which gene) is defective.

## Complementation Analysis of Human Genetic Disease

In the cocultivation experiments just described, the geneticists examined an issue that commonly arises in the study of patients with genetic disease: do two individuals with what appears to be the same disorder have defects in the same gene? Genetic experiments that address this question are called **complementation tests.** If mutual correction of a phenotype occurs in a complementation test, the genetic defects are said to complement one another, the affected genes must be different, and *intergenic complementation* has occurred (but see an exception, intragenic complementation, later). The utility of complementation tests lies in the fact that they require no knowledge of the affected genes or proteins, but only the ability to examine the cells for the correction of a mutant phenotype: in the case of the mucopolysaccharide storage diseases cited earlier, the reduction of mucopolysaccharide accumulation. Complementation analysis has been used to dissect the genetic basis of many human genetic diseases.

If there is doubt that the corrective factor can be transferred through the culture medium, the different cells can be fused to form a heterokaryon, in which both nuclei are inside a single cell (see Chapter 8). Experiments of this type have demonstrated that **xeroderma pigmentosum** (XP), a rare disease associated with a 2000-fold increased frequency of sunlight-induced skin cancer, is caused by mutation in any one of eight genes, seven of which encode proteins required for DNA excision repair. People with mild defects may have only a heightened sensitivity to sunlight, whereas severely affected patients are subject to profound neurological impairment, extreme sun sensitivity in infancy, abnormal freckling and skin atrophy, and ultimately, in the worst cases, various tumors (carcinomas, melanomas, and internal neoplasms) as well.

On occasion, complementation tests in heterokaryons yield positive results even if the mutations in the two groups of mutant cells are known to affect the same gene. In this instance, the complementation is said to be *intragenic* (versus *intergenic*) and demonstrates that the patients have different, but allelic, mutations. Intragenic (or *interallelic*) complementation occurs only when the affected proteins are homomultimers, indicating that the mutant subunit from one allele interacts with the mutant subunit from the other allele in a way that improves the function of the multimeric protein.

#### I-Cell Disease: A Defect in Protein Trafficking

In contrast to mitochondrial and membrane proteins that are directed to their subcellular residence by information contained in the primary amino acid sequence, other proteins are localized on the basis of post-translational modifications (see Table 11–1). This is true of the acid hydrolases found in lysosomes, and, in fact, the existence and the mechanism of this form of cellular trafficking were unrecognized until I-cell disease, a severe autosomal recessive lysosomal storage disease, was investigated in the early 1970s. Cultured skin fibroblasts of patients with I-cell disease contain numerous abnormal lysosomes, or inclusions, throughout the cytoplasm (hence, inclusion-cells or I-cells).

In I-cell disease, many of the acid hydrolases normally present in lysosomes are found in excess in body fluids, while their cellular levels are severely diminished. This unusual situation arises because the lysosomal hydrolases in these patients are abnormal secondary to a failure to be post-translationally modified. A typical hydrolase is a glycoprotein with mannose residues, some of which are phosphorylated. The mannose-6-phosphate residues are essential for recognition of the hydrolases by receptors on the cell and lysosomal membrane surface. In I-cell disease, there is a defect in the enzyme that transfers a phosphate group to the mannose residues. The fact that many enzymes are affected is consistent with the diversity of clinical abnormalities. The disorder has a range of phenotypic effects, involving facial features, skeletal changes, severe growth retardation, and mental retardation. Affected children typically survive for only 5 to 7 years.

### Mutations That Impair the Binding or Metabolism of Cofactors

Certain proteins acquire biological activity only after they associate with nonprotein prosthetic groups or cofactors that play a critical role in the protein's function. The cofactors required for the catalytic activity of some enzymes are one example. Mutations that interfere with ligand binding, synthesis, transport, or removal from a protein (when ligand binding is covalent) are known. Of all genetic disorders, these are among the most responsive to specific biochemical therapy, particularly when the cofactor or its precursor is a water-soluble vitamin that can safely be given in large amounts.

#### Homocystinuria due to Cystathionine Synthase Deficiency: Impaired Cofactor Binding

Homocystinuria due to cystathionine synthase deficiency (Fig. 12–7) was one of the first aminoacidopathies to be recognized. The clinical phenotype of this autosomal recessive condition is often dramatic (and can be confused with the Marfan syndrome, a disorder of connective tissue). The most common features include dislocation of the lens, mental retardation, osteoporosis, long bones, and thromboembolism of both veins and arteries. The accumulation of homocysteine is believed to be central to much, if not all, of the pathology.

Homocystinuria was one of the first genetic diseases shown to be vitamin-responsive: pyridoxal phosphate is the cofactor of the enzyme, and the administration of large amounts of pyridoxine, the

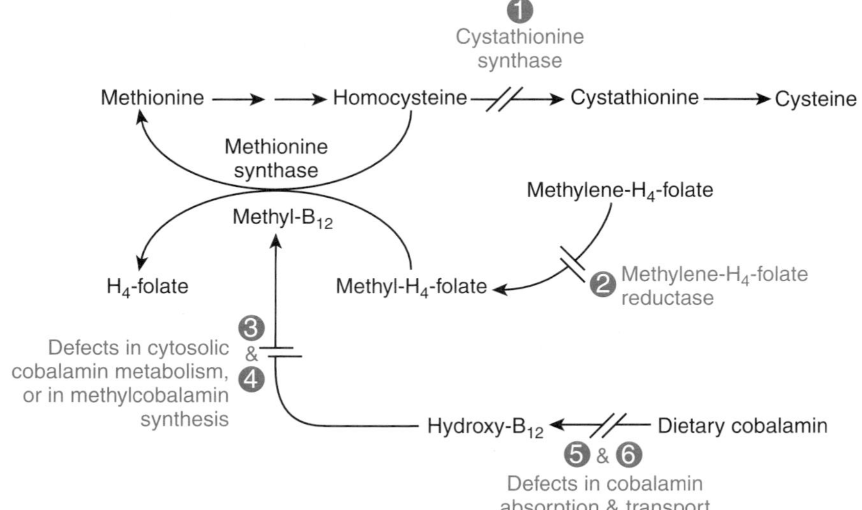


**Figure 12–7.** The six types of genetic defects that can cause homocystinuria. (1) Classical homocystinuria is due to defective cystathionine synthase. (2) In methylene-$H_4$-folate reductase defects, the decrease in methyl-$H_4$-folate impairs the function of methionine synthase. (3) Several different defects in the intracellular metabolism of cobalamins lead to a secondary decrease in the synthesis of methylcobalamin (methyl-$B_{12}$) and thus in the function of methionine synthase. (4) Some disorders directly affect methyl-$B_{12}$ formation. (5) Cobalamin intestinal absorption is abnormal in some patients. (6) Other patients have abnormalities in the major extracellular transport protein, transcobalamin II. Hydroxycobalamin = hydroxy-$B_{12}$.

vitamin precursor of the cofactor, often ameliorates the biochemical abnormality (see Chapter 13) and the clinical disease. In many patients, the affinity of the mutant enzyme for pyridoxal phosphate is reduced, indicating that altered conformation of the protein impairs cofactor binding.

#### Disorders due to Abnormalities in the Metabolism of Cofactors

Loss of protein function is sometimes secondary to decreased availability of an associated molecule, such as an enzyme cofactor. Disorders of this class are well illustrated by types of homocystinuria that result from various secondary defects in another enzyme, methionine synthase, which remethylates homocysteine to form methionine (see Fig. 12–7). As shown, the cofactor of methionine synthase, methylcobalamin, is the product of a complex series of biochemical events. Numerous disorders of vitamin $B_{12}$ (cobalamin) transport or metabolism reduce the availability of methylcobalamin and therefore impair, secondarily, the activity of methionine synthase.

Several defects impair the intestinal absorption of cobalamin or its transport to other cells; others disrupt specific steps in cobalamin metabolism (see Fig. 12–7). The clinical manifestation of these disorders is variable but includes megaloblastic anemia, developmental delay, and failure to thrive. These conditions are often partially or completely treatable with high doses of vitamin $B_{12}$. All are autosomal recessive.

### Alpha$_1$-Antitrypsin Deficiency: Deficiency of a Protease Inhibitor

$\alpha_1$-AT deficiency is an important autosomal recessive condition that leads to chronic obstructive lung disease and cirrhosis of the liver. The $\alpha_1$-AT locus, on chromosome 14, is expressed principally in the liver, which secretes $\alpha_1$-AT into plasma. Although $\alpha_1$-AT inhibits a wide spectrum of proteases, its major physiological role is to bind and inhibit elastase, particularly elastase released from neutrophils in the lower respiratory tract.

Substantial genetic variability has been found in $\alpha_1$-AT, with more than 75 genetic variants, called protease inhibitor types, having been identified (see Chapter 6). Only about a dozen of these alleles lead to an increased risk of lung or liver disease, however, and only the *Z* allele is relatively common. In Caucasian populations, $\alpha_1$-AT deficiency affects about 1 in 2500 persons, and 3 percent are carriers. The reason for the relatively high frequency of the *Z* allele in Caucasian populations is unknown, although analysis of DNA haplotypes suggests a single origin with subsequent spread in northern Europe. Given its increased risk of emphysema, $\alpha_1$-AT deficiency is an important health problem, affecting 100,000 persons in the United States alone.

The mutation in the *Z* allele (Glu342Lys) slows the rate of elastase inhibition by $\alpha_1$-AT. The hepatic pathology of the *Z* protein appears to reflect a novel property, however: its tendency to aggregate in the rough endoplasmic reticulum of hepatocytes.

Whereas normal $\alpha_1$-AT is rapidly secreted from the liver, *Z/Z* patients have only about 15 percent of the normal plasma concentration of $\alpha_1$-AT. The aggregation of the *Z* protein appears to be responsible for its entrapment in the rough endoplasmic reticulum of hepatocytes. The molecular basis of this aggregation or insolubility is unclear, but Glu342 appears to be critical to the normal folding or stability, or both, of the molecule. The presence of stored $\alpha_1$-AT in the liver is believed to be responsible for the liver disease. Consequently, like the sickle cell disease mutation, the *Z* allele is a strong example of a mutation that confers a novel property (see Fig. 11–1) that is responsible for the disease, while disrupting the normal

## Enzyme Deficiencies and Disease: General Concepts

The following concepts are fundamental to understanding and treating enzymopathies:

1. **Enzymopathies are almost always recessive.** Most enzymes are produced in quantities significantly in excess of minimal biochemical requirements, so that heterozygotes with about 50 percent of residual activity are clinically normal. In fact, many enzymes may maintain normal substrate and product levels with activities of less than 10 percent of controls (e.g., hex A). The enzymes of porphyrin synthesis are exceptions (see discussion of acute intermittent porphyria, later in this chapter).
2. **Substrate accumulation or product deficiency.** Because the function of an enzyme is to convert a substrate to a product, all of the pathophysiological consequences of enzymopathies can be attributed either to the accumulation of the substrate, to the deficiency of the product, or to some combination of the two (Fig. 12–8).
3. **Diffusible versus macromolecular substrates.** An important distinction can be made between enzyme defects in which the substrate is a "small" molecule, such as phenylalanine, that can be readily distributed throughout body fluids by diffusion or transport, and defects in which the substrate is a macromolecule, such as a mucopolysaccharide, that remains trapped within its organelle or cell. The pathology of the macromolecular diseases is confined to the tissues in which the substrate accumulates, whereas the site of the disease in the small molecule disorders is often unpredictable because the unmetabolized substrate, or its derivatives, can move freely throughout the body, damaging cells that may normally have no relationship to the affected enzyme.
4. **Loss of multiple enzyme activities.** A single patient may have a loss of function in more than one enyzme. There are several possible mechanisms:
   (a) The enzymes may use the same cofactor (e.g., $BH_4$ deficiency);
   (b) The enzymes may share a common subunit or an activating, processing, or stabilizing protein (e.g., the $G_{M2}$ gangliosidoses);
   (c) The enzymes may be processed by a common modifying enzyme, and, in its absence, they may be inactive or their uptake into an organelle may be impaired (e.g., I-cell disease); and
   (d) A group of enzymes may be absent or ineffective if the organelle in which they are normally found is abnormal (e.g., the disorders of peroxisome biogenesis).
5. **Phenotypic homology.** The pathological and clinical features resulting from an enzyme defect are often shared by (a) diseases due to deficiencies of other enzymes that function in the same area of metabolism (e.g., the mucopolysaccharidoses) and (b) the different diseases that can result from partial and complete defects of the enzyme. Partial defects often manifest with clinical abnormalities that are a subset of those found with the complete deficiency, although the etiologic relationship between the two diseases may not be immediately obvious (e.g., partial Hprt deficiency causing only hyperuricemia versus severe Hprt deficiency causing Lesch-Nyhan syndrome).

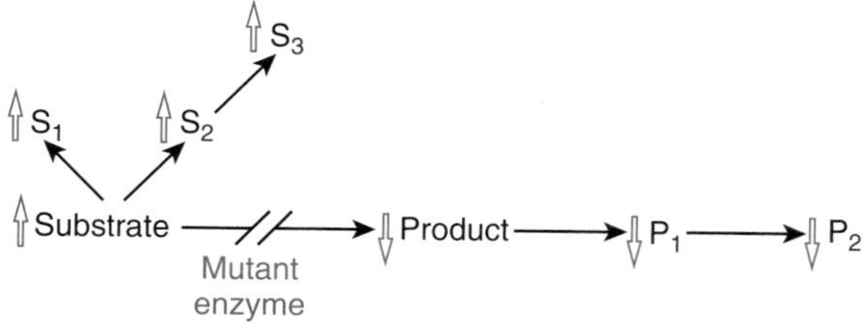


**Figure 12–8.** A model metabolic pathway showing that the potential effects of an enzyme deficiency include accumulation of the substrate (S) or derivatives of it (S1, S2, S3), or deficiency of the product (P) or compounds (P1, P2) made from it. In some cases, the substrate derivatives are normally only minor metabolites that are formed at increased rates when the substrate accumulates (e.g., phenylpyruvate in phenylketonuria).

function of the protein to a much lesser degree. About 17 percent of homozygotes present with neonatal jaundice, and approximately 25 percent of this group subsequently develop cirrhosis.

#### ALPHA$_1$-ANTITRYPSIN DEFICIENCY AS AN ECOGENETIC DISEASE

The lung disease is due to the decreased plasma level of $\alpha_1$-AT, which alters the normal balance between elastase and $\alpha_1$-AT and allows progressive degradation of the elastin of alveolar walls. The progression of the emphysema is greatly augmented by smoking and is a powerful example of the effect that environmental factors may have on the phenotype of a genetic disease. Thus, for persons with the *Z/Z* genotype, survival after 60 years of age is approximately 60 percent in nonsmokers but only about 10 percent in smokers (Fig. 12–9). One molecular explanation for the effect of smoking is that the active site of $\alpha_1$-AT, at methionine 358, is oxidized by both cigarette smoke and inflammatory cells, thus reducing its affinity for elastase by 2000-fold.

The field of **ecogenetics**, illustrated by $\alpha_1$-AT deficiency, is concerned with the interaction between environmental factors and different human genotypes. This area of medical genetics is likely to be one of increasing importance as genotypes are identified that entail an increased risk of disease on exposure to certain environmental agents (e.g., drugs, industrial chemicals, and viruses). In addition, genetic variation that may not by itself produce disease will be subject to increasing scrutiny in the search for the genetic contribution to nonmendelian disorders, such as diabetes mellitus (see Chapter 15). At present, the most highly developed area of ecogenetics is that of pharmacogenetics, which is reviewed at the end of this chapter.

## DEFECTS IN RECEPTOR PROTEINS

The recognition of a class of diseases due to defects in receptor molecules began with the identification, by Goldstein and Brown in 1974, of the low-density-lipoprotein (LDL) receptor as the polypeptide affected in familial hypercholesterolemia. Their discovery has cast much light on normal cholesterol metabolism and on the biology of cell surface receptors in general. LDL receptor deficiency is representative of a number of disorders now recognized to result from receptor defects, a few of which are listed in Table 12–1.

### Familial Hypercholesterolemia: A Genetic Hyperlipoproteinemia

The genetic hyperlipoproteinemias are of clinical significance because of their role in myocardial infarction, a major cause of death and disability. Hyperlipoproteinemias are characterized by elevated levels of plasma lipids (cholesterol, triglycerides, or both) and specific plasma lipoproteins. A number of distinct single-gene forms with different biochemical and clinical phenotypes have been defined, although in some cases the phenotypes have not yet been completely characterized. At each locus, there may well be more than one mutant allele.

**Familial hypercholesterolemia** is one of several disorders grouped as familial type 2 hyperlipoproteinemia. It is characterized by elevation of plasma cholesterol carried by LDL, the principal cholesterol transport protein in plasma. The disease is due to mutations in the structural gene encoding the LDL receptor, a cell surface protein responsible for binding LDL and delivering it to the cell interior. Both heterozygotes and homozygotes develop premature

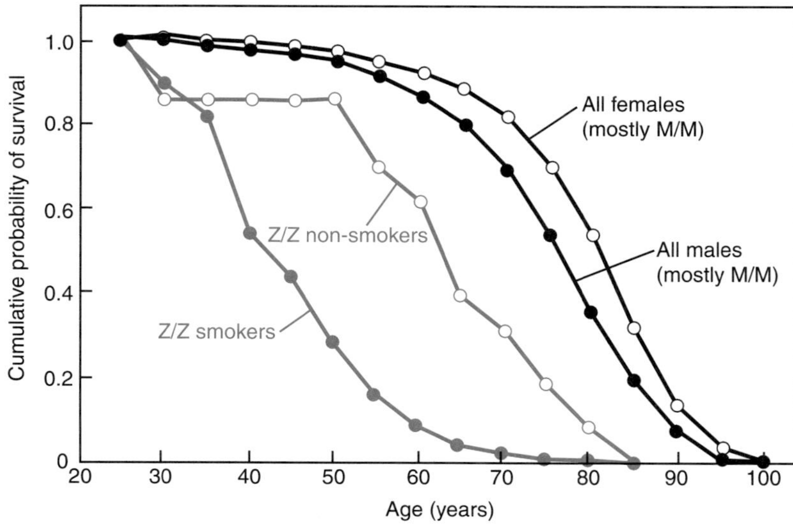


**Figure 12–9.** The effect of smoking on the survival of patients with $\alpha_1$-antitrypsin deficiency. The curves show the cumulative probability of survival to specified ages of smokers, with or without $\alpha_1$-antitrypsin deficiency. (Redrawn from Larrson C [1978] Natural history and life expectancy in severe $\alpha_1$-antitrypsin deficiency, Pi Z. Acta Med Scand 204:345–351.)

heart disease as a result of atheromas (deposits of LDL-derived cholesterol in the coronary arteries), xanthomas (cholesterol deposits in skin and tendons; see Fig. 5–13), and arcus corneae (deposits of cholesterol around the periphery of the cornea). Few diseases have been as thoroughly characterized; the sequence of pathological events from the affected locus to its effect on individuals and populations has been well documented.

**Genetics.** Familial hypercholesterolemia is inherited as an autosomal dominant trait. Both homozygous and heterozygous phenotypes are known, and a clear gene dosage effect is evident: the disease manifests earlier and much more severely in homozygotes than in heterozygotes (see Fig. 5–13), reflecting the greater reduction in the number of LDL receptors and the greater elevation in plasma LDL cholesterol (Fig. 12–10). Homozygotes may have clinically significant coronary heart disease in childhood, and few live beyond the third decade. Although the homozygous form is rare (1 person in 1 million), the heterozygous form, with a population frequency of at least 1 in 500, is one of the most common human single-gene disorders. Heterozygotes have levels of plasma cholesterol that are about twice that of controls (Fig. 12–10). Because of the genetic nature of familial hypercholesterolemia, it is important to make the diagnosis in the approximately 5 percent of survivors of myocardial infarction who are heterozygotes for an LDL receptor defect. Only about 1 in 20 individuals in the general population with increased plasma cholesterol and a type 2 hyperlipoprotein pattern has familial hypercholesterolemia, however, whereas most have an uncharacterized hypercholesterolemia of multifactorial origin.

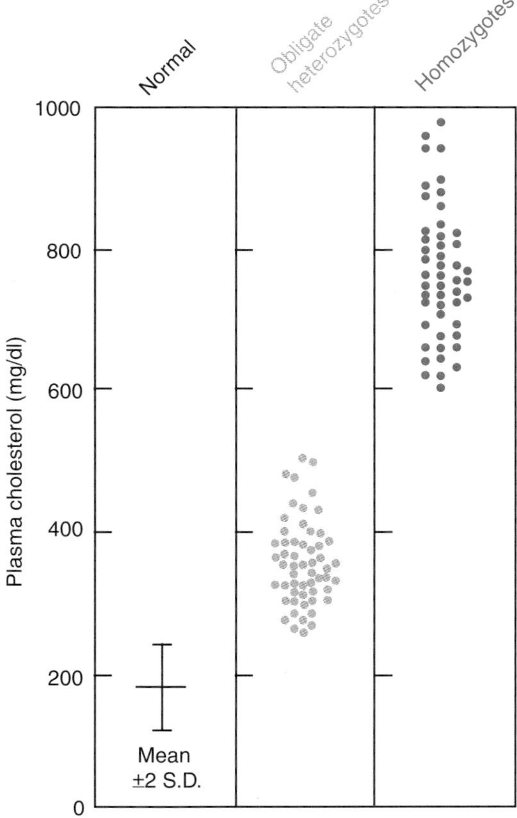


**Figure 12–10.** Gene dosage in low-density-lipoprotein (LDL) deficiency: the distribution of total plasma cholesterol levels in 49 patients homozygous for deficiency of the LDL receptor, in their parents (obligate heterozygotes), and in normal controls. (Redrawn from Goldstein JL, Brown MS [1989] Familial hypercholesterolemia. *In* Scriver CR, Beaudet AL, Sly WS, Valle D [eds] The Metabolic Bases of Inherited Disease, 6th ed. McGraw-Hill, New York, pp. 1215–1250.)

**Cholesterol Uptake by the Low-Density-Lipoprotein Receptor.** Normal cells obtain cholesterol, an essential lipid component of membranes and a precursor of steroid hormones and bile salts, either by de novo synthesis or by the uptake from plasma of exogenous cholesterol bound to LDL. The uptake process is mediated by the LDL receptor, which recognizes apoprotein B-100, the protein moiety of LDL. The LDL receptors on the cell surface are localized to depressed regions (coated pits) lined by the protein clathrin (Fig. 12–11). Receptor-bound LDL is brought into the cell by invagination of the coated pits, which ultimately evolve into lysosomes in which LDL is hydrolyzed to release free cholesterol. The increase in free intracellular cholesterol reduces endogenous cholesterol formation by suppressing the rate-limiting enzyme of the synthetic pathway (3-hydroxy-3-methylglutaryl coenzyme A reductase, or HMG CoA reductase). Cholesterol not required for cellular metabolism or membrane synthesis may be re-esterified for storage as cholesteryl esters, a process stimulated by the activation of acyl CoA: cholesterol acyltransferase (ACAT). The increase in cholesterol also reduces synthesis of the receptor (Fig. 12–11).

The mature LDL receptor has five distinct structural domains that, for the most part, have distinguishable functions. Some of these regions are encoded by single exons or by groups of exons that encode regions that are homologous to domains in other polypeptides (Fig. 12–12). Analysis of the effect on the receptor of mutations in the various domains has played an important part in establishing the function of many of the domains. These studies exemplify the important contribution that genetic analysis can make in determining the structure-function relationships of a protein.

### Classes of Mutations in the Low-Density-Lipoprotein Receptor.

More than 400 different mutations have been identified in the LDL receptor gene, and these are distributed throughout the sequence. Sixteen percent of all

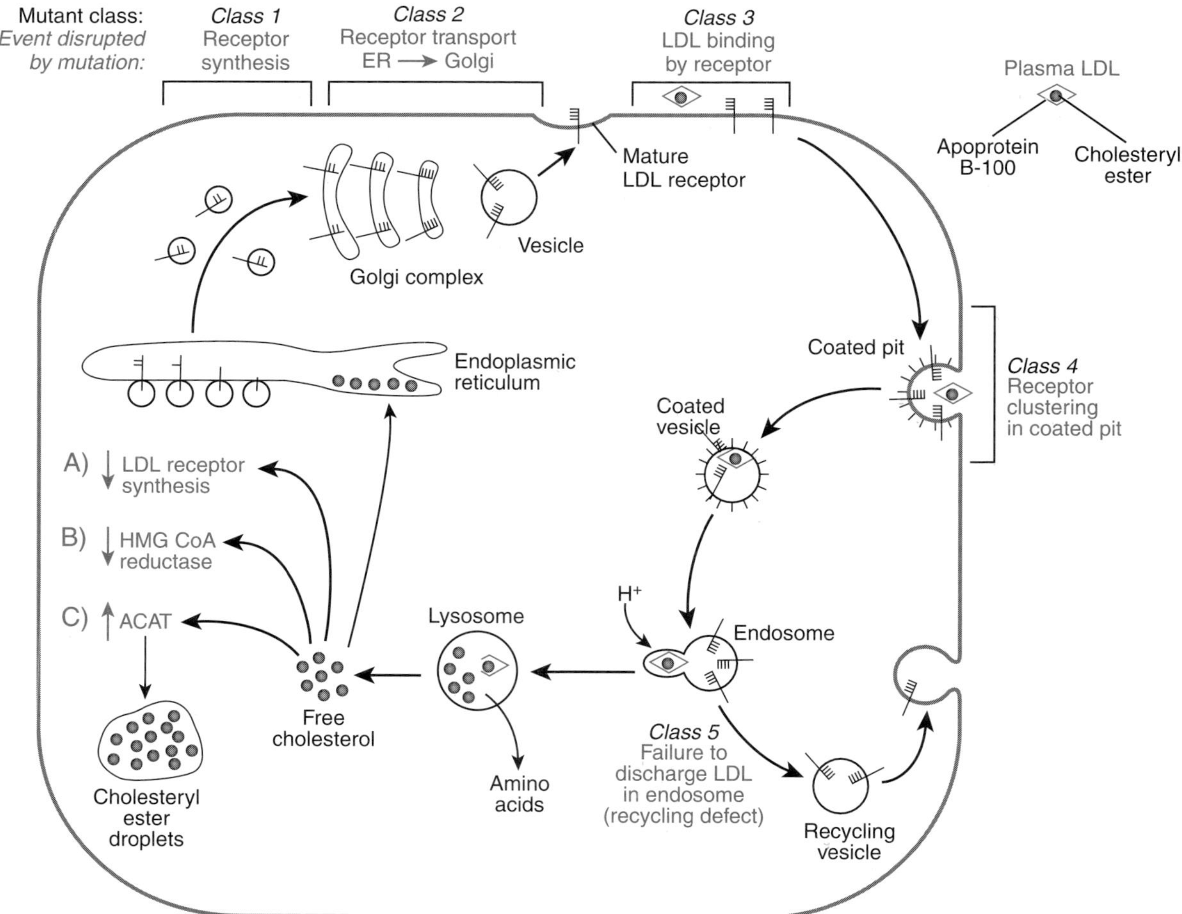


**Figure 12–11.** The cell biology and biochemical role of the low-density-lipoprotein (LDL) receptor and the five classes of mutations that alter its function. After synthesis in the endoplasmic reticulum, the receptor is transported to the Golgi apparatus and subsequently to the cell surface. Normal receptors are localized to clathrin-coated pits, which invaginate, creating coated vesicles and then endosomes, the precursors of lysosomes. Normally, intracellular accumulation of free cholesterol is prevented because the increase in free cholesterol (A) decreases the formation of LDL receptors, (B) reduces de novo cholesterol synthesis, and (C) increases the storage of cholesteryl esters. The biochemical phenotype of each class of mutant is discussed in text. (Modified from Brown MS, Goldstein JL [1985] The LDL receptor and HMG-CoA reductase—two membrane molecules that regulate cholesterol homeostasis. Curr Top Cell Regul 26:3–15.)

mutations documented are large structural rearrangements, but, as is the case with many loci, this type of mutation accounts for only 2 to 10 percent of the LDL receptor alleles in most populations. The remaining alleles are single nucleotide substitutions, small insertions, or deletions. In some inbred populations, specific alleles may account for a large fraction of the mutations, probably reflecting a founder effect (see Chapter 7).

Fibroblasts cultured from affected patients have been used to characterize the mutant receptors and the resulting disturbances in cellular cholesterol metabolism. Mutations in the LDL receptor gene can be grouped into five classes, depending on which step of the normal cellular itinerary of the receptor is disrupted by the mutation (see Fig. 12–11). **Class 1 mutations** are null alleles that prevent the synthesis of any detectable receptor; they are the most common type of disease-causing mutations at this locus. Some class 1 alleles are due to deletions, whereas others produce normal amounts of LDL-receptor mRNA and presumably have defects that impair the formation or stability of the polypeptide. In the remaining four classes, the receptor is synthesized normally, but its function is impaired.

Mutations in classes 2 and 4 (see Fig. 12–11) define features of the polypeptide critical to its subcellular localization. The relatively common **class 2 mutations** are designated *transport-deficient* because the LDL receptors accumulate at the site of their synthesis, the endoplasmic reticulum, instead of being transported to the Golgi complex. These alleles are predicted to prevent proper folding of the protein, an apparent requisite for exit from the endoplasmic reticulum.

**Class 3 mutant receptors** reach the cell surface but are incapable of binding LDL (see Fig. 12–11). Consequently, these alleles have enabled researchers

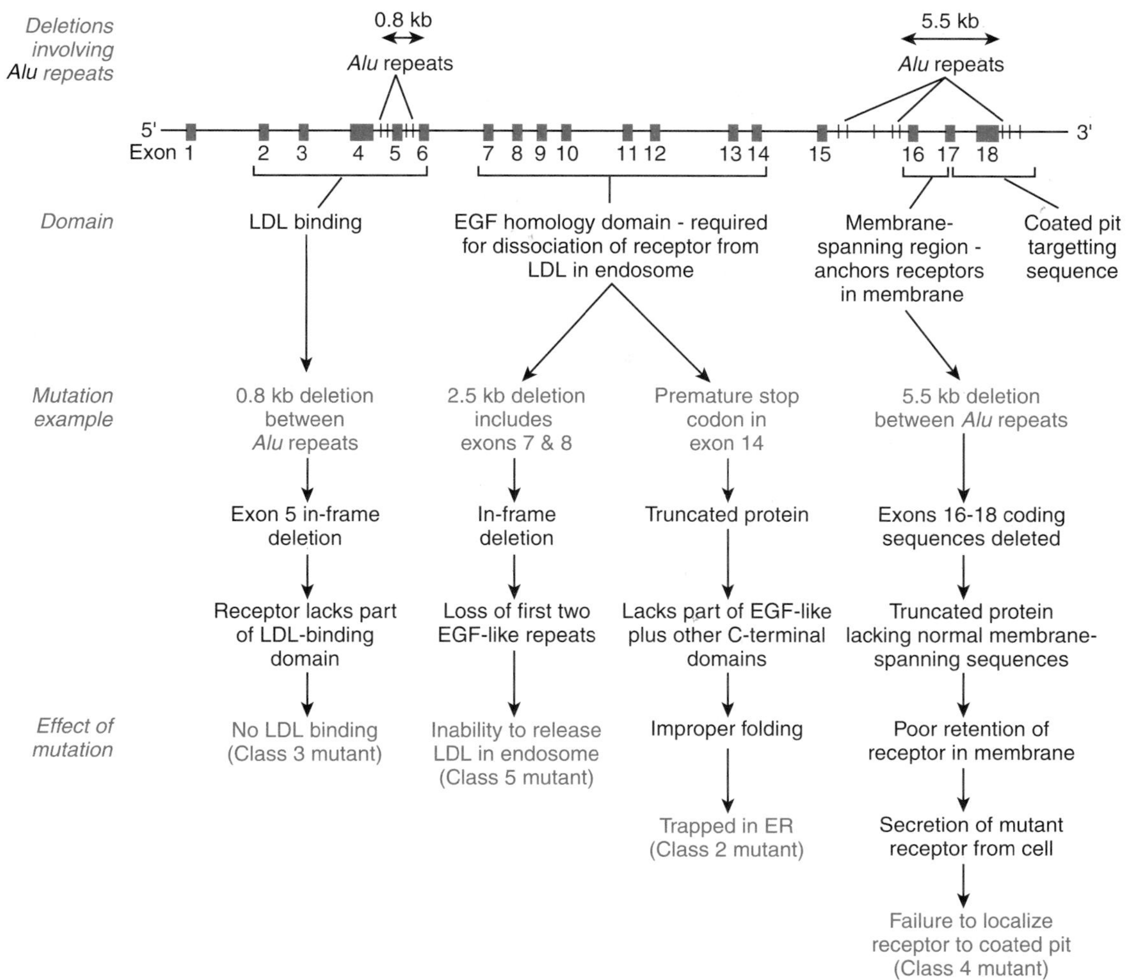


**Figure 12–12.** The structure of the low-density-lipoprotein (LDL) receptor gene showing its five domains and the location of selected mutations leading to familial hypercholesterolemia. The sizes of various deletions are indicated by the horizontal bars above the gene (*with exons indicated in red*). EGF = epidermal growth factor precursor homology domain. ER = endoplasmic reticulum. Exons, introns, and *Alu* repeats are only approximately to scale. (Modified from Goldstein JL, Brown MS [1989] Familial hypercholesterolemia. *In* Scriver CR, Beaudet AL, Sly WS, Valle D [eds] The Metabolic Bases of Inherited Disease, 6th ed. McGraw-Hill, New York, pp. 1215–1250.)

to identify the LDL-binding domain (see Fig. 12–12). In one mutant of this type, an unequal crossover that is due to misalignment and recombination between *Alu* repeat sequences has deleted part of the LDL-binding domain. Homologous unequal recombination between two copies of a repetitive DNA sequence has been found to be a frequent cause of deletions, both in this gene and in others (see Chapter 6).

**Class 4 mutations** impair localization of the receptor to the coated pit, and, consequently, the bound LDL is not internalized (see Fig. 12–11). These mutations alter or remove the cytoplasmic domain at the carboxyl terminus of the receptor, demonstrating that this region normally targets the receptor to the coated pit. One such allele, a cysteine for tyrosine substitution in exon 17 (see Fig. 12–12), is believed to alter the conformation of the cytoplasmic domain of the receptor, thereby interfering with its binding to a protein that directs incorporation into the coated pit.

**Class 5 mutations** are recycling-defective alleles (see Fig. 12–11). Receptor recycling requires the dissociation of the receptor and the bound LDL in the endosome. The dissociation is mediated by the epidermal growth factor precursor homology domain (see Fig. 12–12). Mutations in this domain—both deletions of segments of it, as well as some missense substitutions—prevent the release of the ligand. This failure leads to degradation of the receptor, presumably because it cannot return to the cell surface in an unoccupied state.

**Pathogenesis of Atherosclerotic Plaques in Familial Hypercholesterolemia.** Despite the impressive knowledge of the normal biology of the LDL receptor and its molecular defects in familial hypercholesterolemia, the mechanisms by which the elevation in LDL leads to formation of atherosclerotic plaques in arteries is unclear. In homozygotes, the increased LDL is cleared from the extracellular fluid by *receptor-independent* pathways, including uptake by scavenger cells such as macrophages. Studies of macrophages in vitro show that excess cholesterol is stored as cholesterol ester droplets, producing the foam cell appearance typically seen in xanthomas and atherosclerotic plaques, but the in vivo relevance of this work is uncertain at present.

## TRANSPORT DEFECTS

### Cystic Fibrosis

Since the 1960s, CF has been one of the most publicly visible of all human genetic diseases. It is the most common fatal autosomal recessive genetic disorder of children in Caucasian populations, with an incidence of approximately 1 in 2500 Caucasian births and a carrier frequency of about 1 in 25. The positional cloning (see Chapter 8) of the CF gene (called *CFTR*) in 1989, along with the isolation of the Duchenne muscular dystrophy gene three years previously, were the first major deliveries on the promise that molecular biology would place the genes involved in hereditary diseases into the hands of medical scientists, even if nothing was initially known about the location of the affected locus or the function of its normal product. Shortly after the gene was cloned, physiological analyses demonstrated that the protein encoded by the *CFTR* gene is a regulated $Cl^-$ channel located in the apical membrane of the epithelial cells affected by the disease.

**The Phenotypes of Cystic Fibrosis.** The lungs and exocrine pancreas are the major organs affected by the disease, but a major diagnostic feature is increased sweat $Na^+$ and $Cl^-$ concentrations (often first noted when parents kiss their infants). In most patients with CF, the diagnosis can be based on the pulmonary or pancreatic findings and on an elevated level of sweat chloride (more than 60 mEq/L). Less than 2 percent of patients have normal sweat chloride but an otherwise typical clinical picture; in these cases, molecular analysis can be used to ascertain whether they have mutations at the CF locus.

Chronic obstructive lung disease develops as a result of thick secretions and recurrent infections, and deficiencies of pancreatic enzymes (lipase, trypsin, chymotrypsin) prevent normal digestion. Intense management of the lung disease prolongs life, and digestion and nutrition can be largely restored by pancreatic enzyme supplements. Death results from pulmonary failure and infection. At present, about half the patients survive to 26 years of age, but the clinical course is variable. About 15 percent of patients with CF have enough residual pancreatic exocrine function for normal digestion and are designated *pancreatic sufficient.* Moreover, patients with CF who are pancreatic sufficient have better growth and pulmonary function and a superior overall prognosis than do the majority, who are *pancreatic insufficient.* The clinical heterogeneity of the pancreatic disease is at least partly due to allelic heterogeneity, as discussed later.

Many other phenotypes are observed in patients with CF. For example, postnatal lower intestinal tract obstruction (**meconium ileus**) occurs in 10 to 20 percent of newborns with CF; its presence requires that the diagnosis of CF be excluded. The genital tract is also affected. Although females with CF have some reduction in fertility, more than 95 percent of males with CF are infertile because they lack a vas deferens, a phenotype known as **congenital bilateral absence of the vas deferens** (CBAVD). In a striking example of allelic heterogeneity giving rise to a partial phenotype, it has been found that some infertile males who are otherwise well (i.e., have no other CF phenotypes) have CBAVD associated with specific mutant alleles in the CF gene. Similarly, some individuals with **idiopathic chronic pancreatitis** carry mutations in the CF gene, yet lack other clinical signs of CF.

**The Cystic Fibrosis Gene and the Cftr Protein.** The CF gene on chromosome 7q31 spans about 250 kb of DNA, and the coding region, with 27 exons, is predicted to encode a large integral membrane protein of about 170 kD (Fig. 12–13). On the basis of the physiological abnormalities in transmembrane ion transport observed in CF, the polypeptide encoded by the CF gene has been named the cftr (CF transmembrane conductance regulator) protein. Its primary amino acid sequence indicates that it belongs to the ABC (ATP [adenosine triphosphate]-binding cassette) family of transport proteins. At least seven other diseases have been shown to result from the loss of function of specific ABC transporters.

The cftr $Cl^-$ channel is characterized by five domains, shown in Figure 12–13: two membrane-spanning domains (MSDs), each with six transmembrane sequences; two nucleotide (ATP)-binding domains (NBDs); and a regulatory (R) domain with multiple phosphorylation sites. The importance of each domain is demonstrated by the identification of CF-causing missense mutations in each of them (Fig. 12–13). The pore of the $Cl^-$ channel is formed by the 12 transmembrane segments. ATP is bound and hydrolyzed by the NBDs, and the energy released is used for ion transport. Regulation of the channel is mediated, at least in part, by phosphorylation of the R domain.

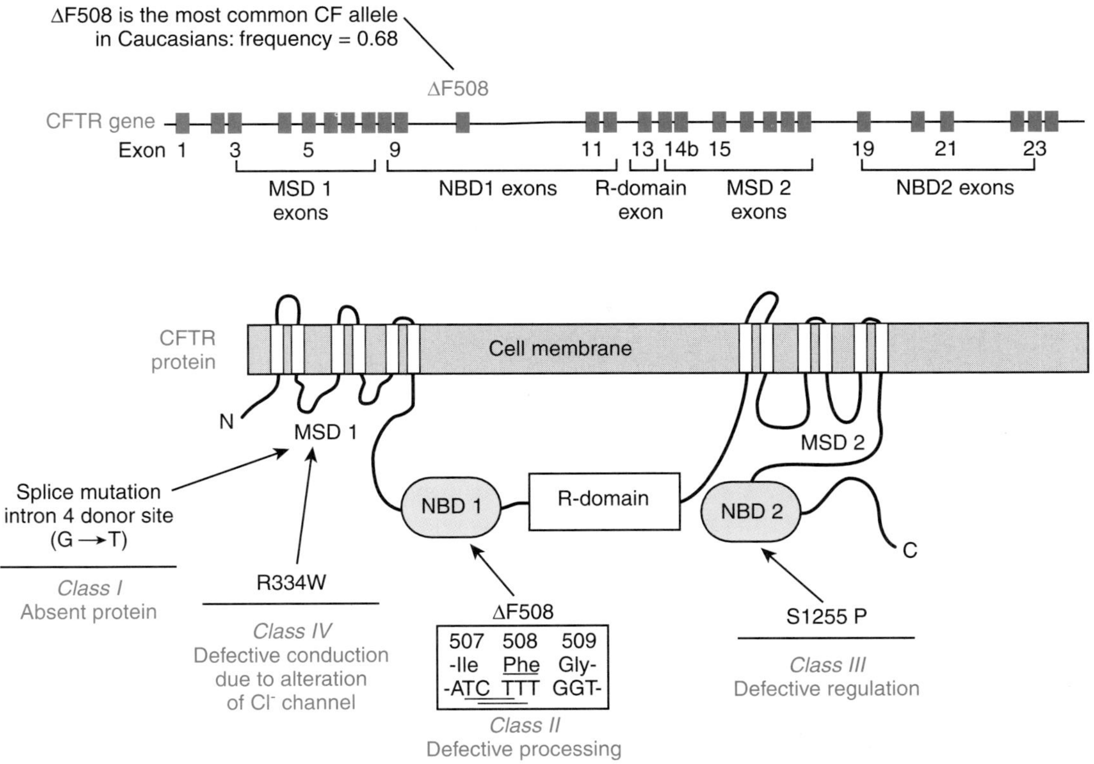


**Figure 12–13.** The structure of the *CFTR* gene and a schematic of the cftr protein. Selected mutations are shown. The exons, introns, and domains of the protein are not drawn to scale. (Based on Zielinski J [2000] Genotype and phenotype in cystic fibrosis. Respiration 67:117–133.)

**The Pathophysiological Defects in Cystic Fibrosis.** As manifested by the increase in sweat $Na^+$ and $Cl^-$ levels, CF is due to abnormal electrolyte transport across epithelial apical membranes. This abnormality leads to pathology in the lung, pancreas, intestine, hepatobiliary tree, and male genital tract. The physiological abnormalities have been most clearly elucidated for the sweat gland: the loss of cftr function means that $Cl^-$ in the duct of the sweat gland cannot flow out of the lumen and through the cells of the duct into the blood stream. As a consequence, the electrochemical gradient that normally drives $Na^+$ entry across the apical membrane is absent or diminished, leading to a secondary increase in $Na^+$ concentration in the sweat duct lumen. The effects on electrolyte transport due to the abnormalities in the cftr protein have also been carefully studied in airway and pancreatic epithelia. In each case, the fundamental defect is in $Cl^-$ transport, but the overall processes are complex, incompletely understood, and beyond the scope of this discussion.

## The Genetics of Cystic Fibrosis

**Mutations in the Cftr Polypeptide.** The first CF mutation identified, a deletion of a phenylalanine residue at position 508 (*ΔF508*) in the first ATP-binding fold (NBD1; Fig. 12–13), is the most common defect, accounting for about 70 percent of all CF alleles in Caucasian populations. In Caucasian populations, only seven other mutations are more frequent

TABLE 12–7

**The Phenotype of Cystic Fibrosis Associated with ΔF508 versus Other Alleles**

| | ΔF508/ΔF508 | ΔF508/Other Allele | Other Allele/Other Allele |
|---|---|---|---|
| Number of patients | 151 | 117 | 25 |
| % of all patients | 52% | 40% | 8% |
| % with PI | 99% | 72% | 36% |
| % with PS | 1% | 28% | 64% |
| Age at diagnosis (±SD) | 1.8 ± 3.3 years | 4.4 ± 5.9 years | 8.4 ± 8.3 years |

PI = pancreatic insufficiency; PS = pancreatic sufficiency.

Adapted from Kerem E, Corey M, Kerem B-S, et al (1990) The relationship between genotype and phenotype in cystic fibrosis: Analysis of the most common mutation (ΔF508). N Engl J Med 323:1517–1522.

than 0.5 percent, and the majority are therefore rare. Mutations of all types have been identified, but the largest single group (nearly half) are missense substitutions. The remainder are point mutations of other types, and less than 1 percent are genomic rearrangements. Although more than 800 CF gene sequence changes have been associated with disease, the actual number of missense mutations that are disease-causing is somewhat uncertain, because few have been subject to functional analysis.

Although the biochemical abnormalities associated with most CF mutations are not known, four general mechanisms of protein dysfunction have been described. Alleles representative of each of these four classes of dysfunction are shown in Figure 12–13. Class I mutations are those that have a defect in protein production, such as those associated with premature stop codons or mutations that generate unstable RNAs. Because cftr is a glycosylated membrane spanning protein, it must be processed in the endoplasmic reticulum (ER) and Golgi to be glycosylated and secreted; class II mutations are a result of defective protein processing due to misfolding of the protein. The *ΔF508* mutant typifies this class; this mutant does not fold normally enough to allow exit from the ER.

The essential functions of the NBDs and the R domain (Fig. 12–13) are illustrated by the occurrence of CF-causing mutations that disrupt regulation of the protein (class III mutations). Class IV mutations are located in the MSDs and, consistent with this localization, have defective chloride conduction.

**Genotype-Phenotype Correlations in Cystic Fibrosis.** Because all patients with CF appear to have mutations in the CF gene, clinical heterogeneity in CF must arise from allelic heterogeneity, the effects of other modifying loci, or nongenetic factors. Two generalizations have emerged from the genetic and clinical analysis of CF patients. First, the *CFTR* genotype is a good predictor of exocrine pancreatic function. For example, patients homozygous for the common *ΔF508* mutation or for predicted null alleles (such as premature stop codons), generally have pancreatic insufficiency (Table 12–7). On the other hand, alleles that allow the synthesis of a partially functional cftr protein, such as Arg334Trp (see Fig. 12–13), tend to be associated with pancreatic sufficiency. Second, there is a poor overall correlation between the pulmonary phenotype and the *CFTR* genotype. For example, among patients homozygous for the *ΔF508* mutation, the severity of lung disease is very variable. The reasons for this poor pulmonary genotype-phenotype correlation are not clear. No modifier genes for the pulmonary phenotype have been identified. A modifier locus for the CF intestinal phenotype of meconium ileus has been mapped to chromosome 19q13, but the gene has not yet been identified.

**The Cystic Fibrosis Gene in Populations.** At present, it is not possible to account for the high CF allele frequency of 1 in 45 that is observed in Caucasian populations (see Chapter 7). The disease is much less frequent in non-Caucasians, although it has been reported in Native Americans, African Americans, and Asians (e.g., approximately 1 in 90,000 Hawaiians of Asian descent). The *ΔF508* allele is the only one found to date that is common in virtually all Caucasian populations. Haplotype analysis of Caucasian populations indicates that the *ΔF508* allele has a single origin. The frequency of this allele, among all mutant alleles, varies significantly in different European populations, from 88 percent in Denmark to 45 percent in southern Italy.

In populations in which the *ΔF508* allele frequency is approximately 70 percent of all mutant alleles, about 50 percent of patients are homozygous for the *ΔF508* allele, and an additional 40 percent have genetic compound genotypes for *ΔF508* and another mutant allele. In addition, approximately 70 percent of CF carriers have the *ΔF508* mutation. Except for *ΔF508*, the CF mutations at the *CFTR* locus are rare, although in specific populations, other alleles may be quite common.

**Population Screening.** The complex issues that are raised by considering population screening for diseases such as CF are discussed in Chapter 20. At present, CF meets most of the criteria for a newborn screening program except it is not yet clear that screening significantly improves long-term prognosis. Furthermore, it is generally agreed that universal screening should not be considered until at least 95 percent of the mutations in carriers can be detected. The fact that many rare mutations make up more than 5 percent of the mutations in most populations is a serious obstacle to screening.

**Genetic Analysis of Families of Patients, and Prenatal Diagnosis.** The high frequency of the *ΔF508* allele is useful when CF patients without a family history present for DNA diagnosis. The identification of the *ΔF508* allele, in combination with haplotype analysis, can be used to predict the status of family members for (1) confirmation of disease status (e.g., in a newborn or a sibling with an ambiguous presentation), (2) carrier detection, and (3) prenatal diagnosis. Given the vast knowledge of CF mutations in many populations, direct mutation detection is the method of choice for genetic analysis. Typically, screening is performed for 10 to 30 of the most common mutations found in the geographic region of origin of the family in question. In principle, accurate diagnosis is possible in virtually all families.

For fetuses with a 1-in-4 risk, prenatal diagnosis by DNA analysis at 8 to 10 weeks, with tissue obtained by chorionic villus biopsy, is the method of choice (see Chapter 18). Biochemical methods of prenatal diagnosis based on the measurement of intestinal enzymes (e.g., intestinal alkaline phosphatase) in amniotic fluid are also reasonably accurate, with a false-positive rate of 2 to 5 percent and a false-negative rate of 2 to 10 percent. This method is now used only when the index case is not available or when time to perform mutational or genetic linkage studies in the family is insufficient.

**Molecular Genetics and the Treatment of Cystic Fibrosis.** At present, the treatment of CF is directed toward controlling pulmonary infection and improving nutrition. Increasing knowledge of the molecular pathogenesis may make it possible to design pharmacological interventions that would directly correct the abnormal biochemical phenotype. Alternatively, gene transfer therapy may be possible in CF, but there are many difficulties, as discussed in Chapter 13.

## DISORDERS OF STRUCTURAL PROTEINS

### Duchenne and Becker Muscular Dystrophies: Defects in Dystrophin

Like CF, DMD has long received attention from the general and medical communities because it is a severe, currently untreatable, relatively common disorder associated with relentless clinical deterioration. The isolation of the gene affected in this X-linked disorder, and the characterization of its protein (named "dystrophin" because of its association with DMD), has given insight into every aspect of the disease, greatly improved the genetic counseling of affected families, and suggested strategies for treatment.

**The Clinical Phenotype of Duchenne Muscular Dystrophy.** Affected boys are normal for the first year or two of life but develop muscle weakness at age 3 to 5 years (Fig. 12–14), when they begin to have difficulty climbing stairs and rising from a sitting position. The child is confined to a wheelchair by the age of 12 and is unlikely to survive beyond the age of 20. Patients die of respiratory failure or, because the myocardial muscle is also affected, of cardiac failure. In the preclinical and early stages of the disease, the serum creatine kinase level is grossly elevated (50 to 100 times the upper limit of normal) because of its release from diseased muscle. The brain is also affected; on average, there is a modest decrease in IQ of about 20 points.

**Becker Muscular Dystrophy.** BMD is also due to mutations in the dystrophin gene, but the Becker alleles produce a phenotype that is much milder. Patients are said to have BMD if they are still walking at the age of 16 years. There is significant variability in the progression of the disease, and some patients remain ambulatory for many years. Generally, patients with BMD carry mutated alleles that maintain the reading frame of the protein and thus express some dystrophin, albeit often an altered product at reduced levels. The presence of dystrophin in the muscle of patients with BMD is generally demonstrable both on Western blots (see Fig. 4–14) and by immunofluorescence (Fig. 12–15). In contrast, patients with DMD have little or no detectable dystrophin using either technique.

#### THE GENETICS OF DUCHENNE MUSCULAR DYSTROPHY AND BECKER MUSCULAR DYSTROPHY

**Inheritance.** DMD has an incidence of about 1 in 3300 live male births, with a calculated mutation rate of $10^{-4}$, an order of magnitude higher than the rate

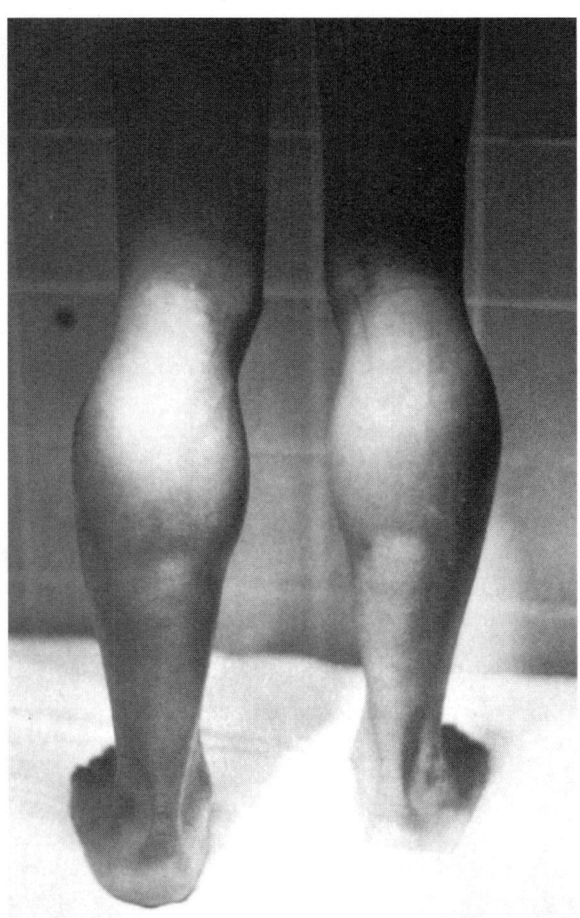

**Figure 12–14.** Pseudohypertrophy of the calves due to the replacement of normal muscle tissue with connective tissue and fat in an 8-year-old boy with Duchenne muscular dystrophy. (Courtesy of R. H. A. Haslam, The Hospital for Sick Children, Toronto.)

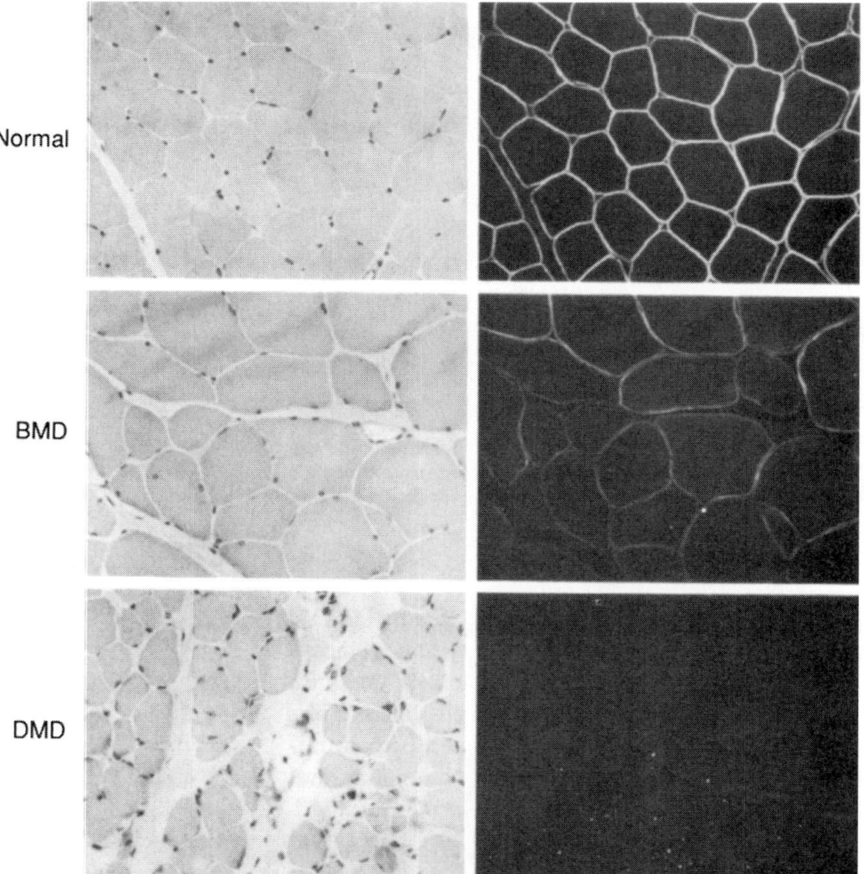


**Figure 12–15.** Microscopic visualization of the effect of mutations in the dystrophin gene in a patient with Becker muscular dystrophy (BMD) and a patient with Duchenne muscular dystrophy (DMD). Left column = hematoxylin and eosin staining of muscle. Right column = immunofluorescence microscopy staining with an antibody specific to dystrophin. Note the localization of dystrophin to the myocyte membrane in normal muscle, the reduced quantity of dystrophin in BMD muscle, and the complete absence of dystrophin from the myocytes of the DMD muscle. The amount of connective tissue between the myocytes in the DMD muscle is increased. (Courtesy of K. Arahata, National Institute of Neuroscience, Tokyo.)

observed in genes involved in most other genetic diseases. In fact, given a production of about $8 \times 10^7$ sperm per day, a normal male produces a sperm with a new mutation in the *DMD* gene every 10 to 11 seconds! In Chapter 5, DMD is presented as a typical X-linked recessive that is lethal in males, so that one third of cases are predicted to be new mutants and two thirds of patients have carrier mothers (see also Chapter 19). The great majority of carrier females have no clinical manifestations, although about 70 percent have slightly elevated levels of serum creatine kinase. In accordance with random inactivation of the X chromosome (see Chapter 5), however, the normal X chromosome appears to be inactivated in a critical proportion of cells in some female heterozygotes; about 8 percent of adult female carriers have significant muscle weakness and, in some instances, serious proximal muscle disability. In rare instances, females have been reported with DMD (Table 12–8); some have X;autosome translocations (see Chapter 10), others have only one X chromosome (Turner syndrome) with a *DMD* mutation on that chromosome, and a rare group consists of heterozygous monozygotic twins.

BMD accounts for about 15 percent of the mutations at the locus. An important genetic distinction between these allelic phenotypes is that whereas DMD is a genetic lethal, the reproductive fitness of males with BMD is quite high (up to about 70 percent of normal), so that they can transmit the gene to their daughters. Consequently, a high proportion of BMD cases are inherited, and few (only about 10 percent) represent new mutations.

**The DMD Gene and Its Product.** The most remarkable feature of the *DMD* gene is its size, estimated to be 2300 kb, or 1.5 percent of the X chromosome. This huge gene, like the gene for neuro-fibromatosis, type 1 (NF1) and a few others, is the largest known in any species, by an order of magnitude. The high mutation rate can therefore be at least partly explained by the fact that the locus is a large target for mutation. The *DMD* gene is structurally complex, with 79 exons, 7 tissue-specific promoters, and differential splicing giving rise to tissue-specific, developmentally regulated isoforms. In muscle, the primary site of pathology, the large (14 kb) dystrophin transcript encodes a huge 427 kD protein (Fig. 12–16). In accordance with the clinical phenotype of the disease, this protein is most abundant in skeletal and cardiac muscle and the brain, although most tissues express at least one dystrophin isoform.

Muscle dystrophin has several domains homologous to other cytoskeletal proteins (Fig. 12–16 and

TABLE 12–8

**Mechanisms of Mutation in Duchenne or Becker Muscular Dystrophy**

| Molecular or Genetic Defect | Frequency | Phenotype |
|---|---|---|
| **In affected males:** | | |
| Gene deletion (1 exon to whole gene) | ~60% | DMD or BMD |
| Point mutations | ~34% | DMD or BMD |
| Partial duplication of the gene | ~6% | DMD or BMD |
| Contiguous gene deletion | Rare | DMD plus other phenotypes, depending on other genes deleted |
| **In affected females:** | | |
| Nonrandom X inactivation | Rare | DMD |
| Turner syndrome (45, X) | Rare | DMD |
| X;autosome translocation | Rare | DMD |

BMD = Becker muscular dystrophy; DMD = Duchenne muscular dystrophy.

Fig. 12–17). Dystrophin appears to be a structural protein, with at least two major roles. First, it is essential for the maintenance of muscle membrane integrity, by linking the actin cytoskeleton to the extracellular matrix. Second, it appears to be required for the assembly of the synaptic junction, because members of the transmembrane complex participate in acetylcholine receptor clustering during development. As indicated in Figure 12–17, mutations in other proteins in the dystrophin glycoprotein complex are responsible for autosomal recessive forms of Duchenne-like muscular dystrophy, limb girdle muscular dystrophies, and other muscular dystrophies.

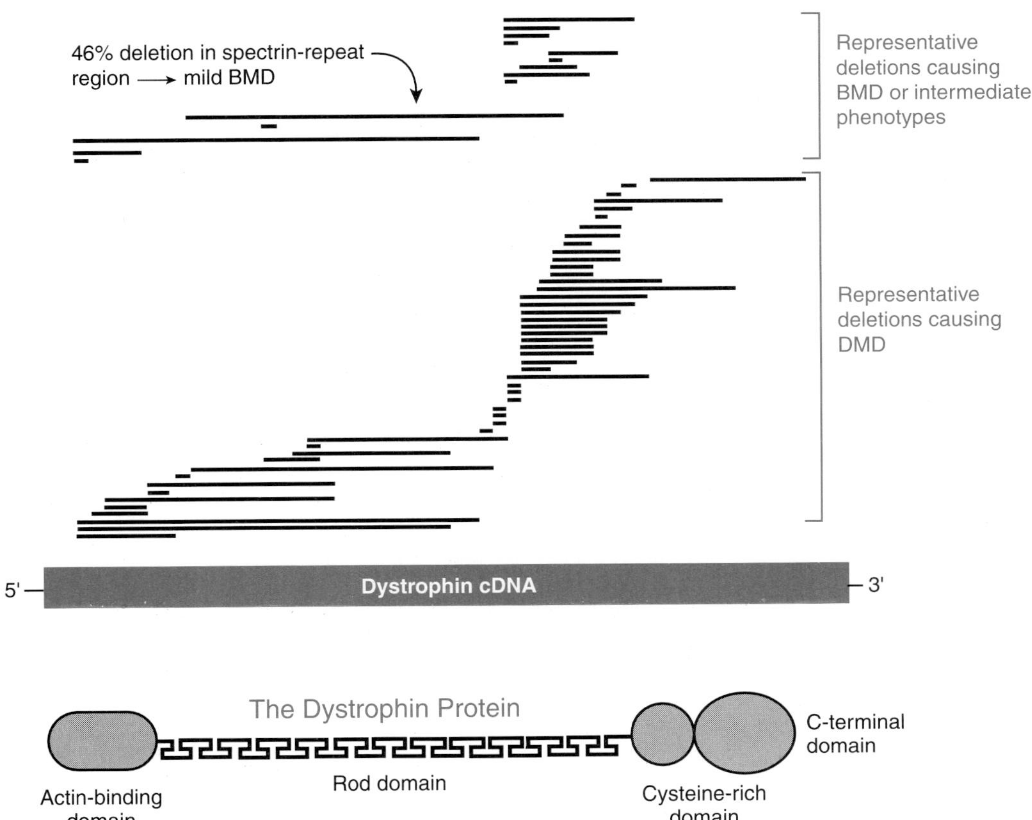


**Figure 12–16.** A representation of the full-length dystrophin protein, the corresponding cDNA and the distribution of representative deletions in patients with Becker muscular dystrophy (BMD) and Duchenne muscular dystrophy (DMD). The actin binding domain links the protein to the filamentous actin cytoskeleton. The rod domain presumably acts as a spacer between the N-terminal and C-terminal domains. The cysteine-rich domain mediates protein-protein interactions. The C-terminal domain, which associates with a large transmembrane glycoprotein complex (see Fig. 12–17), is also found in three dystrophin-related proteins (DRPs): utrophin (DRP-1), DRP-2, and dystrobrevin. The protein domains are not drawn to scale.

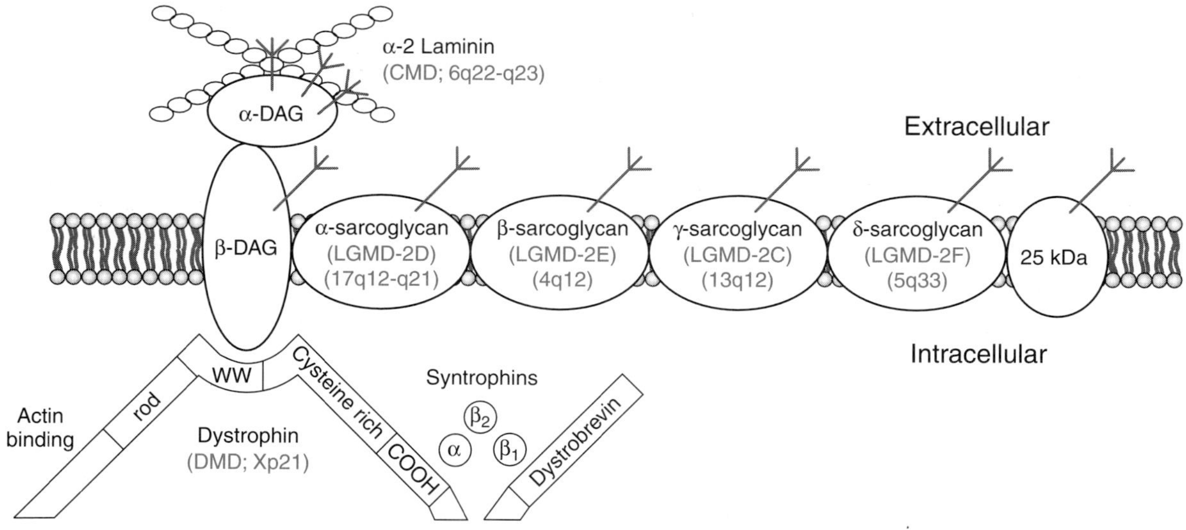


**Figure 12–17.** In muscle, dystrophin links the extracellular matrix (laminin) to the actin cytoskeleton. Dystrophin interacts with a multimeric complex composed of the dystroglycan (DAG), the sarcoglycans, the syntrophins, and dystrobrevin. The $\alpha$, $\beta$-dystroglycan complex is a receptor for laminin and agrin in the extracellular matrix. The function of the sarcoglycan complex is uncertain, but it is integral to muscle function: mutations in the sarcoglycans have been identified in limb girdle muscular dystrophies (LGMD) type 2C, 2D, 2E, and 2F. Mutations in laminin type 2 (merosin) cause a congenital muscular dystrophy (CMD).

**Molecular Analysis of Duchenne Muscular Dystrophy and Becker Muscular Dystrophy.** The most common molecular defects in patients with DMD are deletions (60 percent of alleles) (see Table 12–8, Fig. 12–16, and Fig. 12–18). The distribution of the deletions in the gene is not random; they are clustered in one of two regions within the gene, in the 5′ half or in a central region that appears to encompass a deletion hotspot (see Fig. 12–16). The central deletions presumably result from the slipped mispairing

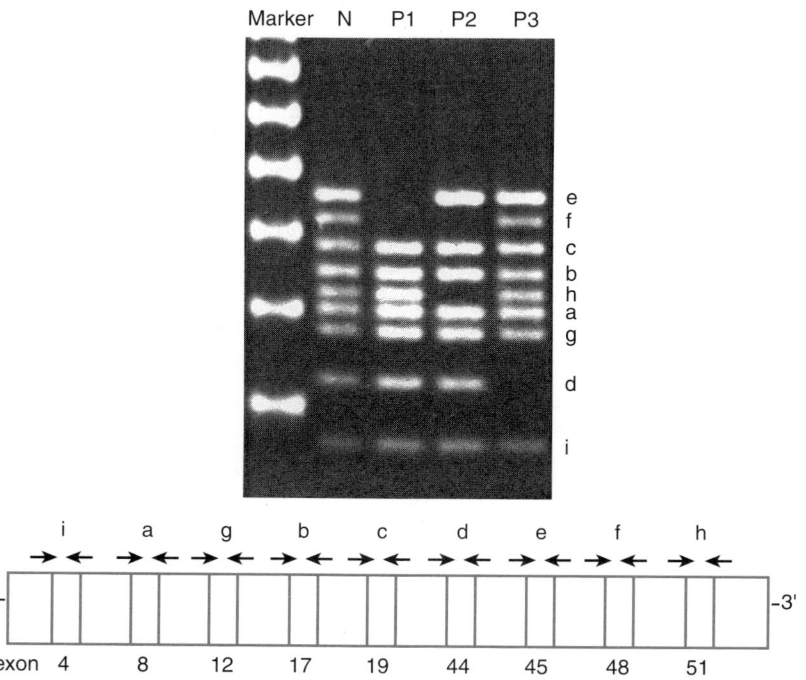


**Figure 12–18.** Diagnosis of Duchenne muscular dystrophy involves screening for deletions and duplications using a procedure called multiplex polymerase chain reaction (PCR). Using primer sets (*pairs of arrows*) that amplify various regions of the gene (*a-i*) in a single reaction, patient DNA is analyzed for aberrant or missing bands by gel electrophoresis. Lane 2 shows the nine PCR products from a normal individual (*N*), indicating the presence of the corresponding exons. Patient 1 (*lane P1*) is missing bands e and f, which identifies a deletion encompassing exons 45–48. Patient 2 (*P2*) is missing bands f and h, which indicates a deletion involving exons 48–51. Patient 3 (*P3*) is missing band d and therefore has a deletion involving exon 44. (Courtesy of P. N. Ray, The Hospital for Sick Children, Toronto.)

mechanism described in Figure 11–8. Point mutations account for approximately one third of the alleles and are randomly distributed throughout the gene.

### The Clinical Application of Molecular Genetics to Muscular Dystrophy

**Prenatal Diagnosis and Carrier Detection.** With molecular techniques, accurate prenatal diagnosis is available for patients with deletions, duplications, and known point mutations in the *DMD* gene. In the 60 to 70 percent of families in whom the mutation results from a deletion or duplication, the presence or absence of the defect can be assessed on examination of fetal DNA by Southern blotting or, more commonly, by multiplex polymerase chain analysis (see Fig. 12–18). In most other families in which the molecular defect has not yet been defined, linked markers allow prenatal diagnosis with an accuracy of about 95 percent. Identification of carrier or noncarrier status is possible in approximately 75 percent of female relatives of an affected boy by using DNA methods and testing for elevated serum creatine kinase.

**Maternal Mosaicism.** If a boy with DMD is the first affected member of his family, and if his mother is not found to carry the mutation in her lymphocytes, the usual explanation is that he has a new mutation at the *DMD* locus. However, about 5 to 15 percent of such cases appear to be due to maternal germline mosaicism, in which case the recurrence risk is significant (see Chapter 5).

**Therapy.** At present, only symptomatic treatment is available for DMD. The possibilities for rational therapy for DMD have greatly increased with the isolation of the dystrophin gene and the understanding of its normal role in the myocyte. Some of the therapeutic considerations are discussed in Chapter 13.

## Mutations in Collagen Genes: Osteogenesis Imperfecta and Ehlers-Danlos Syndrome

### Osteogenesis Imperfecta: Defects in the Collagen Structural Genes

Osteogenesis imperfecta (OI) is a group of inherited disorders of type I collagen that predispose a patient to easy fracturing of bones, even with little trauma, and to skeletal deformity (Fig. 12–19). A remarkable range of clinical variation has been recognized, from a lethal perinatal form to only a mild increase in fracture frequency. The four major phenotypes are outlined in Table 12–9. The clinical heterogeneity can be at least partly explained by locus and allelic heterogeneity: the phenotypes vary according to which chain of type I procollagen is affected and according to the type and location of the mutation in the locus. The combined incidence of all forms of the disease is about 1 in 10,000.

**Normal Collagen Structure in Relation to Osteogenesis Imperfecta.** Certain features of normal type I collagen are essential to appreciating the pathogenesis of this disease. Type I collagen is the major structural protein of bone and other fibrous tissues. The type I procollagen molecule is formed from two pro$\alpha$1(I) chains (encoded on chromosome 17) and one similar but distinct pro$\alpha$2(I) chain (encoded on chromosome 7) (Fig. 12–20).

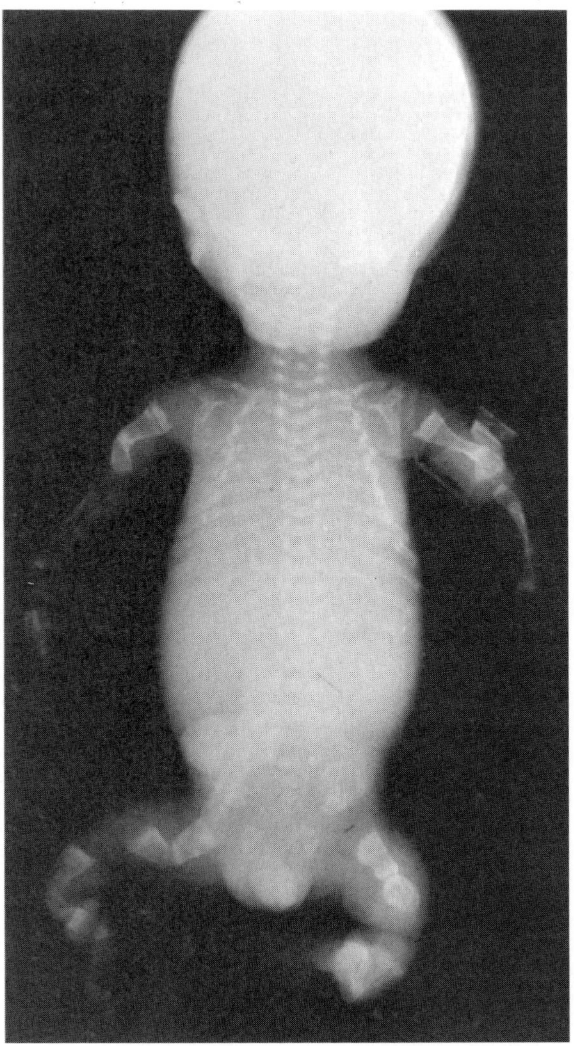

**Figure 12–19.** Radiograph of a premature (26 weeks' gestation) infant with the perinatal lethal form (type II) of osteogenesis imperfecta. The skull is relatively large and unmineralized and was soft to palpation. The thoracic cavity is small, the long bones of the arms and legs are short and deformed, and the vertebral bodies are flattened. All the bones are undermineralized. (Courtesy of T. Costa, The Hospital for Sick Children, Toronto.)

TABLE 12–9

## A Summary of the Genetic, Biochemical, and Molecular Features of the Types of Osteogenesis Imperfecta

| Type | Phenotype | Inheritance | Biochemical Defect | Gene Defect |
|---|---|---|---|---|
| **Defective production of type I collagen*** | | | | |
| Type I | **Mild:** blue sclerae, brittle bones, but no bony deformity; often, presenile deafness | AD | Common: All the collagen made is *normal* (from the normal allele), but the quantity is *reduced* by half. Infrequently, substitutions of gly (see Fig. 12–21) | Common: Null alleles that impair the production of pro $\alpha1$(I) chains, such as defects that interfere with mRNA synthesis |
| **Structural defects in type I collagen** | | | | |
| Type II | **Perinatal lethal:** severe abnormalities (fractures, deformities), dark sclerae, death within 1 month | AD (new mutation) | Common: Production of *abnormal* collagen molecules due to substitution of the gly in Gly-X-Y of the triple helical domain, with some bias toward the COOH-terminal half of the protein (see Fig. 12–22) | Common: Missense skeletal mutations in the glycine codons of the genes for the $\alpha1$ and $\alpha2$ chains |
| Type III | **Progressive deforming:** fractures, often at birth, progressive bony deformity, limited growth, blue sclerae, dentinogenesis imperfecta, hearing loss | AD† | Abnormal collagen molecules: gly substitutions of many types in the triple helix. Located throughout the protein (see Fig. 12–22) | Missense mutations in the glycine codons of the genes for the $\alpha1$ or $\alpha2$ chains |
| Type IV | **Normal sclerae, deforming:** mild to moderate bony deformity, short stature, fractures, hearing loss, dentinogenesis imperfecta | AD | Abnormal collagen molecules: gly substitutions of many types in the triple helix. Located throughout the protein (see Fig. 12–22) | Missense mutations in the glycine codons of the genes for the $\alpha1$ or $\alpha2$ chains |

*A few patients with type I disease have substitutions of glycine in one of the type I collagen chains (see Fig. 12–22).
†Rare cases are autosomal recessive.

Modified from Byers PH (1989) Disorders of collagen biosynthesis and structure. *In* Scriver CR, Beaudet AL, Sly WS, Valle D (eds) The Metabolic Bases of Inherited Disease, 6th ed. McGraw-Hill, New York, pp. 2805–2842; and Byers PH (1990) Brittle bones–fragile molecules: Disorders of collagen structure and expression. Trends Genet 6:293–300.

Proteins composed of subunits, like collagen, are often subject to mutations that prevent subunit association by altering the subunit interfaces (see Table 11–1). The triple helical (collagen) section is composed of 338 tandemly arranged Gly-X-Y repeats; proline is often in the X position, and hydroxyproline or hydroxylysine is often in the Y position. Glycine, the smallest amino acid, is the only residue compact enough to occupy the axial position of the helix, and, consequently, mutations resulting in substitutions to other residues are highly disruptive to the helical structure.

Several features of procollagen maturation are of special significance to the pathophysiology of OI. First, the assembly of the individual chains into the triple helix begins at the C terminus and moves toward the N terminus. Consequently, mutations in the C-terminal part of the molecule are more disruptive because they interfere earlier with the propagation of the triple helix (Fig. 12–21). Second, the post-translational modification (e.g., proline hydroxylation, glycosylation) of procollagen continues on any part of a chain not assembled into the triple helix. Thus, when triple helix assembly is slowed by a mutation, the unassembled sections of the chains that are amino terminal to the defect are modified excessively, which slows their secretion into the extracellular space. Overmodification may also interfere with the formation of collagen fibrils. As a result of all of these abnormalities, not only is the number of fibrils reduced, but many of those that are secreted are defective. In bone, the abnormal chains and their reduced number lead to decreased mineralization (see Fig. 12–19).

### Molecular Abnormalities of Collagen in Osteogenesis Imperfecta

More than 200 different mutations affecting the synthesis or structure of type I collagen have been found in patients with OI. The clinical heterogeneity of this disease has been found to reflect even greater heterogeneity at the molecular level (see Table 12–9). The mutations fall into two general classes. If the mutation decreases the *production* of type I collagen, the relatively mild phenotype of type I OI is the consequence. If the mutation alters the *structure* of the molecule, types II, III, and IV OI are the resulting phenotypes. Thus, to some extent, it is now possible to predict the phenotype that will result from a specific type of molecular defect (Fig. 12–22).

**Type I: Diminished Type I Collagen Production.** The great majority of patients with type I OI have mutations that severely impair the production of type I collagen, represented as the pro$\alpha$1° allele in Figure 12–21. Typically, it is the pro$\alpha$1(I) chain that is affected. The majority of the mutations are either premature stop codons, small insertion or deletion events (usually of 1 to 2 base pairs), or splice site mutations. Missense mutations give rise to this milder form of OI when the amino acid change is located in the N terminus, because substitutions at this location tend to be less disruptive of collagen chain assembly (see Fig. 12–22).

**Types II, III, and IV: Structurally Defective Collagens.** The type II, III, and IV phenotypes of OI result from mutations that produce structurally

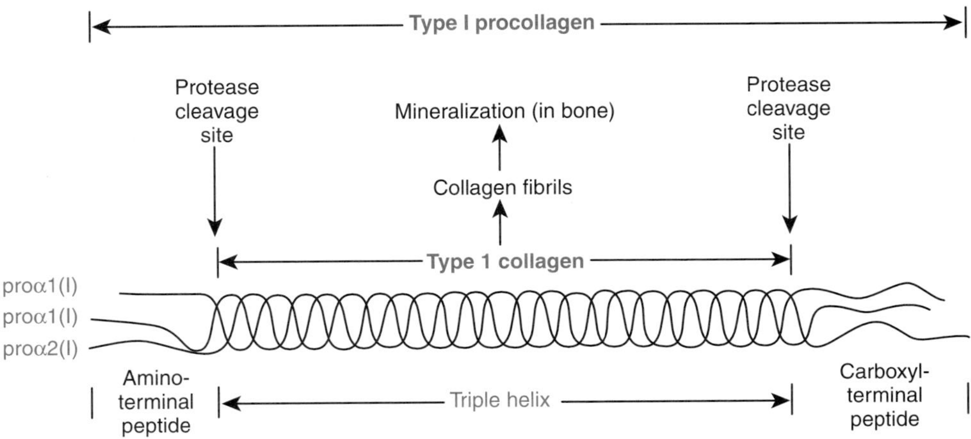


Figure 12–20. The structure of type I procollagen. Each collagen chain is made as a procollagen triple helix that is secreted into the extracellular space. The amino- and carboxyl-terminal domains are cleaved extracellularly to form collagen; mature collagen fibrils are then assembled and, in bone, mineralized. Note that type I procollagen is composed of two pro$\alpha$1(I) chains and one pro$\alpha$2(I) chain. (Redrawn from Byers PH [1989] Disorders of collagen biosynthesis and structure. *In* Scriver CR, Beaudet AL, Sly WS, Valle D [eds] The Metabolic Bases of Inherited Disease, 6th ed. McGraw-Hill, New York, pp. 2805–2842.)

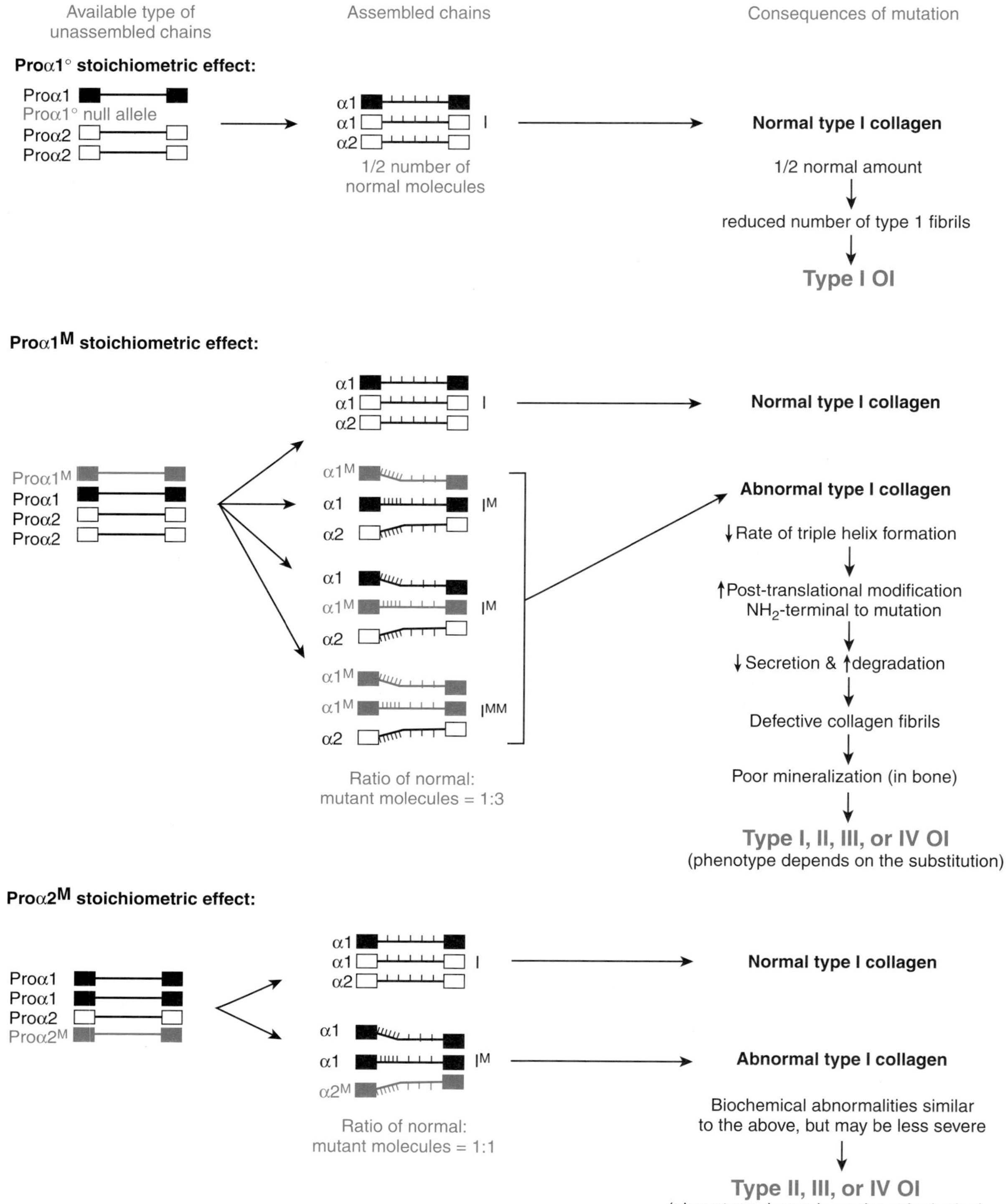


**Figure 12–21.** The pathogenesis of the major classes of type I procollagen mutants. Column 1: the types of procollagen chains available for assembly into a triple helix. Column 2: the effect of type I procollagen stoichiometry on the ratio of normal to defective collagen molecules formed in mutants with pro$\alpha$1 chain versus pro$\alpha$2 mutations. The small vertical bars on each procollagen chain indicate post-translational modifications (*see text*). Column 3: the effect of mutations on the biochemical processing of collagen. Pro$\alpha 1^M$ = a pro$\alpha$1 chain with a missense mutation; pro$\alpha 2^M$ = a pro$\alpha$2 chain with a missense mutation; pro$\alpha 1^0$ = a pro$\alpha$1 chain null allele.

abnormal pro$\alpha$1 chains (see Figs. 12–21 and 12–22) (mutations in the pro$\alpha$2 chain have a comparable effect). The great majority of these patients have substitutions in the triple helix that replace a glycine with a more bulky residue. The gene affected, the location of the substitution, and the substituting residue are all important phenotypic determinants, but some generalizations about the phenotype likely to be associated with a specific substitution are nevertheless possible. Thus, substitutions in the pro$\alpha$1 chain are more prevalent and more often lethal in the population of patients with OI types II, III, or IV. In either chain, replacement of glycine (a neutral residue) with aspartate (an acidic residue) is usually very disruptive and more often associated with a severe (type II) phenotype (see Fig. 12–22). Sometimes, a specific substitution is associated with more than one phenotype, an outcome that is likely to reflect the influence of powerful modifier genes of this monogenic disorder.

### The Genetics of Osteogenesis Imperfecta.

Most of the mutations that cause the disease are dominantly acting, but a few are recessive. At least some of the mechanisms by which different patterns of inheritance arise from different mutations in a single molecule have been revealed by characterization of the biochemical defects. More generally, this disease illustrates the genetic complexities that result when mutations alter structural proteins, particularly those composed of multiple different subunits.

The relatively mild phenotype and dominant inheritance of type I OI are consistent with the fact that although only half the normal number of molecules is made, they are of normal quality (see Fig. 12–21). The more severe consequences of producing structurally defective pro$\alpha$1 chains (compared with producing no chains) partly reflect the stoichiometry of type I collagen, which is two pro$\alpha$1 chains to one pro$\alpha$2 chain (see Fig. 12–21). Accordingly, if one pro$\alpha$1 chain is abnormal, three of four type I

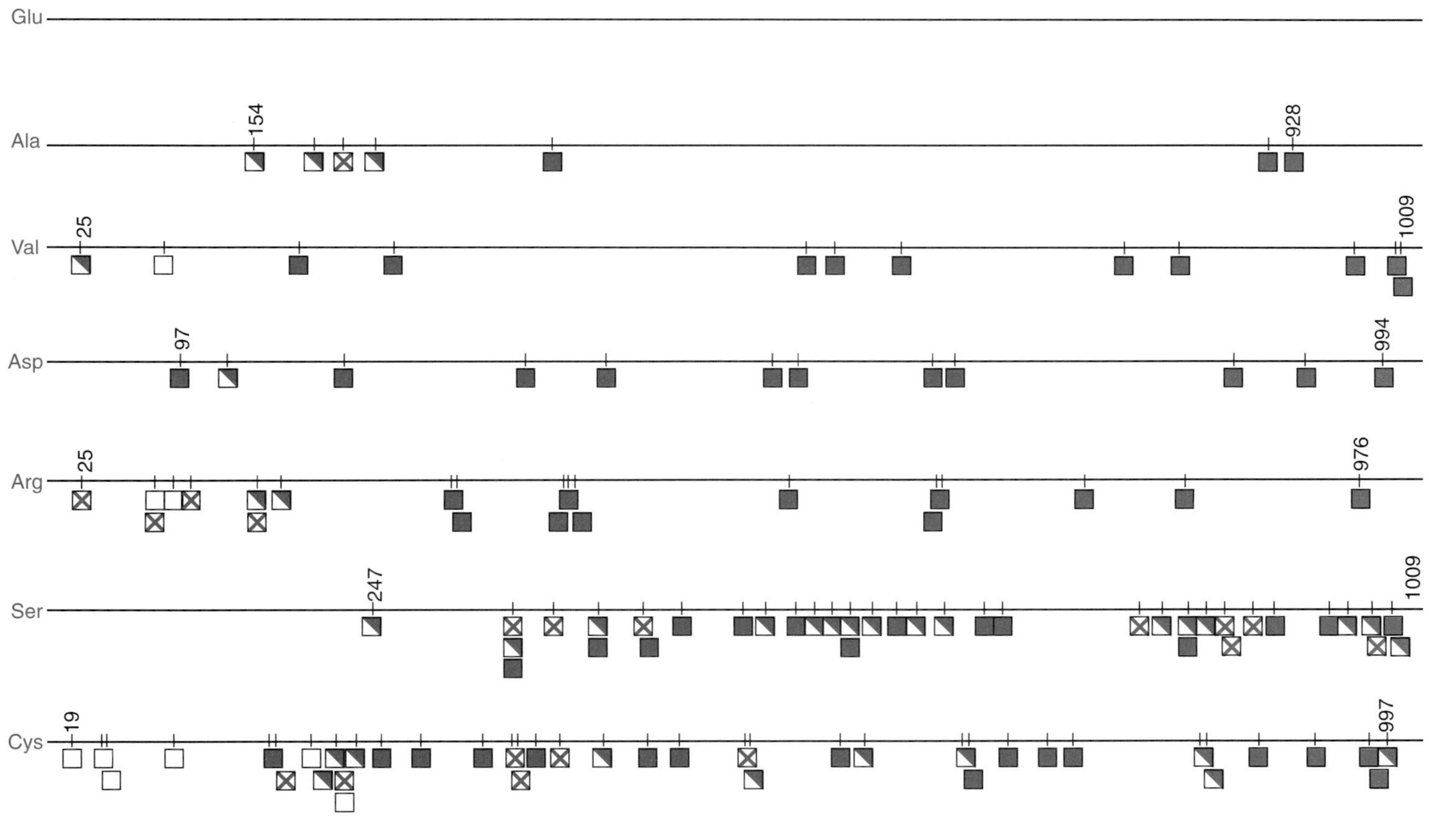


**Figure 12–22.** The phenotypic effect of substitutions in the pro$\alpha$1 chain of type I collagen. I, II, III, and IV = Types I–IV osteogenesis imperfecta. The numbers above the linear representation of the collagen molecules are the glycine residues that have been substituted by the amino acid noted to the left of each line. Note that in general, the phenotypic effect of substitutions near the carboxyl terminus is more severe but that the effect also depends on the nature of the residue that replaces glycine. (Redrawn from Byers PH [1990] Brittle bones—fragile molecules: Disorders of collagen structure and expression. Trends Genet 6:293–300.)

molecules have at least one abnormal chain; in contrast, if a pro$\alpha$2 chain is defective, only one of two molecules is affected. Mutations such as the pro$\alpha$1 missense allele (pro$\alpha 1^M$) shown in Fig. 12–21 are thus **dominant negative alleles** because they impair the contribution of both the normal pro$\alpha$1 allele and the normal pro$\alpha$2 alleles. In other words, the effect of the mutant allele is amplified because of the polymeric nature of the collagen molecule. Consequently, in dominantly inherited diseases such as OI, it is actually better to have a mutation that generates *no* gene product than one that produces an *abnormal* gene product.

Although mutations that produce structurally abnormal pro$\alpha$2 chains reduce the number of normal type I collagen molecules by one half (versus three quarters in structurally abnormal pro$\alpha$1 chains; see Fig. 12–21), this reduction is nevertheless sufficient, in the case of some mutations, to cause the severe perinatal lethal phenotype (see Table 12–9).

Most infants with the type II perinatal lethal form of OI have a *new* dominant mutation, and, consequently, the likelihood of recurrence in the family is very low. In occasional families, however, more than one sibling is affected with the type II disease. Such recurrences seem to be invariably due to parental germline mosaicism (see pedigree in Fig. 5–28). Strong documentation of autosomal recessive forms of type II OI has not been presented, but a few examples of recessive type III OI have been recognized.

**Clinical Management and Prenatal Diagnosis.** The knowledge of OI that is emerging has useful applications to prognosis. If a patient's molecular defect can be determined, it is often possible to predict, at least to some extent, the natural history of the disease. In addition, the demonstration that a defect is inherited from an affected parent (autosomal dominant), from an unaffected parent (with germline mosaicism), from two unaffected but heterozygous parents (autosomal recessive), or as a new mutation will allow accurate recurrence risks to be calculated. Prenatal diagnosis in type II OI, the perinatal lethal form, may be performed by examination of skull and limb length by ultrasonography in the second trimester. For most at-risk pregnancies, however, prenatal diagnosis requires the analysis of collagen synthesized by cells cultured from chorionic villus biopsies or direct analysis of a mutation (or analysis of polymorphic restriction sites) previously identified in the family.

Although the treatment of OI had been restricted to general medical and surgical measures, this situation is changing, owing to the discovery of the beneficial effects of bisphosphonates, a class of drugs that act by decreasing bone resorption. These compounds have been shown to increase both bone density and bone mineral content of patients with severe OI. The more critical issue, whether bisphosphonates reduce the frequency and severity of fractures in OI, is under study.

#### Ehlers-Danlos Syndrome Type VI: Defective Post-translational Modification of Collagen

In some instances, post-translational modification may be a permanent essential feature of a protein's structure or function (see Table 11–1). Defects in post-translational modifications can cause disease. A disorder that results from the deficiency of a permanent post-translational modification of collagen is Ehlers-Danlos syndrome type VI. Ehlers-Danlos syndrome is a heterogeneous group of connective tissue diseases characterized by skin fragility, joint hypermobility, and skin hyperextensibility (Fig. 12–23). In two types, the basic defect has been found to be in the structural gene of the collagen I or III chains, these being the predominant collagens of the affected tissues. In the type VI disorder, however, the disease results from defective post-translational modification of collagens I and III, due to a deficiency of the enzyme lysyl hydroxylase. The hydroxylation of some of the lysine residues of collagen is essential for the formation of normal intermolecular cross links between collagen molecules, a process that stabilizes the collagen fibrillar network.

## NEURODEGENERATIVE DISORDERS

### Alzheimer Disease

Until recently, the biochemical mechanisms underlying almost all adult-onset neurodegenerative diseases were completely obscure. One of the most common of these conditions, AD, affects about 1.4 percent of persons in developed countries and is responsible for 100,000 deaths per year in the United States alone. AD generally manifests in the seventh to ninth decades, but the monogenic forms often present earlier, sometimes as soon as the third decade. The clinical picture is variable, but includes progressive deterioration of memory and of higher cognitive functions, such as reasoning, in addition to behavioral changes. These abnormalities reflect degeneration of neurons in specific regions of the cerebral cortex, particularly the temporoparietal cortex, and the hippocampus.

**The Genetics of Alzheimer Disease.** By 85 years of age, first-degree relatives of patients with AD have a 38 percent final risk of acquiring the disease. Consequently, it appears that most cases with familial aggregation have a complex genetic contribution.

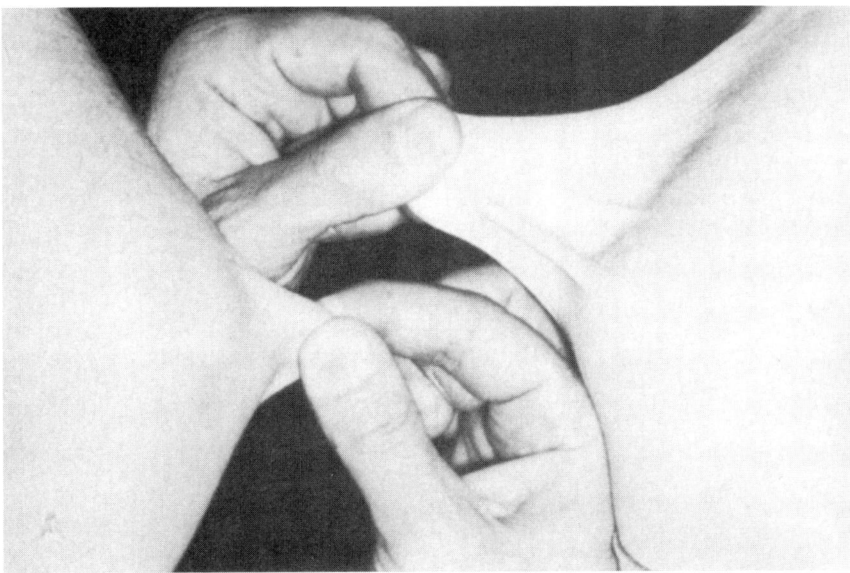

Figure 12–23. The hyperextensible skin of a patient with the Ehlers-Danlos syndrome. (Reproduced from Byers PH, Holbrook KA [1979] Heritable disorders of connective tissue. *In* Cohen AS [ed] The Science and Practice of Clinical Medicine, vol. 4: Rheumatology and Immunology. Grune and Stratton, New York, p. 344.)

This contribution may come from one or more incompletely penetrant genes that act independently, from multiple interacting genes, or from some combination of genetic and environmental factors. About 10 percent of patients have a monogenic form of the disease, familial AD (FAD), with highly penetrant age-related autosomal dominant inheritance. In the 1990s, the identification of four AD genes (Table 12–10) provided insight not only into FAD but also, as is commonly the case in medical genetics, into the biochemical basis of the more common form, sporadic AD.

**Beta-Amyloid Peptide and Tau Protein Deposits Are Central to the Pathogenesis of Alzheimer Disease.** The most important pathological abnormalities of AD are the deposition in the brain of two fibrillary proteins, $\beta$-amyloid peptide (A$\beta$) and Tau protein. The A$\beta$ peptide, which is generated from the protein encoded by one of the FAD susceptibility genes (Table 12–10), is found in amyloid or senile plaques in the cerebral extracellular space of brains with AD. Amyloid plaques contain other proteins besides the A$\beta$ peptide, notably apolipoprotein E (ApoE), also encoded by an AD susceptibility gene (*APOE*) (Table 12–10). Hyperphosphorylated forms of the Tau protein comprise the neurofibrillary tangles that, in contrast to amyloid plaques, are found *within* AD neurons. Tau is a microtubule-associated protein expressed abundantly in neurons of the brain. The protein promotes the assembly and stability of microtubules, functions that are diminished by phosphorylation. Although the formation of Tau neurofibrillary tangles appears to be one of the causes of the neuronal degeneration in AD, mutations in the *TAU* gene are associated not with AD but with a related autosomal dominant disorder, frontotemporal dementia.

**The Amyloid Precursor Protein Gives Rise to the Beta-Amyloid Peptide.** The major features of the amyloid precursor protein ($\beta$APP) and its corresponding gene are summarized in Table 12–10. The protein, which has a single transmembrane domain, is subject to two distinct proteolytic catabolic fates. In its major catabolic pathway, a 40–42 amino acid domain of $\beta$APP, termed the A$\beta$ peptide, is cleaved by a cell surface protease $\alpha$-secretase (Fig. 12–24). This cleavage prevents the formation of the A$\beta$, because it digests the protein within the domain that gives rise to the peptide (Fig. 12–24). A second, minor pathway is involved in the cleavage of $\beta$APP at the N-terminus of the A$\beta$ peptide domain (by $\beta$-secretase) and at the C-terminus of the A$\beta$ peptide domain that lies within the transmembrane region of $\beta$APP (by $\gamma$-secretase). These two cleavage events generate a series of A$\beta$ peptides, 40–42 amino acids in length (A$\beta_{40-42}$), via the joint action of $\beta$-secretase and $\gamma$-secretase. The A$\beta_{42}$ peptide is considered to be the most neurotoxic, because it is the most fibrillogenic. Several of the mutations in the *βAPP* gene selectively increase the production of A$\beta_{42}$, and overproduction of the A$\beta$ peptide appears to be the central pathogenic event in the disease. Consistent with this model is the fact that patients with Down syndrome, with three copies of the *βAPP* gene (which is on chromosome 21), develop the neuropathology of AD by 40 years of age. Moreover, mutations in the AD genes presenilin 1 (*PS1*) and presenilin 2 (*PS2*) (see Table 12–10) also lead to increased production of A$\beta_{42}$.

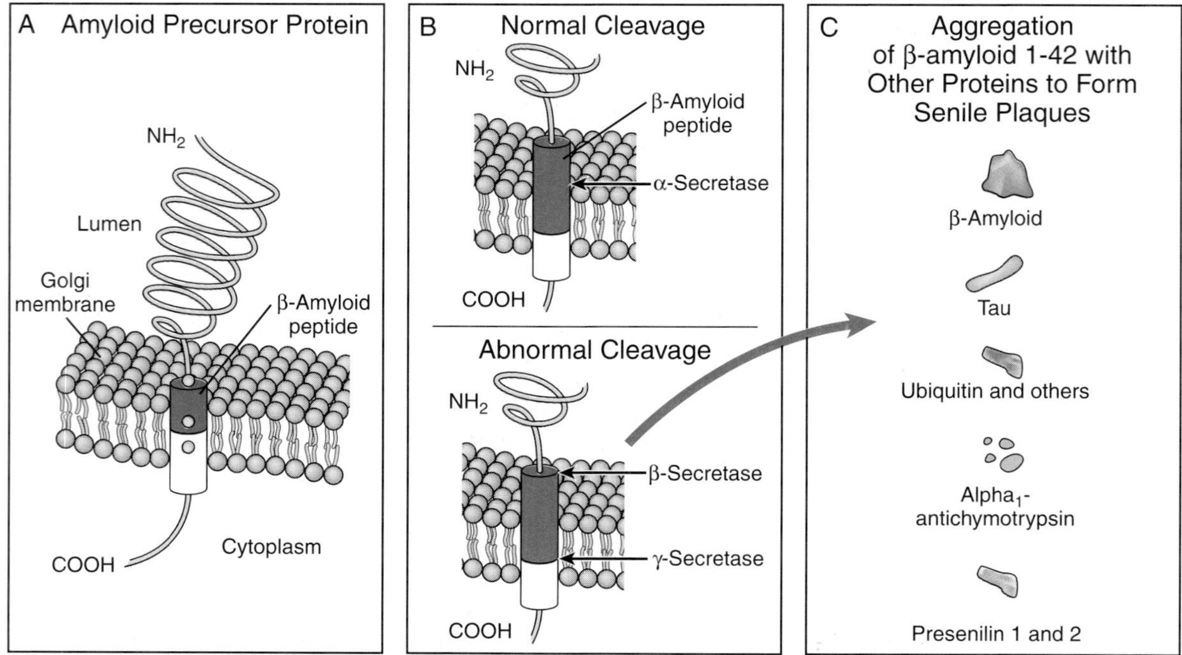


**Figure 12–24.** The topology of the amyloid precursor protein ($\beta$APP), its nonamyloidogenic cleavage by $\alpha$-secretase, and its alternative cleavage by putative $\beta$-secretase and $\gamma$-secretase to generate the amyloidogenic $\beta$ amyloid peptide (A$\beta$). (Reproduced, with permission from Martin JB [1999] Molecular basis of the neurodegenerative disorders. New Engl J Med 340:1970–1980. Copyright © 1999 Massachusetts Medical Society. All rights reserved.)

**The Presenilin 1 and 2 Genes.** The *PS1* and *PS2* genes (see Table 12–10) were identified by positional cloning strategies in families with FAD. The precise normal function of these proteins is unknown, but presenilin 1 is required for $\gamma$-secretase cleavage of $\beta$APP derivatives. Indeed, some evidence has suggested that presenilin 1 may be the $\gamma$-secretase itself. The *PS1* mutations associated with AD are likely to be gain-of-function mutations, a major effect being increased production of the A$\beta_{42}$ peptide. The presenilin 2 protein is 60 percent identical in sequence to presenilin 1, suggesting that the two polypeptides have related functions. A major difference between *PS1* and *PS2* mutations is that the age of onset with the latter is much more variable (*PS1*, 35 to 60 years; *PS2*, 40 to 85 years), and in one family, an asymptomatic octogenarian carrying a *PS2* mutation transmitted the disease to his offspring. The basis of this variation is unknown, but the only known modifier gene of the AD phenotype, the apolipoprotein E (*APOE*) gene (see Table 12–10 and later discussion), has been shown not to be responsible.

**The APOE Gene Is an Alzheimer Disease Susceptibility Locus.** The role of the *APOE* gene as a major susceptibility locus in AD was suggested by four independent lines of evidence: linkage analyses in late-onset families with an aggregation of AD, increased association of the $\varepsilon4$ allele in AD patients compared with controls, the discovery that the ApoE protein is a component of the AD amyloid plaques, and the finding that ApoE binds to the A$\beta$ peptide. The ApoE protein has three common allelic forms (Table 12–11). The $\varepsilon4$ allele is increased in frequency in patients with AD, and is associated with an early onset of AD. Moreover, the relationship between the $\varepsilon4$ allele and the disease is dose-dependent: two copies of $\varepsilon4$ are associated with an earlier age of onset (mean onset before 70 years) than one copy (mean onset after 70 years) (see Fig. 15–6). In contrast, the $\varepsilon2$ allele has a protective effect and, correspondingly, is more common in the general population (Table 12–11). The mechanisms underlying these effects are not known, but ApoE polymorphisms may influence the accumulation of A$\beta$ peptides in the brains of patients with AD. For example, mice without ApoE have a dramatic reduction in the deposition of A$\beta$ peptide generated from a $\beta$APP mutant allele associated with FAD.

## Triplet Repeat Disorders: Unstable, Dynamic Mutations

In all of the types of inheritance presented earlier (see Chapter 5), the responsible mutation is *stable* from generation to generation; that is, all affected members of a family share the identical inherited mutation. In contrast, an entirely new class of genetic disease has been recognized, diseases due to *unstable* **dynamic mutations** in a gene, of which the most common are the **triplet repeat disorders**. By

TABLE 12–10

**The Genes and Proteins Associated with Inherited Susceptibility to Alzheimer Disease**

| Gene | Features of Protein | Normal Function | Role in Familial Alzheimer Disease (FAD) | Chromosome Location | Percentage of FAD | Pattern of Inheritance |
|---|---|---|---|---|---|---|
| **Amyloid precursor protein (*βAPP*)** | A single transmembrane spanning protein, found in endosomes, lysosomes, ER, and Golgi<br>Normally, *βAPP* is cleaved endoproteolytically within the transmembrane domain, so that little of the β-amyloid peptide (Aβ) is formed | Unknown | β-amyloid peptide (Aβ) is the principal component of senile plaques. Increased Aβ production, especially of the $A\beta_{42}$ form, is a key pathogenic event.<br><10 FAD mutations known. They probably increase the production of $A\beta_{42}$. | 21 | <1% | AD |
| **Presenilin 1 (*PS1*)** | A 5–10 membrane spanning domain protein present in many cell types both inside and outside the brain. Located within intracellular membranes in the ER, Golgi, and other uncharacterized cytoplasmic vesicles. | Unknown, but required for γ-secretase cleavage of *βAPP*. Some evidence suggests it may be the γ-secretase. | May participate in the trafficking of *βAPP* and its derivative proteins.<br>More than 40 mutations in FAD. Most are probably gain-of-function, and increase $A\beta_{42}$ production. | 14q24.3 | 50% | AD |
| **Presenilin 2 (*PS2*)** | Structure similar to *PS1*. Maximum expression is outside brain. Similar to *PS1* in localization.<br>May have functions similar to *PS1*. | Unknown | Only two missense mutations identified. | 1q42.1 | <1% | AD |
| **Apolipoprotein E (*APOE*)** | A protein component of several plasma lipoproteins (e.g., VLDL)<br>The *APOE* mRNA is not transcribed in neurons; the protein is imported into the cytoplasm from the extracellular space. | Normal function in neurons unknown<br>Outside the brain, *APOE* participates in lipid transport between tissues and cells. Loss of function causes one form (type III) of hyperlipoproteinemia. | An Alzheimer disease susceptibility gene (see Table 12–11)<br>*APOE* is a component of senile plaques. | 19q13 | <<1% of rate | See Table 12–11 |

FAD = familial Alzheimer disease

Data derived from St George-Hyslop PH, Farrer LA, Goedert M (2001) Alzheimer's disease and the fronto-temporal dementias: Diseases with cerebral deposition of fibrillar proteins. *In* Scriver CR, Beaudet AL, Sly WS, Valle D (eds) The Metabolic and Molecular Bases of Inherited Disease, 8th ed. McGraw-Hill, New York; and Martin JB (1999) Molecular basis of the neurodegenerative disorders. New Engl J Med 340:1970–1980.

TABLE 12–11

**The Amino Acid Substitutions Underlying the Three Common ApoE Alleles**

| Allele | $\varepsilon 2$ | $\varepsilon 3$ | $\varepsilon 4$ |
|---|---|---|---|
| Residue 112 | Cys | Cys | Arg |
| Residue 158 | Cys | Arg | Arg |
| Frequency in Caucasian population | 10% | 75% | 15% |
| Frequency in Alzheimer disease patients | 2% | 58% | 40% |
| Effect on Alzheimer disease | Protective | None known | 30%–50% of the genetic risk of AD |

Data derived from St George-Hyslop PH, Farrer LA, Goedert M (2001) Alzheimer's disease and the fronto-temporal dementias: Disease with cerebral deposition of fibrillar proteins. *In* Scriver CR, Beaudet AL, Sly WS, Valle D (eds) The Metabolic and Molecular Bases of Inherited Disease, 8th ed. McGraw-Hill, New York, pp. 5875–5902.

definition, these conditions are characterized by the expansion, within the affected gene, of a segment of DNA that contains a repeat of three nucleotides (triplet repeats), such as CAGCAGCAG · · · CAG or CCGCCGCCG · · · CCG; as the gene is passed from generation to generation, the number of triplet repeats increases (undergoes **expansion**), leading to abnormalities in gene expression and function.

The recognition of the triplet repeat diseases began in 1991, with reports of unstable triplet repeat expansion both at the fragile X syndrome locus and in the androgen receptor gene in patients with the rare genetic disorder known as Kennedy disease (or spinobulbar muscular atrophy). Shortly thereafter, a similar genetic alteration was found to underlie myotonic dystrophy and Huntington disease, thereby demonstrating the existence of an entirely new mutational mechanism that, remarkably, had never been observed previously in any other genome.

More than a dozen diseases are known to result from triplet repeat expansions. Representative examples of these disorders are summarized in Table 12–12. All of these conditions are primarily neurological. The discovery of this unusual group of conditions has dispelled the orthodox notions of germline stability and provided a biological basis for such eccentric phenomena as anticipation and parental transmission bias.

**Common and Contrasting Features of the Triplet Repeat Disorders.** Although all triplet repeat disorders are caused by dynamic mutations of triplet repeats, there are also significant differences among the various disorders. A dominant inheritance pattern occurs in some, recessive inheritance in others. In general, the wild-type genes associated with these diseases are polymorphic, with variable but relatively low numbers of tandem (i.e., adjacent) repeat units. The degree of expansion of the repeat unit that causes disease is sometimes subtle (as in the rare disorder oculopharyngeal muscular dystrophy) and sometimes explosive (as in congenital myotonic dystrophy or severe fragile X syndrome) (Table 12–12).

Other differences include the base sequence of the repeat; the size of the repeat in normal, presymptomatic and fully affected individuals; the location of the repeat within genes; the pathogenesis of the disease; the degree to which the repeats are unstable during meiosis or mitosis; and parent-of-origin effects on repeat expansion. The four different diseases we review here illustrate the similarities and differences among the triplet repeat diseases described to date (Table 12–12). These four disorders are (1) Huntington disease (HD) (and other progressive neurodegenerative diseases such as spinobulbar muscular atrophy and autosomal dominant spinocerebellar ataxias) due to expansion of tracts of multiple glutamine residues (polyglutamine); (2) fragile X syndrome; (3) myotonic dystrophy; and (4) Friedreich ataxia.

**Slipped Mispairing Underlies Triplet Repeat Expansion.** The biochemical mechanism by which triplet repeat expansions are generated is likely to be the same for all of the triplet repeat diseases. The mechanism considered most likely is slipped mispairing, which was presented in Chapter 11 (see Fig. 11–8) as the explanation for many small deletions in regions of short repeat sequences. Insertions can also arise from slipped mispairing at the replication fork, mediated by direct repeats such as $(CAG)_n$. An insertion occurs when the newly synthesized strand dissociates from the primer strand during replication synthesis. The new strand may slip back to align with a repeat copy other than its cognate copy. Once DNA synthesis is resumed, the misaligned molecule will contain one or more extra copies of the repeat (depending on the number of repeat copies that were skipped over in the misalignment event).

TABLE 12–12

**Four Representative Examples of Triplet Repeat Diseases**

| Disease | Inheritance Pattern | Triplet Repeat | Gene Affected | Location in Gene | Mechanism of Disease | Repeat Number | | |
|---|---|---|---|---|---|---|---|---|
| | | | | | | *Normals* | *Unstable Intermediate* | *Affected* |
| Huntington disease | Autosomal dominant | CAG | huntingtin | coding region | ?toxic effect of glutamines | <36 | 29–35 usually unaffected | >35 |
| Fragile X | X-linked | CGG | *FMR1* | 5′ untranslated | causes excessive methylation leading to reduced *FMR1* expression | <60 | 60–200 usually unaffected | >200 |
| Myotonic dystrophy | Autosomal dominant | CTG | *DMPK* | 3′ untranslated | ?unclear | <30 | 50–80 usually mildly affected | 80–2000 |
| Friedreich ataxia | Autosomal recessive | AAG | frataxin | intron | interferes with RNA processing, leading to reduced frataxin expression | <34 | 36–100 (uninterrupted) | >100 |

### Polyglutamine Disorders

**Huntington Disease. HD** is a well-known disorder that illustrates many of the common genetic and biochemical features of the polyglutamine disorders. HD was first described by the physician George Huntington in 1872 in an American kindred of English descent. The neuropathology is dominated by degeneration of the striatum and the cortex. Patients first present clinically in midlife and manifest a characteristic phenotype of motor abnormalities (chorea, dystonia), personality changes, a gradual loss of cognition, and, ultimately, death.

HD is an autosomal dominant disorder. A loss of function of the mutant allele, causing haploinsufficiency, does not appear to underlie the dominant inheritance in HD, because heterozygous and homozygous patients carrying the mutation have identical phenotypes and because a deletion of one *HD* gene has no phenotype in humans. Rather, as discussed later, the mutant alleles appear to confer novel properties on the protein.

Although initially HD appeared to behave as a straightforward autosomal dominant condition, there were obvious peculiarities in its occurrence that could not be explained. The onset age of HD is variable; only about half the individuals who carry a mutant *HD* allele show symptoms by the age of 40 years. Very early onset disease, beginning during childhood or adolescence, does occur in some families, but only when the mutant gene is paternally inherited. The disease appears to develop at an earlier and earlier age when transmitted through the pedigree, a phenomenon referred to as **anticipation**, but only when transmitted by an affected father and not an affected mother.

The peculiarities of inheritance of HD are now readily explained by the discovery of the mutation: an expansion of a stretch of triplet repeats, CAG, the codon specifying the amino acid glutamine, in the coding region of a gene for a protein of unknown function called huntingtin. Normal individuals carry between 9 and 35 CAG repeats in their *HD* gene, with the average being 18 to 19. Individuals affected with HD have 40 or more repeats, with the average being around 46. A borderline repeat number of 36 to 39, although usually associated with HD, can be found in a few individuals who show no signs of the disease even at a fairly advanced age. Once an expansion increases to greater than 40, however, disease always occurs, and the larger the expansion, the earlier the onset of the disease (Fig. 12–25).

How then does an individual come to have an expanded CAG repeat in his or her *HD* gene (Fig. 12–26)? Most commonly, he or she inherits it as a straightforward autosomal dominant trait from an affected parent who already has an expanded repeat (>36). Unlike stable mutations, however, the size of the repeat may expand on transmission, resulting in earlier onset disease in later generations (thus explaining anticipation); on the other hand, repeat numbers in the 40 to 50 range may not result in disease until later in life, thereby explaining the age-dependent penetrance. In the pedigree shown in Figure 12–26, individual I-1, now deceased, was diagnosed with HD at age 64 and had an expansion of

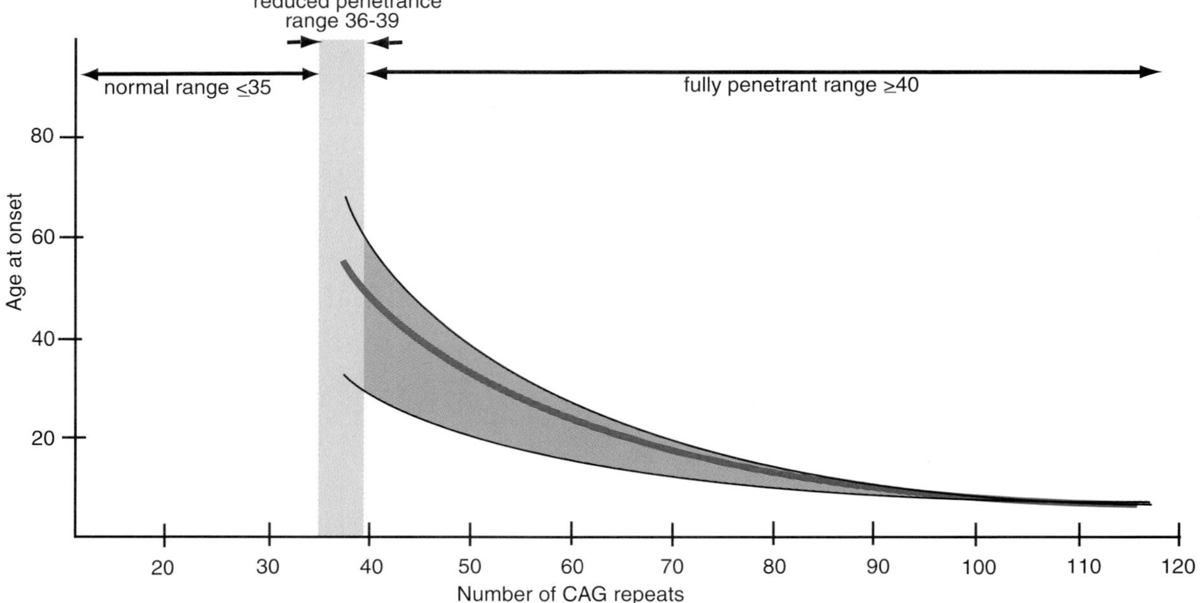


**Figure 12–25.** Graph correlating approximate age at onset of Huntington disease with the number of CAG repeats found in the *HD* gene. Solid line is the average age at onset, and the shaded area shows the range of age at onset for any given number of repeats. (Data courtesy of Dr. M. Macdonald, Massachusetts General Hospital, Boston, Massachusetts.)

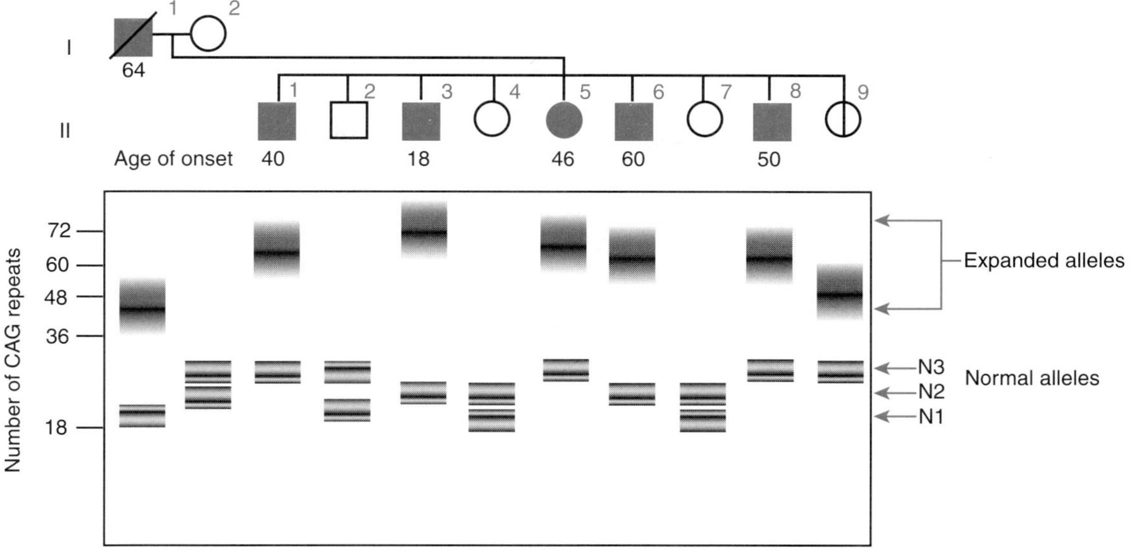


**Figure 12–26.** Pedigree of family with Huntington disease. Below is a schematic diagram of gel electrophoresis. Beneath each individual's symbol are the polymerase chain reaction (PCR) products containing the CAG repeat derived from the individual's two copies of the *HD* gene. Age at first symptoms is shown below each individual's pedigree symbol. Individual I-1 has an expanded repeat that undergoes further expansion when passed on to six of his children. Note that individual II-9 is an asymptomatic carrier of an expanded allele in whom the disease has not yet become penetrant. (The triple banding pattern of the normal alleles and the more diffuse appearance of the bands from expanded alleles result from technical difficulties in PCR amplifications of a triplet repeat as well as from somatic mosaicism in repeat length for the expanded alleles.)

46 CAG repeats. Six of his children inherited the expanded allele, and in five of them, the expansion increased over that found in individual I-1. Individual II-3, in particular, has the largest number of repeats and became symptomatic during adolescence. Individual II-9, in contrast, inherited an expanded allele but remains asymptomatic and will develop the disease sometime later in life.

Occasionally, unaffected individuals carry alleles with repeat lengths at the upper limit of the normal range (29 to 35 CAG repeats) that, however, can expand during meiosis to 40 or more repeats. CAG repeat alleles at the upper limits of normal that do not cause disease, but are capable of expanding into the disease-causing range, are known as **premutations**. Expansion in HD occurs most frequently during male gametogenesis, which is why the severe early-onset juvenile form of the disease, seen with the largest expansions (70 to 121 repeats), is always paternally inherited. Expanded repeats may continue to be unstable during mitosis in somatic cells, resulting in some degree of somatic mosaicism (see later) for the number of repeats in different tissues from the same patient.

The largest group of HD patients known lives in the region of Lake Maracaibo, Venezuela; these patients are descendants of a single individual who introduced the gene into the population early in the 19th century. About 100 living affected persons and another 900 each at 50 percent risk are currently known in the Lake Maracaibo community. High frequency of a disease in a local population descended from a small number of individuals, one of whom carried the gene responsible for the disease, is an example of founder effect (see Chapter 7).

**Ethical and Counseling Issues in Huntington Disease.** Because HD does not usually make its appearance until after the end of the reproductive years, it is likely to be passed on by persons who carry the mutant gene and who are unaware that they are at risk. The discovery first of genetically linked markers for HD (see Chapter 8) and then of the *HD* gene with a CAG expansion as the cause of the disease allows accurate molecular diagnosis based on DNA markers in asymptomatic individuals at risk. Because there is no treatment or cure for HD, however, and because the disease carries such a serious prognosis, there are major ethical implications associated with molecular analysis and genetic counseling for families with the disease. Does an asymptomatic at-risk individual have a duty to undergo testing and learn the result before reproducing? Is it ethical to allow asymptomatic children from families with HD to be tested? Serious psychological trauma, including severe depression and suicide, has resulted from asymptomatic at-risk individuals learning they carry an expanded repeat mutation. In view of these and related problems, approaches to presymptomatic testing in HD are being made with caution and with great concern for the family members who are found to be at risk.

**Spinobulbar Muscular Atrophy and Other Polyglutamine Disorders.** In addition to HD, other diseases are caused by CAG expansions encoding polyglutamine, such as X-linked recessive spinobulbar muscular atrophy (SBMA) and the various autosomal dominant spinocerebellar ataxias. These conditions differ in the gene involved, the normal range of the repeat, the threshold for clinical disease caused by expansion, and the regions of the brain affected; they all share with HD the fundamental characteristic that they result from instability of a stretch of repeated CAG nucleotides leading to expansion of a glutamine tract in a protein.

The normal function of the proteins that may contain expanded CAG repeats is largely unknown, with the exception of SBMA in which expansion occurs in the androgen hormone receptor gene. The example of SBMA is an important one for understanding the pathogenesis of polyglutamine disorders, because it was already known that complete loss of function of the androgen receptor does not lead to SBMA but, instead, causes androgen insensitivity, a defect in male genital development (see Chapter 10). Thus, loss of function of the various proteins with expanded polyglutamine tracts is unlikely to be the pathogenic mechanism in these disorders.

**Disease Pathogenesis due to $(CAG)_n$ Expansions.** It appears that the mutant proteins with expanded polyglutamine are novel property mutants (see Chapter 11), the expanded tract conferring features to the protein that damage specific populations of neurons and produce neurodegeneration by a unique toxic mechanism. Consequently, $(CAG)_n$ expansions are not believed to be pathogenic because of the elongation of the stretch of $(CAG)_n$ repeats in the corresponding gene or its RNA products per se.

The chain of events that leads from an expanded polyglutamine tract—which is present very early in life in the affected neurons—to death of the cells decades later is unknown and, indeed, is one of the most fascinating unsolved problems in human and medical genetics. Several important findings, however, have begun to provide insight into this problem. First, only a subset of neurons is affected, even though the mutant protein (e.g., huntingtin) is often expressed widely in the nervous system as well as in other tissues. This finding suggests that some characteristic(s) of the affected neuronal population makes it uniquely vulnerable to the toxic effects of the mutant protein.

Second, a number of histological abnormalities have been identified in the affected tissues (largely in mouse models of these diseases), but the most striking is the presence of nuclear inclusions in some of the expansion diseases. The inclusions contain, in addition to other proteins, the mutant polyglutamine-expanded protein and may reflect protein misfolding events. Dramatic as these inclusions are, however, it appears that their formation is not essential for neuronal death. In at least some $(CAG)_n$ expansion diseases, nuclear localization of the expanded protein is not required for the pathogenesis. Third, the expanded polyglutamine tract—and not the entire protein with the expanded tract—appears to be sufficient to cause neuronal death. Although a unifying model of neuronal death mediated by polyglutamine expansion is not at hand, it appears likely that the study of animal models of these disorders will provide critical insights in the coming decade. Such insights may well lead to therapies to prevent or reverse the pathogenesis of these slowly evolving disorders.

### Fragile X Syndrome

The **fragile X syndrome** (Fig. 12–27) is the most common heritable form of moderate mental retardation and is second only to Down syndrome among all causes of moderate mental retardation in males. The syndrome is so common that it requires consideration in the differential diagnosis of mental retardation in both males and females and is among the most frequent indications for DNA analysis, genetic counseling, and prenatal diagnosis. The name "fragile X syndrome" refers to a cytogenetic marker on the X chromosome at Xq27.3, a "fragile site" in which the chromatin fails to condense properly during mitosis (Fig. 12–28). The fragile X syndrome, which has a

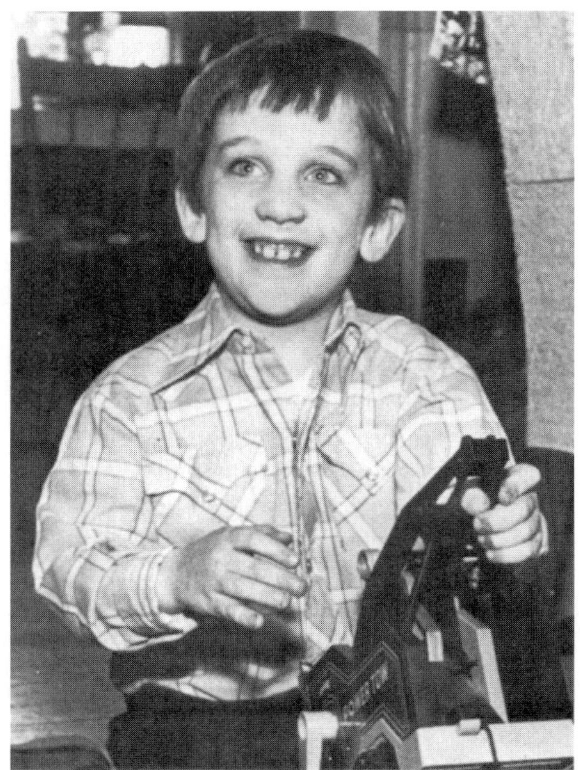

**Figure 12–27.** Characteristic facies of a patient with the fragile X syndrome. (Photograph courtesy of Michael Partington, Queen's University, Kingston, Ontario.)

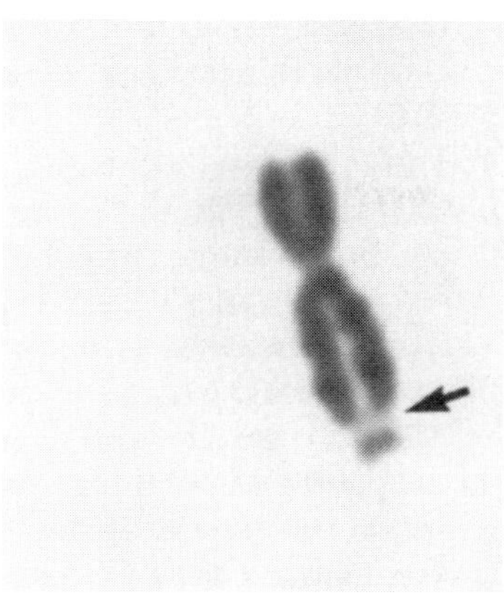

**Figure 12–28.** The fragile site at Xq27.3 associated with X-linked mental retardation.

frequency of at least 1 in 4000 male births, may account for much of the excess of males in the mentally retarded population.

Genetic analysis of the syndrome revealed some unexpected findings that were initially very puzzling but can now be explained by the discovery that the disorder is caused by a dynamic mutation, a massive expansion of another triplet repeat, CGG, located in the 5′ untranslated region of the first exon of a gene called *FMR1* (fragile X mental retardation 1). The normal number of repeats is up to 60, whereas as many as several thousand repeats are found in patients with the full fragile X syndrome. More than 200 copies of the repeat leads to excessive methylation of cytosines in the promoter of *FMR1*, a form of DNA modification that prevents normal promoter function and extinguishes expression of the gene. Massive expansion and methylation also appear to interfere with replication or chromatin condensation or both, producing the characteristic chromosomal fragile site. That loss of function of *FMR1* is the cause of fragile X syndrome is supported by finding a few rare patients with the syndrome in whom deletions or a missense mutation abolish *FMR1* expression or function.

A comparison of HD (and the other polyglutamine neurodegeneration diseases) with the fragile X syndrome reveals some similarities but also many differences. Although triplet repeat expansions are involved in both types of disease, the expansion in the polyglutamine diseases is in the coding region and ranges from 40 up to 120 copies of the CAG, whereas the repeat in fragile X syndrome is a CGG in the 5′ untranslated portion of a gene and expansions of 200 to many thousands are seen in patients affected with the disorder. Second, the polyglutamine neurodegeneration diseases and fragile X syndrome differ in that fragile X syndrome is due to loss of function of a gene and not toxicity of an abnormal protein. Third, asymptomatic individuals carrying premutation expansions and the phenomenon of anticipation are seen in both diseases; however, the number of repeats in premutation alleles of *FMR1* ranges from 60 to 200 copies, much greater than in HD, and the expansion of premutation alleles occurs in the *female*, and not the male, germline. Finally, the degree of mitotic instability in fragile X syndrome is far greater than that seen in HD and results in much greater variability in the numbers of repeats found among cells of the same tissue and between different somatic tissues in a single individual.

### Myotonic Dystrophy

A third triplet repeat expansion disease is **myotonic dystrophy**, an autosomal dominant myopathy characterized by myotonia, muscular dystrophy, cataracts, hypogonadism, frontal balding, and changes in the electroencephalogram. The disease is notorious for lack of penetrance and its variable expression in both clinical severity and age of onset (Fig. 12–29). One form of myotonic dystrophy, the congenital form, is particularly severe and may be life threatening as well as a cause of mental retardation. Virtually every child with the congenital form is the offspring of an affected mother, who herself may have only a mild expression of the disease and may not even know that she is affected. Thus, pedigrees of myotonic dystrophy, like those of HD and fragile X syndrome, show clear evidence of anticipation.

Some, but not all, of the puzzling features of the inheritance of myotonic dystrophy can be explained by the discovery that the disease is associated with amplification of the triplet repeat CTG in the 3′ untranslated region of a protein kinase gene (*DMPK*) on chromosome 19. The normal range for repeats in *DMPK* is from 5 to 30; mildly affected individuals have from 50 to 80 copies, and severely affected individuals have more than 2000 copies. Either parent can transmit an amplified copy, but males can pass on up to 1000 copies of repeat, whereas really massive expansions containing many thousands of repeats occur only in female gametogenesis. Because congenital myotonic dystrophy is due to huge expansions in the many thousands, this form of myotonic dystrophy is therefore almost always maternal in origin. Whether expansion of the CAG in the *DMPK* gene causes disease by interfering with expression of *DMPK* itself, or of other neighboring genes, or both, is not known.

### Friedreich Ataxia

**Friedreich ataxia**, a spinocerebellar ataxia, constitutes a fourth category of triplet repeat disease (see Table 12–12). The disease is autosomal recessive, in contrast to HD, myotonic dystrophy, and fragile

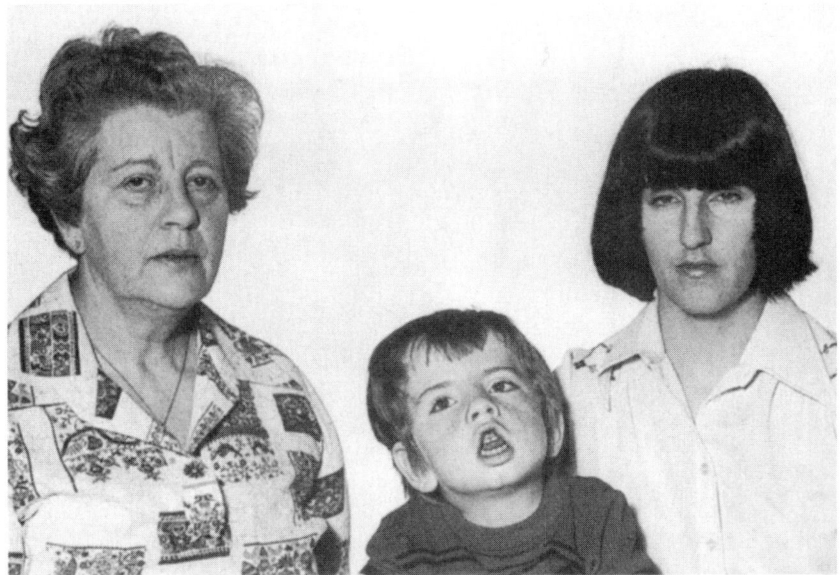

**Figure 12–29.** Myotonic dystrophy, an autosomal dominant condition with variable expression in clinical severity and age at onset. The grandmother in this family (*left*) has had bilateral cataracts but has no facial weakness or muscle symptoms; her daughter was thought to be unaffected until after the birth of her severely affected child, but she now has moderate facial weakness and ptosis, with myotonia, and has had cataract extraction. The child has congenital myotonic dystrophy. (From Harper PS [1989] Myotonic Dystrophy, 2nd ed. WB Saunders, Philadelphia, p. 18.)

X syndrome. The disorder is usually manifested before adolescence and is generally characterized by incoordination of limb movements, difficulty with speech, diminished or absent tendon reflexes, impairment of position and vibratory senses, scoliosis, and foot deformities. In most cases, Friedreich ataxia is caused by amplification of still another triplet repeat, AAG, located this time in an intron of a gene that encodes a mitochondrial protein called frataxin, involved in iron metabolism. In normal individuals, the repeat length varies from 7 to 34 copies, whereas repeat expansions in the patients are typically between 100 and 1200 copies. Expansion within the intron interferes with normal expression of the frataxin gene; because Friedreich ataxia is recessive, loss of expression from both alleles is required to produce the disease. In fact, a few patients are known to be compound heterozygotes in whom one allele is the common amplified intronic AAG repeat mutation and the other a nucleotide mutation.

## Diseases of Mitochondrial DNA and Maternal Inheritance

**The mtDNA Molecule.** As described in Chapter 3, not all the RNA and protein synthesized in a cell are encoded in the DNA of the nucleus; a small but important fraction is encoded by genes within the mitochondrial genome. This genome, whose complete sequence was reported in 1981, is approximately 16.5 kb in size (Fig. 12–30). Mitochondrial DNA (mtDNA) is packaged into a circular chromosome located inside the mitochondrial organelle, not in the nucleus. The compact mtDNA molecule contains 37 genes. The genes encode two types of ribosomal RNA, 22 transfer RNAs, and 13 polypeptides that are subunits of enzymes of oxidative phosphorylation (OXPHOS). The other 74 polypeptides of the OXPHOS complex are encoded by the nuclear genome. Thus, diseases of OXPHOS may be due either to mutations in the mtDNA genome or to mutations in the nuclear genes that encode OXPHOS components. Most cells contain at least 1000 mtDNA molecules, distributed among hundreds of individual mitochondria. A remarkable exception is the mature oocyte, which has more than 100,000 copies of mtDNA, comprising about one third of the total DNA content of these cells.

**Oxidative Phosphorylation Functions and mtDNA Diseases.** The OXPHOS complex is central to three of the major functions of mitochondria. Alteration of these activities, due to mtDNA mutations, is likely to underlie the cell dysfunction and cell death that occurs in mtDNA diseases. The primary function of OXPHOS is the production of much of the energy of the cell; decreased formation of ATP characterizes many diseases of mtDNA. A second OXPHOS function is the generation of reactive oxygen species as a byproduct of OXPHOS; increased production of these species is increased in some defects of OXPHOS, a factor that also contributes to cell death. Third, mitochondria integrate many signals that initiate apoptosis; this process uses some OXPHOS polypeptides, and mtDNA mutations may increase the predilection to apoptosis. The mitochondrial myopathy often associ-

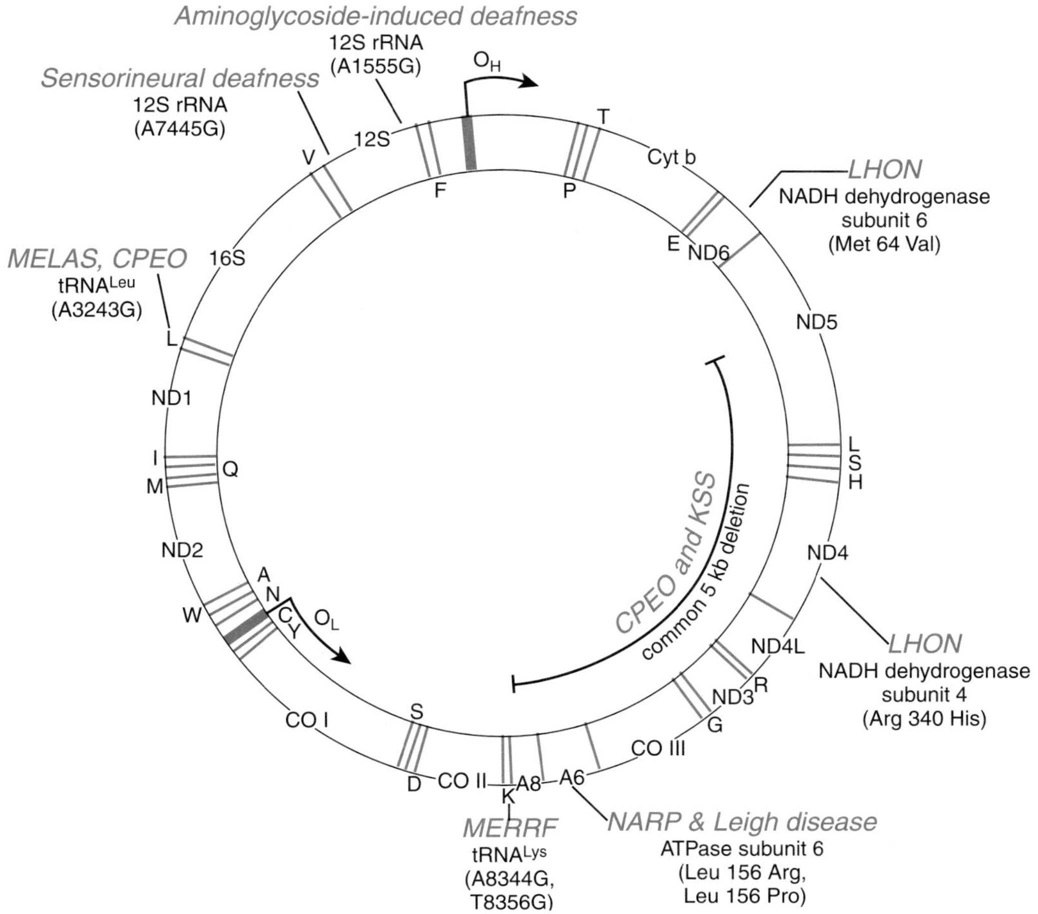


**Figure 12–30.** The human mitochondrial DNA molecule, showing the location of genes encoding 22 tRNAs, two rRNAs, and 13 proteins of the oxidative phosphorylation (OXPHOS) complex. Some of the most common disease-causing substitutions and deletions in the mtDNA genome are also illustrated. $O_H$ and $O_L$ are the origins of replication of the two DNA strands, respectively; 12S = 12S ribosomal RNA; 16S = 16S ribosomal RNA. The tRNAs are indicated by the single letter code for their corresponding amino acids (e.g., L for leucine, K for lysine, and so on). The 13 OXPHOS polypeptides encoded by mtDNA include components of *Complex I*: NADH dehydrogenase (ND1, ND2, ND3, ND4, ND4L, ND5, and ND6); *Complex III*: cytochrome *b* (Cyt *b*); *Complex IV*: cytochrome *c* oxidase I or Cyt *c* (COI, COII, COIII); and *Complex V*: ATPase 6 (ATP-6, ATP-8). The disease abbreviations used in this figure (e.g., MELAS, MERRF) are explained in Table 12–13. (Adapted in part from Shoffner JM, Wallace DC [1995] Oxidative phosphorylation disease. *In* Scriver CR, Beaudet AL, Sly WS, Valle D [eds] The Metabolic and Molecular Bases of Inherited Disease, 7th ed. McGraw-Hill, New York. The concept of illustrating the mutations on the mtDNA molecule arose from Johns DR [1995] Mitochondrial DNA and disease. New Engl J Med 333:638–644.)

ated with mtDNA mutations is characterized by so-called ragged red fibers—a histological phenotype due to the degeneration of muscle fibers and the proliferation of abnormal muscle mitochondria.

### The Genetics of mtDNA Diseases

The first pathogenic mutations in mtDNA were identified in the early 1990s. Unexpected and still unexplained is the fact that the mtDNA genome mutates at a rate about 10-fold greater than does nuclear DNA. The range of clinical disease resulting from mtDNA mutations is diverse (Fig. 12–31), although neuromuscular disease predominates. More than 100 different rearrangements and 50 different point mutations that are disease-related have been identified in mtDNA. Representative mutations and the diseases associated with them are presented in Figure 12–30 and Table 12–13. Three types of mutation have been identified in mtDNA: (1) missense mutations in the coding regions of genes that alter the activity of an OXPHOS protein; (2) point mutations in tRNA or rRNA genes that impair mitochondrial protein synthesis; and (3) rearrangements that generate deletions or duplications of the mtDNA molecule.

As pointed out in Chapter 5, some pedigrees of inherited diseases that could not be explained by typical mendelian inheritance of nuclear genes are now known to be caused by mutations in mtDNA and to manifest maternal inheritance. Disorders caused by mutations in mtDNA demonstrate a number of unusual features that result from the unique characteristics of mitochondrial biology and function.

TABLE 12–13

**Representative Examples of Disorders due to Mutations in Mitochondrial DNA and Their Inheritance**

| Disease | Phenotype | Most Frequent Mutation in mtDNA Molecule | Homoplasmy versus Heteroplasmy | Inheritance |
|---|---|---|---|---|
| Leber's hereditary optic neuropathy | Rapid optic nerve death, leading to blindness in young adult life | Substitution Arg340His in *ND*1 gene of complex I of electron transport chain; other complex I missense mutations | Homoplasmic (usually) | Maternal |
| NARP, Leigh disease | Neuropathy, ataxia, retinitis pigmentosa, developmental delay, mental retardation, lactic acidemia | Point mutations in ATPase subunit 6 gene | Heteroplasmic | Maternal |
| MELAS | Mitochondrial encephalomyopathy, lactic acidosis, and strokelike episodes; may manifest only as diabetes mellitus | Point mutation in $tRNA^{leu}$ | Heteroplasmic | Maternal |
| MERRF | Myoclonic epilepsy, ragged red fibers in muscle, ataxia, sensorineural deafness | Point mutation in $tRNA^{Lys}$ | Heteroplasmic | Maternal |
| Deafness | Progressive sensorineural deafness, often induced by aminoglycoside antibiotics | A1555G mutation in 12S rRNA | Homoplasmic | Maternal |
| | Nonsyndromic sensorineural deafness | A7445G mutation in 12S rRNA | Homoplasmic | Maternal |
| Chronic progressive external ophthalmoplegia (CPEO) | Progressive weakness of extraocular muscles | The common MELAS point mutation in $tRNA^{Lys}$; large deletions similar to KSS | Heteroplasmic | Maternal if point mutations |
| Pearson syndrome | Pancreatic insufficiency, pancytopenia, lactic acidosis | Large deletions | Heteroplasmic | Sporadic, somatic mutations |
| Kearns-Sayre syndrome (KSS) | PEO of early onset with heart-block, retinal pigmentation | The 5 kb large deletion | Heteroplasmic | Sporadic, somatic mutations |

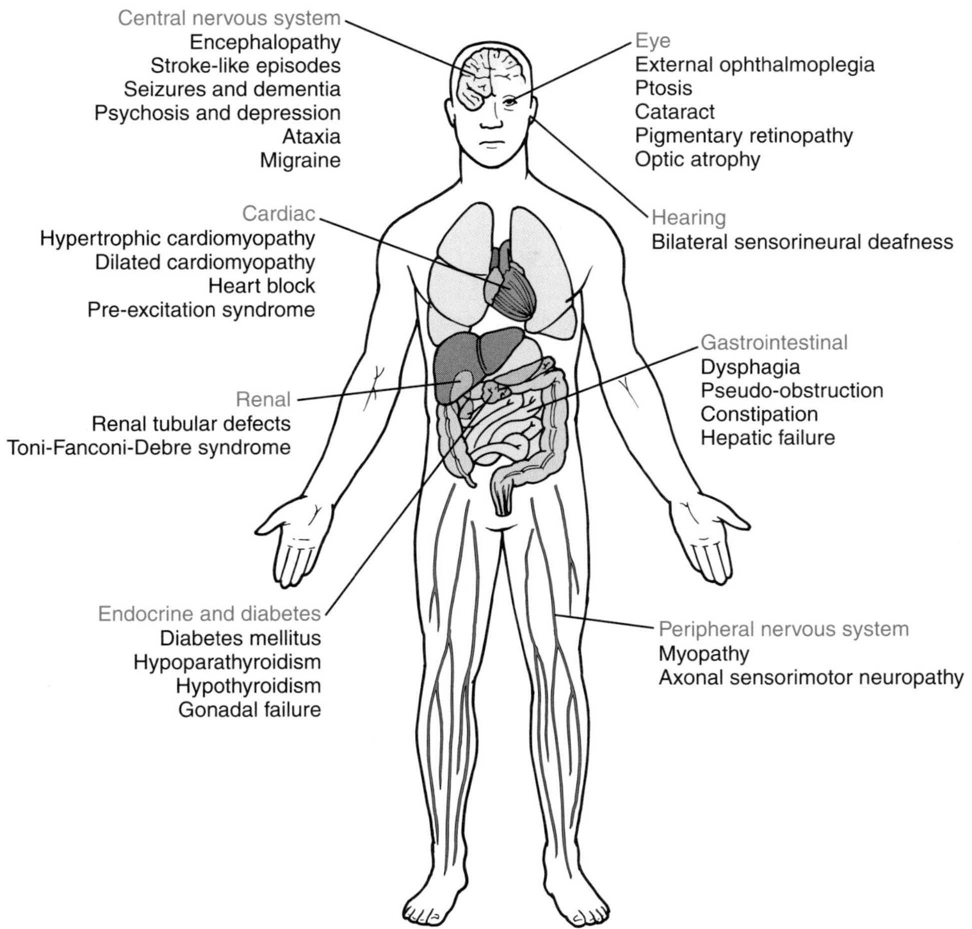


**Figure 12–31.** The range of affected tissues and clinical phenotypes associated with mutations in mtDNA. (Modified from Chinnery PF, Turnbull DM [1999] Mitochondrial DNA and disease. Lancet 354:SI17–SI21.)

### Maternal Inheritance of mtDNA

One defining characteristic of the genetics of mtDNA, compared with the nuclear genome, is its **maternal inheritance**. In contrast to the abundance of mitochondria in each ovum, sperm contain few mitochondria, and even those few do not persist in the offspring. A child, therefore, inherits all his or her mtDNA from the mother and none from the father. Her daughters transmit the mtDNA in their turn, but her sons do not. Thus, all the children of a *female* with a mutation in mtDNA inherit the mutation, whereas none of the offspring of a *male* carrying the same mutation will inherit the defective DNA. An example of a pedigree manifesting maternal inheritance of an mtDNA mutation causing **Leber's hereditary optic neuropathy** (LHON) is shown in Figure 12–32.

### Homoplasmy and Heteroplasmy

A second unique feature of the genetics of mtDNA arises from the fact that most cells contain, as mentioned earlier, more than 1000 mtDNA molecules. When a mutation arises in the mtDNA, it is at first present in only one of the mtDNA molecules in a mitochondrion. When the mitochondrion divides by simple fission, each mtDNA molecule replicates within the mitochondrion. The mtDNA molecules sort randomly among the new organelles, and the mitochondria distribute themselves randomly between the two daughter cells. Thus, when a cell containing a mixture of normal and mutant mtDNAs divides, its daughter cells may, by chance, receive mitochondria that contain only a pure population of normal mtDNA or a pure population of mutant mtDNA (a situation known as **homoplasmy**). Alternatively, the daughter cell may receive a mixture of mitochondria, some with and some without mutation (**heteroplasmy**) (Fig. 12–33). Because the phenotypic expression of a mutation in mtDNA depends on the relative proportions of normal and mutant mtDNA in the cells making up different tissues, reduced penetrance, variable expression, and pleiotropy are all typical features of pedigrees of mitochondrial disorders.

Heteroplasmy is associated with three additional features of mtDNA genetics that are of medical significance. First, deleted mtDNA molecules, a common class of mtDNA mutation that is discussed later,

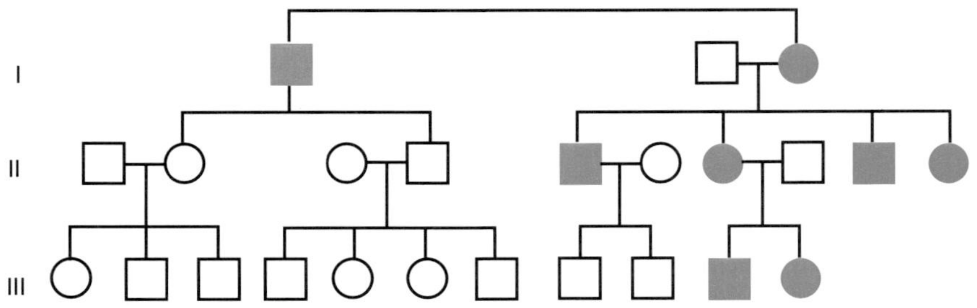


Figure 12–32. Pedigree of Leber's hereditary optic neuropathy, a disorder caused by a defect in mitochondrial DNA. Inheritance is only through the maternal lineage, in agreement with the known maternal inheritance of mitochondrial DNA. No affected male transmits the disease.

are generally not transmitted from clinically affected mothers to their children (the reasons for this exclusion are not clear). On the other hand, female carriers of heteroplasmic mtDNA point mutations, or of mtDNA duplications, usually transmit some mutant mtDNAs to their offspring. Second, the number of mtDNA molecules within each oocyte is reduced before being subsequently amplified to the huge total seen in mature oocytes. This restriction and subsequent amplification of mtDNA during oogenesis is termed the **mitochondrial "genetic bottleneck."** Consequently, the variability in the percentage of mutant mtDNA molecules seen in the offspring of a mother carrying a mtDNA mutation arises, at least in part, from the sampling of only a subset of the mtDNAs during oogenesis. Third, despite the variability in the degree of heteroplasmy arising from the bottleneck, mothers with a high proportion of mutant mtDNA molecules are more likely to have clinically affected offspring than are mothers with a lower proportion.

**Interaction between the Mitochondrial and Nuclear Genomes.** Because both the nuclear and mitochondrial genomes contribute polypeptides to OXPHOS, it is not surprising that the phenotypes associated with mutations in the nuclear genes are often indistinguishable from those due to mtDNA mutations. Genetic evidence has demonstrated, however, that a more direct relationship exists between the nuclear and mtDNA genomes. The first indication of this interaction was provided by the identification of the syndrome of **autosomally transmitted deletions in mtDNA**, whose phenotype resembles chronic progressive external ophthalmoplegia (CPEO) (see Table 12–13). More than one autosomal gene may be required for the integrity of normal mtDNA, because both autosomal dominant as well as

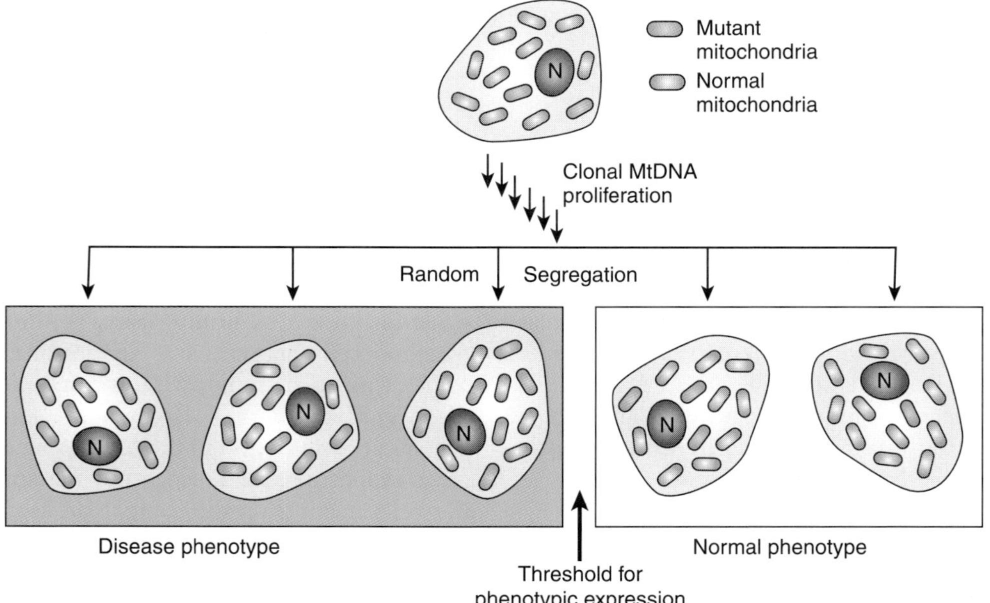


Figure 12–33. Replicative segregation of a heteroplasmic mitochondrial mutation. Random partitioning of mutant and wildtype mitochondria through multiple rounds of mitosis produces a collection of daughter cells with wide variation in the proportion of mutant and wildtype mitochondria carried by each cell. Cell and tissue dysfunction results when the fraction of mitochondria that are carrying a mutation exceeds a threshold level.

autosomal recessive forms of this syndrome have been recognized. A second rare autosomal disease has demonstrated that at least one nuclear gene regulates the abundance of mtDNA molecules. This disorder, called **mtDNA depletion syndrome**, is characterized by a quantitative reduction in the number of copies of mtDNA in various tissues. The clinical phenotype includes myopathy as well as other characteristic features also found in mtDNA diseases.

### Phenotype in Mitochondrial Disorders

Mitochondrial mutations generally affect those tissues that need intact oxidative phosphorylation to satisfy high demands for metabolic energy. Thus, mitochondrial diseases frequently involve the neuromuscular system and produce encephalopathy, myopathy, ataxia, retinal degeneration, and loss of function of the external ocular muscles. The spectrum of mitochondrial disease is very broad, however, and, as illustrated in Figure 12–31, may include liver dysfunction, bone marrow failure, pancreatic islet cell deficiency and diabetes, and deafness, as well as other disorders.

The degree and distribution of heteroplasmy contribute significantly to the pleiotropy and variable expressivity seen with mutations in mtDNA (see Fig. 12–33 and Table 12–13). For example, in a single kindred, one mutant mtDNA population can be associated with diabetes and deafness in one individual and severe encephalopathy with seizures in another. A similar illustration is provided by what appears to be the most common mtDNA mutation (its frequency in the Finnish population is 1/7000 individuals), the A3243G mutation in the $tRNA^{leu}$ gene (the nomenclature refers to the normal nucleotide at position 3243 in the mtDNA molecule, followed by the substituted nucleotide). This mutation is usually associated with the phenotype called MELAS (see Fig. 12–30 and Table 12–13), an acronym for *m*itochondrial *e*ncephalomyopathy with *l*actic *a*cidosis and *s*trokelike episodes. In some families, however, this mutation predominantly causes diabetes and deafness, others have CPEO (see Table 12–13), and yet others present with cardiomyopathy. In addition, between 0.5 to 1.5 percent of diabetes mellitus in the general population has been attributed to the A3243G substitution.

In some mtDNA diseases, such as **myoclonic epilepsy with ragged red fibers** (see Table 12–13), heteroplasmy is common. Maternal inheritance occurs, but now there is added complexity in the inheritance pattern and phenotype because each child will inherit varying numbers of mitochondria carrying the mutation. Finally, heteroplasmy is the rule in the Kearns-Sayre syndrome and Pearson syndrome (see Table 12–13). These disorders occur as sporadic cases in the family, and there is no maternal inheritance of the disorder because every patient represents a new mutation in mitochondrial DNA.

**mtDNA Diseases Are Multifactorial.** Although heteroplasmy is a major source of phenotypic variability in mtDNA diseases, additional factors must also play a role. Strong evidence for the existence of such factors is provided by families carrying mutations associated with LHON, a condition in which the mutations are generally homoplasmic. LHON is expressed phenotypically as rapid, bilateral loss of central vision due to optic nerve death in young adults. Affected individuals may be male or female, but there is a striking and unexplained increase in the penetrance of the disease in males: 80 to 90 percent of carrier males in Caucasian pedigrees develop visual loss, but only 8 to 32 percent of females are affected. The facts that LHON mutations are rarely associated with any phenotype outside eye, as well as the variable sex-influenced penetrance, provide direct evidence that LHON is multifactorial in origin. Furthermore, both alcohol and tobacco use are important ecogenetic factors associated with increased probability of blindness in carriers of LHON mutations.

## PHARMACOGENETIC DISEASES

The overall incidence of adverse drug reactions, at least in American hospitals, is about 6.7 percent; fatal adverse drug reactions occur with an incidence of about 0.3 percent. These unanticipated reactions to medications are largely, if not entirely, genetically determined. **Pharmacogenetics** is the special area of biochemical genetics that deals with the variability in response to drugs that is due to genetic variation. In its narrowest sense, pharmacogenetics can be restricted to those genetic variations that alter the ability of the body to absorb, transport, metabolize, or excrete drugs or their metabolites. In broader and more useful terms, pharmacogenetics encompasses any genetically determined variation in response to drugs. This type of variation includes, for instance, the effect of barbiturates in precipitating clinical disease in persons with acute intermittent porphyria (see later), as well as the effect of alcohol use by pregnant women on the incidence of fetal alcohol syndrome. Five examples of important pharmacogenetic variations are described briefly in this section.

The origin of polymorphisms for drug response and the mechanisms by which they are maintained pose an interesting problem. They obviously have not developed in response to drugs, because they antedate the drugs concerned. The handling of and the response to drugs require many specific biochemical reactions, and the enzymes involved may participate in the metabolism of ordinary food substances. It has been suggested that these polymorphisms arose as the result of different dietary selective pressures in different populations. This view is supported by the geographical distribution of many of these alleles.

Recognizing that there is normal variation in response to drugs, pharmacologists define the "potency" of a drug by the dose that produces a given effect in 50 percent of the population. For genetic traits, continuous variation is usually best explained on the basis of multifactorial inheritance or by a combination of genetic and environmental factors, as discussed in Chapter 15. But response to drugs can also show discontinuous variation, with sharp distinctions between different degrees of response. The finding of a bimodal or trimodal population distribution of activity of a drug-metabolizing enzyme may indicate that the enzyme is encoded by alleles at a single polymorphic locus.

## Genetic Problems in Anesthesia

### Malignant Hyperthermia

Malignant hyperthermia is an autosomal dominant condition in which there may be a dramatic adverse response to the administration of all commonly used inhalational anesthetics (e.g., halothane) and muscle relaxants such as succinylcholine chloride, with development of a very high temperature, sustained muscle contraction, and attendant hypercatabolism. The condition is an important if not a common cause of death in anesthesia, with an incidence that is higher in children (1 in 12,000) than in adults (1 in 100,000). Interestingly, males with malignant hyperthermia outnumber females 2.5 to 1, a difference that is likely to have a hormonal basis.

The fundamental physiological abnormality in the disease is an elevation of the level of ionized calcium in the sarcoplasm of muscle. This increase leads to muscle rigidity, elevation of body temperature, and other abnormalities. Most cases of malignant hyperthermia are associated with mutations in a gene called *RYR1*, encoding the calcium ion release channel. The *RYR1* gene maps to chromosome 19; linkage analysis indicates that mutations in *RYR1* account for only about 50 percent of cases, and, to date, mutations in this gene have been found in 40 percent of families with malignant hyperthermia. Several other loci for malignant hyperthermia loci have now been identified, and in one case, a mutation has been found in the *CACNL1A3* gene, which encodes the $\alpha$-1 subunit of the dihydropyridine receptor.

The need for special precautions when at-risk persons require anesthesia is obvious. Dantrolene sodium is effective in preventing or reducing the severity of the response if an unsuspected attack occurs, and alternative anesthetics can be given to patients at risk.

### Serum Cholinesterase and Succinylcholine Sensitivity

Serum cholinesterase is an enzyme of human plasma that has the property of hydrolyzing choline esters, such as acetylcholine. The normal function of this enzyme is obscure, but its complete absence is fully compatible with normal health; hence, it cannot play a major physiological role. A widely used muscle relaxant, succinylcholine (which is used as an adjunct to general anesthesia), is composed of two molecules of acetylcholine and is normally hydrolyzed by cholinesterase, a process that thereby reduces the amount of succinylcholine that reaches the motor end plates; this hydrolysis is accounted for in the dose given to the average patient. However, at least in European populations, about 1 in 3300 persons is homozygous for an atypical cholinesterase allele. Being unable to degrade succinylcholine at the normal rate, homozygotes respond abnormally to its administration with prolonged apnea (lasting from 1 to several hours) and require artificial respiratory support.

**Genetics.** The gene altered in succinylcholine sensitivity is butyrylcholinesterase (*BCHE*), located on chromosome 3. The major determinants of cholinesterase activity in the plasma are two codominant alleles of the *BCHE* gene, known as the "usual" (*U*) and "atypical" (*A*) alleles; the atypical allele is the result of a missense mutation (Asp70Gly). Another missense substitution allele, the *K* variant, is also common, but *K/K* homozygotes have no increase in succinylcholine sensitivity. Genetic compounds of the *A* and *K* alleles, on the other hand, are sometimes sensitive and sometimes not, but the factors responsible for this variation are unclear. Cholinesterase deficiency is usually due to homozygosity for the atypical allele; the enzyme produced by homozygotes is qualitatively altered and has lower activity than the usual type. Other rare variants of *BCHE* that confer succinylcholine sensitivity have also been identified.

The identification of the specific substitutions that are present in the cholinesterase alleles allows accurate genotyping of patients, determination of the clinical significance of the *K* variant, and improved pedigree analysis and genetic counseling.

## Other Important Pharmacogenetic Diseases

### THE ACETYLATION POLYMORPHISM

This important pharmacogenetic polymorphism was first discovered during the treatment of tuberculosis with the drug isoniazid, when a high incidence of peripheral neuropathy was observed. After a test dose, the rate of disappearance of isoniazid from plasma shows a bimodal distribution in the population, allowing the identification of individuals as rapid or slow acetylators (inactivators of the drug). It is now clear that the slow and rapid inactivation phenotypes are primarily due to allelic differences in an *N*-acetyltransferase gene, *NAT2*, which maps to chromosome 8. Three major slow-acetylator alleles have been described, along with a large number of rare *NAT2* alleles. Slow acetylators have a substantial decrease in the quantity of *N*-acetyltransferase in the liver and are homozygous for recessive alleles at this locus. Rapid inactivators are normal homozygotes or heterozygotes. A second *N*-acetyltransferase gene, *NAT1*, has also been identified on chromosome 8. Only a single slow-acetylator polymorphism has been identified in this gene, however. The frequencies of the slow-acetylator alleles have marked ethnic differences: for example, a minority (5 to 20 percent) of Asians have the slow-acetylation phenotype, whereas 50 percent of African Americans and up to 65 percent of Caucasians are slow-acetylator homozygotes. In some Mediterranean populations, the frequency of slow acetylators is greater than 90 percent.

**Significance.** In addition to its effect on isoniazid inactivation, the acetylation phenotype affects the disposition of a wide variety of other drugs and xenobiotics. For example, rapid acetylators not only have a higher failure rate with weekly isoniazid therapy for tuberculosis but also require larger doses of hydralazine to control hypertension and of dapsone to treat leprosy and other infections. Conversely, slow acetylators are at increased risk of developing a drug-induced systemic lupus erythematosus–like syndrome while receiving hydralazine, hematological adverse drug reactions after isoniazid treatment, and sulfonamide-induced idiosyncratic adverse responses. In addition, slow acetylators exposed to carcinogenic arylamines (e.g., benzidine) have an increased incidence of bladder cancer and, in postmenopausal female smokers, of breast cancer.

### ACUTE INTERMITTENT PORPHYRIA: DRUG-RELATED ALTERATIONS IN THE REGULATION OF GENE EXPRESSION

**Acute intermittent porphyria** is an autosomal dominant disease associated with intermittent neurological dysfunction. The clinical episodes are initiated by a large number of medications, steroid hormones, and starvation. As we will describe, altered regulation of the genes that control the synthesis of heme is responsible for the pathophysiology.

The primary defect in acute intermittent porphyria is a deficiency of porphobilinogen (PBG) deaminase, an enzyme in the biosynthetic pathway of heme (Fig. 12–34). All patients with acute intermittent porphyria, whether their disease is clinically latent (and it remains latent throughout their lifetime in the great majority of patients, about 90 percent) or clinically expressed (about 10 percent), have an approximately 50 percent reduction in the enzymatic activity of PBG deaminase. This reduction is consistent with the autosomal dominant inheritance.

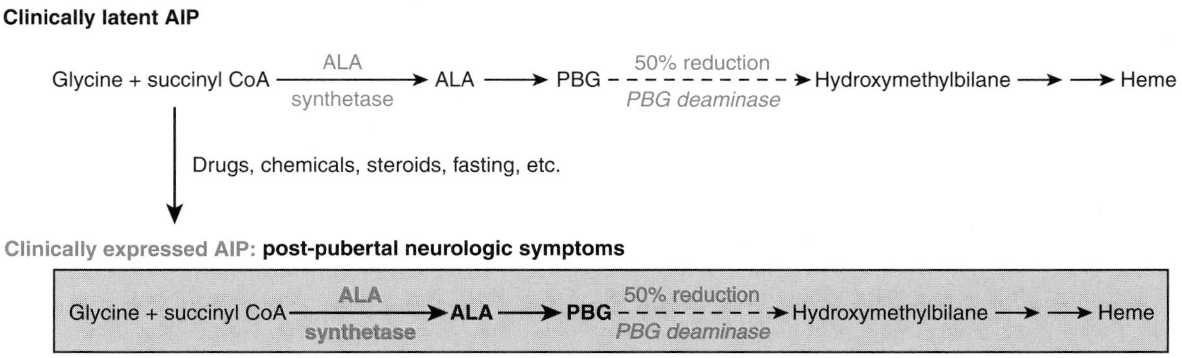

Figure 12–34. The pathogenesis of acute intermittent porphyria (AIP). Patients with AIP who are either clinically latent or clinically affected have about half the control levels of porphobilinogen (PBG) deaminase. When the activity of hepatic δ-aminolevulinic acid (ALA) synthase is increased in carriers by exposure to inducing agents (e.g., drugs, chemicals), the synthesis of ALA and PBG is increased. The residual PBG deaminase activity (approximately 50 percent of controls) is overloaded, and the accumulation of ALA and PBG causes clinical disease. (Redrawn from Kappas A, Sassa S, Galbraith RA, Nordmann Y [1989] The porphyrias. *In* Scriver CR, Beaudet AL, Sly WS, Valle D [eds] The Metabolic Bases of Inherited Disease, 6th ed. McGraw-Hill, New York, pp. 1305–1365.)

Clinical expression of the disease occurs in response to events that decrease the concentration of heme in the liver cell. The drugs that are unsafe for patients include, for example, barbiturates, some steroid hormones, and numerous other chemicals. Exposure to these compounds increases the synthesis of hepatic cytochromes P450, a class of heme-containing proteins. As a result, the cellular level of heme falls, reducing the feedback inhibition of heme on δ-aminolevulinic acid synthase, the rate-limiting step in the heme synthesis pathway (Fig. 12–34). The increased expression of the synthase is achieved by both transcriptional and translational mechanisms. Thus, the relative heme deficiency caused by the reduction in PBG deaminase and the consequent decrease in heme pools is responsible for a *secondary* increase in the synthase to levels greater than the normal range. The fact that half of the normal activity of PBG deaminase is inadequate to cope with the metabolic load in some situations accounts for both the dominant expression of the condition and the episodic nature of the clinical illness. The pathogenesis of the nervous system disease is unknown. The peripheral, autonomic, and central nervous systems are all affected, and the clinical manifestations are diverse. Indeed, this disorder is one of the great mimics in clinical medicine, with manifestations ranging from acute abdominal pain to psychosis.

### Glucose-6-Phosphate Dehydrogenase Deficiency

Deficiency of glucose-6-phosphate dehydrogenase (G6PD), a ubiquitous X-linked enzyme, is the most common disease-producing enzyme defect of humans, estimated to affect 400 million people worldwide; about 10 percent of African-American males are G6PD deficient and are clinically susceptible to drug-induced hemolysis. With more than 400 variants described, G6PD deficiency also appears to be one of the most genetically heterogeneous disorders yet recognized. More than 70 of these variants have been characterized at the molecular level. All but two are point mutations, the exceptions being in-frame deletions of a small number of codons. The high gene frequency of G6PD variants in some populations appears to reflect the fact that G6PD deficiency, like sickle cell hemoglobin and thalassemia, confers some protection against malaria (see Chapter 7). This enzymopathy originally came to attention when the antimalarial drug primaquine was found to induce hemolytic anemia in some African-American males, who were subsequently found to have G6PD deficiency.

The mechanism of the drug-induced hemolysis is reasonably clear. One of the products of G6PD, nicotinamide-adenine dinucleotide phosphate (NADPH), is the major source of reducing equivalents in the red blood cell. NADPH protects the cell against oxidative damage by regenerating reduced glutathione from its oxidized form. In G6PD deficiency, oxidant drugs such as primaquine deplete the cell of reduced glutathione, and the consequent oxidative damage leads to hemolysis. Additional offending compounds include sulfonamide antibiotics, sulfones such as dapsone (widely used in the treatment of leprosy and *Pneumocystis carinii* infections), naphthalene (moth balls), and a few others.

Favism, a severe hemolytic anemia that results from ingestion of the broad bean *Vicia faba* and that has been known since ancient times in parts of the Mediterranean, is due to extreme G6PD deficiency. The enzyme defect makes the cells vulnerable to oxidants in fava beans (Pythagoras, the Greek mathematician, warned his followers of the danger of eating these beans). In areas in which severe deficiency-variants like the Mediterranean allele are prevalent, they are a major cause of both neonatal jaundice and congenital nonspherocytic hemolytic anemia.

## Pharmacogenomics

The Human Genome Project has led to the recognition that genomic information can be beneficially applied to pharmacogenetic problems in a new field of study referred to as **pharmacogenomics.** There are at least two facets to this exciting development. First, and very generally, it is likely that the design of new drugs will be greatly influenced by knowledge of all genes. Second, a pharmacogenetic profile of each individual who is a candidate to receive a medication can be developed, with two possible benefits. The first benefit is that it should be possible to predict, with a high degree of accuracy, individuals who are likely to have an adverse response to a medication, even without specific knowledge of the metabolism of the drug or of the specific alleles that modulate responses to it. Thus, the development of a high-density single nucleotide polymorphism (SNP) map (see Chapter 6) of the human genome could be used to develop an abbreviated SNP profile—a specific pattern of SNP markers—of patients who have responded adversely to a drug. Accordingly, patients with comparable profiles, who are therefore at increased risk of an adverse response, could avoid potentially dangerous medications. In addition, drugs that are highly beneficial and nontoxic to some individuals—even a minority of a population—could be safely administered to patients without the at-risk SNP profile.

A second benefit may come from the development of abbreviated pharmacogenetic SNP profiles: it should be possible to predict the probable efficacy of the medication in an individual before the drug is administered. For example, the abbreviated pharmacogenetic SNP profile of patients who rapidly metabolize a drug—and therefore require higher doses—could be determined (again, even without specific knowledge of the biochemical events involved). Patients with similar SNP profiles would therefore be monitored to be sure that the drug achieves therapeutic levels.

Although the screening programs for abbreviated pharmacogenetic SNP profiles suggested earlier might be costly, the expenses may be more than recouped by the reduction in adverse drug responses and from more effective treatment. In addition, the cost of abbreviated SNP profile chips is likely to fall if large quantities of identical chips are produced. Irrespective of the accuracy of any of these specific predictions, the genome project will have a major impact on drug design and administration, perhaps in ways not yet imagined.

### Pharmacogenetics in Medicine

The preceding examples demonstrate the importance and potential of pharmacogenetics in medicine. Each represents a significant pharmacogenetic problem in which rational therapy must take into account wide, genetically determined individual differences in response. On a broader scale, the role of drug metabolism in many pathophysiological processes, including mutagenesis, carcinogenesis, teratogenesis, cytotoxic damage, and autoimmune diseases, is of great importance. The management of patients with toxic reactions to drugs or chemicals should include, when possible, evaluation of the pharmacogenetic status of both the patient and members of the family and appropriate genetic counseling about potential risks of certain drugs. The application of knowledge from the Human Genome Project to pharmacogenetics should usher in an era of "individualized medicine" in which appropriate medications and therapies are designed for each patient, considering not only the presentation and course of the disease, but also the individual's specific genetic constitution.

## CONCLUSION

As the biochemical pathology of an increasing number of genetic diseases is gradually untangled, and as the genetic components of the common multifactorial diseases are characterized, new and unforeseen pathophysiological mechanisms will be recognized. The understanding of genetic disease at a molecular level not only contributes to the knowledge of normal human biology but is also the foundation of effective treatment for these disorders. The principles applied in the treatment of genetic disease are presented in Chapter 13, with examples that include many of the conditions that have been described here and in Chapter 11.

## General References


Cooper DN, Krawczak M (1993) Human Gene Mutation. Bios Scientific Publishers, Oxford, England.

Harris H (1980) The Principles of Human Biochemical Genetics, 3rd ed. Elsevier North-Holland, Amsterdam.

McKusick VA (1972) Heritable Disorders of Connective Tissue, 4th ed. CV Mosby, St. Louis.

Scriver CR, Beaudet AL, Sly WS, Valle D (eds) (2001) The Metabolic and Molecular Bases of Inherited Disease, 8th ed. McGraw-Hill, New York.

Scriver CR, Childs B (1989) Garrod's Inborn Factors and Disease. Oxford University Press, New York.


## References Specific to Particular Topics


Byers PH (2001) Disorders of collagen biosynthesis and structure. *In* Scriver CR, Beaudet AL, Sly WS, Valle D (eds) The Metabolic and Molecular Bases of Inherited Disease, 8th ed. McGraw-Hill, New York, pp. 5241–5286.

Chillon M, Casals T, Mercier B, et al (1995) Mutations in the cystic fibrosis gene in patients with congenital absence of the vas deferens. N Engl J Med 332:1475–1480.

Chinnery PF, Turnbull DM (1999) Mitochondrial DNA and disease. Lancet 354:SI17–SI21.

Cox DW (2001) $\alpha_1$-Antitrypsin deficiency. *In* Scriver CR, Beaudet AL, Sly WS, Valle D (eds) The Metabolic and Molecular Bases of Inherited Disease, 8th ed. McGraw-Hill, New York, pp. 5559–5586.

Davis L, Britten JJ, Morgan M (1997) Cholinesterase—its significance in anaesthetic practice. Anaesthesia 52:244–260.

Dubowitz V (1997) The muscular dystrophies—clarity or chaos? N Engl J Med 336:650–651.

Glorieux FH, Bishop NJ, Plotkin H, et al (1998) Cyclic administration of pamidronate in children with severe osteogenesis imperfecta [see comments]. N Engl J Med 339:947–952.

Goldstein JL, Hobbs HH, Brown MS (2001) Familial hypercholesterolemia. *In* Scriver CR, Beaudet AL, Sly WS, Valle D (eds) The Metabolic and Molecular Bases of Inherited Disease, 8th ed. McGraw-Hill, New York, pp. 2863–2914.

Hackam AS, Wellington CL, Hayden MR (1998) The fatal attraction of polyglutamine-containing proteins. Clin Genet 53:233–242.

Johns DR (1995) Mitochondrial DNA and disease. New Engl J Med 333:638–644.

Lautenschlager NT, Cupples LA, Rao VS, et al (1996) Risk of dementia among relatives of Alzheimer disease patients in the MIRAGE study: What is in store for the oldest old? Neurology 46:641.

Lightowlers RN, Chinnery PF, Turnbull DM, Howell N (1997) Mammalian mitochondrial genetics: Heredity, heteroplasmy and disease. Trends Genet 13:450–454.

Loke J, MacLennan DH (1998) Malignant hyperthermia and central core disease: Disorders of $Ca^{2+}$ release channels. Am J Med 104:470–486.

Martin JB (1999) Molecular basis of the neurodegenerative disorders. New Engl J Med 340:1970–1980.

Nance MA (1997) Clinical aspects of CAG repeat diseases. Brain Pathol 7:881–900. [This entire volume of the journal is devoted to CAG repeat diseases.]

Nebert DW (1999) Pharmacogenetics and pharmacogenomics: Why is this relevant to the clinical geneticist? Clin Genet 56:247–258.

Nebert DW (1997) Polymorphisms in drug-metabolizing enzymes: What is their clinical relevance and why do they exist? Am J Hum Genet 60:265–271.

Roses AD (2000) Pharmacogenetics and future drug development and delivery. Lancet 355:1358–1361.

Scriver CR, Kaufman S (2001) The hyperphenylalaninemias: Phenylalanine hydroxylase deficiency. *In* Scriver CR, Beaudet AL, Sly WS, Valle D (eds) The Metabolic and Molecular Bases of Inherited Disease, 8th ed. McGraw-Hill, New York, pp. 1667–1724.

Scriver CR, Waters PJ (1999) Monogenic traits are not simple: Lessons from phenylketonuria. Trends Genet 15:267–272.

Shoffner JM (1999) Oxidative phosphorylation disease diagnosis. Ann NY Acad Sci 893:42–60.

St George-Hyslop PH, Farrer LA, Goedert M (2001) Alzheimer's disease and the fronto-temporal dementias: Diseases with cerebral deposition of fibrillar proteins. *In* Scriver CR, Beaudet AL, Sly WS, Valle D (eds) The Metabolic and Molecular Bases of Inherited Disease, 8th ed. McGraw-Hill, New York, pp. 5875–5902.

Wallace DC, Lott MT, Brown MD, Kerstann K (2001) Mitochondria and neuro-ophthalmologic diseases. *In* Scriver CR, Beaudet AL, Sly WS, Valle D (eds) The Metabolic and Molecular Bases of Inherited Disease, 8th ed. McGraw-Hill, New York, pp. 2425–2512.

Warren ST, Nelson DL (1994) Advances in molecular analysis of fragile X syndrome. JAMA 271:536–542.

Welsh MJ, Ramsey BW, Accurso F, Cutting GR (2001) Cystic fibrosis. *In* Scriver CR, Beaudet AL, Sly WS, Valle D (eds) The Metabolic and Molecular Bases of Inherited Disease, 8th ed. McGraw-Hill, New York, pp. 5121–5188.

Worton R (2000) Muscular dystrophies: Diseases of the dystrophin-glycoprotein complex. Science 270:755–756.

Worton RG, Molnan MJ, Brais B, Karpati G (2001) The muscular dystrophies. *In* Scriver CR, Beaudet AL, Sly WS, Valle D (eds) The Metabolic and Molecular Bases of Inherited Disease, 8th ed. McGraw-Hill, New York, pp. 5493–5524.

Zielinski J (2000) Genotype and phenotype in cystic fibrosis. Respiration 67:117–133.

Zielinski J, Corey M, Rozmahel R, et al (1999) Detection of a cystic fibrosis modifier locus for meconium ileus on human chromosome 19q13. Nat Genet 22:128–129.

### URLs for Mutation Database

Collagen mutation database
*http://www.le.ac.uk/genetics/collagen/*

Cystic fibrosis and *CFTR* gene mutation database
*http://www.genet.sickkids.on.ca/cftr/*

Human mitochondrial genome disease database
*http://www.gen.emory.edu/mitomap.html*

Phenylalanine hydroxylase mutation database
*http://www.mcgill.ca/pahdb*

## Problems

1. One mutant allele at the LDL receptor locus (leading to familial hypercholesterolemia) encodes an elongated protein that is about 50,000 daltons larger than the normal 120,000-dalton receptor. Indicate at least three mechanisms that could account for this abnormality. Approximately how many extra nucleotides would need to be translated to add 50,000 daltons to the protein?

2. In discussing the nucleotide changes found to date in the coding region of the CF gene, we stated that some of the changes (the missense changes) found so far are only "putative" disease-causing mutations. What criteria would one need to fulfill before knowing that a nucleotide change is pathogenic and not a benign polymorphism?

3. Johnny, 2 years of age, is failing to thrive. Investigations show that although he has clinical findings of CF, his sweat chloride is normal. The sweat chloride is normal in less than 2 percent of patients with CF. His pediatrician and parents want to know whether DNA analysis can determine whether he indeed has CF.
   (a) Would DNA analysis be useful in this case? Briefly outline the steps involved in obtaining a DNA diagnosis for CF.
   (b) If he has CF, what is the probability that he is homozygous for the $\Delta F508$ mutation? (Assume that 85 percent of CF mutations could be detected at the time you are consulted and that his parents are from northern Europe, where the $\Delta F508$ allele has a frequency of 0.70).
   (c) If he does not have the $\Delta F508$ mutation, does this disprove the diagnosis? Explain.

4. James is the only person in his kindred affected by DMD. He has one unaffected brother, Joe. DNA analysis shows that James has a deletion in the *DMD* gene and that Joe has received the same maternal X chromosome but without a deletion. What genetic counseling would you give the parents regarding the recurrence risk of DMD in a future pregnancy?

5. *DMD* has a high mutation rate but shows no ethnic variation in frequency. Use your knowledge of the gene and the genetics of DMD to suggest why this disorder is equally common in all populations.

6. In patients with osteogenesis imperfecta, explain why the missense mutations at glycine positions in the triple helix of type I collagen are confined to a limited number of other amino acid residues (Ala, Ser, Cys, Arg, Val, Asp).

7. Electrophoresis of red-blood-cell hemolysates shows that some females have two G6PD bands, but males have a single band. Explain this observation and the possible pathological and genetic significance of the finding of two bands in an African-American female.

8. A 2-year-old infant, the child of first-cousin parents, has unexplained developmental delay. A survey of various biochemical parameters indicates that he has a deficiency of four lysosomal enzymes. Explain how a single autosomal recessive mutation might cause the loss of function of four enzyme activities. Why is it most likely that the child has an autosomal recessive condition, if he has a genetic condition at all?

9. The effect of a dominant negative allele illustrates one general mechanism by which mutations in a protein cause dominantly inherited disease. What other mechanism is commonly associated with dominance in genes encoding the subunits of multimeric proteins?

10. The clinical effects of mutations in a housekeeping protein are frequently limited to one or a few tissues, often tissues in which the protein is abundant and serves a specialty function. Identify and discuss examples that illustrate this generalization, and explain why they fit it.

11. The relationship between the site at which a protein is expressed and the site of pathology in a genetic disease may be unpredictable. In addition, the tissue that lacks the mutant protein may even be left unaffected by pathology. Give examples of this latter phenomenon and discuss them.

12. The two pseudodeficiency alleles of hex A are Arg 247 Trp and Arg 249 Trp. What is the probable reason that the missense substitutions of these alleles are so close together in the protein?

13

# The Treatment of Genetic Disease

In the coming decades, molecular biology, protein engineering, and the Human Genome Project will have an enormous impact on the treatment of genetic and other disease. In this chapter, therefore, we not only provide an overview of standard therapies used in the treatment of genetic disease, we also outline new strategies that may be used in the future. In particular, we emphasize therapies that reflect the genetic approach to medicine. As with all therapy, the objective of treating genetic disease is to eliminate or ameliorate the effects of the disorder not only on the patient but also on the family. In addition, the family must be informed about the risk that the disease may occur in other members. The latter responsibility, genetic counseling, is a major component of the management of hereditary disorders and is dealt with separately in Chapter 19. The preferred treatment of some, and perhaps many, single-gene diseases will eventually be gene transfer therapy, if the procedure can be made safe and effective. Initial promising successes with gene therapy have been achieved. However, even when copies of a normal gene can be transferred into the patient to effect permanent cure, the family will need ongoing genetic counseling, carrier testing, and prenatal diagnosis, in many cases over several generations. For single-gene disorders, treatment is generally based on replacing the defective protein, improving its function, or minimizing the consequences of its deficiency.

## THE CURRENT STATE OF TREATMENT OF GENETIC DISEASE

### Multifactorial Diseases

For most multifactorial diseases (see Chapter 15), both the environmental and genetic components of the etiology are poorly understood. When an environmental contribution is recognized, an opportunity for effective intervention is available because exposure to the environmental factor can often be modified. Thus, cigarette smoking is an environmental factor that all patients with emphysema should avoid. At least one mechanism by which cigarette smoke leads to emphysema has been disclosed by the study of the single-gene disorder $\alpha_1$-antitrypsin ($\alpha_1$-AT) deficiency. As described in the preceding chapter, cigarette smoke oxidizes the critical methionine residue at the active site of $\alpha_1$-AT, which reduces by 2000-fold its ability to inhibit elastase. Thus, smoking produces a substantial acquired loss of $\alpha_1$-AT function.

Most diseases with complex inheritance are amenable to some form of medical or surgical treatment, although this treatment may not be particularly "genetic" in its approach. A striking example of a genetically complex disorder for which standard medical therapy is increasingly successful is type 1 diabetes mellitus, in which intensive insulin replacement therapy dramatically improves the outcome (Table 13–1). Surgical treatment of multifactorial disorders can also be highly successful. For example, three structural abnormalities (congenital heart defects, cleft lip and palate, and pyloric stenosis) affect nearly 1.5 percent of all liveborn infants and make up

TABLE 13–1

**The Effect of Intensive Insulin Replacement Therapy on the Rates of Three Common Complications of Type 1 Diabetes Mellitus**

| | Rate/100 Patient Years | | |
|---|---|---|---|
| | *Conventional Treatment* | *Intensive Treatment* | *% of Risk Reduction* |
| Retinopathy | 4.7 | 1.2 | 76 |
| Albuminuria | 3.4 | 2.2 | 34 |
| Neuropathy | 9.8 | 3.1 | 69 |

From the Diabetes Control and Complications Trial Research Group (1993) N Engl J Med 329:977–986. Adapted from Scriver CR, Treacy EP (1999) Is there treatment for "genetic" disease? Mol Gen Metab 68:93–102.

approximately 30 percent of all newborns with genetic disease. Many patients with these conditions can be *cured* by surgery, a form of phenotypic modification. In about half of these patients, the diseases are curable by a single operation; a cure is therefore possible in at least 10 to 15 percent of infants with a genetically determined disorder. Admittedly, the treatment of inherited disease is often not so beneficial, although it frequently improves the quality of life. For multifactorial disorders that typically manifest in adolescence or adult life, such as essential hypertension, diabetes, coronary artery disease, and the major psychoses, the imperfections of treatment reflect our ignorance of the etiology or the complexity of the pathogenesis.

## Single-Gene Diseases

The treatment of single-gene diseases is sadly deficient at present. A survey of 372 mendelian disorders showed that current therapy is completely effective in 12 percent, partially effective in 54 percent, and of no benefit in 34 percent (Fig. 13–1). One strongly encouraging trend identified in several surveys is that treatment is more likely to be successful if the basic biochemical defect is known. For example, in a 1985 study by Hayes and colleagues, life span was increased by treatment in only 15 percent of single-gene diseases studied, but in a subset of 65 inborn errors in which the cause was known, life span was greatly improved in 32 percent; similar increases were observed for other phenotypes, including growth, intelligence, and social adaptation. Thus, research to elucidate the genetic and biochemical basis of hereditary disease has a dramatic impact on the patient. Nevertheless, in general, current therapy fails to restore normal health to the great majority of patients with a monogenic disorder.

The current unsatisfactory state of treatment of genetic disease is due to numerous factors, including the following:

1. **Gene not identified or pathogenesis not understood**. The mutant locus in more than 75 percent of genetic diseases is unknown, and knowledge of the pathophysiology of those diseases in which the affected gene or biochemical abnormality has been defined is inadequate. In phenylketonuria (PKU), for example, despite years of study, the mechanisms by which the elevation in phenylalanine impairs brain development and function are still poorly understood (see Chapter 12). For diseases in which the function of the affected protein has only recently been determined, such as cystic fibrosis and Duchenne muscular dystrophy (DMD) (see Chapter 12), much work is required before this basic knowledge can be translated into effective therapy.
2. **Prediagnostic fetal damage**. Some mutations act early in development or cause irreversible pathology before they are diagnosed. These problems can be anticipated in some cases if there is a family history of a genetic disease or if carrier screening identifies couples at risk. In the latter case, prenatal treatment is sometimes possible for both medical and surgical conditions. Opportunities for prenatal treatment, examples of which are outlined in Table 13–2, will increase as prenatal diagnosis

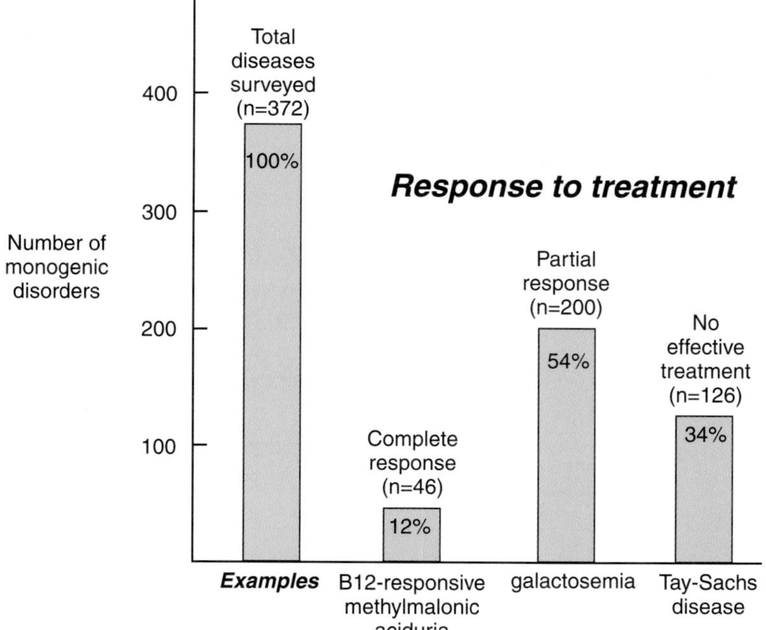


Figure 13–1. The effect of treatment on 372 genetic diseases in which the affected gene or biochemical function is known and for which sufficient information was available for analysis. $B_{12}$-responsive methylmalonic aciduria and Tay-Sachs disease are discussed in Chapter 12, and galactosemia is described in this chapter. (Adapted from Scriver CR, Treacy EP [1999] Is there treatment for "genetic" disease? Mol Gen Metab 68:93–102.)

TABLE 13–2

**Examples of Prenatal Treatment of Inherited and Congenital Disorders**

| Prenatal Medical Treatment | | Prenatal Surgical Treatment | |
|---|---|---|---|
| *Disease* | *Treatment* | *Disease* | *Treatment* |
| Biotinidase deficiency | Maternal biotin administration | Urinary obstruction due to urethral valves → hydronephrosis | Percutaneous catheter or vesicostomy |
| Cobalamin-responsive methylmalonic aciduria | Maternal cobalamin administration | Diaphragmatic hernia → lung hypoplasia | Reduce viscera and repair diaphragm |
| Congenital adrenal hyperplasia | Dexamethasone | Twin-twin transfusion syndrome → vascular steal → fetal hydrops | Divide communicating placental vessels |

(see Chapter 18) becomes feasible for an increasingly broad range of disorders.

3. **Severe phenotypes are the first to be recognized.** The initial cases of a disease to be recognized are usually severely affected ones, which are often less amenable to treatment than are more mildly affected ones. In the milder cases, the mutant protein may retain some residual function that can be increased by one of several strategies, as described later.

## SPECIAL CONSIDERATIONS IN TREATING GENETIC DISEASE

### The Need for Long-Term Assessment of Treatment

In genetic disease, perhaps more than in other areas of medicine, treatment initially judged as successful may eventually be shown to be imperfect. There are at least three facets to this problem. First, treatment may initially appear to be successful, only to be shown by longer observation to have subtle inadequacies. Thus, although well-managed children with PKU have escaped severe retardation and have normal or near-normal IQs (see later), they often manifest subtle learning disorders and behavioral disturbances that impair their academic performance.

Second, successful treatment of the pathological changes in one organ may be followed by unexpected problems in tissues not previously observed to be clinically involved because the patients did not survive long enough. The detection of the later manifestations may require many years of observation after the initial therapy. One disorder that illustrates this point is a well-known inborn error of carbohydrate metabolism, **galactosemia**. This disorder results from the inability to metabolize galactose, a monosaccharide that is a component of lactose (milk sugar). Persons with this autosomal recessive disease completely lack the enzyme galactose-1-phosphate uridyltransferase (GALT), which normally catalyzes the conversion of galactose-1-phosphate to uridine diphosphogalactose (UDPG):

$$\text{galactose-1-phosphate} \xrightarrow{\text{GALT}} \text{UDPG}$$

Infants with galactosemia are usually normal at birth but begin to develop gastrointestinal problems, cirrhosis of the liver, and cataracts in the weeks after they are given milk. If not recognized, galactosemia causes severe mental retardation and is often fatal. Complete removal of milk from the diet, however, can protect against most of the harmful consequences of GALT deficiency, although, as with PKU, learning disabilities are now recognized to be common even in well-treated galactosemia patients. In addition, despite conscientious treatment, most females with galactosemia have ovarian failure that appears to result from continued galactose toxicity.

Another disease that demonstrates this phenomenon is **cystinosis**, which is caused by cystine accumulation in the lysosome due to a defect in cystine efflux (see Table 12–1). The cystine storage initially leads to renal failure. As patients who receive renal transplants grow older, however, morbidity results from hypothyroidism, from islet cell disease that causes diabetes, and from various neurological abnormalities. A final example is provided by mutations in the retinoblastoma gene (see Chapter 16). Patients successfully treated for the eye tumor in the first years of life are at increased risk of developing an independent malignancy, osteosarcoma, after the first decade. Ironically, therefore, treatment that successfully prolongs life provides a new opportunity for the clinical expression of the basic defect, particularly in conditions in which the mutant gene is normally expressed in many tissues, thus providing more potential targets for the development of pathology.

Third, therapy that is believed to be free of side effects in the short term may be associated with serious problems in the long term. For example, clotting factor infusion in hemophilia sometimes results in the formation of antibodies to the infused protein, and blood transfusion in thalassemia invariably produces iron overload, which can be managed but with difficulty.

### Genetic Heterogeneity and Treatment

The optimal treatment of single-gene defects requires an unusual degree of diagnostic precision, often at the level of the affected molecule. As described in early chapters, genetic heterogeneity (allelic heterogeneity or locus heterogeneity) is a common characteristic of genetic diseases. For proper management, it is often critical not simply to treat a biochemical abnormality but to identify precisely the basic biochemical defect, as opposed to a secondary defect (e.g., see Table 11–1). For example, abnormalities in phenylalanine hydroxylase and in the enzymes of biopterin metabolism both produce hyperphenylalaninemia, but the treatment of the two types of defects is quite different. Even allelic mutations may require different management: the clinically distinct $\beta$-globin disorders, thalassemia and sickle cell disease, illustrate this concept.

The study of allelic variants of enzyme defects has shown that alleles that retain small amounts of residual enzyme activity often cause much less severe disease than do null alleles. The contrast between the need for strict dietary phenylalanine restriction in patients with classic PKU (with little or no residual enzyme activity) and the normal diet tolerated by those with benign hyperphenylalaninemia (with approximately 5 percent residual enzyme activity) illustrates this principle. The corollary of this observation is that effective treatment of classic PKU by gene or enzyme transfer would require the production or delivery of only small amounts of phenylalanine hydroxylase.

Allelic heterogeneity has additional implications for therapy. Some alleles produce a protein that is decreased in abundance but has residual function. Strategies designed to increase the expression or stability of the partially functional protein may be effective in correcting the biochemical defect. In contrast, nothing is to be gained by increasing the abundance of a mutant protein with no residual function. In fact, increased expression of a functionless mutant protein may be detrimental because it may exert a dominant negative effect (see Chapter 12) if it interacts with the product of the normal allele, or with other proteins, to impair their function. This consideration is also relevant to efforts to transfer a normal gene into a patient with a genetic disease. For example, in osteogenesis imperfecta, patients with null alleles may be easier to treat eventually by gene transfer than may those with qualitatively abnormal collagen chains that reduce the effective contribution of the transferred gene (see Fig. 12–21).

## TREATMENT STRATEGIES

Genetic disease can be treated at many levels, at various steps away from the mutant gene (Fig. 13–2). In the remainder of this chapter, we describe the rationale used or proposed for treatment at each of these levels. In general, diseases described earlier in the book are used as examples, although other disorders are presented for the first time when necessary to illustrate a specific approach. None of the current treatments is necessarily mutually exclusive, although successful gene therapy would render other therapies superfluous. For diseases in which the biochemical or genetic defect is known, the frequency with which the different strategies are currently used is shown in Figure 13–3.

Treatment "at the level of the clinical phenotype" (see Fig. 13–2) is a category meant to include all the types of medical or surgical intervention that are not unique to the management of genetic disease. Often, this is the only therapy available and, in some cases, may be all that is necessary, as we described earlier for some surgically correctable malformations. Finally, the importance of educating the patient cannot be overemphasized—not only to achieve understanding of the disease, its genetic implications, and its treatment, but also to ensure compliance with therapy that may be inconvenient and lifelong.

### Treatment of Metabolic Abnormalities

The most successful disease-specific approach to the treatment of genetic disease has been at the level of a metabolic abnormality. In fact, this concept is a familiar one because it applies to all of *Homo sapiens*: humans and other primates, in contrast to most mammals, must compensate for their inability to synthesize ascorbic acid (vitamin C) by including this essential vitamin in their diet. The principal strategies used to manipulate metabolism in the treatment of inborn errors are listed in Table 13–3. The necessity for patients with pharmacogenetic diseases, such as glucose-6-phosphate dehydrogenase deficiency, to avoid certain drugs and chemicals is described in Chapter 12.

#### Dietary Restriction

Dietary restriction is one of the oldest and most effective methods of managing genetic disease. Diseases involving more than 24 loci are currently managed in this way. The advantage of this approach is that it can be highly effective; its drawback is that it usually requires lifelong compliance with a restricted and often artificial diet. The dietary constraint is onerous for the family as well as for the patient, especially in ado-

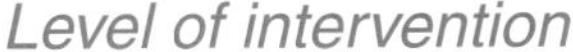

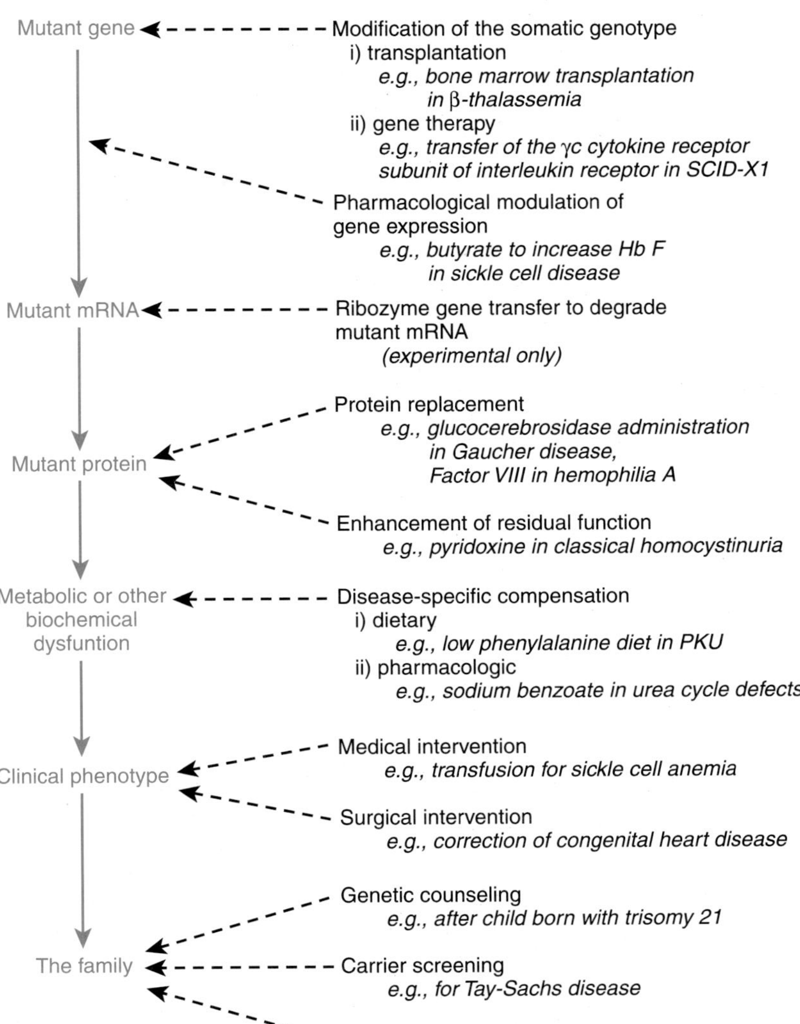


**Figure 13–2.** The various levels of treatment that are relevant to genetic disease, with the corresponding strategies used at each level. For each level, a disease discussed in the text is given as an example. (Adapted from Valle D [1987] Genetic disease: An overview of current therapy. Hosp Pract 22:167–182.)

lescence. Many of the diseases treatable in this manner involve amino acid catabolic pathways, and, therefore, severe restriction of normal dietary protein is usually necessary. Essential nutrients such as amino acids, however, cannot be withheld entirely; their intake must be sufficient for anabolic needs. For that group of patients who have mild enzymatic defects (i.e., "leaky" mutant alleles), some small fraction of the offending compound can often be tolerated; consequently, the diet is less restrictive, and compliance may be better. If the dietary precursor of the offending substrate is not an essential nutrient, it can be eliminated from the diet altogether. An example of such a compound is galactose, which the body can synthesize from glucose in amounts adequate for the small requirements of normal biochemical processes, such as the synthesis of mucopolysaccharides.

A diet restricted in phenylalanine largely circumvents the neurological damage in classic PKU (see Chapter 12). Phenylketonuric children are normal at birth because the maternal enzyme protects them during prenatal life. The results of treatment are best when the diagnosis is made soon after birth and treatment is begun promptly. If the child is fed a normal diet in the first months of life, irreversible mental retardation occurs; the degree of intellectual deficit is directly related to the delay in the institution of the low phenylalanine diet. The normal mental status of patients with benign hyperphenylalaninemia demonstrates that effective treatment of classic PKU can be achieved if the phenylalanine levels can be kept below about 0.4 mM. Without this guidance from nature, many clinical trials would have been required to establish a "safe" plasma phenylalanine level in the classic disease. It is now recommended that patients with PKU remain on a low phenylalanine diet for life because neurological and behavioral abnormalities develop

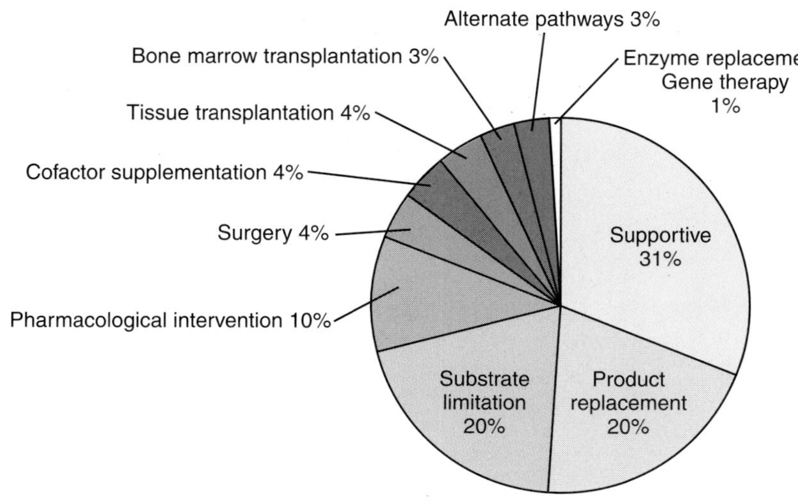


Figure 13–3. The frequency with which various therapeutic and management strategies are currently used in the treatment of 372 metabolic disorders (the same group of disorders referred to in Fig. 13–1). If a disorder is treated using, for example, two strategies, the impact of each strategy on the total treatment was estimated and allocated between each approach. (From Scriver CR, Treacy EP [1999] Is there treatment for "genetic" disease? Mol Gene Metab 68:93–102.)

in many (though not all) patients if the diet is stopped. Even in patients who have been treated throughout life, however, it is now clear that when intelligence (as measured by IQ) is normal or near normal, there are still neuropsychological deficits (e.g., in conceptual, visuospatial, and language skills). Nonetheless, it should be stressed that treatment produces results vastly superior to the outcome without treatment.

### Replacement

The provision of essential metabolites, cofactors, or hormones whose deficiency is due to a genetic disease is simple in concept and often in application. Some of the most successfully treated single-gene defects belong to this category. An important example is provided by **congenital hypothyroidism**, 10 to 15 percent of which is monogenic in origin. This disorder results from a variety of defects in the formation of the thyroid gland or of its major product, thyroxine. Because congenital hypothyroidism is common (about 1/4000 neonates) and treatment can prevent the associated mental retardation, neonatal screening is conducted in many countries so that thyroxine administration may be initiated as soon as possible after birth to prevent the severe intellectual defects that are otherwise inevitable. A second example is provided by **biotinidase deficiency**. The lack of biotinidase activity prevents the recovery of biotin from biotinylated proteins, and, as a result, the recycling of this enzyme cofactor is disrupted. The oral administration of large amounts of biotin is completely corrective if given before serious neurological sequelae develop.

TABLE 13–3
**Treatment of Genetic Disease by Metabolic Manipulation**

| Type of Metabolic Intervention | Substance or Technique | Disease |
|---|---|---|
| Avoidance | Antimalarial drugs<br>Barbiturates | G6PD deficiency<br>Acute intermittent porphyria |
| Dietary restriction | Phenylalanine<br>Galactose | PKU<br>Galactosemia |
| Replacement | Thyroxine<br>Biotin | Congenital hypothyroidism<br>Biotinidase deficiency |
| Diversion | Sodium benzoate<br>Oral resins | Urea cycle disorders<br>Familial hypercholesterolemia heterozygotes |
| Inhibition | Lovastatin | Familial hypercholesterolemia heterozygotes |
| Depletion | LDL apheresis (direct removal of LDL from plasma) | Familial hypercholesterolemia homozygotes |

G6PD = glucose-6-phosphate dehydrogenase; LDL = low-density lipoprotein; PKU = phenylketonuria.
Modified from Rosenberg LE (1990) Treating genetic diseases: Lessons from three children. Pediatr Res 27:S10–S16.

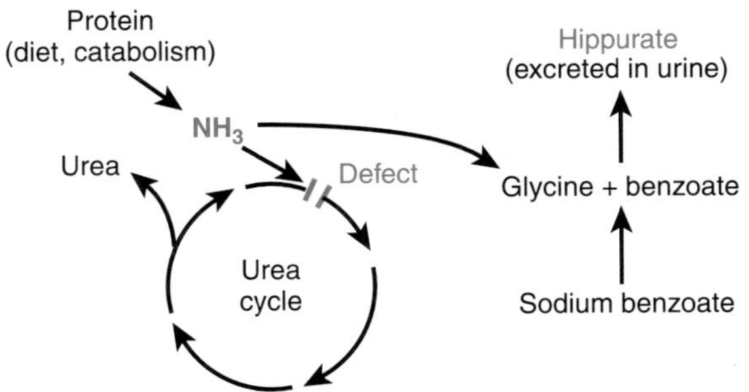


**Figure 13–4.** The strategy of metabolite diversion. In this example, ammonia cannot be removed by the urea cycle because of a genetic defect of a urea cycle enzyme. The administration of sodium benzoate diverts ammonia to glycine synthesis, and the nitrogen moiety is subsequently excreted as hippurate.

### DIVERSION

Diversion therapy is the enhanced use of alternative metabolic pathways to reduce the concentration of a harmful metabolite. The diversion strategy has been successfully applied to the treatment of the **urea cycle disorders** (Fig. 13–4). The function of the urea cycle is to convert ammonia, which is neurotoxic, to urea, which is a benign end product that is excreted. If the cycle is disrupted by an enzyme defect such as argininosuccinate synthetase or lyase deficiency, the consequent hyperammonemia can be only partially controlled by dietary protein restriction. The ammonia can be reduced to normal levels by diversion to metabolic pathways that are normally of minor significance, leading to synthesis of harmless compounds. For example, the administration of large quantities of sodium benzoate forces its ligation with glycine to form hippurate, which is excreted in the urine (see Fig. 13–4). Glycine synthesis is thereby increased, and for each mole of glycine formed, one mole of ammonia is consumed.

A similar approach has been successful in helping to reduce the cholesterol level in *heterozygotes* for **familial hypercholesterolemia (FH)** (reviewed in Chapter 12). By the diversion of an increased fraction of cholesterol to bile acid synthesis, the single normal low-density lipoprotein (LDL) receptor gene of these patients can be stimulated to produce more hepatic receptors for LDL-bound cholesterol (Fig. 13–5). This treatment achieves significant reductions in plasma cholesterol because 70 percent of all LDL-receptor mediated uptake of cholesterol is by the liver. The increase in bile acid synthesis is obtained by the oral administration of nonabsorbable resins such as cholestyramine and colestipol that bind bile acids in the intestine and increase their fecal excretion.

An important principle illustrated by this example is that autosomal dominant diseases may sometimes be treated by increasing the expression of the normal allele. Accordingly, this strategy is generally ineffective in patients without a normal allele, including, for example, FH *homozygotes*. However, patients who are homozygotes for a genetic disease may have some response to the treatments used for heterozygotes (Fig. 13–5) if there is some residual function from either of their two mutant alleles.

### INHIBITION

The pharmacological inhibition of enzymes is sometimes used to modify the metabolic abnormalities of inborn errors. This principle is also effectively exploited in the treatment of patients with FH. If methods are used to decrease the cholesterol load by

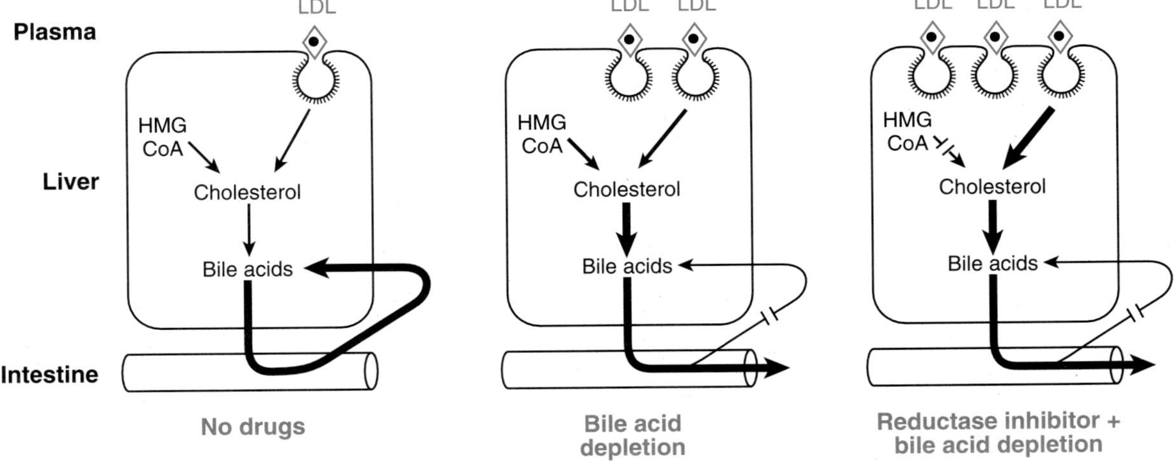


**Figure 13–5.** Rationale for the combined use of a bile acid–binding resin and an inhibitor of 3-hydroxy-3-methylglutaryl coenzyme A (HMG CoA) reductase in the treatment of familial hypercholesterolemia heterozygotes. (From Brown MS, Goldstein JL [1986] A receptor-mediated pathway for cholesterol homeostasis. Science 232:4. Copyright by the Nobel Foundation.)

diverting it to other compounds or by removing it with physical methods, as described in the next section, the liver tries to compensate for the cholesterol deficiency by upregulating cholesterol synthesis. Consequently, the treatment of FH heterozygotes is more effective if hepatic cholesterol synthesis is simultaneously inhibited. The development of statins—powerful competitive inhibitors of the rate-limiting enzyme of cholesterol synthesis, 3-hydroxy-3-methylglutaryl coenzyme A (HMG CoA) reductase—has allowed a rational combined approach that is highly effective. High doses of the statins typically effect a 40 to 60 percent decrease in plasma LDL cholesterol levels in FH heterozygotes; when used together with cholestyramine (Fig. 13–5), the effect is synergistic, and greater decreases can be achieved. The long-term safety of the statins has proved to be remarkably good. Because most FH homozygotes have little or no residual LDL receptor activity, the statins are generally ineffective in the management of these patients.

#### DEPLETION

Genetic diseases characterized by the accumulation of a harmful compound are sometimes treated by direct removal of the compound from the body. This principle is also illustrated by FH. FH homozygotes respond well to the removal of LDL from plasma by a method called LDL apheresis: once a week, for 2 to 3 hours, the patient's plasma is passed continuously over columns that remove apolipoprotein B containing lipoproteins, including LDL. Reductions in LDL cholesterol of up to 70 percent are achieved.

## Treatment at the Level of the Protein

If a mutant protein has some residual function, it may be possible to enhance this activity by increasing the stability of the protein or by increasing the residual working capacity of each abnormal molecule. With enzymopathies, the improvement in function obtained by this approach is usually very small—on the order of a few percent—but this increment is often all that is required to restore biochemical homeostasis. Of course, mutations that prevent the synthesis of any functional protein are not amenable to this approach. Furthermore, most proteins do not interact with "corrective" ligands that can be given in large amounts, and, in these cases, treatment at the protein level can be achieved only by replacement of the protein itself.

#### ENHANCEMENT OF THE FUNCTION OF THE MUTANT PROTEIN

The biochemical abnormalities of a number of metabolic diseases may respond, sometimes dramatically, to the administration of large amounts of the vitamin cofactor of the enzyme impaired by the mutation (Table 13–4). In fact, the **vitamin-responsive inborn errors** are among the most successfully treated of all genetic diseases. The vitamins used are remarkably nontoxic, generally allowing the safe administration of amounts 100 to 500 times greater than those required for normal nutrition. The mechanisms that account for the therapeutic effect vary with the disease. In biotinidase deficiency, for example, the response occurs because the administered biotin replaces the biotin that is not removed and recy-

TABLE 13–4
**Treatment of Genetic Disease at the Level of the Mutant Protein**

| Strategy | Example | Status |
|---|---|---|
| **Enhancement of mutant protein function** | | |
| Cofactor administration to increase enzyme activity | Pyridoxine-responsive homocystinuria | Treatment of choice in the 50% of patients who are responsive |
| **Protein replacement** | | |
| Replacement of an extracellular protein | Factor VIII in hemophilia A | Well established, effective |
| | $\alpha_1$-antitrypsin in $\alpha_1$-AT deficiency | Intravenous (IV) infusion to raise serum/lung levels. Biochemically and clinically beneficial in many patients. Aerosol therapy may supplant IV infusion |
| Extracellular replacement of an intracellular protein | Polyethylene glycol-modified adenosine deaminase (PEG-ADA) in ADA deficiency | Well established, safe and effective, but costly |
| Replacement of intracellular proteins: cell targeting | Modified glucocerebrosidase in Gaucher disease | Established, biochemically and clinically effective, expensive |

cled—because of the biotinidase deficiency—from enzymes to which it is ligated. In **homocystinuria** due to cystathionine synthase deficiency (see Fig. 12–7), the mechanism differs, because the cofactor, pyridoxal phosphate, is not covalently linked to the apoenzyme. About 50 percent of these patients respond to the administration of high doses of pyridoxine (vitamin $B_6$, the precursor of pyridoxal phosphate); in most of these patients, homocystine disappears from the plasma. The increase in hepatic enzyme activity is only a fewfold: in one case, for example, from 1.5 to only 4.5 percent of control activity. The increased pyridoxal phosphate concentrations may overcome reduced affinity of the mutant enzyme for the cofactor (Fig. 13–6). The mutant enzyme may also be stabilized by its association with the cofactor. In any case, pyridoxine treatment substantially improves the clinical course of the disease in responsive patients. Nonresponsive patients generally have no residual cystathionine synthase activity to augment.

## Protein Replacement

The principal types of protein replacement used to date are summarized in Table 13–4. Protein replacement is part of the *routine* therapeutic repertoire in only a few diseases, all of which affect proteins whose principal site of action is in the plasma or extracellular fluid. The prevention or arrest of bleeding episodes in patients with hemophilia by the infusion of plasma fractions enriched for factor VIII is the prime example. The years of experience with this disease also indicate the problems that can be anticipated as new strategies, outlined later, encourage attempts at the replacement of other, particularly intracellular, polypeptides. The problems include the difficulty and cost of procuring sufficient amounts of the protein to treat all patients at the optimal frequency, the need to administer the protein at a frequency consistent with its half-life (only 8 to 10 hours for factor VIII), the formation of neutralizing antibodies in some patients (5 percent of classic hemophiliacs), and the contamination of the protein with foreign agents, particularly viruses (hepatitis, human immunodeficiency virus).

### Replacement of an Extracellular Protein: Alpha$_1$-Antitrypsin Deficiency

$\alpha_1$-AT, as described in Chapter 12, is the major inhibitor of neutrophil elastase, a destructive proteolytic enzyme stored in neutrophils. There are approximately 40,000 *Z/Z* homozygotes in North America alone; thus, $\alpha_1$-AT deficiency is a significant cause of premature death in the adult population (see Fig. 12–9). The most effective treatment for $\alpha_1$-AT deficiency is environmental modification—avoidance of smoking. The object of additional therapy is to redress the imbalance between elastase and $\alpha_1$-AT by delivering $\alpha_1$-AT to the pulmonary epithelium and alveolar interstitial fluid. In $\alpha_1$-AT–deficient patients, human $\alpha_1$-AT can be infused intravenously in doses sufficiently large to maintain the interstitial $\alpha_1$-AT concentration at an effective inhibitory level for 1 week or even longer. A clinically significant effect is observed only in patients with moderate impairment (between 30 and 65 percent of normal) of lung function before treatment; that is, in patients with a greater or lesser reduction in pulmonary function before treatment, no significant slowing of the loss of

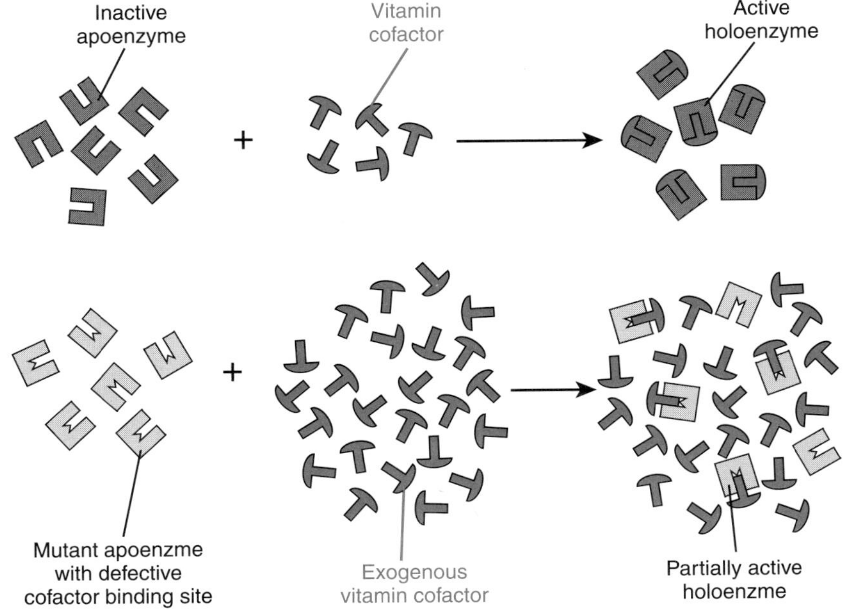


**Figure 13–6.** The mechanism of the response of a mutant apoenzyme to the administration of its cofactor at high doses. Vitamin-responsive enzyme defects are often due to mutations that reduce the normal affinity (*top*) of the enzyme protein (apoenzyme) for the cofactor needed to activate it. In the presence of the high concentrations of the cofactor that result from the administration of up to 500 times the normal daily requirement, the mutant enzyme acquires a small amount of activity sufficient to restore biochemical normalcy. (Redrawn from Valle D [1987] Genetic disease: An overview of current therapy. Hosp Pract 22:167–182.)

pulmonary function is observed. An even more promising approach is offered by the delivery of $\alpha_1$-AT directly to the lungs by aerosol inhalation. This treatment requires only 10 percent of the intravenous dose of $\alpha_1$-AT and achieves effective levels in both lung and plasma with twice-daily inhalations.

### Extracellular Replacement of an Intracellular Enzyme: Adenosine Deaminase Deficiency

Adenosine deaminase (ADA) is a critical enzyme of purine metabolism that catalyzes the deamination of adenosine to inosine and of deoxyadenosine to deoxyinosine (Fig. 13–7). The pathological effects of ADA deficiency, an autosomal recessive disease, result entirely from abnormalities in lymphocytes, in which the enzyme is normally found at its highest level. The resulting lymphotoxicity causes a profound failure of both cell-mediated (T cell) and humoral (B cell) immunity, making ADA deficiency one of the causes of severe combined immunodeficiency (SCID) (see Chapter 14). Untreated patients die of infection within the first 2 years of life. Bone marrow transplantation from a fully HLA-compatible donor is the current treatment of choice. In the absence of an appropriate donor, a highly effective treatment is the administration of bovine ADA that has been modified to increase its efficacy.

**Modified Adenosine Deaminase.** Numerous studies established that the infusion of normal red blood cells into patients with ADA deficiency reduces the levels of toxic metabolites, particularly deoxyadenosine. The response was variable and poorly sustained, however. To circumvent these problems, bovine ADA is modified by the covalent attachment of an inert polymer, polyethylene glycol (PEG). PEG-modified ADA has little immunogenicity, does not enter cells, and has a strikingly long plasma half-life of 3 to 6 days (in comparison with 30 minutes in the normal mouse). PEG-ADA replacement therapy (intramuscular injection once or twice weekly) almost normalizes the metabolic abnormalities in purine metabolism. Although PEG-ADA does not completely correct immune function (most patients remain T lymphopenic), immunoprotection is restored, and dramatic clinical improvement occurs. This approach, although very costly, represents a major new strategy for the treatment of genetic disease.

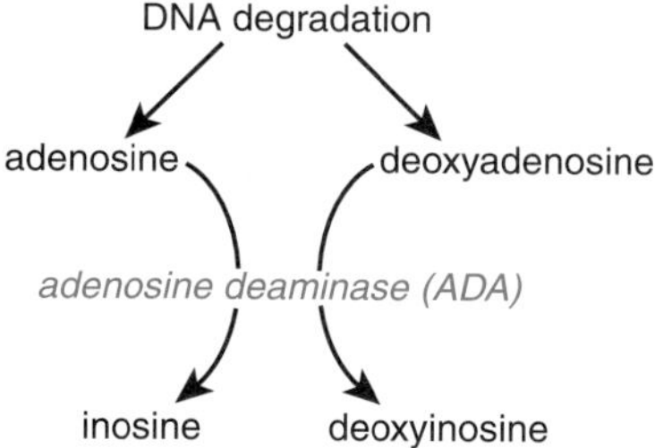


**Figure 13–7.** Adenosine deaminase (ADA) converts adenosine to inosine and deoxyadenosine to deoxyinosine. In ADA deficiency, deoxyadenosine accumulation in lymphocytes is lymphotoxic, killing the cells by impairing DNA replication and cell division to cause severe combined immunodeficiency (SCID).

The general principles exemplified by the use of PEG-ADA are that (1) proteins can be chemically modified to improve their effectiveness as pharmacological reagents, without necessarily interfering with their biological activity; and (2) an enzyme that is normally located inside the cell can be effective extracellularly if its substrate is in equilibrium with the extracellular fluid and if its product can be taken up by the cells that require it. As illustrated in the following section, the strategy of modification can be extended to proteins that can function only intracellularly, by targeting the protein to a specific cell type.

### Replacement of Intracellular Proteins: Targeted Enzymes

The feasibility of directing a polypeptide to a specific cell and a particular intracellular compartment has been demonstrated for **Gaucher disease**, the most prevalent lysosomal storage disorder, affecting up to 1/450 Ashkenazic Jews and 1/40,000 to 1/100,000 individuals in other populations. This autosomal recessive condition is due to a deficiency of the enzyme glucocerebrosidase. Its substrate, glucocerebroside, is a complex lipid normally degraded in the lysosome. The pathology results from glucocerebroside accumulation, particularly in the lysosomes of macrophages in the reticuloendothelial system. The macrophage storage process leads to gross enlargement of the liver and spleen. In addition, bone marrow is slowly replaced by lipid-laden macrophages ("Gaucher cells") that ultimately compromise the production of erythrocytes and platelets, producing anemia and thrombocytopenia. Bone lesions cause episodic pain, osteonecrosis, and much morbidity. A minority of patients have progressive central nervous system degeneration.

Glucocerebrosidase replacement in Gaucher disease illustrates the challenges in targeting a protein both to a particular type of cell and to a specific intracellular address, in this case the macrophage and the lysosome, respectively. Gaucher disease is a suitable model for protein targeting for several reasons. First, because in most patients the central nervous system is not involved, the enzyme must be delivered only to the peripheral reticuloendothelial system. Second, the only alternative therapy at present is bone marrow transplantation, a relatively high-risk procedure. Third, the human enzyme is available in abundance, purified either from placenta or from a recombinant form secreted by cultured cells. Finally, the biology of the macrophage is sufficiently well understood to have suggested a strategy for targeting the enzyme to it.

More than 2500 patients are now being treated worldwide with glucocerebrosidase, with dramatic clinical benefits. The increase in the hemoglobin level of one patient, a response representative of that seen in most patients, is shown in Figure 13–8. Overall, this therapy also reduces the enlargement of liver and spleen, increases the platelet count, accelerates growth, and improves the characteristic skeletal abnormalities. This success depended on a modification of the carbohydrates that normally decorate this glycoprotein: terminal sugars are removed to expose core $\alpha$-mannosyl residues. The exposed mannose sugars target the enzyme to the macrophage, via a mannose receptor on the plasma membrane. Once bound, the enzyme is internalized and delivered to the lysosome. As is PEG-ADA therapy, glucocerebrosidase replacement is currently extremely expensive. Nevertheless, this strategy demonstrates an important principle and illustrates the feasibility of directing an intracellular enzyme to its physiologically relevant location to produce clinically significant effects. For many diseases, it should be possible to use the cloned gene to produce large amounts of the relevant protein in culture and to modify the polypeptide as required for specific cellular and intracellular targeting.

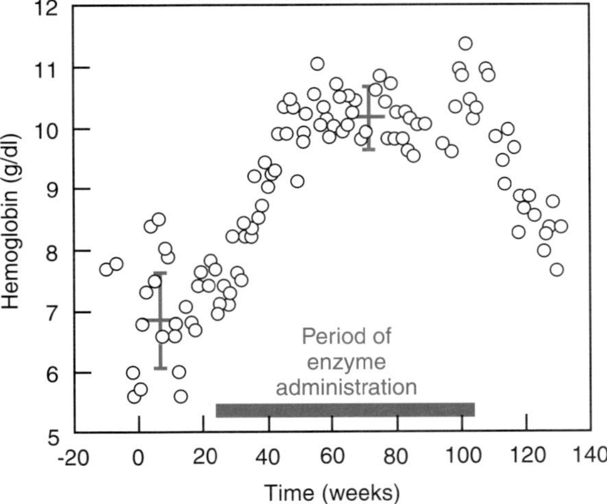


**Figure 13–8.** The effect of weekly intravenous infusions of modified glucocerebrosidase on the hemoglobin concentration of a child with Gaucher disease without neurological involvement. Treatment was begun at 4 years of age and continued for 18 months. The therapy was accompanied by an increased platelet count and radiological improvement in the bony abnormalities. The hematological parameters returned to pretreatment levels when the infusions were stopped. The bar on the abscissa represents the period of enzyme administration. (Redrawn from Barton NW, Furbish FS, Murray GJ, et al [1990] Therapeutic response to intravenous infusions of glucocerebrosidase in a patient with Gaucher disease. Proc Natl Acad Sci USA 87:1913–1916.)

## Modulation of Gene Expression

As the vitamin-responsive inborn errors have demonstrated, even small increases in the function of a mutant protein may be advantageous if it has some residual function. Therapeutic effects could also be obtained, at least in principle, by eliciting small increases in the amount of messenger RNA transcribed from the affected locus (Table 13–5), provided that the mutant protein retained some residual function; at present, no examples exist in which a beneficial therapeutic effect has been demonstrated to result from this mechanism. An alternative strategy, under study for sickle cell disease, is to increase the expression of a normal gene that compensates for the effect of mutation at another locus. This example illustrates a concept that is likely to be applicable to a variety of conditions.

**Butyrate Therapy in Sickle Cell Disease.** Sickle cell disease causes illness both because of the anemia and the sickling of red blood cells (see Chapter 11). Two observations suggested that induction of an increase in the level of hemoglobin (Hb) F ($\alpha_2\gamma_2$) would benefit patients with this disorder. First, HbF is a perfectly adequate oxygen carrier in postnatal life, although its abundance in adult red blood cells of normal humans is low (<1 percent of the total hemoglobin). Second, the polymerization of deoxyhemoglobin S is inhibited by HbF, and the high levels of HbF (to levels in excess of 20 g/100 ml) in sickle cell patients from some parts of India and Saudi Arabia have been shown to ameliorate the clinical severity of the disease. (The genetic basis of their increased $\gamma$-gene expression, a form of hereditary persistence of fetal hemoglobin [see Chapter 11], is unknown.)

The recognition that butyrate might increase the expression of the $\gamma$-globin gene arose from the observation that in infants of diabetic mothers, high plasma concentrations of $\alpha$-amino-n-butyric acid are associated with a delay in the postnatal $\gamma$- to $\beta$-gene switch (see Fig. 11–4). Subsequently, a number of studies of patients with sickle cell disease have shown that butyrate administration does indeed increase $\gamma$-globin gene expression by an unknown mechanism (Fig. 13–9). Further work is required to establish the long-term benefits of this treatment and to identify side effects. At a minimum, these observations demonstrate that, in a clinical setting, it is possible to increase the postnatal expression of genes to a therapeutically significant degree.

## Modification of the Somatic Genome by Transplantation

Transplanted cells retain the genotype of the donor, and, consequently, transplantation can be regarded as a form of gene transfer therapy because it leads to a modification of the somatic genome. Because the

TABLE 13–5
**Treatment by Modification of the Genome or Its Expression**

| Type of Modification | Example | Status |
|---|---|---|
| **Pharmacological modulation of gene expression** | Butyrate therapy to stimulate $\gamma$-globin (and thus HbF) synthesis in sickle cell disease and $\beta$-thalassemia | Investigational |
| **Partial modification of the somatic genotype** | | |
| By transplantation | Bone marrow transplantation in $\beta$-thalassemia | Curative with HLA-matched donor; good results overall |
| | Bone marrow transplantation in storage diseases, e.g., Hurler syndrome | Excellent results in some diseases, even if the brain is affected, such as in Hurler syndrome |
| | Liver transplantation in $\alpha_1$-antitrypsin deficiency | Up to 80% survival over 5 yr for genetic liver disease |
| By gene transfer into somatic tissues | Hemophilia B | Investigational: an initial trial in 3 patients using intramuscular injection of low doses of an adeno-associated virus expressing factor IX led to modest changes in clinical end points |

genome of the recipient remains unchanged in all other cells, the recipient becomes, in effect, a mosaic. There are two general indications for the use of transplantation in the treatment of genetic disease. First, cells or organs may be transplanted *to introduce wild-type copies of a gene* into a patient with mutation(s) in that gene. This indication has the ironic consequence that a grossly normal organ is sometimes removed because its biochemical dysfunction is damaging another tissue. This is the case, for example, in homozygous FH, for which liver transplantation is an effective but high-risk procedure. As experience with partial transplantation (e.g., of liver cells to an ectopic location) grows, however, and once gene transfer therapy is successful, whole organ transplants for this reason may become less frequent. The second and more common indication for transplantation is one of *cell replacement*, to compensate for an organ damaged by genetic disease (e.g., a liver that has become cirrhotic in $\alpha_1$-AT deficiency). Some examples of the uses of transplantation in genetic disease are provided in Table 13–5.

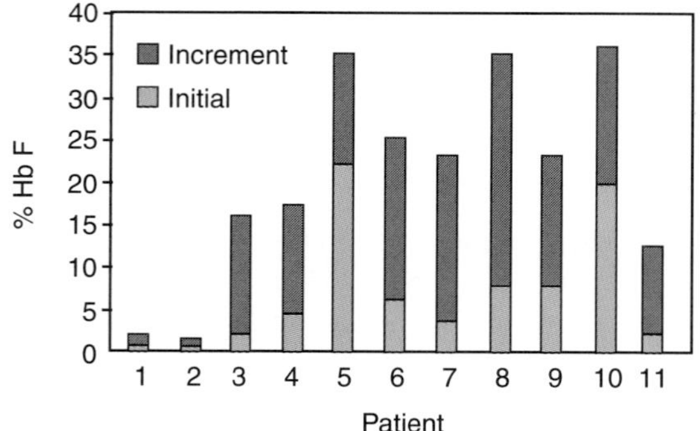


**Figure 13–9.** The effect of pulsed butyrate administration on the percentage of hemoglobin (HbF) in 11 patients with sickle cell disease. Each bar graph shows the initial HbF levels and the increase in HbF during therapy in 11 patients. Each patient received the drug for 4 days (the "pulse"), followed by 10 to 24 days without it. The HbF levels increased from a mean of 7.2 percent to a mean of 21 percent on butyrate. (Adapted from Atweh GF, Sutton M, Nassif I, et al [1999] Sustained induction of fetal hemoglobin by pulse butyrate therapy in sickle cell disease. Blood 93:1790–1797.)

### Bone Marrow Transplantation in Nonstorage Diseases

In addition to its extensive use in the management of cancer, bone marrow transplantation is also the treatment of choice for a selected group of monogenic immune deficiency disorders, including SCID of any type. Apart from a few other conditions with no other effective therapy, its role in the management of genetic disease in general is less certain and under careful evaluation. For example, conventional treatment of patients with thalassemia by means of frequent transfusions and iron chelation has, in some centers, produced excellent results. On the other hand, excellent outcomes have also been obtained with bone marrow transplantation in the treatment of patients with $\beta$-thalassemia younger than 16 years. More than 90 percent of patients with normal liver function and a history of good chelation therapy have 3-year survivals that are free of untoward events. Before any decision can be made concerning the best mode of treatment (standard versus bone marrow transplantation), long-term evaluation must be made of patients who were relatively healthy before the initiation of treatment and then were treated with one or the other approach. The role of bone marrow transplantation in patients with some lysosomal storage diseases is discussed later.

**Transplantation of Hematopoietic Stem Cells from Placental Blood.** Stem cells are self-renewing cells defined by two properties: (1) they can proliferate to make differentiated cell types of a tissue in vivo, and, once developed, (2) they can continue to self-renew for the lifetime of the organism. Embryonic stem cells—which can give rise to the whole organism—are discussed in Chapter 17. At present, the only stem cell of clinical relevance is the hematopoietic stem cell, which can reconstitute the blood system after bone marrow transplantation. Although bone marrow has long been the major source of transplantable hematopoietic stem cells and progenitor cells, the discovery that placental blood (which is readily available) represents a rich source of hematopoietic stem cells is beginning to make a substantial impact on the treatment of malignancy and genetic disease.

The use of placental blood has three great advantages over bone marrow as a source of hematopoietic stem cells. First, recipients are more tolerant of histoincompatible placental blood than of other allogeneic donor cells. Thus, engraftment occurs even if as many as three HLA antigens are mismatched between the donor and the recipient. Second, the wide availability of placental blood, together with the increased tolerance of histoincompatible donor cells, greatly expands the number of potential donors for any recipient. The latter feature is of particular significance to patients from minority ethnic groups, for whom the pool of potential donors is relatively small. Third, the risk of graft-versus-host disease is substantially reduced using placental blood cells as the donor source. It is likely that the isolation and characterization of stem cells from other tissues, including the nervous system, will eventually make cell replacement feasible in a wide variety of malignancies and genetic diseases.

## Bone Marrow Transplantation in Lysosomal Storage Diseases

**Mechanism of Effect.** In the late 1980s, a cautiously encouraging picture began to emerge from animal and human studies of bone marrow transplantation in lysosomal storage diseases. In acting through the two mechanisms depicted in Figure 13–10, bone marrow transplants are effective in correcting lysosomal storage in many tissues, including, in some diseases, the brain. First, the transplanted cells are a source of lysosomal enzymes that can be transferred to other cells through the extracellular fluid, as initially shown by the cocultivation experiments of Neufeld and colleagues with Hurler and Hunter syndrome cells (see Chapter 12). Because bone marrow–derived cells constitute about 10 percent of the total cell mass of the body, the quantitative impact of enzymes transferred from them may be significant. Second, the mononuclear-phagocyte system in most if not all tissues is derived from bone marrow stem cells, so that, after bone marrow transplantation, this system is of donor origin throughout the body. Of special note are the brain perivascular microglial cells, whose marrow origin may partially account for the correction of nervous system abnormalities by bone marrow transplantation in some storage disorders.

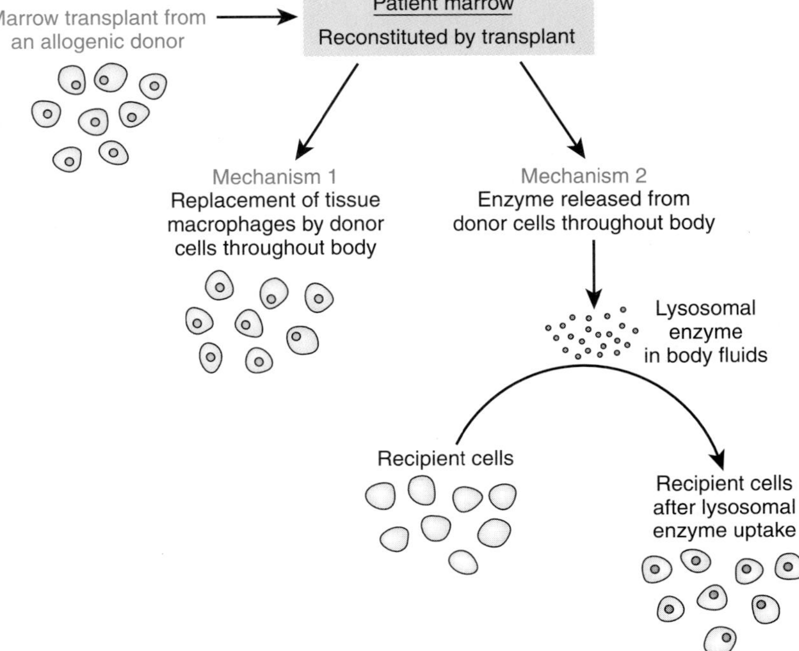


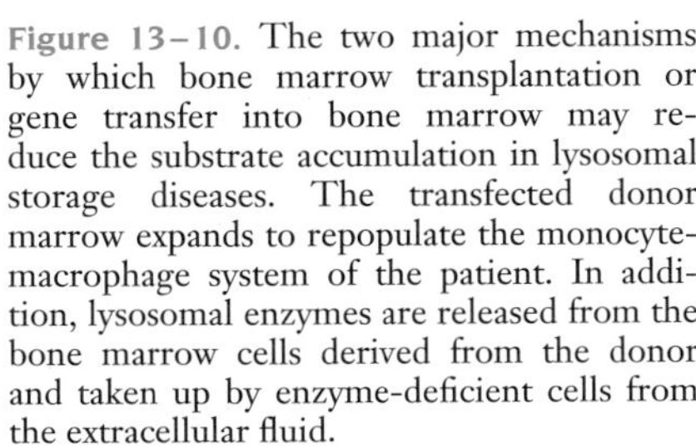
**Figure 13–10.** The two major mechanisms by which bone marrow transplantation or gene transfer into bone marrow may reduce the substrate accumulation in lysosomal storage diseases. The transfected donor marrow expands to repopulate the monocyte-macrophage system of the patient. In addition, lysosomal enzymes are released from the bone marrow cells derived from the donor and taken up by enzyme-deficient cells from the extracellular fluid.

It is now well established that bone marrow transplantation corrects or reduces the visceral abnormalities of many storage diseases. For example, as might be predicted from the efficacy of enzyme therapy (described earlier), patients with Gaucher disease are cured by the enzyme transfer conferred by donor bone marrow cells, with corrections of the growth delay, bone pain, and splenomegaly. A comparable normalization or reduction in the size of the liver, spleen, and heart is also achieved in Hurler syndrome (see Chapter 12), and improvements in upper airway obstruction, joint mobility, and corneal clouding are also obtained. The skeletal abnormalities of Hurler syndrome are generally not corrected by bone marrow transplantation, however, and this lack of effect on the skeletal disease is the case with other storage diseases as well.

The most rewarding outcome after bone marrow transplantation in patients with Hurler disease is the effect of this treatment on the brain. Patients with Hurler syndrome who have good developmental indices before transplantation and who undergo transplantation before 24 months of age continue to develop cognitively after transplantation, in contrast to the inexorable loss of intellectual function that otherwise occurs. Interestingly, a gene dosage effect is manifested in the donor marrow: children who receive cells from homozygous normal donors appear to be more likely to retain fully normal intelligence than the recipients of heterozygous donor cells.

An even more dramatic effect on the neurological component of a storage disease has been observed after bone marrow transplantation of patients with the late-onset form of globoid cell leukodystrophy (or Krabbe disease), a white-matter degenerative disorder. Patients with the late-onset form of this disease, which is due to a deficiency of the enzyme galactocerebrosidase, have a clinical onset at 0.5 to 3 years. The disorder is characterized by a relentless degeneration of central and peripheral myelin, spasticity, dementia, and a peripheral neuropathy. Patients who have undergone transplants have experienced not only an arrest of the disease process but also actual improvement or normalization of tremors, ataxia, motor incoordination, and other abnormalities. Furthermore, the white-matter structural defects in the brains of these patients are often reversible (Fig. 13–11). The success of bone marrow transplantation in the treatment of some storage disorders bodes well for the efficacy of gene transfer therapy in many of these conditions. In this case, the gene of interest will be transferred into the patient's own cultured stem cells, preceding marrow transplantation.

## Liver Transplantation

For some metabolic liver diseases, liver transplantation is the treatment of choice because it is the only treatment of known benefit. For example, the chronic liver disease associated with cystic fibrosis and $\alpha_1$-AT

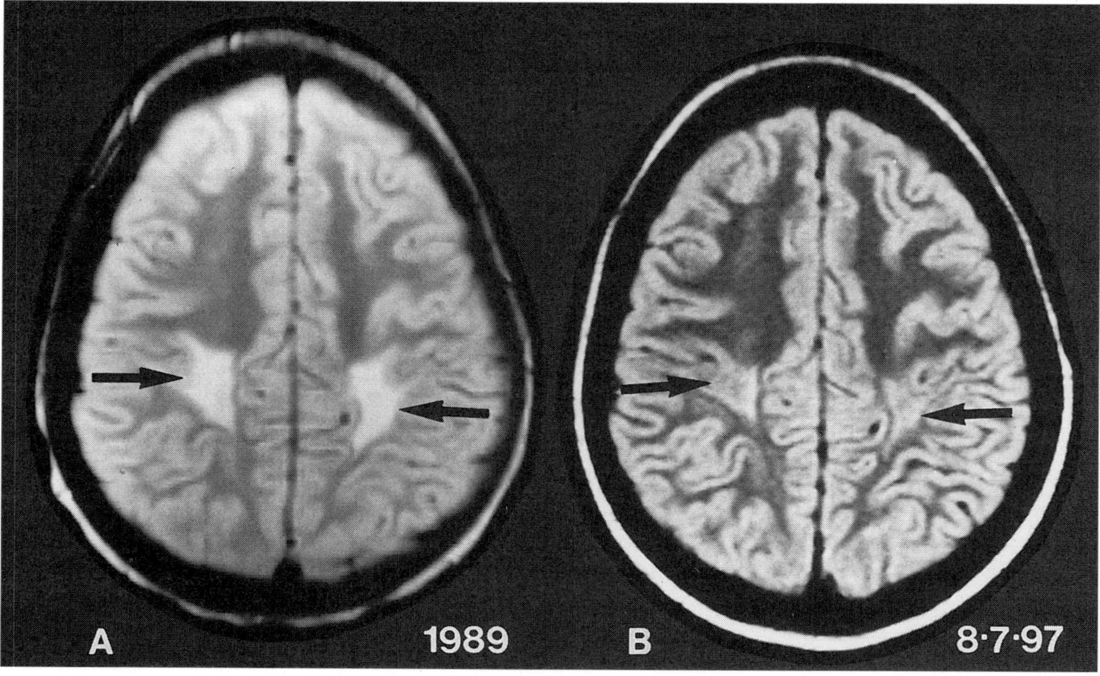


**Figure 13–11.** The effect of bone marrow transplantation on white matter abnormalities in a patient with the late-onset form of globoid cell leukodystrophy. Eight years after transplantation, the increased white matter signal seen pretreatment is greatly reduced. (From Krivit W et al [1998] Hematopoietic stem-cell transplantation in globoid cell leukodystrophy. N Engl J Med 338:1119–1126, copyright © 1998 Massachusetts Medical Society. All rights reserved.)

deficiency can be treated only by liver transplantation, and together these two disorders account for a large fraction of all the liver transplants performed in the pediatric population. Liver transplantation has now been performed for two dozen genetic diseases. At present, the 5-year survival rate of all children who receive liver transplants is in the range of 70 to 85 percent. For almost all of these patients, the quality of life is generally much improved, the specific metabolic abnormality necessitating the transplant is corrected (as in homozygous FH), and, in those conditions in which hepatic damage has occurred (such as $\alpha_1$-AT deficiency), the provision of healthy hepatic tissue restores growth and normal pubertal development.

### The Problems and the Future of Transplantation

There are two major problems limiting the wider use of transplantation. First, the mortality after transplantation is significant, and the morbidity from superimposed infection due to the requirement for immunosuppression and to graft-versus-host disease is substantial. The ultimate goal of transplantation research—transplantation without immunosuppression—comes incrementally closer, and if this is ever achieved, the current therapeutic status of many diseases, both genetic and acquired, will be transformed. The increased tolerance of the recipient to donor stem cells from cord blood (compared with bone marrow–derived donor cells) exemplifies the advances in this area. In addition to the need for immunosuppression, a second problem is the finite supply of organs. For example, for all indications, between 4000 and 5000 liver transplants may be needed annually in the United States alone. In addition, it remains to be demonstrated that transplanted organs are generally capable of functioning normally for a lifetime.

One solution that would circumvent many of the problems associated with allogenic transplantation involves the combination of stem cell and gene therapy. In this situation, a patient's own stem cells would be cultured in vitro, transfected by gene therapy with the gene of interest, and returned to the patient to repopulate the affected tissue with genetically restored cells. The identification of stem cells in a variety of adult human tissues and recent advances in gene transfer therapy offer great promise in this regard.

## Gene Therapy

Recombinant DNA technology has made it possible to consider the correction of genetic disease at the most fundamental level, the gene. Gene therapy is the introduction of a gene into a cell for the purpose of achieving a therapeutic effect. By transferring functional copies of the relevant gene to the patient, correction of the reversible features of the mutant phenotype should, in principle, be possible. The *permanent* genetic cure of an inherited human disease has not yet been demonstrated, but a large number of clinical trials are under way to evaluate both the safety and efficacy of gene transfer therapy. The major conclusions of a 1995 National Institutes of Health panel on the status and promise of gene therapy still hold: progress in this field has been slow, the research emphasis has not always been appropriate, and early claims of efficacy were overstated. Nevertheless, the panel concluded that gene therapy holds great long-term promise for the treatment of human disease.

Preclinical studies in animals and initial trials in humans both suggest that gene therapy will ultimately be successful in numerous diseases, although many difficulties must be overcome. As described later, one trial in two patients with a form of SCID appears to have corrected the disease, at least in the short term. Another study of factor IX gene therapy in three patients with hemophilia B had no untoward effects and a modest clinical improvement. In this section, we outline the potential, methods, and probable limitations of gene transfer for the treatment of human genetic disease. The minimal requirements that must be met before the use of gene transfer can be considered for the treatment of a genetic disorder are presented in the box (next page).

### Gene Therapy: General Considerations

The goal of gene therapy is to improve a patient's health by correction of the mutant phenotype. For this purpose, the delivery of the normal gene to appropriate *somatic* cells (as opposed to the germline) is required. Quite apart from the ethical and technical difficulties involved, it is neither necessary nor desirable to alter the germline of the patient being treated for a genetic disease. One risk is that any effort to integrate a normal copy of a gene into the germline (or into a fertilized egg) would carry a substantial risk of introducing new mutation.

The introduction of a gene into somatic cells may be required for one of three purposes (Fig. 13–12). First, gene therapy may be able to **compensate** for a mutant cellular gene that has a loss-of-function mutation. For such diseases, the introduction of normal functional copies of a gene would suffice to correct a reversible phenotype, such as the increased phenylalanine level in PKU (in this case, the patient's mutant gene or genes are left in place). In these instances, it would generally not be important where in

## Minimal Requirements for Gene Therapy for a Genetic Disorder

1. Identification of the affected locus or at least of the biochemical basis of the disorder.
2. A complementary DNA (cDNA) clone of the gene, the gene itself (particularly if it is not large), or a functional version of the gene from which noncritical components have been removed to reduce its size.
3. A substantial disease burden and a favorable risk-benefit ratio in comparison with alternative therapy.
4. Sufficient knowledge of the molecular basis of the disease to be confident that the gene transfer is likely to ameliorate or correct the biochemical pathology and to prevent or reverse critical phenotypic abnormalities. Whereas loss of function mutations will require replacement with a functional gene, some dominant alleles, such as dominant negative alleles, will require inactivation of the mutant gene or its products.
5. Appropriate regulatory components for the transferred gene. Tight regulation of the level of gene expression is relatively unimportant in some diseases and critical in others. In thalassemia, for example, overexpression of the transferred gene would cause a new imbalance of globin chains, whereas low levels of expression would be ineffective. In contrast, in some enzymopathies, abnormally high levels of expression may have no adverse effect.
6. An appropriate target cell with, ideally, a long half-life or good replicative potential in vivo.
7. Adequate data from cultured cell and animal studies to indicate that the vector, gene construct, and target cell are both efficacious and safe.
8. Protocol review and approval by an Institutional Review Board and, in most countries, an oversight governmental agency.

the genome of a cell the transferred gene inserts. To function in cells into which it is introduced, the product of the transferred gene would need to have access to appropriate cofactors or other molecules essential for its function. For example, the cofactor for phenylalanine hydroxylase, tetrahydrobiopterin or $BH_4$ (see Chapter 12), would have to be given orally if this enzyme were introduced into bone marrow or muscle cells, which do not normally synthesize $BH_4$.

Second, gene therapy may be undertaken to **replace or inactivate** a dominant mutant gene whose abnormal product causes the (generally dominant) disease. Gene replacement of all or part of a mutant gene at the normal locus is much more difficult. This strategy would be required, for example, to replace a Huntington disease gene containing an expanded CAG repeat or at least most of the CAG expansion itself. Alternatively, gene "surgery" of this type could also be achieved by modifying or degrading the mutant RNA rather than the gene that encodes it. For example, selective degradation of a mutant mRNA encoding a dominant negative pro$\alpha_1$(I) collagen that causes osteogenesis imperfecta (see Chapter 12) should, in principle, prevent the bony abnormalities of this disorder. Therapeutic genes that encode RNA enzymes, or ribozymes, designed to degrade only the mRNA from the mutant allele, have shown much promise in laboratory studies. Although such methods are likely to be feasible, this type of gene therapy research is still in its early stages. Third, gene therapy may be most widely used to achieve a **pharmacological effect** to counteract the effects of a mutant cellular gene or genes or to counteract disease pathogenesis in some other way. Patients with acquired diseases, including cancer, are likely to benefit from this strategy (see Fig. 13–12, *B–D*).

In this discussion, we use the term "transferred gene" to refer to any DNA construct that contains the coding sequences of the gene in question, under the control of appropriate regulatory elements. Most often, a transferred gene consists of a cDNA under the control of a promoter that may not necessarily be the natural promoter of the gene (Fig. 13–13). The regulatory elements must be chosen so that the gene is transcribed in the target cells at adequate levels and, if required, is responsive to essential regulatory signals.

### The Target Cell

One of the critical considerations in choosing an appropriate target cell is that it have either a long in vivo half-life or significant replicative potential, so that the biological effect of the transfer can be of useful duration. The ideal target cells are stem cells (which are self-replicating) or progenitor cells with substantial replication potential. Introduction of the gene into stem cells can result in the expression of the transferred gene in a large population of daughter cells. At present, bone marrow is the only tissue for which stem cells or progenitor cells could be used as recipients of transferred genes. Bone marrow transfer will be appropriate both for diseases affecting blood

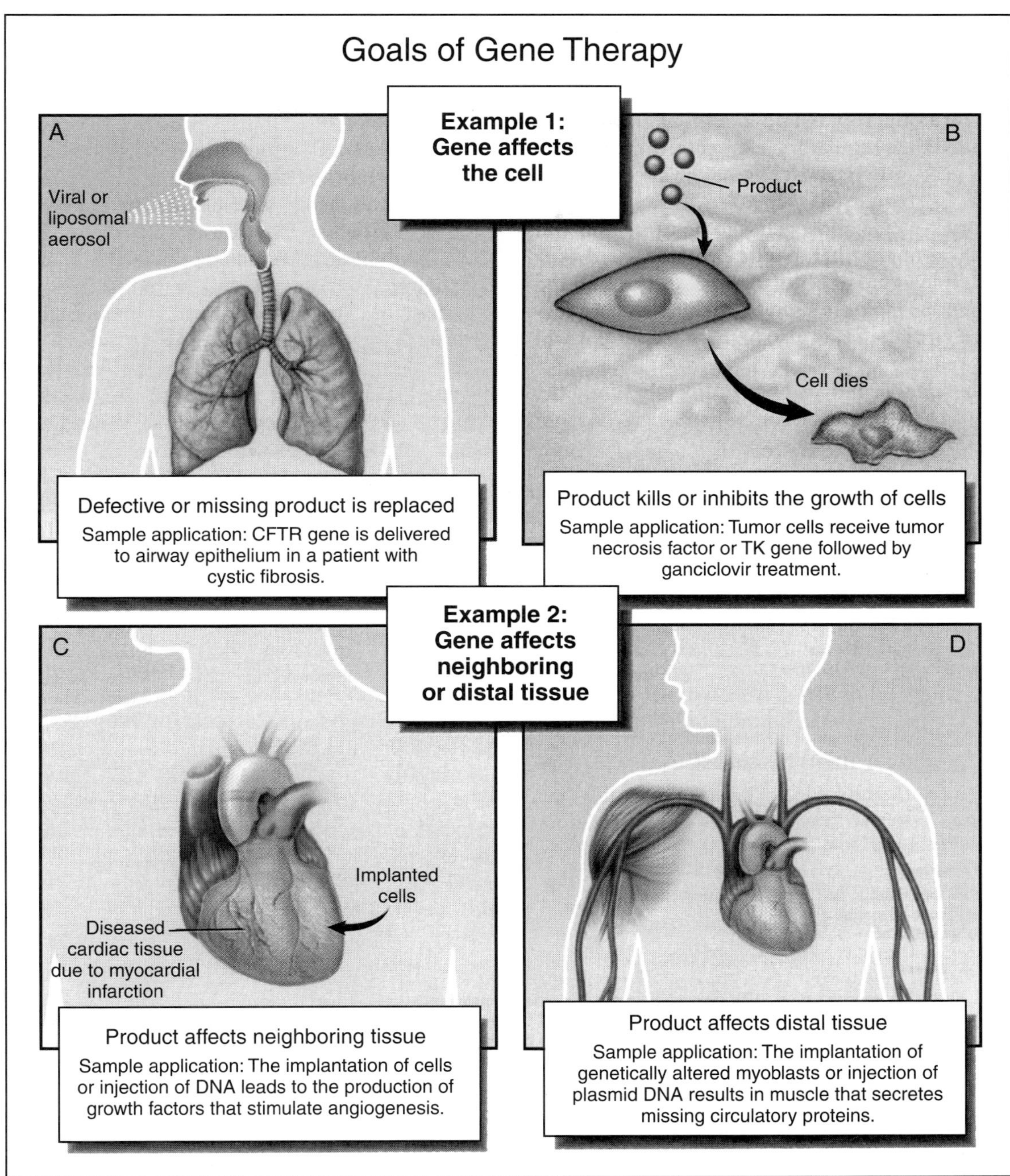


Figure 13–12. Four types of gene therapy. CFTR denotes the cystic fibrosis transmembrane conductance regulator, and TK denotes the herpes simplex virus thymidine kinase. Example D illustrates the strategy used in one of the first human gene therapy experiments shown to have some clinical benefit, the injection and expression of the factor IX gene in muscle of patients with hemophilia B (see text). (Reproduced, with permission, from Blau HM, Springer ML [1995] Gene therapy—a novel form of drug delivery. N Engl J Med 333:1204–1207, copyright © 1995 Massachusetts Medical Society. All rights reserved.)

cells, such as thalassemia and sickle cell disease, and for other diseases that do not involve the blood system per se (e.g., PKU). In the latter instance, the circulation would deliver the substrate to the enzyme in the marrow and also remove the product. Gene transfer therapy into blood stem cells is also likely to be effective for the treatment of storage diseases for which bone marrow transplantation has been effective (see earlier discussion).

Other strategies must be used for cells that cannot divide extensively in culture and then be reimplanted in the patient, or that do not have identifiable stem or progenitor cells in the mature animal. For example, hepatocytes can be briefly maintained in primary culture, transfected with a gene, and then returned to the animal. Alternatively, direct introduction of the gene into the target cells in vivo (e.g., by injection) has been demonstrated with many cell types, includ-

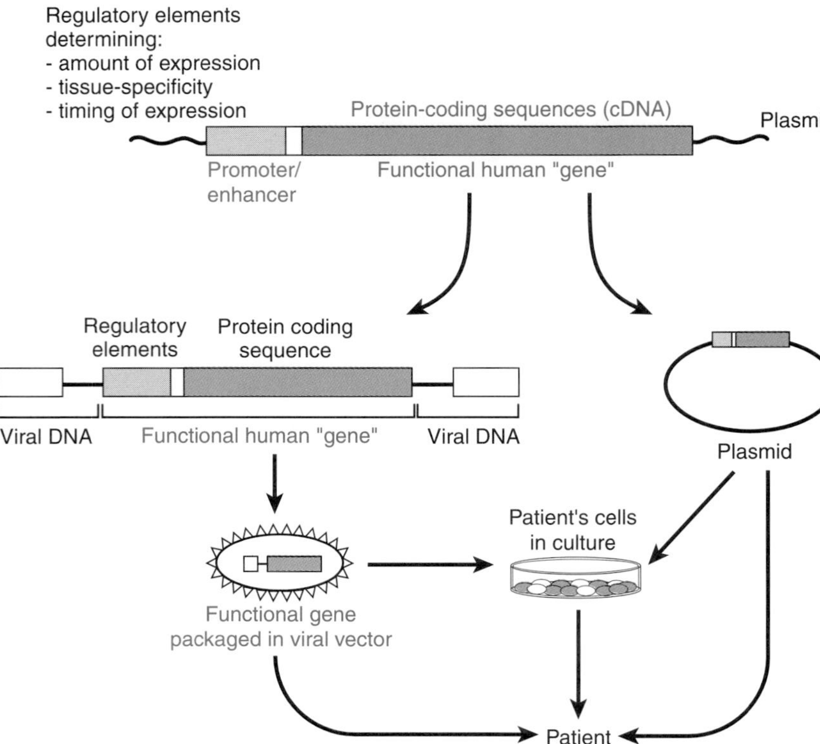


**Figure 13–13.** The two strategies that can be used to transfer a gene to a patient with a genetic disease, based on expression of a human "gene" modified for use in gene transfer using a plasmid vector (*right*) or based on a retroviral vector containing a human cDNA (*left*). The viral components at the ends of the molecule are required for the integration of the vector into the host genome.

ing liver and muscle. Endothelial cells may prove to be particularly useful targets for gene transfer because they line the walls of blood vessels. The protein product of a gene expressed in endothelial cells can be designed for release into the circulation to achieve a systemic effect. An important logistical consideration arises with all of these approaches: the number of cells into which the gene must be introduced may be very large. For example, the approximate number of liver cells into which a gene would have to be transferred to correct a typical inborn error of metabolism, such as PKU, is about 5 percent of the hepatocyte mass, or approximately $10^{10}$ cells (assuming that the level of expression of the transferred gene is similar to wild type).

It should not be forgotten that the target cell must also provide any additional proteins or ligands required for the biological activity of the polypeptide (see Table 11–1).

## Gene Transfer Strategies

An appropriately engineered gene may be transferred into target cells by one of two general strategies (see Fig. 13–13). The first involves ex vivo introduction of the gene into cells that have been cultured from the patient and that are reintroduced after the gene transfer. In the second approach, the gene is injected directly in vivo into the tissue or extracellular fluid of interest (from which it is selectively taken up by the target cells). Targeting of this type is usually achieved by modifying the coat of a viral vector so that only the designated cells bind the viral particles.

## DNA Transfer into Cells: Viral Vectors

The ideal vector for gene therapy would be safe, readily made, easily introduced into the appropriate target tissue, and provide life-long expression of the gene of interest at appropriate levels. At present, no vector—viral or nonviral—has been identified that fulfills all of these criteria. Indeed, no single vector is likely to be satisfactory in all respects for all types of gene therapy (see Fig. 13–12), and a repertoire of vectors will probably be required. Here, we briefly review three of the most widely used classes of viral vectors, those derived from **retroviruses, adenoviruses**, and **adeno-associated virus**.

One of the most widely used classes of vectors is derived from retroviruses, simple RNA viruses with only three structural genes that can be removed and replaced with the gene to be transferred (see Fig. 13–13). A major advantage of viral vectors is that they are capable of entering virtually every cell in the target population. The current generation of retroviral vectors has been engineered to render them incapable of replication. Their other merits include the facts that they are nontoxic to the cell, that only a low number of copies of the viral DNA (with the transferred gene) integrate into the host genome, that the integrated DNA is stable, and that retroviral vectors can accommodate rather large segments of added DNA (up to 8 kb), commodious enough for many genes (but by no means all) that might be transferred. A major limitation of many retroviral vectors is that the viral DNA does not integrate into the host DNA of nondividing cells, precluding the use of such vectors in many tissues. **Lentiviruses**, however, the class of retroviruses that includes the human immunodeficiency virus, may be capable of DNA integration in many slowly dividing or nondividing cells, including neurons. Early experimental work offers hope that these vectors may indeed be suitable for the treatment of neurological disorders.

Adenoviral vectors have the advantages that they can be obtained at high titer; that they will infect a wide variety of cell types, dividing or nondividing; and that they can accommodate inserts of 30 to 35 kb. Their major limitations are that they are episomal and expressed only transiently (weeks) in the target cells and that the viral proteins elicit strong immune and inflammatory responses. The adeno-associated virus, in contrast, is widespread in the human population and has no known adverse effects. Moreover, it infects dividing or nondividing cells on in vivo administration and can exist either episomally or stably integrated into a host chromosome. The disadvantages include the fact that the current adeno-associated virus vectors can accommodate inserts of up to only 5 kb.

### DNA Transfer into Cells: Nonviral Vectors

In principle, nonviral vectors are attractive because they lack the biological risks (e.g., viral contamination) associated with viral vectors and because their preparation, at least theoretically, is more straightforward. Nonviral vectors are of four general types:

1. **Naked DNA**, for example, a cDNA with regulatory elements in a plasmid;
2. **DNA packaged in liposomes**, a continuous lipid bilayer encasing an aqueous volume;
3. **Protein-DNA conjugates**, in which DNA is complexed to a protein—such as a peptide that binds to a cell surface receptor—that facilitates entry of the complex into cells or into a subcellular compartment; and
4. **Artificial chromosomes**, in which the minimal functional components of a natural chromosome (see Chapter 3) are combined with a cDNA or gene of interest, with appropriate regulatory elements.

Although the potential of nonviral vectors is substantial, their overall success has been limited. The major difficulties are twofold: DNA introduced by these vectors tends to be taken up by lysosomes and degraded, and, in addition, DNA that escapes this fate is not taken up efficiently by the nucleus. In addition, each of the nonviral systems has its characteristic problems. For example, the delivery of naked DNA is highly inefficient, although it may be very useful if it can be injected directly into the tissue of interest and when only a transient effect is required, as, for example, in the treatment of malignancy. Liposomes are difficult to target to the tissue of interest, and the design and construction of artificial chromosomes are still at an early stage. Moreover, the introduction of large artificial chromosomes (potentially well over a megabase in size) into a substantial number of cells is difficult, except by direct injection. Thus, the technology and biology of nonviral vectors is still at too early a stage to allow us to define their true potential for the treatment of disease.

### Risks of Gene Therapy

Gene therapy for the treatment of human disease has both demonstrated and theoretical risks that are of three general types. First, at least one patient has died, apparently from an adverse reaction to the adenoviral vector with which he was injected. Thus, principal among the concerns is that the patient will have an adverse reaction to the vector or the transferred gene. Such problems should be largely anticipated with appropriate animal and preliminary human studies. Second is the concern that the transferred gene will integrate into the patient's DNA and activate a proto-oncogene or disrupt a tumor-suppressor gene, leading possibly to malignancy (see Chapter 16). The illicit expression of an oncogene is less likely to occur with the current generation of viral vectors, which have been altered to minimize the ability of their promoters to activate the expression of adjacent host genes. Insertional inactivation of a tumor-suppressor gene is likely to be infrequent and, as such, is an acceptable risk in diseases for which there is no therapeutic alternative.

A third risk—that insertional activation could disrupt an essential gene—will, in general, be without significant effect, because such lethal mutations are rare and will kill only single cells. Because the integration site of a viral vector is more or less random, there is little chance that the same gene will be disrupted in more than one cell. The one exception to this statement applies to the germline: an insertion into a gene in the germline could create a dominant disease-causing mutation. Such events, however, are likely to be rare and the risk acceptable, because it would be difficult to justify withholding carefully planned and reviewed trials of gene therapy from patients who have no other recourse. Moreover, the problem of germline modification by disease treatment is not confined to gene therapy. For example, most chemotherapy used in the treatment of malignancy is mutagenic, but this risk is accepted because of the therapeutic benefits.

### Ethical Considerations

As with any new treatment, proposals for trials of gene transfer into patients must be subjected to rigorous scrutiny by regulatory agencies and hospital ethics committees. However, virtually all governmental and religious agencies that have examined proposals for human gene therapy for the treatment of genetic disease have agreed that this therapeutic opportunity should be pursued. In contrast to the transfer of genes into the germline, somatic gene therapy raises few ethical issues that are not routinely considered when other novel therapy is evaluated (e.g., a new anticancer drug).

### Some Candidate Diseases for Gene Therapy

A large number of single-gene disorders, a few of which have been mentioned in the preceding discussion, are potential candidates for correction by gene therapy. These include hematopoietic conditions such as thalassemia, hemophilia, and various forms of immunodeficiency, as well as disorders such as PKU, urea cycle disorders, FH, and $\alpha_1$-AT deficiency, each affecting proteins made in the liver. Additional considerations relevant to the use of gene therapy for four important disorders are outlined here.

**Severe Combined Immunodeficiency.** The first possible cure of an inherited disease by gene therapy was reported early in 2000. Each of the two treated patients had a form of SCID (see Chapter 14), SCID-X1, due to mutations in the X-linked gene encoding the $\gamma$c cytokine receptor subunit of several interleukin receptors. The receptor deficiency causes an early block in T- and natural killer (NK)–lymphocyte growth, survival, and differentiation. Although a successful bone marrow transplantation can be lifesaving in this disorder, patients with SCID-X1 who receive transplants have extremely poor B-cell function. Careful preclinical studies had suggested that a clinical trial was likely to be safe as well as effective. Bone marrow stem cells from the patients were infected in culture (ex vivo) with a retroviral vector that expressed the $\gamma$c subunit cDNA. A selective advantage was conferred on transduced cells, because the subunit transmits survival signals to T-cell progenitors and proliferative signals to NK-lymphocyte progenitors.

Ten months after the gene transfer, T and NK cells expressing the $\gamma$c subunit transgene were still detected in the patients, and T, B, and NK cell counts and function were restored to the levels of age-matched controls. Moreover, dramatic clinical improvement occurred, with resolution of protracted diarrhea and skin lesions and restoration of normal growth and development. No adverse effects were observed. The critical question now is whether the correction is permanent. The on-going survival of the transduced stem cells apparently responsible for the benefits must be documented, and the expression of the transferred gene must be sustained. Irrespective of the long-term outcome of this early success, however, the results demonstrate the great potential of gene therapy for the correction of inherited human disease.

**Hemophilia B.** This X-linked bleeding disorder, which results from mutations in the factor IX gene, is another monogenic disease for which gene therapy has been convincingly shown to have a clinical effect, albeit a modest one. Factor IX is a proenzyme required for the formation of a fibrin clot. Severe hemophilia B results when the level of circulating factor IX is less than 1 percent of normal; a more modest disease occurs with levels between 1 and 5 percent. The regular infusion of clotting factor concentrates to maintain levels above 1 percent prevents the many complications of bleeding, including joint damage.

The potential of a gene therapy trial in patients with hemophilia B was suggested by studies of animals with factor IX deficiency. In two patients, gene therapy with a factor IX–containing adeno-associated virus vector injected into skeletal muscle effected a very small increase in factor IX levels to about 1 percent in one patient and even less in a second patient. More important, the requirement for factor IX infusions in these two patients fell by 50 percent in one and 80 percent in the other for periods of at least 3 months. No untoward effects were observed, germline transmission did not occur, and inhibitory antibodies to factor IX did not form. Because these patients were the first treated in an experimental design of dose escalation and received the lowest doses of the vector, it is hoped that higher doses will be even more beneficial.

**Duchenne Muscular Dystrophy.** The special problem in DMD is the size (11 kb) of the dystrophin cDNA that encodes the protein, too large to be accommodated by the current generation of retroviral vectors. However, the identification of a patient with Becker muscular dystrophy mild enough to allow him to drive his automobile at age 65 suggests that it may not be necessary to use the whole dystrophin coding region for gene transfer. In this patient, the mutant allele (see Fig. 12–16) lacks nearly half the coding region, so that highly repetitive sequences in the rod domain of dystrophin have been deleted. The shortened dystrophin retains sufficient function to prevent the complete DMD phenotype. These findings emphasize the need for basic research to identify the critical functional domains of a protein so that they can be retained in any therapeutic cDNA. As reported earlier for hemophilia B, the direct injection of vectors into muscle can be effective and indicates a potential approach for placing a dystrophin gene into patients with DMD. A second major difficulty with any gene transfer therapy for DMD, however, is the requirement that the gene be placed into a significant fraction of the skeletal muscle mass (and in some patients, into the cardiac muscle, as well). This is a formidable logistical barrier.

**Adenosine Deaminase Deficiency.** The first gene transfer studies for the treatment of a patient with a monogenic disease were performed in 10 patients with ADA deficiency, another cause of SCID (see Fig. 13–7). This condition was chosen because bone marrow transplantation cures the condition and because it was believed that cells carrying the transferred gene would have a selective survival advantage. Autologous T lymphocytes were treated ex vivo with retroviral vectors expressing the ADA cDNA and then reintroduced into the patient (T cells are very long-lived, some for years). Many of the problems that characterize human gene therapy in general are exemplified by these initial ADA trials. At least two key differences may account for the successful treatment of the patients with SCID-X1 and the lack of success in the initial gene therapy efforts in patients with ADA deficiency. First, in contrast to the powerful selection for transduced cells in the patients with SCID-X1, selective pressure was diminished in patients with ADA deficiency by the concurrent administration of PEG-ADA enzyme replacement therapy, which all of the patients with ADA deficiency continued to receive. Second, the technology of gene transfer improved considerably between the early 1990s, when the ADA trials were done, and the year 2000, when the two SCID-X1 patients were treated. Thus, the efficiency of transduction (transfer of DNA into the target cell) was low in the ADA trial, as were the levels of ADA expression in most cases. Although some circulating T cells continued to express the introduced gene at low levels, no clinical benefit could be attributed to gene therapy.

## Problems

1. X-linked granulomatous disease (CGD) is an uncommon disorder characterized by a defect in host defense that leads to severe, recurrent, and often fatal pyogenic infections beginning in early childhood. The X-linked *CGD* locus encodes the heavy chain of cytochrome-*b*, a component of the oxidase that generates superoxide in phagocytes. Because interferon-γ (IFN-γ) was known to enhance the oxidase activity of normal phagocytes, IFN-γ was administered to boys with X-linked CGD to see whether their oxidase activity increased. Before treatment, the phagocytes of *some* less severely affected patients had small but detectable bursts of oxidase activity (unlike those of severely affected patients), suggesting that increased activity in these less severely affected subjects is the result of greater production of cytochrome-*b* from the affected locus. In these less severe cases, IFN-γ increased the cytochrome-*b* content, superoxide production, and killing of *Staphylococcus aureus* in the granulocytes. The IFN-γ effect was associated with a definite increase in the abundance of the cytochrome-*b* chain. Presumably, the cytochrome-*b* polypeptide of these patients is partially functional, and increased expression of the residual function improved the physiological defect. Describe the genetic differences that might account for the fact that the phagocytes of some patients with X-linked CGD respond to IFN-γ in vitro and others do not.

2. Identify some of the restrictions on the types of proteins that can be considered for extracellular replacement therapy, as exemplified by PEG-ADA. What makes this approach inappropriate for phenylalanine hydroxylase deficiency? For Hurler syndrome? For Lesch-Nyhan syndrome? If Tay-Sachs disease caused only liver disease, would this strategy succeed? If not, why?

3. A 3-year-old girl, Rhonda, has FH due to a deletion of the 5′ end of the gene. The mutation removed the promoter and the first two exons of each allele. (Rhonda's parents are second cousins.) You explain to the parents that she will require plasma exchange therapy every 1 to 2 weeks for years. At the clinic, however, they meet another family with a 5-year-old boy with the same disease. The boy has been treated with drugs with some success. Rhonda's parents want to know why she has not been offered similar pharmacological therapy. Explain.

4. What classes of mutations are likely to be found in homocystinuric patients who are not responsive to the administration of large doses (1000 mg/day) of pyridoxine (vitamin $B_6$)? How might you explain the fact that Tom is completely responsive whereas his first cousin Allan has only a partial reduction in plasma homocystine when given the same amount of vitamin $B_6$?

5. You have just cloned the gene for phenylalanine hydroxylase and wish ultimately to introduce it into patients with PKU. Your approach will be to culture cells from the patient, introduce a functional version of the gene into the cells, and reintroduce the cells into the patient.
   (a) What DNA components do you need to make a functional phenylalanine hydroxylase protein in a gene transfer experiment?
   (b) Which tissues would you choose in which to express the enzyme, and why? How does this choice affect your gene construct in (a)?
   (c) You introduce your version of the gene into fibroblasts cultured from a skin biopsy specimen from the patient. Northern (RNA) blot analysis shows that the messenger RNA is present in normal amounts and is the correct size. However, no phenylalanine hydroxylase protein can be detected in the cells. What kinds of abnormalities in the transferred gene would explain this finding?
   (d) You have corrected all the problems identified in (c). On introducing the new version of the gene into the cultured cells, you now find that the phenylalanine

hydroxylase protein is present in great abundance, and when you harvest the cells and assay the enzyme (in the presence of all the required components), normal activity is obtained. However, when you add $^3$H-labeled phenylalanine to the cells in culture, no $^3$H-labeled tyrosine is formed (in contrast, some cultured liver cells produce a large quantity of $^3$H-labeled tyrosine in this situation). What are the most likely explanations for the failure to form $^3$H-tyrosine? How does this result affect your gene therapy approach to patients?

(e) You have developed a method to introduce your functional version of the gene directly into a large proportion of the hepatocytes of patients with phenylalanine hydroxylase deficiency. Unexpectedly, you find that much lower levels of phenylalanine hydroxylase enzymatic activity are obtained in patients in whom significant amounts of the inactive phenylalanine hydroxylase homodimer were detectable in hepatocytes before treatment than in patients who had no detectable phenylalanine hydroxylase polypeptide before treatment. How can you explain this result? How might you overcome the problem?

## General References


Blau HM, Springer ML (1995) Gene therapy—A novel form of drug delivery. N Engl J Med 333:1204–1207.

Desnick RJ (ed) (1991) Treatment of Genetic Diseases. Churchill Livingstone, New York.

Desnick RJ, Schuchman EH (1998) Gene therapy for genetic diseases. Acta Paed Japonica 40:191–203.

Kay M, Russell DW (2000) Gene therapy. *In* Harrison's Principles of Internal Medicine, 15th ed. McGraw Hill, New York.

Orkin S, Motulsky A (1995) Report and recommendations of the panel to assess the NIH investment in research on gene therapy. See online at *http://www.nih.gov/news/panelrep.html.*

Rosenberg LE (1990) Treating genetic diseases: Lessons from three children. Pediatr Res 27:S10–S16.

Scriver CR, Treacy EP (1999) Is there treatment for "genetic" disease? Mol Gen Metab 68:93–102.

Treacy EP, Childs B, Scriver CR (1995) Response to treatment in hereditary metabolic disease: 1993 survey and 10-year comparison. Am J Hum Genet 56:359–367.

Treacy EP, Valle D, Scriver CR (2001) Treatment of genetic disease. *In* Scriver CR, Beaudet AL, Sly WS, Valle D (eds) The Metabolic and Molecular Bases of Inherited Disease, 8th ed. McGraw-Hill, New York.


## References Specific to Particular Topics


Anderson WF (2000) Perspectives: Gene therapy. The best of times, the worst of times. Science 288:627–629.

Atweh GF, Sutton M, Nassif I, et al (1999) Sustained induction of fetal hemoglobin by pulse butyrate therapy in sickle cell disease. Blood 93:1790–1797.

Cavazzana-Calvo M, Hacein-Bey S, de Saint-Basile G, et al (2000) Gene therapy of human severe combined immunodeficiency (SCID)-X1 disease. Science 288:669–672.

Couture LA, Stinchcomb DT (1996) Anti-gene therapy: The use of ribozymes to inhibit gene function. Trends Genet 12:510–514.

Cox DW (2001) $\alpha_1$-AT deficiency. *In* Scriver CR, Beaudet AL, Sly WS, Valle D (eds) The Metabolic and Molecular Bases of Inherited Disease, 8th ed. McGraw-Hill, New York.

Friedmann T (2000) Medical ethics: Principles for human gene therapy studies. Science 287:2163–2165.

Gage FH (2000) Mammalian neural stem cells. Science 287:1433–1438.

Giardini C (1997) Treatment of $\beta$-thalassemia. Curr Opin Hematol 4:79–87.

Goldstein JL, Hobbs HH, Brown MS (2001) Familial hypercholesterolemia. *In* Scriver CR, Beaudet AL, Sly WS, Valle D (eds). The Metabolic and Molecular Bases of Inherited Disease, 8th ed. McGraw-Hill, New York.

Grabowski GA, Leslie N, Wenstrup R (1998) Enzyme therapy for Gaucher disease: The first 5 years. Blood Rev 12:115–133.

Hayes A, Costa T, Scriver CR, Childs B (1985) The effect of mendelian disease on human health. II: Response to treatment. Am J Med Genet 21:243–255.

Hershfield MS (1998) Adenosine deaminase deficiency: Clinical expression, molecular basis, and therapy. Semin Hematol 35:291–298.

Hollon T (2000) Researchers and regulators reflect on first gene therapy death. Nat Med 6:6.

Hoogerbrugge PM, Brouwer OF, Bordigoni P, et al (1995) Allogenic bone marrow transplantation for lysosomal storage diseases. Lancet 345:1398–1402.

Kay MA, Manno CS, Ragni MV, et al (2000) Evidence for gene transfer and expression of factor IX in haemophilia B patients treated with an AAV vector. Nat Genet 24:257–261.

Kelly DA (1998) Current results of evolving indications for liver transplantation in children. J Pediatr Gastroenterol Nutr 27:214–221.

Krivit W, Shapiro EG, Peters C, et al (1998) Hematopoietic stem cell transplantation in globoid-cell leukodystrophy. N Engl J Med 338:1119–1126.

Miano M, Porta F, Locatellie F, et al (1998) Unrelated donor marrow transplantation for inborn errors. Bone Marrow Transplant 21:(Suppl 2) S37–S41.

Oliveri NF (1999) The $\beta$-thalassemias. N Engl J Med 341:99–109.

Parkman R (1998) The future of placental-blood transplantation. N Engl J Med 339:1627–1629.

Peters C, Shapiro EG, Anderson J, et al (1998) Hunter syndrome: II. Outcome of HLA-genotypically identical sibling and HLA-haploidentical related donor bone marrow transplantation in fifty-four children. Blood 91:2601–2608.

Rosenberg LE, Schechter AN (2000) Gene therapist, heal thyself. Science 287:1751.

Scriver CR, Kaufman S (2001) The hyperphenylalaninemias: Phenylalanine hydroxylase deficiency. *In* Scriver CR, Beaudet AL, Sly WS, Valle D (eds). The Metabolic and Molecular Bases of Inherited Disease, 8th ed. McGraw-Hill, New York.

Starzl TE, Demetris AJ (1990) Liver transplantation: A 31-year perspective. Part I. Curr Probl Surg 27:49–116.

Weissman IL (2000) Translating stem and progenitor cell biology to the clinic: Barriers and opportunities. Science 287:1442–1446.

Van der Kooy D, Weiss S (2000) Why stem cells? Science 287:1439–1441.

# 14

# Genetics of the Immune System

The organization and control of the immune system demonstrate several unusual genetic phenomena that are distinctive from other systems: extensive polymorphism of expressed proteins, an obvious evolutionary relationship among its various components, and, especially, a unique system of generating great diversity utilizing relatively few loci. The genes of the immune system are clinically important in relation to transplantation, autoimmune disease, and response to infection; they are also the loci responsible for a number of single-gene disorders. The application of molecular techniques has greatly expanded the understanding of the immune response while at the same time revealing new layers of complexity that remain to be explored.

Higher organisms are unique in their ability to distinguish between "self" and "nonself" and to mount a reaction selectively against a very broad spectrum of foreign antigens. This reaction is mediated by the complex interactive network of cells and cellular cytokines of the immune system and is referred to as the **immune response**. Genetic factors play a key role not only in the generation of the normal immune response but also in the development of aberrant immune reactions and consequent immune-mediated disease. In this chapter we describe the genetic basis of the immune response and discuss a number of diseases in which immune-related genes, such as those of the **major histocompatibility complex** (MHC), contribute to disease susceptibility.

The discussion here is not intended to provide a comprehensive review of immunology or immunogenetics, for which the reader is directed to the General References listed at the end of the chapter. Rather, we introduce some of the gene systems that govern immune function, and we reinforce the concept that, with the exception of monozygotic twins (or identical triplets and other multiple births), each person is genetically unique. Much of human immunological uniqueness depends on the expression of the genes of the MHC, and, thus, in the discussion that follows, we highlight this gene system, as well as two others within the same superfamily that encode additional key components of the immune response: **immunoglobulins** (Igs) and **T-cell antigen receptors** (TCRs).

## THE MAJOR HISTOCOMPATIBILITY COMPLEX

The MHC is composed of a large cluster of genes located on the short arm of chromosome 6 (Fig. 14–1). On the basis of structural and functional differences, these genes are categorized into three classes, each of which is highly complex and polymorphic. Two of the three classes, class I and class II, correspond to the human leukocyte antigen (HLA) genes, originally discovered by virtue of their importance in tissue transplantation between unrelated individuals. These antigens are involved in transplant rejection and are also critical to immunocompetence; they are intricately involved in antigen recognition, lymphocyte interactions, and the development of self-tolerance. The HLA class I and class II genes encode cell surface proteins that play a critical role in the initiation of an immune response and specifically in the "presentation" of antigen to $CD4^+$ helper T lymphocytes and $CD8^+$ cytotoxic T lymphocytes, which cannot recognize and respond to an antigen unless it is complexed with an HLA molecule on the surface of an antigen presenting cell.

The class I genes (*HLA-A*, *HLA-B*, and *HLA-C*) encode antigens that are an integral part of the plasma membrane of nucleated cells (Fig. 14–2). A class I antigen consists of two polypeptide subunits, a variable heavy chain encoded within the MHC, and a nonpolymorphic polypeptide, $\beta_2$-microglobulin, which is encoded by a gene outside the MHC, mapping to chromosome 15. The immune system generally recognizes and responds not to an entire

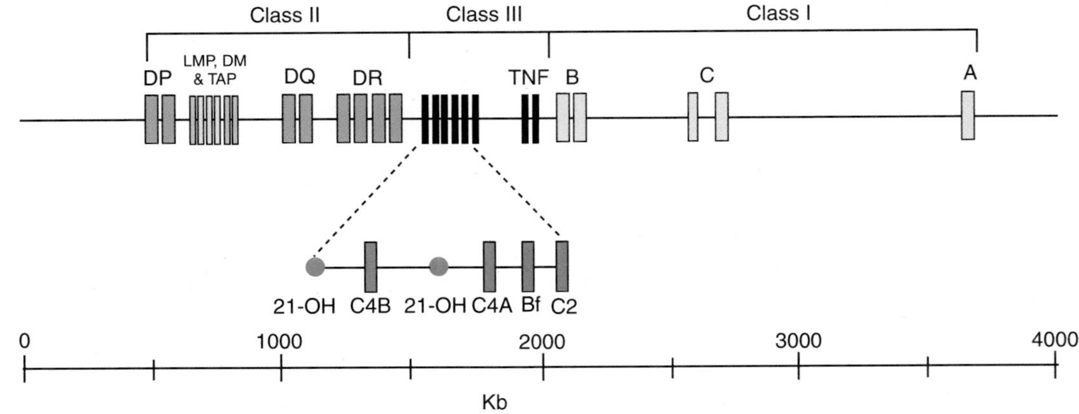


**Figure 14–1.** A schematic of the major histocompatibility complex on chromosome 6p. DP, DQ, and DR = class II antigen genes; B, C, and A = class I antigen genes; LMP = genes encoding components of large multifunctional protease; DM = heterodimer of *DMA* and *DMB* genes encoding antigen-processing molecule required for binding peptide to MHC class II antigens; TAP = transporter associated with antigen processing; TNF = tumor necrosis factor; Bf = properdin factor B; C2, C4A; C4B = complement components; 21-OH = 21-hydroxylase. (One of the 21-OH loci is a pseudogene.) For discussion, see text.

protein but to peptide fragments derived from the protein. Peptide antigens derived from intracellular proteins are generated by proteolytic degradation by a large multifunctional protease (LMP); the peptides are then transported by a transporter associated with antigen processing (TAP) to the cell surface and bound to a class I molecule that displays the peptide antigen to cytotoxic T cells (see Fig. 14–2).

The class II locus is composed of several subregions that encode cell surface antigens, such as *HLA-DP*, *HLA-DQ*, and *HLA-DR*, as well as other polymorphic proteins such as TAP and LMP, which are not cell surface molecules but are involved in processing antigens into peptides for presentation. Like the class I antigens, class II molecules are integral to the cell membrane. Class II molecules are expressed primarily on B lymphocytes, macrophages, and activated T lymphocytes, but under certain conditions they may be expressed by other cell types as well. Each class II molecule is a heterodimer, composed of $\alpha$ and $\beta$ subunits, both of which are encoded by the MHC. Synthesized in the endoplasmic reticulum and released into endosomes, class II heterodimers are bound to an invariant protein, Ii, which must be removed by the DM protein for the class II molecule to bind peptide antigens located within endosomes that were originally derived from endocytosed proteins.

The class III genes are not HLA genes but include genes for polymorphic serum proteins and membrane receptors closely involved in immune function, such as properdin factor Bf and complement proteins C2 and C4 (see Fig. 14–1). A number of other gene loci within the MHC are genetically linked to the HLA

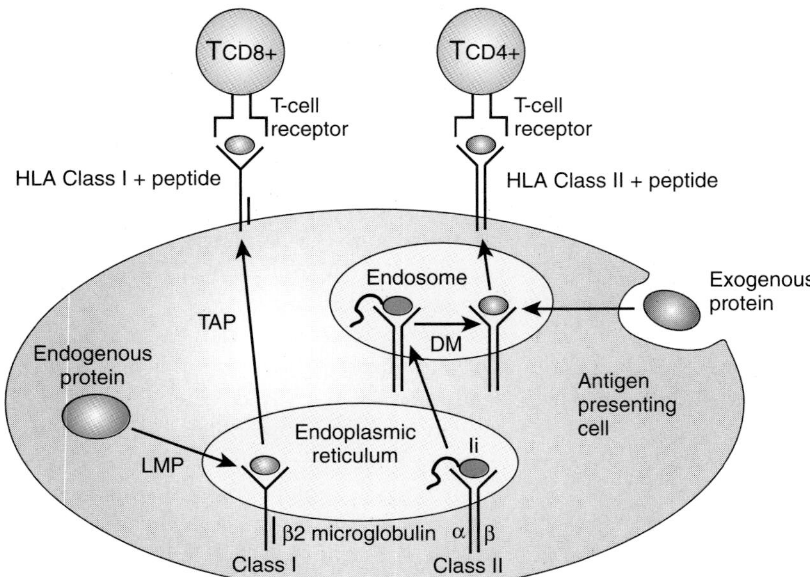


**Figure 14–2.** Schematic representation of the interaction between MHC class I and class II molecules, foreign proteins, and T-cell receptors. LMP = large multifunctional protease; TAP = transporter associated with antigen processing; Ii = invariant chain; DM = heterodimer encoded by the *DMA* and *DMB* genes; $CD8^+$ = cytotoxic T cells; $CD4^+$ = helper T cells. (Adapted, with permission of Elsevier Science, from Thorsby E [1997] HLA associated diseases. Hum Immunol 53:1–11, copyright 1997 by the American Society of Histocompatibility and Immunogenetics.)

genes but are functionally unrelated to them. These include the genes for the tumor necrosis factors, as well as other genes that when defective cause diseases, such as the gene for 21-hydroxylase, involved in **congenital adrenal hyperplasia,** and the gene for **hemochromatosis,** a liver disease caused by iron overload. These genes appear not to function in determining histocompatability or immune responsiveness.

There is a striking similarity, both in organization and in DNA sequence, between HLA class I and class II genes and between the HLA genes and the immunoglobulin and T-cell receptor genes described in the following sections. The similarity among these genes and a number of other genes encoding cell surface molecules has led to their classification into a gene family designated the **immunoglobulin gene superfamily**. The members of the family appear to be evolutionarily related genes, whose products serve a wide variety of functions beyond the immunological role of HLA molecules, immunoglobulins, and T-cell receptors.

## Polymorphism and the Inheritance of HLA Haplotypes

The HLA system is extraordinarily polymorphic. Numerous distinct antigenic variants have already been recognized at the *HLA-A*, *HLA-B*, *HLA-C*, *HLA-DP*, *HLA-DQ*, and *HLA-DR* loci. Table 14–1 indicates the complexity and extensive polymorphism of the system. According to the traditional system of HLA nomenclature, the different alleles were distinguished from one another based on their reaction to a panel of antisera obtained from multiparous females who had naturally developed antibodies against the paternal HLA antigens expressed by their fetuses. Some of these antigenic variants (specificities) are the direct result of amino acid differences in particular $\alpha$ or $\beta$ chains; other variants result from changes in both $\alpha$ and $\beta$. As the genes responsible for encoding the class I and class II MHC antigens were identified and sequenced, the number of HLA alleles has mushroomed enormously. As a result, many HLA alleles initially defined serologically can be shown to consist of two or more alleles because DNA sequence variants were found; for example, 12 different nucleic acid sequence variants of the *HLA-B* gene exist in what was previously defined as a single B27 allele by serological testing! Thus, the MHC consists of a group of the most polymorphic genes in the genome; a large number, but by no means all, of these polymorphisms result in structural (and therefore antigenic) variants of cell surface proteins that are crucially involved in immune defenses.

TABLE 14–1
**Protein and DNA Variation at HLA Loci**

| HLA Locus | Antigenic Variants | DNA Variants |
|---|---|---|
| HLA-A | 25 | 83 |
| HLA-B | 53 | 186 |
| HLA-C | 11 | 42 |
| HLA-DR ($\beta$ chain only) | 20 | 221 |
| HLA-DQ ($\alpha$ and $\beta$ chains) | 9 | 49 |
| HLA-DP ($\alpha$ and $\beta$ chains) | 6 | 88 |

The HLA alleles on a given chromosome are so closely linked that they are transmitted together as a **haplotype** (see Chapter 8). The alleles are codominant; each parent has two haplotypes, expresses both, and, as shown in Figure 14–3, transmits one or the other to each child. As a result, parent and child share only one haplotype, and there is a 25 percent chance that two sibs inherit matching HLA haplotypes. Because acceptance of transplanted tissues largely correlates with the degree of similarity between donor and recipient HLA haplotypes (and ABO blood groups), the favored donor for bone marrow or organ transplantation is an ABO-compatible and HLA-identical sibling of the recipient.

Considerable variation in the profile and frequency of HLA variants exists among different populations. HLA-A2, for example, is among the most frequent *HLA-A* specificities in all populations, whereas

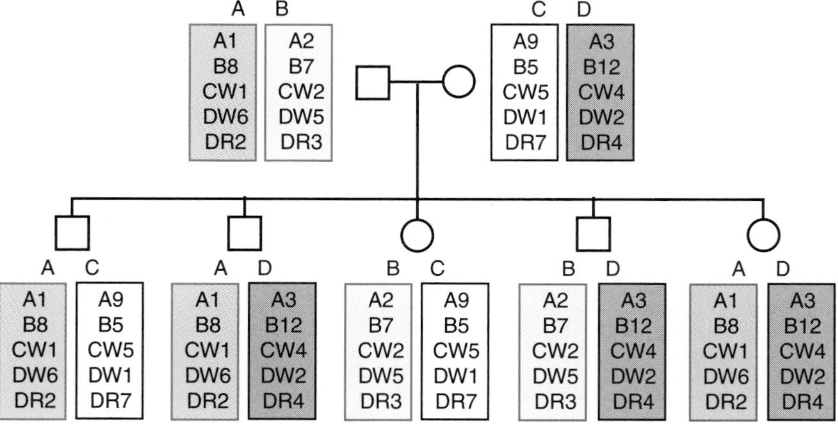


Figure 14–3. The inheritance of HLA haplotypes. Usually a haplotype is transmitted, as shown in this figure, as a unit. In extremely rare instances, a parent will transmit a recombinant haplotype to the child.

HLA-A24 is found in Caucasians but not in African Americans or Asians. The HLA haplotypes also show marked linkage disequilibrium. Certain haplotypes are much more frequent than expected, whereas others are exceptionally rare, and most of the $3 \times 10^7$ phenotypic combinations theoretically possible among Caucasians have never been observed. Sometimes the search for a suitable bone-marrow donor is unsuccessful despite a wide search. In addition to the ethnic distribution of single HLA alleles, there is also a striking ethnic distribution of haplotypes.

## HLA and Disease Association

With the increasing delineation of HLA alleles has come an appreciation of the association between certain diseases and specific HLA antigens or haplotypes. The etiologic basis for most of the HLA-disease associations remains obscure. As is apparent from Table 14–2, most, but not all, of these disorders are **autoimmune**—that is, associated with an abnormal immune response apparently directed against one or more self-antigens that is thought to be related to variation in the immune response resulting from polymorphism in immune response genes. For example, there is a very strong association between HLA-B27 and **ankylosing spondylitis**, a chronic inflammatory disease of the spine and sacroiliac joints. Whereas only 9 percent of Norwegians, for example, are B27-positive, more than 95 percent of those with ankylosing spondylitis are B27-positive. Thus, the relative risk of developing ankylosing spondylitis is at least 150 times higher for people who have HLA-B27 than for those who do not. Even so, less than 5 percent of B27-positive individuals develop the disease, although as many as 20 percent of B27-positive individuals may have very subtle, subclinical manifestations of the disease without any symptoms or disability. Similarly, **Reiter syndrome**, a condition that closely resembles ankylosing spondylitis, is also strongly associated with the B27 antigen.

In other cases, the association between a particular HLA allele or haplotype and a disease is not due to variation in immune response genes but is instead due to linkage disequilibrium between certain MHC alleles and mutations in closely linked genes situated within the MHC complex. For example, the autosomal recessive disorders congenital adrenal hyperplasia due to 21-hydroxylase deficiency and primary hemochromatosis result from mutations in genes that lie within the MHC. Analysis of the various 21-hydroxylase mutations responsible for adrenal hyperplasia has revealed that different mutations at this locus originally occurred on different haplotype backgrounds and have remained in linkage disequilibrium with these specific haplotype markers. Hemochromatosis is a common autosomal recessive disorder of iron overload that was found to be strongly associated with the HLA-A3 allele. More than 80 percent of patients with hemochromatosis are homozygous for a common mutation in the hemochromatosis gene (*HFE*) that is located near to *HLA-A* (see Fig. 14–1) and is in strong linkage disequilibrium with the HLA-A3 allele. *HFE* does not encode an immune response or MHC class I protein; instead, it appears to be involved with iron transport or metabolism in the intestine.

Finally, in still other cases, it is unclear whether a particular HLA haplotype is associated with a disease

TABLE 14–2
**HLA Alleles with Striking Disease Associations**

| Disease | HLA Allele | *Frequency (%) | | |
|---|---|---|---|---|
| | | *Patients* | *Controls* | †*Odds Ratio* |
| Ankylosing spondylitis | B27 | >95 | 9 | >150 |
| Reiter syndrome | B27 | >80 | 9 | >40 |
| Acute anterior uveitis | B27 | 68 | 9 | >20 |
| Subacute thyroiditis | B35 | 70 | 14 | 14 |
| Psoriasis vulgaris | Cw6 | 87 | 33 | 7 |
| Narcolepsy | DQ6 | >95 | 33 | >38 |
| Grave disease | DR3 | 65 | 27 | 4 |
| Rheumatoid arthritis | DR4 | 81 | 33 | 9 |
| Juvenile rheumatoid arthritis | DR8 | 38 | 7 | 8 |
| Celiac disease | DQ2 | 99 | 28 | >250 |
| Multiple sclerosis | DR2, DQ6 | 86 | 33 | 12 |
| Insulin-dependent diabetes | DQ8 | 81 | 23 | 14 |
| Insulin-dependent diabetes | DQ6 | <1 | 33 | 0.02 |
| Hemochromatosis | A3 | 75 | 13 | 20 |
| Congenital adrenal hyperplasia (21-OH deficiency) | Bw47 | 25 | 0.2 | 80–150 |

* Frequency data are for Norwegian populations and are approximate; †The odds ratio is approximate and is calculated as ad/bc where a = number of patients with the antigen, b = number of controls with the antigen, c = number of patients without the antigen, d = number of controls without the antigen. Adapted from Fugger L, Tisch R, Libau R, et al (1995) The role of human major histocompatibility complex (HLA) genes in disease. *In* Scriver CR, Beaudet AL, Sly WS, Valle D (eds) The Metabolic and Molecular Bases of Inherited Disease, 7th ed. McGraw-Hill, New York, pp. 555–585; and Bell JI, Todd JA, McDevitt HO (1989) The molecular basis of HLA-disease association. Adv Hum Genet 18:1–41; and adapted, with permission of Elsevier Science, from Thorsby E (1997) HLA associated diseases. Hum Immunol 53:1–11, copyright 1997 by the American Society of Histocompatibility and Immunogenetics.

because of variation in immune response or because of simple linkage disequilibrium (i.e., because a disease gene not involved in the immune response happens to be embedded within the HLA complex). For example, one of the strongest HLA-disease associations known is that between **narcolepsy** and HLA-DQ6; almost 100 percent of Norwegian patients with narcolepsy express this class II antigen, compared with only about 33 percent of healthy controls. Only a small percentage of persons with HLA-DQ6 develop narcolepsy, however, and the odds ratio of narcolepsy in those persons, compared with persons who do not have HLA-DQ6, is only approximately 40 (see footnote of Table 14–2).

Even though the basis of most HLA-disease associations is unknown, the evidence to date suggests that the HLA genes are not solely responsible for specific diseases but instead may simply contribute, along with other genetic or environmental factors, to disease predisposition. Because the HLA molecules are integral to T-cell antigen recognition, it is speculated that their role in disease pathogenesis may relate to differences in the capacity of these polymorphic proteins to interact with antigen and the T-cell receptor in the initiation of an immune response (see Fig. 14–2). This hypothesis, which implies a direct pathogenetic role for the HLA molecule, is supported by the finding, described in some detail in Chapter 15, that the association between HLA-DQ and insulin-dependent diabetes mellitus is related to a single amino acid change in one of the external domains of the HLA-DQ $\beta$ chain. The precise mechanism whereby this substitution confers disease susceptibility is still unknown, however.

## IMMUNOGLOBULINS

Antibodies are immunoglobulins that are elicited in response to a stimulus by a foreign antigen and can recognize and bind that antigen and facilitate its elimination. They are mediators of the immune response in the HLA-related diseases just described, as well as in response to foreign antigens. A number of genetic diseases are due to deficiencies of immunoglobulins. However, the primary significance of immunoglobulins from the perspective of genetics is that they exhibit a unique property, **somatic rearrangement**, by which cutting and pasting of DNA sequences in lymphocyte precursor cells is used to rearrange genes in somatic cells to generate diversity.

Antibodies exist in two forms: a membrane-bound form, on B lymphocytes, and a soluble or secreted form. Secreted antibodies are produced by plasma cells, which are derived from B lymphocytes by proliferation and maturation. This process, known as B-cell activation, is initiated by interaction between a specific antigen and a suitable antibody molecule on the B-cell membrane. Such an interaction results in the clonal expansion and differentiation of the B cell, with consequent formation of both plasma cells, which secrete antibodies specific for the inciting antigens, and memory B cells capable of responding promptly and strongly to any later challenge by the same antigen.

### Immunoglobulin Structure and Diversity

One of the most fascinating aspects of immunogenetics is the mechanism whereby a seemingly infinite number of different antibodies could be encoded in the germline DNA of any one individual. It is estimated that each human being can generate a repertoire of about $10^{11}$ different antibodies, yet the genome is composed of only $6 \times 10^9$ base pairs of DNA. This seeming disparity has been reconciled by the demonstration that antibodies are encoded in the germline by a relatively small number of genes that, during B-cell development, undergo a unique process of somatic rearrangement and somatic mutation that allows for the generation of enormous diversity. The potential to create such huge numbers of different antibodies appears to have evolved as a mechanism for protection against the large array of environmental infectious organisms, toxic agents, and autologous malignant cells to which a person may be exposed.

Immunoglobulin molecules are composed of four polypeptide chains, two identical heavy (H) chains and two identical light (L) chains, that are held together by interchain disulfide bonds (Fig. 14–4). Intrachain disulfide bonds subdivide each chain into a series of homologous domains. On the basis of structural differences at the carboxyl-terminal portion, the H chains are subdivided into five classes or isotypes, $\gamma$, $\alpha$, $\mu$, $\delta$, and $\varepsilon$, and the corresponding immunoglobulins are accordingly named IgG, IgA, IgM, IgD, and IgE. As indicated in Table 14–3, the different immunoglobulin classes differ functionally as well as structurally. The L chains of immunoglobulin molecules may also be of two types, $\kappa$ and $\lambda$, but not both in the same antibody. Therefore, the antibody produced by a single B cell contains only a single H-chain isotype and a single L-chain subtype, a phenomenon known as **isotypic exclusion**. Moreover, unlike most other autosomal loci (imprinted loci being the exception; see Chapter 5), only one of the pair of parental alleles for each H-chain and L-chain is expressed within a single cell: either the paternal or the maternal allele, but not both. Restricted expression to only one of two alleles, **allelic exclusion**, is still not fully understood.

Each H and L chain of an immunoglobulin protein consists of two segments, the constant (C)

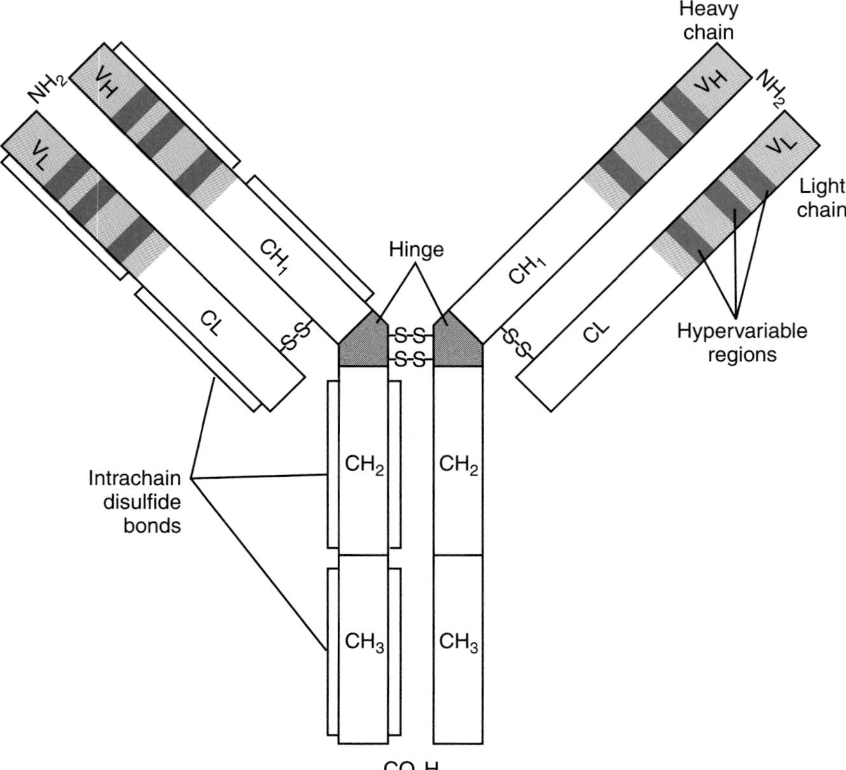


**Figure 14–4.** Basic structure of an immunoglobulin molecule, consisting of two identical light chains and two identical heavy chains. Each chain consists of a variable region (V) and a constant region (C). $NH_2$ = amino terminus. $CO_2H$ = carboxyl terminus.

and the variable (V) regions (see Fig. 14–4). The constant region, which determines the class of the immunoglobulin molecule, is located at the carboxyl terminus, and its amino acid sequence is relatively conserved among immunoglobulins of the same class. By contrast, the V region is located at the amino terminus and its amino acid sequence shows wide variation among different antibodies. The V regions of the H and L chains form the antigen-binding site and determine the antibody specificity.

The genes encoding the H chains (all five isotypes) and both the κ and λ L chains are located in three unlinked chromosomal regions (Fig. 14–5). The κ L-chain genes are on chromosome 2 at band 2p13, λ L-chain genes are on chromosome 22 at band 22q11, and the H-chain genes for all five isotypes are on chromosome 14 at band 14q32. Each H and L chain is encoded by multiple genes that are widely separated by hundreds of kb *in germline DNA*. The κ L-chain locus contains approximately 100 individual V genes, five joining (J) segments, and a single constant domain gene; the λ L-chain locus contains a similar number of individual V genes and joining (J) segments but has six genes capable of encoding the constant domain of the light chain. The H-chain V region is made up of three domains: the V and J segments and a third unit, the diversity (D) segment (see Fig. 14–5). More than 200 different V-segment genes are present in the H-chain locus; further down the chromosome are approximately 20 D-segment genes and six J-segment genes, followed by the various constant segment genes for each of the immunoglobulin isotypes. In total, each cluster of immunoglobulin genes spans many millions of base pairs.

During differentiation of antibody producing cells, but not in any other cell lineages, DNA at the immunoglobulin loci undergoes **somatic rearrangement** catalyzed by **recombinases.** As shown schematically in Figure 14–6, a recombinase creates a complete variable region gene by generating double-strand DNA breaks in the L-chain locus and religating the free DNA ends, resulting in the juxtaposition of one of the approximately 100 $V_\kappa$ segments to one of the $J_\kappa$ regions and deletion of the intervening DNA. This rearranged segment is then transcribed, and the intronic sequences between the $J_\kappa$ and $C_\kappa$

TABLE 14–3

## Generation of Primary Antibody Diversity in Humans

| Germline Genes | H | κ | λ |
|---|---|---|---|
| V | 200 | 100 | 100 |
| J | 6 | 5 | 6 |
| D | 20 | — | — |
| Somatic rearrangement V×J (×D) | $2.4 \times 10^4$ | 500 | 600 |
| H-L chain dimerization | | | |
| H×κ | $1.2 \times 10^7$ | | |
| H×λ | $1.4 \times 10^7$ | | |
| Total potential repertoire with junctional diversity | $\sim 10^{11}$ | | |

Numbers of gene segments and the contribution of junctional diversity are estimates. Somatic mutation increases further the degree of diversity in secondary responses to antigens.

H chain locus (chromosome 14)

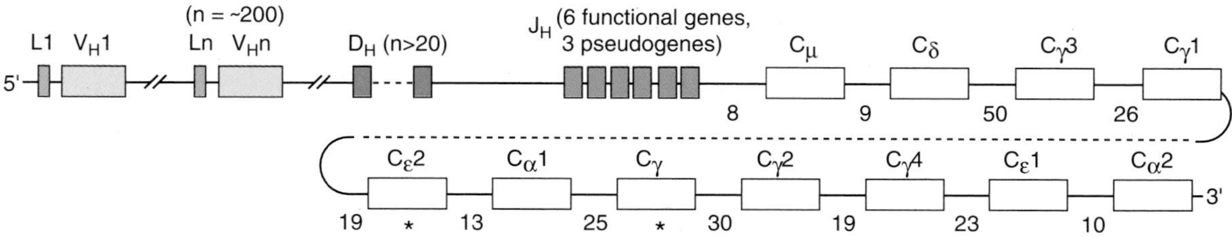


κ chain locus (chromosome 2)

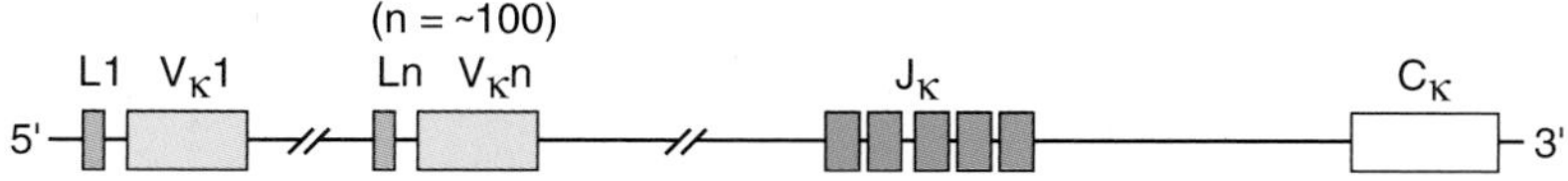


λ chain locus (chromosome 22)

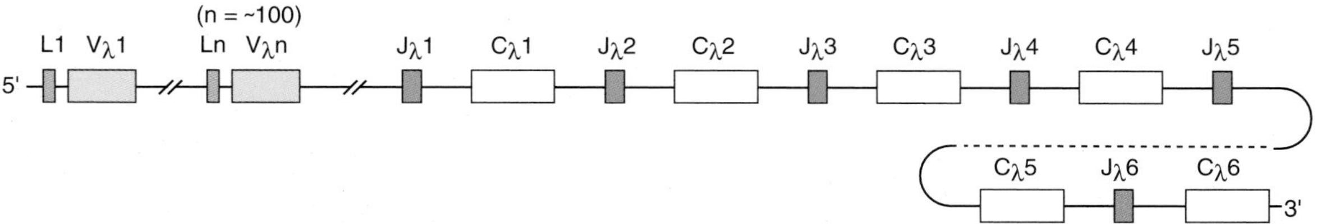


**Figure 14–5.** Structure of the immunoglobulin gene clusters. Coding and noncoding regions are not drawn to scale. Asterisks indicate pseudogenes. The exact number of genes and the overall size of the gene clusters are not known. (Reproduced, with permission, from Abbas AK, Lichtman AH, Pober JS [1997] Cellular and Molecular Immunology, 3rd ed. WB Saunders, Philadelphia.)

segments are removed, as usual, by RNA splicing to generate a mature messenger RNA (mRNA) for translation into a specific $\kappa$ light chain. The $\lambda$ light chain undergoes a similar process of DNA rearrangement before transcription but has a somewhat different germline organization; each J segment is associated with one of six different $C_\lambda$ segment (see Figs. 14–5 and 14–6). Similarly, for the heavy chains, a D segment and a J segment are juxtaposed and then fused to a V segment by somatic rearrangement catalyzed by recombinases. The additional use of one of multiple D segments in the formation of the H-chain variable region generates even greater diversity in the H-chain variable region (see Fig. 14–5).

Another source of antibody diversity is generated by deletions caused by imprecise joining of the V and J gene segments (L-chain) or the V, D, and J segments (H-chain) during the DNA rearrangement process. Insertions at the site of joining can also occur when nucleotides (so-called N sequences that are added by a terminal transferase that are not present in the original germline DNA) are inserted at the site of religation. Loss or gain of a few nucleotides produces frameshifts that encode different amino acids in the final rearranged gene.

The diversification possibilities provided by pairing different H and L chains and by DNA rearrangements that join together different germline V, D, and J gene segments occur during development of B cells before any antigen stimulation. They create the basic repertoire of antibodies that B cells are capable of producing. Once antigen stimulation occurs, however, B-cells that produce antibodies with some affinity for the antigen are stimulated and undergo frequent point mutations within their rearranged VJ or VDJ coding sequences. This rate of spontaneous mutation (one mutation per $10^3$ DNA base pairs per cell division) is strikingly high, 100 to 1000 times greater than the average mutation rate elsewhere in the genome. These spontaneous mutations change the amino acid sequence within the variable (antigen-recognition) domain of antibody molecules and are a "fine-tuning" mechanism for improving the affinity of an antibody through a positive feedback mechanism. If a mutation within a B cell increases the affinity of an antibody molecule for an antigen, that B cell receives additional stimulation and expands its production of the improved antibody. Somatic mutation provides another important mechanism for great expansion of the potential repertoire of antibody specificities.

Antibody diversity is therefore generated by several molecular mechanisms, including the following:

1. The possibility of pairing between any of the H-chain isotypes and L-chain subtypes.
2. The availability of different V, D, and J genes.
3. Junctional diversity, created by imprecise joining and random insertion of nucleotides between recombining V and D elements or D and J elements.

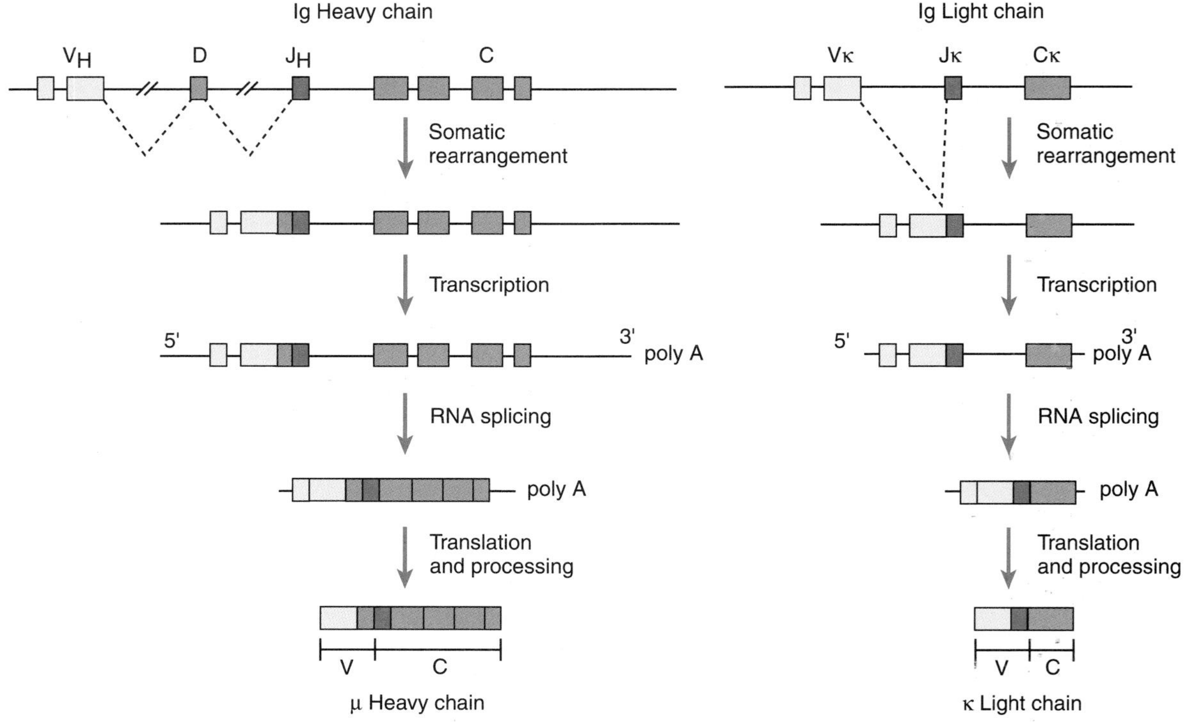


**Figure 14–6.** Schematic of rearrangement of the heavy chain and light chain immunoglobulin genes in antibody formation.

4. Elevated rates of somatic mutation within the V region segments to increase the affinity of an antibody for its antigen.

As shown in Table 14–3, the molecular diversity in antibodies generated by all of these mechanisms is truly astonishing and makes it possible for humans to respond to a vast array of antigens.

## THE T-CELL ANTIGEN RECEPTOR

The mechanism of generation of diversity characteristic of the immunoglobulins is shared by another member of the immunoglobulin gene superfamily, the TCR. The TCR represents the T-cell analog of membrane-bound immunoglobulin on B cells (see Fig. 14–2). The receptor is a highly variable transmembrane heterodimeric glycoprotein that plays a key role in antigen recognition and in the genesis of T-cell helper or cytotoxic activity. Unlike immunoglobulin, the TCR has no soluble form. The TCR resembles the immunoglobulin molecule structurally, however; all chains have both constant and variable sections, the variable sections being generated by an assortment of V, D, and J segments. Thus, the TCR genes, which are encoded in three separate chromosomal regions (Fig. 14–7), appear to be members of the immunoglobulin gene superfamily, sharing ancestry with the immunoglobulin genes.

One significant difference between antibodies and the TCR is the prerequisite role for MHC molecules in T-cell antigen recognition. The T-cell receptor cannot recognize an antigen unless the antigen is presented as a processed peptide complexed with a class I or class II MHC molecule (see Fig. 14–2). Thus, the T-cell receptor on the T cells of an individual is specific for the combination of antigenic peptide and that individual's own surface MHC antigens, a phenomenon known as **MHC restriction**.

Just as there is an orderly succession of expression of embryonic, fetal, and adult hemoglobins through development (see Chapter 11), different T-cell receptors are expressed during development. During initial T-cell development in the thymus, at or about 9 weeks' gestation in humans, T-cell precursors express heterodimers of the $\gamma$ and $\delta$ chains of the TCR. The $\gamma\delta$ TCRs are thought to be important in generating self-tolerance within the immune system by allowing selection *against* cells that react to self. Within one or two weeks, $\gamma\delta$ expression fades to much lower levels, and mature T cells appear carrying heterodimers of $\alpha$ and $\beta$ chains on their surface.

Just as for the immunoglobulin genes, the recombination of multiple germline elements, imprecision of joining, and the possibility of various chain combinations create extensive diversity in TCR genes. Unlike immunoglobulins, however, the genesis of TCRs does not involve somatic mutation. Even without somatic mutation generating diversity, there is a much greater junctional diversity in TCR genes due

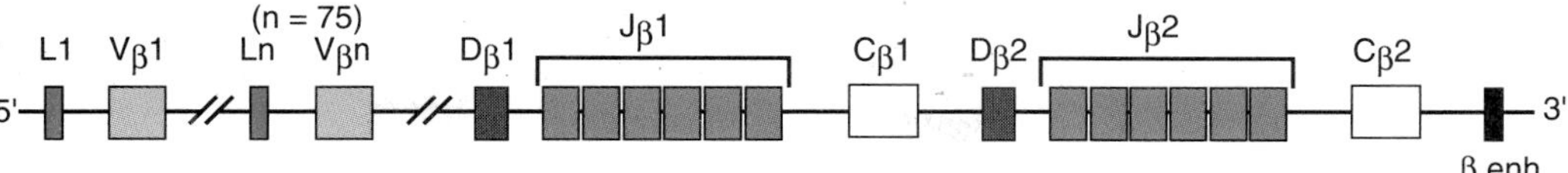


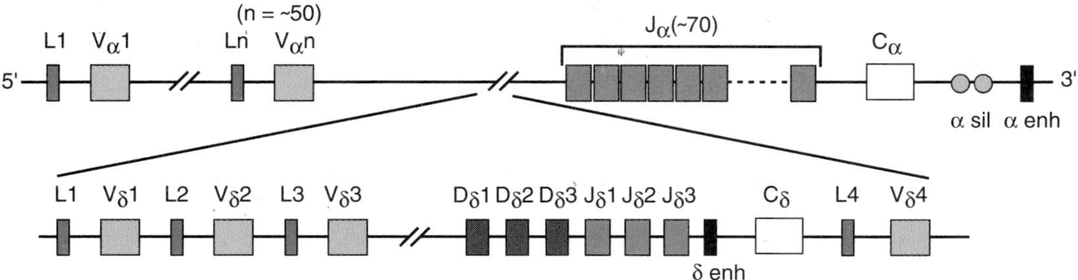


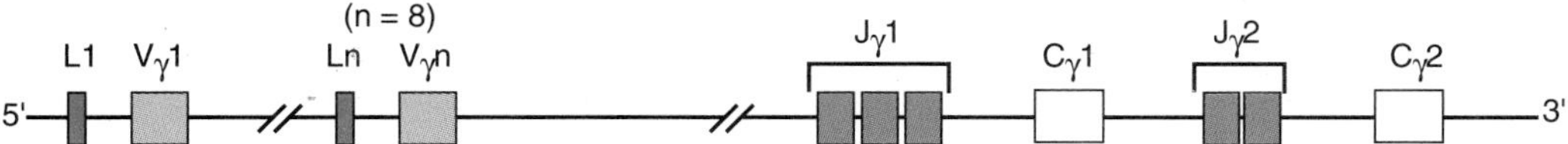


Figure 14–7. Germline arrangement of human *TCR* genes. Sizes of exons and introns are not shown to scale. The $\beta$-chain gene cluster consists of 75 variable (V) gene segments and two sets of diversity (D), joining (J), and constant (C) region gene segments. The $\alpha$ chain gene cluster contains $\sim$50 V gene segments, $\sim$70 J segments, and a single C gene segment. The $\gamma$ chain gene cluster has $\sim$8 V segments, along with two sets of J and C gene segments. The $\delta$ chain gene cluster is embedded within the $\alpha$ cluster on chromosome 14. Sequences termed enhancer (enh) and silencer (sil) are involved in control of gene expression by increasing or shutting off transcription respectively. (Reproduced, with permission, from Abbas AK, Lichtman AH, Pober JS [1997] Cellular and Molecular Immunology, 3rd ed. WB Saunders, Philadelphia.)

to insertion of extra nucleotides at VJ and VDJ junctions. Through this mechanism, truly staggering levels of diversity are generated in the TCR genes: estimates are that $10^{16}$ different $\alpha\beta$ and $10^{18}$ different $\gamma\delta$ T-cell receptors are possible.

The somatic rearrangement that occurs during B- and T-cell development, along with the high rate of somatic mutation in B cells responding to an antigen, occur only in the immunoglobulin and TCR gene clusters in the B- and T-cell lineages, respectively. Such behavior is unique to these gene families and cell lineages and makes the immune system a fascinating subject for the study of gene structure, gene expression, and development.

## SINGLE-GENE DISORDERS OF THE IMMUNE SYSTEM

With so complex a system as the immune system, it is not surprising that a large number of genetic defects can occur to produce highly pleiotropic phenotypes of variable severity. A large number and variety of single-gene disorders of the immune system have been described and an increasing number of the genes responsible identified (see examples in Table 14–4). Some immunodeficiency genes are involved in the cellular signaling pathways involved in lymphocyte maturation. One example is the gene encoding a subunit ($\gamma$) of the receptor for interleukin-2, a T-cell growth factor; mutations in this gene are responsible for the X-linked form of **severe combined immunodeficiency**. Another example are the genes (*RAG1* and *RAG2*) that encode the recombinases responsible for the somatic DNA rearrangements that occur during T-cell and B-cell development; total loss of function of either of these genes causes severe combined immunodeficiency, whereas less deleterious mutant alleles cause **Omenn syndrome**. Other causes of immunodeficiency result from enzyme deficiencies that impair cellular function, such as defective phagocytosis in cytochrome oxidase deficiency, or defective complement-mediated bacterial killing due to complement deficiencies.

Isolation of the genes underlying the various primary immunodeficiency disorders also makes possible their potential treatment by somatic cell gene therapy. The immunodeficiency diseases are particularly appropriate candidates for this therapeutic approach, both because of their considerable morbidity and mortality and because the defects underlying the abnormal phenotypes are largely restricted to hematopoietic cells and could therefore be corrected by introduction of a normal gene into the patient's bone marrow cells as a replacement. As

TABLE 14–4

**Genetic Immunodeficiency Diseases**

| Category | Designation | T-Cell Numbers | B-Cell Numbers | Ig Levels | Gene Defect; Pathogenesis | Genetic Locus |
|---|---|---|---|---|---|---|
| Combined T- and B-lymphocyte defects | X-linked severe combined immunodeficiency (SCID) | Low | Normal to high | Low | Defect of $\gamma$ chain of IL-2 receptor and receptors for other cytokines, IL-4, 7, 9, 15 | *IL2RG (SCIDX1)* Xq13.1 |
| | JAK3 deficiency | Low | Normal to high | Low | *JAK3* intracellular signaling kinase defect | *JAK3* 19p13.1 |
| | Adenosine deaminase (ADA) deficiency | Progressive decrease | Progressive decrease | Low | Selective lymphocyte toxicity of purine pathway intermediates | *ADA* 20q13.11 |
| | Purine nucleoside phosphorylase (PNP) deficiency | Progressive decrease | Normal | Normal or low | Lymphocyte toxicity of purine pathway intermediates | *PNP* 14q13 |
| | MHC class II deficiency | Low CD4 | Normal | Normal or low | Mutation in factors controlling *MHC II* gene expression | *CIITA* 16p13 *RFX5* 1q |
| | ZAP 70 kinase deficiency | Low CD8 | Normal | Normal | Thymocyte intracellular kinase defect; blocked maturation of T cells | *ZAP70* 2q12 |
| | Recombinase activating gene (*RAG1*, *RAG2*) deficiency | Low | Absent | Absent | No T-cell or B-cell receptor rearrangement; blocked lymphocyte development | *RAG1*, *RAG2* 11p13 |
| | Omenn's syndrome | Low | Low | Low | Defective T-cell or B-cell receptor rearrangement | *RAG1*, *RAG2* |
| | X-linked Hyper IgM syndrome | Normal | Normal | Normal to high IgM; low IgA, IgG | Defect of *CD40* ligand, expressed on T cells; block in B-cell isotype switch | *HIGMX* Xq25-q26 |
| | DiGeorge syndrome | Normal to low | Normal | Normal to low | Embryological defect of thymic development; variable associated defects of heart, parathyroid, face | 22q11.2 and other loci |
| Antibody deficiencies | X-linked agammaglobulinemia | Normal | Very low to absent | Low to absent | Defect of B-cell specific Bruton's tyrosine kinase (BTK) | *XLA* Xq22 |
| | $\mu$ heavy chain deficiency | Normal | Absent | Absent | Defect of cell surface $\mu$ chain expression | *IGH$\mu$* 14q32.3 |

| | | | | | | |
|---|---|---|---|---|---|---|
| Other distinctive syndromes with immune defects | Wiskott-Aldrich syndrome | Normal to low | Normal | Normal (some low IgM) | Defect of *WASP* gene involved in cytoskeleton; sparse, small platelets; eczema | *WASP* Xp11.23 |
| | Ataxia telangiectasia | Normal | Normal | Normal | DNA repair defect in *ATM* gene; ataxia, progressive neurodegeneration; cancer; radiation sensitivity | *ATM* 11q22-q23 |
| | Bloom syndrome | Normal | Normal | Normal | DNA repair defect in *BLM* gene; progressive neurodegeneration; cancer; radiation sensitivity | *BLM* 15q26.1 |
| | Autoimmune lymphoproliferative syndrome | Normal to high; elevated CD4-/CD8- T cells | High | High | Impaired Fas-mediated apoptosis of B and T cells; lymphadenopathy, autoimmunity | *FAS* 10q24 |
| Phagocyte disorders | Chronic granulomatous disease (CGD) | Normal | Normal | Normal | Impaired killing of ingested organisms due to defects in 4 genes encoding enzymes of cytochrome oxidase system | *CYBB* (gp91$^{phox}$), Xp21.1<br>*CYBA* (p22$^{phox}$), 16q24.1<br>*NCF1* (p47$^{phox}$), 7q11.23<br>*NCF2* (p67$^{phox}$), 1q25 |
| | Leukocyte adhesion deficiency (LAD) | Normal | Normal | Normal | Defects of CD18 or other leukocyte surface proteins required for motility, adherence and endocytosis | *CD18* 21q22.3 |
| | Chediak-Higashi syndrome | Normal | Normal | Normal | Defect of *CHS1* gene causing faulty lysosomal assembly, giant cytoplasmic granules | *CHS1*, 1q42-q44 |
| Complement disorders | Individual component deficiencies | Normal | Normal | Normal | C1, C2, C4, C3 deficiencies associated with autoimmunity and pyogenic infections; C3, C5-9 and properdin deficiencies with neisserial infections | Many |

described in Chapter 13, an X-linked recessive form of severe combined immunodeficiency, was the first human immunodeficiency disease successfully treated by somatic gene therapy.

## General References

Abbas AK, Lichtman AH, Pober JS (1997) Cellular and Molecular Immunology, 3rd ed. WB Saunders, Philadelphia.

Ochs HD, Smith E, Puck JM (1998) Primary Immunodeficiency Disease: A Molecular and Genetic Approach. Oxford University Press, Oxford, England.

## References Specific to Particular Topics

Bell JI, Todd JA, McDevitt HO (1989) The molecular basis of HLA-disease association. Adv Hum Genet 18:1–41.

Bodmer JG, Marsh SGE, Albert ED, et al (1997) Nomenclature for factors of the HLA system, 1996. Hum Immunol 53:98–128.

Fugger L, Tisch R, Libau R, et al (1995) The role of human major histocompatibility complex (HLA) genes in disease. *In* Scriver CR, Beaudet AL, Sly WS, Valle D (eds) The Metabolic and Molecular Bases of Inherited Disease, 7th ed. McGraw-Hill, New York, pp. 555–585.

Puck JM (1997) Primary immunodeficiency diseases. JAMA 278:1835–1841.

deVries RRP, van Rood JJ (1992) Immunogenetics and disease. *In* RA King, JL Rotter, AG Motulsky (eds) The Genetic Basis of Common Diseases. Oxford University Press, New York, pp. 92–114.

## Problems

1. Ankylosing spondylitis and HLA-B27 are closely *associated*. The *HLA-B* locus and the locus for 21-hydroxylase (mutations at which lead to congenital adrenal hyperplasia) are closely *linked*. Distinguish between these two concepts.

2. Arrange the following family members in order of their probability of sharing two HLA haplotypes with the recipient and thus being suitable donors of tissues or organs: sib, father, monozygotic twin, dizygotic twin, half-sib, mother, unrelated person, first cousin.

   Why is a monozygotic twin of a recipient not necessarily the donor of choice?

3. How does somatic rearrangement of immunoglobulin and T-cell receptor genes differ from the splicing of introns and exons that is characteristic of most genes?

4. How does expression of immunoglobulin genes differ from the expression of most other autosomal loci?

5. For some X-linked immunodeficiencies, such as Wiskott-Aldrich syndrome, agammaglobulinemia, and severe combined immunodeficiency (SCID), certain cell populations in carrier females show nonrandom X inactivation; that is, all cells contain the X with the normal allele active, unlike other tissues that show random X inactivation in the same women. The affected cell population is characteristic of each disorder; that is, B cells in agammaglobulinemia, B and T cells in SCID, and T cells in Wiskott-Aldrich syndrome. Explain. Would you expect to find random or nonrandom X inactivation in cells from carriers of autosomal forms of immunodeficiency?

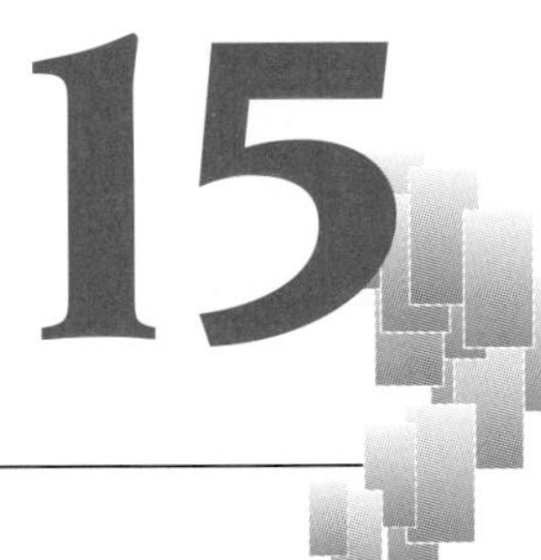

# Genetics of Disorders with Complex Inheritance

Heredity contributes to most common human diseases. Diseases such as congenital birth defects, myocardial infarction (MI), cancer, mental illness, diabetes, and Alzheimer disease (AD) cause morbidity and premature mortality in nearly two of every three individuals during their lifetimes (Table 15–1). Although these illnesses may be caused by a mutation in a single gene in a few families, they are not, in general, single-gene disorders. Rather, these disorders result from complex interactions between a number of predisposing factors, including the genotype at one or more loci and a variety of environmental exposures that trigger, accelerate, or exacerbate the disease process. In this situation, disease occurrence in families will not match one of the simple mendelian patterns of inheritance and instead is said to follow a **complex** or **multifactorial** inheritance pattern.

A genetic disease trait that is either present or absent is referred to as a **discrete** or **qualitative** trait; one has the trait or not. In contrast are **quantitative** traits, which are measurable characteristics (physiological or biochemical quantities) such as height, blood pressure, serum cholesterol, and body mass index (weight in kilograms divided by the square of height in meters, a measure of obesity). The genetic basis for variability in quantitative traits is central to understanding how genes contribute to many common and devastating illnesses in the population.

In this chapter, we address the question of how we determine that genes contribute to common disease traits and to variability in quantitative physiological traits. We describe studies of twins and case-control methods used by geneticists to determine the relative contributions of genes and environment to qualitative and quantitative traits. We then explain the methods used to ascertain how many genes, if any, contribute to the phenotype and how the genomic location of such genes is determined. Finally, we present a number of examples of diseases in which we have begun to understand the mechanisms by which alleles at more than one locus confer disease susceptibility or contribute to phenotypic variation. The field is developing rapidly, and it is clear that the genetic basis of many more complex diseases in humans will be elucidated soon. Identification of both genetic and environmental factors that result in common diseases will allow the development of rational preventive and therapeutic measures.

## GENETIC ANALYSIS OF QUALITATIVE DISEASE TRAITS

### Familial Aggregation of Disease

Because relatives share a greater proportion of their genes with one another than with unrelated individu-

TABLE 15–1

**Frequency of Different Types of Genetic Disease**

| Type | Incidence at birth (per 1000) | Prevalence at Age 25 Years (per 1000) | Population Prevalence (per 1000) |
|---|---|---|---|
| Disorders due to genome and chromosome mutations | 6 | 1.8 | 3.8 |
| Disorders due to single-gene mutations | 10 | 3.6 | 20 |
| Disorders with multifactorial inheritance | ~50 | ~50 | ~600 |

Data adapted from Rimoin DL, Connor JM, Pyeritz RE (1997) Emery and Rimoin's Principles and Practice of Medical Genetics, 3rd ed. Churchill Livingstone, Edinburgh.

als in the population, a primary characteristic of diseases with complex inheritance is that affected individuals tend to cluster in families (**familial aggregation**). The converse, however, is not necessarily true: familial aggregation of a disease does not mean that a disease must have a genetic contribution. Family members may develop the same disease or trait by chance alone, particularly if it is a common one in the population. Even if familial aggregation is not due to chance, families share more than their genes: for example, they often have cultural attitudes and behaviors, diet, and environmental exposures in common. It is the task of the genetic epidemiologist to determine whether familial aggregation is coincidental or the result of factors common to members of the family and to assess the extent to which those common factors are genetic and environmental. Ultimately, gene mapping studies to locate and identify the particular loci and alleles involved provide the definitive proof of a genetic contribution to multifactorial disease.

## Concordance and Discordance

When two related individuals in a family have the same disease, they are called **concordant** for the disorder. Conversely, when only one member of the pair of relatives is affected and the other is not, the relatives are **discordant** for the disease. Diseases with complex inheritance result from the impact of environmental factors on individuals with certain genotypes. Discordance for phenotype between relatives who share a genotype at loci that predispose to disease can be explained if the unaffected individual has not experienced the other factors (environmental or chance occurrences) necessary to trigger the disease process and make it manifest. Conversely, concordance for a phenotype may occur even when the two affected relatives have different predisposing genotypes, if the disease in one relative is a **genocopy** or **phenocopy** of the disease in the other relative. Lack of penetrance and frequent genocopies and phenocopies all contribute to obscuring the inheritance pattern in multifactorial genetic disease.

## Measuring Familial Aggregation

### RELATIVE RISK $\lambda_r$

The familial aggregation of a disease can be measured by comparing the frequency of the disease in the relatives of an affected proband with its frequency (prevalence) in the general population. The **relative risk ratio $\lambda_r$** is defined as

$$\lambda_r = \frac{\text{prevalence of the disease in a relative "r" of an affected person}}{\text{population prevalence of the disease}}$$

(The subscript r for $\lambda$ is used here generically; in practice, one measures $\lambda$ for a particular class of relatives, e.g., r = s for sibs, r = p for parents.) The value of $\lambda_r$ is a measure of familial aggregation that depends both on the risk of the disease recurring in the family and on the population prevalence: the larger $\lambda_r$ is, the greater the familial aggregation. The population prevalence enters into the calculation because the more common a disease, the greater is the likelihood that aggregation may be just a coincidence rather than a result of sharing the alleles that predispose to disease. A value of $\lambda_r = 1$ indicates that a relative is no more likely to develop the disease than is any individual in the population. Examples of $\lambda_r$ values greater than 1 for various diseases are shown in Table 15–2.

### CASE-CONTROL STUDIES

Another approach to assessing familial aggregation is the **case-control study** in which patients with a disease (the cases) are compared with suitably chosen individuals without the disease (the controls) with respect to family history of disease (as well as other factors, such as environmental exposures, occupation, geographical location, parity, and previous illnesses). To assess a possible genetic contribution to familial aggregation of a disease, the frequency with which the disease is found in the extended families of the cases (**positive family history**) is compared with the frequency of positive family history among suitable controls, matched for age and ethnicity, but who do not have the disease. Spouses are often used as controls in this situation because they usually match the

TABLE 15–2

**Risk Ratios $\lambda_r$ for Relatives of Probands with Diseases with Familial Aggregation and Complex Inheritance**

| Disease | Relationship | $\lambda_r$ |
|---|---|---|
| Schizophrenia | MZ twins | 48 |
| | Siblings | 12 |
| Autism | MZ twins | 2000 |
| | Siblings | 150 |
| Manic-depressive (bipolar) disorder | MZ twins | 60 |
| | Siblings | 7 |
| Type 1 diabetes mellitus | MZ twins | 80 |
| | Siblings | 12 |
| Crohn's disease | MZ twins | 840 |
| | Siblings | 25 |
| Multiple sclerosis | MZ twins | 800 |
| | Siblings | 24 |

MZ = Monozygotic.

Data adapted from Rimoin DL, Connor JM, Pyeritz RE (1997) Emery and Rimoin's Principles and Practice of Medical Genetics, 3rd ed. Churchill Livingstone, Edinburgh; King RA, Rotter JI, Motulsky AG (1992) The Genetic Basis of Common Diseases. Oxford University Press, Oxford, England.

cases in age and ethnicity and share the same household environment. Other frequently used controls are patients with unrelated diseases matched for age, occupation, and ethnicity. Thus, for example, in a study of **Parkinson disease** (PD), 6.3 percent of first- and second-degree living relatives of patients with PD also had PD, a prevalence that was significantly higher than the 1.2 percent prevalence of PD among the relatives of matched controls with other neurological diseases but not PD. One can conclude, therefore, that a family history of PD is found more frequently among patients with PD than in controls, indicating that some familial aggregation is occurring in PD.

Case-control studies for familial aggregation are subject to many different kinds of errors. One of the most troublesome is **ascertainment bias**, a difference in the likelihood that affected relatives of the cases will be reported to the epidemiologist as compared with the affected relatives of controls. A proband's relatives may be more likely than a control's relatives to know of other family members with the same disease or may be more motivated to respond to a questionnaire because of familiarity with the disease (**recall bias**). Another confounding factor is the choice of controls. Controls should differ from the cases only in their disease status and not in ethnic background, occupation, gender, or socioeconomic status, any of which may distinguish them as being different from the cases in important ways that have little or nothing to do with the fact that they are not affected by the disease. Finally, an association found in a case-control study does not prove causation. For example, if two factors are not independent of each other, such as ethnic background and dietary consumption of certain foods, a case-control study may find a significant association between the disease and ethnic background when it is actually the dietary habits associated with ethnic background that are responsible. For example, the lower frequency of coronary artery disease (CAD) among Japanese compared with that among North Americans becomes less pronounced in first-generation Japanese who emigrated to North America and adopted the dietary customs of their new home.

## Assessing the Relative Contributions of Genes and Environment to Complex Disease Traits

### Concordance and Allele-Sharing among Relatives

The more closely related two individuals are in a family, the more alleles they have in common, inherited from their common ancestors. Conversely, the more distantly related the relative is to the proband, the fewer the alleles shared between the proband and the relative. One approach to dissecting the contribution of genetic influences from environmental effects in multifactorial disease is to compare disease concordance in relatives who are more or less closely related to the proband. When genes are important contributors to a disease, the frequency of disease concordance increases as the degree of relatedness increases. The most extreme examples of two individuals having alleles in common are identical (**monozygotic [MZ]**) twins (see later in this chapter) who have the same alleles at every locus. The next most closely related individuals in a family are first-degree relatives, such as a parent and child or a pair of sibs, including fraternal (**dizygotic [DZ]**) twins. In a parent-child pair, the child has one allele in common with each parent at every locus—that is, the allele the child inherited from that parent. For a sibpair (including DZ twins), the situation is slightly different. A pair of sibs inherits the same two alleles at a locus 25 percent of the time, no alleles in common 25 percent of the time, and only one allele in common 50 percent of the time (Fig. 15–1).

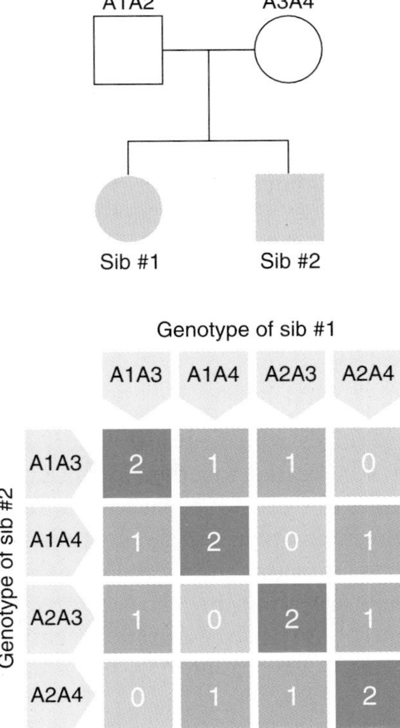


**Figure 15–1.** Allele-sharing at an arbitrary locus between sibs concordant for a disease. The parents' genotypes are shown as *A1A2* for the father, *A3A4* for the mother. All four possible genotypes for sib #1 are given across the top of the table, and all four possible genotypes for sib #2 are given along the left side of the table. The numbers inside the boxes represent the number of alleles both sibs have in common for all 16 different combinations of genotypes for both sibs. For example, the upper left hand corner has the number 2 because sib #1 and sib #2 both have the genotype *A1A3* and so have both *A1* and *A3* alleles in common. The bottom left hand corner contains the number 0 because sib #1 has genotype *A1A3* whereas sib #2 has genotype *A2A4*, so there are no alleles in common.

At any one locus, the average number of alleles one sibling shares with another is therefore given by

$$0.25 \text{ (2 alleles)} + 0.5 \text{ (1 allele)} + 0.25 \text{ (0 alleles)} = 1 \text{ allele}$$

For example, if genes predispose to a disease, one would expect $\lambda_r$ to be greatest for MZ twins (see Table 15–2), then decrease for first-degree relatives such as sibs or parent-child pairs, and continue to decrease as allele-sharing decreases among the more distant relatives in a family (Table 15–3).

#### SEPARATING GENETIC AND ENVIRONMENTAL FACTORS

The more closely related two individuals are, the more likely they are to share home environment as well. One way to separate family environment from genetic influence is to compare the incidence of disease in unrelated family members (adoptees, spouses) to that in biological relatives. In one study of multiple sclerosis, for example, $\lambda_r = 20$ to 40 in first-degree biological relatives (parents, children, and sibs) but $\lambda_r = 1$ for siblings or children adopted into the family, suggesting that most familial aggregation in multiple sclerosis was genetic rather than environmental in origin.

### Twin Studies

Another common method for separating genetic from environmental influences on disease is to study twins, both MZ and DZ. Twins are "experiments of nature" that come closest to providing an opportunity to assess environmental and genetic influences separately in humans. DZ twins reared together allow geneticists to measure disease concordance in relatives who grow up in similar environments but do not share all their genes, whereas MZ twins provide an opportunity to compare relatives with identical genotypes who may or may not be reared together in the same environment. Studies of twins have played a significant role in helping geneticists to assess the relative contributions of genes and environment to disease causation.

MZ twins arise from the cleavage of a single fertilized zygote into two separate zygotes early in embryogenesis. As a result, MZ twins have identical genotypes at every locus and are always of the same gender. They occur in approximately 0.3 percent of all births, without significant differences among different ethnic groups. DZ twins arise from the simultaneous fertilization of two eggs by two sperm; genetically, DZ twins are siblings who share a womb and, like all siblings, share, on average, 50 percent of the alleles at all loci. DZ twins are of the same sex half the time and of opposite sex the other half. DZ twins occur with a frequency that varies as much as fivefold in different populations, from a low of 0.2 percent among Asians to more than 1 percent of births in parts of Africa and among African Americans, suggesting that there may be a heritable basis for differences in the frequency of DZ twinning.

TABLE 15–3
**Degree of Relationship and Alleles in Common**

| Relationship to Proband | Proportion of Alleles in Common with Proband |
|---|---|
| Monozygotic twins | 1 |
| First-degree relative | 1/2 |
| Second-degree relative | 1/4 |
| Third-degree relative | 1/8 |

See Chapter 5, Figure 5–2, for description of degrees of relationship.

#### DETERMINING ZYGOSITY IN TWINS

Determining whether same-sex twins are MZ or DZ used to require careful examination of many characteristics, such as the appearance of the placenta, the number of amniotic and chorionic membranes surrounding the newborns, physical characteristics such as hair and eye coloration, fingerprints, and blood groups and other serological markers (see Chapters 6 and 14). The advent of highly polymorphic DNA markers (see Chapter 6, Fig. 6–6) now provides reliable determination of zygosity with extremely high probability and has superseded older methods.

#### DISEASE CONCORDANCE IN MONOZYGOTIC TWINS

An examination of how frequently MZ twins are concordant for a disease is a powerful method for determining whether genotype alone is sufficient to produce a particular disease. For example, if one MZ twin has sickle cell anemia, the other twin will also have sickle cell anemia. In contrast, when one MZ twin has type 1 diabetes mellitus (previously known as insulin-dependent or juvenile diabetes), only about 40 percent of the other twins will also have type 1 diabetes. *Disease concordance less than 100 percent in MZ twins is strong evidence that nongenetic factors play a role in the disease.* Such factors could include environmental influences, such as exposure to infection or diet, as well as other effects, such as somatic mutation, effects of aging, or differences in X-inactivation in one twin compared with the other.

#### COMPARING CONCORDANCE OF MONOZYGOTIC VERSUS DIZYGOTIC TWINS

MZ and same-sex DZ twins share a common intrauterine environment and sex and are usually reared together in the same household by the same parents.

Thus, a comparison of concordance for a disease between MZ and same-sex DZ twins shows how frequently disease occurs when relatives who experience the same prenatal and, possibly, postnatal environment have all their genes in common compared with only 50 percent of their genes in common. *Greater concordance in MZ versus DZ twins is strong evidence of a genetic component to the disease* (Table 15–4). This conclusion is strongest for conditions with early onset, such as birth defects. For late-onset diseases, such as neurodegenerative disease of late adulthood, the assumption that MZ and DZ twins are exposed to similar environments throughout their adult lives becomes less valid, and, thus, a difference in concordance provides less strong evidence for genetic factors in disease causation.

#### Twins Reared Apart

If MZ twins are separated at birth and raised apart, geneticists have the opportunity to observe disease concordance in individuals with identical genotypes reared in different environments. Such studies have been used primarily in research in psychiatric disorders, substance abuse, and eating disorders, in which strong environmental influences within the family are believed to play a role in the development of disease. For example, in one study of alcoholism, five of six MZ twin pairs reared apart were concordant for alcoholism, a concordance rate at least as high as what is seen among MZ twins reared together, suggesting that shared genetic factors are far more important than shared environment.

### Limitations of Twin Studies

As useful as twin studies are for dissecting genetic and environmental factors in disease, they must be interpreted with care for several reasons. First, MZ twins do not have precisely identical gene expression despite having identical genotypes: for example, on the X chromosome, random X-inactivation after cleavage into two female MZ zygotes produces significant differences in the expression of alleles of X-linked genes in different tissues (see Chapter 5, Fig. 5–16). Somatic rearrangements in the immunoglobulin and T-cell receptor loci will also differ between MZ twins in various lymphocyte subsets (see Chapter 14). Second, environmental exposures may not be the same for twins, especially once the twins reach adulthood and leave their childhood home. Even intrauterine environment may not be the same. For example, MZ twins frequently share a placenta, and there may be a disparity between the twins in blood supply, intrauterine development, and birth weight. Third, it is important to note that measurements of disease concordance in MZ twins give an average estimate that may not be accurate if the relevant predisposing alleles or environmental factors are different in different twin pairs. Suppose the genotype of one pair of twins generates a greater risk for disease than does the genotype of another pair; the observed concordance will be an average that really applies to neither pair of twins. As a more extreme example, the disease may not always be genetic in origin—that is, nongenetic phenocopies may exist. If genotype alone causes the disease in some pairs of twins (MZ twin concordance 100 percent) and a nongenetic phenocopy affects one twin of the pair in another group of twins (MZ twin concordance 0 percent), twin studies will show an intermediate level of concordance greater than 0 percent and less than 100 percent that really applies to neither form of the disease. Finally, ascertainment bias is a problem, particularly when one twin with a particular disease is asked to recruit the other twin to participate in a study (**volunteer-based ascertainment**), rather than if they are ascertained first as twins and only then is their health status examined (**population-based ascertainment**). Volunteer-based ascertainment can give biased results because twins, particularly MZ twins who may be emotionally close, are more likely to volunteer if they are concordant than if they are not, which inflates the concordance rate. To a first approximation, however, twins offer an unusual opportunity to study disease occurrence when genetic influences are held constant (measuring disease concordance in MZ twins reared together or apart) or when genetic differences are present but environmental influences are similar (comparing disease concordance in MZ versus DZ twins).

TABLE 15–4

**Concordance Rates in MZ and DZ Twins**

| Disorder | Concordance (%) MZ | DZ |
|---|---|---|
| Nontraumatic epilepsy | 70 | 6 |
| Multiple sclerosis | 17.8 | 2 |
| Type 1 diabetes | 40 | 4.8 |
| Schizophrenia | 53 | 15 |
| Osteoarthritis | 32 | 16 |
| Rheumatoid arthritis | 12.3 | 3.5 |
| Psoriasis | 72 | 15 |
| Cleft lip with/without cleft palate | 30 | 5 |
| Systemic lupus erythematosus | 22 | 0 |

Data adapted from Rimoin DL, Connor JM, Pyeritz RE (1997) Emery and Rimoin's Principles and Practice of Medical Genetics, 3rd ed. Churchill Livingstone, Edinburgh; King RA, Rotter JI, Motulsky AG (1992) The Genetic Basis of Common Diseases. Oxford University Press, Oxford, England; Tsuang MT (1998) Recent advances in genetic research on schizophrenia. J Biomed Sci 5:28–30.

## GENETIC ANALYSIS OF QUANTITATIVE TRAITS

Measurable physiological quantities, such as blood pressure, serum cholesterol, and body mass index (as a measure of obesity), vary among different individuals and are important determinants of health and disease in the population. Such variation is usually due to differences in genotype as well as nongenetic (i.e., environmental) factors. The challenge to geneticists is to determine the extent to which genes contribute to this variability, to identify these genes, and to ascertain the alleles responsible.

## Normal Distribution

As is often the case with physiological quantities measured in a population, a graph of the number of individuals in the population (y-axis) having a particular quantitative value (x-axis) produces the familiar bell-shaped curve known as the **normal (gaussian)** distribution (Fig. 15–2). In a graph of the population frequency of a normally distributed value, the position of the peak of the graph and the shape of the graph are governed by two quantities: the **mean** ($\mu$) and the **variance** ($\sigma^2$), respectively. The mean is the arithmetic average of the values, and, because more people have values for the trait near the average, the curve has its peak at the mean value. The **variance** (or its square root, the **standard deviation**, $\sigma$), is a measure of the degree of spread of values to either side of the mean and therefore determines the breadth of the curve. Any physiological quantity that can be measured is a **quantitative phenotype**, with a mean and a variance. The variance of a measured quantity in the population is therefore called the **total phenotypic variance**.

## The Normal Range

The concept of the normal range of a physiological quantity is fundamental to clinical medicine. For example, extremely tall or short stature, hypertension, hypercholesterolemia, and obesity are all considered abnormal when a value sits clearly outside the normal range. In assessing health and disease in children, height, weight, head circumference, and other measurements are compared with the "normal" expected measurements for a child's sex and age. But how is the "normal range" determined? In many situations in medicine, a particular measured physiological value is "normal" or "abnormal" depending on how far it is above or below the mean. The normal distribution provides guidelines for setting the limits of the normal range. Basic statistical theory states that when a quantitative trait is normally distributed in a population, only approximately 5 percent of the population will have measurements more than 2 standard deviations above or below the population mean. (Note that the word "normal" is used here in two different ways. Asserting that a physiological quantity has a normal distribution in the population and stating that an individual's value is in the normal range are different uses of the same word.)

## Familial Aggregation of Quantitative Traits

Just as familial aggregation, as measured by $\lambda_r$ and case-control studies, is used to assess the role of heredity in qualitative disease traits, family studies can also be used to determine the role of heredity in quantitative traits. Quantitative traits, however, are not either present or absent; they are measurements. Consequently, one cannot simply compare the prevalence of disease in relatives versus controls or the degree of concordance in twins. Instead, geneticists measure the **correlation** of particular physiolog-

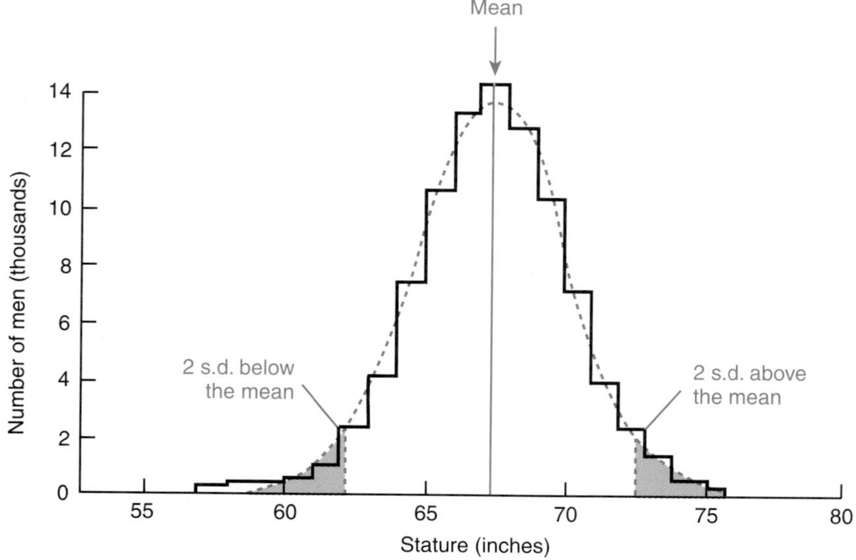


**Figure 15–2.** Distribution of stature in a sample of 91,163 young English males in 1939. The red line is a normal (gaussian) curve with the same mean and standard deviation (s.d.) as the observed data. The shaded areas indicate persons of unusually tall or short stature (greater than two s.d. above or below the mean). (Adapted from Harrison GA, Weiner JS, Tanner JM, et al [1977] Human Biology, 2nd ed. Oxford University Press, Oxford, England.)

ical quantities among relatives, that is, the tendency for the actual values of a physiological measurement to be more similar among relatives than among the general population. The **coefficient of correlation** (symbolized by the letter **r**) is a statistical measure applied to a pair of measurements, such as, for example, a person's blood pressure and the mean blood pressures of that person's siblings. Accordingly, a **positive correlation** exists between the blood pressure measurements in a group of patients and the blood pressure measurements of their relatives if it is found that the higher a patient's blood pressure, the higher are the blood pressures of the patient's relatives. (A **negative correlation** exists when the greater the increase in the patient's measurement, the lower the measurement is in the patient's relatives. The measurements are still correlated, but in the opposite direction.) The value of r can range from 0 when there is no correlation to +1 for perfect positive correlation and to −1 for perfect negative correlation.

Figure 15–3 shows a graph of the average height of more than 200 parent couples plotted against the average height of their nearly 1000 adult children. There is a positive but not perfect correlation ($r = \sim 0.6$) between the average parental height and the mean height of their children.

The correlation among relatives can be used to estimate genetic influence on a quantitative trait if you assume that the degree of similarity in the values of the trait measured among relatives is proportional to the number of alleles they share at the relevant loci for that trait. The more closely related the individuals are in a family, the more likely they are to share alleles at loci that determine a quantitative trait and the more strongly correlated will be their values. However, just as with disease traits that are found to aggregate in families because relatives share genes and environmental factors, correlation of a particular physiological value among relatives reflects the influence of both heredity and common environmental factors. A correlation does not indicate that genes are wholly responsible for whatever correlation there is.

## Heritability

The concept of **heritability** (symbolized as $\boldsymbol{h^2}$) was developed to quantify the role of genetic differences in determining variability of quantitative traits. Heritability is defined as the fraction of the total phenotypic variance of a quantitative trait that is caused by genes and is, therefore, a measure of the extent to which different alleles at various loci are responsible for the variability in a given quantitative trait seen across a population. The higher the heritability, the greater is the contribution of genetic differences among people in causing variability of the trait. The value of $h^2$ varies from 0, if genes contribute nothing

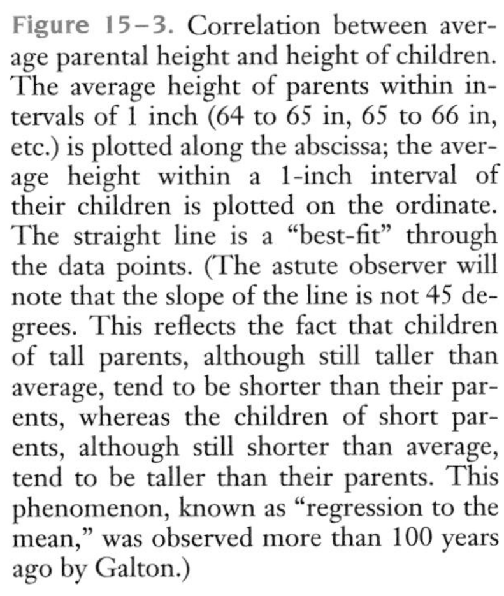
Figure 15–3. Correlation between average parental height and height of children. The average height of parents within intervals of 1 inch (64 to 65 in, 65 to 66 in, etc.) is plotted along the abscissa; the average height within a 1-inch interval of their children is plotted on the ordinate. The straight line is a "best-fit" through the data points. (The astute observer will note that the slope of the line is not 45 degrees. This reflects the fact that children of tall parents, although still taller than average, tend to be shorter than their parents, whereas the children of short parents, although still shorter than average, tend to be taller than their parents. This phenomenon, known as "regression to the mean," was observed more than 100 years ago by Galton.)

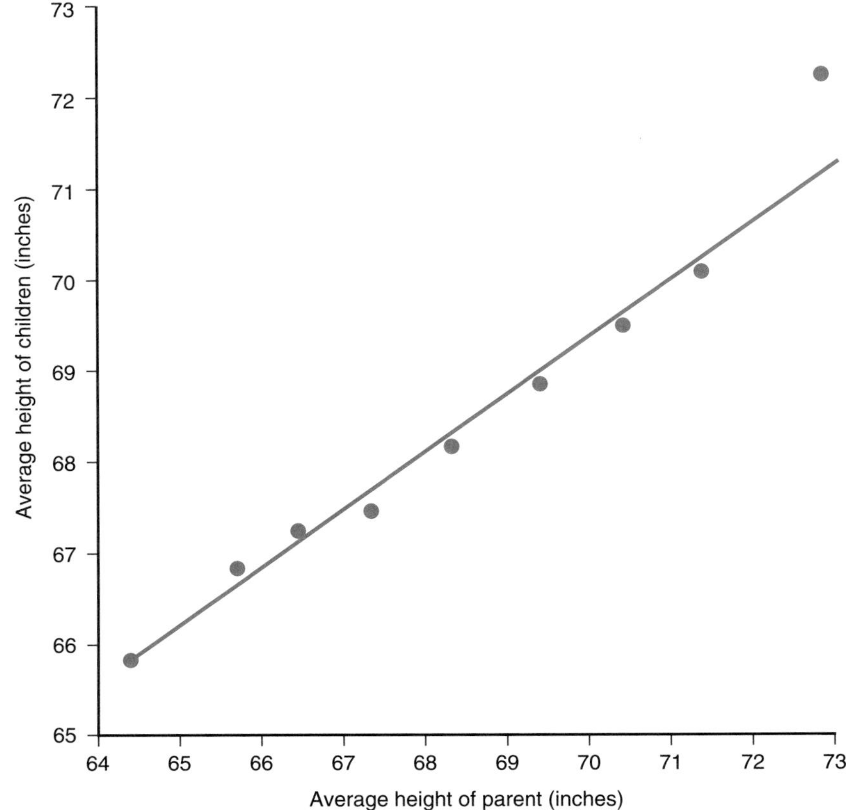

to the total phenotypic variance, to 1, if genes are totally responsible for the phenotypic variance.

Heritability of a trait is a somewhat theoretical concept that is estimated from the correlation between measurements of that trait among relatives of known degrees of relatedness, such as parents and children, siblings, or, as described next, MZ and DZ twins. There are, however, a number of practical difficulties in measuring and interpreting $h^2$. One is that relatives share more than their genes; they also share environmental exposures, and so the correlation between relatives may not reflect simply their familial genetic relationship. Even when the heritability of a trait is high, it does not reveal the underlying mechanism of inheritance of the trait, such as the number of loci involved or how the various alleles at those loci interact. Finally, as tempting as it is to think of heritability as an intrinsic quality of a particular quantitative trait, it cannot be considered in isolation from the population group and living conditions in which the estimate is being made.

### Estimating Heritability from Twin Studies

Just as twin data may be used to assess the separate roles of genes and environment in qualitative disease traits, they can also be used to estimate the heritability of a quantitative trait. The variance in the values of a physiological measurement made in a set of MZ twins (who share 100 percent of their genes) is compared with the variance in the values of that measurement made in a set of DZ twins (who share 50 percent of their genes, on average). The formula for calculating $h^2$ is given by

$$h^2 = \frac{\text{variance in DZ pairs} - \text{variance in MZ pairs}}{\text{variance in DZ pairs}}$$

(The derivation of this equation is beyond the scope of this book.) If the variability of the trait is determined chiefly by environment, the variance within pairs of DZ twins will be very similar to that seen within pairs of MZ twins, and the numerator, and therefore $h^2$ itself, will approach 0; if the variability is determined exclusively by genetic makeup, variance of MZ pairs is zero, and $h^2$ is 1.

Adult stature has been studied by geneticists for decades as a model of how genetic and environmental contributions to a quantitative trait can be apportioned. Large numbers of measurements have been collected (from military recruits, for example). A graph of the frequency of various heights in the population (see Fig. 15–2) demonstrates a bell-shaped curve that fits the normal distribution. Using the twin method in samples of Northern European extraction, $h^2$ for stature is estimated to be approximately 0.8, indicating that most of the variability in height among individuals is due to genotypic differences between them, not differences in environmental exposures. Thus, genes play a far greater role in determining adult height than does environment.

As another example, a comparison of MZ twins reared together or apart with DZ twins reared together or apart is a classic way of measuring heritability of complex traits. Studies of the body mass index of twins showed a high heritability value, indicating that there is a strong influence of heredity on the body mass index ($h^2$ = .70 to .80).

One has to make a number of simplifying assumptions when using twins to estimate heritability. The first is that MZ and same-sex DZ twins reared together differ only in that they share all (MZ) or, on average, half (DZ) of their genes although their experiences and environmental exposures are identical. In analyzing the heritability of stature, such assumptions may not be too far off the mark, but they are much more difficult to justify when estimating the heritability of more complicated quantitative measurements, such as body mass index or scores on personality profiles and IQ tests. Another important caveat is that one may not always be able to extrapolate heritability estimated from twins to the population as a whole, to different ethnic groups, or even to the same group if socioeconomic conditions change over time.

#### Characteristics of Inheritance of Complex Diseases

1. Diseases with complex inheritance are not single-gene disorders and do not demonstrate a simple mendelian pattern of inheritance.
2. Diseases with complex inheritance demonstrate familial aggregation, because relatives of an affected individual are more likely to have disease-predisposing alleles in common with the affected person than are unrelated individuals.
3. Pairs of relatives who share disease-predisposing genotypes at relevant loci may still be discordant for phenotype (show lack of penetrance) because of the crucial role of nongenetic factors in disease causation. The most extreme examples of lack of penetrance despite identical genotypes are discordant monozygotic (MZ) twins.
4. The disease is more common among the close relatives of the proband and becomes less common in relatives who are less closely related. Greater concordance for disease is expected among MZ versus dizygotic (DZ) twins.

## GENETIC MAPPING OF COMPLEX TRAITS

Once a disease inherited as a complex trait is shown to have a significant hereditary component, the next step is to map the genes involved and identify them. Two major approaches have been used to locate and identify genes that predispose to complex diseases or contribute to the genetic variance of quantitative traits. The first is a type of linkage analysis that relies on pairs of family members, such as siblings, who are concordant for the phenotype (**affected pedigree member method**). As shown in Figure 15–1, siblings have, on average, 50 percent of their alleles in common (identical by descent from their common parents) at any one locus. If a region of the genome is shared more frequently than expected by relatives concordant for a particular phenotype, the inference is that there are alleles that predispose to that phenotype at one or more loci in this region. The second approach is **association**, which looks for increased frequency of particular alleles in affected compared with unaffected individuals in the population. Both approaches have advantages and disadvantages in particular situations, as described later.

### Model-Free Linkage Analysis of Complex Disease Traits

Standard linkage analysis, as described in Chapter 8, is a powerful method for mapping single-gene disorders, but it is rarely applicable to complex traits. Linkage analysis depends on assuming a mode of inheritance and then counting nonrecombinant and recombinant offspring in families to (1) determine whether there is evidence for a genetic locus that recombines with the disease locus with a frequency $\theta$ that is less than the 50 percent expected with unlinked loci, and (2) estimate the value of the parameter $\theta$ that gives the highest lod score, $\theta_{max}$ (see Chapter 8). This approach to linkage analysis is called **model-based** (or **parametric**) **linkage analysis** because it assumes that there is a particular mode of inheritance (autosomal dominant, autosomal recessive, or X-linked) that explains the inheritance pattern. By their very nature, diseases inherited as complex traits are not usually amenable to an analysis that depends on knowing that a mutation in a single gene, inherited in a specific mendelian inheritance pattern, causes the disease. Instead, **model-free** (or **nonparametric**) **methods** have been developed that make no assumption concerning the number of loci or the role of environment and chance in causing lack of penetrance. Rather, model-free methods depend solely on the assumption that two affected relatives will have disease-predisposing alleles in common.

One type of model-free analysis is the **affected sibpair method**. Only siblings concordant for a disease are used, thereby eliminating the problem of determining whether an unaffected individual is a nonpenetrant carrier of the alleles that predispose to disease or simply did not inherit them. No assumptions need be made about the number of loci involved or the inheritance pattern. Instead, sibs are analyzed to determine whether there are loci at which affected sibpairs share alleles more frequently than the 50 percent expected by chance alone (see Fig. 15–1). What happens if hundreds of sibpairs concordant for the disease are systematically studied for allele-sharing at loci throughout the genome? Bear in mind that there may be multiple loci that predispose to the disease, so not all pairs of sibs concordant for a disease will share alleles at the same loci; however, if a particular locus is an important contributor to the disease, significantly more than the expected degree of allele-sharing will be seen at that locus in the collection of sibpairs. Whether the degree of allele-sharing diverges significantly from the 50 percent expected by chance alone can be assessed by using a maximum likelihood odds ratio, just as model-based linkage analysis uses a lod score to assess whether a recombination frequency less than 50 percent is significant (see Chapter 8).

In the affected sibpair method, DNA of affected sibs is systematically analyzed using hundreds of polymorphic markers throughout the entire genome (**a genome scan**) in a search for regions that are shared by the two sibs significantly more frequently than expected on a purely random basis. When elevated degrees of allele-sharing are found at a polymorphic marker, it suggests that a locus involved in the disease is located close to the marker. However, consider that the more polymorphic loci studied, the more likely it is that a locus will show what looks like significantly elevated allele-sharing by chance alone. To understand why, consider the example of coin tossing. Although it is unlikely that a single experiment of tossing a coin five times will give five heads, it is very likely that, if the experiment is repeated hundreds of times, at least one of those hundreds of experiments will yield five heads. Significance levels and a corresponding lod score (see Chapter 8) for increased allele-sharing in a genome scan using approximately 400 markers have been proposed to reduce the risk of inappropriately assigning significance to what is only random fluctuation from expected allele-sharing levels. In this setting, a lod score greater than approximately 3.6 for allele-sharing at a locus would occur with a probability of less than 1 in 20 by chance alone; a lod score greater than 5.4 would occur by chance only once in 1000 studies.

Although the affected sibpair method avoids making possibly incorrect assumptions about how many loci are involved and how alleles at these various loci interact to cause disease, it does so at the cost of being insensitive and imprecise. Its insensitivity is reflected in the fact that large numbers of sibpairs are required to detect a significant deviation from the expected 50 percent allele-sharing. Suppose, for example, an allele at a disease locus has a frequency of 10 percent in the population and increases disease risk fourfold in heterozygotes and 16-fold in homozygotes. In this situation, under the best of circumstances, it is estimated that it would take 185 sibpairs to detect an elevation of allele-sharing to nearly 60 percent. If the locus is a relatively infrequent contributor to the disease or causes much less of an increase in disease risk than the fourfold in heterozygotes, elevation of allele-sharing greater than 50 percent would be proportionately less, and many, many more sibpairs, numbering in the thousands or tens of thousands, would be needed to detect the locus. Thus, practically speaking, affected sibpair methods are unlikely to identify loci in which only a few rare alleles make only minor contributions to a disease.

Model-free methods are also imprecise. Because one is not assuming that a single gene or a particular inheritance pattern is involved, one cannot determine definitively whether a recombination has occurred between a possible disease-predisposing locus and the disease phenotype. In model-based linkage strategy for fine mapping of a single-gene disease (see Chapter 8), finding the closest markers on either side of the disease gene that *do* recombine at least once with the disease gene defines the boundaries of a narrow, critical interval in which the disease gene must reside. Model-free methods can only identify broad regions of increased allele-sharing and not a narrow, critical region delimiting the location of a gene contributing to a complex trait.

## Model-Free Linkage Analysis of Quantitative Traits

Model-free linkage methods based on allele-sharing can also be used to map loci involved in quantitative complex traits. Although a number of approaches are available, one interesting example is the **highly discordant sibpair method**. Once again, no assumptions need be made about the number of loci involved or the inheritance pattern. Sibpairs highly discordant for the quantitative trait—that is, with values of a physiological measurement that are at opposite ends of the bell-shaped curve, are assumed to be less likely to share alleles at loci that contribute to the trait. The DNA of highly discordant sibs is then systematically analyzed using polymorphic markers throughout the entire genome in a search for regions that are shared by the two sibs significantly *less* frequently than expected on a purely random basis. When reduced levels of allele-sharing are found at a polymorphic marker, it suggests that the marker is linked to a locus whose alleles contribute to whatever physiological measurement is under study.

## Disease Association

The fact that a particular allele at a locus is present at increased frequency in affected individuals compared with controls is known as a **disease association**. Association methods are a form of case-control study in which the frequency of a *particular allele* (such as for an HLA antigen) at a locus is compared among affected and unaffected individuals in the population (see Chapter 14). The strength of an association is measured by the **odds ratio**, which is calculated from the frequency of a specific allele in patients and controls.

| | With allele | Without allele |
|---|---|---|
| **Patients** | a | c |
| **Controls** | b | d |

a = number of patients with the allele; b = number of controls with the allele; c = number of patients without the allele; d = number of controls without the allele.

Odds ratio is then = ad/bc. If the frequency of the allele in question were the same in patients and controls, the odds ratio would be 1.

For example, in one study of a group of 120 patients with cerebral or deep vein thrombosis (discussed later in this chapter) and 120 controls, a particular mutation in the prothrombin gene was found in 23 of the patients and four of the controls. The odds ratio then = (23)(116)/(4)(97) = ~7. This means that the odds of developing thrombosis are seven times higher in individuals who carry the prothrombin gene mutation than in those who do not carry the prothrombin gene mutation.

A different but related measure of association is the **relative risk** (RR), which compares the risk of developing a disease when one carries a specific allele relative to the risk if one does not carry it. RR = (a/(a + c))/(b/(b + d)), approximately equal to the odds ratio when the disease allele is rare (i.e., $b < d$ and $a < c$). In the case of the mutant prothrombin allele and thrombosis, RR = (23/120)/(4/120) = 5.75. (Do not confuse RR with $\lambda_r$, the relative risk ratio, discussed previously in the chapter. $\lambda_r$ is the prevalence of a particular disease phenotype in an affected individual's relatives versus the general population.)

#### Strengths and Weaknesses of Association Studies

Association methods are powerful tools for pinpointing precisely the genes that contribute to genetic disease by demonstrating not only the genes but also the particular alleles responsible. They are also relatively easy to perform because one needs samples only from a set of affected individuals and controls and does not have to carry out laborious family studies and collection of samples from members of a pedigree. Association studies must be interpreted with caution, however, because an increased odds ratio for an allele at a particular locus does not prove that the allele or even the locus at which the allele resides is involved in disease pathogenesis.

*There are two ways that the odds ratio for carrying a particular allele may be increased in patients with a disease, without that allele being involved in the disease at all.* First, the allele in question may be in linkage disequilibrium (see Chapter 8) with a quite different allele at another unknown but nearby locus that is actually involved in the pathogenesis of the disease. Any alleles at loci that are in linkage disequilibrium with the allele and locus involved in the disease will show an apparently increased odds ratio and a positive association. A second, and even more serious, limitation of association studies is that they are sensitive to the effect of population stratification (see Chapter 7). If a population is stratified into separate subpopulations (such as by ethnicity and religion) and members of one subpopulation rarely mate with members of other subpopulations, then a disease that happens to be more common in one subpopulation can appear (incorrectly) to be associated with any alleles that also happen to be more common in that subpopulation than in the population as a whole. Factitious association due to population stratification can be minimized, however, by careful selection of controls as well as by using more sophisticated, family-based methods of testing for association between a disease and particular alleles.

## DISEASES WITH COMPLEX INHERITANCE

The common multifactorial disorders that account for much morbidity and mortality in children and adults have always been a problem to geneticists. Using familial aggregation, relative risk ratios, twin studies, and estimates of heritability and concordance, the genetic contribution to diseases or quantitative traits with complex inheritance can be inferred and even quantified without specifying precisely how many loci are involved or how a particular genotype and set of environmental influences result in a disease or in a particular value of a quantitative trait. This lack of precision is an accurate reflection of our current state of knowledge. In stark contrast to mendelian single-gene defects, *there are only a handful of multifactorial diseases or quantitative human traits for which the underlying genetic models (the number of loci, the nature of environmental factors, and the interaction between them) are known.* This lack of knowledge severely hampers our ability to understand the role of heredity in multifactorial disease and to make accurate predictions of the risk for disease in relatives for the purpose of genetic counseling.

Historically, geneticists have attempted to understand the underlying mechanisms by which complex diseases or quantitative traits are inherited by creating theoretical models. In these models, geneticists would specify a set of alleles at various loci, a number of environmental factors, and the nature of the interactions among these factors and then test the models for how well they could predict the inheritance pattern of a disease observed in actual families and patients. A good match between theoretical prediction and observation would suggest that the theoretical model is a good approximation of the true underlying mechanism of disease. Unfortunately, many different models can result in nearly identical inheritance patterns, making it difficult to know which model was closest to the correct underlying mechanism. With advances in gene mapping technology, a second, more empiric approach is becoming possible. By applying model-free linkage analysis and association studies in actual families, the loci and alleles responsible for diseases inherited as complex traits are being determined. In the following, we stress the empiric rather than theoretical approach. We describe a number of complex diseases, in which the genetic contributions have begun to be identified, as examples of the genetic mechanisms responsible for complex diseases. We present these diseases in order of increasing complexity, with the best understood disorders discussed first.

### Digenic Retinitis Pigmentosa

A simple example of a trait determined by the additive effect of multiple loci (**multigenic**) has been found in a few families of patients with a form of retinal degeneration called retinitis pigmentosa (Fig. 15–4). Two rare mutations in two different unlinked genes encoding proteins found in the photoreceptor are present in the family. Patients heterozygous either for a particular missense mutation in one gene, encoding the photoreceptor membrane protein peripherin, or for a null allele in the other gene, encoding a related photoreceptor membrane protein called

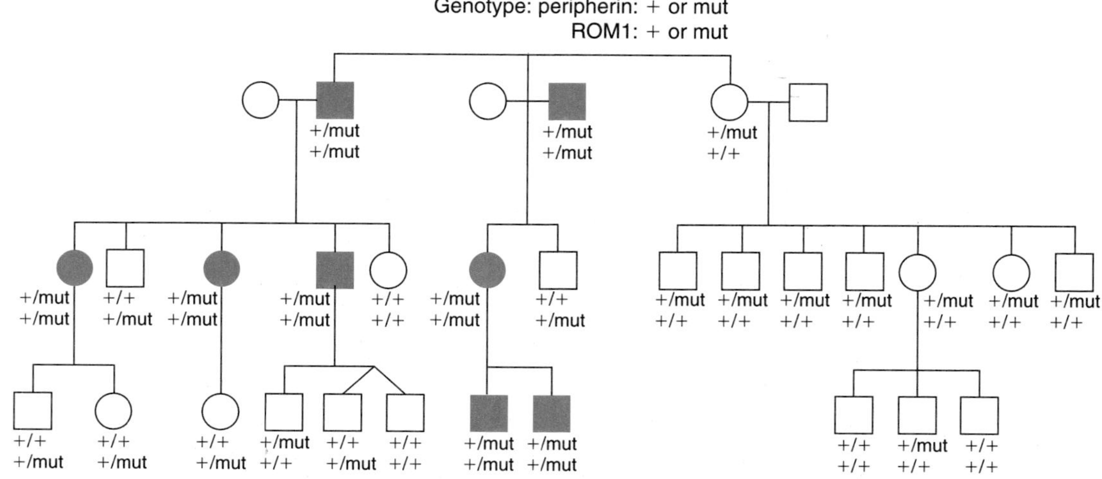


**Figure 15–4.** Pedigree of a family with retinitis pigmentosa due to digenic inheritance. Filled symbols are affected individuals. Each individual's genotypes at the peripherin locus (*first line*) and *ROM1* locus (*second line*) are written below each symbol. The normal allele is +; the mutant allele is mut. (From Kajiwara K, Berson EL, Dryja TP [1994] Digenic retinitis pigmentosa due to mutations at the unlinked peripherin/RDS and ROM1 loci. Science 264:1604–1608.)

Rom1, do not develop the disease. Patients heterozygous for both mutations do develop the disease, however. Thus, inheritance of this disease is caused by the simplest form of multigenic inheritance, digenic inheritance. These two photoreceptor proteins are associated noncovalently in the stacks of membranous disks containing the visual pigments. It is hypothesized that the deleterious effect of each mutation alone is insufficient to cause disease, but their joint presence is sufficient to cross a threshold of cell damage, photoreceptor death, and loss of vision.

## Cerebral Venous Thrombosis

Another example of two mutant alleles that interact to predispose to a disease is found in the disorder known as **idiopathic cerebral thrombosis**. In this case, however, there is a third factor, an environmental influence that, in the presence of the predisposing genetic factors, increases the risk of disease even more. Idiopathic cerebral thrombosis is a catastrophic occlusion of cerebral veins in the absence of an inciting event such as infection or tumor. It affects young adults, and, although quite rare (<1 per 100,000 in the population), it carries with it a high mortality rate (5 to 30 percent). Three factors (two genetic and one environmental) that lead to abnormal coagulability of the clotting system are each known to individually increase the risk for this illness: a common missense mutation in a clotting factor, factor V, another common variant in the clotting factor prothrombin, and the use of oral contraceptives.

A mutant allele of factor V (**factor V Leiden**), in which arginine is replaced by glutamine at position 506 (Arg506Gly), has an allele frequency of approximately 2.5 percent in Caucasians but is rarer in other population groups. Heterozygous carriers of factor V Leiden have a risk of thrombosis that is seven times higher than that in the general population; homozygotes have a risk that is 80 times higher. A mutation in the prothrombin gene that changes a G to an A at position 20210 (G20210A) in the 3′ untranslated region has a frequency of approximately 2.4 percent in Caucasians but is rare in other groups. The G20210A mutation raises the risk of venous thrombosis three- to sixfold. Finally, the use of oral contraceptives increases the risk of thrombosis 22-fold, independent of genotype at the factor V and prothrombin loci, probably by increasing the levels of many clotting factors in the blood. Using oral contraceptives and being heterozygous for factor V Leiden cause a modest increase in risk compared with either factor alone. If a woman uses oral contraceptives and is a heterozygote for the prothrombin mutation, her relative risk rises to 149! Thus, each of these three factors, two genetic and one environmental, on its own increases the risk for an abnormal hypercoagulable state; having two or three of these factors at the same time raises the risk for a devastating illness of the cerebral vascular system even more.

These alleles at the factor V and prothrombin loci, as well as an allele for a heat-sensitive methylene tetrahydrofolate reductase (see later discussion), have also been implicated as serious predisposing genetic risk factors for **placental artery thrombosis**. Carrying one of these mutations raises the risk an average of fivefold over the general population risk for this severe obstetrical complication. The resulting placental dysfunction is associated with severe pre-eclampsia, premature separation of the placenta from the uterine wall, intrauterine growth retardation, and stillbirth.

The interaction of these genetic factors with the use of oral contraceptives has led to a proposal that physicians screen women for the predisposing factor V and prothrombin gene mutations before prescribing birth control pills.

## Hirschsprung Disease

A more complicated set of interacting genetic factors has been described in the pathogenesis of a developmental abnormality of the parasympathetic nervous system in the gut known as **Hirschsprung disease** (HSCR). In HSCR, there is complete absence of some or all of the intrinsic ganglion cells in the myenteric and submucosal plexuses of the colon. An aganglionic colon is incapable of peristalsis, resulting in severe constipation, symptoms of intestinal obstruction, and massive dilatation of the colon (megacolon) proximal to the aganglionic segment. The absence of ganglion cells generally occurs in a single continuous segment that can vary in length from just a few inches at the distal end of the colon to the entire length of the colon. The disorder affects approximately 1 in 5000 newborns. HSCR occurs most commonly as an isolated defect involving only a short segment of colon, but it can also involve long colonic segments and can also occur as one element of a broader constellation of congenital abnormalities including deafness and pigmentary abnormalities of hair and eyes (the Waardenburg-Shah syndrome).

The hereditary pattern of HSCR has many of the characteristics of a disorder with complex genetics. The relative risk ratio for sibs, $\lambda_s$, is very high (approximately 200), but MZ twins do not show perfect concordance. HSCR can occur through multiple generations or can affect multiple siblings in a family, or both, suggesting an autosomal dominant or recessive disorder, but recurrence risks are not strictly 50 percent or 25 percent as one might expect for autosomal dominant or autosomal recessive disease traits. Males have a twofold higher risk of developing HSCR as compared with females within the same family.

Linkage and DNA sequence analysis in families with multiple probands with HSCR have revealed that mutations in many different genes may cause the disease. The condition is most commonly due to mutations in the *RET* gene located at 10q11.2, encoding ret, a tyrosine kinase receptor. A small minority of individuals with HSCR have mutations in the gene encoding one of the ligands that binds to ret, the glial cell line-derived neurotrophic factor (gdnf), whereas still other individuals have been described with mutations in either of a pair of genes, the endothelin B receptor (*EDNRB*) at 13q22, and the *EDN3* gene encoding its ligand, endothelin 3, at 20q13. The involvement of endothelin 3 and its receptor in HSCR came as a surprise because these molecules were thought to play a role in blood vessel formation, not autonomic nervous system development. The relationship between the *EDNRB* and *RET* signaling pathways is also quite obscure, but both pathways seem to function in parallel, rather than in series, to promote development of colonic ganglion cells.

Although mutations in *RET* are the most common cause of HSCR affecting multiple individuals in a family, the penetrance of these *RET* alleles is far from complete. In some families, the penetrance is increased if these individuals also have a mutation in the gene for one of the ligands that signals through ret, such as gdnf; in other families, alleles at an as-of-yet unidentified locus at 19q31 were shown by linkage analysis to increase the penetrance. The most likely explanation for these observations is that some mutant alleles of *RET* still provide residual function sufficient to prevent development of the disease unless additional dysfunction in other components of relevant signaling pathways also occurs.

Similarly, in one large inbred Mennonite family, linkage analysis revealed that expression of the HSCR phenotype due to a mutation in *EDNRB* was strongly influenced by an individual's genotype at the *RET* locus. Despite this genetic evidence implicating *RET* in the penetrance of an *EDNRB* mutation, however, the sequence of the coding region of *RET* in these patients failed to reveal an obvious deleterious mutation. The failure to find an obvious mutation in the coding region of *RET* serves to illustrate that the mutations or polymorphisms responsible for modifying expression of a multifactorial trait may be quite subtle in how they exert their effects on gene expression and, as a consequence, disease penetrance and expressivity.

The multifactorial nature of HSCR was brought into even sharper focus when the genetic basis of the most common form of HSCR, involving only a short segment of colon, was analyzed in sibpairs concordant for HSCR in families that did not show any obvious dominant inheritance pattern. Non–model-based linkage analysis (see earlier) in 67 sibpairs concordant for HSCR revealed significant allele-sharing at three loci: the 10q11.2 region, where *RET* is located, and two unidentified loci in 3p21 and 19q12. Most of the 67 sibpairs concordant for HSCR (55 of 67) were found to share alleles at all three loci, whereas only 12 concordant sibpairs were found to share alleles at two of the three loci. No concordant affected sibpairs shared alleles at only one or none of the loci (Fig. 15–5). The most likely model to explain these observations is that certain alleles of *RET*, the chromosome 3p21 locus, and the chromosome 19q12 locus confer some susceptibility to HSCR but do not cause the disease by themselves. Rather, HSCR is a multifactor-

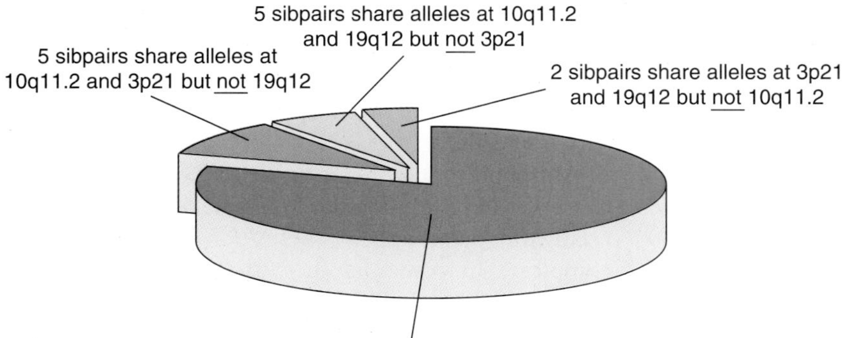


Figure 15–5. Pie chart of 67 sibpairs concordant for Hirschsprung disease, divided according to the number of loci for which the sibs show allele-sharing. The three loci are located at 10q11.2 (*RET*), 3p21, and 19q12. (Data provided by A. Chakravarti, Johns Hopkins University, Baltimore.)

ial disease that results from the additive effects of susceptibility alleles at a number of loci. Thus, the underlying genetic mechanisms for this relatively well-defined congenital malformation have turned out to be surprisingly complex; still, they are likely to be far simpler than are the mechanisms involved in the more common complex diseases, such as diabetes.

## Diabetes Mellitus

There are two major types of diabetes mellitus: **type 1 (insulin-dependent)** and **type 2 (non–insulin-dependent)**, representing about 10 percent and 88 percent of all cases, respectively. They differ in typical onset age, MZ twin concordance, and HLA associations. Familial aggregation is seen in both types of diabetes, but, in any given family, one generally sees either type 1 or type 2 but not both.

### Type 1 Diabetes Mellitus

Type 1 diabetes has an incidence in the Caucasian population of about 1 in 200 (0.5 percent) and usually manifests in childhood or adolescence. It results from autoimmune destruction of the $\beta$ cells of the pancreas, which normally produce insulin.

**MHC Association in Type 1 Diabetes.** Genetic factors alone do not cause type 1 diabetes, because the MZ twin concordance rate for type 1 diabetes is only approximately 40 percent. Nevertheless, there is strong evidence for genetic factors in type 1 diabetes: concordance among MZ twins far exceeds the concordance in DZ twins, and the risk for type 1 diabetes in siblings of an affected proband is approximately 6 percent, resulting in an estimated $\lambda_s = 6\%/0.5\% = 12$. That the MHC locus is a major genetic factor in type 1 diabetes was first shown when an association study revealed that about 95 percent of all patients with type 1 diabetes (in comparison with about half the normal population) are heterozygous for *HLA-DR3* or *HLA-DR4; DR3/DR4* heterozygotes are particularly susceptible to type 1 diabetes. This is one of the strongest MHC-disease associations known (see Chapter 14).

Because the $\beta$-cell destruction responsible for type 1 diabetes appears to be an autoimmune process, it makes sense that there is an association between certain alleles (*DR3* and *DR4*) in a locus known to regulate immune response and liability to autoimmune disease. Further insights into the underlying mechanism of the *DR3* and *DR4* association with type 1 diabetes have come from molecular analysis of different *DR* haplotypes containing various alleles of the HLA class II genes, especially *DQ* (see Chapter 14). The presence of aspartic acid (Asp) at position 57 of the *DQ* chain (see Fig. 14–1) is closely associated with resistance to type 1 diabetes, whereas other amino acids at this position (alanine, valine, or serine) confer susceptibility. About 90 percent of patients with type 1 diabetes are homozygous for *DQ*$\beta$ genes that do not encode Asp at position 57. Given that the *DQ* molecule, and position 57 of the $\beta$ chain in particular, is critical to peptide antigen binding and presentation to the T cell for response, it is very likely that the *DQ* molecule, especially amino acid 57 of its $\beta$ chain, contributes directly to the autoimmune response that destroys the insulin-producing cells of the pancreas.

**Genes Other than Class II MHC Loci in Type 1 Diabetes.** Family studies in type 1 diabetes (Table 15–5) suggest that even when siblings share the same *DR* haplotypes, the risk of disease is approximately 13 percent, still well below the MZ twin concordance rate of approximately 40 percent. This discrepancy indicates that the MHC haplotype alone accounts for only a third (13 percent/40 percent) of the genetic

TABLE 15–5

**Risk for Type 1 Diabetes in Siblings of Probands with Type 1 Diabetes**

| Extent of MHC Haplotype Sharing | Risk of Type 1 Diabetes in Sib of Type 1 Diabetes Patient (%) |
|---|---|
| Proband and sib both share *DR3/DR4* | 20 |
| Proband and sib share any two haplotypes | 13 |
| Proband and sib share any one haplotype | 5 |
| Proband and sib share no haplotype | 2 |

MHC = Major histocompatibility complex.

contribution to the risk for type 1 diabetes in siblings of a proband. Thus, there must be other genes, elsewhere in the genome, that also predispose to the development of type 1 diabetes, assuming MZ twins and sibs have similar environmental exposures. Finding these predisposing genes is the goal of large mapping studies that are using model-free sibpair linkage methods (described earlier in this chapter) to scan the genome. As many as 13 additional loci have been proposed for type 1 diabetes based on genome-wide scans; of these, the best evidence is for a susceptibility locus located at or near a variable number tandem repeat polymorphism (see Chapter 6) in the promoter of the insulin gene itself. Identification of other susceptibility genes for type 1 diabetes, both within and outside the MHC, remains the target of intensive investigation. At present, the nature of the nongenetic risk factors in type 1 diabetes is largely unknown.

## Alzheimer Disease

**AD** is a fatal neurodegenerative disease that affects 1 to 2 percent of the United States population. Patients experience a chronic, progressive loss of memory and other intellectual functions, associated with death of neurons and development of extracellular protein aggregates called amyloid plaques throughout the cerebral cortex. The most important constituent of these plaques is a small (39 to 42 amino acid) peptide, A$\beta$, derived from cleavage of a normal neuronal protein, the amyloid protein precursor. The secondary structure of A$\beta$ gives the plaques the staining characteristics of amyloid proteins (see also Chapter 12). In addition to three rare autosomal dominant forms of the disease (see Table 12–10), in which disease onset is in the third to fifth decade, there is a common form of AD with onset after age 60 years (late onset). This form has no obvious mendelian inheritance pattern but does show familial aggregation and an elevated relative risk ratio ($\lambda_r$) typical of disorders with complex inheritance.

**The $\varepsilon$4 Allele of Apolipoprotein E.** The first significant genetic factor associated with common late-onset AD is the **apolipoprotein E** (*APOE*) locus. ApoE is a protein component of the low-density lipoprotein (LDL) particle and is involved in clearing LDL through an interaction with high-affinity receptors in the liver. ApoE is also a constituent of amyloid plaques in AD and is known to bind the A$\beta$ peptide. The *APOE* gene maps to chromosome 19 and has three alleles, $\varepsilon 2$, $\varepsilon 3$, and $\varepsilon 4$, owing to substitutions of arginine for two different cysteine residues in the protein.

Model-free linkage analysis in sibpairs concordant for AD initially revealed excess allele-sharing in a region of chromosome 19 that included the locus for apoE. With this result in mind, an association study between specific *APOE* alleles and AD was performed in AD patients versus controls appropriately matched for age, gender, and ethnicity. When the frequency of the $\varepsilon 2$, $\varepsilon 3$, and $\varepsilon 4$ genotypes was compared with the frequency of genotypes without $\varepsilon 4$ in patients with AD, a genotype with at least one $\varepsilon 4$ allele was found two to three times more frequently among the patients compared with controls (Table 15–6) in both the general U.S. and Japanese populations. There seems to be much less of an association in the Hispanic and African-American populations. Even more striking is that the risk for AD appears to increase as the number of $\varepsilon 4$ alleles increases, through an effect on the age of onset: the more $\varepsilon 4$ alleles one has, the earlier the onset of AD. In a study of patients with

TABLE 15–6

**Association of *APOE* $\varepsilon$4 Allele with Alzheimer Disease: Frequency of Genotypes with and without the $\varepsilon$4 Allele among AD Patients and Controls from the United States and Japan**

| | Frequency | | | |
|---|---|---|---|---|
| Genotype | *AD (United States)* | *Control (United States)* | *AD (Japan)* | *Control (Japan)* |
| $\varepsilon 4/\varepsilon 4$; $\varepsilon 4/\varepsilon 3$; or $\varepsilon 4/\varepsilon 2$ | 0.64 | 0.31 | 0.47 | 0.17 |
| $\varepsilon 3/\varepsilon 3$; $\varepsilon 2/\varepsilon 3$; or $\varepsilon 2/\varepsilon 2$ | 0.36 | 0.69 | 0.53 | 0.83 |

AD = Alzheimer disease.

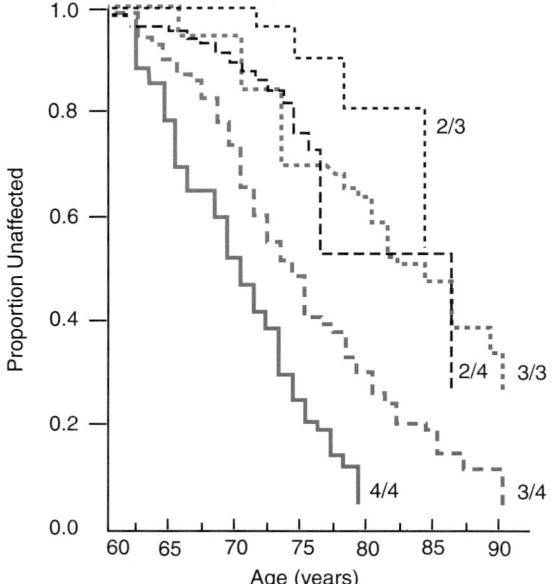


**Figure 15–6.** Chance of remaining unaffected by Alzheimer disease as a function of age for different *APOE* genotypes. At one extreme is the $\varepsilon4/\varepsilon4$ homozygote who has a less than 10 percent chance of remaining free of the disease by age 80, whereas an $\varepsilon2/\varepsilon3$ heterozygote has a more than 90 percent chance of remaining disease-free at age 80. (Modified, with permission, from Strittmatter WJ, Roses AD [1996] Apolipoprotein E and Alzheimer's disease. Annu Rev Neurosci 19:53–77. ©1996, by Annual Reviews.)

AD and both unrelated and family unaffected controls (Fig. 15–6), the age at which the AD developed in the affected patients was earliest for $\varepsilon4/\varepsilon4$ homozygotes, next for $\varepsilon4/\varepsilon3$ heterozygotes, and significantly less for the other genotypes.

In the population in general, the $\varepsilon4$ allele is clearly a predisposing factor that increases the risk of developing AD by shifting the age of onset to an earlier age so that the disease becomes evident before most patients die from other life-threatening illnesses of the elderly. Despite this increased risk, other genetic and environmental factors must be important because many $\varepsilon4/\varepsilon4$ homozygotes live to extreme old age with no evidence for AD, and 50 to 75 percent of all heterozygotes carrying one $\varepsilon4$ allele never develop AD. A role for other genes received further support from a model-free linkage analysis on pairs of siblings affected with AD when a region with elevated allele sharing was found on chromosome 12. There is also an association between the presence of the $\varepsilon4$ allele and neurodegenerative disease following head injury (as seen in professional boxers), indicating that at least one environmental factor interacts with the $\varepsilon4$ allele in the pathogenesis of neurodegenerative disease. Thus, the $\varepsilon4$ variant of *APOE* represents a prime example of a predisposing allele: it predisposes to a complex trait in a powerful way but does not predestine any individual carrying the allele to developing the disease. Additional genes as well as environmental effects are also clearly involved but remain to be definitively elucidated. Testing asymptomatic people for the $\varepsilon4$ allele remains controversial, because knowing that one is a heterozygote or homozygote for the $\varepsilon4$ allele does not mean one will develop AD nor is there any intervention currently known that can affect the chance one will or will not develop AD (see Chapters 12 and 20).

TABLE 15–7
**Some Common Congenital Malformations with Multifactorial Inheritance**

| Malformation | Population Incidence (per 1000) (approximate) |
|---|---|
| Cleft lip with/without cleft palate | 0.4–1.7 |
| Cleft palate | 0.4 |
| Congenital dislocation of hip | 2* |
| Congenital heart defects | 4–8 |
| Ventricular septal defect | 1.7 |
| Patent ductus arteriosus | 0.5 |
| Atrial septal defect | 1.0 |
| Aortic stenosis | 0.5 |
| Neural tube defects | 2–10 |
| Anencephaly | Variable |
| Spina bifida | Variable |
| Pyloric stenosis | 1†<br>5* |

*Per 1000 males; †per 1000 females.

*Note*: Many of these disorders are heterogeneous and are usually but not invariably multifactorial.

Data from Carter CO (1976) Genetics of common single malformations. Br Med Bull 32:21–26; Nora JJ (1968) Multifactorial inheritance hypothesis for the etiology of congenital heart diseases: The genetic environmental interaction. Circulation 38:604–617; Lin AE, Garver KL (1988) Genetic counseling for congenital heart defects. J Pediatr 113:1105–1109.

## Multifactorial Congenital Malformations

Several common congenital malformations, occurring as isolated defects and not as part of a syndrome, seem to recur in families. The familial aggregation and elevated risk of recurrence in relatives of an affected individual are all characteristic of a complex trait (Table 15–7). Some of the more important congenital malformations with complex inheritance are **neural tube defects**, **cleft lip** with or without **cleft palate**, and **congenital heart malformations**.

### Neural Tube Defects

**Anencephaly** and **spina bifida** are neural tube defects (NTDs) that frequently occur together in families and are considered to have a common pathogenesis (Fig. 15–7). In anencephaly, the forebrain, overlying meninges, vault of the skull, and skin are all absent. Many infants with anencephaly are stillborn, and

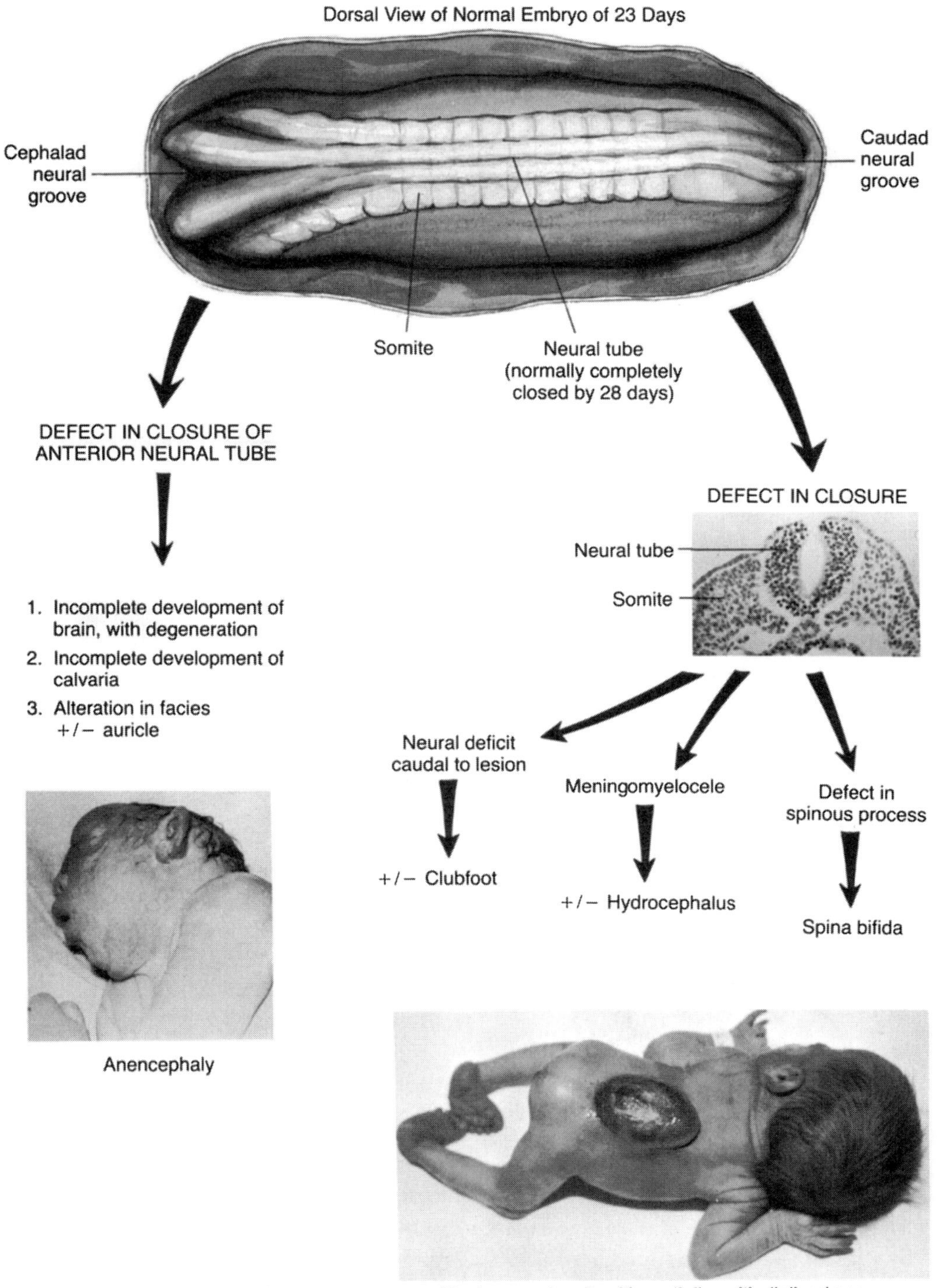


**Figure 15–7.** The origin of the neural tube defects anencephaly and spina bifida. (From Jones KL [1988] Smith's Recognizable Patterns of Human Malformation, 4th ed. WB Saunders, Philadelphia.)

those born alive survive a few hours at most. About two thirds of affected infants are female. In spina bifida, there is failure of fusion of the arches of the vertebrae, typically in the lumbar region. There are varying degrees of severity, ranging from spina bifida occulta, in which the defect is in the bony arch only, to spina bifida aperta, in which a bony defect is also associated with meningocele (protrusion of meninges) or meningomyelocele (protrusion of neural elements as well as meninges through the defect; see Fig. 15–7).

As a group, NTDs are a leading cause of stillbirth, death in early infancy, and handicap in surviving children. Their incidence at birth is variable, ranging from almost 1 percent in Ireland to 0.2 percent or less in the United States. The frequency also appears to vary with social factors and season of birth, and oscillates widely over time (with a marked decrease in recent years; see later discussion).

A small proportion of NTDs have specific causes: for example, amniotic bands (fibrous connections between the amnion and fetus caused by early rupture of the amnion, which may disrupt structures during their embryological development), some single-gene defects with pleiotropic expression, some chromosome disorders, and some teratogens. Most NTDs, however, are isolated defects.

**Maternal Folic Acid Deficiency and Neural Tube Defects.** NTDs were long believed to follow a multifactorial inheritance pattern determined by multiple genetic and environmental factors. It was, therefore, a stunning discovery to find that the single greatest factor in causing NTDs is a vitamin deficiency. The risk of NTDs was found to be inversely correlated with maternal serum folic acid levels during pregnancy, with a threshold of 200 $\mu$g/L, below which the risk of NTD becomes very significant. Along with reduced blood folate levels, elevated homocysteine levels were also seen in the mothers of children with NTDs, suggesting that a biochemical abnormality was occurring at the step of recycling of tetrahydrofolate to methylate homocysteine to methionine (Fig. 15–8). Folic acid levels are strongly influenced by dietary intake and can become depressed during pregnancy even with a typical intake of approximately 230 $\mu$g/day. The impact of folic acid deficiency is exacerbated by a genetic variant of the enzyme 5,10-methylenetetrahydrofolate reductase (MTHFR), caused by a common missense mutation that makes the enzyme less stable than normal. Instability of this enzyme hinders the recycling of tetrahydrofolate and interferes with the methylation of homocysteine to methionine. The mutant allele is so common in many populations that between 5 and 15 percent of the population is homozygous for the mutation. In studies of infants with NTDs and their mothers, it was found that mothers of infants with NTDs were twice as likely to be homozygous for the mutant allele encoding the unstable enzyme as controls. Not all mothers of NTD infants with low folic acid levels are homozygous for the mutant allele of MTHFR, however, indicating that low folic acid levels may be caused by other unknown genetic factors or by simple dietary deficiency alone. How this enzyme defect contributes to NTDs and whether the abnormality is a direct result of elevated homocysteine levels, depressed methionine levels, or some other metabolic derangement remains undefined.

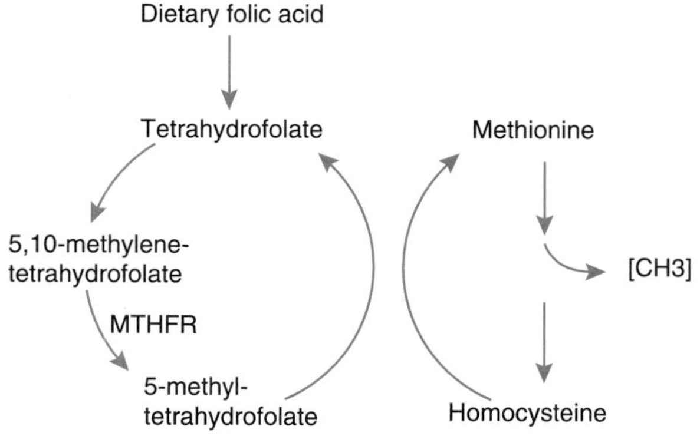


**Figure 15–8.** Metabolic pathway for recycling folic acid, a one-carbon donor used to generate methionine from homocysteine.

**Prevention of Neural Tube Defects.** The discovery of folic acid deficiency in NTDs has led to a remarkable public health initiative to educate women to supplement their diets with folic acid 1 month before conception and continuing for 2 months after conception during the period when the neural tube forms. Dietary supplementation with 400 to 800 $\mu$g of folic acid/day for women who plan their pregnancies has been shown to reduce the incidence of NTDs by more than 75 percent. Much active discussion is ongoing as to whether the entire food supply should be supplemented with folic acid as a public health measure to avoid the problem of women failing to supplement their diets individually during pregnancy.

Parents of children with an NTD are at increased risk for a recurrence in future pregnancies. Recurrence risks within families are given in Table 15–8. NTD also rank high among the conditions for which prenatal diagnosis is possible; anencephaly and most cases of open spina bifida can be identified prenatally by detection of excessive levels of **alpha-fetoprotein** (AFP) and other fetal substances in the amniotic fluid and by **ultrasonographic scanning** (see Chapter 18 for further discussion). Less than 5 percent of all patients with NTDs are born to women with previous affected children, however. For this reason, screening of all pregnant women for NTDs using measurements of AFP and other fetal substances in maternal serum is becoming more widespread. Thus, we can anticipate that a combination of preventive folic acid therapy and maternal AFP screening will provide major public health benefits by drastically reducing the incidence of NTDs.

## Congenital Heart Defects

Congenital heart defects (CHDs) are very common, with a frequency of about four to eight cases/1000 births. They are a heterogeneous group, caused in some cases by single-gene or chromosomal mechanisms and in others by exposure to teratogens, such as rubella infection or maternal diabetes. The cause is

TABLE 15–8

**Recurrence Risks (%) for Cleft Lip with or without Cleft Palate and for Neural Tube Malformations**

| Affected Relatives | Cleft Lip with/ without Cleft Palate | Anencephaly and Spina Bifida |
|---|---|---|
| No sibs | | |
| Neither parent | 0.1 | 0.3 |
| One parent | 3 | 4.5 |
| Both parents | 34 | 30 |
| One sib | | |
| Neither parent | 3 | 4 |
| One parent | 11 | 12 |
| Both parents | 40 | 38 |
| Two sibs | | |
| Neither parent | 8 | 10 |
| One parent | 19 | 20 |
| Both parents | 45 | 43 |
| One sib and one second-degree relative | | |
| Neither parent | 6 | 7 |
| One parent | 16 | 18 |
| Both parents | 43 | 42 |
| One sib and one third-degree relative | | |
| Neither parent | 4 | 5.5 |
| One parent | 14 | 16 |
| Both parents | 44 | 42 |

From Bonaiti-Pellié C, Smith C (1974) Risk tables for genetic counselling in some common congenital malformations. J Med Genet 11:374–377.

usually unknown, and the majority of cases are believed to be multifactorial in origin.

There are many types of CHDs, with different population incidences and empiric risks. It is known that when heart defects recur in a family, however, the affected children do not necessarily have exactly the same anatomical defect but, instead, show recurrence of lesions that are similar with regard to developmental mechanisms. Using developmental mechanism as a classification scheme, five main groups of CHDs can be distinguished: flow lesions, defects in cell migration or in cell death, abnormalities in extracellular matrix, and defects in targeted growth. A familial pattern is found primarily in the group with flow lesions, a large category that includes hypoplastic left heart syndrome, coarctation of the aorta, atrial septal defect of the secundum type, pulmonary valve stenosis, a common type of ventricular septal defect, and other forms. Some of this familial pattern is explainable by deletion in the region of chromosome 22q11, as is seen in the **velocardiofacial syndrome** associated with tetralogy of Fallot and other flow lesions (see Chapter 10).

Are isolated CHDs inherited as multifactorial traits? The relative risk ratios for sibs, $\lambda_s$, for flow lesions support familial aggregation for this class of CHD (Table 15–9). Until more is known, the figures given can be used as estimates of the recurrence risk for flow lesions in first-degree relatives. There is, however, a rapid fall-off in risk (to levels not much higher than the population risk) in second- and third-degree relatives of index patients with flow lesions. Similarly, relatives of index patients with types of CHDs other than flow lesions can be offered reassurance that their risk is no greater than that of the general population. For further reassurance, many CHDs can now be assessed prenatally by ultrasonography (see Chapter 18).

### CLEFT LIP AND CLEFT PALATE

Cleft lip with or without cleft palate, or CL(P), is one of the most common congenital malformations. CL(P), which is etiologically distinct from isolated cleft palate without cleft lip, originates as a failure of

TABLE 15–9

**Population Incidence and Recurrence Risks for Various Flow Lesions**

| Defect | Population Incidence (%) | Frequency in Sibs (%) | $\lambda_{sib}$ |
|---|---|---|---|
| Ventricular septal defect | 0.17 | 4.3 | 25 |
| Patent ductus arteriosus | 0.083 | 3.2 | 38 |
| Atrial septal defect | 0.066 | 3.2 | 48 |
| Aortic stenosis | 0.044 | 2.6 | 59 |

fusion of the frontal process with the maxillary process at about the 35th day of gestation. About 60 to 80 percent of those affected are males. CL(P) is heterogeneous and includes isolated single-gene forms, numerous single-gene syndromes, forms associated with chromosomal disorders (especially trisomy 13), cases resulting from teratogenic exposure (rubella embryopathy, thalidomide, or anticonvulsants), and forms that appear in nonfamilial syndromes. In the past, almost every conceivable mode of inheritance has been proposed for CL(P) to explain its complex inheritance pattern.

There is considerable variation in frequency in different racial groups: about 1.7 per 1000 in Japanese, 1.0 per 1000 in Caucasians, and 0.4 per 1000 in African Americans. Relatively high rates are also seen in some North American populations of Asian descent—for example, in Indians of the southwest United States and the west coast of Canada. The concordance rate is about 30 percent in MZ twins and about 5 percent (the same as the risk for nontwin sibs) in DZ twins (see Table 15–4).

One of the predictions of complex inheritance is that the recurrence risk in relatives of probands that are severely affected is greater than the risk to relatives of mildly affected probands. The explanation for this phenomenon is that more severe disease indicates a greater load of alleles predisposing to disease in the family. Accordingly, family studies of CL(P) have shown an increase in recurrence risk with severity, from unilateral to bilateral and from cleft lip alone (CL) to cleft lip with cleft palate (CLP). Until better insight into the basis of these abnormalities is gained, however, the empiric risk figures (see Tables 15–8, 15–10, and 15–11) are the only guidelines available for genetic counseling.

## Coronary Artery Disease

Coronary artery disease (CAD) kills 500,000 individuals in the United States yearly and is the number 1 cause of morbidity and mortality in the developed world. CAD due to atherosclerosis is the major cause of the nearly 1,500,000 cases of myocardial infarction (MI) occurring annually. In the aggregate, CAD costs more than $100 billion in health care expenses and lost productivity each year in the United States. Family and twin studies have repeatedly supported a role for heredity in MI occurring in younger age groups. For example, a study of 21,004 twins in Sweden revealed that, after controlling for risk factors such as diabetes, smoking, and hypertension, if one male twin experienced an MI before age 65, the other twin's risk for MI was increased six- to eightfold if he was an MZ twin and threefold if a DZ twin. Among female twins, the increase in risk for MI in MZ twins compared with that in DZ twins was even greater: 15-fold for an MZ twin and only 2.6-fold for a DZ twin when one twin experienced an MI before age 65. The older the first twin was at time of MI, the less increased was the risk to the other twin. Thus, the younger the person, the more important are genetic factors in MI, particularly for females.

TABLE 15–10

**Empiric Risks for Cleft Lip with/without Cleft Palate in Relatives of Affected Probands**

| Population Affected | Incidence Cleft Lip with/without Cleft Palate (%) | $\lambda_{relative}$ |
|---|---|---|
| General population | 0.1 | — |
| First-degree relatives | 4.0 | 40 |
| Second-degree relatives | 0.7 | 7 |
| Third-degree relatives | 0.3 | 3 |

TABLE 15–11

**Risk for Cleft Lip with/without Cleft Palate in Siblings of Proband Affected with Clefts of Increasing Severity**

| Phenotype of Proband | Incidence in Sibs of Cleft Lip with/without Cleft Palate (%) |
|---|---|
| Unilateral cleft lip without cleft palate | 4.0 |
| Unilateral cleft lip and palate | 4.9 |
| Bilateral cleft lip without cleft palate | 6.7 |
| Bilateral cleft lip and palate | 8.0 |

There are many stages in the evolution of atherosclerotic lesions in the coronary artery at which genetic differences may predispose or protect from CAD. What begins as a fatty streak in the intima of the artery evolves into a fibrous plaque containing smooth muscle, lipid, and fibrous tissue. These intimal plaques become vascular and may bleed, ulcerate, and calcify, thereby causing severe vessel narrowing as well as providing fertile ground for thrombosis resulting in sudden, complete occlusion and MI. A large number of genes and gene products have been suggested and, in some cases, implicated in promoting one or more of the developmental stages of CAD. These include genes encoding proteins involved in the following:

1. Serum lipid transport and metabolism (apoE, C-III, the LDL receptor, and lipoprotein[a]), as well as total cholesterol level, which, itself, is a quantitative trait with a substantial heritability;
2. Vasoactivity, such as angiotensin-converting enzyme;
3. Blood coagulation, platelet adhesion, and fibrinolysis, such as plasminogen activator inhibitor-1, and the platelet surface glycoproteins Ib and IIIa.

Familial hypercholesterolemia, an autosomal dominant defect of the LDL receptor discussed in Chapter 12, accounts for only about 5 percent of survivors of MI. Although there are other single-gene causes, most cases of CAD are thought to show multifactorial inheritance, with both nongenetic and genetic predisposing factors.

The risk factors for CAD include several other multifactorial disorders with genetic components: hypertension, obesity, and diabetes mellitus. In this context, the metabolic and physiological derangements represented by these disorders also contribute to enhancing the risk of CAD.

One feature of CAD that is consistent with multifactorial inheritance is that although males are at higher risk of death from MI both in the population and within affected families, the recurrence risk in relatives is somewhat greater when the proband is female or when the proband is young, or both. This increased risk suggests that there is a greater load of alleles that predispose to MI in the family, thereby increasing the risk for disease in the proband's relatives.

CAD is often an incidental finding in family histories of patients with other genetic diseases. In view of the high recurrence risk, physicians and genetic counselors may need to consider whether first-degree relatives of patients with CAD should be evaluated further and offered counseling, even when CAD is not the primary genetic problem for which the patient or relative has been referred.

## CONCLUSION

Diseases inherited as complex traits represent one of the greatest challenges facing medical geneticists today. Many of these diseases are common and cause substantial morbidity and mortality. Families and patients dealing with these diseases deserve accurate genetic counseling concerning recurrence risks in the relatives and offspring of affected individuals. Yet, our ability to provide such counseling is severely hampered by our lack of knowledge of the number of genes, the nature of the variant alleles, and the underlying mechanisms of how these variant alleles contribute to disease causation or predisposition. Diseases with complex inheritance are being actively studied, and much is being learned. We hope that as the information being gained by the Human Genome Project is applied to the problem of diseases with complex inheritance, physicians

### Genetic Counseling of Families of Patients with Multifactorial Traits

The underlying mechanisms by which genes and environment interact to cause diseases with complex inheritance are largely unknown. For genetic counseling, we are dependent on measuring actual recurrence risks in collections of families to generate average **empiric estimates** of the recurrence risks. Of course, the actual risk for an individual family may be larger or smaller than the average. For now, these population-based empiric risks, although often inadequate, are the only source available for genetic prediction. Certain general principles must be considered, however, when providing genetic counseling for multifactorial disorders.

1. The recurrence risk is much higher for first-degree relatives of affected family members than for more distant relatives.
2. The best estimate of the recurrence risk is the empiric risk, which is simply the recurrence risk, observed in similar families, for a relative with the same degree of relationship. It is often useful to state the empiric risk as a multiple of the population risk of the defect. The empiric risk is based entirely on past experience and does not imply that the genetic and environmental factors in the pathogenesis of the malformation are understood. An empiric risk is an average for the population and is not necessarily accurate for a specific family.
3. The recurrence risk is increased by:
   a. the presence of more than one affected relative;
   b. a severe form, or early onset of the disorder;
   c. an affected person of the sex less likely to be affected; and
   d. consanguineous parentage.
4. Two common errors in risk calculation should be avoided:
   a. If the parent of a child with a multifactorial birth defect has another child by a different partner, the children are second-degree, not first-degree, relatives, and the empiric risk for the second child is much lower than if the children had both parents in common (usually, the risk is approximately 1 percent instead of approximately 5 percent).
   b. When an unaffected uncle or aunt of a child with a multifactorial defect inquires about the risk of the same defect in his or her offspring, the relevant risk is not the risk to the aunt or uncle (a second-degree relative to the proband) but the risk to the offspring of the aunt or uncle (a third-degree relative).

and genetic counselors in the years ahead will get the information they need to provide accurate molecular diagnosis and risk assessment for an increasing number of these diseases.

## General References

King RA, Rotter JI, Motulsky AG (1992) The Genetic Basis of Common Diseases. Oxford University Press, Oxford, England.

Rimoin DL, Connor JM, Pyeritz RE (1997) Emery and Rimoin's Principles and Practice of Medical Genetics, 3rd ed. Churchill Livingstone, Edinburgh.

## References Specific to Particular Topics

Ebers GC, Sadovnick AD, Risch NJ, et al (1995) A genetic basis for familial aggregation in multiple sclerosis. Nature 377:150–151.

Foy CA, Grant PJ (1997) Genes and the development of vascular disease. Postgrad Med J 73:271–278.

Hawkes CH (1997) Twin studies in medicine—what do they tell us? Q J Med 90:311–321.

Kajiwara K, Berson EL, Dryja TP (1994) Digenic retinitis pigmentosa due to mutations at the unlinked peripherin/RDS and ROM1 loci. Science 264:1604–1608.

Lander E, Kruglyak L (1995) Genetic dissection of complex traits: Guidelines for interpreting and reporting linkage results. Nat Genet 11:241–247.

Lander ES, Schork NJ (1994) Genetic dissection of complex traits. Science 265:2037–2048.

Lin AE, Garver KL (1988) Genetic counseling for congenital heart defects. J Pediatr 113:1105–1109.

Marenberg ME, Risch N, Berkman LF, et al (1994) Genetic susceptibility to death from coronary heart disease in a study of twins. N Engl J Med 330:1041–1046.

Martinelli I, Sacchi E, Landi G, et al (1998) High risk of cerebral-vein thrombosis in carriers of a prothrombin-gene mutation and in users of oral contraceptives. N Engl J Med 38:1793–1797.

Mein CA, Esposito L, Dunn MG, et al (1998) A search for type 1 diabetes susceptibility genes in families from the United Kingdom. Nat Genet 19:297–300.

Peyser PA (1997) Genetic epidemiology of coronary artery disease. Epidemiol Rev 19:80–90.

Risch N (1990) Linkage strategies for genetically complex traits. I. Multilocus models. Am J Hum Genet 46:222–228.

Risch N, Merikangas K (1996) The future of genetic studies of complex human diseases. Science 273:1516–1517.

Risch N, Zhang H (1995) Extreme discordant sib pairs for mapping quantitative trait loci in humans. Science 268:1584–1589.

Strittmatter WJ, Roses AD (1996) Apolipoprotein E and Alzheimer's disease. Annu Rev Neurosci 19:53–77.

Todd JA, Bell JI, McDevitt HO (1988) A molecular basis for genetic susceptibility to insulin-dependent diabetes mellitus. Trends Genet 4:129–134.

Tsuang MT (1998) Recent advances in genetic research on schizophrenia. J Biomed Sci 5:28–30.

## Problems

1. For a certain malformation, the recurrence risk in sibs and offspring of affected persons is 10 percent, the risk in nieces and nephews is 5 percent, and the risk in first cousins is 2.5 percent.
   (a) Is this more likely to be an autosomal dominant trait with reduced penetrance or a multifactorial trait? Explain.
   (b) What other information might support your conclusion?
2. A large sex difference in affected persons is often a clue to X-linked inheritance. How would you establish that pyloric stenosis is multifactorial rather than X-linked?
3. A series of children with a particular congenital malformation includes both boys and girls. In all cases, the parents are normal. How would you determine whether the malformation is more likely to be multifactorial than autosomal recessive?

# 16

# Genetics and Cancer

Cancer is one of the most common and severe diseases seen in clinical medicine. Statistics show that cancer in some form strikes more than one third of the population, accounts for more than 20 percent of all deaths, and, in developed countries, is responsible for more than 10 percent of the total cost of medical care. Cancer is invariably fatal if not treated. Early diagnosis and early treatment are vital, and identification of persons at increased risk of cancer before its development is an important objective of cancer research.

In this chapter, we emphasize that *cancer is fundamentally a genetic disease* (Box). We describe the kinds of genes that have been implicated in initiating cancer and the mechanisms by which dysfunction of these genes can result in the disease. We describe a number of heritable cancer syndromes and demonstrate how insights gained into their pathogenesis have illuminated the basis of cancer in general. We also describe some of the special challenges that such syndromes present for medical genetics and genetic counseling.

## CANCER BIOLOGY

Cancer is not a single disease but rather a name used to describe the more virulent forms of **neoplasia**, a disease process characterized by uncontrolled cellular proliferation leading to a mass or tumor (**neoplasm**). For a neoplasm to be a cancer, however, it must in addition be **malignant**, which means its growth is no longer controlled and the tumor is capable of invading neighboring tissues or spreading (**metastasizing**) to more distant sites, or both. (Tumors that do not metastasize are not cancerous but are referred to as **benign** tumors, although their size and location may make them anything but benign to the patient.) There are three main forms of cancer: **sarcomas**, in which the tumor has arisen in mesenchymal tissue, such as bone, muscle, or connective tissue; **carcinomas**, which originate in epithelial tissue, such as the cells lining the intestine, bronchi, or mammary ducts; and **hematopoietic** and **lymphoid** malignancies, such as leukemias and lymphomas, which spread throughout the bone marrow, lymphatic system, and peripheral blood. Within each of the major groups, tumors are classified by site, tissue type, histological appearance, and degree of malignancy.

### The Genetic Basis of Cancer

1. Regardless of whether a cancer occurs sporadically in an individual or repeatedly in many individuals in a family as a hereditary trait, cancer is a genetic disease.
2. Different kinds of genes have been implicated in initiating the cancer process. These include genes encoding
   * proteins in signaling pathways for cell proliferation;
   * cytoskeletal components involved in maintenance of contact inhibition;
   * regulators of the mitotic cycle;
   * components of programmed cell death machinery;
   * proteins responsible for detecting and repairing mutations.
3. Different types of mutations are responsible for causing cancer. These include mutations such as
   * activating gain-of-function mutations of one allele of a **proto-oncogene**;
   * loss of function of both alleles or dominant negative mutation of one allele of a **tumor-suppressor gene**;
   * **chromosomal translocations** that cause misexpression of genes or create chimeric genes encoding proteins that have gained novel functional properties.
4. Once initiated, a cancer evolves by accumulating additional genetic damage through mutations or epigenetic silencing of the genes that encode the cellular machinery that repairs damaged DNA and maintains cytogenetic normality.

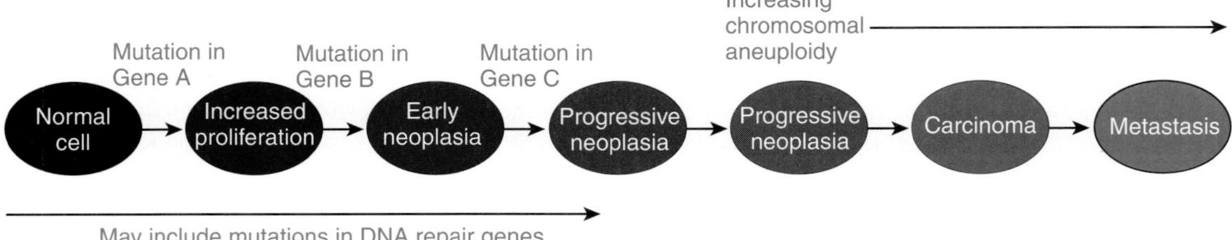


**Figure 16–1.** Stages in the evolution of cancer. Increasing degrees of abnormality are associated with sequential loss of tumor-suppressor genes from several chromosomes and activation of proto-oncogenes, with or without a concomitant defect in DNA repair. For example, sporadic cancer with DNA repair defects is less common than are cancers without abnormal repair but, when present, may develop along a somewhat different, but parallel, pathway leading to the final common end point of malignancy.

Neoplasia, an abnormal accumulation of cells, occurs because of an imbalance between cellular proliferation and cellular attrition. Cells proliferate as they pass through the cell cycle and undergo mitosis, whereas attrition, due to programmed cell death, removes cells from a tissue through a normal process of DNA fragmentation and cellular suicide referred to as **apoptosis** (Fig. 16–1).

## GENETIC BASIS OF CANCER

The processes of cell division and cell death are regulated by a vast array of genes. Extensive research during the past few decades has revealed that *mutations in the genes controlling proliferation and death are responsible for cancer*. In most cancers, the mutations occur in a single somatic cell that then divides and proceeds to develop into the cancer. More rarely, when cancer occurs as part of a hereditary cancer syndrome, the initial cancer-causing mutations are inherited through the germline and are therefore already present in every cell of the body. With either mechanism, once initiated, a cancer evolves by accumulating additional genetic damage through mutations in the genes that encode the cellular machinery that repairs damaged DNA and maintains cytogenetic normality. Damage to these genes produces an ever worsening cascade of mutations in an increasing assortment of the genes that control cellular proliferation and repair DNA damage. In this way, the original clone of neoplastic cells can evolve into multiple sublineages of varying degrees of malignancy, each carrying a set of mutations that are different from, but overlap with, mutations carried in other sublineages. The paradigm illustrated in Figure 16–1 is a general one that, although best elucidated in the case of colon cancer (see later in this chapter), likely applies to many, if not most, cancers. It is a useful conceptual model that provides a framework for considering the role of genetic changes in cancer, as we emphasize throughout this chapter.

It is useful to separate the genes involved in cancer into two distinct categories: **oncogenes** and **tumor-suppressor genes** (Fig. 16–2). Oncogenes are most often mutant ("activated") alleles of a class of normal cellular genes known as **proto-oncogenes** but can also be genes such as those encoding telomerase or

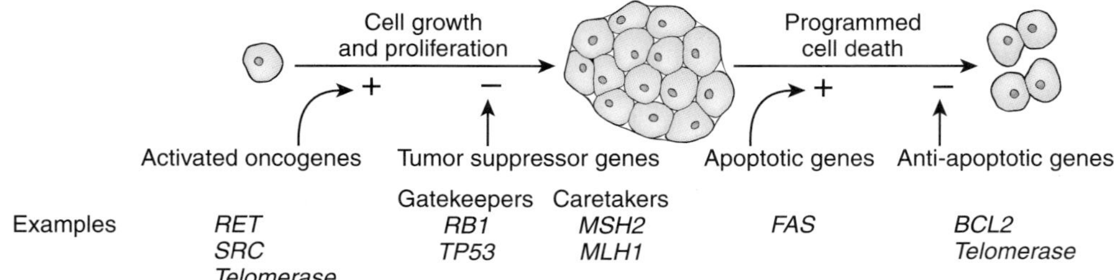


**Figure 16–2.** General scheme for mechanisms of oncogenesis by proto-oncogene activation, mutation or loss of tumor-suppressor genes, activation of antiapoptotic genes, or loss of proapoptotic genes. The effect of genes that enhance a process is shown as +, whereas the effect of genes that suppress a process is shown as −. Cell division and proliferation are stimulated (+) by the products of proto-oncogenes. Some tumor-suppressor genes directly regulate proto-oncogene function (*gatekeepers*); others act more indirectly by maintaining genome integrity and correcting mutations during DNA replication and cell division (*caretakers*). Activation of an antiapoptotic gene allows excessive accumulation of cells, whereas loss of function of apoptotic genes has the same effect. Activation of oncogenes or antiapoptotic genes is dominant and requires only a single mutant allele. Action of tumor-suppressor genes is recessive; when both alleles are mutated or lost, cell growth is unregulated or genomic integrity is compromised. Loss of proapoptotic genes may occur through loss of both alleles or through a dominant negative mutation in one allele.

genes that block apoptosis (see later). Oncogenes are usually due to *gain-of-function* mutations (see Chapter 11) that facilitate malignant transformation by mechanisms such as stimulating proliferation, increasing blood supply to the tumor, and inhibiting apoptosis. Tumor-suppressor genes, as the name implies, block tumor development by regulating cell growth. *Loss of function* of proteins encoded by tumor-suppressor genes leads to uncontrolled cell division and abnormal cell growth or defective apoptosis.

Mutations occur continuously during cell division (see Chapter 6), and oncogenes and tumor-suppressor genes are generally not inherently more mutable than other genes. What makes the mutations in cancer different from other mutations is the strong positive selection for cell proliferation or survival caused by the mutations. It is precisely the phenotype of a cancer cell—namely, uncontrolled and excessive proliferation—that ultimately allows even one mutant cell to develop into a life-threatening disease. In contrast, mutations that cause one cell among many to lose function or die have no phenotypic effects because the loss of the cell is masked by the vast majority of healthy cells in an organ or tissue.

### Cancer in Families

Many forms of cancer have a higher incidence in relatives of patients than in the general population. Most prominent among these familial forms of cancer are the nearly 50 mendelian disorders in which the risk of cancer is very high (Table 16–1), indicating that in some cancers mutations in a single gene can be the predominant contributory factor to disease causation. Extensive epidemiological studies have shown, however, that some families have an above-average risk of cancer even in the absence of an obvious mendelian inheritance pattern of cancer. For example, an increased incidence of cancer, in the range of two- to threefold, has been observed in first-degree relatives of probands, which suggests that many cancers are complex traits resulting from both genetic and environmental factors (see Chapter 15). Thus, a family history of cancer in a first-degree or second-degree relative of a patient should arouse the physician's suspicion of increased cancer risk in the patient.

Although individuals with a strong hereditary predisposition to cancer represent probably less than 5 percent of all patients with cancer, identifying a genetic basis for their disease has great importance both for providing clinical management in these families and for understanding cancer in general. First, the relatives of individuals with strong hereditary predispositions, which are most often due to mutations in a single gene, can be offered testing and counseling, to provide appropriate reassurance or more intensive monitoring and therapy, depending on the results of testing. Second, as is the case with many common diseases, understanding the hereditary forms of the disease provides crucial insights into disease mechanisms that go far beyond the rare hereditary forms themselves. If a series of mutations is required for a malignancy to develop (see Fig. 16–1), an inherited mutation at any one of the critical genes would be expected to have a dramatic impact on the predisposition of carriers to cancer and could account for a substantial portion of all cancers. Carriers of such genes could account for the vast majority of cancers that are not recognized as "familial."

## ONCOGENES

An **oncogene** is a mutant gene whose altered function or expression results in abnormal stimulation of cell division and proliferation. The activating mutation can be in the oncogene itself, in its regulatory elements, or even in its genomic copy number, leading to unregulated function or overexpression of the oncogene product. Oncogenes have a dominant effect at the cellular level; that is, when activated or over-expressed, a single mutant allele is sufficient to change the phenotype of a cell from normal to malignant.

### Hereditary Syndromes Due to Activated Oncogenes

#### Multiple Endocrine Adenomatosis, Type 2

Multiple endocrine adenomatosis, type 2 (MEN2), in its more common type A variant, is an autosomal dominant disorder characterized by a high incidence of medullary carcinoma of the thyroid (a thyrocalcitonin-producing tumor of parafollicular cells of the thyroid) that is often, but not always, associated with pheochromocytoma or benign parathyroid adenomas, or both. The rarer type B variant, termed MEN2B, has, in addition to the tumors seen in patients with MEN2A, thickening of nerves and the development of benign neural tumors, known as **neuromas**, on the mucosal surface of the mouth and lips. The mutations responsible for MEN2 are in the *RET* gene, which encodes a receptor tyrosine kinase that serves as a receptor for two ligands, the glial cell-line–derived growth factor (gdnf) and neurturin, and is the same gene implicated in Hirschsprung disease (see Chapter 15). Tyrosine kinase receptors transduce an external signal, such as the binding of the receptor's ligand, by undergoing conformational change, such as dimerization. Conformational change in the receptor activates an intrinsic kinase activity that phosphorylates other cellular proteins, thereby initiating a cascade of changes in protein-protein and DNA-protein interac-

TABLE 16–1

**Familial Cancer Syndromes with Mendelian Inheritance**

| Syndrome | Primary Tumor | Associated Cancers and Other Traits | Gene | Chromosomal Location | Proposed Function of Gene Product |
|---|---|---|---|---|---|
| **Autosomal Dominant Inheritance—Activated Oncogene** | | | | | |
| Multiple endocrine neoplasia 2 | Medullary thyroid cancer | Type 2A pheochromocytoma, parathyroid hyperplasia Type 2B pheochromocytoma, mucosal hamartomas | *RET* | 10q11.2 | Transmembrane tyrosine kinase receptor for glial cell-line derived neurotrophic factor |
| Hereditary papillary renal carcinoma | Renal-cell cancer | | *MET* | 7q31 | Transmembrane receptor for hepatocyte growth factor |
| **Autosomal Dominant Inheritance—Loss of a Tumor-Suppressor Gene** | | | | | |
| Familial retinoblastoma | Retinoblastoma | Osteosarcoma | *RB1* | 13q14.3 | Cell cycle and transcriptional regulator |
| WAGR | Wilms' tumor | Contiguous gene syndrome including ambiguous genitalia, mental retardation | *WT1* | 11p13 | Repressor of transcription |
| Von Hippel-Lindau | Renal cancer (clear cell) | Pheochromocytomas, retinal angiomas, hemangioblastomas | *VHL* | 3p25 | Regulator of RNA transcription |
| Nevoid basal cell carcinoma | Basal cell skin cancer | Jaw cysts, palmar and plantar pits, medulloblastoma, ovarian fibromas | *PTCH* | 9q22.3 | Transmembrane receptor for signaling by the hedgehog molecule |
| Cowden disease | Breast cancer, thyroid cancer (follicular) | Intestinal polyps | *PTEN* | 10q23.3 | Protein and lipid phosphatase |
| Peutz-Jeghers | Gastrointestinal cancer | Ovarian, testicular cancer | *STK11* | 19p13.3 | Serine/threonine protein kinase |
| Familial melanoma | Melanoma | Pancreatic cancer, dysplastic nevi, atypical moles | *CDKN2* | 9p21 | Inhibitor of CDK4 and CDK6, kinases that promote transition from $G_1$ into S phase of cell cycle |
| | | | *CDK4* | 12q14 | Protein kinase that signals cell division |
| Neurofibromatosis, type 1 | Neurofibromas | Neurofibrosarcomas, brain tumors | *NF1* | 17q11.2 | Regulation of *RAS*-like G proteins |
| Neurofibromatosis, type 2 | Acoustic neuromas, meningiomas | Gliomas, ependymomas, mesothelioma | *NF2* | 22q12.2 | Link between membrane proteins and cellular cytoskeleton |
| Familial adenomatous polyposis | Colorectal cancer | Duodenal and gastric tumors, retinal abnormalities, jaw osteomas and desmoid tumors, medulloblastoma, glioblastoma (Turcot syndrome) | *APC* | 5q21-q22 | Regulation of $\beta$-catenin, a component of cellular cytoskeleton |
| Familial gastric cancer | Gastric cancer | | *CDH1* | 16q22 | E-cadherin, involved in cell adhesion |
| Multiple endocrine neoplasia, type 1 | Pancreatic islet cell | Parathyroid hyperplasia, pituitary adenomas | *MEN1* | 11q13 | Unknown |
| **Autosomal Dominant Inheritance—Loss of DNA Repair Genes** | | | | | |
| Li-Fraumeni | Sarcomas, breast cancer | Brain tumors, leukemias | *TP53* | 17p13.1 | Transcription factor p53 that responds to DNA damage to induce apoptosis |
| Familial breast cancer, type 1 | Breast cancer | Ovarian cancer | *BRCA1* | 17q21 | Repair of double-strand DNA breaks? |

TABLE 16–1 *Continued*

**Familial Cancer Syndromes with Mendelian Inheritance**

| Syndrome | Primary Tumor | Associated Cancers and Other Traits | Gene | Chromosomal Location | Proposed Function of Gene Product |
|---|---|---|---|---|---|
| **Autosomal Dominant Inheritance—Loss of DNA Repair Genes *(continued)*** | | | | | |
| Familial breast cancer, type 2 | Breast cancer | Pancreatic cancer, breast cancer in males | *BRCA2* | 13q12 | Repair of double-strand DNA breaks? |
| Hereditary nonpolyposis colorectal cancer | Colorectal cancer | Endometrial, ovarian, hepatobiliary, and bladder cancer, glioblastoma (Turcot syndrome) | *MSH2*<br>*MLH1*<br>*PMSL1*<br>*PMSL2*<br>*MSH6* | 2p22-p21<br>3p21<br>2q31.1<br>7p22<br>2p16 | Repair of DNA base-pair mismatches. Maintains stability of simple tandem repeats of DNA |
| **Autosomal Dominant Inheritance—Interference with Apoptosis** | | | | | |
| Autoimmune lympho-proliferative syndrome | Hodgkin and non-Hodgkin lymphoma | Massive lymphadenopathy and splenomegaly, hemolytic anemia and thrombocytopenia | *TNFRSF6* (*FAS*)<br>*TNFSF6* (*FASL*) | 10q24.1<br>1q23 | Receptor that transduces apoptotic signal from fas ligand<br>Fas ligand |
| **Autosomal Recessive Inheritance—Abnormal Genome Integrity** | | | | | |
| Ataxia telangiectasia | Lymphoma | Cerebellar degeneration, sterility | *ATM* | 11q22-q23 | DNA repair |
| Bloom | Solid tumors | Immunodeficiency, short stature, pigmentary abnormalities, sun sensitivity, infertility, chromosome instability | *BLM* | 15q26.1 | ?DNA helicase |
| Xeroderma pigmentosa (total of seven complementation groups, named A–G. All seven genes have been cloned) | Skin cancer | Sun sensitivity, hypogonadism, occasional mental retardation and neurodegeneration | *XPB*<br>*XPD*<br>*XPA*<br>*XPC*<br>*XPF*<br>*XPE*<br>*XPG* | 2q21<br>19q13<br>9q22.3<br>3p25<br>16p13<br>11p11-p12<br>13q33 | Components of DNA repair machinery involved in excising and repairing ultraviolet light damage |
| Fanconi anemia (total of eight complementation groups, A–H) | Leukemia | Pancytopenia, hypoplasia of radial bone/thumb, chromosome instability, occasional cardiac and renal anomalies | *FANCA*<br>*FANCC*<br>*FANCD*<br>*FANCE* | 16q24.3<br>9q22.3<br>3p25.3<br>11p15 | Components of DNA repair machinery |

tions, and in the enzymatic activity of many proteins. As opposed to the *loss-of-function* mutations in *RET* found in Hirschsprung disease, the *RET* mutations in MEN2A and MEN2B are specific point mutations that *activate* the receptor and cause it to phosphorylate tyrosines even in the absence of binding by gdnf or neurturin. Individuals who inherit an activating mutation in *RET* have an approximately 60 percent chance of developing symptomatic medullary carcinoma of the thyroid, although more sensitive tests, such as blood tests for thyrocalcitonin or urinary catecholamines synthesized by pheochromocytomas, are abnormal in well over 90 percent of heterozygotes for MEN2.

### Hereditary Papillary Renal Carcinoma

Comprising approximately 15 percent of all renal-cell neoplasms, papillary renal carcinomas contain vascularized stems of connective tissue surrounded by neoplastic cells. In some families, papillary renal carcinoma is inherited as an autosomal dominant trait due to a mutation in the gene for *MET*, another tyrosine kinase receptor. As with *RET* in MEN2, the mutations in *MET* in hereditary papillary renal carcinoma (HPRC) are activating mutations that cause the receptor to function as an active tyrosine kinase even in the absence of its normal ligand, hepatocyte growth factor.

### Clonality and Tissue Specificity of Multiple Endocrine Adenomatosis Type 2 and Hereditary Papillary Renal Carcinoma

Although we know from the hereditary nature of medullary thyroid carcinoma and HPRC that mutations in *RET* or *MET* are the underlying cause of the cancers, not all of the parafollicular cells of the thyroid or the renal papillary cells actually become cancerous, indicating that the oncogenes themselves are not sufficient to cause the disease. Other genome and chromosome mutations are known to occur, such as loss of a portion of chromosome 1p in the medullary thyroid carcinomas in MEN2A and trisomy 7 due to duplication of the chromosome 7 bearing the activated *MET* oncogene in renal carcinoma tissue in HPRC. These second events arise at multiple sites in individual cells, each of which then divides and develops into a tumor that originates from a single cell and is thus said to be **clonal**.

Both *RET* and *MET* are expressed in many tissues of the body and are required, in the case of *RET*, for normal embryonic development of autonomic ganglia and kidney and, in the case of *MET*, for normal development of liver, muscle, and placenta. It remains completely unknown why germline activating mutations in these two proto-oncogenes result in particular cancers of distinct histological type restricted to specific tissues, because other tissues in which the oncogene is expressed do not develop tumors. Perhaps, in those tissues in which the oncogene is expressed, activation of *RET* or *MET* does not confer a growth advantage.

## Activation of Oncogenes in Sporadic Cancer

Well before the discovery of hereditary cancer syndromes due to autosomal dominant inheritance of activated proto-oncogenes, many mutated oncogenes, including *RET* and *MET*, had been identified in sporadic cancers. These oncogenes were first discovered using a powerful assay known as **DNA-mediated transformation** (Fig. 16–3). Human DNA, extracted and purified from sporadic cancer cell lines, was introduced into a nontumorigenic mouse cell line in culture to generate colonies of cells that were **transformed,** that is, had acquired tumorigenic properties. DNA containing a portion of the original tumorigenic DNA, including the responsible oncogene, was isolated from a colony of transformed mouse cells, transferred again into the nontumorigenic mouse cell and transformed colonies identified. This process was repeated until, eventually, the only human DNA present in the transformed cells was the small segment containing the activated human oncogene derived initially from the human cancer cell line. Using the human-specific *Alu* repeat (see Chapter 3) as a hybridization probe, scientists could identify and clone the human genomic DNA encoding the transforming oncogene from a library made from the transformed mouse cell (see Chapter 4).

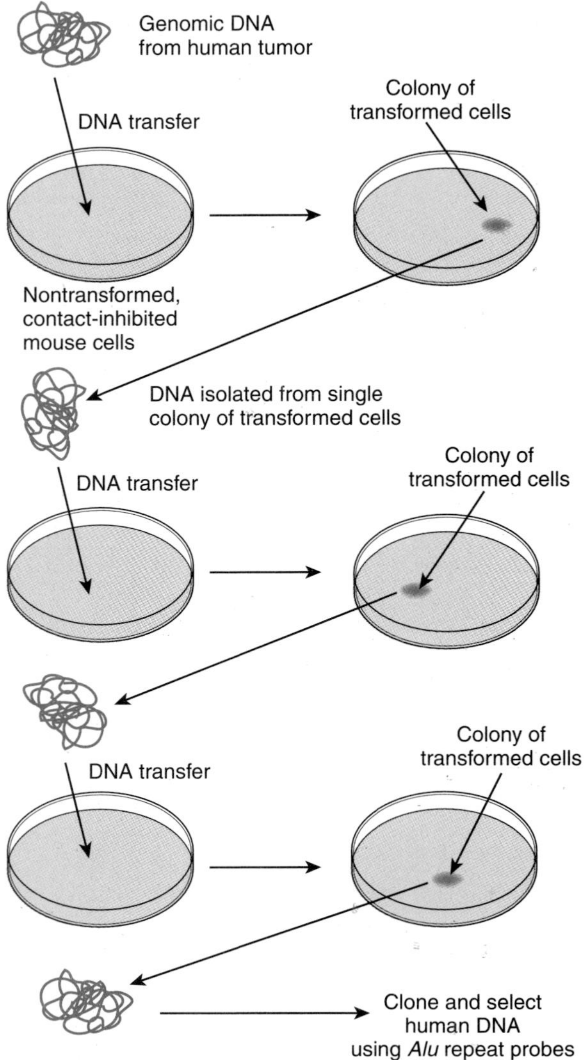


**Figure 16–3.** DNA-mediated transformation assay. High-molecular-weight DNA from a tumor cell line is applied to a lawn of nontransformed mouse cells, and the cells are allowed to take up the DNA. A few colonies of transformed cells appear. A single colony is isolated, its DNA isolated, and the process of applying the DNA to nontransformed mouse cells is repeated. After a few cycles, the only human DNA within a transformed colony will be the DNA containing an activated oncogene present in the original tumor cell line. Human-specific repeat sequences (such as *Alu*) can be used to identify and clone the human DNA sequences containing the activated oncogene from a genomic library made from the DNA of the transformed mouse cells.

One of the first activated oncogenes discovered by the transformation assay was a mutant *RAS* gene derived from a bladder carcinoma cell line. *RAS* encodes one of a large family of small guanosine triphosphate (GTP)–binding proteins (**G proteins**). G proteins serve as molecular "on-off" switches that activate or inhibit downstream molecules when bound to GTP but then terminate their effect when the bound GTP is cleaved to guanosine diphosphate (GDP) by an intrinsic GTPase enzymatic activity. Remarkably, the activated oncogene and its normal counterpart proto-oncogene differed in only a single base pair. The alteration, a point mutation in a somatic cell of the tumor, led to synthesis of an abnormal ras protein that was able to signal continuously, even in the absence of bound GTP, to stimulate the growth of the cell line, thus changing it into a tumor.

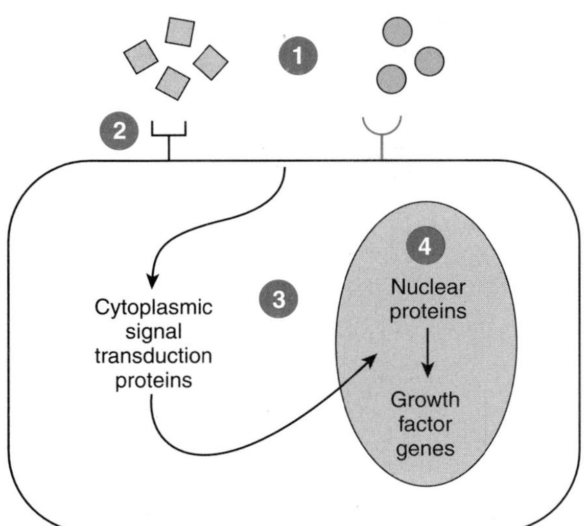


Figure 16–4. Signal transduction and growth regulation by products of proto-oncogenes, classified by their location and function in the cell. Deregulation of a proto-oncogene can lead to malignant transformation. *1*, Secreted growth factors, such as embryonic growth factor (EGF) and platelet-derived growth factor (PDGF). *2*, Specific receptors for the secreted growth factors, such as *RET*. *3*, Cytoplasmic signal transduction proteins, such as the G-protein encoded by RAS and the protein kinase encoded by *ABL*. *4*, Nuclear proteins, such as the transcription factor encoded by *MYC* that binds to DNA and modifies transcription.

*RAS* point mutations are observed in many tumors, and the *RAS* genes have been shown experimentally to be the mutational target of known carcinogens, a finding that supports a role for mutated *RAS* genes in the development of many cancers.

To date, more than 50 human oncogenes (and thus their normal proto-oncogenes) have been identified, largely on the basis of DNA transformation studies with genomic DNA from human tumors. Examples of some of these oncogenes are given in Table 16–1. The various roles of several classes of proto-oncogenes in growth regulation are illustrated in Figure 16–4.

### Activation of Oncogenes by Chromosome Translocation

Gene mutation is only one of several mechanisms that can induce activation of proto-oncogenes (Table 16–2). In some instances, a proto-oncogene is activated by a chromosome mutation, usually through translocation (Table 16–3). More than 40 oncogenic chromosome translocations have been described, primarily in sporadic leukemias and lymphomas, but also in a few rare connective-tissue sarcomas. In some cases, the translocation breakpoints are within the introns of two genes, thereby producing a chimeric protein with novel properties (gain-of-function) that are oncogenic. The best known example is the translocation between chromosomes 9 and 22 that is seen in chronic myelogenous leukemia (CML). In others, the translocation activates an oncogene by placing it downstream of a strong, constitutive promoter belonging to another gene. Two well-known examples are the translocation between chromosomes 8 and 14 in Burkitt lymphoma and the translocation involving chromosome 18 in B-cell lymphoma.

**Chronic Myelogenous Leukemia.** In CML, the cytogenetic abnormality seen, the so-called Philadelphia chromosome ($Ph^1$), is the product of a translocation between chromosomes 9 and 22 (Fig. 16–5). The translocation moves the proto-oncogene *ABL*, a tyrosine kinase, from its normal position on chromosome 9q to the "breakpoint cluster region" gene (*BCR*), a gene of unknown function on chromosome 22q. The juxtaposition of *BCR* sequences and *ABL* sequences allows the synthesis of a chimeric protein that is longer than the normal abl protein and has increased tyrosine kinase activity. Although the function of the normal abl and bcr proteins is not yet clear, the enhanced tyrosine kinase activity of the novel protein encoded by the chimeric gene is the primary event causing the chronic leukemia.

**Burkitt Lymphoma.** Burkitt lymphoma is a B-cell tumor of the jaw that has an unusual geographic distribution: it is the most common tumor of children in equatorial Africa but is rare elsewhere. In most tumors of this type, the *MYC* proto-oncogene is translocated from its normal chromosomal position at 8q24 to a position distal to the immunoglobulin heavy-chain locus at 14q32. Cytogenetically, this is seen as an apparently balanced 8;14 translocation. The translocation presumably brings enhancer or other transcriptional activating sequences, normally associated with the immunoglobulin genes, near to the *MYC* gene. Supporting this hypothesis is the

TABLE 16–2

**Mechanisms of Activation of Proto-Oncogenes**

| Mechanism | Type of Gene Activated | Result |
|---|---|---|
| Regulatory mutation | Growth factor genes | Increased expression or secretion |
| Structural mutation | Growth factor receptors, signal transducing proteins | Allows autonomy of expression |
| Translocation, retroviral insertion, gene amplification | Nuclear oncogenes | Overexpression |

From Miller DM, Blume S, Borst M, et al (1990) Oncogenes, malignant transformation, and modern medicine. Am J Med Sci 300:59–69.

TABLE 16–3

**Characteristic Chromosome Translocations in Selected Human Malignancies**

| Neoplasm | Chromosome Translocation | % of Cases | Proto-Oncogene Affected |
|---|---|---|---|
| Burkitt lymphoma | t(8;14)(q24;q32) | 80% | *MYC* |
| | t(8;22)(q24;q11) | 15% | |
| | t(2;8)(q11;q24) | 5% | |
| Chronic myelogenous leukemia | t(9;22)(q34;q11) | 90%–95% | *BCR-ABL* |
| Acute lymphocytic leukemia | t(9;22)(q34;q11) | 10%–15% | *BCR-ABL* |
| Acute lymphoblastic leukemia | t(1;19)(q23;p13) | | *PRL* homeobox gene |
| Acute promyelocytic leukemia | t(15;17)(q22;q11) | | retinoic acid receptor |
| Chronic lymphocytic leukemia | t(11;14)(q13;q32) | 10%–30% | *BCL-1* |
| Follicular lymphoma | t(14;18)(q32;q21) | | *BCL-2* |

Based on Croce CM (1987) Role of chromosome translocations in human neoplasia. Cell 49:155–156; Park M, van de Woude GF (1989) Oncogenes: Genes associated with neoplastic disease. In Scriver CR, Beaudet AL, Sly WS, Valle D (eds) The Molecular and Metabolic Bases of Inherited Disease, 6th ed. McGraw-Hill, New York, pp. 251–276; Nourse J, Mellentin JD, Galili N et al (1990) Chromosomal translocation t(1;19) results in synthesis of a homeobox fusion mRNA that codes for a potential chimeric transcription factor. Cell 60:535–545; Borrow J, Goddard AD, Sheer D, Solomon E (1990) Molecular analysis of acute promyelocytic leukemia breakpoint cluster region on chromosome 17. Science 249:1577–1580.

finding that other translocations observed in a smaller proportion of Burkitt lymphoma cases involve translocating immunoglobulin light-chain genes on chromosomes 22 or 2 near to the *MYC* gene (see Table 16–3). In either case, these translocations clearly have an important effect on the *MYC* gene, allowing its unregulated expression and resulting in uncontrolled cell growth. The function of the myc protein is still not entirely known, but it appears to be a transcription factor with powerful effects on the expression of a number of genes involved in cellular proliferation as well as on telomerase expression (see later discussion).

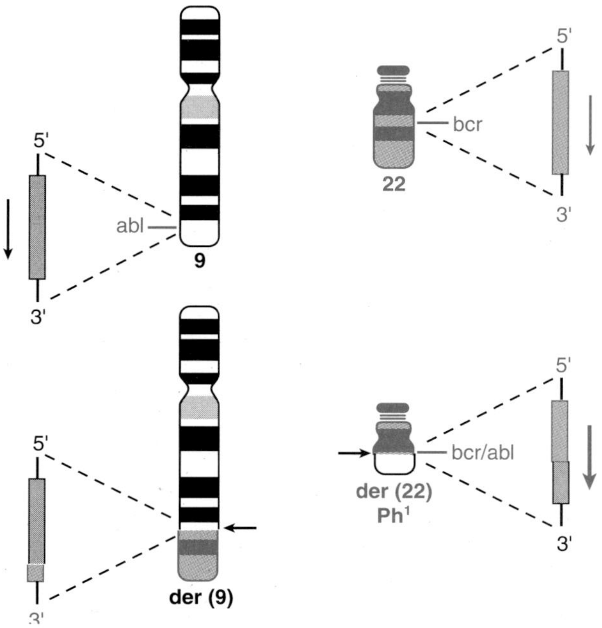

**Figure 16–5.** The Philadelphia chromosome translocation, t(9;22)(q34;q11). The Philadelphia chromosome (Ph[1]) is the derivative chromosome 22, which has exchanged part of its long arm for a segment of material from chromosome 9q that contains the *ABL* oncogene. Formation of the chimeric *BCR-ABL* gene on the Ph[1] chromosome is the critical genetic event in the development of chronic myelogenous leukemia.

**Follicular B-Cell Lymphoma.** Apoptosis, or programmed cell death, is a normal cellular process in which cells are induced to undergo a stereotypic form of suicide characterized by fragmentation of cellular DNA and activation of a family of cysteine proteases, known as caspases, inside cells. Apoptosis plays a critical role in normal development; it is particularly prominent in the development of the immune system, in which the vast majority of developing lymphocytes must be destroyed to protect against cells that might react to one's own antigens. Overexpression of an anti-apoptotic protein in lymphocyte lineages could result in vast expansion of lymphocyte populations, thereby contributing to the pathogenesis of lymphoma.

The first apoptotic gene implicated in cancer was identified in sporadic B-cell lymphoma. In nearly all B-cell lymphomas of the follicular type, a gene, *BCL2*, located at 18q21, was found to be activated by a t(14;18) chromosomal translocation that placed the gene under the strong promoter and enhancer of the immunoglobulin heavy-chain gene located at 14q32. The protein encoded by *BCL2* is a mitochondrial inner membrane protein with powerful antiapoptotic effects in B-cells. Inappropriate, prolonged expression of this gene driven by the immunoglobulin promoter results in a massive expansion of B-cells, not because of increased proliferation but because normal apoptosis of these cells is inhibited.

## TELOMERASES AS ONCOGENES

Another type of oncogene that has recently been discovered is the gene encoding **telomerase**, a reverse transcriptase responsible for lengthening telomeres at the ends of chromosomes. DNA is a double-stranded structure, with the two strands running in an antiparallel direction with respect to the phosphodiester backbone (see Chapter 3). Thus, one of the strands (called the "lagging strand") at a replication fork must replicate discontinuously, because DNA polymerase can only add to the 3′ end of a growing DNA strand. The cell accomplishes lagging strand synthesis by synthesizing fragments of DNA off the 3′ end of RNA primers made to be complementary to the DNA located 5′ of the forks. Replicating the strand when its 5′ end is at a telomere, however, is a problem because there is no DNA to serve as a template

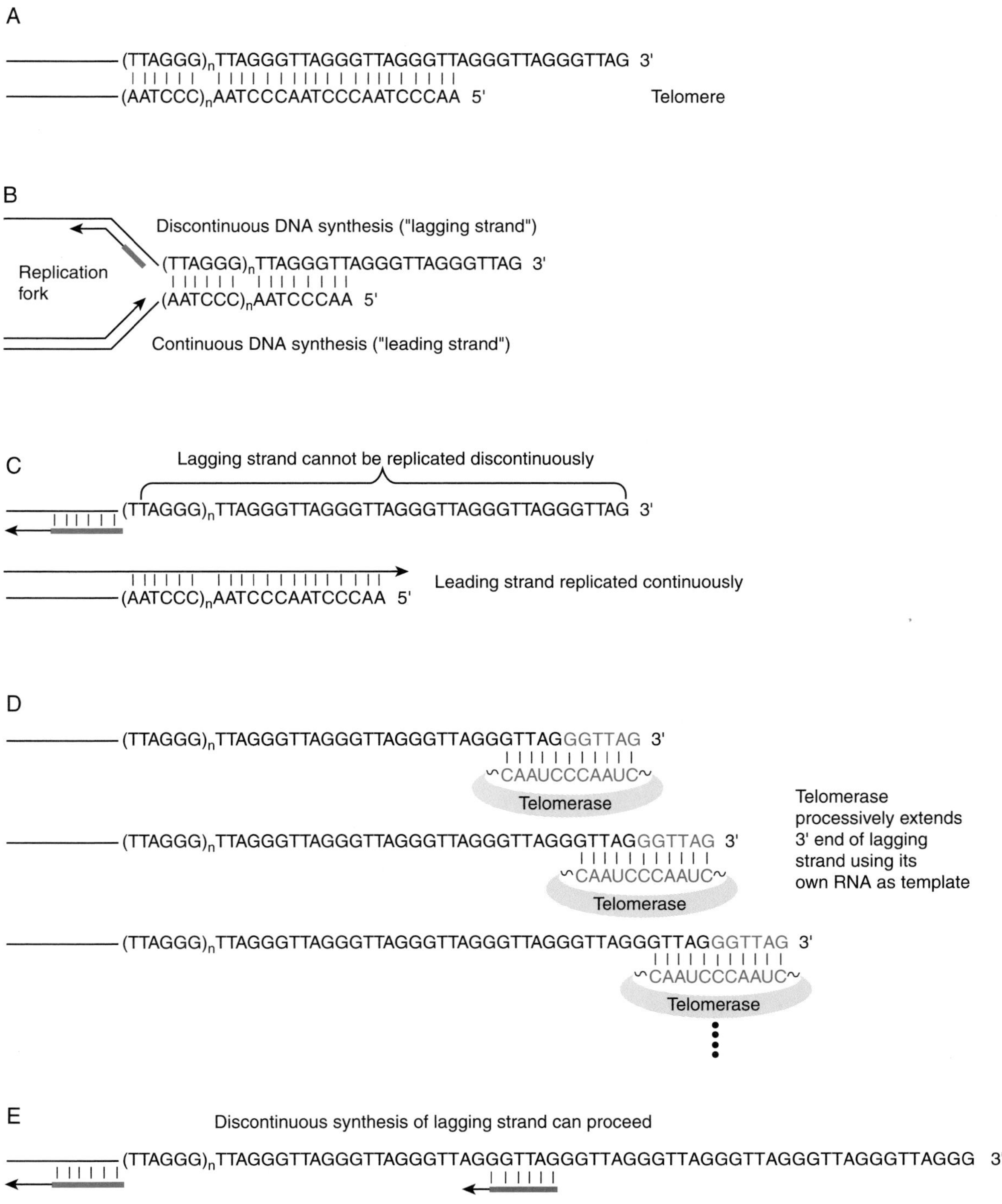


**Figure 16–6.** Diagram of telomere replication and the role of telomerase. *A*, the hexameric repeat sequence found at telomere ends in human chromosomes. *B* and *C*, a replication fork attempting to replicate the telomere. The Okazaki fragment (*red arrow*) allows replication of all but the most terminal portion of the lagging strand. *D* and *E*, telomerase, carrying its own RNA template (5′-CUAACCCUAAC-3′), extends the lagging strand at the end of the chromosome and allows replication.

for the RNA primers beyond the end of the chromosome. Under these conditions, with each round of replication, the lagging strand cannot replicate out to the end of the chromosome, and the telomere therefore gets shorter and shorter. Maintaining telomeres during cell division is the job of a special ribonucleoprotein, the enzyme telomerase, which provides its own RNA as a template for the addition of a repetitive DNA at telomeres. Different species have different repeats at their telomeres; in humans, telomerase adds a hexameric DNA repeat, TTAGGG (Fig. 16–6).

In human germline cells, telomeres contain approximately 15 kb of telomeric hexamer repeat. During development, as cells differentiate, telomerase function declines and telomeres shorten, ultimately leading to a loss of approximately 35 base pairs of telomeric repeat DNA with each cell division. After hundreds of cell divisions, the chromosome ends will become damaged, and genes located near telomeres may be deleted. DNA damage, in turn, causes cells to stop dividing and to enter $G_0$ of the cell cycle by means of the p53 and Rb1 pathway (see next section). It has been suggested that **cellular senescence**, the inability of normal cells to divide indefinitely in culture, may be a manifestation of the loss of telomerase function.

In contrast, telomerase expression reappears in transformed cells in culture and in many tumors, thereby enhancing the ability of the tumor cells to proliferate indefinitely. In some cases, the appearance of telomerase activity results from chromosome or genome mutations that directly upregulate the telomerase gene; in others, telomerase may be only one of many genes whose expression is altered by a transforming transcription factor oncogene, such as *MYC*. In either case, the reappearance of telomerase activity is now being used as a diagnostic tool for cancer in cells obtained by biopsy or needle aspiration of suspected cancerous lesions. Even more important, the role of telomerases in enhancing cellular proliferation suggests that inhibition of telomerase could be a significant new potential target for cancer treatment.

## TUMOR-SUPPRESSOR GENES

Whereas the proteins encoded by oncogenes promote cancer, generally through gain-of-function mutations or through increased or inappropriate expression of one allele of the gene, there are many other genes in which mutations contribute to malignancy by a different mechanism, that is, through loss of function of both alleles of the gene. Such genes are referred to as **tumor-suppressor genes** (see Fig. 16–2). Tumor-suppressor genes are highly heterogeneous. Some are truly tumor suppressors in the sense that they are directly involved in regulation of the cell cycle or in growth inhibition by cell-to-cell contact; tumor suppressors of this type have been referred to as "**gatekeepers**" because they *directly* regulate cell growth. Other genes, referred to as "**caretakers**," are involved in repairing DNA damage and maintaining genomic integrity. Loss of both alleles of genes that are involved in repairing DNA damage or chromosome breakage leads to cancer *indirectly* by allowing additional secondary mutations to accumulate either in proto-oncogenes or in other tumor-suppressor genes. The products of many tumor-suppressor genes have been isolated and characterized (Table 16–4). Because tumor-suppressor genes and their products are by nature protective against cancer, it is hoped that understanding them will eventually lead to improved methods of anticancer therapy.

### The Two-Hit Origin of Cancer

The existence of tumor-suppressor gene mutations leading to cancer was originally proposed in the 1960s, when it was suggested that some forms of hereditary cancer might be initiated when a cell in a person heterozygous for a germline mutation undergoes a second, somatic mutation, thus rendering the cell homozygous for loss-of-function mutations in a tumor-suppressor gene and giving rise to a tumor. Loss of both alleles of a tumor-suppressor gene also plays an important role in the pathogenesis of many common sporadic cancers, although in this instance, both alleles are inactivated by two somatic events occurring in the same cell. This **"two-hit" hypothesis** was first applied to explain how cancers such as retinoblastoma can occur in both hereditary and sporadic forms, but it has now been widely accepted as an important model in many familial cancers, including familial polyposis coli; familial breast cancer; neurofibromatosis, type 1 (NF1); hereditary nonpolyposis colon carcinoma; and the rare form of familial cancer known as Li-Fraumeni syndrome. Although in each of these disorders autosomal dominant inheritance of one mutated gene is generally the rule, loss of function of both copies of the responsible tumor-suppressor gene is required for tumor development. The explanation of this seeming paradox is that cells heterozygous for a mutation still have a single functional copy of a tumor-suppressor gene, which is enough to provide a normal cellular phenotype; however, a cell in which one copy is already altered or lost by inheritance of a germline mutation will lose its ability to suppress tumor development if by chance it loses function of the other, remaining allele. This "second hit" is most often a somatic mutation, although loss of function without mutation,

TABLE 16–4

**Products of Selected Tumor-Suppressor Genes**

| Tumor-Suppressor Gene | Gene Product and Possible Function | Disorders in which Gene Affected | |
|---|---|---|---|
| | | Familial | Sporadic |
| *RB1* | p110<br>Cell-cycle regulation | Retinoblastoma | Retinoblastoma; small-cell lung carcinomas |
| *TP53* | p53<br>Cell-cycle regulation | Li-Fraumeni syndrome | Lung cancer, breast cancer |
| *BRCA1, BRCA2* | Brca1, Brca2<br>Participate in response to double-stranded DNA breaks | Familial breast cancer | Breast cancer, ovarian cancer |
| *NF1* | neurofibromin<br>GTPase activating protein | Neurofibromatosis, type 1 | Unknown |
| *NF2* | merlin<br>Links cell surface molecules to cytoskeleton | Neurofibromatosis, type 2 | Sporadic schwannomas and meningiomas |
| *DCC* | Dcc<br>Receptor for axonal guidance molecules (netrins) | Not known | Colorectal cancer |
| *VHL* | Vhl<br>Part of a transcriptional elongation complex | Van Hippel-Lindau | Clear cell renal carcinoma |
| *MLH1, MSH2* | Mlh1, Msh2<br>Repair nucleotide mismatches between strands of DNA | Hereditary nonpolyposis colon cancer | Colorectal cancer |

such as occurs with transcriptional silencing, has also been observed in some cancer cells (see below). The second hit can cause a tumor whenever it occurs in one of the numerous cells of a tissue. For this reason, the initial tumors in the hereditary syndromes associated with loss of tumor-suppressor genes often arise multiple times in the same tissue. In contrast, in the sporadic forms of cancers due to loss of a tumor-suppressor gene, only a single cell is likely to suffer so rare an event as two hits in the same cell; the cancers are usually monoclonal, and the original tumor arises at a single location in the affected tissue, although it may metastasize widely later.

The two-hit model is now widely accepted as the basis for both hereditary and sporadic cancers arising from mutations that cause loss of function of both copies of a tumor-suppressor gene within a cell. The theory has had to be expanded, recently, when it was discovered that a second hit in the normal allele is not always necessarily a mutation. Silencing due to excessive DNA methylation, associated with a closed chromatin configuration and loss of accessibility of the DNA to transcription factors (see Chapters 3 and 10), has been found to be an important, alternative molecular mechanism for loss of function of a tumor-suppressor gene. Because an alteration in gene function due to methylation is stably transmitted through mitosis, it behaves like a mutation; because there is no change in the DNA itself, however, it is referred to as an **epigenetic** rather than a genetic change. Epigenetic silencing of gene expression is a normal phenomenon that explains such widely diverse phenomena as X inactivation (see Chapters 5 and 10), genomic imprinting (see Chapter 5), and maintenance of a specialized repertoire of gene expression in the development and maintenance of differentiation of specific tissues (see Chapter 17).

## Tumor Suppressor Genes in Autosomal Dominant Cancer Syndromes

### Retinoblastoma

Retinoblastoma, the prototype of diseases caused by mutation in a tumor-suppressor gene, is a rare malignant tumor of the retina in infants, with an incidence of about 1 in 20,000 births (Fig. 16–7). Diagnosis of a retinoblastoma must usually be followed by removal of the affected eye, although smaller tumors, diagnosed at an early stage, can be treated by local therapy so that vision can be preserved.

About 40 percent of cases of retinoblastoma are of the heritable form, in which the child inherits one mutant allele at the retinoblastoma locus (*RB1*) through the germline. A somatic mutation or other alteration in a single retinal cell leads to loss of function of the remaining normal allele, thus initiating development of the tumor (Fig. 16–8). The disorder is inherited as a dominant trait, because the large number of primordial retinoblasts and their rapid rate of proliferation make it very likely that a somatic mutation will occur in one or more of the more than $10^6$ retinoblasts. Thus, heterozygotes for the disorder are

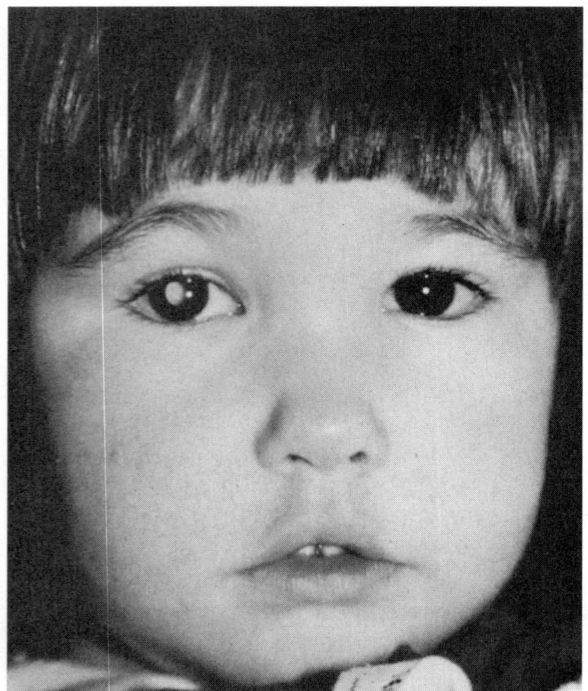

**Figure 16–7.** Retinoblastoma in a young girl, showing as a white reflex in the affected eye when light reflects directly off the tumor surface. (Photograph courtesy of B. L. Gallie, The Hospital for Sick Children, Toronto.)

often affected with multiple tumors, often affecting both eyes. Nevertheless, the penetrance of retinoblastoma, although high, is not complete, because the occurrence of the second hit is a matter of chance.

The other 60 percent of cases of retinoblastoma are nonheritable (sporadic); in these cases *both RB1* alleles in a single retinal cell have been inactivated by independent somatic mutations. Because this is a rare event, there is usually only a single clonal tumor (the retinoblastoma is unilateral), and the average age of onset is later than in infants with the heritable form (see Fig. 16–8). For genetic counseling, an important further point is that 15 percent of patients with unilateral retinoblastoma have the heritable type but by chance develop a tumor in only one eye.

Infants with heritable retinoblastoma have a greatly increased (400-fold) risk of developing mesenchymal tumors such as osteogenic sarcomas, fibrosarcomas, and melanomas in early adult life. The risk is much higher if the child has received radiotherapy.

The *RB1* gene has been mapped to chromosome 13, in band 13q14. In a small percentage of patients with retinoblastoma, the inherited mutation is due to a cytogenetically detectable deletion or translocation of this portion of chromosome 13, a finding that was instrumental in assigning the *RB1* gene to this location. Such chromosomal changes, if they also disrupt genes adjacent to *RB1*, may lead to dysmorphic features in addition to retinoblastoma.

The *RB1* gene is expressed in many tissues other than retina, although loss of *RB1* initiates tumors only in the retina and, later in life, at a small number of secondary sites (leading to osteogenic sarcoma, fibrosarcoma, and melanoma). The reason for this tis-

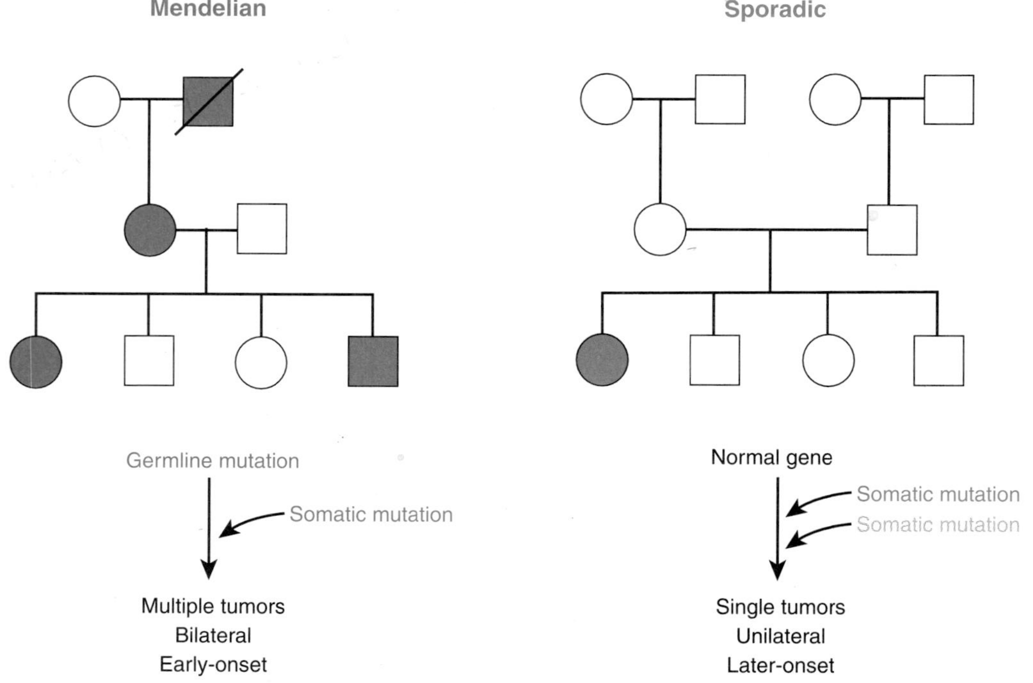


**Figure 16–8.** Comparison of mendelian and sporadic forms of cancers such as retinoblastoma and familial polyposis of the colon. Mechanisms of somatic mutation are presented in Figure 16–9. See text for discussion.

sue specificity is unknown. The *RB1* gene product, described as p110 Rb1 (a protein 110 kilodaltons in size), is also absent or mutant in a number of cell lines derived from certain other tumors during their progression (see Table 16–4).

The p110 Rb1 protein is a phosphoprotein that is hypophosphorylated and then hyperphosphorylated at different stages of the cell cycle. In its hypophosphorylated state, it blocks cell cycle progression at the boundary between $G_1$ and S, thereby inhibiting entry into S phase, by binding to and inactivating transcription factors that promote DNA synthesis. As p110 Rb1 becomes progressively more heavily phosphorylated, it releases its protein-binding partners, allowing entry of the cell into S phase; it is then progressively dephosphorylated over the course of the cell cycle, allowing it to function again to block entry into S phase of the next cell cycle. Loss of the *RB1* gene deprives cells of an important mitotic checkpoint and allows uncontrolled proliferation. The *RB1* gene is a prototypical gatekeeper tumor-suppressor gene.

**Loss of Heterozygosity.** Geneticists studying DNA polymorphisms in the region close to the *RB1* locus made an unusual but highly significant genetic discovery when they analyzed the alleles seen in tumor tissue from heritable and sporadic retinoblastoma patients. Individuals with retinoblastoma who were heterozygous in normal tissues, such as in their white blood cells, had tumors that contained alleles from only one of their two chromosome 13 homologs, revealing **a loss of heterozygosity** (LOH) for portions of 13q in the region of the gene. In familial cases, the retained chromosome 13 markers were the ones inherited from the affected parent—that is, the one with the abnormal *RB1* allele. Thus, LOH represented the second hit of the remaining allele. LOH may occur by interstitial deletion, but there are other mechanisms, such as mitotic recombination or nondisjunction (Fig. 16–9). LOH is the most common mutational mechanism by which the remaining normal *RB1* allele is lost in heterozygotes. When LOH is not seen, the second hit is usually a second somatic gene mutation or, occasionally, transcriptional inactivation of a nonmutated allele through methylation. LOH is a feature of a number of other tumors, both heritable and sporadic, and is often considered evidence for the existence of a tumor-suppressor gene, even when that gene is unknown (Table 16–5).

### Li-Fraumeni Syndrome

There are rare "cancer families" in which there is a striking history of many different forms of cancer (including several kinds of bone and soft-tissue sarcoma, breast cancer, brain tumors, leukemia, and adrenocor-

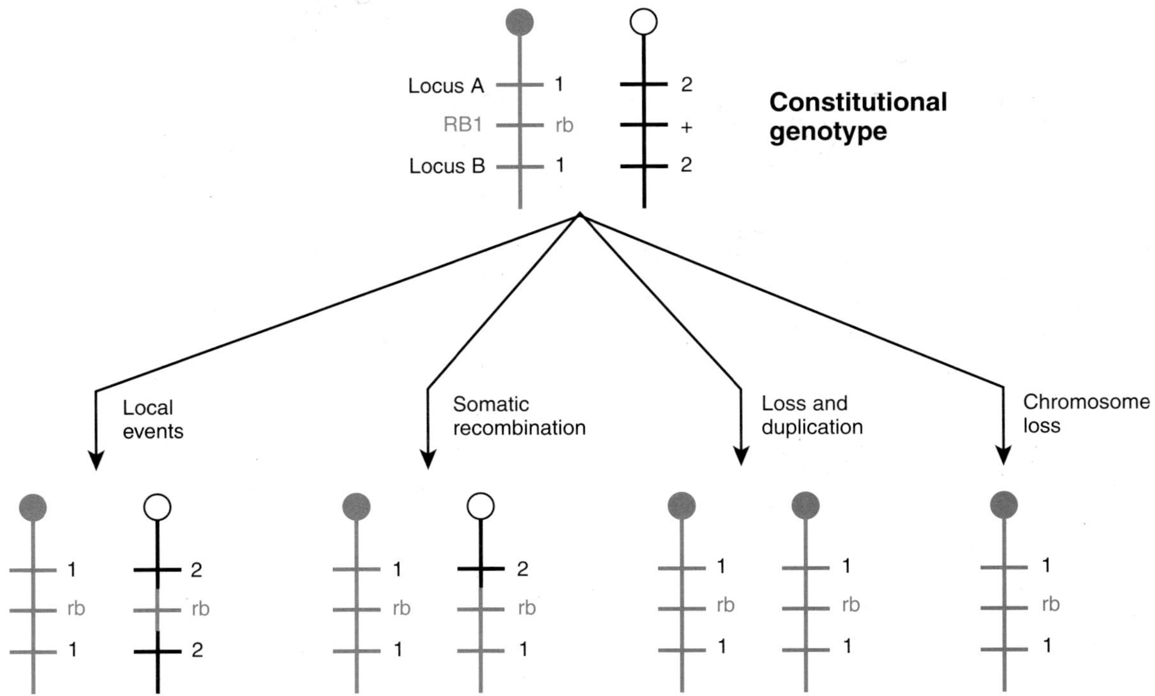


Figure 16–9. Chromosomal mechanisms that could lead to loss of heterozygosity for DNA markers at or near a tumor-suppressor gene in an individual heterozygous for an inherited germline mutation, illustrated in the case of the retinoblastoma gene on chromosome 13q. Local events such as mutation, gene conversion, or transcriptional silencing, however, could cause loss of function of both *RB1* genes without producing LOH. *RB1* + is the normal allele, rb the mutant allele.

TABLE 16–5

**Examples of Chromosomal Regions That Show Frequent, Repeated LOH in Particular Tumors**

| Chromosomal Region | Disorder(s) | Associated Tumor-Suppressor Gene |
|---|---|---|
| 1q | Breast carcinoma | Unknown |
| 3p | Small-cell lung carcinoma | Unknown |
| 5q | Familial polyposis coli; colorectal carcinoma | *APC* |
| 13q | Retinoblastoma; breast carcinoma; osteosarcoma | *RB1* |
| 17p | Colorectal carcinoma; breast carcinoma | *TP53* |
| 18q | Colorectal carcinoma | *DCC* |

tical carcinoma), affecting a number of family members at an unusually early age, inherited in an autosomal dominant pattern (Fig. 16–10). This highly variable phenotype is known as the **Li-Fraumeni syndrome** (LFS). Because the tumor-suppressor gene *TP53* encoding the protein p53 is inactivated in the sporadic forms of many of the cancers found in LFS, *TP53* was considered a candidate for the gene defective in LFS. DNA analysis of several families with LFS has now confirmed this hypothesis; affected members in more than 70 percent of families with LFS carry a mutant form of the *TP53* gene as a germline mutation. Thus, LFS is an extreme form of a group of cancers that occurs in both a sporadic and a familial form; as seen also in retinoblastoma, one of the two mutations necessary to inactivate the *TP53* gene is present in the germline in familial LFS, whereas in the sporadic form, both mutations are somatic events.

The p53 protein is a DNA-binding protein that appears to be an important component of the cellular response to DNA damage. In addition to being a transcription factor that activates the transcription of genes that stop cell division and allow repair of DNA damage, p53 also appears to be involved in inducing apoptosis in cells that have experienced irreparable DNA damage. Loss of p53 function, therefore, allows cells with damaged DNA to survive and divide, thereby propagating potentially oncogenic mutations.

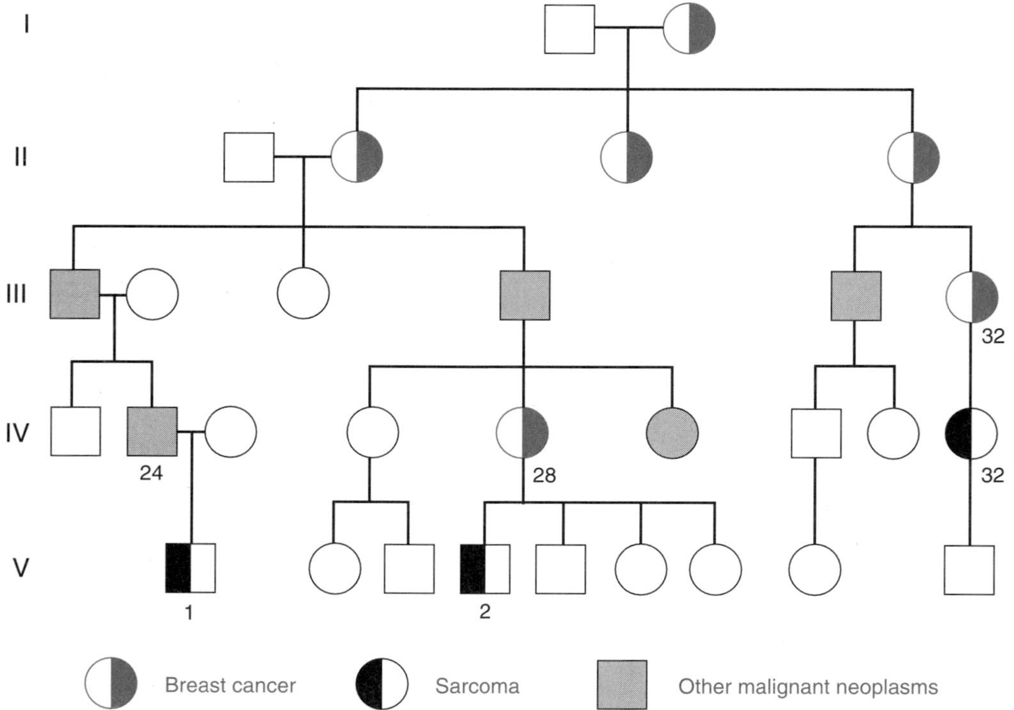


**Figure 16–10.** A pedigree of the Li-Fraumeni syndrome, in which breast cancer, sarcomas, and other malignant tumors have occurred. Ages at diagnosis are shown. (Redrawn from Li FP [1988] Cancer families: Human models of susceptibility to neoplasia—the Richard and Hinda Rosenthal Foundation award lecture. Cancer Res 48:5381–5386.)

## Neurofibromatosis, Type 1

NF1 is a relatively common autosomal dominant disorder that primarily affects the peripheral nervous system and is often characterized by large numbers of neurofibromas (see Chapter 5). Although these growths are benign, a minority of patients with NF1 also show an increased incidence of malignancy, such as neurofibrosarcoma, astrocytoma, Schwann cell cancers, and childhood CML. The abnormal cell growth observed in NF1 suggests that the normal gene may function in the regulation of cell division in neural tissue.

The *NF1* gene was mapped to the proximal long arm of chromosome 17 by family linkage studies and was subsequently cloned by application of several of the positional cloning strategies presented in Chapter 8. Inspection of the sequence of the *NF1* gene and its protein product demonstrated significant homology to proteins that activate the GTPase activity of the *RAS* oncogene product (see earlier). This finding strongly suggests that the normal *NF1* product interacts with a member of the *RAS* gene family to regulate proliferative activity in normal cells. The mutant *NF1* gene, then, may fail to regulate growth in the normal cells from which neurofibromas are derived, leading to inappropriate growth and tumor formation.

This model suggests that *NF1* is a tumor-suppressor gene. By analogy with other dominantly inherited tumor-suppressor gene mutations, loss or inactivation of the remaining normal allele at the *NF1* locus would be required to explain the development of tumors in patients with NF1. In some, but not all, cases of malignant Schwann cell tumors and juvenile myelogenous leukemia, LOH of the normal *NF1* allele has been demonstrated in the tumor tissues but not in surrounding normal tissues. The finding of LOH for the normal *NF1* gene in some of these tumors does not preclude a role for multiple mutations in other genes leading to unregulated cell division (see Fig. 16–1).

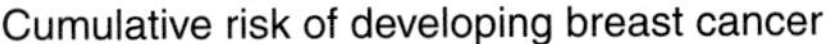


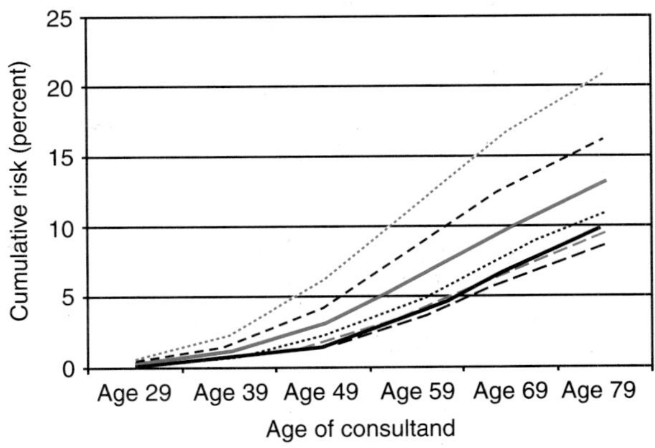


**Figure 16–11.** Breast cancer risks. Cumulative risk, with age, of a female consultand developing breast cancer when a first-degree relative has breast cancer. The risk for the consultand increases directly with her own age and inversely with the age at which the first-degree relative was first diagnosed with breast cancer. (Adapted from Claus EB, Risch N, Thompson WD [1994] Autosomal dominant inheritance of early-onset breast cancer. Implications for risk prediction. Cancer 73:643–651.)

## Familial Breast Cancer Due to Mutations in BRCA1 and BRCA2

Breast cancer is common. Population-based epidemiological studies have shown that up to 10 percent of all women in North America will develop breast cancer in their lifetime. Breast cancer has long been recognized to have a strong genetic component; a woman's risk of developing breast cancer is increased up to threefold if one first-degree relative is affected and up to 10-fold if more than one first-degree relative is affected. These familial risks are increased even more if the onset of disease in the affected first-degree relative is at 40 years of age or younger (Fig. 16–11). Although as much as 20 percent of all breast cancer cases may have a significant genetic component as part of a polygenic or multifactorial mode of inheritance (see Chapter 15), a small proportion of cases appears to be due to a dominantly inherited mendelian predisposition to breast cancer. These families share features characteristic of familial (as opposed to sporadic) cancer: multiple affected individuals in a family, earlier age of onset, and frequent bilateral disease.

Genetic linkage studies in families with early-onset familial breast cancer have led to the discovery of mutations in two genes that increase susceptibility to breast cancer, *BRCA1* on chromosome 17q21 and *BRCA2* on chromosome 13q12.3. Together, these two loci account for about one half and one third of autosomal dominant familial breast cancer, respectively, but less than 5 percent of all breast cancer in the population. Many mutant alleles of both genes have now been catalogued. Mutations in *BRCA1* and *BRCA2* are also associated with a significant increase in the risk for ovarian cancer in female heterozygotes; mutations in *BRCA2*, but not *BRCA1*, also account for 10 to 20 percent of all *male* breast cancer, a rare disease affecting less than 0.1 percent of males.

The gene products of *BRCA1* and *BRCA2* are nuclear proteins contained within the same multiprotein complex. This complex has been implicated in the cellular response to double-strand DNA breaks, such as occurs normally during homologous recombination or abnormally as a result of damage to DNA. As might be expected with any tumor-suppressor gene, tumor tissue from heterozygotes for *BRCA1* and *BRCA2* mutations demonstrate LOH with loss of the normal allele.

**Penetrance of BRCA1 and BRCA2 Mutations.** Presymptomatic detection of women at risk for developing breast cancer as a result of any of these susceptibility genes is an important aim of current research, both in familial cases and in the larger number of sporadic cases. For the purposes of patient management and counseling, it would obviously be extremely helpful to know the lifetime risk of developing breast cancer in patients carrying particular mutations in the *BRCA1* and *BRCA2* genes, compared with the risk in the general population (Fig. 16–12). Initial studies have shown a more than 80 percent risk of breast cancer by age 70 in women heterozygous for *BRCA1* or *BRCA2* mutations. These estimates relied on estimates of the risk of developing cancer in female relatives within families ascertained because breast cancer had already occurred many times in family members; that is, the *BRCA1* or *BRCA2* mutation was highly penetrant in the carriers. When similar risk estimates were made from population-based studies, however, in which women carrying *BRCA1* and *BRCA2* mutations were not selected because they were members of families in which many cases of breast cancer had already developed, the risk estimates were lower and ranged from 45 to 60 percent by age 70. The discrepancy between studies based on families with multiple occurrences of the disease due to high penetrance of mutant alleles and studies of women identified by population screening and not by family history suggests that other genetic or environmental factors may play a role in the ultimate penetrance of *BRCA1* and *BRCA2* mutations in women heterozygous for these mutations.

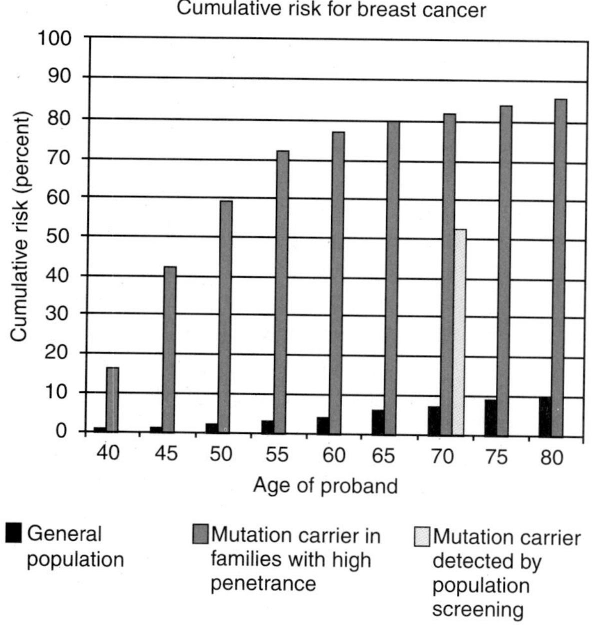


Figure 16–12. Cumulative risk for breast cancer, with age, in women carrying a mutation in *BRCA1* or *BRCA2*, calculated using data from families with high penetrance for the mutation (*red bars*). The risk is compared with the risk for breast cancer in the general population (*black bars*), as well as the estimated risk (~52 percent) at age 70 for breast cancer in a mutation carrier for *BRCA*1 or *BRCA*2 identified through population surveys (*stippled pink bar*) rather than in families with high penetrance. See text. (Adapted from King MC, Rowell S, Love SM [1993] Inherited breast and ovarian cancer. What are the risks? What are the choices? JAMA 269:1775–1980; Ford D, Easton DF, Stratton M, et al [1998] Genetic heterogeneity and penetrance analysis of the *BRCA1* and *BRCA2* genes in breast cancer families. The Breast Cancer Linkage Consortium. Am J Hum Genet 62:676–689; Brody LC, Biesecker BB [1998] Breast cancer susceptibility genes *BRCA1* and *BRCA2*. Medicine [Baltimore]. 77:208–226.)

## Familial Colon Cancer

**Familial Polyposis Coli.** Colorectal cancer, a malignancy of the epithelium of the colon and rectum, is one of the most common forms of cancer. It affects more than 150,000 individuals per year in the United States alone and is responsible for about 15 percent of all cancer. A small proportion of colon cancer cases are due to the autosomal dominant condition **familial polyposis coli** (also known as familial adenomatous polyposis or FAP) and its subvariant, the Gardner syndrome. FAP has an incidence of about 1 in 10,000.

In FAP heterozygotes, numerous adenomatous polyps, which themselves are benign growths, develop in the colon during the first 2 decades of life. In almost all cases, one or more of the polyps becomes malignant. Surgical removal of the colon (colectomy) prevents the development of malignancy. Because this disorder is autosomal dominant, relatives of affected persons must be examined periodically by colonoscopy. The responsible gene, *APC*, was isolated by positional cloning after the disease locus was mapped to chromosome 5q, both by genetic linkage studies in affected families (see Chapter 8) and by demonstration of loss of heterozygosity in colon tumors. Gardner syndrome is also due to mutations in *APC* and is therefore allelic to FAP. Patients with Gardner syndrome have, in addition to the adenomatous polyps with malignant transformation seen in FAP, other anomalies, including osteomas of the jaw and desmoids, which are tumors arising in the muscle of the abdominal wall.

*APC* encodes a cytoplasmic protein that regulates the bifunctional protein known as $\beta$-catenin. $\beta$-catenin serves both as a link between the cytoplasmic portion of transmembrane cell adhesion molecules, such as the cadherins, and the actin cytoskele-

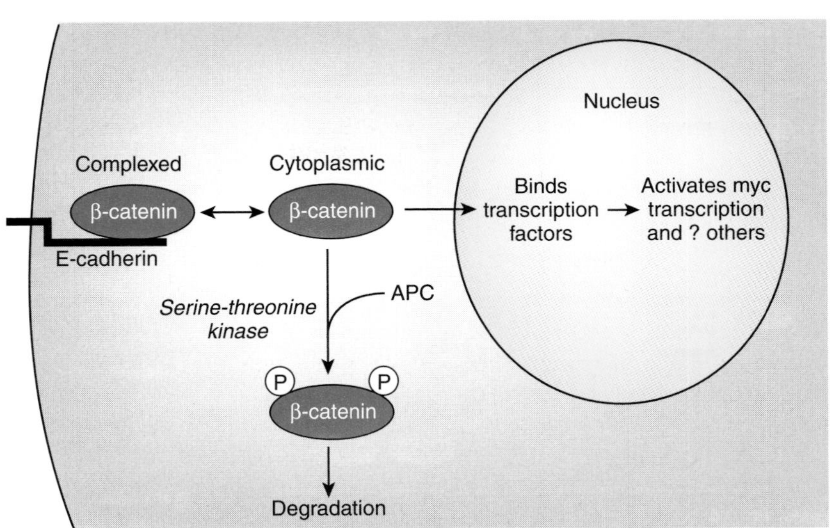


Figure 16–13. Schematic diagram of interaction between the product of the *APC* gene and β-catenin. β-catenin forms a complex with the cell adhesion molecule E-cadherin. β-catenin also exists free in cytoplasm, where it is either targeted by the *APC* gene product for degradation through phosphorylation by a serine/threonine kinase or enters the nucleus and activates transcription of oncogenic genes, such as *MYC*.

ton, and as an activator of transcription (Fig. 16–13). Under normal conditions, when the colonic epithelial layer is intact and no cellular proliferation is required, most β-catenin is present in a large protein complex with E-cadherin. *APC* induces the phosphorylation and subsequent degradation of any unbound β-catenin, thereby keeping free β-catenin levels low in the cell. Loss of *APC* leads to accumulation of free cytoplasmic β-catenin that is translocated into the nucleus and activates transcription of cellular proliferation genes, including *MYC*, the same gene that is overexpressed in Burkitt lymphoma.

**Hereditary Nonpolyposis Colon Cancer.** Approximately 2 to 4 percent of cases of colon cancer are attributable to a group of familial cancer syndromes known as **hereditary nonpolyposis colon cancer** (HNPCC). HNPCC is characterized by autosomal dominant inheritance of colon cancer occurring during adulthood, but at a relatively young age and without the adenomatous polyps seen with FAP. Male heterozygotes for a mutant HNPCC gene have an approximately 90 percent lifetime risk of developing cancer of the colon; female heterozygotes have a somewhat smaller risk, approximately 70 percent, but have an approximately 40 percent risk for endometrial cancer. There are also additional risks of 10 to 20 percent for cancer of the biliary or urinary tract, and the ovary.

HNPCC is a group of five similar familial cancer syndromes (HNPCC1 through HNPCC5) caused by mutations in one of five distinct DNA repair genes responsible for repairing DNA segments in which correct DNA base pairing (A with T, C with G) has been violated (see Chapters 6 and 8). These genes, known as *MLH1*, *MSH2*, *PMSL1*, *PMSL2*, and *MSH6*, are all named because of their sequence similarity to a group of microbial genes that encode the enzymes responsible for repairing mismatches between two complementary strands of DNA. Although all five of these genes have been implicated in HNPCC in different families, *MLH1* and *MSH2* are together responsible for approximately 60 to 70 percent of HNPCC, whereas the others have been found in only a few very rare patients and are often associated with a lesser degree of mismatch repair deficiency. The HNPCC genes are prototypical caretaker tumor-suppressor genes.

As with other tumor-suppressor genes, the autosomal dominant inheritance pattern of HNPCC comes about through inheritance of one mutant allele followed by mutation or inactivation of the remaining normal allele in a somatic cell. At the cellular level, the most striking phenotype of cells lacking both alleles of one of these genes is an enormous increase in point mutations and in instability of DNA segments containing simple sequence repeats, such as $(dA)_n$ or microsatellite polymorphisms (see Chapter 6). Microsatellite DNA is believed to be particularly vulnerable to mismatch because slippage of the strand being synthesized on the template strand can occur more readily when short tandem DNA repeats are synthesized. Such instability, referred to as the **replication error positive** (or **RER+**) phenotype, occurs at two orders of magnitude higher frequency in cells lacking both copies of a mismatch repair gene. The RER+ phenotype is easily seen in DNA as three, four, or even more alleles of a microsatellite polymorphism in a single individual's tumor DNA (Fig. 16–14). It is estimated that cells lacking both copies of a mismatch repair gene may carry 100,000 mutations within simple repeats throughout the genome. Oncogenic mutations secondary to the repeat instability could occur in any number of genes: at least two such genes have been isolated and characterized. The first is *APC*, whose normal function and role in FAP were described previously. The second is the gene encoding transforming growth factor beta receptor II (TGF-βII). TGFβII, a serine/threonine kinase that has a

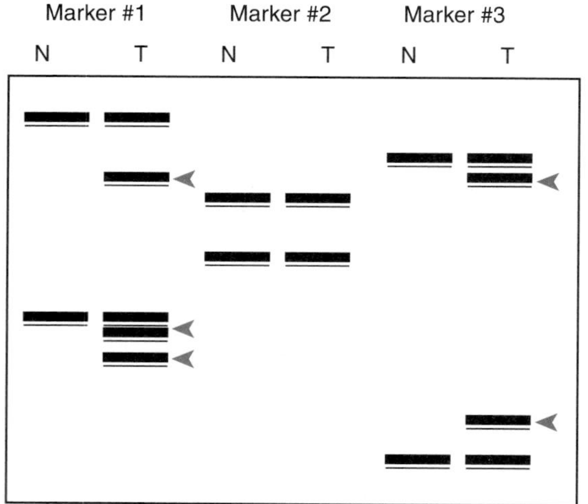


Figure 16–14. Gel electrophoresis of three different microsatellite polymorphic markers in normal (*N*) and tumor (*T*) samples from a patient with a mutation in *MSH2* and microsatellite instability. Although marker #2 shows no difference between normal and tumor tissues, genotyping at markers #1 and #3 reveals extra alleles, some smaller, some larger, than the alleles present in normal tissue (*red arrows*).

growth-controlling activity through phosphorylation of downstream signaling molecules, has a stretch of 10 adenines encoding three lysines within its coding sequence; deletion of one or more of these adenines in both alleles of the gene occurs with high frequency in RER+ cells and results in frameshift and loss of function of this receptor. As illustrated generally in Figure 16–1, oncogenic mutations due to repeat instability could produce many of the mutations that allow a normal cell to become a fully malignant, metastatic cancer cell.

### Hereditary Lymphoma with Loss of Expression of Proapoptotic Tumor-Suppressor Genes

**Autoimmune lymphoproliferative syndrome** (ALPS) is a rare autosomal dominant condition characterized by massive lymphadenopathy and splenomegaly, particularly in childhood, and the development of autoimmune phenomena such as antibody-mediated thrombocytopenia or hemolytic anemia. Although the manifestations of this condition are primarily those of autoimmunity, B-cell and Hodgkin lymphomas have both been described with an increased frequency of 14-fold and 50-fold, respectively.

In ALPS, the primary abnormality is in the mechanism for lymphocyte apoptosis mediated by the fas receptor and its ligand, fas-ligand. Both fas-ligand and fas are homotrimers. Dominant negative mutations (see Chapter 12) in one allele of either of the genes encoding these molecules causes loss of function of the receptor or its ligand, resulting in deficiency of apoptotic signaling and a massive expansion of immature T lymphocytes known as double-negative cells (because they lack both the T-helper [T4] and T-suppressor [T8] cell-surface markers). Precisely how this defect in apoptosis of T lymphocytes can lead to an increased frequency of various kinds of lymphomas is unknown but may be due to the markedly increased number of cells that can serve as targets for mutation and, therefore, malignant transformation.

## Chromosome Instability Syndromes

Four rare autosomal recessive chromosome instability syndromes mentioned in Chapter 9—**ataxia telangiectasia, Fanconi anemia, Bloom syndrome**, and **xeroderma pigmentosum**—are all associated with an increased risk of malignancy, particularly leukemia, or, in the case of xeroderma pigmentosum, skin cancers in sun-exposed areas (see Table 9–6). Clinically, radiography must be used with extreme caution if at all in patients with ataxia telangiectasia, Fanconi anemia, and Bloom syndrome. Furthermore, exposure to sunlight must be avoided in patients with xeroderma pigmentosum.

Although the susceptibility to chromosome and DNA damage by X-irradiation, ultraviolet light, or certain chemical agents and the susceptibility to malignancy seen in these syndromes is not fully explained, the genes for many of them have been isolated and have been shown to encode proteins that are intimately involved in DNA repair and the maintenance of chromosome and genome integrity. Thus, the genes that are defective in the chromosome instability syndromes may be viewed as caretaker tumor-suppressor genes (see Table 16–1).

Although the chromosome instability syndromes are rare autosomal recessive disorders, heterozygotes for these gene defects are much more common and may also be at an increased risk of malignancy. Heterozygous female relatives of ataxia telangiectasia homozygotes may have a four- to sixfold increased risk of breast cancer compared with spouse controls, for example. Should this finding be definitively confirmed, it would become possible to identify, preclinically, a class of individuals with a dramatic genetic predisposition to at least one of the common cancers.

## Loss of Tumor-Suppressor Genes in Sporadic Cancer

### TP53 Mutations in Sporadic Cancers

Although LFS, which is caused by the inheritance of germline mutations in *TP53*, is a rare familial syndrome, somatic mutation causing a loss of function of both alleles of *TP53* turns out to be one of the most

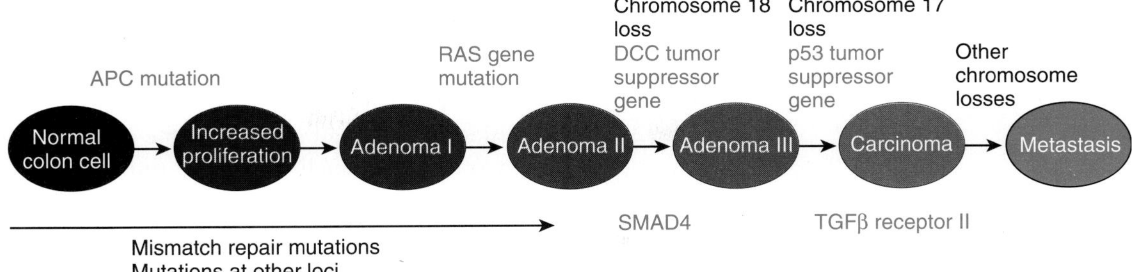


**Figure 16–15.** Stages in the evolution of colon cancer, serving as a model more generally for cancer evolution (see Fig. 16–1). Increasing degrees of abnormality are associated with sequential loss of tumor-suppressor genes from several chromosomes and activation of the *RAS* proto-oncogene, with or without a concomitant defect in mismatch repair. The order of events is usually, but not always, as shown here. For example, sporadic cancer with abnormal mismatch repair is less common than are cancers without abnormal repair but, when present, may operate along a somewhat different, but parallel, pathway leading to malignancy as the final common end point. (Adapted from Kinzler KW, Vogelstein B [1996] Lessons from hereditary colorectal cancer. Cell 87:159–170.)

common genetic alterations seen in sporadic cancer. Mutations of the *TP53* gene or deletion of the segment of chromosome 17p (band p13.1) that includes *TP53*, or both, are frequently and repeatedly seen in a wide range of sporadic cancers, including breast, ovarian, bladder, cervical, esophageal, colorectal, skin, and lung carcinomas, glioblastoma of the brain, osteogenic sarcoma, and hepatocellular carcinoma. The central role of p53 as a tumor suppressor was underscored by its designation as "Molecule of the Year" by *Science* magazine in 1993.

### BRCA1 and BRCA2 in Sporadic Breast and Ovarian Cancer

Mutations in *BRCA1* and *BRCA2* have been found in a small percentage of patients with breast or ovarian cancer without family history. In some cases, the mutations are constitutional, but no family history was apparent; in others, analysis of the tumor itself revealed a somatic mutation in one allele of either *BRCA1* or *BRCA2* along with LOH for the corresponding genomic region containing the other, normal allele. Comparative genome hybridization (see Chapter 4) has been a particularly powerful method used to scan for LOH in breast tumor tissue versus normal tissue from the same woman. LOH has been found in a number of chromosomal regions, including 1p, 3p, 11p, 13q, 16q, and 17p, which suggests that there may be many genes important for breast tumor progression. Although the gene on chromosome 17p is likely to be *TP53*, the other genes have not been identified.

### Hereditary Nonpolyposis Colon Cancer and Familial Adenomatous Polyposis Genes in Sporadic Colon Cancer

In contrast to the low frequency with which *BRCA1* and *BRCA2* are found to be mutated in most sporadic breast cancer, there is ample evidence to support a major involvement of the genes responsible for familial colon cancer, such as HNPCC and FAP, in sporadic colon cancer (Fig. 16–15). In nearly 70 percent of adenomatous polyps in individuals without FAP, the two-hit model for tumorigenesis has been confirmed by finding loss of both copies of *APC* in the adenoma but not in the surrounding normal tissues. In the remaining 30 percent, in which *APC* is normal, mutations in $\beta$-catenin that block its phosphorylation and degradation have been found in nearly half. The RER+ phenotype, with associated mutation or transcriptional silencing of both alleles of one or more of the mismatch repair genes, has been reported in up to 12 percent of sporadic colon cancer in individuals without an obvious family history for HNPCC. Activating mutations of one member of the *RAS* gene family (*KRAS*), as well as loss of both copies of *TP53*, are also frequently seen in sporadic colon cancer. Loss of expression of a gene on 18q21, called *DCC* (for deleted in colon carcinoma), is observed in more than 70 percent of cases of colorectal cancer; this gene encodes a receptor for molecules involved in axonal guidance during normal development of the nervous system. In another 15 percent of sporadic colon cancers, the *SMAD4* gene, which is involved in signaling downstream from the TGF$\beta$II receptor, is mutated.

As important as defects in mismatch repair are in HNPCC and some sporadic colon cancers, most sporadic colon cancer has no RER+ phenotype. Instead, these tumors generally have chromosome and genome mutations that reflect defects either in double-stranded break repair or maintenance of the fidelity of how chromosomes align on the mitotic spindle during mitosis. Defects in the former generate chromosome translocations, whereas abnormalities in the latter can lead to nondisjunction and aneuploidy. In summary, there are many ways for cell division and growth to become dysregulated, and many more undoubtedly are waiting to be discovered and elucidated.

## TUMOR PROGRESSION BY CLONAL EVOLUTION

In familial cancer syndromes, the pattern of inheritance implies that a defect in a single gene, inherited in the germline, is capable of initiating a multistep process that leads to cancer. Although many of these same genes are found to be mutated in sporadic cancers, such cancers may take decades to develop to the point at which they are clinically evident, and, therefore, it is far more difficult to determine which of these mutations actually initiated the malignant process. Furthermore, the paradigms used to explain hereditary cancer syndromes, whereby the development of malignancy requires the activation of a proto-oncogene, loss of function of both alleles of a tumor-suppressor gene, or dysregulation of apoptotic processes, are necessarily oversimplified. Tumor formation is clearly a multistep process involving a succession of genetic changes in the evolving tumor cell population (see Fig. 16–1). The steps to malignancy may also not fall into a single linear pathway because different genetic changes, driven by defects either in DNA repair or maintenance of genomic integrity, can occur as different malignant sublineages branch off during evolution and progression of the tumor.

### Cytogenetic Changes in Cancer

#### Aneuploidy and Aneusomy

Cytogenetic changes are hallmarks of cancer, particularly in later and more malignant or invasive stages of tumor development. Such cytogenetic alterations suggest that an important element of cancer progression includes defects in genes involved in maintaining chromosome stability and integrity and ensuring accurate mitotic segregation.

Initially, most of the cytogenetic studies of tumor progression were carried out in leukemias, because the tumor cells were amenable to being cultured and karyotyped by standard methods. For example, when CML, with a 9;22 Philadelphia chromosome, evolves from the typically indolent chronic phase to a severe, life-threatening blast crisis, there may be several additional cytogenetic abnormalities, including numerical or structural changes, such as a second copy of the 9;22 translocation chromosome or an isochromosome for 17q. In advanced stages of other forms of leukemia, other translocations are common.

Comparative genome hybridization (CGH) (see Chapter 4) has allowed cancer cytogeneticists to analyze tumor tissues for genome and chromosome mutations without having to propagate the tumor cells themselves for karyotyping. When the tumor cells can be karyotyped, spectral karyotyping (see Chapters 4 and 9) has also revealed a far greater range of abnormalities than was visible by earlier methods of karyotyping and chromosome identification by banding (see Fig. 9–5, *color insert*). A vast array of abnormalities is seen in all cancers. Some abnormalities are seen only occasionally in some tumor samples and may be random aberrations, and others are found repeatedly in cancers of the same histological type. This suggests that these mutations are involved in some way in the evolution of the malignancy. Still other changes are found only in metastases of a cancer but not in the original primary tumor. A focus of cancer research is the cytogenetic and molecular definition of these abnormalities, many of which are already known to be related to proto-oncogenes or tumor-suppressor genes and presumably allow enhanced proto-oncogene expression or represent loss of tumor-suppressor gene alleles.

#### Gene Amplification

In addition to translocations and other rearrangements, another cytogenetic aberration seen in many cancers is **gene amplification**, a phenomenon in which there are many additional copies of a segment of the genome present in the cell. Gene amplification is common in many cancers, including neuroblastoma, squamous cell carcinoma of the head and neck, colorectal cancer, and malignant glioblastomas of the brain. Amplified segments of DNA are readily detected by CGH and appear as two types of cytogenetic change in routine chromosome analysis: **double minutes** (very small accessory chromosomes) and **homogeneously staining regions** (HSRs) that do not band normally and contain multiple, amplified copies of a particular DNA segment. How and why double minutes and HSRs occur are poorly understood, but amplified regions are known to include extra copies of proto-oncogenes, such as the genes encoding myc, ras, and epithelial growth-factor receptor, which stimulate cell growth or block apoptosis, or both. For example, amplification of the *MYCN* proto-oncogene encoding n-myc is an important clinical indicator of prognosis in the childhood cancer **neuroblastoma** (Fig. 16–16). *MYCN* is amplified more than 200-fold in 40 percent of advanced stages of neuroblastoma; despite aggressive treatment, only 30 percent of patients with advanced disease survive 3 years. In contrast, *MYCN* amplification is found in only 4 percent of early-stage neuroblastoma, and the 3-year survival is 90 percent. Amplification of genes encoding the targets of chemotherapeutic agents has also been implicated as a mechanism for the development of drug resistance in patients previously treated with chemotherapy.

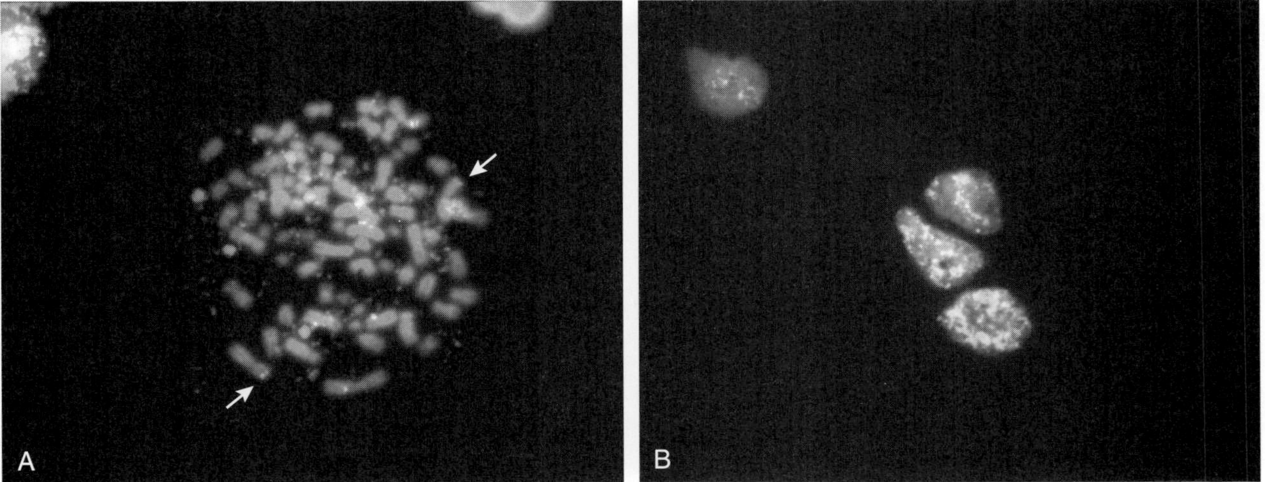


Figure 16–16. Fluorescence in situ hybridization with *MYCN* probe in advanced neuroblastoma. *A*, Metaphase spread of a tetraploid neuroblastoma cell showing double minutes. Intensity of fluorescent signal varies according to the size of the double minute and the number of *MYCN* copies it contains. White arrows point to fluorescent signal arising from the normal *MYCN* locus on distal chromosome 2p. *B*, Interphase nuclei of neuroblastoma cells showing varying degrees of fluorescent intensity arising from double-minute chromosomes. (Photograph courtesy of J. Biegel, Children's Hospital of Philadelphia.)

## CANCER AND THE ENVIRONMENT

The risk of cancer shows significant variation among different populations and within the same population in different environments. For example, gastric cancer is almost three times as common among Japanese in Japan as among Japanese living in Hawaii or Los Angeles. Thus, it appears that a considerable proportion of the risk must depend on exposure to mutagens and carcinogens in the environment. The nature of environmental carcinogens, assessment of the additional risk associated with exposure, and ways of protecting the population from such hazards are matters of strong public concern.

The theme of this chapter is that cancer is a genetic disease, but there is no contradiction in considering the role of environment in carcinogenesis. Environmental agents act as mutagens that cause somatic mutations; the somatic mutations, in turn, are responsible for carcinogenesis. According to some estimates based chiefly on data from the aftermath of the atomic bombings of Hiroshima and Nagasaki, as much as 75 percent of the risk of cancer may be environmental in origin.

### Radiation

Ionizing radiation is known to cause an increased risk of cancer. The data for survivors of the Hiroshima and Nagasaki atomic bombings and other exposed populations show a long latency period, in the 5-year range for leukemia but up to 40 years for some tumors. The risk is age-dependent, being greatest for children younger than 10 years and for the elderly. As noted earlier, radiation is much more damaging to persons with inborn defects of DNA repair than to the general population. Everyone is exposed to some degree of ionizing radiation through background radiation (which varies greatly from place to place), medical exposure, and nuclear energy. Unfortunately, there are still large areas of uncertainty about the magnitude of the effects of radiation, especially low-level radiation, on cancer risks.

### Chemical Carcinogens

Interest in the carcinogenic effect of chemicals dates back at least to the 18th century, when the high incidence of scrotal cancer in young chimney sweeps was noticed. Today, there is concern about many possible chemical carcinogens, especially tobacco, components of the diet, industrial carcinogens, and toxic wastes. Documentation of the risk of exposure is often difficult, but the level of concern is such that all clinicians should have a working knowledge of the subject and be able to distinguish between well-established facts and areas of uncertainty and debate.

One important area in which environment and genetic factors can interact to either enhance or prevent the carcinogenic effects of chemicals is in the genes encoding enzymes that metabolize exogenous drugs and chemicals. A class of drug-metabolizing enzymes, encoded by the family of **cytochrome P450** genes (*CYP*) (of which there are dozens and perhaps even hundreds in the human genome), is responsible for the detoxification of foreign chemicals. A number of *CYP* genes are polymorphic and underlie variation in drug metabolism (see discussion of pharmacogenetics in Chapter 12). One well-studied genetic polymorphism has been associated with susceptibility to lung cancer. The enzyme **aryl hydrocarbon hydroxylase** (AHH) is an inducible protein involved in the metabolism of polycyclic hydrocarbons, such as those found in cigarette smoke. AHH converts hydrocarbons into an epoxide form that is more easily excreted by the body but that also happens to be carcinogenic. The extent of hydrocarbon metabolism is genetically controlled and shows polymorphic variation in the normal population. People who carry a "high-inducibility" allele, particularly those who are smokers, appear to be at an increased risk of lung cancer. Data indicate that cigarette smoke itself induces expression of the *CYP1A1* gene (which encodes AHH) in persons with a high-inducibility allele. On the other hand, homozygotes for the recessive "low-inducibility" allele appear to be less likely to develop lung cancer, possibly because their AHH is less effective at converting the hydrocarbons to highly reactive carcinogens.

A second cytochrome P450 enzyme polymorphism, controlling the ability to metabolize the compound debrisoquin (a beta-adrenergic blocking agent), has also been associated with an increased susceptibility to lung cancer. A small proportion of people are "poor metabolizers" of debrisoquin and are homozygous for a recessive allele at the *CYP2D6* gene on chromosome 22. These persons appear to be more resistant to the potential carcinogenic effects of cigarette smoke or occupational lung carcinogens (such as asbestos or polycyclic aromatic hydrocarbons). "Extensive metabolizers" (homozygotes for a fully functional *CYP2D6* allele) have a fourfold greater risk for lung cancer than do "poor metabolizers." This risk increases to 18-fold among persons exposed routinely to lung carcinogens. A similar association has been reported for bladder cancer.

Although the precise genetic and biochemical basis for the apparent differences in cancer susceptibility within the normal population remains to be determined, these associations could have significant public health consequences and may point eventually to a way of identifying persons who are genetically predisposed to developing cancer.

## CONCLUSION

Cancer is a genetic disorder in which the control of cell proliferation is lost. The basic mechanism in all cancers is mutation, either in the germline or, much more frequently, in somatic cells. Much remains to be learned about the genetic processes of carcinogenesis and about the environmental factors that can alter DNA and thus lead to malignancy. It is likely that new insights into the fundamental role of DNA changes in carcinogenesis will lead in the near future to improved and more specific ways of early detection, prevention, and treatment of malignant disease.

## General References

Fearon ER (1999) Cancer progression. Curr Biol 9:R873–R875.
Fearon ER (1997) Human cancer syndromes: Clues to the origin and nature of cancer. Science 278:1043–1049.
Kinzler KW, Vogelstein B (1996) Lessons from hereditary colorectal cancer. Cell 87:159–170.
Kinzler KW, Vogelstein B (1997) Cancer susceptibility genes. Gatekeepers and caretakers. Nature 386:761–763.
Knudson AG (1996) Hereditary cancer: Two hits revisited. J Cancer Res Clin Oncol 122:135–140.
Knudson AG (1997) Hereditary predisposition to cancer. Ann NY Acad Sci 833:58–67.
Look AT (1997) Oncogenic transcription factors in the human acute leukemias. Science 278:1059–1063.
Lengauer C, Kinzler KW, Vogelstein B (1998) Genetic instabilities in human cancers. Nature 396:643–649.
Mitelman F (1998) Catalogue of Chromosome Aberrations in Cancer, 6th ed. on CD-ROM. John Wiley & Sons, New York.
Nowell PC, Rowley JD, Knudson AG Jr (1998) Cancer genetics, cytogenetics—defining the enemy within. Nat Med 4:1107–1111
Offit K (1997) Clinical Cancer Genetics: Risk Counseling and Management. Wiley-Liss, New York.
Perera FP (1997) Environment and cancer: Who are susceptible? Science 278:1068–1073.
Vogelstein B, Kinzler KW (1998) The Genetic Basis of Human Cancer. McGraw Hill, New York.

## References Specific to Particular Topics

Burke W, Daly M, Garber J, et al (1997) Recommendations for follow-up care of individuals with an inherited predisposition to cancer II. BRCA1 and BRCA2. JAMA 277:997–1003.
Cahill DP, Lengauer C, Yu J, et al (1998) Mutations of mitotic checkpoint genes in human cancers. Nature 392:300–303.
Eshleman JR, Markowitz SD (1995) Microsatellite instability in inherited and sporadic neoplasms. Curr Opin Oncol 7:83–89.
Fearon ER, Dang CV (1999) Cancer genetics: Tumor-suppressor meets oncogene. Curr Biol 9:R62–R65.
Holt SE, Shay JW (1999) Role of telomerase in cellular proliferation and cancer. J Cell Physiol 180:10–18.
Ivanovich JL, Read TE, Ciske DJ, et al (1999) A practical approach to familial and hereditary colorectal cancer. Am J Med 107:68–77.
Jones PA, Laird PW (1999) Cancer epigenetics comes of age. Nat Genet 21:163–167.
Morin PJ (1999) β-catenin signaling and cancer. Bioessays 21:1021–1030.
Rowley JD (1990) The Philadelphia chromosome translocation: A paradigm for understanding leukemia. Cancer 65:2178–2184.
St. John DJ, McDermott FT, Hopper JL, et al (1993) Cancer risk in relatives of patients with common colorectal cancer. Ann Intern Med 118:785–790.
Weinberg RA (1990) The genetic basis of cancer. Arch Surg 125:257–260.

## Problems

1. A patient with retinoblastoma has a single tumor in one eye; the other eye is free of tumors. What steps would you take to try to determine whether this was sporadic or heritable retinoblastoma? What genetic counseling would you provide? What information should the parents have before a subsequent pregnancy?

2. Discuss possible reasons why colorectal cancer is an adult cancer, whereas retinoblastoma affects children.

3. Many tumor types are characterized by the presence of an isochromosome for the long arm of chromosome 17. Provide a possible explanation for this finding.

4. Many children with Fanconi anemia have limb defects. If an affected child requires surgery for the abnormal limb, what special considerations arise?

5. Wanda, whose sister has premenopausal bilateral breast cancer, has a greater risk of developing breast cancer herself (30 to 50 percent) than does Wilma, whose sister has premenopausal breast cancer in only one breast (10 to 15 percent). Both Wanda and Wilma, however, have a greater risk than does Winnie, who has a completely negative family history (about 5 to 10 percent). Considering the information in this chapter and in Chapter 15, provide an explanation for these empiric risk figures.

17

# Genetic Aspects of Development

There is an intricate relationship between genetics and embryonic development that has both fundamental and practical implications for human health and disease. Congenital abnormalities such as cleft palate, intestinal aganglionosis, and cardiovascular malformations occur in approximately 1 of 200 liveborn infants and account for about 25 percent of deaths in a neonatal intensive care setting. Comprehending the genetic programs that guide normal development is a prerequisite for understanding and designing treatments for human birth defects. The interface between developmental biology and genetics is also the testing ground for technologies based on stem cells, tissue engineering, and cell cloning, which hold tremendous promise for treating adult-onset diseases such as Parkinson disease, leukemia, and spinal cord injury. Finally, the principles that guide normal development are those on which modern techniques of prenatal diagnosis are based.

In this chapter, we first review general principles of developmental genetics using as examples several important human malformation syndromes. We then discuss how these principles are applied by practicing physicians in caring for patients and their families affected with, or at risk for, serious birth defects. Finally, we discuss how recent advances in experimental embryology offer new opportunities and new challenges for the treatment of human disease.

## INTRODUCTION TO DEVELOPMENTAL BIOLOGY

We begin by describing the origins and concepts of developmental biology and the relevance of developmental mechanisms to human disease.

### What Is Developmental Biology?

Developmental biology refers to the processes—genetic, biochemical, cellular, and physiological—whereby a one-cell embryo gives rise to an entire organism. The field had its origins when embryos could first be observed using the microscope, but the 20th century saw the transformation of embryology, a descriptive science, into developmental biology, an integrative science based on experimental manipulation. This transformation came initially in the form of studies carried out on the embryos of model organisms: labeling cells so they could be tracked during embryogenesis, explanting embryonic tissues into tissue culture, and transplanting embryonic tissues from one region of an embryo to another region. Such microsurgical manipulation of embryos provided a foundation for viewing embryonic development in terms of key processes and mechanisms (Fig. 17–1 and Box). More recently, developmental biology has become a thoroughly modern science through the introduction of the concepts and tools of molecular genetics. The study of mutations that cause developmental abnormalities and the ability to ablate or alter the expression of genes in model organisms allow developmental biologists to identify the genes important for normal development and the pathways these genes regulate.

### Developmental Biology and Human Disease

Normal developmental mechanisms and the ways in which they go awry form a conceptual basis for understanding many different types of human disease; knowledge of these mechanisms provides a cornerstone in caring for affected patients and their families. The

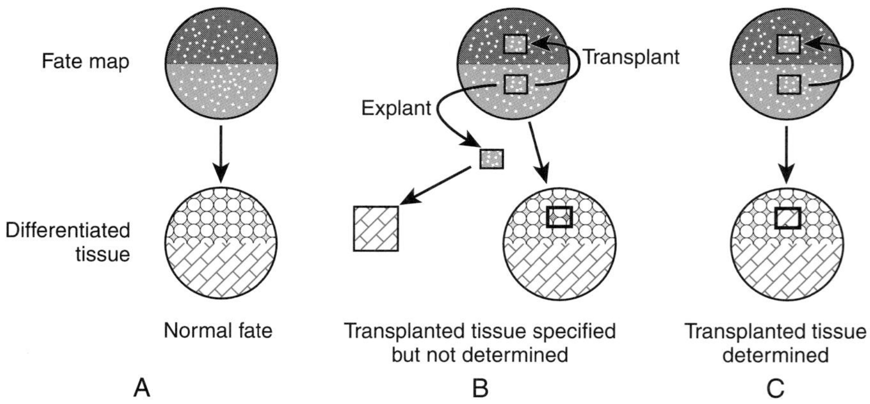


**Figure 17–1.** Operational concepts of experimental embryology. Two diagrammatic embryonic regions in the upper and lower halves of the embryo are depicted arbitrarily as black and red, respectively. In the actual embryo, the cells can be distinguished only by their position, but, after differentiation, the two cell types give rise to different tissues (as indicated by pattern, rectangular versus circular). Thus, a fate map can be drawn wherein the upper part of the embryo gives rise to circular cells and the lower part gives rise to rectangular cells (*A*). If labeled cells from the lower half (*red*) are explanted and retain their original fate when grown autonomously, they are said to have undergone **specification.** If these same cells, when transplanted to the upper half, take on the fate of the upper half, then the cells were not yet **determined** (*B*). If cells are transplanted and retain their original fate, they are said to have become determined prior to the transplantation (*C*).

clinical spectrum of human developmental abnormalities is extremely broad (Table 17–1). Although most developmental abnormalities come to clinical attention at birth or within the first few months of life, some—situs inversus or a bicuspid aortic valve, for example—may not be apparent until adolescence or adult life. Some developmental abnormalities are caused by mutations in single genes required for key morphogenetic events and therefore occur in inheritance patterns predicted by classical mendelian inheritance (Table 17–1). In other instances, abnormalities are caused by chromosomal imbalance, as in trisomy 21 (see Chapter 10), and occur sporadically. Finally, as with many common genetic disorders (see Chapter 15), human developmental abnormalities can be caused by a combination of genetic or environmental factors, or both, and therefore occur in patterns more typical of multifactorial inheritance. Even when the initiating event for a human developmental abnormality is completely environmental, however, such as in fetal dilantin syndrome or fetal alcohol syndrome, the pathophysiological sequence is mediated by alterations in gene expression. Thus, comprehending the morphogenetic programs that guide normal development is a prerequisite for understanding and designing treatments for all developmental abnormalities, regardless of their primary cause.

## GENES IN DEVELOPMENT

### The Importance of Model Organisms for Human Developmental Genetics

Model organisms, such as fruitflies, worms, and fish, have been used for many years to study development. One approach is to carry out **mutagenesis screens** in which a large number of animals are exposed to a mutagen and then bred and their offspring analyzed for abnormalities in embryonic development. Genetic or physical mapping (see Chapter 8) of animals exhibiting abnormal development allowed researchers to identify and isolate numerous genes required for normal embryogenesis. Such screens have indicated that a large proportion of genes in all multicellular animals carry out functions directly related to morphogenetic programs. What is important for human geneticists, however, is that many if not most of these genes exhibit amazing evolutionary conservation. In the fruitfly *Drosophila melanogaster* in particular, developmental genetic studies have revealed a number of developmental control genes conserved and used throughout the animal kingdom to establish the body plan during embryogenesis. Virtually all of these developmental control genes are used during human development and, when mutated, give rise to abnormalities recognized as human birth defects (Table 17–2).

#### Example: The PAX6 Gene Is a Conserved Regulator of Eye Development

A telling example of the principles just outlined is evident from humans with mutations in the *PAX6* gene, in which early studies based on experimental embryology later intersected with those based on developmental genetics in fruitflies and humans.

The vertebrate lens develops from a specialized area of surface ectoderm that becomes thickened into a **placode** (the optic placode) and overlies an outgrowth of neurectoderm known as the **optic cup** (Fig. 17–2). Signals from the optic cup **induce** overlying cells in the placode to initiate a program of gene

## Concepts in Modern Developmental Biology

1. **Morphogenesis** refers to the process whereby changes in cell shape, cell adhesion, cell movement, cell proliferation, and/or cell death give rise to a specific three-dimensional *structure*. By contrast, **differentiation** refers to the process whereby one or more cells acquire a specific pattern of gene and protein expression characteristic of a particular *cell type or tissue*.
2. When a specific region of the embryo regularly gives rise to the same structure or structures in the context of normal development, the region is said to have a specific **fate**; a compendium of how all the different regions of an embryo develop is described as a **fate map**, and the process by which a cell achieves its fate is called its developmental **program**. For example, the outer cells of a human blastocyst regularly give rise to tissues of the placenta and related structures, whereas the inner cells regularly give rise to the embryo proper (see main text).
3. If a region of the embryo can give rise to multiple structures when exposed to different environments, the region is termed **pluripotent**.
4. During the course of normal development, particular embryonic regions become **committed** to their fate in a two-stage process of **specification** followed by **determination**. Initially, commitment is labile. Early in commitment, if a region of the embryo is removed and grown in vitro, free of influences from surrounding embryonic tissues (*explanted*), it will usually develop into the same tissues it would have become if it had not been explanted. However, if the same region is *transplanted*, that is, moved to another location in the embryo, it can acquire a different fate. This phenomenon is termed specification. After the initial phase of specification, however, commitment becomes irreversible and cell fate can no longer be influenced by different embryonic environments. This phenomenon is termed determination. Understanding and manipulating the mechanisms that govern developmental commitment are the focus of attempts to develop transplantable replacements for a variety of human tissues.
5. A **lineage** refers to the progeny of a particular cell that has been experimentally labeled. Progeny of a cell that can be easily identified later in development, for example because they remain physically adjacent, are referred to as a **clone**. Cell migration or fate, or both, may depend on cell lineage; for example, the progeny of somitic and neural crest cells give rise to a segmental distribution of dermatomyotomes and melanocytes, respectively. In other instances, cell fate depends not on lineage but on environment; for example, precursors of the neural retina give rise to different types of retinal neurons depending on the identity of neighboring cells. These different patterns of development are sometimes described as "**lineage versus position**–dependent development." A related set of concepts is **cell autonomy** or **cell nonautonomy**, terms used to refer to whether the fate of a particular cell depends on genes expressed within that cell or on signals from other cells.
6. **Embryonic induction** is the process whereby the fate of one embryonic region depends on receiving an extracellular signal from a second, usually adjacent, region. By definition, the first region must not have been fully determined and therefore must be **competent** to respond to the **inductive signal** provided by the second region.
7. **Regulative development** describes the process in which removal or destruction of a region of the embryo destined to assume a particular fate is compensated for by other embryonic regions. By contrast, **mosaic development** describes a process whereby different regions of the embryo develop independently from surrounding regions. The transition from regulative to mosaic development helps to explain the pattern of birth defects caused by environmental or pharmaceutical agents (see main text).

expression leading to lens development and differentiation. However, the identity of the genes that initiate this hypothetical morphogenetic program of eye development proved elusive until it was found that humans (and mice) with a genetic form of abnormal eye development had mutations in a gene named *PAX6*. The *PAX6* gene encodes a transcription factor that contains two types of DNA binding domains (a **paired domain** and a **homeodomain**, see later) and can initiate an entire array of changes in gene and protein expression (see later). Humans heterozygous for *PAX6* loss-of-function mutations have several eye abnormalities, including **aniridia**, or absence of the iris; rare homozygotes have complete absence of eye structures. Recognition that mutations in *PAX6* caused aniridia or anophthalmia led to subsequent experiments proving that *PAX6* normally initiates and orchestrates programs of eye development in both the optic cup and the lens placode, therefore providing a key link between experimental embryology and genetics.

TABLE 17–1

**Examples of Human Developmental Abnormalities According to Primary Cause**

| Condition | Clinical Findings | Genetics and Pathogenesis |
|---|---|---|
| | *Single Gene* | |
| Aniridia | Reduced or absent iris, frequent retinal, lens, and/or corneal abnormalities | Autosomal semidominant loss-of-function mutations in the pairedlike transcription factor *PAX6*; also observed along with Wilms' tumor and genitourinary abnormalities as part of the 11p13 WAGR deletion syndrome (Wilms' tumor, aniridia, ambiguous genitalia) |
| Rubenstein-Taybi syndrome | Mental retardation, broad thumbs and toes, downslanting palpebral fissures, hypoplastic maxilla, prominent nose, congenital heart disease | Heterozygosity for loss-of-function mutations in the autosomal gene encoding CREB-binding protein (CBP), a transcriptional coactivator for many different target genes |
| Waardenburg syndrome | Deafness, white forelock, pale and/or asymmetrical eye pigmentation. Cases due to *PAX3* mutations have abnormally wide space between the inner eyelids and occasional upper-limb defects | Autosomal semidominant loss-of-function mutations in one of two different genes: *PAX3*, which encodes a pairedlike transcription factor expressed in the neural tube and somites, or *MITF*, which encodes a bHLH transcription factor expressed in developing pigment cells |
| Synpolydactyly | Interphalangeal webbing and extra digits in hands and feet | Semidominant gain-of-function mutation in *HOXD13* |
| Holoprosencephaly | Defective morphogenesis and bilateral cleavage of the forebrain and midface causes manifestations ranging from mild (single central incisor) to severe (microcephaly, cyclopia) | Approximately 10% of cases caused by heterozygosity for loss-of-function mutations in *SHH*, which encodes a dosage-sensitive paracrine signaling molecule; other etiologies include single-gene loci, multifactorial causes, and chromosomal imbalance syndromes |
| Cornelia de Lange syndrome | Growth and mental retardation, upper-limb deficiencies, synophrys, depressed nasal bridge, anteverted nares, thin upper lip | Usually sporadic and probably new dominant mutation of unknown gene; rare sibling recurrence may be germline mosaicism |
| | *Multifactorial and/or Teratogenic* | |
| Cleft lip with or without cleft palate | Absence of midline tissue from the upper lip, may extend posteriorly to involve the hard and soft palate | Isolated occurrences usually polygenic and associated with recurrence risks of 3%–5%; less frequently, associated findings suggest syndromic cause (Chapter 15) |
| Fetal alcohol syndrome | Microcephaly, optic nerve hypoplasia, developmental delay, facial abnormalities, hyperactive behavior | Prenatal exposure to ethanol during critical periods of brain development directly causes death of developing neurons |
| Retinoic acid embryopathy | Microtia (small ears), conotruncal cardiac malformations, posterior fossa malformations, thymus and parathyroid abnormalities | Exposure to isotretinoin causes abnormalities of neural crest– and branchial arch–derived structures |
| | *Chromosomal Imbalance* | |
| Trisomy 21 | Growth and mental retardation, abnormal facial features, hypotonia, endocardial cushion defect, duodenal atresia | 50% increase in dosage for 250 genes on chromosome 21 |
| Velocardiofacial syndrome | Cleft palate, prominent pear-shaped nose, conotruncal heart malformations, learning disabilities | Heterozygous microdeletion in 22q11 that contains 20 genes; individual genes responsible for morphogenetic abnormalities not yet identified |

TABLE 17–2

**Homologs of *Drosophila* Developmental Control Genes as Causes of Human Abnormalities**

| Condition | Gene | Clinical Findings |
|---|---|---|
| Nevoid basal cell carcinoma syndrome | *Drosophila patched* gene required for embryonic segmentation; human *PTC* gene is 29% similar | Overgrowth, skeletal abnormalities, increased susceptibility to basal cell carcinoma and medulloblastoma |
| Greig syndrome; Pallister-Hall syndrome; postaxial polydactyly | *Drosophila cubitus interruptus* gene required for embryonic segmentation; human *GLI3* gene is 22% identical | Extra digits (polydactyly), fusion of bony sutures in skull (craniosynostosis), hypothalamic tumors (in Pallister-Hall syndrome) |
| Holoprosencephaly (HPE3) | *Drosophila hedgehog* gene required for embryonic segmentation; human *SHH* gene is 38% identical | Reduced or absent development of forebrain and midline facial structures |
| Saethre-Chotzen syndrome | *Drosophila twist* gene required for mesoderm development; human *TWIST* gene is 32% similar | Craniosynostosis and abnormal facial features |
| Townes-Brock syndrome | *Drosophila spalt* gene required for specification of head and tail embryonic regions; human *SALL1* gene is 21% identical | Limb deficiency, ear abnormalities, anal atresia or stenosis |

One of the most important aspects of the role of *PAX6* in mammalian eye development is that the gene was named by virtue of its sequence similarity and evolutionary conservation to the gene *paired* in the fruitfly *Drosophila*. Described for the way mutations affect pairs of embryonic segments, paired is one of many embryonic lethal mutations in *Drosophila* (see Table 17–2) that control developmental programs. Including *PAX6*, there are a total of nine human genes related to the fly *paired* gene, and evidence to date suggests that each of them controls specific aspects of human embryonic development. In a remarkable footnote, it has turned out that there are additional *Drosophila* genes similar to *paired*, and one of them, the one most closely similar to *PAX6*, is named *eyeless* (Ey) because mutant fruitflies lack eyes. Targeted ectopic expression of the Ey gene causes eyes to develop in locations such as legs or antennae. *Thus, even though many aspects of eye structure and development differ enormously between insects and humans, closely related genes initiate the developmental program for the same organ in animals separated by 500 million years of evolution.*

## EARLY DEVELOPMENT: FERTILIZATION TO GASTRULATION

One of the best understood aspects of human development is the phase that takes place between fertilization and uterine implantation. Early studies of preimplantation development were carried out primarily in

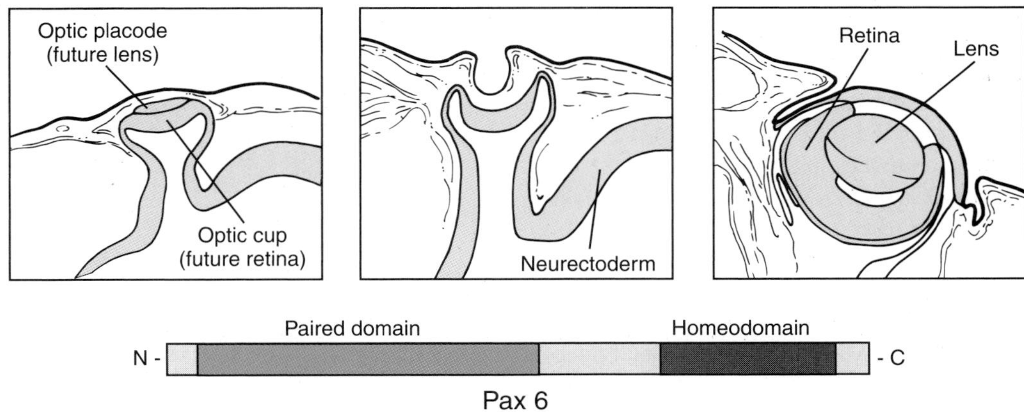


Figure 17–2. Embryonic induction and *PAX6* expression during eye development in the mouse. Proximity to the newly formed optic cup causes overlying ectodermal cells to thicken into the optic placode, which later differentiates into the lens. *PAX6* is expressed at high levels in the nascent optic placode and is required for placode formation. *PAX6* is also expressed at lower levels in the optic cup and the differentiating lens, retina, and iris. Heterozygosity for a *PAX6* loss-of-function mutation causes several eye abnormalities including hypoplasia or aplasia of the iris (aniridia); homozygosity causes absence of the optic placode and central-nervous-system abnormalities. (Reprinted by permission from Grindley JC, Davidson DR, Hill RE [1995] The role of Pax-6 in eye and nasal development. Development 121:1433–1442. Copyright 1995, The Company of Biologists Limited.)

mice, because a preimplantation embryo can be removed from the reproductive tract, specific cells labeled, and the embryo then returned to the fallopian tube or uterus and allowed to develop normally. Such studies have helped us to not only understand normal human development but also to develop approaches and methods such as in vitro fertilization and preimplantation diagnosis for treating a variety of abnormalities in human reproduction (see later).

A general principle of mammalian embryogenesis is that the first cells to differentiate are those that give rise to extraembryonic tissues required for implantation and formation of the placenta (Fig. 17–3). Before implantation, definitive embryonic tissues have not yet been formed, and the mammalian zygote is sometimes referred to as a conceptus or pre-embryo. The definitive embryo arises from a small group of cells within the blastocyst; this region is described initially as the **inner cell mass** (ICM) and later as the **primitive ectoderm** or **epiblast** (when internal cell layers form within the blastocyst and the amniotic cavity appears). One of the earliest tissues formed by the definitive embryo are germ cells, which later give rise to oocytes or spermatocytes.

## Early Mammalian Development Is Mostly Regulative

In the mammalian blastocyst, substantial portions of a particular region can be removed, and the conceptus is able to develop normally. For example, division of an early blastocyst into two equal parts gives rise to normal-sized monozygotic twins (see later). A second illustration is the fact that a normal embryo can be formed from just a single cell of the ICM. This ability to compensate for regions that are injured or removed is described as **regulative development** and has important consequences for human reproduction. In tissues subject to regulative development, cells can be removed or damaged without harm. For example, prenatal diagnosis carried out via biopsy of a preimplantation embryo is made possible by regulative development of the ICM. In addition, exposure to potential teratogens in the 2 weeks after conception carries a very low risk of causing birth defects, in part because tissues of the early embryo are capable of regulative development.

**Mosaic development** lies at the opposite end of the spectrum from regulative development and refers to a situation wherein the fate of a particular cell is specified independently of its environment. In this case, if parts of a developing tissue are removed or destroyed, what remains continues to develop as it otherwise would without compensating for the missing cells. In mammalian embryos, mosaic development generally occurs in developing organs for a short phase before overt differentiation. Mosaic development, or, more properly, absence of regulative development, underlies the harmful effects of terato-

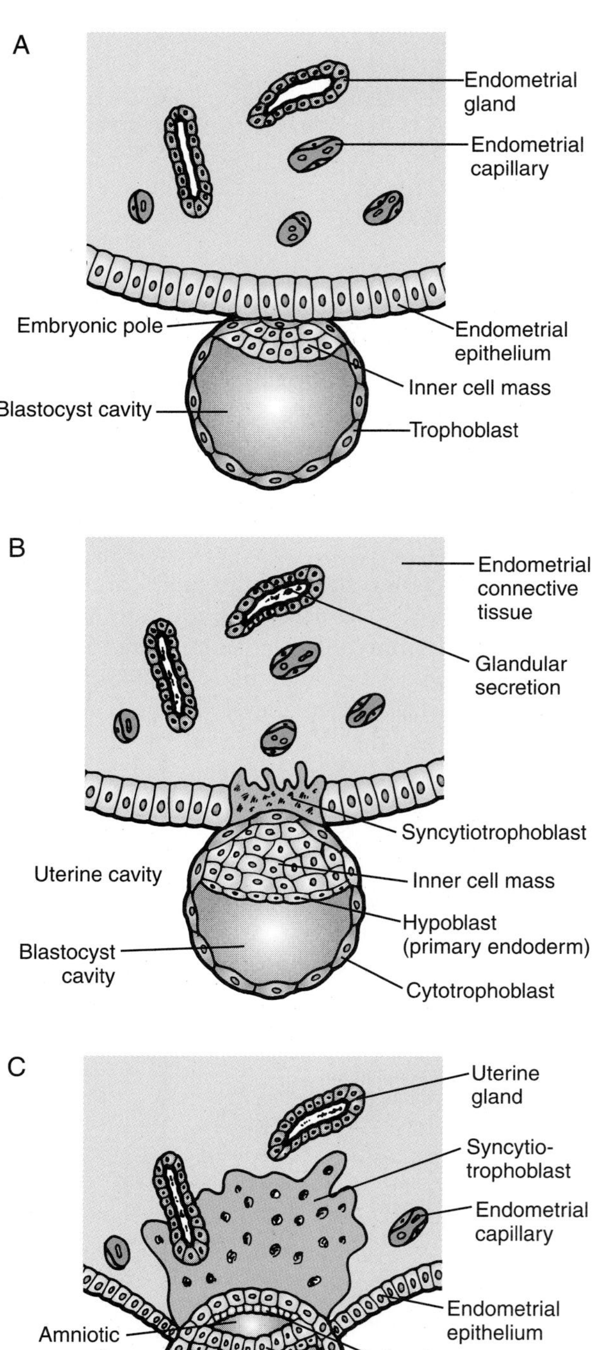


**Figure 17–3.** Cell lineage and fate during preimplantation development. Embryonic age is given in time post fertilization in humans: *A*, 6 days; *B*, 7 days; *C*, 8 days post fertilization. (Reprinted by permission from Moore KL, Persaud TVN [1998] The Developing Human: Clinically Oriented Embryology, 6th ed. WB Saunders, Philadelphia.)

genic agents that act by causing susceptible cells to die, as in the loss of cells in the fetal lens during exposure to rubella virus, leading to congenital cataracts and microphthalmia.

#### Gastrulation and Developmental Abnormalities

Shortly after a mammalian conceptus attaches to the lining of the uterus and implantation begins, about day 6 after conception, cells that will ultimately give rise to the embryo lie in a single tissue, the primitive ectoderm or epiblast. The three primary germ layers—definitive **ectoderm**, definitive **endoderm**, and **mesoderm**—then arise from the epiblast by a process known as gastrulation, a highly orchestrated series of signals and cell movements. (A complete description of gastrulation is beyond the scope of this text.) Primordia for several major organ systems become apparent after gastrulation, including the heart, brain and spinal cord, skeletal system, and gastrointestinal tract. Gastrulation is not only the starting point for organogenesis but also marks the beginning of a period in which the embryo can no longer easily compensate for damaged or lost cell groups; in other words, regulative development is no longer operative. *For these reasons, and because several organ primordia are allocated from relatively small groups of cells, the period of organogenesis after gastrulation is one in which developmental defects are most likely to occur.*

## GENE EXPRESSION DURING DEVELOPMENT

As with all other aspects of cellular function, it is the set of genes expressed within a cell that ultimately control that cell's function. In development, however, there is an additional (and essential) level of complexity. Different cells in an embryo express different sets of genes at different times. We first consider the more general question of how the genome controls gene expression and then discuss how gene expression programs in different cells interact to carry out morphogenesis and differentiation programs.

### Cellular Differentiation, the Genome, and Gene Expression

To understand how a single genome sequence encodes instructions for multiple different cell types, it is essential to know how patterns of gene expression become altered during cellular differentiation. The differences between a neuron, a keratinocyte, and an osteoblast are, to a large extent, the result of differential expression of a small number of "master genes," developmental regulatory genes that are also often required to maintain the differentiated state. In contrast, the majority of genes expressed in a cell are also widely expressed in other cell types. This common set of genes is required for basic cellular metabolic functions such as nucleic acid and protein synthesis, nutrient transport and utilization, and cytoskeletal and organelle biogenesis. For the most part, these **housekeeping** genes are expressed ubiquitously and may comprise 80 to 90 percent of the genes expressed in a particular cell type. The remainder of expressed genes vary; they are **specialty** genes that define the unique features of different cell types (see Chapter 12).

The regulation of gene expression is an essential aspect of developmental biology. As described in Chapter 3, this regulation is mediated by a class of proteins—transcription factors—that bind to regulatory elements adjacent to the transcribed sequences. These regulatory elements are essential components of every gene and are as critical to the normal function of a gene as are the coding sequences (Fig. 17–4). Regulatory sequences immediately adjacent to the start site that are required for general aspects of transcription are often described as **promoter** elements. Promoter elements are to be contrasted with **silencer** or **enhancer** elements, which facilitate tissue-specific transcription and may lie some distance away from the start site. Silencer and enhancer elements are bound by specialized transcription factors that help to inhibit or activate, respectively, patterns of gene expression that define particular cell types.

#### Example: Mutations in a Transcriptional Coactivator Cause Rubenstein-Taybi Syndrome

Ultimately, the actions of tissue-specific and general transcription factors intersect to allow initiation of mRNA synthesis. The biochemical mechanisms by which this occurs, and the importance of transcriptional regulation for development, are underscored by genotype-phenotype correlations for a molecule named CBP, or CREB-binding protein. CBP serves as a molecular bridge, or coactivator, between several different types of tissue-specific transcription factors and the so-called general transcriptional machinery (Fig. 17–4*A*). Loss-of-function mutations in CBP cause a dominant condition, **Rubenstein-Taybi syndrome**, in which mental retardation with broad thumbs and toes is accompanied by hirsutism, cryptorchidism, congenital heart defects, and characteristic facial features with downslanting palpebral fissures, hypoplastic maxilla, and a prominent nose

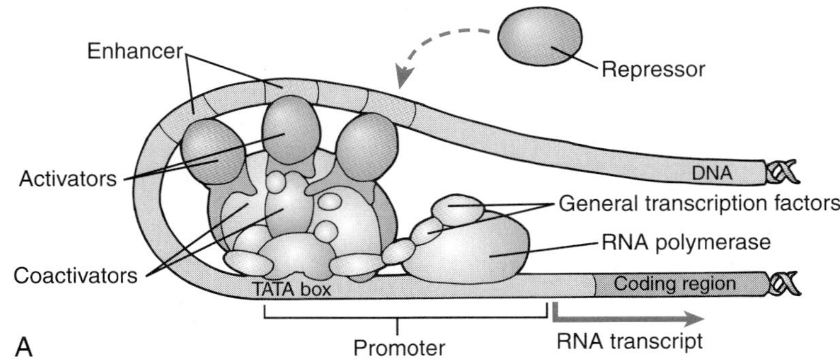

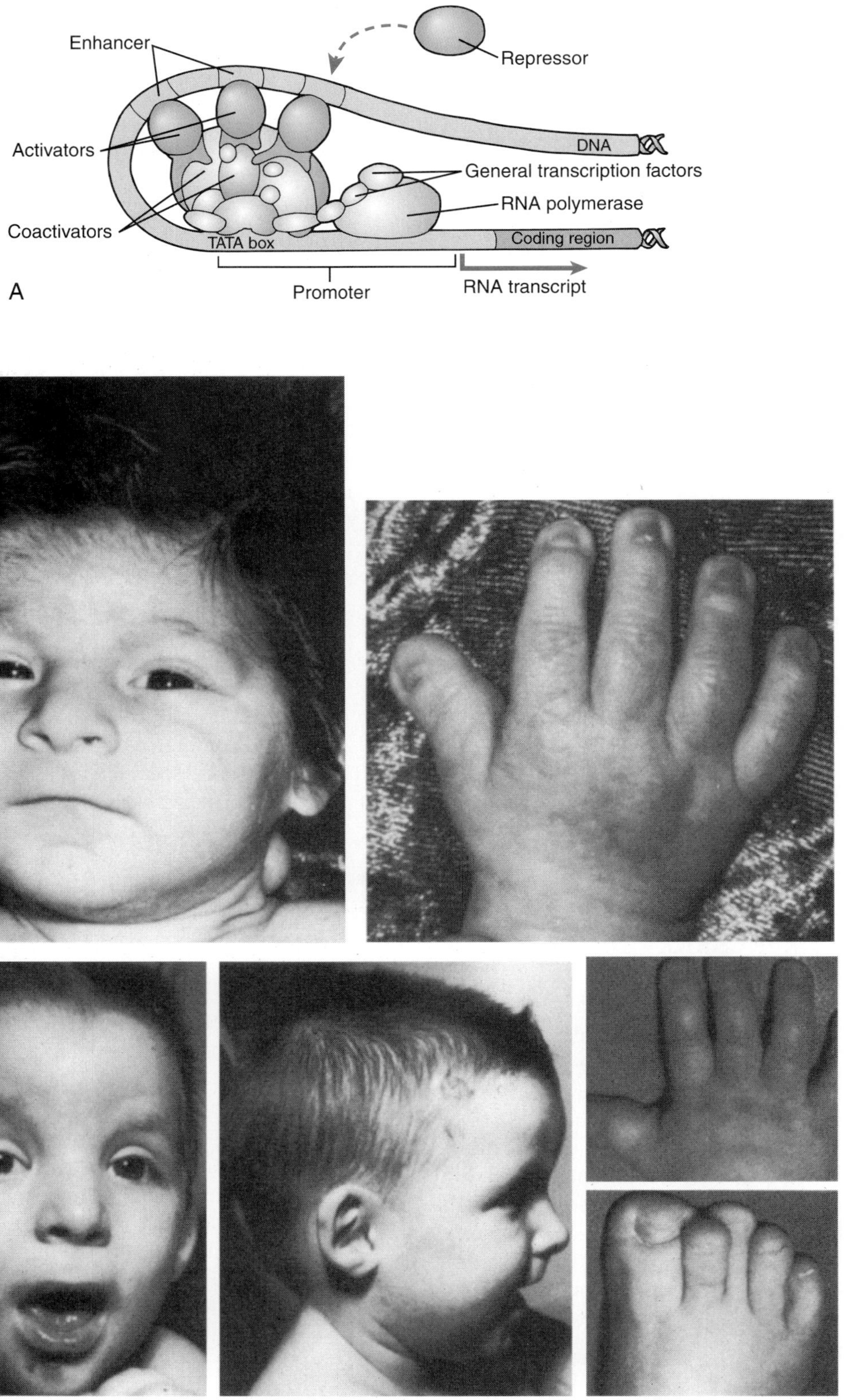

B

**Figure 17–4.** Mutations of a transcriptional coactivator cause pleiotropic abnormalities. *A*, RNA polymerase and general transcription factors, shown in green, bind to cis-acting sequences closely adjacent to the mRNA transcriptional start site; these cis-acting sequences are collectively referred to as the promoter. More distal enhancer and/or silencer elements bind specialized and/or tissue-specific transcription factors. Coactivator proteins such as CBP facilitate a biochemical interaction between specialized and general transcription factors. (From Tijian R [1995] Molecular machines that control genes. Sci Amer 272:54–61.) *B*, Heterozygosity of a CBP loss-of-function mutation causes Rubenstein-Taybi syndrome, in which pleiotropic abnormalities reflect the multitude of genes for which CBP is required to achieve proper transcriptional regulation. (Figure reprinted by permission from Jones KL [1998] Smith's Recognizable Patterns of Human Malformation. WB Saunders, Philadelphia.)

(Fig. 17–4*B*). The widespread or **pleiotropic** nature of the abnormalities seen in patients with Rubenstein-Taybi syndrome illustrate the diversity of cell types that use a common molecular pathway for transcriptional regulation.

## Stability of the Differentiated Phenotype and Cell Lineage

Once activated, maintenance of the differentiated phenotype is usually stable throughout subsequent cell divisions, thereby establishing a **cell lineage**. For example, skin fibroblasts and keratinocytes from a single individual express high levels of collagen and keratin, respectively, yet their genome sequences are identical. When these cell types are cultured outside the body, not only are characteristic patterns of gene expression maintained, but such cultures can be used to provide skin grafts. Stable transmission of gene expression patterns to daughter cells, in the absence of any change in DNA content or sequence, is one form of **epigenetic** regulation, whereby changes in phenotype are transmitted without a change in genotype. At the molecular level, maintenance of the differentiated phenotype is the consequence of an alteration in chromatin structure or DNA modification, or both (see Chapters 3 and 10). Such alterations do not affect the DNA sequence per se, but are preserved through mitosis so that stable patterns of gene expression are maintained and a cell lineage perpetuated.

## Stem Cells and Regeneration

For some cell types, acquisition of a normal differentiated phenotype is associated with a loss of proliferative ability. Neurons, erythrocytes, and platelets, for example, are highly differentiated cells that carry out essential functions but do not divide. Replacement of erythrocytes and platelets occurs on a regular basis, however, and depends on **stem cells**. Undifferentiated cells that are capable of extensive proliferation, stem cells may give rise to additional stem cells (self-renewal) or to progenitor cells committed to forming differentiated derivatives (Fig. 17–5). Most stem cells are said to be **pluripotent**, meaning that they give rise to multiple different types of cells after subsequent rounds of division. The entire program of blood cell development is based on a lineage that makes use of stem cells and pluripotent precursors (Fig. 17–5). Besides their relevance to the pathogenesis of genetic disease, the programs that create and maintain hematopoietic stem cells have provided the basis for using bone marrow transplantation to treat diseases such as aplastic anemia, leukemia, and lymphoma (see Chapter 13).

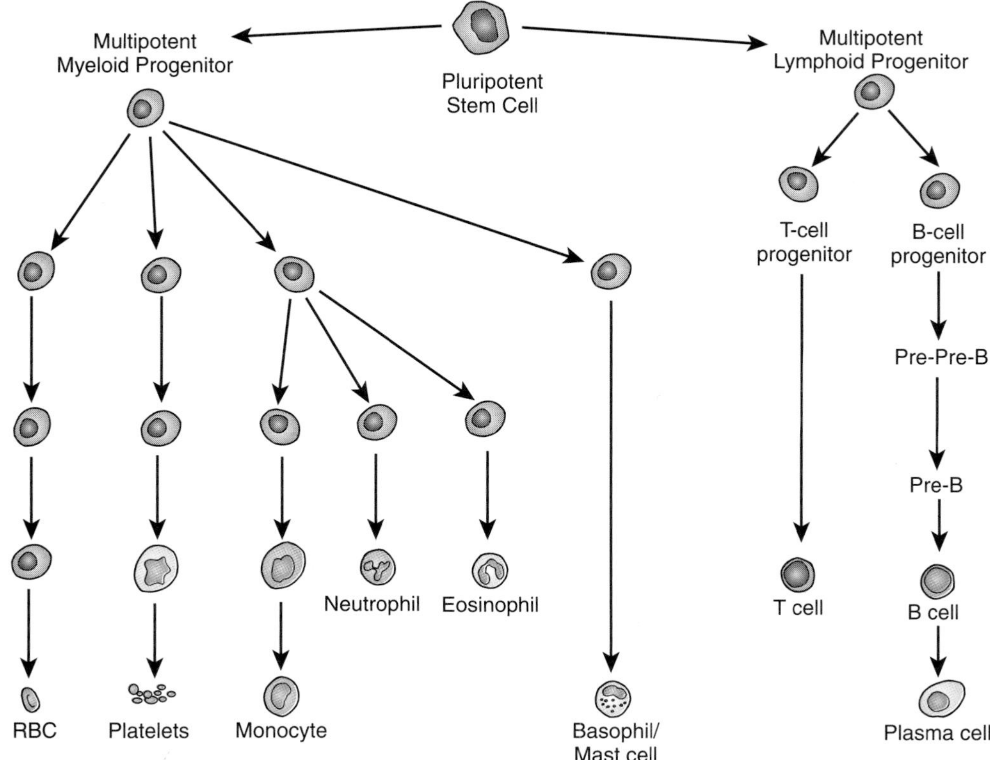


Figure 17–5. Development of hematopoietic cells. (Figure reprinted by permission from Stamatoyannopoulos G, Nienhuis AW, Majerus PW, Varmus H [1987] The Molecular Basis of Blood Diseases, 2nd ed. WB Saunders, Philadelphia.)

Unlike erythrocytes or platelets, some differentiated cells that lack proliferative capacity, such as neurons or endocrine secretory cells, can live for decades without being replaced. Studies carried out during the past several years, however, have demonstrated that stem cells for neurons and other differentiated tissues are present not only during development but remain, in some cases, in adult tissues. Remarkably, these stem cells can often be transplanted—as in the case of bone marrow transplantation—to divide and contribute differentiated derivatives in a manner similar to what normally pertains during development. Most studies of fetal stem cells have been carried out in animal models, but this area of research offers tremendous potential for treating a variety of human diseases, such as Parkinson disease, type 1 diabetes mellitus, and cirrhosis (see later).

## Hierarchies of Developmental Programs and Progressive Restrictions of Cell Fate

Patterns of gene expression characteristic of highly differentiated cells such as melanocytes, fibroblasts, and keratinocytes are acquired relatively late in development, after the body axes and major germ layers have been laid down and rudiments for the major organ systems are established. However, precursors for these cell types develop in a specific and orchestrated pattern that often depends on cell lineage. For example, melanocytes develop from the neural crest, which also gives rise to the adrenal medulla, the autonomic nervous system, sensory neurons, and connective tissue of the head and face. The neural crest is itself a product of neurectoderm, which also gives rise to the brain, the posterior pituitary gland, and the optic cup. Thus, cell fate during development is acquired in a hierarchical fashion that depends on cell lineage (see Fig. 17–5). What are the genetic mechanisms that account for progressive specification and determination of cell fate during early development? Although comprehensive answers are not yet available, a general theme based on studies in model organisms indicates that tissue-specific transcription factors act in a hierarchical and combinatorial network to specify different cell fates.

### Example: Waardenburg Syndrome and Mutations of Tissue-Specific Transcription Factors

The relationship between hierarchies of cell lineage during development and networks of tissue-specific transcription factors is exemplified by the molecular pathogenesis of **Waardenburg syndrome,** which, in some cases, results from mutations in a gene related to *PAX6* (see earlier discussion) called *PAX3*. *PAX3* is expressed in the developing neural crest and also in the dermatomyotomal component of somites, which are mesoderm-derived cells that give rise to skeletal muscle and dermis (Fig. 17–6*A*). Heterozygosity for *PAX3* loss-of-function mutations causes type I Waardenburg syndrome, characterized by a reduction or deficiency of neural crest derivatives such as melanocytes in the hair, eyes, and inner ear, leading to a white forelock, pale and often asymmetrically colored eyes, and sensorineural deafness (Fig. 17–6*B*). In addition, patients with *PAX3* mutations exhibit an abnormally wide space between the inner parts of their eyes and occasionally have upper-extremity limb defects (a condition known as type III Waardenburg syndrome). By contrast, abnormalities in patients with type II Waardenburg syndrome are limited to derivatives of pigment cells—the white forelock, eye color changes, and deafness—due to mutations in a different gene called *MITF*, for microphthalmia-associated transcription factor (because it was first discovered as the cause of a mouse mutation named Microphthalmia). *MITF* encodes a specialized transcription factor that binds to and activates target genes required for development of pigment cells. Expression of *MITF* is limited to pigment cells and their precursors and is believed to depend, in part, on transactivation by *PAX3*. Thus, clinical features of Waardenburg syndrome caused by melanocyte abnormalities can be traced back to a tissue-specific transcription factor, *MITF*, in which defects are caused either by mutations in the *MITF* gene itself or in *PAX3*, one of its upstream regulators. In contrast, the facial or upper-extremity abnormalities seen in addition to pigment cell abnormalities in patients with types I and III Waardenburg syndrome reflect a role of *PAX3* in neural crest–derived connective tissue of the face and head, and in somite-derived tissue of the upper limbs.

## Cell Migration and Mixing during Development

The extensive cell movement exhibited by neural crest derivatives is a characteristic feature of several tissues, including germ cells and hematopoietic cells. The biochemical mechanisms that facilitate cell migration during development are not well understood but are likely to involve programmed changes in cell adhesion as well as short- and long-range diffusible signaling molecules (see later).

Early in embryogenesis before definitive germ layers have been formed, extensive mixing occurs, and cells related by a common lineage generally are scattered throughout the embryo. Shortly after organogenesis begins, however, cell mixing becomes less extensive, and in many adult tissues, cells related by

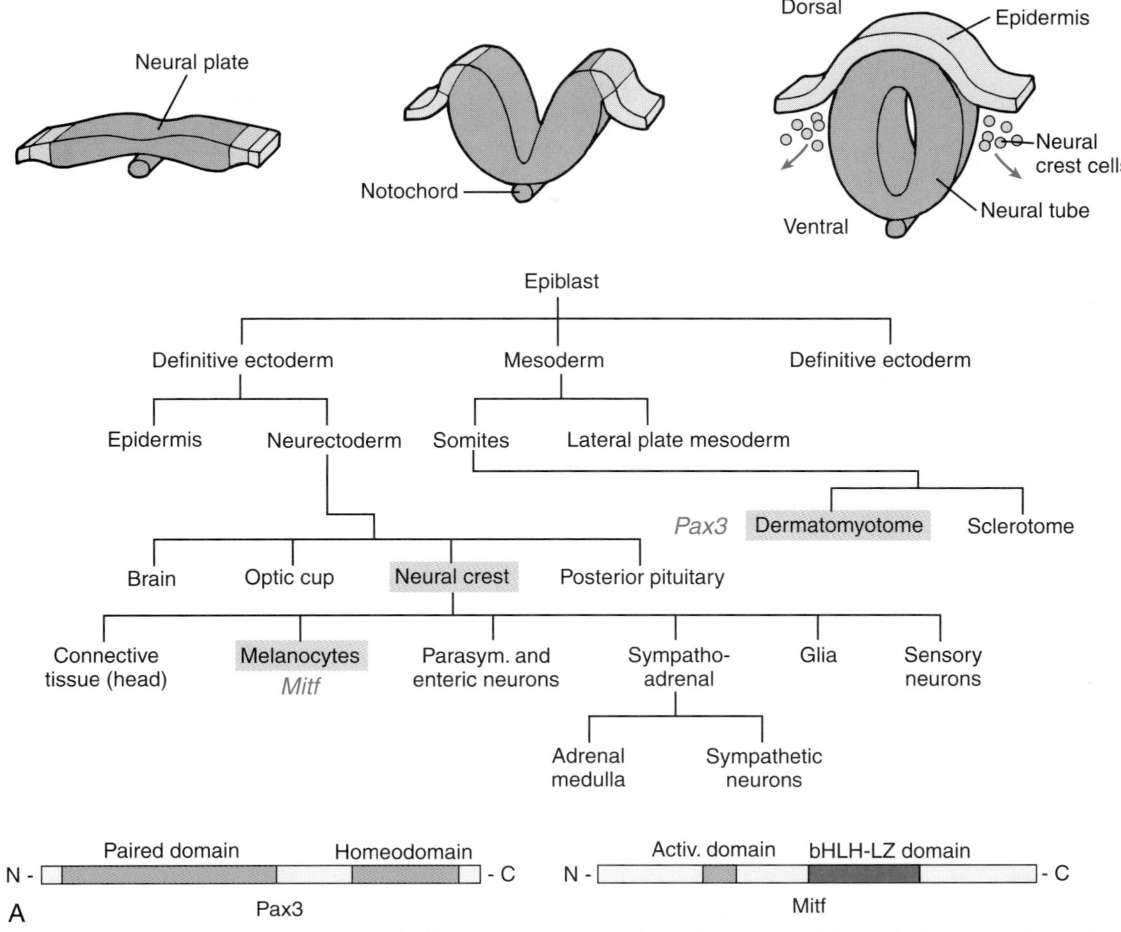


**Figure 17–6.** *A*, Neural crest formation and cell lineage and the positions of *PAX6* and *MITF* in the heirarchy of neural crest and melanocyte development. The neural crest forms from the edges of the neural tube as it closes underneath the ectoderm; the neural tube itself (neurectoderm) is a derivative of definitive ectoderm. Somites are segmented condensations of mesoderm that occur adjacent to the neural tube and give rise to skeletal precursors (sclerotome) and precursors of dermis and muscle (dermatomyotome). (Figure reprinted by permission from Wolpert L, Beddington R, Brockes J, et al [1998] Principles of Development. Copyright 1998, Oxford University Press, Oxford, England.) *PAX3* and *MITF* encode transcription factors required for neural crest and melanocyte development as described in the text. *PAX3* is expressed in the neural tube, in neural crest cells, and in the dermatomyotome; *MITF* is expressed in the subset of neural crest cells that give rise to melanocytes.

*Illustration continued on following page*

lineage remain adjacent to one another. This can create a mosaic pattern composed of patches or **clones** of cells that have descended from a common precursor. As described in Chapter 5, this pattern is often readily apparent in females heterozygous for X-linked mutations that cause changes in cell appearance, such as X-linked ocular albinism or incontinentia pigmenti.

## Morphogenesis: Cell-Autonomous and Cell-Nonautonomous Morphogenetic Programs

There are two fundamentally different ways in which mutations can affect morphogenetic processes. Processes governed by intrinsic changes in gene expression are described as **cell-autonomous**; when changes induced by extrinsic factors affect morphogenesis, the process is described as **cell-nonautonomous**. For example, anophthalmia caused by mutations of the transcription factor *PAX6* is cell-autonomous because cells that normally express *PAX6* fail to develop properly (see Fig. 17–2). By contrast, a common cause of ambiguous genitalia in newborn females is an inborn error of metabolism known as 21-hydroxylase deficiency, in which an inability to produce cortisol or aldosterone, or both, leads to compensatory congenital adrenal hyperplasia and increased production of adrenal androgens (see Chapter 10). The consequent masculinization of female external genitalia is a morphogenetic change that is cell-nonautonomous because it is caused by genes expressed in the adrenal gland rather than in the sex organs themselves.

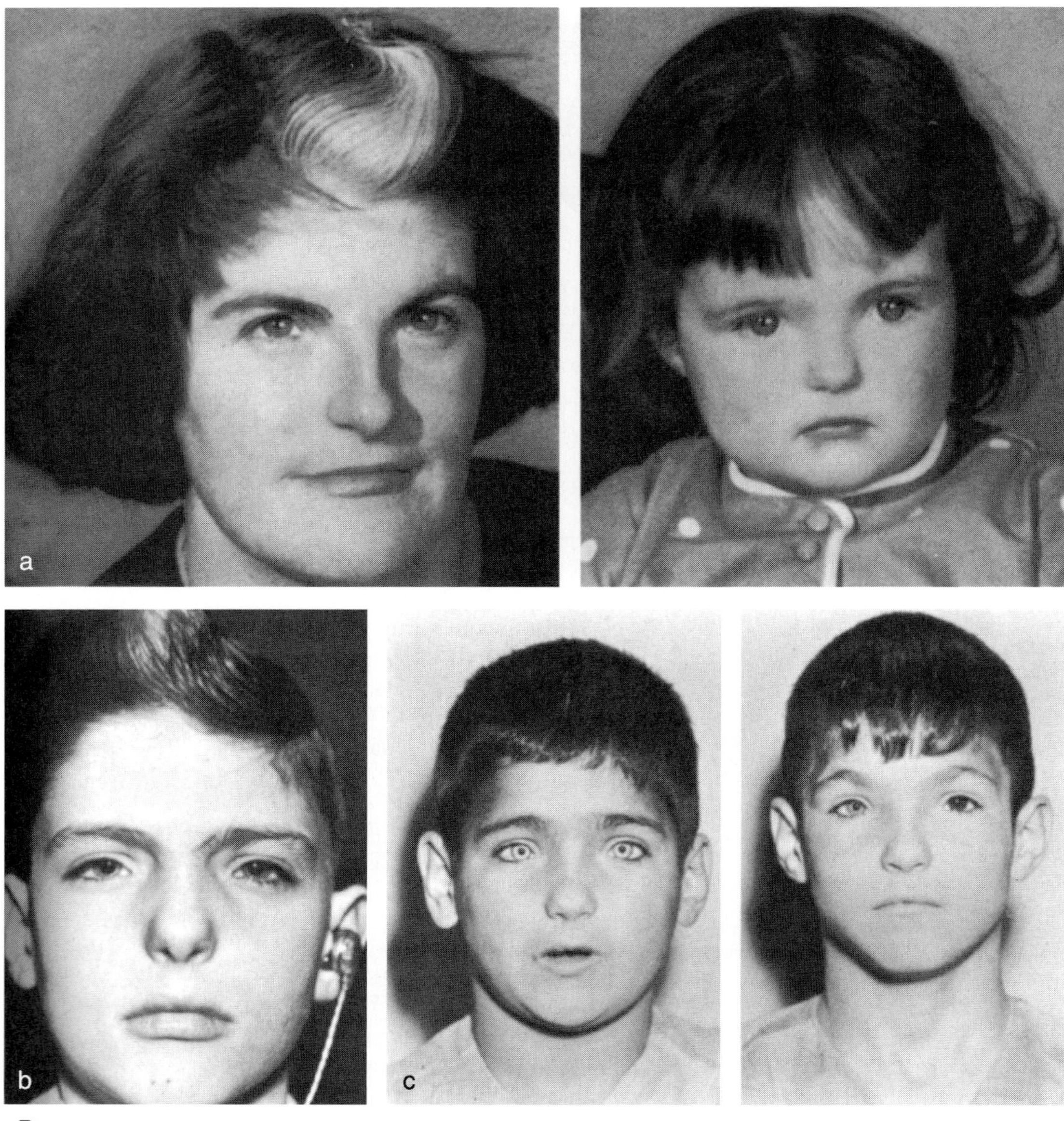

Figure 17–6 *Continued. B*, Patients with type I Waardenburg syndrome. a, Mother and daughter with white forelocks. (From Partington MW [1959] Arch Dis Child 34:1542.) b, Ten-year-old with congenital deafness and white forelock. (From DiGeorge AM et al [1960] J Pediatric 57:649.) c, Brothers, one of whom is deaf. There is no white forelock but boy on the right has heterochromatic irides. Mutations of *PAX3* cause type I Waardenburg syndrome. (From Jones KL [1998] Smith's Recognizable Patterns of Human Malformation. WB Saunders, Philadelphia.)

## HOX Genes: Transcription Factors Code for Developmental Identity

As described earlier for *MITF* (see Fig. 17–6), defects in tissue-specific transcription factors often cause abnormalities of an entire cell lineage or program of gene expression. The *HOX* genes, short for "homeotic selector," encode a special class of transcription factors originally discovered in *Drosophila*, in which they are named homeotic (*HOM*) genes because of their ability to transform one part of the body into another. For example, mutations of one *HOM* gene, the *Antennepedia* gene, cause legs to grow where there should be antennae. Thus, *HOM* transcription factors regulate a large set of downstream genes that are ultimately responsible for the morphogenesis of different body parts. When first identified, *Drosophila HOM* genes were found to share a protein motif, named the **homeodomain**, that binds to DNA. The homeodomain has now been discovered in many other transcription factors including *PAX3* and *PAX6*. However, human *HOX* genes are most closely related to the *Drosophila HOM* genes in both sequence and arrangement (see later). Remarkably, not only the structure but also the action of *HOX* genes have been conserved for hundreds of millions of years.

In *Drosophila*, there is a single cluster of eight *HOM* genes; in humans and other mammals, there

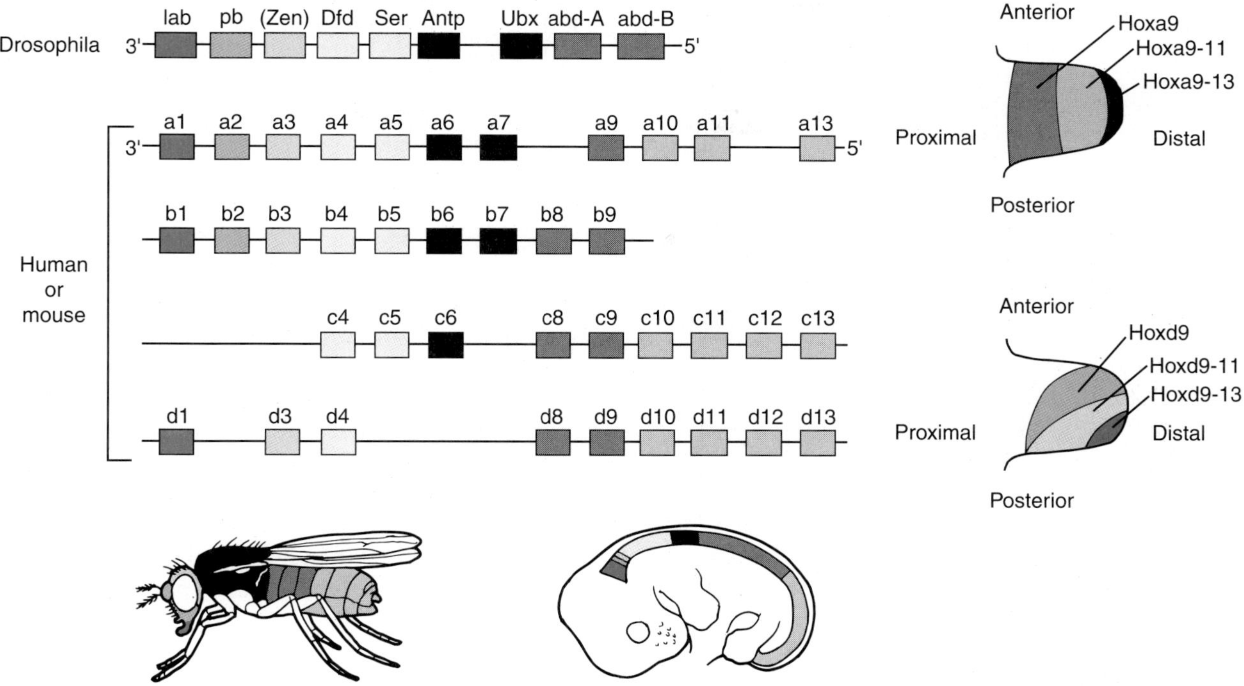


**Figure 17–7.** Action and arrangement of *HOX* genes. An ancestral *HOX* cluster in a common ancestor of vertebrates and invertebrates has been quadruplicated in mammals, and individual members of the ancestral cluster have been lost. The combination of *HOX* genes expressed in adjacent regions along the anteroposterior axis of developing embryos select a unique developmental fate. In the developing limbs, different combinations of *HOXA* and *HOXD* genes are expressed in adjacent zones that help select developmental fate along the proximal-distal and anterior-posterior axes. (Figure reprinted by permission from Wolpert L, Beddington R, Brockes J, et al [1998] Principles of Development. Copyright 1998, Oxford University Press, Oxford, England.)

are four clusters named *HOXA*, *HOXB*, *HOXC*, and *HOXD*, in which each cluster contains up to 11 individual genes (Fig. 17–7). Unique combinations of *HOX* gene expression in small groups of cells that make up particular regions of the embryo help to select the developmental fate of those regions. The *HOXA* and *HOXB* clusters, for example, act along the rostral-caudal axis to determine the identity of individual vertebrae and somites, whereas the *HOXA* and *HOXD* clusters determine regional identity along the axes of the developing limb (Fig. 17–7).

### Example: HOXD13 Mutations and Synpolydactyly

In mice, loss-of-function mutations have been generated for nearly all of the *HOX* genes, and homeotic transformations of vertebral or spinal segments, or both, are often observed for members of the *HOXA*, *HOXB*, or *HOXC* clusters. In humans (and in mice), an unusual mutation of *HOXD13* causes synpolydactyly, a semidominant condition in which heterozygotes have interphalangeal webbing and extra digits in their hands and feet. Rare homozygotes have similar but more severe abnormalities and also have bony malformations of the hands, wrists, feet, and ankles (Fig. 17–8). The *HOXD13* mutation responsible for synpolydactyly in humans and in mice is caused by expansion of a polyalanine tract in the amino-terminal domain of the protein; the normal protein contains 15 alanines, although the mutant protein contains 22 to 24 alanines. *HOXD13* loss-of-function mutations have only a mild effect on limb development; therefore, the polyalanine expansion that causes synpolydactyly must act by a gain-of-function mechanism. Intriguingly, mice that have multiple loss-of-function mutations in *HOXD11*, *HOXD12*, and *HOXD13* exhibit abnormalities very similar to those caused by the *HOXD13* polyalanine expansion, which suggests that the hoxd11, hoxd12, and hoxd13 proteins may normally act as heterodimeric complexes and that the *HOXD13* polyalanine expansion interferes with the function of all three proteins. Regardless of the exact mechanism, a general function for *HOX* genes in all animals is to determine regional identity along specific body axes during development.

## Paracrine Signals in Development

Hox proteins and other transcription factors that affect development do so in a cell-autonomous manner: the immediate targets of their action are the cells within which they are expressed. A critical and essential aspect of development, however, is an instructional interaction between cells, whereby a protein secreted from one group of cells alters the pattern of gene expression in adjacent cells, a process that is

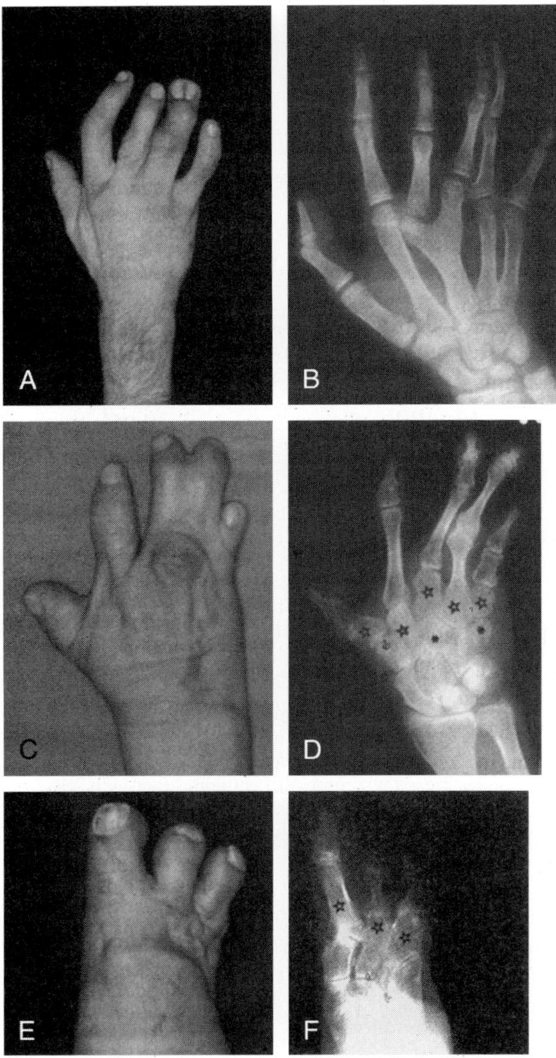


**Figure 17–8.** An unusual gain-of-function mutation in *HOXD13* creates an abnormal protein that has a semidominant effect. (Figure reprinted by permission from Muragaki Y, Mundlos S, Upton J, Olsen B [1996] Altered growth and branching patterns in synpolydactyly caused by mutations in HOXD13. Science 272: 548–551. Copyright 1996, American Association for the Advancement of Science.)

clearly not cell-autonomous. Some short-range extracellular or **paracrine** signals control simple on or off switches; others, termed **morphogens**, can elicit multiple responses depending on their level along a concentration gradient. In this way, a cell or group of cells that secretes a morphogen can initiate several types of developmental programs in surrounding cells, depending on their location along the morphogen gradient.

### Example: The Sonic Hedgehog Morphogen and Holoprosencephaly

One of the best examples of a developmental morphogen is the *hedgehog* gene, originally discovered in *Drosophila* and named for its ability to alter the orientation of epidermal bristles. Diffusion of the hedgehog protein creates a gradient in which different concentrations of the protein cause surrounding cells to assume different fates. In humans, several genes closely related to *Drosophila hedgehog* also encode developmental morphogens; one example is the gene whimsically named *Sonic hedgehog* (*SHH*). Although the specific programs controlled by *hedgehog* in *Drosophila* are very different from those controlled by its mammalian counterparts, the underlying themes are very similar. For example, secretion of Sonic hedgehog protein by the notochord and the floorplate of the developing neural tube results in a gradient that induces and organizes the different types of cells and tissues in the developing brain and spinal cord (Fig. 17–9). Sonic hedgehog is also produced by a small group of cells in the limb bud to create what is known as the **zone of polarizing activity**, which is responsible for the asymmetrical pattern of digits within individual limbs.

Mutations that inactivate *SHH* in humans are inherited in a dominant manner, which demonstrates that a 50 percent reduction in gene expression is sufficient to produce an abnormal phenotype, presumably by altering the magnitude of the hedgehog protein gradient. Affected individuals usually exhibit **holoprosencephaly**, or failure of the midface and forebrain to develop, leading to cleft lip and palate, hypotelorism (eyes that are closely spaced together), and absence of forebrain structures. Occasionally, however, the clinical findings are very mild or subtle, such as, for example, a single central incisor or partial absence of the corpus callosum (Fig. 17–10). Because variable expressivity has been observed in members of the same family, it cannot be due to different mutations and instead must reflect the action of modifier genes at other loci, or chance, or both. Liability of a genetic process to factors that modify the mutant phenotype is an important characteristic not only of the *SHH* pathway and holoprosencephaly but also of other pathways in which developmental morphogens are implicated, such as fusion of endocardial cushions, and branching of epithelial tubules that occurs during the development of organs such as the lungs and the kidneys.

## Integration of Signaling Pathways in Development

As described earlier, transcription factors that control the expression of multiple downstream genes provide a molecular basis for carrying out cell-autonomous developmental programs; in contrast, paracrine signaling molecules provide a molecular basis whereby one group of cells controls the devel-

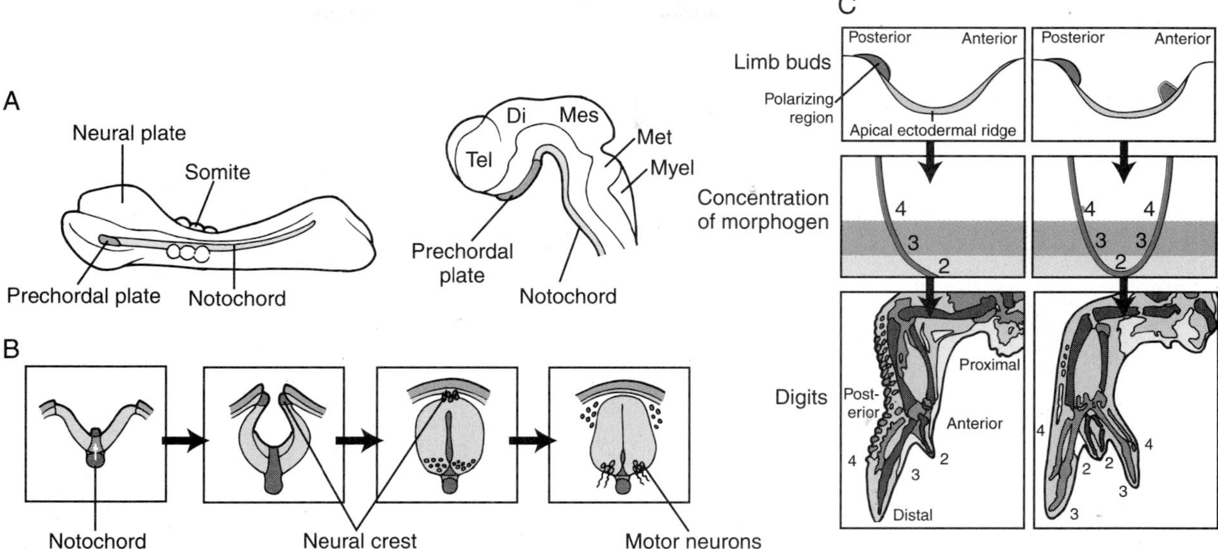


Figure 17–9. Action of morphogens during neural tube and limb formation. *A*, Development of the neural tube during the third through fifth week of development. Folding and fusion of the neural fold into the neural tube is quickly followed by the development of brain vesicles from which the brain will ultimately develop. *B*, Transverse section of developing neural tube. Sonic hedgehog protein released from the notochord diffuses upward to the ventral portion of the developing neural tube (dark gray); high concentrations immediately above the notochord induce the floorplate, whereas lower concentrations more laterally induce motor neurons. Ectoderm above (dorsal to) the neural tube releases bone morphogenetic proteins (BMPs) that help to induce neural crest development at the dorsal edge of the closing neural tube. (Figures reprinted by permission from Muenke M, Beachy PA [2000] Genetics of ventral forebrain development and holoprosencephaly. Curr Opin Genet Dev 10:262–269. Copyright 2000 Elsevier Science; and from Lumsden A, Graham A [1995] Neural Patterning: A forward role for hedgehog. Curr Biol 5:1347–1350. Copyright 1995 Elsevier Science.) *C*, Morphogenetic action of the sonic hedgehog protein during limb bud formation, where it is released from the polarizing region in the posterior limb known as the zone of polarizing activity to produce a gradient (shown with its highest levels as 4 declining to 2). Mutations or transplantation experiments that create an ectopic polarizing region in the anterior limb bud cause a duplication of posterior limb elements. (Figure reprinted by permission from Wolpert L, Beddington R, Brockes J, et al [1998] Principles of Development. Copyright 1998, Oxford University Press, Oxford, England.)

opmental program of an adjacent group. From a biochemical perspective, a paracrine signaling molecule must have a specific receptor on its target cell, that receptor must couple to one or more intracellular effectors, and those effectors must lead to changes in the activity of the target transcription factor or factors. An underlying theme of developmental genetics is that entire signaling pathways are conserved, from paracrine signaling molecules to transcription factor targets. Such **developmental signaling pathways** are used repeatedly for different morphogenetic programs within an embryo and for homologous morphogenetic programs in embryos of different species.

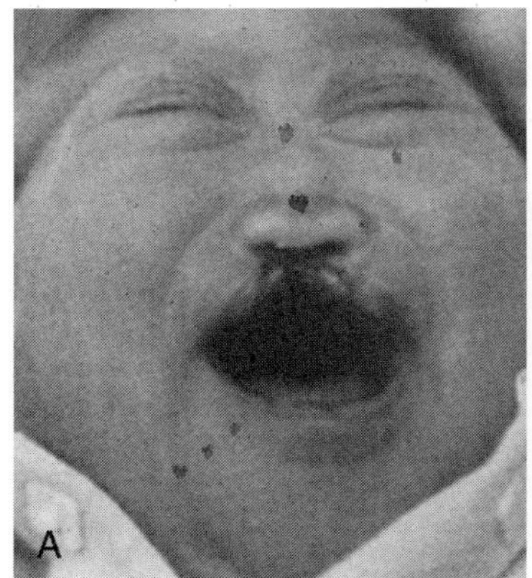


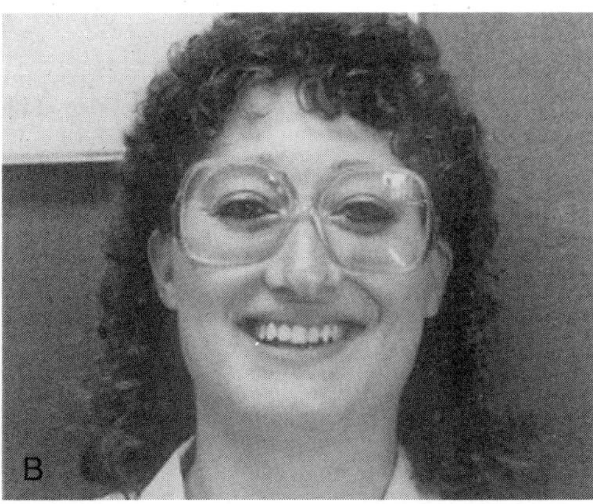


Figure 17–10. Variable expressivity of an *SHH* mutation. The mother and her daughter carry the same missense mutation in *SHH*, but the daughter is severely affected with microcephaly, hypotelorism, and a cleft palate, whereas the only manifestation in the mother is a single central upper incisor. (Reprinted by permission from Roessler E, Belloni E, Gaudenz K, et al [1996] Mutations in the human sonic hedgehog gene cause holoprosencephaly. Nat Genet 14:357–360, copyright 1996 Macmillan Ltd.)

## DEVELOPMENTAL GENETICS IN CLINICAL PRACTICE

Principles of developmental genetics are used implicitly by any health care professional who cares for children with birth defects. Among major birth defects, chromosomal imbalance accounts for about 25 percent, exposure to a known teratogen accounts for about 5 percent, and single genes cause about 20 percent (Fig. 17–11). Many of the latter class represent autosomal dominant conditions with relatively high rates of new mutation, such as type 1 neurofibromatosis, Marfan syndrome, and achondroplasia (see Chapter 5), and only a small proportion is due to mendelian abnormalities in developmental control genes such as *SHH* and *PAX6*. Nonetheless, major birth defects with no identifiable cause occur in a familial pattern similar to that of multifactorial diseases such as diabetes and mental illness (see Chapter 15). Whole genome association studies that will be carried out in the next several years may well reveal single nucleotide polymorphisms in developmental control genes that partially alter their function and thus reveal polygenic etiologies for the 50 percent of birth defects whose specific cause is currently unknown.

### Dysmorphology

**Dysmorphology** is the branch of clinical genetics that specializes in birth defects and combines a knowledge of genetic principles, developmental mechanisms, and the natural history of a wide variety of congenital abnormalities. In some settings, dysmorphologists work closely with specialists in pediatric surgery, rehabilitation medicine, and the allied health professions to provide ongoing care for children with serious birth defects.

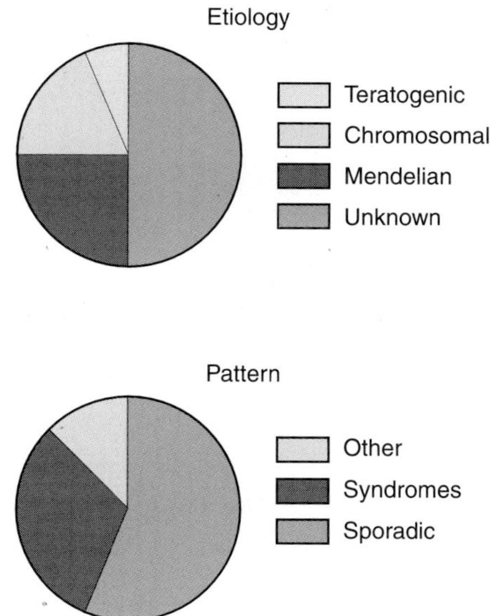


**Figure 17–11.** Causes and phenotypic patterns of birth defects.

#### Isolated Birth Defects, Syndromes, and Sequences

About 60 percent of major birth defects affect a single organ system, such as the heart (e.g., ventricular septal defects) or lip (e.g., cleft lip with or without cleft palate). Specific causes for these so-called isolated birth defects are the ones most difficult to identify. Of the remainder, many occur in recognizable patterns that point to a single etiology and represent so-called **malformation syndromes** (see Table 17–1). Like chromosomal imbalance, which represents a special class of malformation syndromes, different individuals affected with the same syndrome rarely have the same set of birth defects, and it is only in the context of many affected individuals that the patterns become apparent. For example, a condition whose cause is unknown, **Cornelia de Lange syndrome**, is characterized by growth retardation, mental retardation, hirsutism, cryptorchidism, upper-limb deficiencies, and characteristic facial features with synophrys (excessive growth of the eyebrows toward the center of the face), a depressed nasal bridge, anteverted nares, a long philtrum, and a thin upper lip with downturned corners of the mouth (Fig. 17–12). Most children affected with Cornelia de Lange syndrome or with Rubenstein-Taybi syndrome (discussed previously; see Fig. 17–4) manifest only a subset of findings, each of which can be variably expressed. Yet individuals with either condition are nearly always recognized by their constellation of features, and the two syndromes are easily distinguished.

Some birth defects occur in patterns pointing to a common pathophysiological mechanism, even though they may be due to more than one cause. Such conditions are often described as **sequences** or **associations**, to distinguish them from malformation syndromes that each have a single cause. For example, a restriction of mandibular growth before the ninth week of gestation can cause the tongue to lie more posteriorly than is normal, interfering with normal closure of the palatal shelves (Fig. 17–13). The constellation of a U-shaped cleft palate and a small mandible is described as **Robin sequence**. This phenotype can represent an isolated birth defect of unknown cause, can be due to extrinsic impingement on the developing mandible by a twin, or can be one of several features of a condition known as **Stickler syndrome**, often caused by an underlying abnormality of type II collagen. The clefting occurs via a common pathophysiological mechanism. However, a knowledge of dysmorphology and developmental genetic

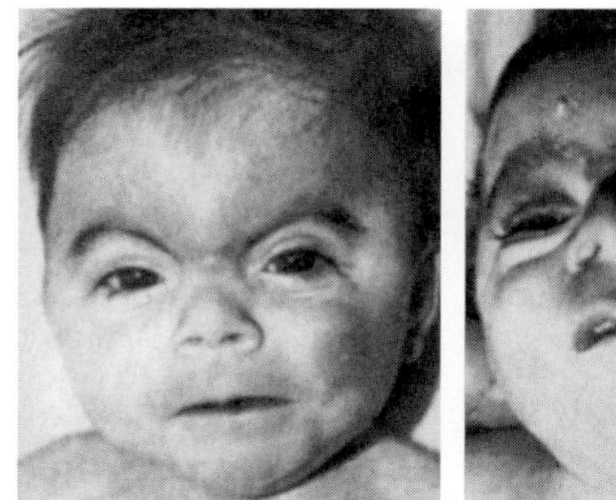
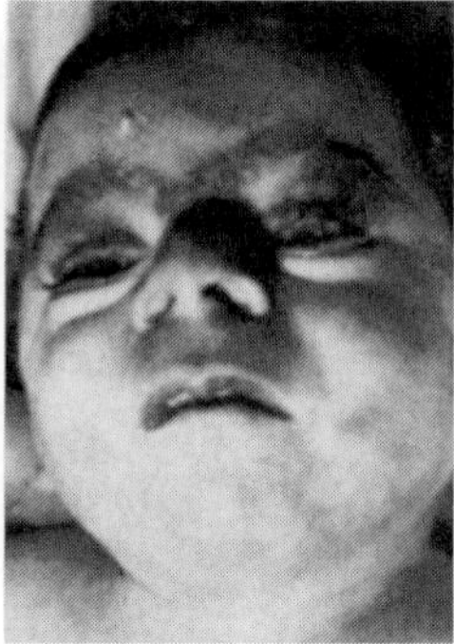
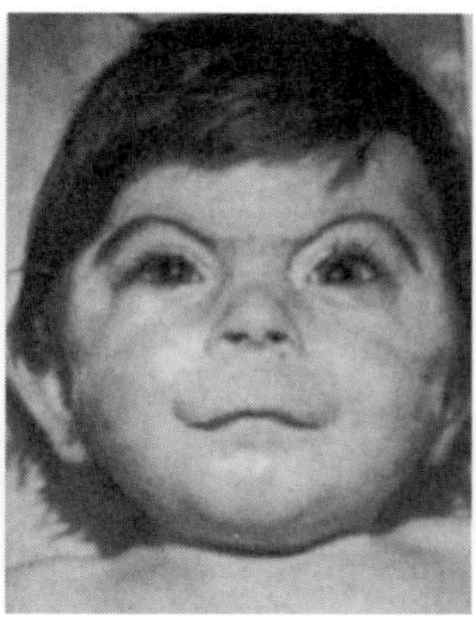
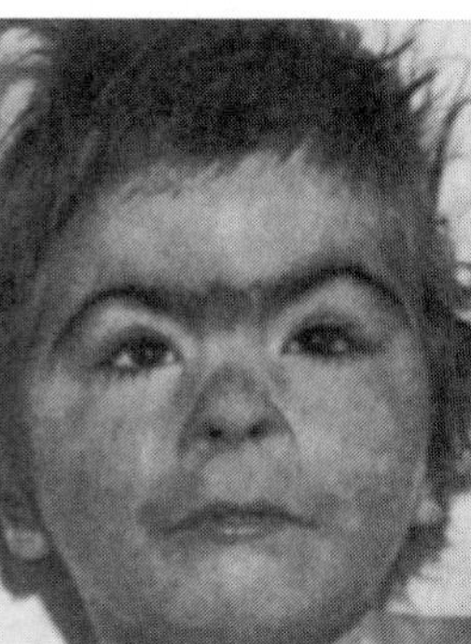

Figure 17–12. In Cornelia de Lange syndrome, affected individuals can usually be recognized by a characteristic facial appearance, but other manifestations of the condition, such as upper limb deformities, are variably expressed. (From Ptacek LJ et al [1963] J Pediatric 63:1000.)

principles is necessary to properly diagnose the conditions and to recognize that different prognoses depend on the primary etiology.

## Malformations, Deformations, and Disruptions

Malformations represent intrinsic abnormalities in development and can often be distinguished from abnormalities caused by extrinsic factors or so-called **deformations** (Fig. 17–14*A*). Deformations are especially common during the second trimester of development when the fetus is constrained within the amniotic sac and uterus. Certain types of deformations occur more commonly than do others, and can be recognized by their patterns. For example, contractions of the lower limbs, or **arthrogryposes**, in combination with deformation of the developing skull, occasionally accompany constraint of the fetus due to multiple births or prolonged leakage of amniotic fluid.

Most deformations apparent at birth either resolve spontaneously or can be treated by external fixation devices to reverse the effects of the instigating cause. Another type of birth defect, resulting from **disruption** of developing tissue, is more difficult to treat because normal tissue is destroyed (Fig. 17–14*A*). Although deformations and disruptions both occur in recognizable patterns, their manifestations tend to be

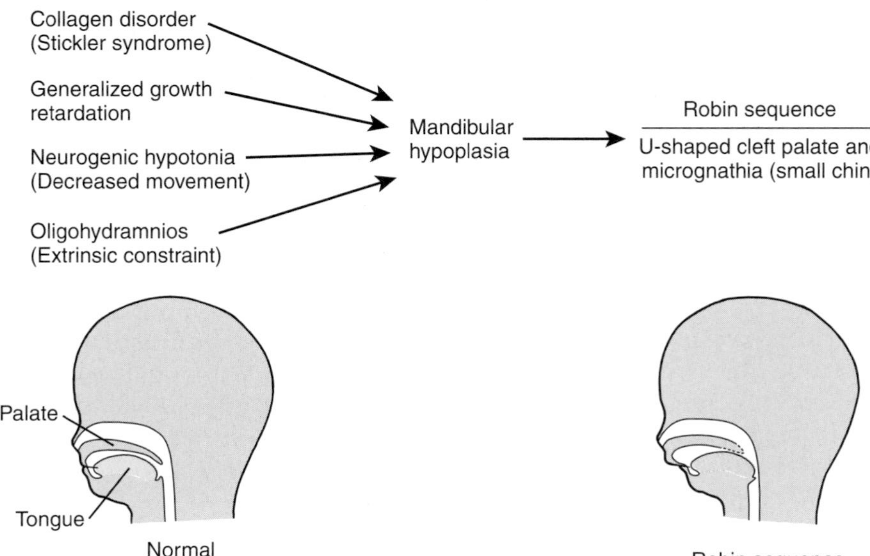


Figure 17–13. The Robin anomaly as an example of a dysmorphologic sequence. Different primary abnormalities can lead to a restriction of mandibular growth in which posterior displacement of the tongue obstructs palatal closure, leading to the constellation of a U-shaped cleft palate and a small chin (cleft palate not caused by mandibular hypoplasia is often V-shaped). If the primary etiology of micrognathia (a small chin) in children with Robin sequence is caused by external deformation, such as oligohydramnios, the mandible often shows postnatal "catch-up" growth.

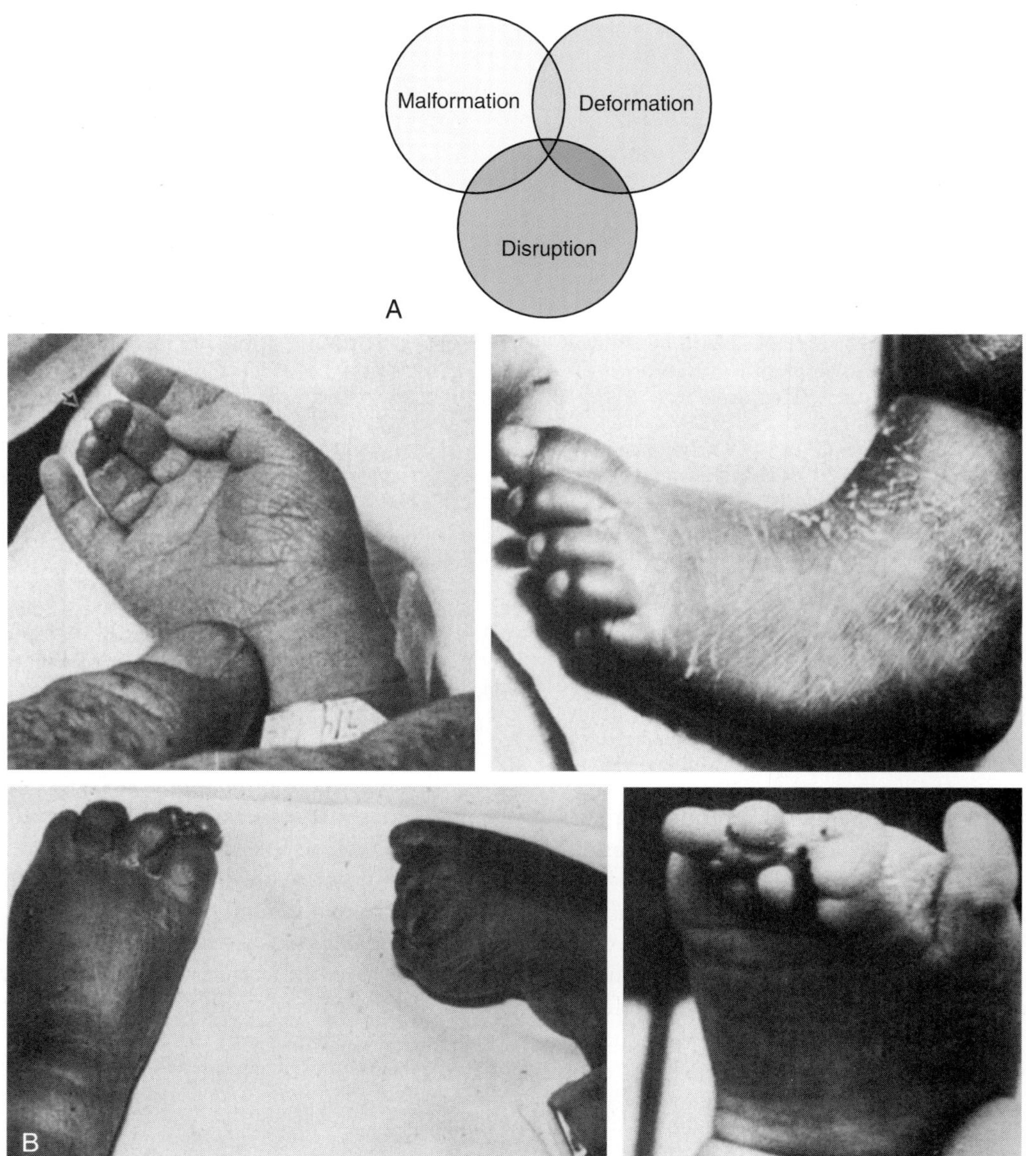


Figure 17–14. *A*, Amnion disruption sequence may involve several pathogenetic pathways. As described in the text, malformations, deformations, and disruptions are useful clinical guides to explain the pathophysiology of birth defects, but the concepts occasionally overlap. *B*, Early amnion rupture sequence. The consequences of amnion disruption sequence can be recognized by an asymmetrical and irregular pattern of anomalies, the absence of normal tissue, and the consequences of external compression or constriction in utero. Variable limb anomalies secondary to bands including pseudosyndactyly, ankle constriction, and amputation with disrupted toe development. (B from Jones KL et al [1974] J Pediatric 84:90.)

irregular and asymmetrical compared with those of malformation syndromes. For example, partial rupture of the amniotic sac can cause fragments of the amniotic membrane to impair or constrict developing limbs or, occasionally, the orofacial region. Amniotic disruption sequence is often recognized clinically by the presence of partial and irregular digit amputations in conjunction with constriction rings (Fig. 17–14*B*). The pathophysiological concepts of malformations, deformations, and disruptions are useful clinical guides to the recognition, diagnosis, and treatment of birth defects, but they sometimes overlap. For example, rupture of the amnion may be caused by an intrinsic abnormality of connective tissue and may lead to destruction of fetal tissue in some regions but deformation in others.

## TERATOLOGY

Identifying and understanding the mechanism of so-called **teratogens**—drugs, infections, or environmental agents that cause birth defects—has important implications for both clinical medicine and basic science. Recognizing teratogenic effects of drugs or environmental toxins has obvious ramifications for public health, and understanding the mechanisms of teratogenicity can provide insight into the underlying developmental pathways that have gone awry. Because many molecular and cellular pathways used during development are unique, teratogens that cause serious birth defects may have few or no side effects in adult patients. One of the best examples is thalidomide, a sedative widely used in the 1950s that was later found to cause a very high incidence of limb reduction defects in fetuses exposed between 4 and 8 weeks of gestation. Thalidomide appears to act not by interfering with the number or pattern of digits, but by damaging tissue within the proliferating center, or **progress zone**, of the developing limb bud (Fig. 17–15). This effect is specific; thalidomide is a relatively safe drug outside of its teratogenic effects and, in fact, is very useful for treating certain abnormalities of the immune system associated with excessive cell proliferation. Similarly, exposure to some derivatives of retinoic acid in utero can cause a variety of serious birth defects, probably because endogenous retinoids are a fundamental component of signaling pathways used to pattern the branchial arches. Retinoids have few nonteratogenic side effects, however, and are extremely useful for treating certain skin diseases or rare forms of leukemia.

A fundamental distinction between birth defects caused by teratogens and mutagens is that mutagens cause damage by creating heritable alterations in genetic material, whereas teratogens act directly and transiently on developing embryonic tissue. Thus, exposure to a mutagen can cause an increased risk of birth defects throughout the life of the exposed individual, whereas exposure to a teratogen increases the risk of birth defects for current but not for subsequent pregnancies.

Different teratogens often cause very specific patterns of birth defects, the risk of which depends critically on the time and level of exposure during pregnancy. Thus, dysmorphologists or clinical geneticists can often diagnose teratogen-induced birth defects by the pattern of abnormalities, explain their causes and consequences, give accurate recurrence risk counseling to families in which an affected child has already been born, and, for pregnant couples who may have been inadvertently exposed to a teratogen, provide likelihood counseling based on the level and time of exposure.

## Reproductive Genetics

Many birth defects become apparent during gestation because of reduced fetal growth or abnormalities detected on routine sonography (see Chapter 18). Clinical geneticists and dysmorphologists often work closely with obstetricians and specialists in maternal-fetal medicine to evaluate abnormalities detected in utero. The involvement of clinical geneticists is especially important for cases of unexplained spontaneous abortion, because a large proportion is caused by chromosomal aneuploidy (see Fig. 17–11). Recognition that a

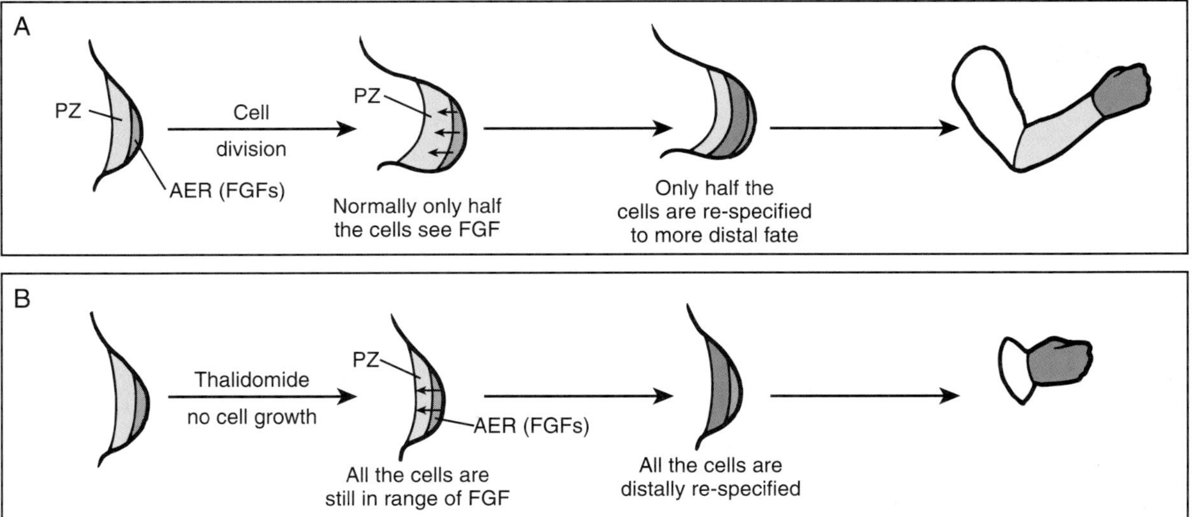


Figure 17–15. A developmental mechanism for thalidomide-induced embryopathy. A model for specification of limb identity along the proximal-distal axis posits that diffusible signals including fibroblast growth factors (FGFs) released from the apical ectodermal ridge (AER) at the tip of the developing limb bud act locally to specify the fate of underlying mesenchymal cells in the progress zone (PZ). If growth within the progress zone is impaired by thalidomide, the entire progress zone is subject to the action of AER-induced signals leading to "distal respecification." This mechanism manifests clinically as the absence of proximal but not distal limb elements. (Reprinted by permission from Tabin CJ [1998] A developmental model for thalidomide defects. Nature 396:322–323. Copyright 1998 Macmillan Magazines Ltd.)

spontaneous abortion or stillbirth has been caused by a malformation syndrome or chromosome abnormality can provide accurate recurrence risk counseling for family members, alleviate unjustified personal guilt that may accompany spontaneous abortions or stillbirths, and, in some cases, allow the opportunity for early prenatal diagnosis in future pregnancies. Even in cases in which a spontaneous abortion or stillborn child is known to have a normal karyotype—for instance, when amniocentesis or chorionic villus sampling has been carried out owing to advanced maternal age—examination of the fetus and placenta by a clinical geneticist may be very helpful, for example, for diagnosing obvious abnormalities such as holoprosencephaly or amniotic disruption.

Among the more common abnormalities that develop in utero are those secondary to monozygotic twinning. About one third of the time, the twinning event is relatively early, before trophoblast formation, such that each zygote forms its own set of extraembryonic tissues and the twins are said to be dichorionic (Fig. 17–16). The remainder of the time, the twinning event involves only the inner cell mass and occurs after trophoblast formation, in which case the twins share a common placenta and are said to be monochorionic (but diamniotic). Rarely, twinning occurs at or just after implantation and involves only the primitive ectoderm, in which case the twins may share amniotic as well as chorionic membranes. Monochorionic twins (both diamniotic and monoamniotic) have a common placental circulation and, therefore, are at risk for a variety of abnormalities caused by thromboembolic events or by an uneven distribution of blood volume, or both. Monoamniotic twins are at additional risk for birth defects caused by deformation or uneven allocation of cells during gastrulation. Twinning events that occur during gastrulation are extremely rare and are probably responsible for various types of conjoined twins.

## Genetic Determinism and Stochastic Processes in Development

"Why did this happen?" is one of the first questions asked by most families when a child has been born with a birth defect, but medical genetics can provide a general answer only about half the time (see Fig. 17–11). Even for birth defects in which the etiology is known, expressivity can vary widely, and the search for an underlying explanation can be frustrating to both patient and physician. An unstated assumption in such a "search" is that an explanation actually exists; in other words, that sufficient knowledge of genetic or environmental parameters, or both, for a cell, organ, or embryo would allow a deterministic prediction of the eventual phenotype. A certain level of determinism is, of course, the foundation of genetics; the notion that a combination of genotypic and environmental variables predicts phenotypic variation and disease is a fundamental tenet of all biology. Nonetheless, such predictions are not always absolute, particularly when it comes to developmental variation. The effect of chance on development is most easily grasped by considering human twins or inbred animals in a situation in which little or no environmental variation occurs. Monozygotic twins are almost always more similar to each other than are

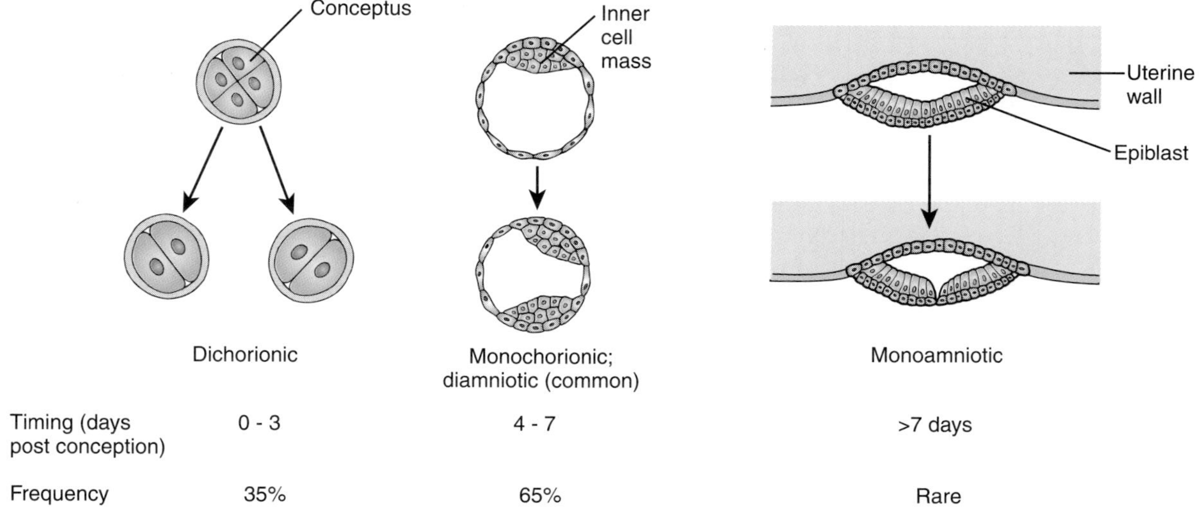


**Figure 17–16.** The arrangement of placental membranes in monozygotic twins depends on the timing of the twinning event. Dichorionic twins result from a complete splitting of the entire embryo, leading to duplication of all extraembryonic tissues. Monochorionic diamniotic twins are caused by division of the inner cell mass at the blastocyst stage. Monoamniotic twins are caused by division of the epiblast at the egg cylinder stage.

dizygotic twins, but obvious residual differences—fingerprints and birthmarks, for example—can be explained only by chance.

Fingerprints and birthmarks are probably representative of many developmental processes when viewed from a cellular perspective. Thus, the ability to predict a cell's phenotype or phenotypic potential in a developing embryo is often, but not always, a function of that cell's genotype and its position in space and time, that is, its environment (see Fig. 17–1). For example, it is impossible to predict which of the cells in a four-cell embryo will give rise to the inner cell mass or the trophoblast (see Fig. 17–3), and it is impossible to predict which cells of the inner cell mass in a female embryo will inactivate the paternally derived or the maternally derived X chromosome (see Chapter 10). A process that cannot be predicted from the events that preceded it is said to be **stochastic** and characterizes many aspects of early mammalian development. Understanding the stochastic nature of these processes is essential in caring for patients affected with developmental abnormalities whether caused by genes, environment, or chance.

## RECENT ADVANCES IN DEVELOPMENTAL GENETICS AND POTENTIAL APPLICATIONS

Much of our understanding of the mechanisms that guide human embryonic development depends on studies carried out in model organisms. Invertebrate model organisms such as fruitflies or worms are very useful because of the powerful genetic and embryological experimental methods that can be brought to bear and because many of the molecular and cellular mechanisms operating during human development are also used during invertebrate development. Mammalian model organisms such as mice and rats are also useful because actual tissue interactions and movements are conserved; development of the heart, brain, liver, and lungs in mouse embryos, for example, occurs in nearly the exact same way (but on a longer time scale) in human embryos. Model organisms not only provide tools for understanding human development but are also the platform and proving ground for development of new therapies relevant to organ transplantation and regeneration. Two areas in which progress has been especially notable are embryonic stem cells and cloning.

### Embryonic Stem Cells

Technology for producing animals from undifferentiated embryonic cells grown in culture is an outgrowth of studies carried out on mouse and human teratocarcinomas. These unusual tumors were originally recognized because they consist of both undifferentiated cells and multiple types of differentiated cells. Undifferentiated cells from teratocarcinomas can be grown in culture and are pluripotent because multiple tissues reappear after the cultured teratocarcinoma cells are injected back into embryos or adult animals (Fig. 17–17).

The ability of an undifferentiated tumor cell to both self-renew and give rise to different types of committed progenitor cells is reminiscent of normal stem cell behavior as described previously. In fact, undifferentiated teratocarcinoma cells share many characteristics with normal embryonic cells from the inner cell mass or primitive ectoderm; not only will teratocarcinoma cells occasionally contribute to differentiated adult tissues after injection into embryos, but normal inner cell mass injected into adult tissues will occasionally give rise to teratocarcinomas (Fig. 17–17).

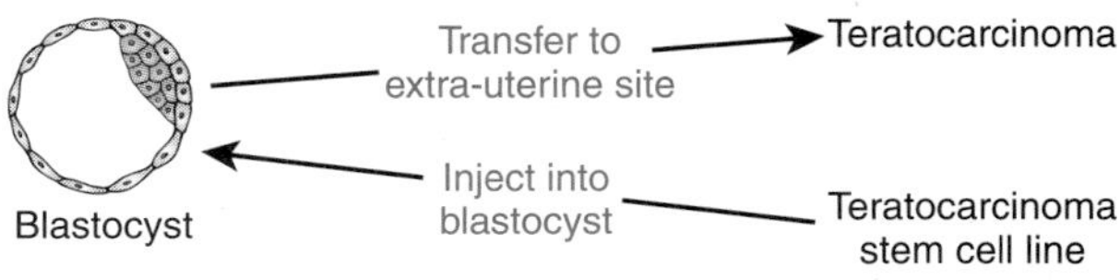


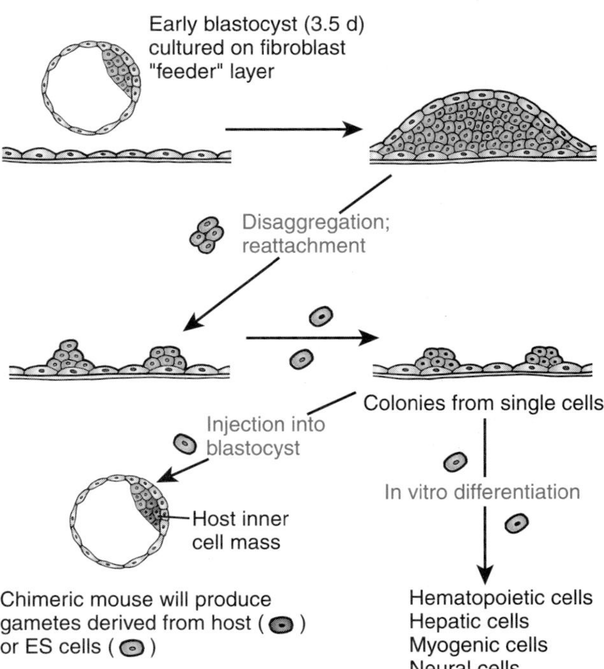


**Figure 17–17.** Teratocarcinomas and embryonic stem cells. Cells from teratocarcinomas can be grown in culture and injected into a blastocyst and will give rise to many different tissue types. Embryonic stem cells share many features with teratocarcinoma cells but are derived directly from the inner cell mass or primitive ectoderm and, in contrast to teratocarcinoma cells, are often euploid and can therefore contribute to the germline. Cultured embryonic stem cells differentiated in vitro can give rise to a variety of different cell types.

Teratocarcinoma cells are usually aneuploid. Under appropriate conditions, however, the normal inner cell mass can be explanted and maintained in culture in an undifferentiated euploid state. Cells derived in this way are referred to as **embryonic stem cells**. They can be cultured for many generations, manipulated in culture, and later injected into normal embryos to produce a **chimera**, a single animal with contributions from more than one zygote. Because gametes produced by a chimeric animal can be derived either from the host embryo or from the embryonic stem cell, this set of procedures can be used to create animals with precise alterations of gene arrangement, gene number, or gene structure.

Embryonic stem cell technology provides a mechanism for creating animal models of important human genetic diseases and, in many cases, has provided unexpected insight into the role such genes play in normal development. For example, the breast cancer susceptibility gene *BRCA1* is required both for early embryonic development and for proper branching and architecture of developing mammary ducts. Creating animal models for diseases like hemophilia or cystic fibrosis is a prerequisite for developing and testing gene therapy; in addition, embryonic stem cell technology provides a testing ground for efforts to correct genetic defects in utero.

## Animal Cloning

Attempts to bypass fertilization by reproducing whole organisms from diploid somatic cells lie at the heart of one of the oldest questions in developmental biology: is the program for embryogenesis encoded in DNA, and is that code preserved in the differentiated cells of adult animals? Studies carried out in the past several years have answered both questions affirmatively in several different mammals, with important implications for many aspects of biology and medicine. In most studies, a nucleus from a differentiated diploid cell such as a fibroblast, a breast epithelial cell, or an ovarian cumulus cell is transplanted into an oocyte from which the original nucleus has been removed. The newly constructed zygote is allowed to undergo several divisions in culture and is then transferred to a uterus and allowed to implant and develop. The cytoplasmic environment of the oocyte is believed to provide essential components required for the first few embryonic cell divisions, but other than mitochondria, all components of a cloned animal are genetically encoded by the transplanted nucleus. Although only a small fraction of zygotes constructed by nuclear transplantation develop successfully, animals have been successfully cloned using diploid nuclei from mammary cells, cumulus cells of the ovary, and embryonic stem cells grown in culture. Thus, epigenetic changes required for organogenesis, differentiation, X inactivation, and gametic imprinting do not represent an insurmountable obstacle to recapitulating the entire program of embryonic development.

## Developmental Genetics, Medicine, and Society

One of the most far-reaching implications of embryonic stem cell and animal cloning technology is the potential to change how tissue and organ trans-

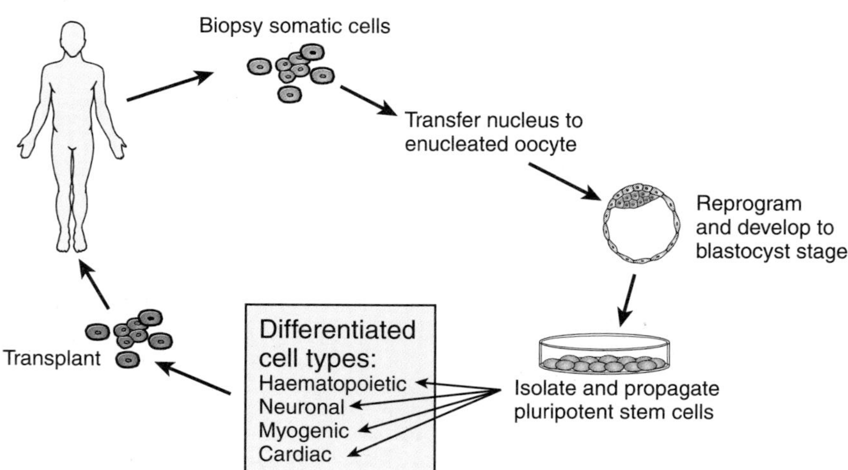


**Figure 17–18.** Potential application of cell cloning and embryonic stem cell technology to organ and tissue transplantation. (Figure reprinted from Smith A [1998] Cell therapy: In search of pluripotency. Curr Biol 8:R802–804. Copyright 1998, with permission from Elsevier Science.)

plantation is carried out (Fig. 17–18). For example, controlled differentiation of embryonic stem cells into hematopoietic or hepatic cells could provide a source of bone marrow or liver transplants that do not require individual donors, whereas the ability to produce neurons in cell culture might provide new ways of treating many different neurodegenerative conditions. A key scientific problem is how potential immune rejection of transplanted animal cells might be overcome, because live tissue or organ replacements developed from animal embryonic stem cells will be much more immunogenic than, for example, chemically treated porcine cardiac valves. One possible solution to this problem is to develop human embryonic stem cells from which major histocompatibility-encoding genes have been removed. A second possibility is to "humanize" animal embryonic stem cells by removing all genes that encode immunogenic proteins. A third possibility is to use cell cloning to develop embryonic stem cells (and their differentiated derivatives) from the individual in need of transplantation (Fig. 17–18). All of these approaches raise important ethical and public health questions that must be considered carefully. For example, transplantation of live animal cells into humans is associated with a potential risk for transmission of infectious agents across species boundaries. In addition, certain types of experiments may be associated with a risk of gametic mutations, and there is widespread consensus that either accidental or deliberate alteration of human germ cells runs counter to modern moral and ethical principles. As with many areas of science, developmental genetic technology not only offers the potential for dramatic improvements in human health, but also confronts us with new concepts and challenges that require education, discussion, and consensus among scientists, health professionals, patients, and society at large.

## General References


Epstein CJ (1991) Aneuploidy and morphogenesis. Prog Clin Biol Res 373:1–18.

Epstein CJ (1995) The new dysmorphology: Application of insights from basic developmental biology to the understanding of human birth defects. Proc Natl Acad Sci U S A 92:8566–8573.

Gilbert SF (1997) Developmental Biology. Sinauer Associates, Sunderland, Massachusetts.

Gurdon J (1999) Developmental biology and the redirection or replacement of cells. Philos Trans R Soc Lond B Biol Sci 354:1967–1976.

Jones KL, Smith DW (1997) Smith's Recognizable Patterns of Human Malformation. WB Saunders, Philadelphia.

Moore KL, Persaud TVN (1998) The Developing Human: Clinically Oriented Embryology, 6th ed. WB Saunders, Philadelphia.

Slack JMW (1991) From Egg to Embryo: Regional Specification in Early Development. Developmental and Cell Biology Series. Cambridge University Press, Cambridge, England and New York.

Wilkins AS (1993) Genetic Analysis of Animal Development. Wiley-Liss, New York.

Wolpert L, Beddington R, Brockes J, et al (1998) Principles of Development. Oxford University Press, Oxford, England.


## References Specific to Particular Topics


Angrist M, Bolk S, Halushka M, et al (1996) Germline mutations in glial cell line-derived neurotrophic factor (GDNF) and RET in a Hirschsprung disease patient. Nat Genet 14:341–344.

Baloh RH, Enomoto H, Johnson EM Jr, Milbrandt J (2000) The GDNF family ligands and receptors—Implications for neural development. Curr Opin Neurobiol 10:103–110.

Capecchi MR (1997) Hox genes and mammalian development. Cold Spring Harb Symp Quant Biol 62:273–281.

Conway SJ, Henderson DJ, Copp AJ (1997) PAX3 is required for cardiac neural crest migration in the mouse: Evidence from the splotch (Sp2H) mutant. Development 124:505–514.

Dale JK, Vesque C, Lints TJ, et al (1997) Cooperation of BMP7 and SHH in the induction of forebrain ventral midline cells by prechordal mesoderm. Cell 90:257–269.

Doray B, Salomon R, Amiel J, et al (1998) Mutation of the RET ligand, neurturin, supports multigenic inheritance in Hirschsprung disease. Hum Mol Genet 7:1449–1452.

Dlugosz A (1999) The hedgehog and the hair follicle: A growing relationship [comment]. J Clin Invest 104:851–853.

Ezer S, Bayes M, Elomaa O, et al (1999) Ectodysplasin is a collagenous trimeric type II membrane protein with a tumor necrosis factor-like domain and co-localizes with cytoskeletal structures at lateral and apical surfaces of cells. Hum Mol Genet 8:2079–2086.

Gehring WJ, Ikeo K (1999) Pax 6: Mastering eye morphogenesis and eye evolution. Trends Genet 15:371–377.

Grindley JC, Davidson DR, Hill RE (1995) The role of Pax-6 in eye and nasal development. Development 121:1433–1442.

Lumsden A, Graham A (1995) Neural patterning: A forward role for hedgehog. Curr Biol 5:1347–1350.

Mansouri A, Hallonet M, Gruss P (1996) Pax genes and their roles in cell differentiation and development. Curr Opin Cell Biol 8:851–857.

Ming JE, Roessler E, Muenke M (1998) Human developmental disorders and the sonic hedgehog pathway. Mol Med Today 4:343–349.

Muenke M, Beachy PA (2000) Genetics of ventral forebrain development and holoprosencephaly. Curr Opin Genet Dev 10:262–269.

Muragaki Y, Mundlos S, Upton J, Olsen B (1996) Altered growth and branching patterns in synpolydactyly caused by mutations in HOXD13. Science 272:548–551.

Opdecamp K, Nakayama A, Nguyen MT, et al (1997) Melanocyte development in vivo and in neural crest cell cultures: Crucial dependence on the MITF basic-helix-loop-helix-zipper transcription factor. Development 124:2377–2386.

Radhakrishna U, Bornholdt D, Scott HS, et al (1999) The phenotypic spectrum of GLI3 morphopathies includes autosomal dominant preaxial polydactyly type-IV and postaxial polydactyly type-A/B; No phenotype prediction from the position of GLI3 mutations. Am J Hum Genet 65:645–655.

Roessler E, Belloni E, Gaudenz K, et al (1996) Mutations in the human sonic hedgehog gene cause holoprosencephaly. Nat Genet 14:357–360.

Smith A (1998) Cell therapy: In search of pluripotency. Curr Biol 8:R802–804.

Tabin CJ (1998) A developmental model for thalidomide defects. Nature 396:322–323.

Thesleff I, Vaahtokari A, Vainio S, Jowett A (1996) Molecular mechanisms of cell and tissue interactions during early tooth development. Anat Rec 245:151–161.

Wilmut I, Young L, Campbell KH (1998) Embryonic and somatic cell cloning. Reprod Fertil Dev 10:639–643.

Xu X, Wagner KU, Larson D, et al (1999) Conditional mutation of Brca1 in mammary epithelial cells results in blunted ductal morphogenesis and tumour formation. Nat Genet 22:37–43.

## *Problems*

1. What are the two steps by which the cells in an embryo undergo commitment to a particular fate? How are these steps distinguished experimentally? What is the significance of separating these two steps for reproductive genetics?

2. Match the terms in the left-hand column with the terms that best fit in the right-hand column.

| | |
|---|---|
| A. Lineage-dependent development | 1. Pluripotency |
| B. Position-dependent development | 2. Morphogen |
| C. Regulative development | 3. Epigenetic regulation of gene expression |
| D. Embryonic stem cells | 4. Monozygotic twinning |

3. What distinguishes a morphogen from a paracrine signal?

4. Match the terms in the left-hand column with the terms that best fit in the right-hand column.

| | |
|---|---|
| A. Amniotic band | 1. U-shaped cleft palate |
| B. Aniridia | 2. Thalidomide |
| C. Inadequate amniotic fluid | 3. *PAX6* mutation |
| D. Limb reduction | 4. Disruption |
| E. Robin sequence | 5. Deformation |

5. What type of diploid cells would not be appropriate nucleus donors in an animal cloning experiment and why?

6. For discussion: In Chapter 12, we learned of many mutations that cause disease inherited in an autosomal recessive manner. Why do some mutations in transcription factors result in developmental defects even when present in the heterozygous state?

# 18

# Prenatal Diagnosis

Prenatal diagnosis had its beginning in 1966, when Steele and Breg showed that the chromosome constitution of a fetus could be determined by analysis of cultured cells from the amniotic fluid. Because the association between late maternal age and an increased risk of Down syndrome was already well known, their report led directly to the development of prenatal diagnosis as a medical service. This service requires the collaboration of a number of disciplines: obstetrics; ultrasonography; clinical genetics, for the purpose of assessment, diagnosis, and genetic counseling; and laboratory services. Because of the complexity of integrating these functions, prenatal diagnosis is usually arranged by referral to a multidisciplinary program in which genetics plays an essential part. Prenatal diagnosis has already been referred to in the context of many specific genetic disorders, and in this chapter, its scope, methodology, and limitations are considered in further detail.

The purpose of prenatal diagnosis is not simply to detect abnormalities in fetal life and allow termination of pregnancy when the fetus is found to have a defect. Rather, the goals of prenatal diagnosis are the following:

1. To provide a range of informed choice to couples at risk of having a child with an abnormality.
2. To provide reassurance and to reduce anxiety, especially among high-risk groups.
3. To allow couples at risk of having a child with a specific birth defect, who might otherwise forego having children, to begin a pregnancy with the knowledge that the presence or absence of the disorder in the fetus can be confirmed by testing. Many couples at risk of having a child with a severe genetic disorder have been able to have healthy children because of the availability of prenatal diagnosis.
4. To allow couples the option of appropriate management for the impending birth of a child with a genetic disorder in terms of psychological preparation, pregnancy/delivery management, and postnatal care.
5. To enable prenatal treatment of the affected fetus. This is now possible for a very small but growing number of congenital disorders. For example, severe fetal bladder outlet obstruction can be detected by fetal ultrasound. If untreated, the consequent reduction in urine production would cause severe oligohydramnios and consequent poor lung development (Potter syndrome). Relief of the bladder obstruction by shunting procedures in utero may prevent irreversible damage to the developing lungs and may also ameliorate renal abnormalities.

## INDICATIONS FOR PRENATAL DIAGNOSIS

By far the leading indication for prenatal diagnosis is late maternal age. In North America and Western Europe, according to statistical data for maternal age at birth in comparison with the number of prenatal diagnoses, at least half of all pregnant women older than 35 years present for amniocentesis. In the United States, courts have considered a physician to be negligent if he or she fails to offer prenatal diagnosis to women considered to be of advanced maternal age.

The chief condition for which pregnant women of advanced age are at risk is Down syndrome (Fig. 18–1). Despite the widespread availability of prenatal diagnosis to older women, most fetuses with Down syndrome are not identified prenatally because the majority of such pregnancies are in mothers younger than 35 years of age who are thus too young to be eligible for **amniocentesis** or **chorionic villus sampling** (CVS) on a routine basis. For women younger than 35 years, new noninvasive testing may help to identify a larger proportion of the fetuses at risk. Such noninvasive testing includes **maternal serum screening** (MSS) together with ultrasonographic examination to screen for fetuses with Down syndrome, neural tube defects (NTDs), and other abnormalities; these tests are described later.

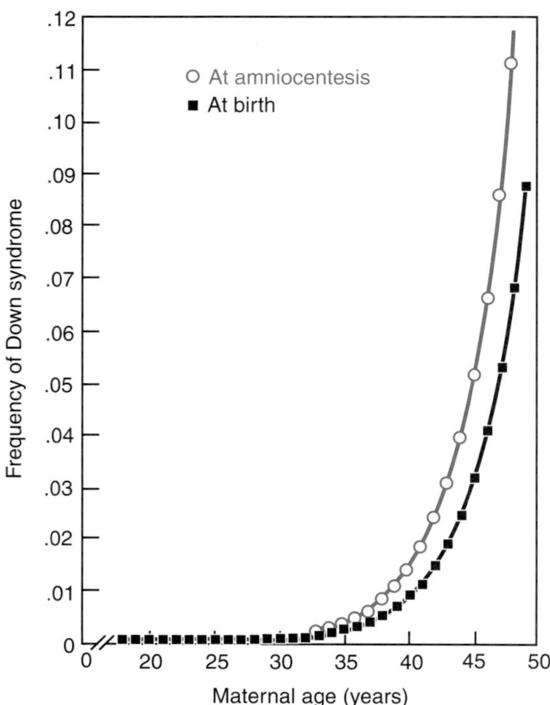


**Figure 18–1.** Maternal age dependence of incidence of trisomy 21 at birth and at time of amniocentesis. See also Chapter 10. (Data from Hook EB, Cross PK, Schreinemachers DM [1983] Chromosomal abnormality rates at amniocentesis and in live-born infants. JAMA 249:2034–2038.)

Prenatal diagnosis cannot be used to rule out all possible fetal abnormalities. It is limited to determining whether the fetus has (or probably has) a designated condition for which an increased risk is indicated by late maternal age, family history, or other well-defined risk factors. If amniocentesis is performed for any reason, both the amniotic fluid alpha-fetoprotein (AFAFP) level (discussed later) and the karyotype are determined to screen for open NTDs and chromosomal abnormalities, respectively. Other tests are performed only for specific indications.

## GENETIC COUNSELING FOR PRENATAL DIAGNOSIS

Parents considering prenatal diagnosis need information that will allow them to understand their situation and to give or withhold consent for the procedure. In addition, the professional staff of the prenatal diagnosis program (physician, nurse, and genetic counselor) must assess the situation, determine the genetic risk, and learn whether other genetic problems should also be considered. Ethnic background or family history may indicate the need for carrier tests of the parents in advance of prenatal diagnostic testing. For example, one must consider the risk of Tay-Sachs disease in the fetus of an Ashkenazic Jewish couple referred for any reason.

Preliminary genetic counseling of candidates for prenatal diagnosis usually deals with the following: (1) the risk that the fetus will be affected; (2) the nature and probable consequences of the specific problem; (3) the risks and limitations of the procedures to be used; (4) the time required before a report can be issued; and (5) the possible need for a repeat procedure in the event of a failed attempt. In addition, the couple must be advised that a result may be difficult to interpret, that further tests and consultation may be required, and that even then the results may not necessarily be definitive.

Finally, although the great majority of prenatal diagnoses end in reassurance, options available to parents in the event of an abnormality—of which termination of pregnancy is only one—should be discussed. *Above all, the parents must understand that in undertaking prenatal diagnosis, they are under no implied obligation to terminate a pregnancy in the event that an abnormality is detected.* The objective of prenatal diagnosis is to determine whether the fetus is affected or unaffected with the disorder in question. Diagnosis of an affected fetus may, at the least, allow the parents to prepare emotionally and medically for the management of a newborn with a disorder.

Numerous diseases cannot yet be diagnosed prenatally, but every month additional disorders are added to the list of conditions for which prenatal diagnosis is possible (e.g., see Table 18–1). Keeping up with the rapid changes and serving as a central source of information about the current status of prenatal testing is one of the contributions of genetics clinics to medical practice in general.

## METHODS OF PRENATAL DIAGNOSIS

The methods currently used for prenatal diagnosis, both invasive and noninvasive, are shown in Table 18–2. Both amniocentesis and CVS are invasive procedures associated with a small risk of fetal loss. Thus, the use of amniocentesis or CVS is indicated for only a small percentage of pregnant women who meet the criteria for prenatal diagnosis as outlined earlier. In contrast, a combination of MSS or triple screening (discussed later) and ultrasonographic scanning can be used for fetal evaluation in low-risk as well as in *some* high-risk pregnancies because both are noninvasive and without risk to the fetus. MSS can help to identify fetuses at increased risk of open NTDs, some chromosomal abnormalities including Down syndrome, and other disorders, as described later in this

## The Principal Indications for Prenatal Diagnosis by Invasive Testing

The generally accepted guidelines for eligibility of pregnant women for prenatal diagnosis by amniocentesis or CVS are based on evidence that the risk for fetal abnormality is at least as great as the risk of miscarriage from the procedure itself. Currently, more than 200 genetic disorders* can be diagnosed prenatally using amniocentesis or CVS. As the scope of prenatal diagnosis expands and technology improves, the guidelines are sure to change, but at present, the chief indications for prenatal diagnosis are the following:

1. **Advanced maternal age.** The definition of advanced maternal age varies somewhat among prenatal genetics centers but is usually at least 35 years at the expected date of confinement. This age has been selected because at 35 years, the risk of a fetus with a chromosome abnormality is approximately equal to the risk of miscarriage associated with amniocentesis (see Table 10–1 for maternal age–specific risks of a fetus with a chromosomal abnormality).
2. **Previous child with a de novo chromosome abnormality.** Although the parents of a child with a chromosome abnormality may have normal chromosomes themselves, in some situations there may still be an increased risk of a chromosomal abnormality in a subsequent child. For example, if a woman at 30 years of age has a child with Down syndrome, the recurrence risk for *any* chromosomal abnormality is about 1/100, in comparison with the age-related population risk of about 1/390. Parental mosaicism is one possible explanation of the increased risk, but in the majority of cases, the mechanism of the increase in risk is unknown.
3. **Presence of structural chromosome abnormality in one of the parents.** Here, the risk of a chromosome abnormality in a child varies depending on the type of abnormality and sometimes on the parent of origin. The greatest risk, 100 percent for Down syndrome, occurs only if either parent has a 21q21q Robertsonian translocation or isochromosome (see Chapter 10).
4. **Family history of a genetic disorder that may be diagnosed or ruled out by biochemical or DNA analysis.** Most of the disorders in this group are caused by single-gene defects and therefore have recurrence risks of 25 percent or 50 percent. Cases in which the parents have been diagnosed as carriers after a population screening test, rather than after the birth of an affected child, are also in this category. Even before DNA analysis became available, numerous biochemical disorders could be identified prenatally, and DNA analysis has greatly increased this number. Table 18–1 provides some examples of relatively common single-gene disorders for which prenatal diagnosis can be performed by DNA analysis (either by mutation analysis or linkage analysis).
5. **Family history of an X-linked disorder for which there is no specific prenatal diagnostic test.** When there is no alternative method, the parents of a boy affected with an X-linked disorder may use fetal sex determination to help them decide whether to continue or terminate a subsequent pregnancy because the recurrence risk may be as high as 25 percent. For X-linked disorders, such as Duchenne muscular dystrophy and hemophilia A and B, however, in which prenatal diagnosis by DNA analysis is available, the fetal sex is first determined and DNA analysis is then performed if the fetus is male. In either of the situations mentioned, preimplantation genetic diagnosis (see later discussion) may be an option for allowing the transfer to the uterus of only those embryos determined to be unaffected for the disorder in question.
6. **Risk of a neural tube defect.** First-degree relatives (and second-degree relatives at some centers) of patients with NTDs are eligible for amniocentesis because of an increased risk of having a child with an NTD (see Table 15–8); many open NTDs can now be detected by other noninvasive tests, however, as described later.
7. **Maternal serum screening and ultrasound.** Genetic assessment and further testing are recommended when fetal abnormalities are detected by routine screening of low-risk pregnancies by MSS or by fetal ultrasound (see later).

* The figure of approximately 200 disorders is derived from those listed on the Genetests web site (*http://www.genetests.org*) and does not include tests that may be available in other laboratories.

TABLE 18–1

**Selected Common Single-Gene Disorders for Which Prenatal Diagnosis by DNA Analysis Is Possible in Many Families**

| Disorder | Inheritance |
|---|---|
| Achondroplasia | AD |
| Autosomal dominant polycystic kidney disease | AD |
| Huntington disease | AD |
| Myotonic dystrophy | AD |
| Neurofibromatosis, type 1 | AD |
| Retinoblastoma | AD |
| Cystic fibrosis | AR |
| Congenital adrenal hyperplasia | AR |
| Friedreich ataxia | AR |
| Phenylketonuria | AR |
| Sickle cell disease | AR |
| Spinal muscular atrophy | AR |
| Tay-Sachs disease | AR |
| $\alpha$- and $\beta$-thalassemias | AR |
| Duchenne and Becker muscular dystrophy | X-linked |
| Fragile X syndrome | X-linked |
| Hemophilia A and B | X-linked |
| Ornithine transcarbamylase deficiency | X-linked |

AR = autosomal recessive; AD = autosomal dominant.

chapter. Ultrasonography, in addition to its function in assessment of gestational age and fetal growth, enables the diagnosis of a number of morphological abnormalities, many of which are genetic in origin, at early gestational ages (see later).

## Invasive Testing

### AMNIOCENTESIS

Amniocentesis refers to the procedure of removing a sample of amniotic fluid transabdominally by syringe (Fig. 18–2*A*). The amniotic fluid contains cells of fetal origin that can be cultured for diagnostic tests. Before amniocentesis, ultrasonographic scanning is routinely used to confirm fetal viability, gestational age (by measuring the fetal biparietal diameter and femoral length), the number of fetuses, structural normality, and the optimal position for needle insertion by establishing the position of the fetus and placenta. Amniocentesis is performed on an outpatient basis typically at the 15th to 16th week after the first day of the last menstrual period; however, the procedure has been performed at a much earlier stage in pregnancy, as early as 10 to 14 weeks in some centers.

In addition to fetal chromosome analysis, the concentration of AFP can be assayed in amniotic fluid to detect open NTDs. AFP is a fetal glycoprotein produced mainly in the liver, secreted into the fetal circulation, and excreted through the kidneys into the amniotic fluid via fetal urine. AFP enters the maternal blood stream via the placenta, amniotic membranes, and the maternal-fetal circulation. It can therefore be assayed either in amniotic fluid (AFAFP) or in maternal serum (MSAFP). Both assays are extremely useful in prenatal diagnosis, chiefly for assessing the risk of an open NTD but also for other reasons (see later discussion).

AFP concentration is measured by immunoassay, a relatively simple and inexpensive method that can be applied to all amniotic fluid samples regardless of the specific indication for the amniocentesis. When the AFAFP assay is used in conjunction with ultrasonographic scanning at 18 to 19 weeks' gestation, about 99 percent of fetuses with open spina bifida and virtually all fetuses with anencephaly can be identified. To interpret the findings, the normal range must be established in relation to gestational age and to factors other than an open NTD that can increase the AFAFP level. Factors potentially leading to abnormally high concentrations of AFP in amniotic fluid include the following:

1. Underestimation of gestational age. The AFP concentration is higher at about the 12th to the 14th week of pregnancy than at the 16th week, when amniocentesis is most often performed.
2. Fetal blood contamination.
3. Fetal death.
4. Twin pregnancy.
5. Fetal abnormalities, including omphalocele and at least one form of congenital nephrosis, as well as other rare problems.
6. Other unexplained variation in the normal AFP concentration of amniotic fluid.

Some of these causes of an elevated AFAFP level can be identified by ultrasonographic examination.

The major complication associated with midtrimester amniocentesis is a 0.5 to 1 percent risk of inducing miscarriage over the baseline risk of approximately 2 to 3 percent for any pregnancy at this stage of gestation. Other complications are rare, including leakage of amniotic fluid, infection, and injury to the fetus by needle puncture. As mentioned previously, amniocentesis can be performed as early as 10 to 14 weeks. One randomized study comparing the safety and fetal outcome of early amniocentesis versus midtrimester amniocentesis demonstrated an in-

TABLE 18–2

**Methods of Prenatal Diagnosis**

**Invasive Testing**
Amniocentesis
Chorionic villus sampling
Cordocentesis
Preimplantation genetic diagnosis

**Noninvasive Testing**
Maternal serum alpha-fetoprotein
Maternal serum screen
Ultrasonography
Isolation of fetal cells from maternal circulation

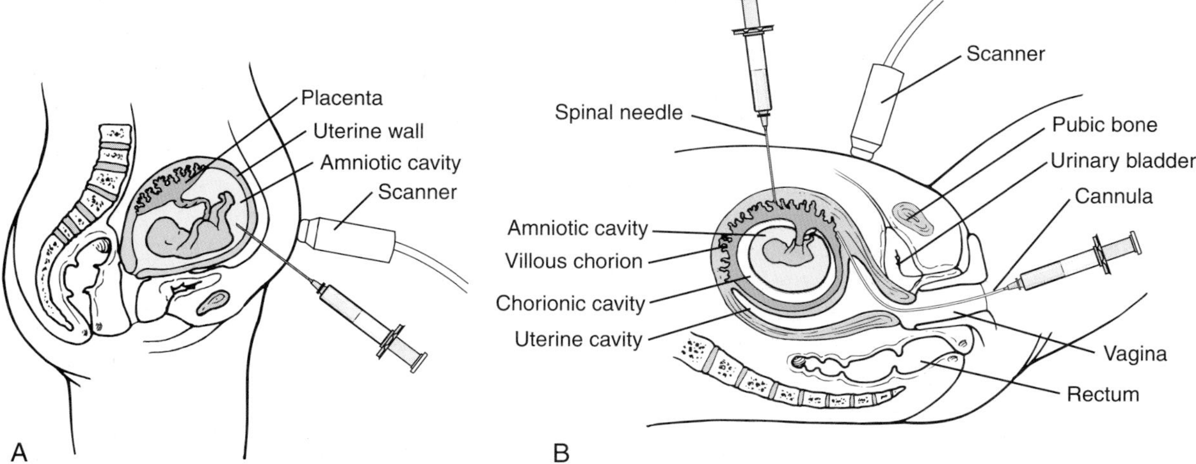


Figure 18–2. *A*, Amniocentesis. A needle is inserted transabdominally into the amniotic cavity, and a sample of amniotic fluid (usually about 20 ml) is withdrawn by syringe for diagnostic studies (e.g., chromosome studies, enzyme measurements, or DNA analysis). Ultrasonography is routinely performed before or during the procedure. *B*, Chorionic villus sampling. Two alternative approaches are drawn: transcervical (by means of a flexible cannula) and transabdominal (with a spinal needle). In both approaches, success and safety depends on use of ultrasound imaging (scanner). (From Moore KL and Persaud TVN [1998] The Developing Human: Clinically Oriented Embryology, 6th ed. WB Saunders, Philadelphia.)

creased risk of spontaneous abortion of 2.6 percent in the early group versus 0.8 percent in the midtrimester group. The only congenital anomaly found to be increased with early amniocentesis is talipes equinovarus (club feet), with an incidence of 1.3 percent versus the general population risk of 0.1 to 0.3 percent (a risk that is not increased with midtrimester amniocentesis). To prevent Rh immunization of the mother (see Chapter 14), administration of Rh immune globulin is routine for Rh-negative women after any invasive procedure (including amniocentesis and the two procedures described in the next sections, CVS and cordocentesis).

### Chorionic Villus Sampling

**Embryological Development of the Chorionic Villi.** A brief review of the early development of the chorionic villi helps to clarify the basis of the CVS technique (Fig. 18–3). The villi are derived from the trophoblast, the extraembryonic part of the blastocyst. During implantation, the trophoblast differentiates into the cytotrophoblast and the syncytiotrophoblast. The syncytiotrophoblast invades the uterine wall and eventually forms lacunae in which maternal blood is pooled. At the end of the second week, the **primary chorionic villi** are formed as proliferations of the cytotrophoblast

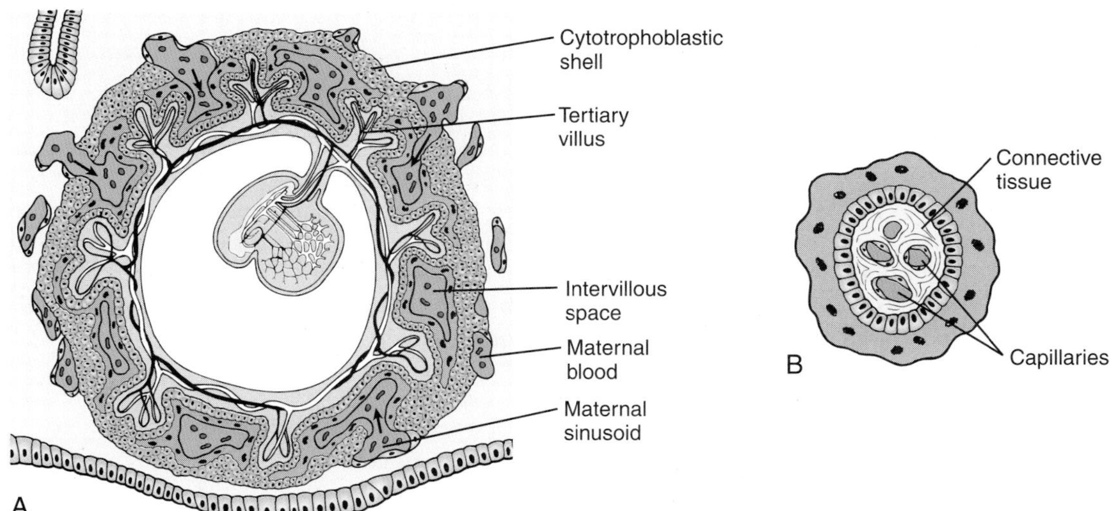


Figure 18–3. Development of the tertiary chorionic villi and placenta. *A*, Diagrammatic cross-section of an implanted embryo and placenta at about 21 days. *B*, Cross-section of a tertiary villus showing establishment of circulation in mesenchymal core, cytotrophoblast, and syncytiotrophoblast. (From Moore KL [1988] The Developing Human: Clinically Oriented Embryology, 4th ed. WB Saunders, Philadelphia.)

that protrude into the syncytiotrophoblast. The villi soon begin to branch, and mesenchyme grows into them to form a core; the formation of a core characterizes the **secondary villi**. Networks of capillaries develop in the mesenchymal core, and circulation is established; the villi are then **tertiary villi**. The tertiary villi branch profusely, and by the end of the eighth week they cover the entire surface of the chorionic sac as the **chorion frondosum**. Part of the chorion subsequently becomes the **smooth chorion (chorion laeve)** as the villi in that area degenerate. The villi that are sampled for prenatal diagnosis are tertiary villi from the chorion frondosum and are composed of mesenchymal core, cytotrophoblast, and an outer layer of syncytiotrophoblast.

**Advantages and Risks of Chorionic Villus Sampling.** CVS involves the biopsy of tissue from the villous area of the chorion transcervically or transabdominally, generally between the 10th and 12th week of pregnancy (see Fig. 18–2*B*). The major advantage of CVS compared with midtrimester amniocentesis is that CVS allows the results to be available at an early stage of pregnancy, thus reducing the period of uncertainty and allowing termination, if elected, to be performed in the first trimester and on an outpatient basis. However, AFP cannot be assayed at this stage (in contrast to 15 to 16 weeks when amniocentesis is performed), and screening for open NTDs should be performed by MSS at approximately 16 weeks of gestation. As with amniocentesis, ultrasound is used before CVS to determine the best approach for sampling. The increase in the rate of fetal loss due to CVS is approximately 1 percent, in addition to the baseline risk of 2 to 5 percent after 7 to 12 weeks of gestation. The success of chromosome analysis is the same as with amniocentesis (i.e., more than 99 percent). However, about 2 percent of CVS samplings yield ambiguous results due to chromosomal mosaicism (including true and pseudomosaicism—see later); in these situations, follow-up with amniocentesis is recommended to establish whether the fetus has a chromosomal abnormality.

### Cordocentesis

Cordocentesis is a procedure used to obtain a sample of fetal blood directly from the umbilical cord with ultrasonographic guidance. The fetal blood sample requires only a few days in culture to provide cells suitable for chromosome analysis or hematological studies. Cordocentesis is used to follow up an ultrasonographic examination that has shown some fetal abnormality, when culture of amniotic fluid cells has failed or yielded ambiguous results, or when DNA diagnosis is not possible for a disorder that can be identified by biochemical tests of fetal plasma or blood cells. Cordocentesis is usually performed at 19 to 21 weeks of pregnancy, and the incidence of fetal loss due to the procedure is approximately 2 to 3 percent.

## Noninvasive Testing

### Maternal Serum Screen for Alpha-Fetoprotein Assay at 16 Weeks

When the fetus has an open NTD, the concentration of AFP is likely to be higher than normal in the maternal serum as well as in the amniotic fluid. This observation is the basis for the use of MSAFP measurement at 16 weeks as a test for open NTDs. Because an estimated 95 percent of infants with NTDs are born into families with no known history of this malformation, a relatively simple test that can be followed by more specific tests constitutes an important screening tool. As shown in Figure 18–4, there is considerable overlap between the normal range for MSAFP and the range of concentration found when the fetus has an open NTD. If an elevated concentration is defined as two multiples of the median, one can estimate that 20 percent of fetuses with open NTDs remain undetected.

**Combined Use of Maternal Serum Screen for Alpha-Fetoprotein and Ultrasound.** The combined use of the MSAFP assay with detailed diagnostic ultrasonography (see later discussion) approaches the accuracy of AFAFP and ultrasound for the detection of open NTDs. Because the assay of MSAFP is not invasive, its measurement, together with ultrasonography, is preferred for the diagnosis of open NTDs in many centers. Thus, in many prenatal diagnosis programs, first-degree, second-degree, or more remote relatives of patients with NTDs may have an MSAFP assay (at 16 weeks) followed by detailed ultrasound (at 18 weeks).

Periconceptional supplementation with folic acid (i.e., at least 1 month before conception and continuing through the first trimester of pregnancy) has been shown to decrease the incidence of NTDs by nearly 75 percent (see Chapter 15). Reductions in the incidence of other birth defects has also been demonstrated. All pregnant women should be given this information. The recommended dosage of folic acid increases with the estimated risk for NTD (i.e., a higher dose is given to women at increased risk based on a positive family history).

### Maternal Serum Screening (Triple Screen)

MSS—sometimes called triple screen—measures three blood markers and is made available to most pregnant women at 15 to 20 weeks' gestation to identify those at increased risk for Down syndrome, tri-

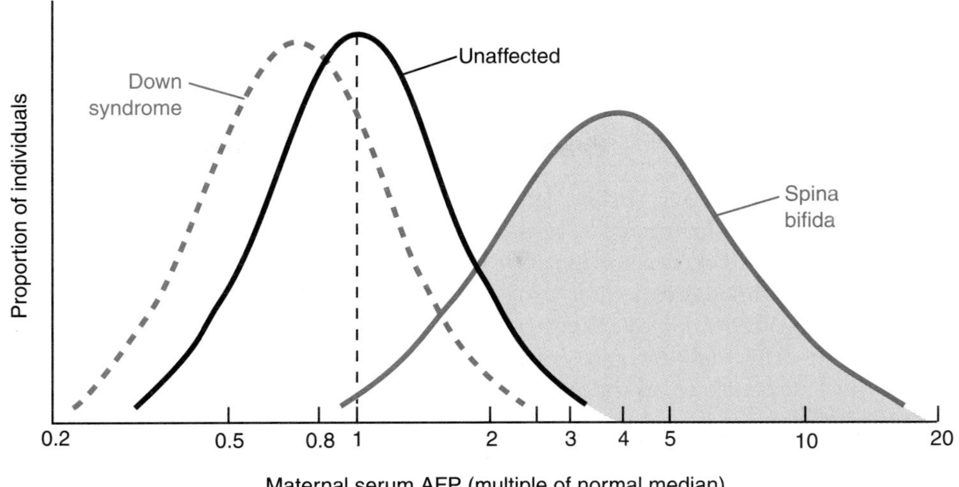


Figure 18–4. Maternal serum alpha-fetoprotein (AFP) concentration, expressed as multiples of the median, in normal fetuses, fetuses with open neural tube defects, and fetuses with Down syndrome. (Redrawn from Wald NJ, Cuckle HS [1987] Recent advances in screening for neural tube defects and Down syndrome. *In* Rodeck C [ed] Prenatal Diagnosis. Baillière Tindall, London, pp. 649–676.)

somy 18, and NTD (the latter by specifically measuring AFP as discussed earlier).

| | AFP | uE3 | HCG |
|---|---|---|---|
| Increased risk of Down syndrome | ↓ | ↓ | ↑ |
| Trisomy 18 | ↓ | ↓ | ↓ |
| NTD | ↑ | not applicable | not applicable |

The three serum components measured in this screening test include AFP, unconjugated estriol (uE3), and human chorionic gonadotrophin (HCG). In pregnancies with Down syndrome, the levels of AFP and uE3 are *reduced* in maternal serum, with median values of approximately 0.72 and 0.73 multiples of the median, respectively, in comparison with controls. (By definition, the control multiple of the median is 1.0.) The concentration of uE3 is also reduced in women who are smokers and, in general, in cases of fetal immaturity; extremely low levels may be indicative of steroid sulfatase deficiency or the Smith-Lemli-Opitz syndrome. HCG in maternal serum is significantly *higher* than normal when the fetus has Down syndrome, with a median value of two multiples of the median. Screening using maternal age alone detects approximately 30 percent of pregnancies with Down syndrome, whereas, by assaying all three biochemical markers and also considering maternal age, the detection of pregnancies with Down syndrome is improved to approximately 60 percent.

When the level of all three of these biochemical markers is low, the risk for trisomy 18 is significantly increased; in fact, the detection rate for trisomy 18 is believed to be greater than 80 percent. Other second trimester markers are being investigated to enhance this form of screening. In addition, several studies are under way to identify and evaluate the use of biochemical markers, including free $\beta$-HCG and pregnancy-associated placental protein (PAPP-A), for the prediction of Down syndrome and trisomy 18 in the first trimester of pregnancy.

It is critical that women and their partners be informed that MSS, either in the first or second trimester, is only a *screening* test and not a diagnostic tool. An MSS test is considered to be "screen positive" for Down syndrome once an ultrasound has confirmed fetal age and once the estimated risk is equivalent to or greater than the risk for a 35-year-old woman. Further counseling and diagnostic testing (e.g., amniocentesis) should be offered to women whose MSS screening test result is positive. Women whose MSS screening test result is considered to be "negative" must also be aware that their risk of having a child with Down syndrome, trisomy 18, or an NTD, although greatly reduced, is not zero (i.e., the result is only a risk estimate).

In many clinical practices, MSS has already become a standard test offered to all pregnant women; thus, this test is even more closely related to the everyday concerns of primary physicians than are the rare abnormalities or even the common genetic conditions that form so much of the subject matter of medical genetics. Health care professionals must be aware of the limitations and benefits of MSS and must be knowledgeable about the correct management in the event of a screen-positive result.

### ULTRASONOGRAPHY

High-resolution, real-time scanning is increasingly important in prenatal diagnosis for fetal assessment and for the detection of morphological anomalies (Fig. 18–5). It permits accurate determination of fetal age, identifies multiple pregnancies, and verifies fetal viability. It can even be used in midtrimester to identify fetal sex with a high degree of accuracy. Transabdominal ultrasound, the traditional method, is now supplemented with increasing frequency by transvaginal ultrasound to evaluate fetal viability and gestational dating and, in the first trimester, to detect several major types of anomalies, such as anencephaly and cystic hygroma (Table 18–3). Thus, many malformations are now detectable in the first instance by routine ultrasonography, even without a family history to indicate an increased risk. Long-term follow-up assessments have failed to provide any evidence that ultrasonography is harmful to the fetus or the mother.

**Prenatal Ultrasound for Chromosomal Aneuploidy.** A number of fetal abnormalities that can be detected by ultrasound are associated with chromosomal aneuploidy. Table 18–4 lists the prevalence of fetal chromosomal defects in fetuses with selected isolated and with multiple abnormalities detected by ultrasound. An example of a useful ultrasound marker for evaluating the risk of fetal aneuploidy is the measurement of fetal nuchal translucency (NT), which quantifies the subcutaneous translucency between the skin and the soft tissue overlying the cervical spine. NT can be increased because of an abnormal accumulation of fluid behind the fetal neck in the first trimester (10 to 14 weeks). The risk for aneuploidy, which varies with maternal age and gestational age, is also dependent on the degree of NT. Screening for increased NT requires highly skilled operators because caliper placement can result in significant variation in measurement. This screening test detects up to 80 percent of pregnancies with Down syndrome. In addition to chromosomal aneuploidy, increased NT can also be indicative of an underlying cardiac defect or genetic syndrome. When the possibility of a chromosome defect has been raised, it can be confirmed or ruled out by fetal chromosome analysis. Determination of the fetal karyotype is important for decision making about the continuation of pregnancy,

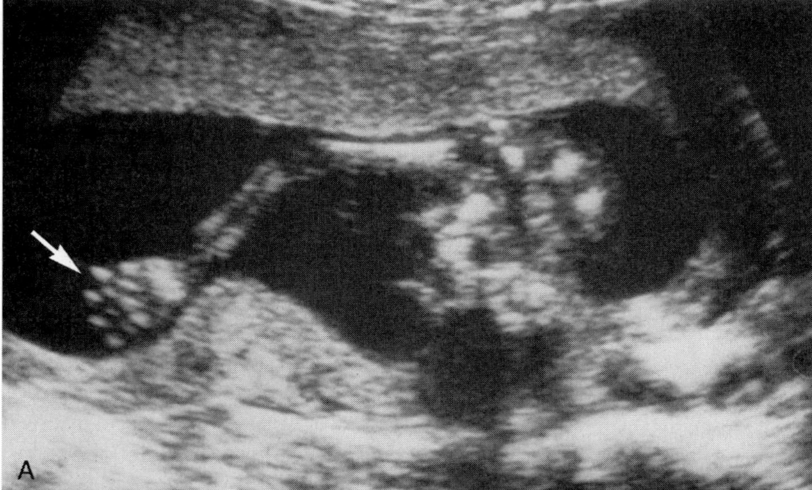


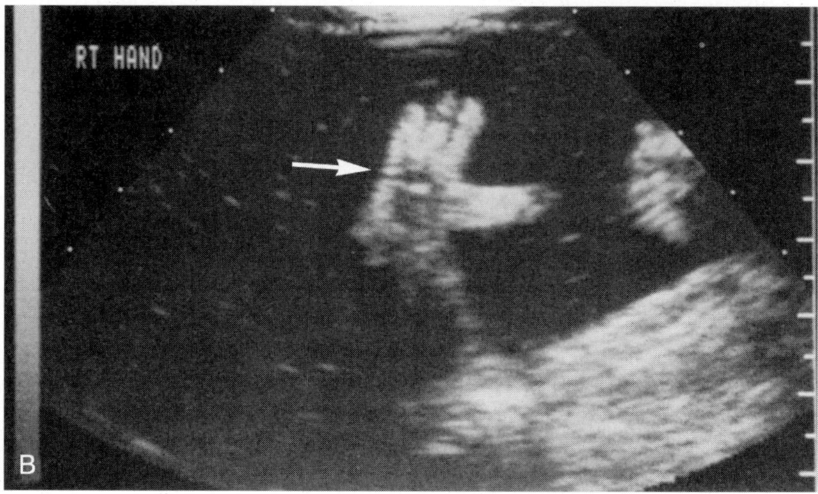


**Figure 18–5.** Ultrasonograms of hands (*arrows*) of normal fetus (*A*) and fetus with Holt-Oram syndrome (*B*), an autosomal dominant defect with heart and variable limb abnormalities. Hand picture (*B*) shows that there are only three obvious fingers and a thumb. The thumb is abnormal in shape (large and thick) and in position. (Photographs courtesy of A. Toi, Toronto General Hospital.)

TABLE 18–3

**Examples of Defects That Can Be Diagnosed or Ruled Out by Prenatal Diagnostic Ultrasound**

**Single-gene disorders**
Holoprosencephaly
Infantile polycystic kidney disease
Meckel-Gruber syndrome (an autosomal recessive disorder with encephalocele, polydactyly, and polycystic kidneys)
Fryns syndrome (an autosomal recessive disorder, generally perinatally lethal, with abnormalities of the face, diaphragm, limbs, genitourinary tract, and central nervous system)

**Disorders usually thought of as multifactorial**
Cleft lip
Club foot
Congenital heart defects
Neural tube defects

**Anomalies that may indicate a syndrome**
Abnormal genitalia
Cystic hygroma
Polydactyly
Omphalocele
Radial ray defects

management of the pregnancy, and delivery if the pregnancy is continued, and for genetic counseling with respect to future pregnancies.

**Prenatal Ultrasound for Single-Gene Disorders.** When a fetus is at risk for a single-gene disorder for which the precise genetic lesion is not known, detailed ultrasonography may sometimes be the only method of prenatal diagnosis possible. For example, the prenatal diagnosis of Meckel-Gruber syndrome (see Table 18–3) can at present be made only by ultrasound. Although the detection of a specific structural anomaly (e.g., encephalocele) signals the recurrence of this syndrome, the absence of detectable abnormalities does not entirely exclude the disorder, because structural abnormalities may be missed, owing either to variability in clinical presentation or the limitations of the procedure. Once the genes associated with this disorder have been identified, specific DNA testing will replace ultrasonography in the prenatal diagnosis of this condition.

In some cases for which DNA testing is possible but a blood or tissue sample is unavailable for DNA or protein studies, diagnostic ultrasonography can be appropriate even if the risk of recurrence is low. For example, a woman may present at 16 weeks' gestation stating that her previous pregnancy resulted in a stillbirth with features highly suggestive of the severe bone disorder osteogenesis imperfecta, type II (see Chapter 12); no autopsy was performed, and no tissue samples are available from the stillbirth. Osteogenesis imperfecta, type II, is usually due to a new dominant mutation, with an empiric recurrence risk of 6 percent due to germline mosaicism. In approximately 5 percent of families, however, the condition may be inherited in an autosomal recessive manner. Given that there is an increased recurrence risk of the disorder for this woman's current pregnancy, diagnostic ultrasonography is indicated. The finding of a normal fetus would be very reassuring, whereas the identification of a fetus with multiple fractures would guide the management of the remainder of the pregnancy. It should also be noted that some laboratories may be prepared to undertake collagen testing in such situations if the couple chooses to have earlier, although invasive, testing.

**Prenatal Ultrasound for Multifactorial Disorders.** A number of isolated abnormalities that may recur in families and that are believed to have multifactorial inheritance can also be identified by ultrasonography (see Table 18–3), including neural tube malformations (Fig. 18–6). Fetal echocardiography is offered at an increasing number of centers for a detailed assessment of pregnancies at risk for a congenital heart defect (Table 18–5).

**Determination of Fetal Sex.** Ultrasound can be used from 15 weeks of gestation onward to determine fetal sex. This determination may be an important prelude or adjunct in the prenatal diagnosis of X-linked disorders (e.g., hemophilia) for those women identified to be at increased risk. A couple may decide not to proceed with invasive testing if a female (and therefore unaffected) fetus is identified by ultrasound.

The equipment and techniques used by ultrasonographers now allow the detection of many malformations by routine ultrasonography. Once a malformation has been detected or is suspected on routine ultrasound, a detailed ultrasound study should be organized for further evaluation. In addition, a consultation with a clinical genetics unit/perinatal unit should be initiated for counseling and further investigation. The finding of a normal fetus can be cautiously reassuring, whereas the identification of a fetus with an abnormality allows the couple the option of either appropriate pregnancy and delivery management or pregnancy termination.

TABLE 18–4

**Prevalence of Fetal Chromosomal Defects in Fetuses with Selected Isolated and Multiple Sonographically Detected Abnormalities***

| | Chromosomal Defects (%) | |
|---|---|---|
| **Abnormality** | *Isolated Finding* | *Multiple Findings* |
| Ventriculomegaly | 2 | 17 |
| Choroid plexus cysts | 1 | 48 |
| Cystic hygroma | 52 | 71 |
| Nuchal edema | 19 | 45 |
| Diaphragmatic hernia | 2 | 49 |
| Heart defects | 16 | 66 |
| Duodenal atresia | 38 | 64 |
| Exomphalos | 8 | 46 |
| Renal abnormalities | 3 | 24 |

* These common ultrasound abnormalities are most typically associated with trisomy 21, trisomy 18, trisomy 13, or 45,X but can be associated with any chromosome abnormality. Adapted from Snijders RJM, Nicolaides KH (1996) Ultrasound Markers for Fetal Chromosomal Defects. The Parthenon Publishing Group, New York.

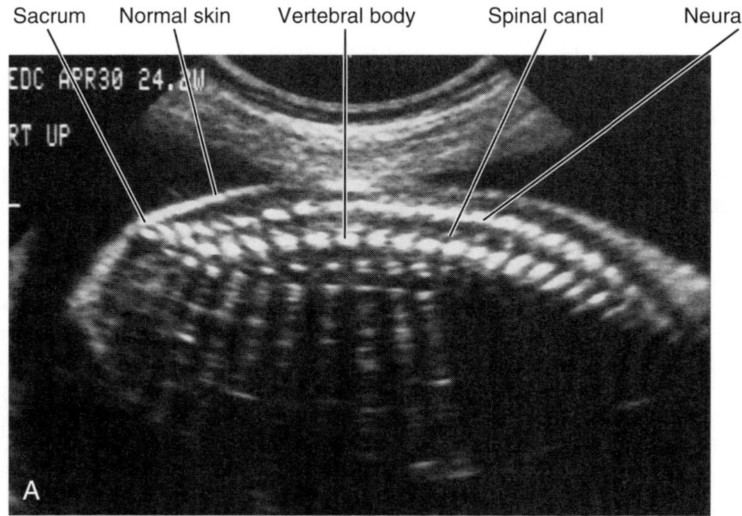


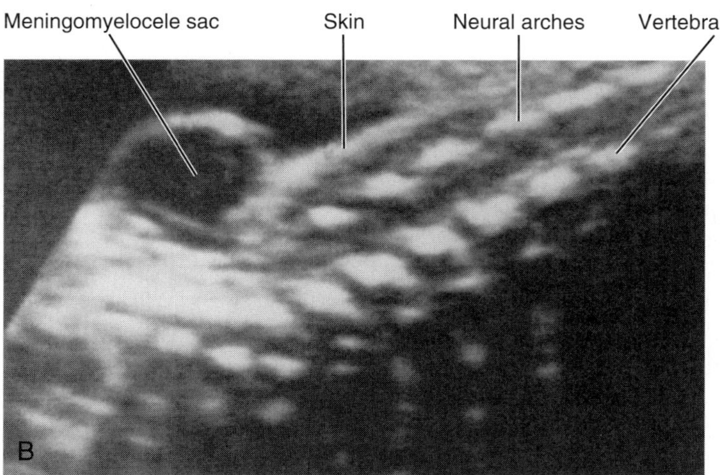


**Figure 18–6.** Ultrasonograms of spinal canal and neural tube in a normal fetus at 24 weeks' gestation (*A*) and a fetus with a neural tube defect (*B*). The *A* view is a longitudinal midline view, with the sacrum to the left, thoracic spine to the right. Note the two parallel rows of white echos that represent the neural arches. Also shown are echos of the vertebral bodies and the overlying intact skin. The *B* figure clearly shows the meningomyelocele sac protruding through the skin. Compare with Figure 15–7. (Photographs courtesy of A. Toi, Toronto General Hospital.)

TABLE 18–5
**Some Examples of Indications for Fetal Echocardiography***

**Maternal Indications** (% risk for congenital heart defect)
- Maternal disease
  - insulin dependent diabetes mellitus (3%–5%)
  - phenylketonuria (15%)
- Teratogen exposure
  - thalidomide (10% if 20–36 days post conception)
  - phenytoin (2%–3%)
  - alcohol (25% with fetal alcohol syndrome)
- Maternal heart disease (5%–10% risk for most lesions)
- Abnormal maternal triple screen

**Fetal Indications**
- Abnormal general fetal ultrasound
- Arrhythmia
- Chromosomal abnormalities
- Nuchal thickening
- Nonimmune hydrops fetalis

**Familial Indications**
- Mendelian syndromes (e.g., tuberous sclerosis, Noonan syndrome, velo-cardiofacial syndrome, Holt-Oram syndrome, Williams syndrome)
- Paternal heart disease (2%–5%)
- Previously affected child (2%–4%, higher for certain lesions)

* This list is not comprehensive, and indications vary between centers.

## EMERGING TECHNOLOGIES FOR PRENATAL DIAGNOSIS

### Preimplantation Genetic Diagnosis

Preimplantation genetic diagnosis is the use of molecular or cytogenetic techniques during **in vitro fertilization** (IVF) to select embryos free of a specific genetic condition for transfer to the uterus. This technology was developed in an effort to offer an alternative option to those couples opposed to pregnancy termination and at significant risk for a specific genetic disorder or aneuploidy in their offspring. Preimplantation genetic diagnosis can be performed using micromanipulation techniques to remove a polar body (see Chapter 2) or by biopsy of a single cell from a 6- to 8-cell blastomere after IVF. Molecular analysis using the polymerase chain reaction has been undertaken for a number of single-gene disorders and appears to give accurate results; chromosome abnormalities have also recently been diagnosed using fluorescence in situ hybridization (FISH) (see Chapters 4 and 9). The transfer of unaffected embryos is then undertaken after molecular or chromosomal analyses establish that the blastomere does not carry the genetic abnormality in question. The few data currently available on this technology suggest that there are no detrimental effects to embryos that have undergone biopsy. Affected embryos are discarded, although this latter practice has raised ethical concerns.

### Fetal Cells in Maternal Blood

As early as 1969, it was shown that the maternal circulation contained fetal cells at very low abundance. This discovery led to the realization that the isolation of fetal cells from maternal blood could be used as a noninvasive means of providing prenatal diagnosis of certain single-gene disorders as well as for chromosome analysis. Several fetal cell types can be separated from maternal blood by a variety of techniques and then selected using monoclonal antibodies. Enriched fetal cells can be used for chromosome analysis, sex determination, and molecular diagnosis of single-gene disorders. This technology is still at an early stage of development, and many important questions must be answered before this approach can be widely applied. One of the major scientific issues that must be addressed is identification of the ideal fetal target cell type for study. Although fetal lymphocytes may persist for many years in maternal blood, nucleated erythrocytes and trophoblast sprouts have been shown not to persist. The persistence of fetal lymphocytes in the maternal circulation may confound the use of fetal cell sampling in subsequent pregnancies. Other issues include the most appropriate time during gestation for sampling of maternal blood for fetal cells and determination of the fraction of fetal cells in these samples. It has been shown that there is an increased number of fetal cells in the maternal circulation in many cases of aneuploidy, especially trisomy 21, which may allow improved detection of such pregnancies.

## LABORATORY STUDIES

### Cytogenetics in Prenatal Diagnosis

Either amniocentesis or CVS can provide fetal cells for karyotyping, as well as for biochemical or DNA analysis. Preparation and analysis of chromosomes from cultured amniotic fluid cells or cultured chorionic villi require 1 to 2 weeks. Chorionic villi can be used for karyotyping after either short-term incubation or long-term culture. Short-term incubation, although providing a result more quickly, yields relatively poor-quality preparations in which the banding resolution is inadequate for detailed analysis. Most laboratories use both techniques, but if only one is used, long-term culture of the cells of the mesenchymal core is the technique of choice at present.

FISH (see Chapters 4 and 9) makes it possible to screen interphase nuclei in fetal cells for the common aneuploidies of chromosomes 13, 18, 21, X, and Y immediately after amniocentesis or CVS. This approach for rapid prenatal cytogenetic assessment is still being evaluated as a diagnostic tool.

#### Chromosome Analysis after Ultrasonography

Because some birth defects detectable by ultrasonography are associated with chromosome abnormalities, karyotyping of amniotic fluid cells, chorionic villus cells, or fetal blood cells obtained by cordocentesis may be indicated after ultrasonographic detection of such an abnormality. Chromosome abnormalities are more frequently found when multiple rather than isolated malformations are detected (see Table 18–4). The karyotypes most often seen in fetuses ascertained by abnormal ultrasonographic findings are the common autosomal trisomies (21, 18, and 13), 45,X (Turner syndrome), and unbalanced structural abnormalities. The presence of a cystic hygroma can indicate a 45,X karyotype, but it can also occur in Down syndrome and trisomy 18 as well as in fetuses with normal karyotypes. Thus, complete chromosome analysis is indicated.

#### Problems in Prenatal Chromosome Analysis

**Mosaicism.** Mosaicism refers to the presence of two or more cell lines in an individual or tissue sample. When mosaicism is found in cultured fetal cells, there may be problems in interpretation, regarding whether the fetus is truly mosaic and regarding the clinical significance of the observation.

Cytogeneticists distinguish three levels of mosaicism in amniotic fluid or CVS cell cultures:

(1) **True mosaicism**—detected in multiple colonies from several different primary cultures. Postnatal studies have confirmed that true mosaicism in culture is associated with a high risk that mosaicism is truly present in the fetus. The probability varies with different situations, however; mosaicism for structural aberrations of chromosomes, for example, is hardly ever confirmed.
(2) **Pseudomosaicism**—a single unusual cell, which can usually be disregarded.
(3) Mosaicism involving several cells or colonies of cells in a single primary culture only, which is difficult to interpret but is generally thought to reflect pseudomosaicism that has arisen in culture.

Maternal cell contamination is a possible explanation of some cases of apparent mosaicism with both XX and XY cell lines. It is more common in long-term CVS cultures than in amniotic fluid cell cultures, as a consequence of the intimate association between the chorionic villi and the maternal tissue (see Fig. 18–3). To minimize the risk of maternal cell contamination, any maternal decidua present in a chorionic villus sample must be carefully dissected and removed, although even the most careful dissection of chorionic villi does not eliminate every cell of maternal origin. When maternal cell contamination is suspected and cannot be disproved (e.g., by DNA genotyping using polymorphisms), amniocentesis is recommended to allow a second chromosome analysis.

In CVS studies, discrepancies between the karyotypes found in cytotrophoblast, villous stroma, and fetus have been reported in about 2 percent of pregnancies studied at 10 to 11 weeks' gestation. Mosaicism is sometimes present in the placenta but not present in the fetus, a situation termed **confined placental mosaicism** (Fig. 18–7). Occasionally, placental mosaicism with a normal cell line and a trisomic cell line has been reported when a liveborn infant or fetus has nonmosaic trisomy 13 or trisomy 18, the percentage of placental cells with a normal karyotype ranging from 12 to 100 percent. This finding suggests that when the zygote is trisomic, a normal placental cell lineage established by postzygotic loss of the additional chromosome in a progenitor cell of the cytotrophoblast can improve the probability of intrauterine survival of a trisomic fetus.

Confined placental mosaicism for any chromosome, but particularly for trisomy 15, raises the additional concern that the fetal diploidy may have actually arisen by "trisomy rescue." This term refers to the loss of an extra chromosome post-zygotically, an event that presumably allows fetal viability. If the fetus has retained two copies of chromosome 15 from one parent, however, the result is uniparental disomy (see Chapters 5 and 9). Because some genes on chromosome 15 are imprinted, uniparental disomy of this chromosome must be excluded because two maternal copies of chromosome 15 cause Prader-Willi syndrome and two paternal copies are associated with Angelman syndrome (see Chapter 5).

Confirming and interpreting mosaicism are among the most difficult challenges in genetic counseling for prenatal diagnosis because, at present, clinical outcome information on the numerous possible types and extents of mosaicism is inadequate. Further studies (amniocentesis that follows CVS, or cordocentesis that follows amniocentesis) and the medical literature may provide some guidance, but sometimes the interpretation still remains uncertain. Ultrasonographic scanning may provide some reassurance if normal growth is observed and if no congenital anomalies can be demonstrated.

Parents should be counseled in advance of the possibility that mosaicism may be found and that the interpretation of mosaicism may be uncertain. After birth, an effort should be made to verify any abnormal chromosome findings suspected on the basis of prenatal diagnosis. In the case of termination, verification should be sought by analysis of fetal tissues. Confirmation of mosaicism, or lack thereof, may prove helpful with respect to medical management issues, as well as for genetic counseling of the specific couple and for other family members.

**Culture Failure.** If couples are to have an opportunity to consider termination of a pregnancy when

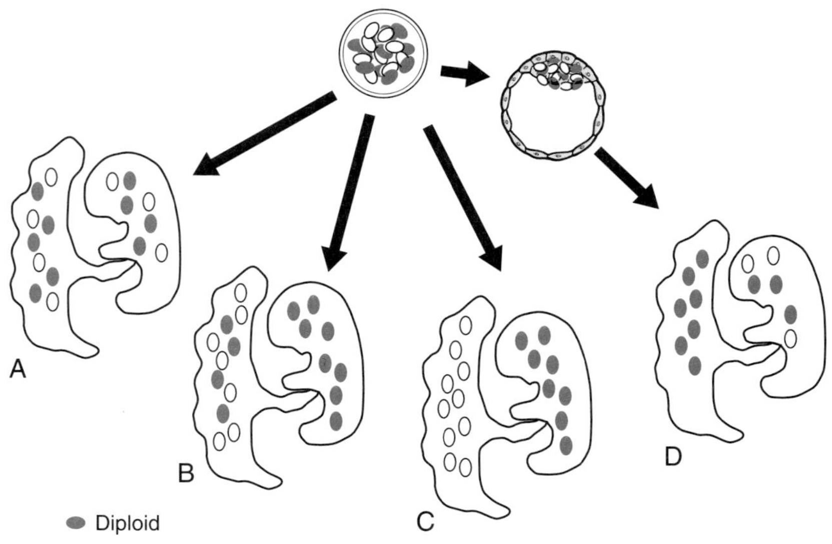


Figure 18–7. The different types of mosaicism that may be detected by prenatal diagnosis. *A*, Generalized mosaicism affecting both the fetus and placenta. *B*, Confined placental mosaicism with normal and abnormal cell lineages present. *C*, Confined placental mosaicism with only an abnormal cell lineage present. *D*, Mosaicism confined to the embryo. (Adapted from Kalousek DK [1994] Current topic: Confined placental mosaicism and intrauterine fetal development. Placenta 15: 219–230.)

an abnormality is found in the fetus, they need to be provided with the information at the earliest possible time. Because prenatal diagnosis is always a race against time, the rate of culture failure can be a concern; fortunately, this rate is low. When a CVS culture fails to grow, there is time to repeat the chromosome study with amniocentesis. If an amniotic fluid cell culture fails, either a repeat amniocentesis or a cordocentesis can be offered, depending on fetal age.

**Unexpected Adverse Findings.** Occasionally, prenatal chromosome analysis performed primarily to rule out aneuploidy reveals some other unusual chromosome finding: for example, a normal chromosome number but a common variant, a rare rearrangement, or a marker chromosome. In such a case, because the significance of the finding in the fetus cannot be assessed until the parental karyotypes are known, both parents should be karyotyped to determine whether the finding seen in the fetus is de novo or inherited. Unbalanced or de novo structural rearrangements may cause serious fetal abnormalities. If one parent is found to be a carrier of a structural rearrangement seen in unbalanced form in the fetus, the consequences for the fetus may be serious. On the other hand, if the same finding is seen in a normal parent, it is likely to be a benign change without untoward consequences. Potential exceptions to this guideline include the possibility of uniparental disomy (see Chapter 5) in a region of the genome that contains imprinted genes (see Fig. 9–13). In this situation, an inherited balanced rearrangement may cause serious fetal abnormalities. This possibility can be excluded if there has been a previous transmission of the same balanced rearrangement from a parent of origin of the same sex as the transmitting parent in the current pregnancy.

## Biochemical Assays for Metabolic Diseases

More than 100 metabolic disorders can be diagnosed prenatally in chorionic villus tissue or cultured amniotic fluid cells (Table 18–6), and a few rare conditions can even be identified directly by assay of a substance in amniotic fluid. Most metabolic disorders are rare in the general population but have a high recurrence risk (usually 25 percent within sibships, because most are autosomal recessive conditions). Because each condition is rare, the experience of the laboratory performing the prenatal diagnostic testing is very important; thus, referral to specialized centers is often desirable. Whenever possible, biochemical assay on direct CV tissue—as opposed to cultured tissue—is preferred, to avoid misinterpretation of results due to the expansion in culture of the number of contaminating maternal cells.

TABLE 18–6

**Examples of Metabolic Disorders Diagnosed by Enzyme Assay or DNA Analysis in Chorionic Villi or Cultured Amniotic Fluid Cells**

| |
|---|
| **Amino acid and organic acid disorders** |
| Phenylketonuria |
| Homocystinuria |
| Maple syrup urine disease |
| Methylmalonic acidemia |
| Propionic acidemia |
| **Carbohydrate disorders** |
| Galactosemia |
| Glycogen storage diseases, types II, III, IV |
| **Cholesterol and steroid metabolism disorders** |
| Smith-Lemli-Opitz syndrome |
| X-linked ichthyosis |
| **Lysosomal disorders** |
| Hurler syndrome |
| Krabbe disease |
| Niemann-Pick disease |
| Tay-Sachs disease |
| **Metal metabolism disorders** |
| Menkes syndrome |
| **Peroxisomal disorders** |
| Chondrodysplasia punctata |
| Zellweger syndrome |
| X-linked adrenoleukodystrophy |
| **Purine and pyrimidine disorders** |
| Adenosine deaminase deficiency |

Biochemical tests have one significant advantage over DNA analysis in some cases: whereas DNA analysis by direct detection of a mutation is accurate only for that mutation and not for other alleles at the locus, biochemical testing can detect abnormalities caused by any mutant allele that has a significant effect on the function of the protein. This advantage is particularly significant for disorders characterized by a high degree of allelic heterogeneity or by a high proportion of new mutations (i.e., X-linked recessive lethal disorders, see Chapter 5).

## DNA Analysis

Numerous disorders, many of which were not previously detectable prenatally, can now be diagnosed by DNA analysis (see Table 18–1). DNA analysis can be performed either by means of closely linked markers or by direct detection of the mutation. Any technique used for direct mutation screening (see Chapter 4) can be used for prenatal diagnosis. The number of disorders that can be diagnosed and the precision and efficiency of analysis are increasing rapidly as new approaches are developed, as new mutations are characterized, and as additional genetic diseases are mapped.

When possible, direct methods of detecting a particular mutation are preferred. Because the spectrum of mutations varies from disorder to disorder and often varies between racial and ethnic groups within a particular disorder, the application of DNA analysis to prenatal diagnosis remains highly specialized, except for common diseases such as cystic fibrosis and fragile X syndrome; specific diagnostic laboratories develop particular expertise for the subset of genetic disorders most often manifesting in their practice or research. The degree of certainty of the diagnosis approaches 100 percent when direct detection of a mutation is possible. As noted earlier, however, if the disorder in the patient is due to a different mutation from the one that is being sought, DNA analysis may fail to detect it. Furthermore, prenatal diagnosis by DNA analysis may not be predictive of the exact clinical presentation in an affected pregnancy; for example, in neurofibromatosis, type I, a specific mutation may lead to a severe clinical manifestation in one family member and a mild manifestation in another.

When application of direct methods of DNA diagnosis is impossible or impractical, the indirect approach of genetic linkage analysis can be used. If linked DNA markers are available, the accuracy of diagnosis depends on how closely linked the markers are to the disease gene and on whether appropriate family studies can be performed and are informative (see Chapters 8 and 19).

## THE EFFECT OF PRENATAL DIAGNOSIS ON THE PREVENTION AND MANAGEMENT OF GENETIC DISEASE

In the vast majority of cases, the findings in prenatal diagnosis are normal, and parents are reassured that their baby will be unaffected by the condition in question. Unfortunately, in a small proportion of cases, the fetus is found to have a serious genetic defect. Because effective prenatal therapy is not available for most disorders, the parents may then choose to terminate the pregnancy. Few issues today are as hotly debated as elective abortion, but despite legal restrictions in some areas, elective abortion is widely used. Among all elective abortions, those performed because of prenatal diagnosis of an abnormality in the fetus account for only a very small proportion. Without a means of legal termination of pregnancy, prenatal diagnosis would not have developed into the accepted procedure that it has become.

Some pregnant women who would not consider termination nevertheless request prenatal diagnosis to reduce anxiety or prepare for the birth of a child with a genetic disorder. The question then is whether the request is justified, because invasive techniques have an associated risk of fetal loss. In practice, the use of prenatal diagnosis by invasive techniques appears to be increasing because the risks are low compared with the couple's a priori risk and because many health care providers believe that parents are entitled to the information. This information may be used for psychological preparation as well as for management of the delivery and of the newborn infant.

At the population level, prenatal diagnosis combined with elective abortion has led to a major decline in the incidence of a few serious disorders, namely Tay-Sachs disease and $\beta$-thalassemia, in designated population groups. Prenatal diagnosis cannot reduce the gene frequency of these disorders, however (see Chapter 7). In fact, there is a possibility that the frequency of some deleterious genes will increase in the population if couples compensate for the loss of homozygotes by having additional children, who have a two-thirds risk of being heterozygotes.

The principal advantage of prenatal diagnosis is not to the population but to the immediate family. Parents at risk of having a child with a serious abnormality can undertake pregnancies that they may otherwise not have risked, with the knowledge that they can learn early in a pregnancy whether the fetus has the abnormality.

Parents and health professionals must give consideration to the ethical issues involved in prenatal diagnosis. New reproductive technologies have added to the ethical concerns. The difficulty, as always, is to balance the benefits to individuals against the interests of society as a whole. Health professionals, bioethicists, and the families with whom they work must remain aware of new developments in both applied and basic genetic research to make the most informed and ethically well-defined decisions possible. Indeed, the application of genetic knowledge to the improvement of human health is the ultimate goal of genetics in medicine (see Chapter 20).

## CONCLUSION

Prenatal diagnosis is a constantly changing field, with expanding knowledge and new technologies; thus, any attempt to define the state of the art rapidly becomes outdated. Health care providers must be aware of the likelihood of changes and the importance of obtaining access to the latest information, which should be available to them through prenatal diagnosis programs or genetic clinics. By the same token, genetic clinics must accept the responsibility of keeping current with new developments and the practicalities of obtaining access to them. Families who may use prenatal diagnosis should also be made aware of the importance of obtaining the latest information before undertaking a pregnancy or before making an irrevocable decision not to reproduce. Many couples at risk of having a child with a severe genetic disorder have been able to have healthy children because of prenatal diagnosis.

## General References


Brock DJH, Rodeck CH, Ferguson-Smith MA (1992) Prenatal Diagnosis and Screening. Churchill Livingstone, Edinburgh.

Canadian guidelines for prenatal diagnosis of genetic disorders: An update (1993) J Soc Obstet Gynaecol Can 15 Suppl:15–39.

Dimmick JE, Kalousek DK (1992) Developmental Pathology of the Embryo and Fetus. JB Lippincott, Philadelphia.

Harrison MR, Golbus MS, Filly RA (1991) The Unborn Patient, Prenatal Diagnosis and Treatment, 2nd ed. WB Saunders, Philadelphia.

Milunsky A (1998) Genetic Disorders and the Fetus: Diagnosis, Prevention, and Treatment, 4th ed. Johns Hopkins University Press, Baltimore.


## References Specific to Particular Topics


Brambati B, Tului L, Cislaghi C, et al (1998) First 10,000 chorionic villus samplings performed on singleton pregnancies by a single operator. Prenat Diagn 18:255–266.

Copel JA, Bahado-Singh RO (1999) Prenatal screening for Down's Syndrome—A search for the family's values. N Engl J Med 341:521–522.

Friedman AH, Copel JA, Kleinman CS (1993) Fetal echocardiography and fetal cardiology: Indications, diagnosis and management. Semin Perinatol 17:76–88.

Handyside AH (1996) Preimplantation genetic diagnosis today. Hum Reprod 11(Suppl 1):139–151.

Rhoads GG, Jackson LG, Schlesselman SE, et al (1989) The safety and efficacy of chorionic villus sampling for early prenatal diagnosis of cytogenetic abnormalities. N Engl J Med 320: 609–617.

Snijders RJM, Nicolaides KH (1996) Ultrasound Markers for Fetal Chromosomal Defects. Parthenon Publishing Group, New York.

The Canadian Early and Midtrimester Amniocentesis Trial (CEMAT) Group (1998) Randomised trial to assess safety and fetal outcome of early and midtrimester amniocentesis. Lancet 351:242–247.

Wald NJ, Watt HC, Hackshaw AK (1999) Integrated screening for Down's syndrome based on tests performed during the first and second trimesters. N Engl J Med 341:461–467.


## URLs for Web Resources Related to Prenatal Diagnosis

New York OnLine Access to Health (NOAH)
*http://www.noah-health.org/english/providers/mod.html#* TESTING
*http://www.noah-health.org/english/providers/mod.html#* POTENTIAL PROBLEMS AND RISKS
A joint effort by The City University of New York, The Metropolitan New York Library Council, The New York Academy of Medicine, and The New York Public Library to provide health information online. Includes information on prenatal diagnosis from the March of Dimes Birth Defects Foundation.

Society of Obstetricians and Gynaecologists of Canada *http://www.sogc.org/SOGCnet/sogc docs/common/guide/pdfs/ps75.pdf*
Practice guidelines for health care providers involved in prenatal screening and diagnosis

Genetests *http://www.genetests.org/* A US government supported website maintained by the University of Washington and Seattle Children's Hospital providing information on testing laboratories as well as educational material on genetic testing, including prenatal diagnosis.

## Problems

1. Match the term in the top section with the appropriate comment in the bottom section.
   (a) Rh immune globulin
   (b) 10th week of pregnancy
   (c) Cordocentesis
   (d) Mosaicism
   (e) 16th week of pregnancy
   (f) Alpha-fetoprotein in maternal serum
   (g) Aneuploidy
   (h) Cystic hygroma
   (i) Chorionic villi
   (j) Amniotic fluid
   _______ Method of obtaining fetal blood for karyotyping
   _______ Usual time at which amniocentesis is performed
   _______ Increased level when fetus has neural tube defect
   _______ Contains fetal cells viable in culture
   _______ Major cytogenetic problem in prenatal diagnosis
   _______ Ultrasonographic diagnosis indicates possible Turner syndrome
   _______ Risk increases with maternal age
   _______ Usual time at which CVS is performed
   _______ Derived from extraembryonic tissue
   _______ Used to prevent immunization of Rh-negative women
2. A couple has a child with Down syndrome, who has a 21q21q translocation inherited from the mother. Could prenatal diagnosis be helpful in the couple's next pregnancy? Explain.
3. Cultured cells from a chorionic villus sample show two cell lines: 46,XX and 46,XY. Does this necessarily mean the fetus is abnormal? Explain.
4. What two chief types of information about a fetus can be indicated (though not proved) by assay of alpha-fetoprotein, human chorionic gonadotrophin, and unconjugated estriol in maternal serum?
5. If all fetuses with the following disorders could be identified and the pregnancies were terminated, what would be the effect on the population frequency of the disease? On the population frequency of mutant alleles at the locus?
   (a) PKU
   (b) Neurofibromatosis, type 1
   (c) Huntington disease
6. A couple has had a first-trimester spontaneous abortion in their first pregnancy and requests counseling.
   (a) What proportion of all pregnancies abort in the first trimester?
   (b) What is the most common genetic abnormality found in such cases?
   (c) Assuming that there are no other indications, should this couple be offered prenatal diagnosis for their next pregnancy?
7. A young woman consults a geneticist during her first pregnancy. Her brother was previously diagnosed with

Duchenne muscular dystrophy and had since died. The woman had been tested biochemically and found to have elevated creatine kinase levels indicating she is a carrier of the disease.

Unfortunately, no DNA analysis had been conducted on the woman's brother to determine whether the mutation in his *DMD* gene was a deletion. The woman was investigated by molecular analysis and found to be heterozygous (A1/A2) for a microsatellite marker closely linked to the *DMD* gene. No relatives except the parents of the woman were available for analysis.

(a) Can the phase of the mutation in the woman be determined from analysis of the available individuals?
(b) Can this information be used to diagnose her pregnancy?
(c) What other molecular analysis could be performed on the fetus?

8. Discuss the relative advantages and disadvantages of the following diagnostic procedures and cite types of disorders for which they are indicated or not indicated: amniocentesis, CVS, and maternal serum screening.

19

# Genetic Counseling and Risk Assessment

## GENETIC COUNSELING

Clinical genetics is concerned with the diagnosis and management of the medical, social, and psychological aspects of hereditary disease. As in all other areas of medicine, it is essential to make a correct diagnosis and provide appropriate treatment, which must include helping the affected person and family members understand and come to terms with the nature and consequences of the disorder. When a disorder is suspected of being heritable, however, there is an added dimension: the need to inform other family members of their risk and the means available to them to modify these risks. Just as the unique feature of genetic disease is its tendency to recur within families, the unique aspect of genetic counseling is its focus, not only on the original patient, but also on members of the patient's family, both present and future. Genetic counseling, a core activity in medical genetics, is concerned not only with informing the patient and family but also with providing psychologically oriented counseling to help individuals adapt and adjust to the impact and implications of the disorder in the family.

This chapter focuses on the role of the genetic counselor in providing information and risk assessment. The much broader topic of the psychological aspects of counseling is beyond the scope of this chapter, and the reader is referred to the General References listed at the end of the chapter.

### Common Indications for Genetic Counseling

Table 19–1 lists some of the most common situations that lead people to pursue genetic counseling. Often, the persons seeking genetic counseling (the **consultands**) are the parents of a child with a potential or known genetic condition, but the consultand may be an adult with an abnormality or a family history of an abnormality. Genetic counseling is also an integral part of prenatal testing (see Chapter 18) and of genetic testing and screening programs (discussed in Chapter 20).

TABLE 19–1

**Common Indications for Referral**

1. Previous child with multiple congenital anomalies, mental retardation or an isolated birth defect, such as neural tube defect, cleft lip and palate
2. Family history of a hereditary condition, such as cystic fibrosis, fragile X syndrome, or diabetes
3. Prenatal diagnosis for advanced maternal age or other indication
4. Consanguinity
5. Teratogen exposure, such as to occupational chemicals, medications, alcohol
6. Repeated pregnancy loss or infertility
7. Newly diagnosed abnormality or genetic condition
8. Before undertaking genetic testing and after receiving results, particularly when testing for susceptibility to late-onset disorders, such as cancer or neurological disease
9. As follow-up for a positive newborn test, as with PKU, or a heterozygote screening test, such as Tay-Sachs

### The Process of Genetic Counseling

Established standards of medical care require that providers of genetic services obtain a history that includes family and ethnic information, advise patients of the genetic risks to them and other family members, offer genetic testing or prenatal diagnosis when indicated, and outline the various treatment or management options for reducing the risk of disease. Generally, patients are not told what decisions to make with regard to the various testing and management options but, instead, are provided information and support; this approach to counseling, referred to as **nondirective counseling**, has been adopted widely as the standard of practice in this field. It should be emphasized that genetic counseling is not limited to the provision of information and calculation of the risk for disease, but is rather a communication process. The ability to define and address the complex psychosocial issues associated with a genetic disorder in a family is central to this practice. Addressing these issues may be most effectively accomplished over time through periodic contact with the family as the medical or social issues become relevant to the lives of those involved.

## The Role of Genetic Counselors

Genetic counseling in the past was often provided by a physician as an integral part of the clinical management of the patient and family; indeed, genetic counseling still remains an important component of medical genetics practice. As the body of genetic knowledge and the extent and sophistication of laboratory diagnosis have expanded, so has the demand for education and counseling to help patients and their families deal with the many complex issues raised by genetic disease. Clinical genetics is particularly time-consuming in comparison with other clinical fields because it requires extensive preparation and follow-up in addition to direct patient contact. Increasingly, genetic counseling services are being provided by **genetic counselors**, qualified professionals trained in genetics *and* counseling who serve as members of a health care team along with physician geneticists or other physician specialists (e.g., in an obstetrical practice, orthopedic clinic, or cancer clinic). Genetic counseling in the United States and Canada is a self-regulating health profession with its own board (the American Board of Genetic Counselors) that oversees the accreditation of training programs and certification of practitioners.

Genetic counselors play an essential role in clinical genetics, participating in many aspects of the investigation and management of genetic problems. A genetic counselor is often the first point of contact that a patient makes with clinical genetic services, provides genetic counseling directly to consultands, helps patients and families deal with the many psychological and social issues that arise during genetic counseling, and continues in a supportive role and as a source of information after the clinical investigation and formal counseling have been completed. Counselors are also very active in the field of genetic testing; they provide close liaison among the referring physicians, the diagnostic laboratories, and the families themselves. Their special expertise is invaluable to clinical laboratories, because explaining and interpreting genetic testing to patients and referring physicians often requires a sophisticated knowledge of genetics and genomics, as well as good communication skills.

## Prevention of Recurrence in Families

For many families seeking genetic counseling, one of the major goals is to ascertain the risk for heritable disease in their children and to learn what options are available for preventing recurrence of the particular genetic disorder in question. Although prenatal diagnosis is one approach that can often be offered to families, it is by no means a universal solution to the risk of genetic problems in offspring. There are many disorders for which prenatal diagnosis is not feasible, and for many parents, it is not an acceptable option even if available. Other measures available for management of recurrence include the following:

1. Genetic laboratory tests (karyotyping, biochemical analysis, or DNA analysis) sometimes reassure couples with a family history of a genetic disorder that they themselves are *not* at increased risk of having a child with a specific genetic disease. In other cases, such tests indicate that the couple is at increased risk. Genetic counseling is recommended both before and after such testing to assist consultants in making an informed decision to undergo testing as well as to understand and use the information gained through testing.
2. If the parents plan to have no more children or no children at all, **contraception or sterilization** may be their choice, and they may need information about the possible procedures or an appropriate referral.
3. For parents who want a child or more children, **adoption** is a possibility.
4. **Artificial insemination** may be appropriate if the father has a gene for an autosomal dominant or X-linked defect or has a heritable chromosome defect, but it is obviously not indicated if it is the mother who has such a defect. Artificial insemination is also useful if both parents are carriers of an autosomal recessive disorder. In vitro fertilization with a **donated egg** may be appropriate if the mother has a gene for an autosomal defect or carries an X-linked defect. In either case, genetic counseling and appropriate genetic tests of the sperm or egg donor should be part of the process.
5. In some disorders, DNA analysis of embryos in the preimplantation stage can be carried out using the polymerase chain reaction of a single cell obtained from an early embryo generated by in vitro fertilization (see Chapters 17 and 18). For some parents, a decision to not implant an embryo found to be abnormal would be much more acceptable than abortion at a later stage.

If the parents decide to terminate a pregnancy, provision of relevant information and support is an appropriate part of genetic counseling. Periodic follow-up through additional visits or by telephone is often arranged for a year or more after a pregnancy termination.

### Psychological Aspects

Patients and families dealing with a risk for a genetic disorder or coping with the actual occurrence of the disorder are subject to varying degrees of emotional and social stress. Although this is also true of nongenetic disorders, the concern generated by knowledge that the condition might recur, the guilt or censure felt by some individuals, and the need for reproductive decisions can give rise to severe distress. Many persons have the strength to deal personally with such problems; they prefer receiving even bad news to remaining uninformed, and they make their own decisions on the basis of the most complete and accurate information they can obtain. Other persons require much more support and may need referral for psychotherapy. The psychological aspects of genetic counseling are beyond the scope of this book, but several books cited in the General References at the end of this chapter give an introduction to this important field.

### Support Organizations

Organizations devoted to self-help are used by many families. These organizations, usually focused on a single disease or a group of diseases, can help those concerned to share their experience with others facing the same problem, to learn how to deal with the day-to-day problems caused by the disorder, to hear of new developments in therapy or prevention, and to promote research into the condition. Many support groups have Internet sites and electronic chat rooms through which patients and families give and receive information and advice, ask and answer questions, and obtain much-needed emotional support. Referral to support groups is often undertaken by genetics centers. A coalition known as the Genetic Alliance has been formed to coordinate the activities of the many individual groups.

## CASE MANAGEMENT IN GENETIC COUNSELING

Although genetic counseling case management must be individualized for each patient's needs and situation, a generic approach can be summarized as shown in Table 19–2.

**Genetic Counseling**

The purpose of genetic counseling is to provide information and support to families at risk for having or who already have members with birth defects or genetic disorders. Genetic counseling helps the family or individual to:

1. Comprehend the medical facts, including the diagnosis, the probable course of the disorder, and the available management;
2. Understand the way heredity contributes to the disorder and the risk of recurrence for themselves and other family members;
3. Understand the options for dealing with the risk of recurrence;
4. Identify those values, beliefs, goals, and relationships affected by the risk for or presence of hereditary disease;
5. Choose the course of action that seems most appropriate to them in view of their risk, their family goals, and their ethical and religious standards; and
6. Make the best possible adjustment to the disorder or to the risk of recurrence of that disorder, or both, by providing supportive counseling to families and making referrals to appropriate support services or groups, or both.

### An Example of Genetic Case Management

To provide an appreciation of the process of genetic counseling, we consider a hypothetical referral for prenatal counseling as an example of one of the more common situations faced by counselors.

B.D. is referred to the genetics clinic at 16.5 weeks' gestation because of a positive maternal serum screen (MSS) for Down syndrome (see Chapter 18); she is 30 years of age, and her MSS result indicates that her risk for having a baby with Down syndrome is now increased to that of a 37-year-old.

#### Preassessment

##### Family History

B.D.'s concerns and the quality of any previous information she has received must first be assessed. She, and her partner if he is present, would then be given an idea of what to expect during the process of genetic counseling (this may be done either by telephone or in person). The next step would be to take a detailed pedigree (Fig. 19–1), which reveals that B.D.'s brother is developmentally delayed.

TABLE 19–2

**Genetic Counseling Case Management**

| |
|---|
| **Collection of information** |
| Family history (questionnaire) |
| Medical history |
| Tests and/or additional assessments |
| **Assessment** |
| Physical examination |
| Validation or establishment of diagnosis—if possible |
| **Counseling** |
| Nature and consequence of disorder |
| Recurrence risk |
| Availability of further or future testing |
| Decision making |
| Referral to other specialists, health agencies, support groups |
| **Follow-up** |
| Continuing clinical assessment, especially if no diagnosis |
| Psychosocial support |

### MEDICAL HISTORY

B.D.'s pregnancy history would first be obtained; it has been uncomplicated to this point. In an attempt to then determine the etiology of the developmental delay in B.D.'s brother (see pedigree, Fig. 19–1), one would request medical records and attempt to schedule an assessment for him. Although there is not a great deal of time to sort out a potential risk for B.D.'s pregnancy, the request for outside records might still be undertaken, because accuracy in establishing a diagnosis is critical to the provision of genetic counseling. B.D. tells you that her family has never discussed her brother's problems, and she was always given to understand that he "was born normal" and then experienced brain damage due to a fever. He is not known to have any congenital anomalies; she will bring in some family photographs.

### ASSESSMENT AND INVESTIGATIONS

Because B.D. and her partner are not consanguineous, autosomal recessive etiologies should not pose an increased risk to this pregnancy. The genetics team would then consider possible causes of developmental delay in B.D.'s brother that might pose a risk for the pregnancy. Such causes would likely include chromosome abnormality due to a heritable structural rearrangement, fragile X syndrome, and other X-linked causes of mental retardation. Specific testing is available for the first two potential causes.

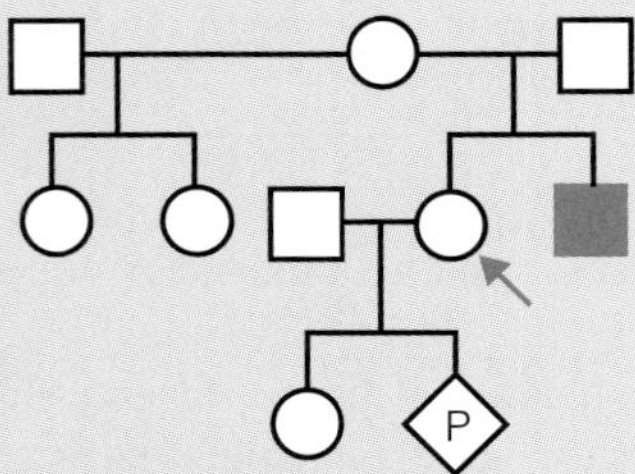


**Figure 19–1.** Pedigree of family of consultand. The consultand has been referred for an elevated maternal serum screen and reports that she has a brother with developmental delay (*filled-in symbol*). Notation is as in Bennett RL, Steinhaus KA, Urich SB, et al (1996) Recommendations for standardized pedigree nomenclature. J Genet Counsel 4:26.

## Genetic Counseling

In approaching the case at hand, the genetic counselor might begin by outlining the two primary issues to be discussed: the MSS results and the family history of developmental delay. A discussion of the MSS results would include reviewing the limitations of this testing, the risk estimate and how this couple personally interprets risks, a brief discussion of Down syndrome, and the options available for them with respect to the pregnancy. These options include amniocentesis to determine the fetal karyotype, continuing the pregnancy without invasive testing, or perhaps if they remain undecided, detailed ultrasound to provide additional, although limited, information.

At this point, the genetic counselor could bring B.D.'s family history into the discussion and B.D.'s concern about having a child with the same disorder as her brother. The options available for providing further clarification would be reviewed (i.e., examining B.D.'s blood to rule out a structural chromosome rearrangement and to allow molecular testing for fragile X carrier status). In addition, if this couple feels strongly about proceeding with amniocentesis because of the MSS result, the amniocytes could also be sent to a laboratory for molecular testing for fragile X syndrome if B.D. proves to be a carrier. The discussion would also involve the specific tests to be undertaken, including an assessment of *FMR1* trinucleotide expansion size and methylation (see Chapter 12) and the difficulty inherent in determining a phenotype in the event that the fetus is female and carries an expanded repeat. One would also explore how the parents might feel about such a result and how they view their options, that is, continuing or terminating the pregnancy. Finally, the genetic counselor must not leave the impression that if the amniocentesis reveals neither a chromosome abnormality nor a fragile X mutation, the fetus will be free of any genetic disease or birth defects. The residual risk for a birth defect (2 to 3 percent) faced by *all* pregnant couples should still be reviewed with the consultands.

## Follow-up

B.D. is, in fact, found to be a heterozygote for an expanded fragile X syndrome repeat, and her amniocentesis reveals a male fetus with a normal karyotype and with a CGG repeat length in the normal range. Knowing her carrier status leads to the likely conclusion that B.D.'s brother has fragile X syndrome and that their mother is a carrier. Again, this finding has implications for B.D.'s half-sisters because they may also be carriers (see Fig. 19–1). B.D. would be encouraged to share this information with her sisters, and the counselor would recommend that they seek genetic counseling and, if desired, testing. The responsibility of the physician and genetic counselor to inform, however, does not extend beyond the consultand to other family members. Many geneticists and counselors involve bioethicists to obtain guidance in establishing guidelines for appropriate practice. It is generally accepted that the consultand is entitled to confidentiality and that this confidentiality cannot be broken without the consultand's consent, unless exceptional circumstances indicate that the harm from failing to disclose greatly outweighs the harm caused by disclosure of confidential information (see Chapter 20).

As B.D. is a carrier of fragile X syndrome, she may return to raise the issue of testing for her daughter. Most geneticists and genetic counselors counsel against carrier testing for young children at an age when they are incapable of offering informed assent, because this interferes with the child's own autonomy and confidentiality. There are, however, circumstances in which the testing could have immediate medical or psychosocial benefits to the child and her family, benefits that outweigh the potential harm caused by testing.

## DETERMINING RECURRENCE RISKS

The estimation of recurrence risks is a central concern in genetic counseling. Ideally, it is based on knowledge of the genetic nature of the disorder in question and on the pedigree of the particular family being counseled. The family member whose risk of a genetic disorder is to be determined is usually a relative of a proband, such as a sib of an affected child or a living or future child of an affected adult. In some families, especially for some autosomal dominant and X-linked traits, it may also be necessary to estimate the risk for more remote relatives.

When a disorder is known to have single-gene inheritance, the recurrence risk for specific family members can usually be determined from basic mendelian principles discussed in Chapter 5 (Fig. 19–2). On the other hand, risk calculations may be less than straightforward if there is reduced penetrance or variability of expression or if disease is frequently the result of new mutation, such as in many X-linked and autosomal dominant disorders. Laboratory tests that give equivocal results can add further complications. Under these circumstances, mendelian risk estimates can sometimes be modified by means of **Bayesian analysis** of the pedigree (see later), which takes into account information about the family that may increase or decrease the previous mendelian risk.

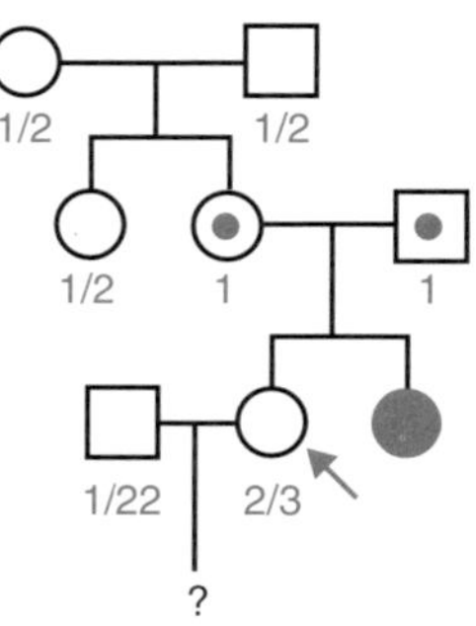


Figure 19–2. Mendelian risk estimates in genetic counseling. The consultand's sister is affected with an autosomal recessive condition, in this example cystic fibrosis (CF). The risk of other family members being carriers can be determined through mendelian principles and is indicated in the pedigree. The risk of the consultand having an affected child is $2/3 \times 1/22 \times 1/4$, or less than 1 percent.

In contrast to single-gene disorders, the underlying mechanisms of inheritance for most chromosomal disorders and complex traits are unknown, and estimates of recurrence risk are based on previous experience (Fig. 19–3). This approach is all very well if there are good data on the frequency of recurrence of the disorder in families and if the phenotype is not heterogeneous. However, when a particular phenotype has an undetermined risk or can result from a variety of causes with different frequencies and with widely different risks, estimation of the recurrence risk is hazardous at best. In a later section, the estimation of recurrence risk in some typical clinical situations, both straightforward and more complicated, is considered.

### Risk Estimation When Genotypes Are Known

The simplest risk estimates apply to families in which the relevant genotypes of all family members are known or can be inferred. For example, if both mem-

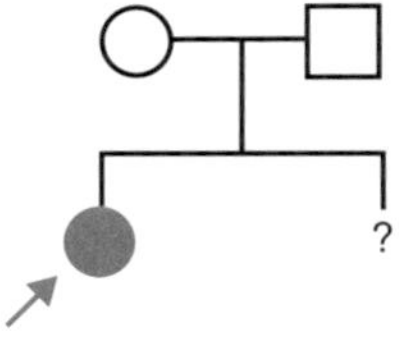


Figure 19–3. Empiric risk estimates in genetic counseling. A family with no other positive family history has one child affected with a disorder known to be multifactorial or chromosomal. What is the recurrence risk? If the child is affected with spina bifida, the empiric risk to a subsequent child is approximately 4 percent (see Chapter 15). If the child has Down syndrome, the empiric risk of recurrence would be approximately 1 percent if the karyotype were trisomy 21, but it might be substantially higher if one of the parents were a carrier of a Robertsonian translocation involving chromosome 21 (see Chapter 10).

bers of a couple are known to be heterozygous carriers of an autosomal recessive condition, and one is interested in the chance of the couple having another affected child, the risk (probability) is one in four with each pregnancy that the child will inherit the disease. Even if the couple has had six unaffected children subsequent to the affected child, the risk in the 8th, 9th, or 10th pregnancy is still one in four for each pregnancy.

Even when all the relevant genotypes are not completely known, the risk of being a carrier can be estimated from the Hardy-Weinberg equation (see Chapter 7). For example, the chance that a known carrier of cystic fibrosis (CF) might have an affected child depends on the chance that the other partner in the mating is a carrier. The risk of the partner being a carrier depends on the ethnic background (see Chapters 6 and 7). For the general Caucasian population, this chance is 1/22. Because the chance that the child of two carriers would be homozygous for the mutant CF allele is 1/4, the chance that a known carrier and his unrelated partner would have an affected first child is the product of these probabilities, or $1/22 \times 1/4 = 1/88$ (about 1 percent). In this discussion, it is assumed, of course, that there is no way to determine whether the other partner is a heterozygote at the locus in question; although this is true for most autosomal recessive conditions, most (although not yet all) carriers for CF can be readily identified by DNA testing.

## Risk Estimation When Alternative Genotypes Are Possible

In contrast to the simple case described, situations arise in which the genotypes of the relevant individuals in the family are not definitively known; the risk of recurrence will be very different depending on whether or not the consultand is a carrier of an abnormal allele of a disease gene. Obviously, if one can test directly for the mutant allele, the uncertainty of carrier status can be resolved. In other situations, however, (thankfully, fewer and fewer because of progress in molecular genetics), one cannot test carrier status directly. **Bayesian analysis** (based on Bayes' theorem on probability, published in 1763) is a method of using *phenotypic* information in a pedigree to assess the relative probability of two or more alternative possibilities; for example, whether an individual does or does not carry a particular mutant allele. Some examples of the use of Bayesian analysis for risk assessment in pedigrees are examined in this section.

### X-Linked Pedigrees

To illustrate the value of Bayesian analysis, consider the pedigrees shown in Figure 19–4. In Family A, the mother II-1 is an **obligate carrier** for hemophilia A because her father was affected. Her risk of transmitting the hemophilia gene is 1/2, and the fact that she has already had four unaffected sons does *not* reduce this risk. Thus, the risk that the consultand (III-5) is a carrier is 1/2, and the overall risk of her having an affected child is 1/2 (the risk she is a carrier) $\times$ 1/2 (the risk of transmitting the gene) $\times$ 1/2 (the chance of having a son) = 1/8. In Family B, however, the consultand's mother (individual II-2) may or may not be a carrier depending on whether she has inherited the hemophilia A allele from her mother I-1. If III-5 were the only child of her mother, her risk of having an affected child would be 1/2 (her mother's risk of being a carrier) $\times$ 1/2 (her risk of inheriting the mutant allele from her mother) = 1/4 (25 percent), and her risk of having an affected child would be 1/4 (her carrier risk) $\times$ 1/4 (the risk of transmitting the gene to an affected son) = 1/16 (approximately 6 percent). Short of testing III-5 directly for the mutant allele, we cannot tell whether she is a carrier. In this case, however, the fact that III-5 has four unaffected brothers is relevant; one begins to suspect that maybe her mother is not a carrier. Before her childbearing, there is no additional information of any kind to indicate whether II-2 is or is not a carrier; because II-2 is the daughter of a female carrier, both possibilities are

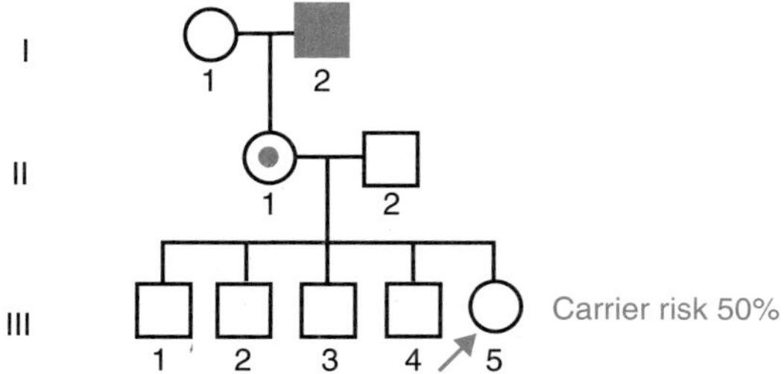


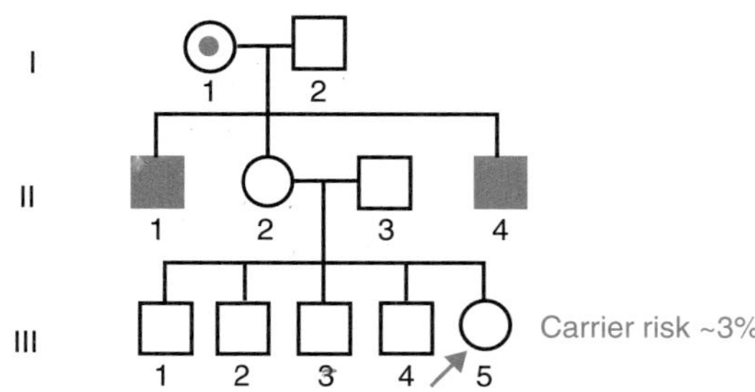


**Figure 19–4.** Modified risk estimates in genetic counseling. The consultands in the two families are at risk for having a son with hemophilia A. In Family A, the consultand's mother is an obligate heterozygote; in Family B, the consultand's mother may or may not be a carrier. Application of Bayesian analysis reduces the risk of being a carrier to only approximately 3 percent for the consultand in Family B but not the consultand in Family A. See text for derivation of the modified risk.

equally likely. Every time II-2 has a son, however, the chance that the son would be unaffected is only 1/2 if II-2 *were* a carrier, whereas it is a near certainty (probability = 1) that the son would be unaffected if II-2 were, in fact, *not* a carrier at all. With each son, II-2 has, in effect, tested her carrier status by placing herself at a 50 percent chance of having an unaffected son; it would seem intuitively obvious that having four unaffected sons must shift the odds in favor of her not being a carrier. Bayesian analysis allows one to take this kind of indirect information into account when calculating whether or not II-2 is a carrier, thus modifying the consultand's risk of being a carrier and of having an affected child. Indeed, overall, the consultand's risk of being a carrier of the hemophilia gene is only about 3 percent rather than 25 percent. Consequently, her risk of having an affected child is less than 1 percent, not 6 percent.

How did we arrive at these figures for Family B? To translate this intuition into actual risk calculation, we use a Bayesian probability calculation. Identify the alternative hypotheses and label one column (see below) for each hypothesis. In each column, fill in the appropriate probability values as follows. "Prior probability" is the initial chance of each hypothesis being correct without knowing anything more about the family pedigree. The "conditional probability" in each column is the probability, under the hypothesis for that column, that events that you know have already occurred (i.e., facts you have obtained about the pedigree) could occur under the assumption that the hypothesis at the top of that column is correct. (The conditional probabilities in each of the columns do NOT have to add up to 1 because they represent probabilities of events occurring under very different assumptions and they do not cover all possibilities.) The "joint probability" is the product of the prior and conditional probabilities. All of these different probabilities allow us to make the calculation we really want: the relative probability of one hypothesis versus the other, taking all the available conditional information into account. This calculation is called the "posterior probability," in which one joint probability is weighed against the other.

| | **Hypothesis 1** | **Hypothesis 2** |
|---|---|---|
| | *II-2 Is a Carrier* | *II-2 Is NOT a Carrier* |
| Prior probability | 1/2 | 1/2 |
| Conditional probability | $(1/2)^4 = 1/16$ | 1 |
| Joint probability | $1/2 \times 1/16 = 1/32$ | $1/2 \times 1 = 1/2$ |
| Posterior probability | $\frac{1/32}{1/32 + 1/2} = 1/17$ | $\frac{1/2}{1/32 + 1/2} = 16/17$ |

In Family B, we must first determine the risk that her mother (II-2) is a carrier before calculating the modified risk for the consultand (III-5). II-2 is the daughter of an obligate female carrier of the hemophilia A gene. *There are two alternative hypotheses*: either II-2 *is* a carrier or II-2 is *not* a carrier. Her mendelian risk that she is a carrier (called the **prior probability**) is 1/2; the prior probability that she is *not* a carrier is, of course, also 1/2. We label two columns: II-2 is a carrier and II-2 is not a carrier.

Next, we consider the probabilities that all four unaffected sons would inherit a normal allele at the X-linked factor VIII locus from their mother, given the two hypothetical conditions, that she *is* a carrier and that she is *not* a carrier; these are called the **conditional probabilities.** If II-2 is a carrier, the chance that all four sons would be unaffected is $(1/2)^4$, or 1/16. If, on the other hand, she is not a carrier, the probability that her sons would be unaffected is essentially 1.

We next consider the **joint probability**, which is the product of the prior and conditional risks. The joint probability assuming II-2 *is* a carrier with four normal sons is 1/2 (her prior risk of being a carrier) × 1/16 (the conditional risk of having four normal sons in such a case), or 1/32. The joint probability assuming II-2 is *not* a carrier is 1/2 × 1, or 1/2.

Now we can calculate the **posterior probability** that II-2 is a carrier. Given that her four sons are normal, there is a 1/32 chance that she is a carrier and a 1/2 chance that she is not; therefore, the posterior probability, expressed as a fraction that II-2 is a carrier, is

$$\frac{1/32}{(1/2 + 1/32)} = 1/17$$

and the final probability that she is *not* a carrier is 16/17.

Finally, then, the consultand's risk of being a carrier is half her mother's risk, which is 1/2 × 1/17 = 1/34, or approximately 3 percent. Thus, application of Bayes' theorem to modify the mendelian risk has reduced the consultand's prior risk of being a carrier from 25 percent to a final risk of only 3 percent.

For every additional child without disease born to II-2 in Family B, the probability that III-5 is a carrier falls, not because the independent assortment of chromosomes and the laws of mendelian inheritance are changing, but because the joint, and therefore the posterior, probability that II-2 is a carrier is changing. Similarly, if III-5 also has unaffected sons, her carrier risk could also be modified downward using a Bayesian calculation. If II-2 were to have an affected child, then she would have proved herself a carrier, and III-5's risk in Family B would become the same as it is in Family A = 1/2. Of course, if III-5 were to have an affected child, then she must be a carrier, and Bayesian analysis would no longer be necessary because there would only be one possible hypothesis: III-5 is a carrier.

Bayesian analysis may seem like mere statistical maneuvering. However, the analysis allows genetic counselors to quantify what seemed to be intuitively likely from inspection of the pedigree: the fact that the consultand had four unaffected brothers provides support for the hypothesis that her mother is not a carrier. The analysis having been performed, the final risk that III-5 is a carrier can be used in genetic counseling. The risk that her first child will have hemophilia A is 1/34 × 1/4, or less than 1 percent. This risk is appreciably below the prior probability estimated without taking into account the genetic evidence provided by her brothers.

### Isolated Cases of X-Linked Disorders

Because any severe X-linked disorder is manifested in the hemizygous male, an isolated case (no family history) of such a disorder may represent either a new gene mutation (in which case the mother is not a carrier) or may represent inheritance of a mutant allele from his unaffected carrier mother (we ignore the small but real chance of mosaicism for the mutation in the mother). Estimating the recurrence risk depends on knowing the chance she could be a carrier. Bayesian analysis can be used to estimate carrier risks in X-linked lethal disease such as Duchenne muscular dystrophy (DMD) or ornithine transcarbamylase (OTC) deficiency.

Consider the family at risk for DMD shown in Figure 19–5. There are three possible explanations for this isolated case of DMD, each with dramatically different risk estimates for the family:

A. III-1's condition may be the result of a new mutation. In this case, none of his female relatives will be at significant risk of being a carrier.
B. His mother, II-1, is a carrier, but her condition is the result of a new mutation. In this case, her daughter (III-2) has a 1/2 risk of being a carrier, and her granddaughter (IV-1) has a 1/4 risk. None of the other female relatives would be at significant risk, however.
C. His mother inherited a mutant allele from her mother (I-1), who is also a carrier. In this case, all of the female relatives have either a 1/2 or a 1/4 risk of being carriers.

The prior probability that each woman is or is not a carrier can be calculated under certain simple assumptions about the mutation rate, $\mu$ (see Box).

Now, Bayesian analysis can be applied.

**Bayesian Calculations for Mothers of Isolated Cases of X-Linked Lethal Disorders**

| | Hypothesis 1<br>*II-1 Is a Carrier* | Hypothesis 2<br>*II-1 Is NOT a Carrier* |
|---|---|---|
| Prior probability | $4\mu$ | $1 - 4\mu \approx 1$ |
| Conditional probability | 1/2 | $\mu$ |
| Joint probability | $4\mu \times 1/2 = 2\mu$ | $1 \times \mu$ |
| Posterior probability | $\frac{2\mu}{2\mu + \mu} = 2/3$ | $\frac{\mu}{2\mu + \mu} = 1/3$ |

Thus, the final probability that the mother of an isolated case of an X-linked lethal disorder is a carrier is 2/3, and the corresponding probability that the patient represents a new mutation must be 1/3. We are ignoring the small but very real possibility of germline mosaicism in these calculations (see Chapter 5).

Finally, the probability that the maternal grandmother of an isolated case (e.g., see I-1 in Fig. 19–5) is a carrier can be calculated in a similar way, except the conditional probabilities are now different. If I-1 is a carrier, the probability of having an affected grandson is 1/2 (the chance II-1 inherits the mutant allele) × 1/2 (the chance III-1 inherits the mutant al-

Suppose $f_{current}$ is the probability that any female in the current generation is a carrier of an X-linked lethal disorder. Then $f_{current}$ is the chance that she inherited a mutant allele from her mother *plus* the chance that she received a newly mutated gene from her mother *plus* the chance that she received a newly mutated gene from her father. If the mutation rate is the same in males and females, the last two factors are each equivalent to the mutation rate, $\mu$, and the prior risk then becomes the chance that she inherited a mutant allele from her mother *plus* $2\mu$. The chance that she inherited a mutant allele from her mother is $1/2 \times f_{previous}$, the probability that any female in the previous generation is a carrier of an X-linked disorder. So,

$$f_{current} = (1/2 \times f_{previous}) + 2\mu$$

Assuming the frequency of the disease, f, is unchanging from one generation to the next ($f_{current} = f_{previous} = f$) and solving for f yields $f = 4\mu$.

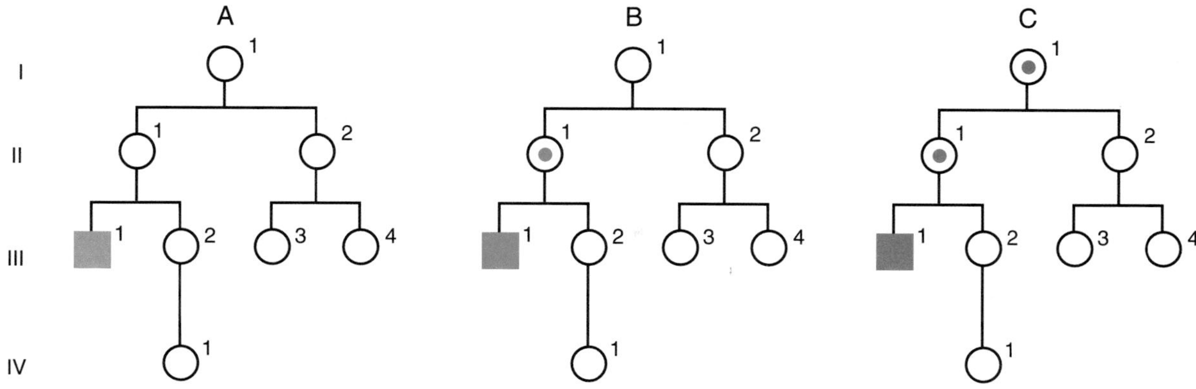


Figure 19–5. Three possible explanations for the occurrence of an isolated case of Duchenne muscular dystrophy (DMD): *A*, The affected boy might have a new mutant gene; *B*, his mother might be a carrier due to a new mutant gene; or *C*, both his mother and his grandmother might be carriers. Determination of which explanation is correct has significant implications for estimating risks for the boy's other relatives.

lele) = 1/4. The probability of having an affected grandson if I-1 is *not* a carrier is $\mu$ (a new mutation in the egg that went to make III-1) plus 1/2 (the chance III-1 inherits a mutant allele) $\times$ $2\mu$ (the chance II-1 is a carrier through a new mutation in either of the gametes that went to make her) $= \mu + 1/2 \times (2\mu) = 2\mu$.

**Bayesian Calculations for Grandmothers of Isolated Cases of X-Linked Lethal Disorders**

| | Hypothesis 1 | Hypothesis 2 |
|---|---|---|
| | *I-1 Is a Carrier* | *I-1 Is NOT a Carrier* |
| Prior probability | $4\mu$ | $1 - 4\mu \approx 1$ |
| Conditional probability | 1/4 | $2\mu$ |
| Joint probability | $4\mu \times 1/4 = \mu$ | $1 \times 2\mu$ |
| Posterior probability | $\frac{\mu}{2\mu + \mu} = 1/3$ | $\frac{2\mu}{2\mu + \mu} = 2/3$ |

The risk that the grandmother I-1 in the family shown in Fig. 19–5 is a carrier is therefore 1/3 (Fig. 19–6).

## Disorders with Incomplete Penetrance

To estimate the recurrence risk of disorders with incomplete penetrance, the probability that an apparently normal person actually carries the mutant gene in question must be considered.

Figure 19–7 shows a pedigree of split-hand deformity, an autosomal dominant abnormality with incomplete penetrance discussed in Chapter 5. An estimate of penetrance can be made from a single pedigree if it is large enough or from a review of published pedigrees; we use 70 percent in our example.

The pedigree shows several people who must carry the mutant gene but do not express it (i.e., in whom the defect is not penetrant): I-1 or I-2 (assuming no somatic or germline mosaicism) and II-3. The other unaffected family members may or may not carry the mutant gene.

If III-4 is the consultand, her risk of having a child with split-hand deformity can be estimated as follows: first, determine the chance that III-4 is a carrier, and then, calculate the chance of having an affected child.

**Bayesian Calculations for an Autosomal Dominant Disorder with Incomplete Penetrance**

| | Hypothesis 1 | Hypothesis 2 |
|---|---|---|
| | *III-4 Is Heterozygous* | *III-4 Is Homozygous Normal* |
| Prior probability | 1/2 | 1/2 |
| Conditional probability | 3/10 | 1 |
| Joint probability | $1/2 \times 3/10 = 3/20$ | $1/2 \times 1 = 1/2$ |
| Posterior probability | $\frac{3/20}{1/2 + 3/20} = 3/13$ | $\frac{1/2}{1/2 + 3/20} = 10/13$ |

This calculation means that the prior probability that a child born to III-4 will inherit the split-hand deformity allele $= 1/2 \times 3/13 = 3/26$ and, if inherited, the probability the abnormal allele will be penetrant = 7/10, leading to the final risk that III-4 will have a child affected with the split-hand deformity $= 3/26 \times 7/10 \approx 8$ percent.

## Disorders with Late Age of Onset

Many autosomal dominant conditions characteristically show a late age of onset, beyond the age of reproduction. Thus, it is not uncommon in genetic counseling to ask whether or not a person of reproductive age who is at risk for a particular autosomal

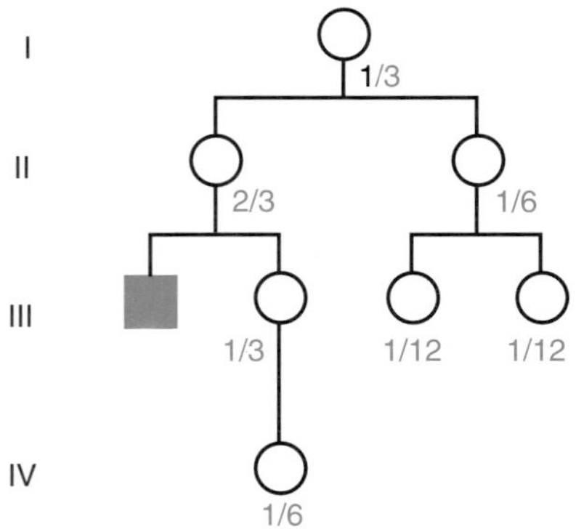


Figure 19–6. Overall carrier risk estimates for females in the family depicted in Figure 19–5. These risk estimates, based on genetic principles, can be further modified by considering information obtained from family history, carrier detection testing, or molecular genetic methods for direct detection of the mutation in the affected boy, using Bayesian calculations.

dominant disorder carries the gene. One example of such a disorder is a rare, familial form of Parkinson disease (PD) inherited as an autosomal dominant condition.

Consider the dominant PD pedigree in Figure 19–8 in which the consultand, an asymptomatic 35-year-old man, wishes to know his risk for PD. His prior risk of having inherited the *PD* gene from his affected grandmother is 1/4. Considering that perhaps only 5 percent of persons with this rare form of PD show symptoms at his age, he would not be expected to show signs of the disease even if he had inherited the mutant allele. The more significant aspect of the pedigree, however, is that the consultand's father (II-2) is also asymptomatic at age 60, an age by which perhaps two thirds of persons with this form of PD show symptoms and one third would not.

As is frequently done in Bayesian analysis, we do not immediately calculate the consultand's risk. Instead, we take a step back to a previous generation, make the calculation for an ancestor, and use that calculation as the basis for a prior probability for the consultand himself.

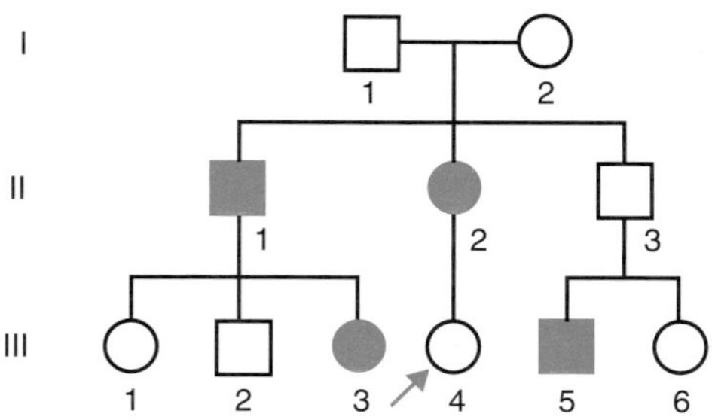


Figure 19–7. Pedigree of family with split-hand deformity and lack of penetrance. The consultand's risk of having a clinically affected child can be calculated to be approximately 8 percent. For discussion, see text.

**Bayesian Calculation for Disorders with Late Age of Onset**

| | Hypothesis 1 | Hypothesis 2 |
|---|---|---|
| | *II-2 Is a Heterozygote* | *II-2 Is NOT a Heterozygote* |
| Prior probability | 1/2 | 1/2 |
| Conditional probability | 1/3 | 1 |
| Joint probability | 1/2 × 1/3 = 1/6 | 1/2 |
| Posterior probability | $\frac{1/6}{1/6 + 1/2} = 1/4$ | $\frac{1/2}{1/6 + 1/2} = 3/4$ |

According to Bayesian analysis, the *father's* risk of carrying the *PD* gene, considering that he is asymptomatic at age 60, is 1/4. Using this information, we can modify the consultand's risk of inheriting the *PD* gene down to 1/2 × 1/4 = 1/8 or 12.5 percent. Because the penetrance is only approximately 5 percent at age 35, the fact that the consultand is asymptomatic has very little effect and lowers his risk of carrying the *PD* gene by only a percent to about 11.5 percent. Whether he develops the disease and at what age depends on knowing the age-specific penetrance for this disorder. For example, his chance of developing the disease by age 60 is 2/3 × 11.5 percent = 7.7 percent.

Providing these recurrence risks in genetic counseling requires careful follow-up. If, for example, the consultand or his father were to develop symptoms of PD, the risks change dramatically.

## Empiric Recurrence Risks

Genetic counselors deal with many disorders that are not single-gene disorders. Instead, counselors may be called on to provide risk estimates for complex trait disorders with a strong genetic component and familial clustering, such as cleft lip and palate, congenital heart disease, and meningomyelocele (see Tables

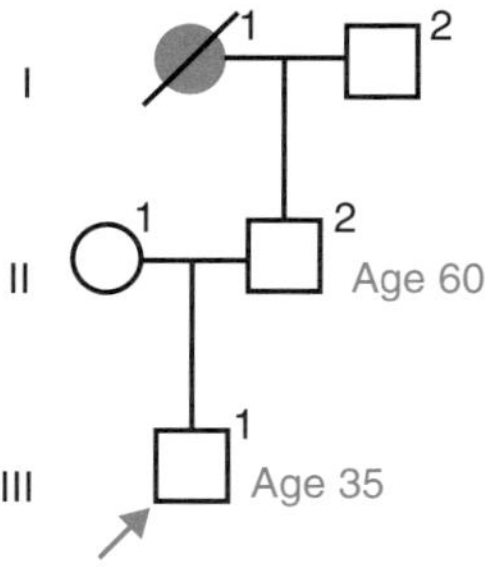


Figure 19–8. Age-modified risks for genetic counseling in dominant PD. That the consultand's father is asymptomatic at age 60 reduces the consultand's final risk of carrying the gene to approximately 12.5 percent. That the consultand himself is asymptomatic reduces the risk only slightly, because most patients carrying the mutant allele for this disorder will be asymptomatic at age 35.

15–8, 15–9 and 15–10 in Chapter 15). In these situations, the risk of recurrence in first-degree relatives of affected individuals may be increased over the background incidence of the disease in the population but is not at the level expected with autosomal dominant or recessive disorders. In these situations, recurrence risks are estimated empirically by studying as many families with the disorder as possible and observing how frequently recurrences of the disorder occur. The observed frequency of a recurrence is taken as an **empiric recurrence risk**.

Genetic counselors must use caution when applying empiric risk figures to a particular family. First, empiric estimates are an average over what is undoubtedly a group of heterogeneous disorders with different mechanisms of inheritance. In any one family, the real recurrence risk may actually be higher or lower than the average. Second, empiric risk estimates use history to make predictions about future occurrences; if the underlying biological causes are changing through time, data from the past may not be accurate for the future. Finally, figures are derived from a particular population, and so the data from one ethnic group, socioeconomic class, or geographic location may not be accurate for an individual from a different background. Nonetheless, such figures are useful when patients ask genetic counselors to give a best estimate for recurrence risk for disorders with complex inheritance.

For example, neural tube defects (NTDs) (myelomeningocele and anencephaly) occur in approximately 0.3 percent of births in the U.S. Caucasian population. If, however, a couple has a child with an NTD, the risk in the next pregnancy is 4 percent (13 times higher) (see Table 15–8). If these risk figures are calculated for different genders, the figures are even more striking: the sister of a girl with an NTD has a 6 percent chance of also having an NTD. The risks remain elevated compared with the general population risk for more distantly related individuals: a second-degree relative (such as a nephew or niece) of an individual with an NTD is at a 1.7 percent chance of having a similar birth defect. With folate supplementation before conception and during early pregnancy, however, these recurrence risk figures fall dramatically (see Chapter 15).

## Genetic Counseling for Consanguinity

Consanguineous couples sometimes request genetic counseling before they have children because an increased risk of birth defects in their offspring is widely appreciated. Two main points are to be explained to such couples. First, the relative risk of abnormal offspring is higher for related than for unrelated parents but is still quite low: baseline risk figures for any abnormality are up to 3 percent for any child of any parents, and the risk increases only slightly to approximately 4.5 to 5 percent for the offspring of first cousins. This increased risk is not exclusively for single-gene autosomal recessive disorders but includes the entire spectrum of single-gene and complex trait disorders. Second, any couple, consanguineous or not, who produces a child with an autosomal recessive disorder then faces a 25 percent recurrence risk in their future pregnancies, regardless of what their risk was before they had an affected child. This risk applies, of course, only to offspring of the same couple. Because both parents of affected children must be carriers, and because carriers are rare in comparison with normal homozygotes, a parent of a child with an autosomal recessive disorder is less likely to have another affected child with a different partner, depending on the carrier frequency.

## Application of Molecular Genetics to Determining Recurrence Risks

Many disease genes can now be detected directly in carriers and affected persons by means of DNA analysis. This represents a major improvement in carrier detection and prenatal diagnosis, in many cases allowing determination of the presence or absence of a particular gene with essentially 100 percent accuracy.

There are two chief approaches to risk estimation by DNA analysis. The first method is by **direct detection of the mutation**, using gene, cDNA, or synthetic probes to detect a mutation in a patient's or other family member's genomic DNA. As described in Chapter 4, such methods are quick, accurate, and relatively noninvasive. Obviously, direct tests can be used only when the mutation or mutations responsible for a particular disorder are known. The second is the method of using **closely linked markers**, preferably markers flanking the gene (see Chapter 8). This method is indirect, but it works well if the following relatively rigid requirements can be met:

1. There is close linkage between the mutation and the marker, so that recombination is unlikely.
2. The family is "informative"; that is, crucial family members are available for the study and are heterozygous for the markers.
3. The linkage phase is known or can be reasonably inferred.
4. No recombination has occurred between the markers being followed and the disease gene.

In favorable cases, at least some information can be obtained to modify the risk of certain family members' being carriers of the mutation in question.

## Direct Detection of Mutations

### Deletion Analysis in Duchenne Muscular Dystrophy

About 60 percent of patients with DMD have deletions within the gene (see Chapter 12), and many of these deletions can be detected by Southern blot analysis with a series of cDNA probes or by a set of polymerase chain reactions designed to amplify the parts of the gene most frequently deleted in affected patients (see Fig. 12–18). In the pedigree shown in Figure 19–9*A*, if the patient with DMD (II-4) had an identifiable deletion, DNA from the fetus (obtained by methods described in Chapter 18) could be examined directly for the presence or absence of the deletion, and a diagnosis could be made with certainty. Another valuable way to identify deletions is when the probe detects a restriction fragment that is formed by the junction of the two segments of DNA on either side of the deletion. Such fragments are generally altered in size compared with the normal fragment and are therefore diagnostic of the deletion allele.

At present, detection of a deletion in a heterozygous female (III-1 in Figure 19–9*A*) is challenging but feasible because the absence of the deleted segment is obscured by the normal, undeleted chromosome. Finding a junction fragment with a shifted band is diagnostic of a heterozygote for a deletion, however. In the absence of a junction fragment, identification of the mutant gene in female family members is often still done by the use of linked markers (see Fig. 19–9*B*).

### Detection of Mutations in Cystic Fibrosis

Most mutations in CF are single base mutations or deletions or duplications of a small number of nucleotides (see Chapter 12). Carrier detection and prenatal diagnosis in CF make use of the enormous amount of information that has been accumulated on the types of mutations that cause the disease. More than 900 different mutations have been described in this gene. Some are rare, occurring in only a few families. Others are much more common, but their frequency can vary enormously in different ethnic groups. As discussed in Chapter 12, in individuals of northern European descent, about 70 percent of the CF mutations are due to the three base-pair deletion that removes the phenylalanine at position 508 (Δ*F508*). The Δ*F508* mutation is less common or even totally absent in other ethnic groups, in which mutations other than Δ*F508* are more frequent. As additional mutations in different patients are identified, laboratories have begun to offer a battery of mutation detection tests in which dozens of the more common mutations in a population can be identified. The polymerase chain reaction and hybridization with oligonucleotides specific for each mutation are

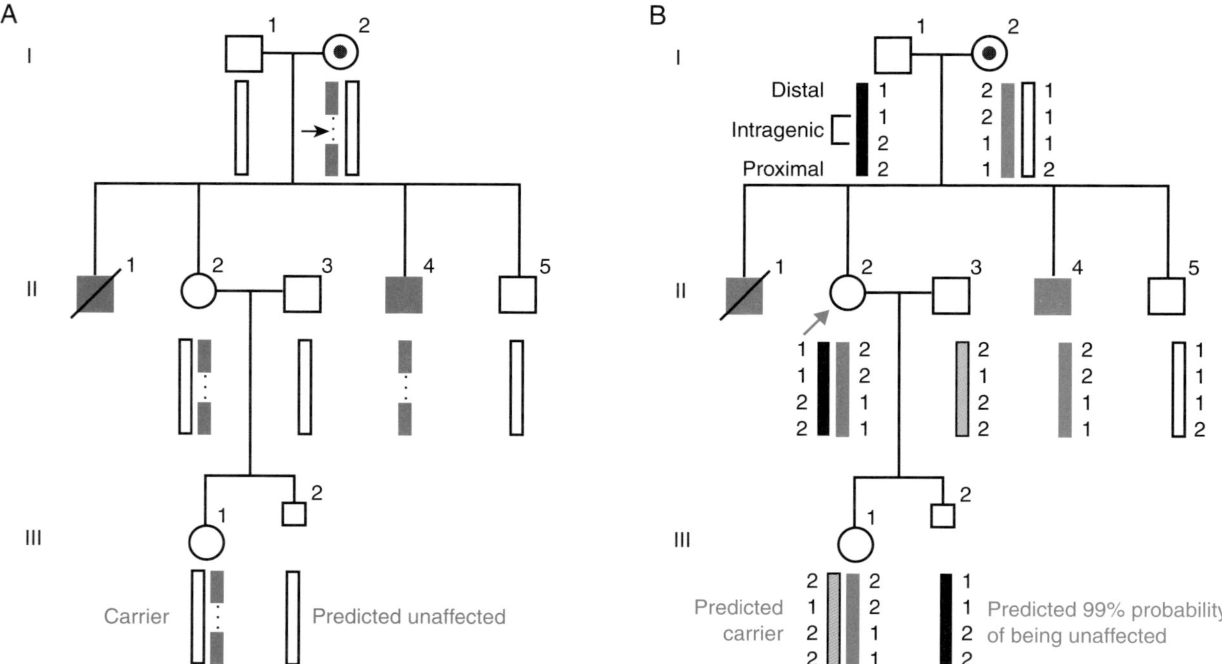


**Figure 19–9.** Use of direct mutation detection and genetic linkage analysis for genetic counseling in a family with DMD. *A.* The proband has a deletion mutation indicated by the broken red bar. Normal *DMD* genes are symbolized by open bars. *B.* The proband's mutation is unknown. Four polymorphic markers were tested, two within the *DMD* gene and one on each side, flanking it. The overall frequency of recombination between the farthest markers is 5 percent. Haplotypes observed in the family are shown. The haplotype indicated in red contains the mutant *DMD* allele. Predicted genotypes of the consultand's daughter and male fetus are based on the DNA data.

used to identify heterozygous carriers and homozygous affected fetuses easily and rapidly. For the minority of families in whom the mutations are unknown, DNA markers very closely linked to the CF locus are available for diagnosis by linkage analysis.

### Application of Linked Markers to Molecular Diagnosis

The first DNA polymorphism applied to clinical diagnosis was a restriction fragment length polymorphism 3′ of the β-globin gene used to diagnose cases of sickle cell disease by linkage analysis (see Fig. 11–7). Although the distance between the polymorphic site and the site of the sickle cell mutation in the β-globin gene was so small as to make the frequency of recombination between them negligible, it is important to recognize that the linkage approach to mutation detection, even when one is using informative polymorphisms in the gene that is responsible for a genetic defect, is *indirect.* Using a linked marker to track the inheritance of a mutant gene carries a risk of recombination between the genetic marker and the actual mutation. In most instances, this risk is probably very low. Very large genes, such as the *DMD* gene, provide exceptions to this generalization because crossing over within the gene occurs at a detectable frequency. In Figure 19–10, we illustrate the use of cloned genes as polymorphic markers for disease diagnosis, using as an example β-thalassemia. The examples illustrate, once again, the requirements that a genetic marker must be informative and that it must be possible to assign phase in order to perform linkage analysis.

The accuracy of diagnosis by using genetically linked markers with an appreciable recombination frequency between the marker and the disease locus can be increased markedly by using two informative genetic markers that flank the disease gene. In this instance, the chance of a misdiagnosis is reduced significantly, because misdiagnosis will result only if *two* crossovers occur, one on each side of the disease gene. For example, for flanking markers that each show 10 percent recombination with a disease gene, diagnosis by genetic linkage will be 99 percent accurate (instead of 90 percent for a single marker). The benefit of using flanking markers reinforces the value of an accurate genetic linkage map, with well-mapped markers of known order and distance.

**Linkage Analysis in Duchenne Muscular Dystrophy.** The hypothetical DMD pedigree shown in Figure 19–9*B* illustrates the use of linked markers to detect a carrier and to diagnose a fetus prenatally. In this family, the maternal grandmother I-2 is clearly a carrier, because she has had two affected sons. She is informative for DNA markers that flank the *DMD* gene (and that are known to have about a 5 percent chance of recombination) and for one of two markers within this large gene. The linkage phase in the maternal grandmother can be inferred from her two living sons II-4 and II-5, because any phase other than that indicated in Figure 19–9*B* would require two recombination events (i.e., in the meioses leading to her two living sons). The consultand II-2 has inherited the same maternal haplotype as her affected brother. The markers of her father I-1 are known, and she herself is informative at all four loci. Her linkage phase is known with certainty, and thus her risk of transmitting the affected haplotype to her offspring can be determined. The risk of a double recombination occurring in a meiosis in the consultand, which would have allowed her to transmit her mother's *DMD* gene with her father's flanking markers, is less than 1 percent, so the probability that the fetus III-2 is unaffected is greater than 99 percent. Moreover, because the consultand's husband's markers are known, it can be predicted that her daughter III-1 has inherited the *DMD* gene and is a carrier.

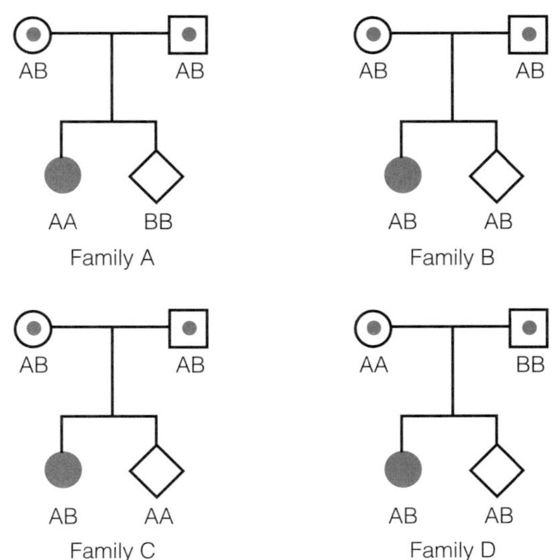


**Figure 19–10.** Examples of molecular diagnosis in β-thalassemia, with polymorphisms in the β-globin locus. The chance of recombination between the polymorphic marker and the mutation is assumed to be negligible. In Family A, phase can be determined from the affected sibling, and a diagnosis of unaffected is possible. In Family B, phase cannot be determined completely; no diagnosis is possible, because the second child could be either affected (50 percent chance) or unaffected (50 percent chance). In Family C, phase cannot be determined completely, but it is possible to provide a diagnosis that the second child will be an unaffected heterozygous carrier. In Family D, no diagnosis is possible; the family is uninformative.

## Risk Estimates When the Gene Has Not Been Identified

The examples given stress two relatively common conditions for which the responsible gene has been cloned and extensively characterized. In these conditions, many mutations have been directly analyzed, and many DNA polymorphisms are available for performing linkage analyses when direct detection is not possible. In other disorders, however, the gene for which a given family is at risk has not yet been identified. In these cases, the role of DNA diagnostic services is somewhat more complicated and expensive. Even when the chromosomal location of a gene is known with some precision because of successful linkage studies (see Chapter 8), there may be considerable uncertainty about the exact genetic distances between the disease gene and linked DNA markers used for diagnosis. There may also be some uncertainty as to possible locus heterogeneity. Determination of risk estimates for the purpose of providing accurate genetic counseling may involve extensive studies of many family members with many different DNA probes to attempt to collect definitive information about location, phase, and the presence of possible recombination events. This task, however, is becoming less and less burdensome as the Human Genome Project provides more and more detailed and dense genetic and physical maps.

## CONCLUSION

In the future, as the knowledge base of medical genetics expands, the scope of genetic counseling will increase proportionately. For physicians, the challenge is to appreciate the importance of genetic counseling in medical practice, to understand its scientific basis, and to be aware of the limitations of our knowledge. To quote Sir William Osler, who wrote in a clinical context but could well have been discussing genetic risks, "Errors of judgment are bound to occur in the practice of an art that consists largely in balancing probabilities."

## General References

Andrews L, Fullarton J, Holtzman N, Motulsky A (1994) Institute of Medicine. Assessing Genetic Risks: Implications for Health and Social Policy. National Academy Press, Washington DC.

Baker DL, Schuette JL, Uhlmann WR (1998) A Guide to Genetic Counseling. John Wiley, New York.

Bennett RL, Steinhaus KA, Uhrich SB, et al (1995) Recommendations for standardized pedigree nomenclature. J Genet Counsel 4:267–279.

Burnard P (1994) Counseling Skills for Health Professionals, 2nd ed. Singular Pub Group, London.

Clarke A (ed) (1994) Genetic Counseling: Practice and Principles. Routledge Press, New York.

Croyle R (ed) (1995) Psychosocial Effects of Screening for Disease Prevention and Detection. Oxford University Press, Oxford, England.

Emery AEH, Pullen I (eds) (1984) Psychological Aspects of Genetic Counseling. Academic Press, London.

Gardner RJM, Sutherland GR (1996) Chromosome Abnormalities and Genetic Counseling, 2nd ed. Oxford University Press, Oxford, England.

Harper PS (1998) Practical Genetic Counseling, 5th ed. Butterworth-Heinemann Medical, Oxford, England.

Kessler S (1979) Genetic Counseling: Psychological Dimensions. Academic Press, London.

Mahowald MB, Verp MS, Anderson RR (1998) Genetic counseling: Clinical and ethical challenges. Annu Rev Genet 32: 547–549.

Marteau T, Richards M (eds) (1996) The Troubled Helix: Social and Psychological Implications of the New Human Genetics. Cambridge University Press, Cambridge, England.

Marks JH, Heimler A, Reich E, Wexler NS (1990) Genetic Counseling Principles in Action: A Casebook. (Birth Defects) Original Article Series 25(5), March of Dimes Birth Defects.

## URLs for Web Resources Related to Genetic Counseling

The Genetic Alliance
An international organization of consumers, professionals, laboratories, hospitals, companies, and not-for-profit foundations dedicated to improving the life of people affected by genetic disease.
*www.geneticalliance.org/*

GeneClinics
A website supported by the Federal government and maintained by the University of Washington and Seattle Children's Hospital providing information on diagnosis, management, and counseling for specific disorders.
*www.geneclinics.org/*

OMIM–Online Mendelian Inheritance in Man
Online database of human genes and genetic diseases maintained by the Johns Hopkins University School of Medicine and supported by the National Library of Medicine, National Institutes of Health.
*www3.ncbi,nlm.nih.gov/Omim/*

## Problems

1. You are consulted by a couple, Dorothy and David, who tell the following story: Dorothy's maternal grandfather, Bruce, had congenital stationary night blindness, which also affected Bruce's maternal uncle, Arthur; in other words, the family history appears to fit the X-linked pattern. (There is also an autosomal dominant form.) Dorothy and David have three unaffected children: a daughter, Elsie, and two sons, Edward and Eliot. Elsie is planning to have children in the near future. Dorothy wonders whether she should warn Elsie about the risk that she might be a carrier of a serious eye disorder. Sketch the pedigree and answer the following:
   (a) What is the chance that Elsie is heterozygous?
   (b) An ophthalmologist traces the family history in further detail and finds evidence that in this pedigree the disorder is not X-linked but autosomal dominant. There is no evidence that Dorothy's mother Cecile was affected. On this basis, what is the chance that Elsie is heterozygous?

2. A deceased boy, Nathan, was the only member of his family with DMD. He is survived by two sisters, Norma (who has a daughter, Olive) and Nancy (who has a daughter, Odette). His mother Molly has two sisters, Maud and Martha. Martha has two unaffected sons and two daughters, Nora and Nellie. Maud has one daughter, Naomi. No carrier tests are available because the mutation in the affected boy remains unknown.

(a) Sketch the pedigree, and calculate the posterior risks for all these females, using information provided in this chapter.
(b) In many molecular diagnosis laboratories, prenatal diagnosis by DNA analysis is available only to women with more than a 2 percent risk that a pregnancy will result in a son with DMD. Which of these women would not qualify?

3. In a village in Wales in 1984, 13 boys were born in succession before a girl was born. What is the probability of 13 successive male births? The probability of 13 successive births of a single sex? What is the probability that after 13 male births the 14th child will be a boy?

4. Let $H$ be the population frequency of carriers of hemophilia A. The incidence of hemophilia A in males ($I$) equals the chance a maternal *F8* gene has a new mutation ($\mu$) *plus* the chance it carries a pre-existing mutation ($1/2H$). Thus, $I = \mu + 1/2H$. Hemophilia A has a fitness ($f$) of ~0.70, i.e., hemophiliacs have ~70 percent as many offspring as do controls. $H$ is then the chance a carrier inherits the mutation from an affected father ($I \times f$) *plus* the chance of a new paternal mutation ($\mu$) *plus* the chance of inheriting it from her mother. $H = If + \mu + \mu + 1/2H$.
(a) For hemophilia A, what is the incidence of affected males? Of carrier females? (Answer parts [a] and [b] in terms of multiples of the mutation rate.) If a woman has a son with an isolated case of hemophilia A, what is the relative risk that she is a carrier? What is the chance that her next son will be affected?
(b) For DMD, $f = 0$. What is the population frequency of affected males? Of carrier females?
(c) Color blindness is thought to have normal fitness ($f = 1$). What is the incidence of carrier females if the frequency of color-blind males is 8 percent?

5. Match terms in section **B** with explanations or definitions in section **A**.

| *A* | | *B* |
|---|---|---|
| a. The probability that any woman in the population is a carrier of DMD. | ____ | Consultand |
| b. Carrier testing in the sister of a boy with a partial duplication in the factor VIII gene. | ____ | 2/3 |
| c. Used with DNA markers as an approach to risk estimation. | ____ | Obligate heterozygote |
| d. Mutation detection by an allele-specific oligonucleotide. | ____ | Prior probability |
| e. The mendelian risk that a person is a carrier of a certain disorder. | ____ | Nonsense mutation in cystic fibrosis gene |
| f. The person seeking or receiving genetic counseling. | ____ | Direct detection of a mutation by Southern blot test |
| g. A person who on the basis of family history must be a heterozygote. | ____ | Informative family |
| h. The probability that the mother of a child with an isolated case of DMD is a carrier. | ____ | $4\mu$ |
| i. A family in which markers linked to a locus of interest allow a mutation to be traced through a family. | ____ | First-degree relative |
| j. Parent, full sib, or offspring (but not a monozygotic twin). | ____ | Linkage analysis |

6. Ira and Margie each has a sibling affected with CF.
(a) What are their prior risks of being carriers?
(b) What is the risk of their having an affected child in *any* pregnancy?
(c) They have had three unaffected children and now wish to know their risk of having an affected child. Using Bayesian analysis to take into consideration that they have already had three unaffected children, calculate the chance that their next child will be affected.

7. A 30-year-old woman with myotonic dystrophy comes in for counseling. Her son, aged 14, shows no symptoms, but she wishes to know whether he will be affected with this autosomal dominant condition later in life. Approximately half of individuals carrying the mutant gene are asymptomatic before age 14. What is the risk that the son will eventually develop myotonic dystrophy? Should you test the child for the expanded repeat in the gene for myotonic dystrophy?

8. A couple arrives in your clinic with their 7-month-old son, who has been moderately developmentally delayed from birth. The couple is contemplating having additional children, and you are asked whether this could be a genetic disorder.
(a) Is this possible, and, if so, what pattern or patterns of inheritance would fit this story?
(b) On taking a detailed family history, you learn that both parents' families were originally from the same small village in northern Italy. How might this fact alter your assessment of the case?
(c) You next learn that the mother has two sisters and five brothers. Both sisters have developmentally delayed children. How might this alter your assessment of the case?

9. You are addressing a Neurofibromatosis Association parents' meeting. A severely affected woman, 32 years old, comments that she is not at risk of passing on the disorder because her parents are not affected and her neurofibromatosis, therefore, is due to a new mutation. Comment.

# 20

# Genetics and Society

The ultimate goal of medical genetics is to improve the health and well-being of individuals, their families, their communities, and society. In this chapter, we expand the discussion of medical genetics beyond the individual patient and his or her family and examine the role of genetics in the society at large. The application of medical genetic testing to an ethnic group or to an entire population is already occurring in a few, selected circumstances. With the information coming from the Human Genome Project, we can anticipate that medical genetic technology, particularly in the areas of testing and screening for hereditary disorders and genetic predisposition, will have an even greater impact on the health and well-being of the population at large. On the other hand, ethical values and societal concerns must help shape how medical genetics knowledge will be applied so that we maximize the benefits and minimize any harm.

## POPULATION SCREENING FOR GENETIC DISEASE

**Genetic screening** is a population-based method for identifying persons with certain genotypes known to be associated with a genetic disease or predisposition to a genetic disease. The disorder that is the target of screening may affect either the individuals being screened or their descendants. Screening at the population level is not to be confused with testing for affected persons or carriers within families already identified because of family history. Rather, the objective of population screening is to examine all members of a designated population, regardless of family history. Genetic screening is an important public health activity that will become more significant as more and better screening tests become available for hereditary diseases and for other conditions with an identifiable genetic component.

### Screening of Newborns

The best-known public health efforts in genetics are the government programs that carry out population screening of all newborns to identify infants with genetic disorders for which early treatment can prevent, or at least ameliorate, the consequences. A determination of the suitability and cost-effectiveness of newborn screening for any particular condition is usually based on criteria similar to those listed in Table 20–1.

The validity of test results is particularly important; false-positive results cause unnecessary concern to the parents, whereas false-negative results vitiate the whole objective of the program.

Two heritable conditions clearly satisfy all of these criteria: phenylketonuria (PKU) and galactosemia. The prototype of such disorders is PKU; routine neonatal screening for PKU is mandated by law in all but one state in the United States and in almost all developed countries. Galactosemia screening is less common. (Screening for congenital hypothyroidism, a disorder that is not usually genetic but is treatable, is also routine in many countries.) A number of other disorders—such as sickle cell anemia, biotinidase

TABLE 20–1

**Criteria for Effective Newborn Screening Programs**

1. Treatment is available.
2. Early institution of treatment before symptoms become manifest has been shown to reduce or eliminate the severity of the illness.
3. Routine observation and physical examination will not reveal the disorder in the newborn—a test is required.
4. A rapid and economical laboratory test is available that is highly sensitive (no false-negatives) and reasonably specific (few false-positives).
5. The condition is frequent and serious enough to justify the expense of screening; that is, screening is cost-effective.
6. The societal infrastructure is in place to inform the newborn's parents and physicians of the results of the screening test, confirm the test results, and institute appropriate treatment and counseling.

deficiency, congenital adrenal hyperplasia, and various abnormalities of amino acid metabolism—are less commonly part of neonatal screening programs because their incidence is lower or because completely effective treatment is not available. Screening is not performed for many other conditions for which it is possible because of very low incidence or lack of an effective method of treatment.

Not everyone agrees that screening should be performed only for highly treatable conditions. It has been argued, for example, that newborn screening for cystic fibrosis (CF) would benefit the newborn by allowing the institution of treatment for pancreatic insufficiency while the newborn is relatively well, before the onset of malabsorption, failure to thrive, and infection. For many conditions, even ones like Duchenne muscular dystrophy (DMD), for which treatment is only palliative, early diagnosis can allow prompt genetic counseling before the birth of more affected children to help parents in their planning for prenatal diagnosis in any future pregnancies.

## Adult Screening

The concepts of newborn screening have been extended to include a proposal for population screening of adults for hemochromatosis, a relatively common autosomal recessive disorder in which a total body overload of iron leads, in some individuals, to permanent liver, pancreatic, and cardiac damage. Nearly 3 per 1000 individuals in the United States have two mutant alleles in the hemochromatosis gene, and one particular mutant allele, a substitution of tyrosine for cysteine at position 282, is responsible for the vast majority of all cases of the disease. Many homozygotes are asymptomatic, particularly women, for whom penetrance of the condition is lower. Screening could be performed either by direct detection of the mutant alleles or by measuring a biochemical parameter, such as transferrin saturation, depending on which test proves to be most cost-effective. Treatment by repeated phlebotomy to remove red blood cells (or, rather, the iron in the hemoglobin they contain) is highly effective in preventing organ damage if initiated before symptoms develop. Thus, population screening could identify asymptomatic homozygotes at risk for developing disease early enough to begin therapy that can prevent serious morbidity and mortality.

## Heterozygote Screening

In contrast to screening for genetic disease in newborns and adults, screening for carriers has, as its main purpose, the identification of individuals who are themselves healthy but at risk for having children with a severe autosomal recessive or X-linked illness. The principles of heterozygote screening are outlined in Table 20–2.

TABLE 20–2
**Criteria for Heterozygote Screening Programs**

1. High frequency of carriers, at least in a specific population.
2. Availability of an inexpensive and dependable test with very low false-negative and false-positive rates.
3. Access to genetic counseling for couples identified as heterozygotes.
4. Availability of prenatal diagnosis.
5. Acceptance and voluntary participation by the population targeted for screening.

Current heterozygote screening programs have focused on particular ethnic groups in which the frequency of the disorder is high enough to justify screening (see Table 7–1). Heterozygote screening has so far been used routinely only for Tay-Sachs disease (the prototype of carrier screening) and Canavan disease, both in the Ashkenazic Jewish population, sickle cell anemia in the African-American population of North America, and $\beta$-thalassemia in high-incidence areas, especially in Cyprus and Sardinia or among emigrants from those areas. Heterozygote screening is voluntary and focuses on individuals who identify themselves as being members of a particular high-risk ethnic group.

The impact of carrier screening in lowering the incidence of a genetic disease can be dramatic. Carrier screening for Tay-Sachs disease in the Ashkenazic Jewish population has been carried out on a massive scale since 1969. Screening followed by prenatal diagnosis, when indicated, has already lowered the incidence of Tay-Sachs disease by 65 to 85 percent in this ethnic group. Prevention of $\beta$-thalassemia by carrier detection and prenatal diagnosis has brought about a similar drop in the incidence of the disease in Cyprus and Sardinia. In contrast, attempts to screen for carriers of sickle cell disease in the U.S. African-American community have been less effective and have had little impact on the incidence of the disease so far. The success of carrier screening programs for Tay-Sachs disease and $\beta$-thalassemia, as well as the relative failure for sickle cell anemia, underscores the importance of community consultation, community education, and the availability of genetic counseling and prenatal diagnosis as critical requirements for an effective program.

The feasibility of direct detection of the common *CFTR* mutations has led to serious consideration of the possibility of population-based heterozygote screening for CF among Caucasian populations of North America. At present, diagnostic laboratories test for the *ΔF508* mutation plus a few dozen additional mutant alleles; testing for these mutations can identify nearly 90 percent of all carriers of CF mutations and, therefore, about 80 percent of the couples at risk (those in which both partners are heterozygous for a *CFTR* mutation) in the general U.S. population. Other couples at risk, in which only one member or neither has an identifiable mutation, would be indistinguishable from other couples in the population (see Chapter 12).

In the U.S. Caucasian population, the incidence of CF is approximately 1 in 2000, the allele frequency of all CF mutations is .0224, and the 30 most common mutations account for 90 percent of all mutations. Screening for these 30 mutations in a population of 1000 would identify 40 and miss 4 of the expected 44 carriers. It should be emphasized that these calculations are true only for U.S. Caucasians. In the Ashkenazic Jewish population, in contrast, the incidence of CF is 1 in 3300, and the frequency of all mutant alleles is therefore $\sqrt{1/3300} = .0174$. Because only 5 mutations account for 97 percent of mutant *CFTR* alleles in this ethnic group, screening for these 5 mutations would identify 33 of the 34 carriers among 1000 Ashkenazic individuals screened.

Heterozygote testing of persons with a family history of CF, and of their partners, is already widely used. The prospect of population screening for CF heterozygotes has been widely discussed and remains controversial. Many medical geneticists believe that heterozygote testing should begin now. Others argue that additional data on ethnic differences in mutant allele frequencies must be obtained to develop more complete panels of mutations to reduce the false-negative rate of carrier screening. As experience is gained and additional mutations are identified, screening for CF heterozygotes in the general population is likely to become standard practice.

### Prenatal Screening

Two tests are commonly used for population screening in fetal life: chromosome analysis for advanced maternal age and maternal serum alpha-fetoprotein or triple-screens for neural tube defects and chromosome aneuploidies. This topic is discussed in the context of prenatal diagnosis in Chapter 18. It has been argued, however, that once the pregnancy has been exposed to the risk of prenatal diagnosis of chromosomal aneuploidy because of advanced maternal age, additional testing, such as alpha-fetoprotein levels in amniotic fluid or mutation screening for CF and other common disorders, should also be offered.

## ETHICAL ISSUES IN MEDICAL GENETICS

The successes of medical genetics have been accompanied by a parallel growth in the level of concern and anxiety that our knowledge be used judiciously for the benefit, and not to the detriment, of individuals, their families, and society as a whole. With the initiation of the Human Genome Project in the United States, the U.S. Congress recognized the ethical dilemmas and the potential for serious societal harm from the misuse of this vastly expanded knowledge of human genetics. Congress responded by mandating that a portion of the U.S. Human Genome Project budget be used to support research and education in the Ethical, Legal, and Social Implications (ELSI) of the Project. Similar programs exist in other countries as well. The ELSI effort is designed to study the effect of the knowledge gained by the Human Genome Project in many areas, including the practice of medicine and other health care professions, the formulation and administration of public policy, the law, and education. In this section, we focus our discussion on some of the ethical dilemmas arising in medical genetics, dilemmas that will become only more difficult and complex as the Human Genome Project and genetics research in general expand our genetic knowledge (Table 20–3). The list is by no means exhaustive, and the various issues are not independent of one other.

In any discussion of ethical issues in medicine, three cardinal principles are frequently cited: **beneficence** (doing good for the patient), **respect for individual autonomy** (safeguarding an individual's rights to control his or her medical care and be free of coercion), and **justice** (ensuring that all individuals are treated equally and fairly). Complex ethical issues arise when these three cardinal principles are perceived to be in conflict with one another. The role of ethicists working at the interface between society and medical genetics is to weigh and balance conflicting demands, each of which has a claim to legitimacy based on one or more of these cardinal principles.

### Ethical Dilemmas in Genetic Testing

#### Prenatal Genetic Testing

Geneticists are frequently asked to help couples use prenatal diagnosis or assisted reproductive technology to avoid having offspring with a serious hereditary disorder. It should be recognized that for some

TABLE 20–3

**Some Critical Ethical Issues in Medical Genetics**

| |
|---|
| **Genetic Testing** |
| Prenatal diagnosis, especially for nondisease traits or sex |
| Testing for genes that predispose to late-onset disease |
| Testing children for a carrier state |
| **Privacy of Genetic Information** |
| Access to an individual's genetic information |
| **Misuse of Genetic Information** |
| Discrimination in employment based on an employee's genotype |
| Discrimination in life insurance underwriting |
| Discrimination in health insurance underwriting |
| **Genetic Screening** |
| Stigmatization and privacy |

hereditary disorders, prenatal diagnosis remains controversial, particularly when the diagnosis leads to a decision to abort the pregnancy for a disease that, unlike Tay-Sachs disease, is not an untreatable, fatal disease of infancy. A debate is ongoing in the community of disabled, mentally retarded, and deaf patients and their families, to name only a few examples, about whether prenatal diagnosis and abortion for these disorders are justified. The ethical dilemma is in attempting to balance respect for the autonomy of parents' reproductive decision-making with an assessment of whether aborting a fetus affected with a disability compatible with life is either fair or beneficial to disabled persons.

The dilemma is even more acute when a couple makes a similar request for a pregnancy that is not at risk for a serious disease or disability. The motivation for seeking prenatal diagnosis might include avoiding recurrence of a disorder associated with a mild or cosmetic defect or for selection of sex. The issue of sex selection for reasons other than reducing the risk for sex-limited or X-linked disease is a very contentious one. Many genetics professionals are concerned that couples are using assisted reproductive technologies, such as in vitro fertilization and blastomere biopsy or prenatal sex determination and abortion, for balancing the sex of the children in their family or avoiding having children of one or the other sex for social and economic reasons prevalent in their societies.

In the future, particular alleles and genes that contribute to complex traits such as intelligence, personality, stature, and other physical characteristics may possibly be identified during the course of the Human Genome Project. Will such nonmedical criteria be viewed as a justifiable basis for prenatal diagnosis? Some might argue that parents are, to varying extents, already expending tremendous effort and resources on improving the *environmental* factors that contribute to healthy, successful children. They might therefore ask why not improve the *genetic* factors as well? Others consider prenatal selection for particular desirable genes as a dehumanizing step that treats children simply as commodities fashioned for their parents' benefit. Once again, the ethical dilemma is in attempting to balance respect for the autonomy of parents' reproductive decision-making with an assessment of whether terminating a pregnancy of a fetus for a cosmetic problem, or for what are perceived to be undesirable alleles, or even for the "wrong" sex, is either fair or beneficial. Does a health professional have, on the one hand, a responsibility and, on the other hand, the right to decide for a couple when a disorder is not serious enough to warrant prenatal diagnosis and abortion or assisted reproduction? The debate continues about *where* or even *whether* one can draw the line in deciding what constitutes a serious enough trait to warrant the application of prenatal testing technology.

### Genetic Testing for Predisposition to Disease

Another area of medical genetics in which ethical dilemmas frequently arise is genetic testing for diseases that may have an onset much later in life than when the molecular testing is being performed. The ethical principles of respect for individual autonomy and beneficence are central to testing in this context. At one end of the spectrum is testing for late-onset neurological disorders, such as Huntington Disease (see Chapter 12). In such diseases, individuals carrying a mutant allele may be presymptomatic but will certainly develop a devastating illness later in life for which there is currently little or no treatment. For any one presymptomatic individual, is knowledge of the test result more beneficial than harmful, or vice versa? How does the balance shift when testing for predisposing mutations that predispose to disease but may not inevitably cause disease? For example, in autosomal dominant hereditary breast cancer (see Chapter 16), individuals carrying various mutations in *BRCA1* or *BRCA2* have a 50 to 90 percent chance of developing breast or ovarian cancer. Identifying heterozygote carriers could have benefits, because individuals at risk could choose to undergo more frequent surveillance or preventive surgery such as mastectomy and oophorectomy, or both, while recognizing that these measures can only reduce but not eliminate the increased risk of cancer. On being tested for a predisposing gene mutation, these individuals incur the risk of serious psychological damage, stigmatization in their social lives, and discrimination in insurance and employment (see later). What if surveillance and preventive measures were more effective, as they are in hereditary nonpolyposis colorectal cancer (see Chapter 16)? Does the ethical balance shift between respect for autonomy and beneficence? The ethical decision to be tested or not is not an absolute decision made in a vacuum. The patient must make an informed decision using all available information concerning the risk for and severity of the disease, the effectiveness of preventive and therapeutic measures, and the potential harm that could arise from testing.

### Genetic Testing of Children

Additional ethical problems arise when genetic testing involves children. As with adults, testing healthy children for genes that predispose to late-onset disease could be beneficial if interventions that decrease morbidity or increase longevity are available. Testing children, however, carries the same risks of serious psychological damage, stigmatization, and insurance and employment discrimination (see later). In addition to insisting that we always seek to do more good than harm, another ethical principle, that of respect for autonomy, must be considered. Children's autonomy, their ability to make decisions for themselves about their own genetic constitution, must be balanced with the desire of parents to obtain such information. There are several reasons why parents may wish to have their children tested. Some have argued that even if there are no clear medical interventions that might benefit the child, it is the parents' duty to inform and prepare their children for the future possibility of developing a serious illness. The parents may also seek this information for their own family planning or to avoid what some parents consider the corrosive effects of keeping important information about their children from them.

A different but related issue arises when testing children for the carrier state of a disease that poses no threat to their health but places them at risk for having affected children. (Once again, the debate centers on the balance between respect for children's autonomy as regards their own procreation and the desire on the part of well-meaning parents to educate and prepare children for the difficult decisions and risks that lie ahead once they reach child-bearing age.)

The preponderance of opinion among bioethicists is that unless there is a clear benefit to the child, testing for a late-onset disease or for the carrier state should be done only when the child is sufficiently old and mature enough, such as in late adolescence or on reaching adulthood, to decide whether to seek such testing.

## Ethical Dilemmas in Genetic Screening

Although the ultimate objective of genetic screening is to improve the public health, there may also be unintended negative consequences. As with genetic testing, abnormal screening results may lead to stigmatization, adverse psychological consequences, or discrimination in the workplace or the insurance market (see later). Additional, special problems arise from screening programs, however. Because genetic screening is performed on a very large number of persons, there is a greater danger than with genetic testing that the screening will not conform to the highest standards of informed consent or may be the result of compulsion, overt or implied, to have the screening done. The right of individuals not to know about their deleterious genes may be compromised once a widespread screening program is in operation. The privacy issue of unauthorized access to the data collections or even to the samples themselves is an even greater concern because the persons being screened have generally not sought the testing because of an affected individual in the family. For example, who will have access to samples and data, and how can we make sure that samples, such as DNA, are not used for purposes other than the screening tests for which they were collected and for which consent was given? It is clear that these matters must be considered in the planning of screening programs, which require an ethical review to ensure that concerns are addressed and appropriate safeguards are in place.

## Privacy of Genetic Information and Its Misuse

A third major ethical principle, along with beneficence and respect for autonomy, is justice—the requirement that everyone be able to benefit equally from progress in medical genetics. Justice is a major concern in the area of the use of genetic information in employment and insurance. Is it fair to stigmatize people who, through no fault of their own, are found to carry a genetic predisposition to disease?

As regards employment, should employers be able to obtain genetic information in making hiring decisions if that information helps them choose dependable and healthy employees with low absenteeism? In particular, some have argued that an employer who funds an employee health care plan must have access to such information in making hiring decisions so that he or she can refuse to hire individuals at risk for developing a serious illness later in life that could bankrupt the employee health plan.

In the area of life insurance, insurers insist that they must have access to all pertinent genetic information about an individual that the individual himself or herself has. Life insurance companies calculate their premiums based on actuarial tables of age-specific survival averaged over the population; premiums will not cover losses if individuals with private knowledge that they are at higher risk for disease conceal this information and buy extra life insurance.

The issue of the availability of health insurance for persons carrying alleles for genes that predispose to disease is another vexing problem in societies that lack universal health coverage, such as the United States. Health insurers routinely obtain family history data and smoking history and request blood pressure, serum cholesterol, or urine glucose testing when deciding on availability and setting the premiums for health insurance. Insurers ask why they should be constrained from testing for genes that increase disease risk. Is one's genetic makeup any different from historical and phenotypic data? Many would argue that there *is* a clear distinction between what are already phenotypic manifestations of a disease, such as hypertension, hypercholesterolemia, and diabetes mellitus, and predisposing alleles, such as *BRCA1* mutations (see Chapter 16) and *APOE* $\varepsilon4$ alleles (see

Chapter 15), that may never result in overt disease in the individual who carries them.

As can be seen from these examples, medical genetics will have a profound impact beyond the narrow confines of medical practice, and integrating this knowledge into sound public policy will require the coordinated efforts of government, business, and the public.

## EUGENIC AND DYSGENIC EFFECTS ON GENE FREQUENCIES

### The Problem of Eugenics

The term **eugenics**, introduced by Darwin's cousin Francis Galton in 1883, refers to the improvement of a population by selection of only its "best" specimens for breeding. Plant and animal breeders have followed this practice since ancient times. In the late 19th century, Galton and others began to promote the idea of using selective breeding to improve the human species, thereby initiating the so-called eugenics movement, which was widely advocated for the next half-century. The so-called ideal qualities that the eugenics movement sought to promote through the encouragement of certain kinds of human breeding were more often than not defined by social, ethnic, and economic prejudices and fed by anti-immigrant and racist sentiments in society. For example, egregious excesses were committed in the United States during the first half of the 20th century when involuntary sterilization was carried out under laws passed in support of eugenics. What we now would consider a lack of education was described then as familial "feeble-mindedness"; what we now would call rural poverty was considered by eugenicists to be hereditary "shiftlessness." Although many scientists began to appreciate the theoretical and practical difficulties of carrying out eugenics programs, eugenics became totally discredited when it came to be used in Nazi Germany as a justification for mass murder.

There are two major difficulties in planning a eugenics program: (1) the scientific problem of determining which characteristics are truly heritable and to what extent heredity is contributory to the trait, and (2) the insoluble ethical issues involved in determining who will decide when one trait is more desirable than another and how reproductive behavior can be influenced to further a eugenics program. As described in Chapter 15, the vast majority of human traits, even those with some genetic component, are complex in their inheritance pattern and are influenced strongly by environmental factors. A purely genetic approach to modifying the incidence of such diseases that ignores environmental factors is far too narrow in scope. It is also quite likely that, as illustrated by autosomal recessive conditions, simply restricting the reproduction of individuals with undesirable phenotypes that are complex in their inheritance pattern can have little if any demonstrable effect on the frequency of the contributing alleles or, more important, on the undesirable phenotype. Equally important, it is not clear how we might balance individual autonomy and privacy rights with legitimate public health concerns without subordinating the individual to a theoretical societal goal of "improving the gene pool"; this latter concept is a totalitarian goal not far removed from the Nazi doctrine of racial hygiene.

### The Problem of Dysgenics

The opposite of eugenics is **dysgenics**, a deterioration in the health and well-being of a population by practices that allow the accumulation of deleterious alleles. In the case of some single-gene defects, medical treatment can have a dysgenic effect by reducing selection against a particular genotype, thereby allowing the incidence of harmful genes to increase. The effect of relaxed selection is more striking for autosomal dominant and X-linked disorders than for autosomal recessive disorders, in which the vast majority of mutant alleles are in silent heterozygous carriers. For example, if all persons affected with CF could survive and reproduce at a normal rate, the incidence of the disease would rise from 1 in 2000 to only about 1 in 1550 over 200 years. In contrast, if successful treatment of DMD were to be achieved, therapy for DMD could cause the incidence of the disease to rise sharply because the *DMD* genes of the affected males would then be transmitted to all their daughters. The effect of this transmission would be to greatly increase the proportion of carriers in the population.

Common genetic disorders with complex inheritance, discussed in Chapter 15, could also become more common if selection is removed. Congenital heart malformations and cleft lip and palate are multifactorial traits that limited reproductive fitness in the past but are now often treated successfully by surgery. Similarly, the discovery of insulin, a major medical advance, could lead to an increase in the incidence of type 1 diabetes mellitus by allowing juvenile diabetics to survive and reproduce. A similar situation may occur with neural tube defects, in which folic acid supplementation during pregnancy can have a significant and rapid impact on reducing the incidence of the disorder. To the extent that common, complex disorders are caused by genetic factors, the incidence of these disorders may increase somewhat, although it is likely that, as with autosomal recessive diseases, most of the susceptibility alleles are distributed among unaffected individuals. Consequently, reproduction by affected persons would have little effect on the allele's frequency.

On the other hand, genetic counseling and parental decisions to limit reproduction can greatly reduce the incidence of some diseases, particularly those with an X-linked or autosomal dominant pattern. If no one at risk for Huntington disease in their offspring reproduced, for example, there would be a large effect on the incidence of the responsible gene. Other late-onset autosomal dominant diseases, such as myotonic dystrophy, would also become less common if at-risk family members were identified and chose not to reproduce or chose to have prenatal diagnosis and then ensured that the disease gene was not transmitted. In the case of autosomal recessive conditions, however, the effect on the frequency of the mutant allele of aborting all homozygous affected pregnancies would be small, because most of these alleles are carried silently by heterozygotes.

The long-term impact of activities in medical genetics that can affect gene frequencies may be difficult to predict. As prenatal diagnosis (see Chapter 18) becomes widespread, significant numbers of pregnancies in which the fetus has a genetic defect are terminated, with the potential outcome of reducing the frequency of the disorders. At present, however, no one has measured the extent to which pregnancy termination for genetic reasons is followed by **reproductive compensation**—that is, by the birth of additional, unaffected children, many of whom are carriers of the deleterious gene. Some families with X-linked disorders have chosen to terminate pregnancies in which the fetus was male, but, of course, daughters in such families, although unaffected, may be carriers. Thus, reproductive compensation has the potential long-term consequence of increasing the frequency of the genetic disorder that led to the loss of an affected child.

Population screening for carriers of autosomal recessive disorders can alter the incidence of disease by alerting couples at risk for having affected children to the need for genetic counseling. Heterozygote screening programs would also have some impact on X-linked and dominant disorders, but the most severe disorders in these two classes of heritable disease would continue to recur, owing to new mutations.

## CONCLUSION

The last half of the 20th century will be remembered as the era in which the study of human and medical genetics was revolutionized by molecular biology, particularly recombinant DNA technology, leading to an explosion in our knowledge of the molecular basis of human heredity. Genes ceased to be theoretical information-carrying units, whose existence had to be inferred through the study of the patterns of transmission of various traits, and instead became material objects, segments of DNA, in which the information was encoded by rules that could be discovered and understood. The ultimate expression of the human genetics revolution is the Human Genome Project. At the beginning of the 21st century, the human species has, for the first time, a complete representative sequence of its own DNA, a comprehensive inventory of its genes, a vigorous ongoing effort to identify and characterize variation at the level of DNA sequence, and a rapidly expanding knowledge base in which various traits and disease predispositions will be attributable to DNA sequence variation. Human genetics has already begun to have a major impact in many areas of medicine—the knowledge gained from the Human Genome Project will revolutionize clinical medicine as profoundly as did the earlier demonstration that the laws of chemistry were the same whether a reaction takes place in a test tube or in the cells of the body. The challenge confronting us all is to make sure that the advances in human genetic knowledge and technology are used responsibly, fairly, and humanely. In the end, **Genetics in Medicine** is not about knowledge for its own sake but for the sake of improving health, relieving suffering, and enhancing human dignity.

## General References


Andrews LB, Fullarton JE, Holtzman NA, Motulsky AG (1994) Assessing Genetic Risks: Implications for Health and Social Policy. National Academy Press, Washington, DC.

Beauchamp TL, Childress JF (1994) Principles of Biomedical Ethics, 4th ed. Oxford University Press, New York.

Chadwick RF (1999) The Ethics of Genetic Screening *In* The Library of Medical Ethics and Theoretical Medicine, Vol 1. Kluwer Academic Publishers, Dordrecht, the Netherlands.

Harper PS (1997) Genetic testing, life insurance, and adverse selection. Philos Trans R Soc Lond B Biol Sci 352:1063–1066.

Hudson KL, Rothenberg KH, Andrews LB, et al (1995) Genetic discrimination and health insurance: An urgent need for reform. Science 270:391–393.

Kevles D (1995) In the Name of Eugenics: Genetics and the Uses of Human Heredity. Harvard University Press, Cambridge, Massachusetts.

Lapham EV, Kozma C, Weiss JO (1996) Genetic discrimination: Perspectives of consumers. Science 274:621–624.

Mahowald MB, Verp MS, Anderson RR (1998) Genetic counseling: Clinical and ethical challenges. Annu Rev Genet 32:547–549.

Murray TH (1991) Ethical issues in human genome research. FASEB J 5:55–60.

Pokorski RJ (1997) Insurance underwriting in the genetic era. Am J Hum Genet 60:205–216.

Web sites of the American Society of Human Genetics, the American College of Medical Genetics, the American Board of Genetic Counseling, and the National Human Genome Research Institute all carry policy statements on various aspects of medical genetics:
*http://www.faseb.org/genetics/ashg/ashgmenu.htm*
*http://www.faseb.org/genetics/acmg/acmgmenu.htm*
*http://www.faseb.org/genetics/abgc/abgcmenu.htm*
*http://www.nhgri.nih.gov/ELSI/*

## Problems

1. A couple with two children is referred for genetic counseling because their younger son, an 8-year-old boy, has a movement disorder for which testing for juvenile Huntington disease is being considered. What are the ethical considerations for the family in testing?

2. Do a literature search and investigate the history of newborn sickle cell screening programs in the United States. What potential benefits might accrue from such testing? What harms? Consider the historical context in which screening was undertaken and the extent to which the African-American community was involved in planning and implementing testing.

3. A research project screened more than 40,000 consecutive, unselected births for the number of X chromosomes and the presence of a Y chromosome and correlated the sex-chromosome karyotype with the sex assigned by visual inspection in the newborn nursery. The purpose of the project was to follow infants with sex-chromosome abnormalities (see Chapter 10) prospectively for developmental difficulties. What are the ethical considerations in carrying out this project?

4. A state health department proposes carrying out a screening test for profound deafness among newborns. Discuss the appropriateness of such a screening program, applying the criteria commonly used for deciding whether or not to implement a particular newborn screening test.

# Glossary

**Acceptor splice site** The boundary between the 3′ end of an intron and the 5′ end of the following exon. Also called *3′ splice site*.

**Acrocentric** A type of chromosome with the centromere near one end. The human acrocentric chromosomes (13, 14, 15, 21, and 22) have satellited short arms that carry genes for ribosomal RNA.

**Affected pedigree member method** A model-free method of linkage analysis that systematically measures whether relatives affected with a disease share alleles at a locus more frequently than would be predicted by chance alone from their familial relationship. If the relatives are sibs, referred to as *affected sibpair method* of linkage analysis.

**Allele** One of the alternative versions of a gene that may occupy a given locus.

**Allele-specific oligonucleotide (ASO)** An oligonucleotide probe synthesized to match a particular DNA sequence precisely and allow the discrimination of alleles that differ by only a single base.

**Allelic exclusion** In immunogenetics, the observation that only one of the pair of parental alleles for each H-chain and L-chain of an immunoglobulin molecule is expressed within a single cell.

**Allelic heterogeneity** In a population, there may be a number of different mutant alleles at a single locus. In an individual, the same or similar phenotypes may be caused by different mutant alleles rather than by identical alleles at the locus.

**Allogenic** In transplantation, denotes individuals (or tissues) that are of the same species but that have different antigens. *Alternative spelling: allogeneic.*

**Alpha-fetoprotein (AFP)** A fetal glycoprotein excreted into the amniotic fluid, which reaches abnormally high concentration in amniotic fluid (and maternal serum) when the fetus has certain abnormalities, especially an open neural tube defect.

***Alu* repeat sequence** In the human genome, about 10 percent of the DNA is made up of a set of about 1,000,000 dispersed, related sequences, each about 300 base pairs long, so named because they are cleaved by the restriction enzyme *Alu*I.

**Amniocentesis** A procedure used in prenatal diagnosis to obtain amniotic fluid, which contains cells of fetal origin that can be cultured for analysis. Amniotic fluid is withdrawn from the amniotic sac by syringe after insertion of a hollow needle into the amnion through the abdominal wall and uterine wall.

**Amplification** In molecular biology, the production of multiple copies of a sequence of DNA. Also, in cytogenetics, refers to multiple copies of a sequence in the genome that are detectable by comparative genomic hybridization (CGH).

**Aneuploidy** Any chromosome number that is not an exact multiple of the haploid number; or an individual with an aneuploid chromosome number. The common forms of aneuploidy in humans are *trisomy* (the presence of an extra chromosome) or *monosomy* (the absence of a single chromosome).

**Anticipation** The progressively earlier onset and increased severity of certain diseases in successive generations of a family. Caused by expansion of the number of triple repeats within or associated with the gene responsible for the disease.

**Anticodon** A three-base unit of RNA complementary to a codon in mRNA.

**Antisense strand of DNA** The noncoding DNA strand, which is complementary to mRNA and serves as the template for RNA synthesis. Also called the *transcribed strand.*

**Apoptosis** Programmed cell death characterized by a stereotypic pattern of mitochondrial breakdown and chromatin degradation.

**Ascertainment** The method of selection of individuals for inclusion in a genetic study.

**Ascertainment bias** Difference in the likelihood that affected relatives of affected individuals will be identified, as compared with similarly affected relatives of controls. A possible source of error in family studies.

**Association** In human genetics, describes the situation in which a particular allele is found either significantly more or significantly less frequently in a group of affected individuals than would be expected from the frequency of the allele in the general population from which the affected individuals were drawn. Not to be confused with *linkage*.

**Assortative mating** Selection of a mate with preference for a particular genotype; that is, nonrandom mating. Usually positive (preference for a mate of the same genotype), less frequently negative (preference for a mate of a different genotype).

**Assortment** The random distribution of different combinations of the parental chromosomes to the gametes. Nonallelic genes assort independently, unless they are linked.

**Autoimmune disorder** A disease characterized by an abnormal immune response apparently directed against antigens of the individual's own tissues; thought to be related to variation in the immune response resulting from polymorphism in immune-response genes.

**Autologous** Refers to grafts in the same animal from one part to another, or to malignant cells and the cells of the individual in which they have arisen.

**Autonomy** A situation during embryonic development when a cell's fate is independent of the genes expressed by its neighboring cells.

**Autosome** Any nuclear chromosome other than the sex chromosomes; 22 pairs in the human karyotype. A disease caused by mutation in an autosomal gene or gene pair shows *autosomal inheritance*.

**B-cell activation** The process resulting in the production of secreted antibodies by plasma cells, initiated by antigen-antibody interaction on the B-cell membrane, followed by clonal expansion and differentiation of B cells.

**Bacterial artificial chromosomes (BACs)** Vectors capable of carrying 100 to 300 kb of cloned human DNA; propagated in bacteria and used in high-resolution gene mapping and DNA sequencing.

**Bacteriophage lambda** A virus that infects bacteria; used in molecular biology as a vector for cloning DNA sequences up to 20 kb in length.

**Balanced polymorphism** A polymorphism maintained in the population by heterozygote advantage, allowing an allele, even one that is deleterious in the homozygous state, to persist at a relatively high frequency in the population.

**Banding** One of several techniques that stain chromosomes in a characteristic pattern, allowing identification of individual chromosomes and structural abnormalities. See *C bands*, *G bands*, *Q bands*, *R bands* in text.

**Barr body** The sex chromatin as seen in female somatic cells, representing an inactive X chromosome.

**Base pair (bp)** A pair of complementary nucleotide bases, as in double-stranded DNA. Used as the unit of measurement of the length of a DNA sequence.

**Bayesian analysis** A mathematical method widely used in genetic counseling to calculate recurrence risks. The method combines information from several sources (genetics, pedigree information, and test results) to determine the probability that a specific individual might develop or transmit a certain disorder.

**Benign polymorphism** A polymorphism for which the different phenotypes are all clinically normal, e.g., the ABO blood group polymorphism.

**Benign trait** A variant trait with no clinical significance.

**Binomial theorem** When there are two alternative classes, one with probability $p$ and the other with probability $1 - p = q$, the frequencies of the possible combinations of $p$ and $q$ in a series of $n$ trials is $(p + q)^n$.

**Bioinformatics** Computational analysis and storage of biological and experimental data, widely applied to genomic and proteomic studies.

**Birth defect** An abnormality present at birth, not necessarily genetic.

**Bivalent** A pair of homologous chromosomes in association, as seen at metaphase of the first meiotic division.

**Blood group** The phenotype produced by genetically determined antigens on a red blood cell. The antigens formed by a set of allelic genes make up a blood group system.

**Candidate gene** In a search for a disease gene, a candidate gene is a gene whose product has biochemical or other properties suggesting that it may prove to be the disease gene being sought.

**Cap** A modified nucleotide added to the 5′ end of a growing mRNA chain, required for normal processing, stability, and translation of mRNA.

**Caretaker genes** Tumor-suppressor genes that are indirectly involved in controlling cellular proliferation by repairing DNA damage and maintaining genomic integrity, thereby protecting proto-oncogenes and gatekeeper tumor-suppressor genes from mutations that could lead to cancer.

**Carrier** An individual heterozygous for a particular mutant allele. The term is used for heterozygotes for autosomal recessive alleles, for females heterozygous for X-linked alleles, or, less commonly, for an individual heterozygous for an autosomal dominant allele but not expressing it (e.g., a heterozygote for a Huntington disease allele in the presymptomatic stage).

**Case-control study** An epidemiological method in which patients with a disease (the cases) are compared with suitably chosen individuals without the disease (the controls) with respect to the relative frequency of various putative risk factors.

**cDNA** See *complementary DNA*.

**Cell cycle** The stages between two successive mitotic divisions, described in the text. Consists of the $G_1$, S, $G_2$, and M stages.

**CentiMorgan (cM)** The unit of distance between genes along chromosomes, named for Thomas Hunt Morgan. Two loci are 1 cM apart if recombination is detected between them in 1 percent of meioses.

**Centromere** The primary constriction on the chromosome, a region at which the sister chromatids are held quired and at which the kinetochore is formed. Required for normal segregation in mitosis and meiosis.

**Centrosomes** A pair of centers that organize the growth of the microtubules of the mitotic spindle; visible at the poles of the dividing cell in late prophase.

**CG (or CpG) island** Any region of the genome containing an unusually high concentration of the dinucleotide sequence 5′-CG-3′.

**Chain termination mutation** A mutation that generates a stop codon, thus preventing further synthesis of the polypeptide chain.

**Checkpoint** Positions in the cell cycle, usually at the junction between the $G_1$ and S or the $G_2$ and M stages, at which the cell determines whether to proceed to the next stage of the cycle.

**Chiasma** Literally, a cross. The term refers to the crossing of chromatid strands of homologous chromosomes, seen at the diplotene of the first meiotic division. Chiasmata are thought to be evidence of interchange of chromosomal material (crossovers) between members of a chromosome pair.

**Chimera** An individual composed of cells derived from two genetically different zygotes. In humans, *blood group chimeras* result from exchange of hematopoietic stem cells by dizygotic twins in utero; *dispermic chimeras,* which are very rare, result from fusion of two zygotes into one individual. Chimerism is also an inevitable result of transplantation.

**Chorionic villus sampling (CVS)** A procedure used for prenatal diagnosis at 8 to 10 weeks' gestation. Fetal tissue for analysis is withdrawn from the villous area of the chorion either transcervically or transabdominally, under ultrasonographic guidance.

**Chromatids** The two parallel strands of chromatin, connected at the centromere, that constitute a chromosome following DNA synthesis.

**Chromatin** The association of DNA and proteins of which chromosomes are composed. See also *nucleosome.*

**Chromosomal disorder** A clinical condition caused by an abnormal chromosome constitution in which there is duplication, loss, or rearrangement of chromosomal material.

**Chromosomal satellite** A small mass of chromatin containing genes for ribosomal RNA, at the end of the short arm of each chromatid of an acrocentric chromosome. Not to be confused with *satellite DNA.*

**Chromosome** One of the threadlike structures in the cell nucleus; consists of chromatin and carries the genetic information (DNA).

**Chromosome mutation** A change in the genetic material at the chromosome level.

**Chromosome painting probe** A multilocus probe designed for fluorescence in situ hybridization (FISH) that hybridizes to only one particular chromosome or chromosome arm.

**Chromosome segregation** The separation of chromosomes or chromatids in cell division so that each daughter cell gets an equal number of chromosomes.

**Chromosome spread** The chromosomes of a dividing cell as seen under the microscope in metaphase or prometaphase.

**Clinical heterogeneity** The term describing the occurrence of clinically different phenotypes from mutations in the same gene.

**Clonal evolution** The multistep process of successive genetic changes that occur in a developing tumor cell population.

**Clone** (1) A cell line derived by mitosis from a single ancestral diploid cell; in embryology, a cell lineage in which the cells have remained geographically close to each other. (2) In molecular biology, a recombinant DNA molecule containing a gene or other DNA sequence of interest. Also, the act of generating such a cell line or clone.

**Cloning, molecular** Transfer of a DNA sequence into a single cell of a microorganism, followed by culture of the microorganism to produce large quantities of the DNA sample for analysis.

**Coding strand** In double-stranded DNA, the strand that has the same 5′-to-3′ sense (and sequence, except that, in mRNA, U substitutes for T) as does mRNA. The coding strand is the strand that is *not* transcribed by RNA polymerase. Also called the *sense strand.*

**Codominant** If both alleles of a pair are expressed in the heterozygous state, then the alleles (or the traits determined by them, or both) are codominant.

**Codon** A triplet of three bases in a DNA or RNA molecule, specifying a single amino acid.

**Coefficient of inbreeding (F)** The probability that an individual homozygous at a locus received both alleles from one ancestor (i.e., the alleles are *identical by descent*).

**Cofactor-responsive disease** A genetic disease in which a specific biochemical abnormality affecting a single mutant protein (usually an enzyme) is corrected by the administration of pharmacological amounts of the specific cofactor of the mutant protein (e.g., vitamin $B_6$-responsive homocystinuria).

**Colinearity** The parallel relationship between the base sequence of the DNA of a gene (or the RNA transcribed from it) and the amino acid sequence of the corresponding polypeptide.

**Commitment** The transition of an embryonic cell from pluripotency to its particular fate.

**Comparative genome hybridization (CGH)** A fluorescence in situ hybridization (FISH) technique used to compare two different DNA samples in terms of gene dosage, especially useful in the study of chromosomal changes in cancer cells.

**Complementarity** The complementary nature of base pairing in DNA.

**Complementary DNA (cDNA)** DNA synthesized from a messenger RNA template, through the action of the enzyme reverse transcriptase. See *genomic DNA* for comparison.

**Complementation** In genetics, the ability of cells from patients with two different genetic defects to correct one another, thus demonstrating that the defects are not identical. The complementation may be intergenic or intragenic.

**Complex inheritance** A pattern of inheritance that is not mendelian. A trait with complex inheritance usually results from alleles at more than one locus interacting with environmental factors.

**Compound (compound heterozygote)** An individual, or a genotype, with two different mutant alleles at the same locus. Not to be confused with *homozygote,* in which the two mutant alleles are identical.

**Concordance** Describes a pair of relatives in which (1) both members of the pair have a certain qualitative trait, or (2) both members have values of a quantitative trait that are similar in magnitude. See *discordant*.

**Conditional probability** In bayesian analysis, this is the chance of an observed outcome given that a consultand has a particular genotype. The product of the prior and conditional probabilities is the joint probability.

**Confined placental mosaicism** Mosaicism in a chorionic villus sampling (CVS) specimen obtained from the placenta that is not present in the fetus itself.

**Congenital** Present at birth; not necessarily genetic.

**Consanguineous** Related by descent from a common ancestor.

**Consensus sequence** In genes or proteins, an idealized sequence in which each base or amino acid residue represents the one most frequently found at that position when many actual sequences are compared; for example, the consensus sequence for splice donor or acceptor sites.

**Consultand** In genetic counseling, anyone who consults a genetic counselor for genetic information.

**Contig** A set of overlapping large DNA fragments, usually of cloned human DNA, that spans a segment of DNA containing a gene of interest and the nearby genetic markers. Used in high-resolution physical mapping.

**Contiguous gene syndrome** A syndrome resulting from a *microdeletion* of chromosomal DNA extending over two or more contiguous loci. Also called *segmental aneusomy*.

**Cordocentesis** A procedure used in prenatal diagnosis to obtain a sample of fetal blood directly from the placenta.

**Correlation** A statistical tool applied to a set of paired measurements. A positive correlation exists when the larger the first measurement in the pair is, the larger the second measurement of the pair is. A negative correlation is the opposite, that is, the larger the first measurement, the smaller the second.

**Correlation coefficient (r)** A measure of correlation that varies from 1 for perfect positive correlation, −1 for perfect negative correlation, and 0 when there is no correlation between pairs of measurements.

**Coupling** When two nonallelic mutations are carried on the same chromosome, the two mutations are said to be in coupling; if on opposite members of a homologous chromosome pair, they are in *repulsion*.

**Crossover, crossing over** The reciprocal exchange of segments between chromatids of homologous chromosomes, a characteristic of prophase of the first meiotic division. See also *recombination*. *Unequal crossing over* between misaligned chromatids can lead to duplication of the involved segment on one chromatid and deletion on the other, and is a frequent cause of mutation.

**Cryptic splice site** A DNA sequence similar to the consensus splice site but not normally used. Used when the normal splice site is altered by mutation or when a mutation in the cryptic site increases its use by the splicing apparatus. May be in a coding or a noncoding sequence.

**Cytotrophoblast** The fetal cells of the chorionic villi that are sampled for karyotyping and DNA analysis.

**Daughter chromosomes** The two individual chromosomes formed when a single chromosome composed of paired chromatids separates at the centromere in anaphase of cell division.

**Deformation syndrome** A recognizable pattern of dysmorphic features caused by extrinsic factors that affect the fetus in utero.

**Degeneracy of the code** The genetic code is described as degenerate because most of the 20 amino acids are specified by more than 1 of the 64 codons.

**Deletion** The loss of a sequence of DNA from a chromosome. The deleted DNA may be of any length, from a single base to a large part of a chromosome.

**Denaturation (of DNA)** The conversion of DNA from the double-stranded to the single-stranded state, usually accomplished by heating to destroy chemical bonds involved in base pairing.

**Deoxyribonucleic acid** See *DNA*.

**Determination** During development, the second stage of commitment in which a cell follows its developmental program regardless of whether it is transplanted to a different region of the embryo.

**Developmental program** The process by which a cell in an embryo achieves its fate.

**Dicentric** A structurally abnormal chromosome with two centromeres.

**Dictyotene** The stage of the first meiotic division in which a human oocyte remains from late fetal life until ovulation.

**Differentiation** The process whereby a cell acquires a tissue-specific pattern of expression of genes and proteins and a characteristic phenotype.

**Diploid** The number of chromosomes in most somatic cells, which is double the number found in the gametes. In humans, the diploid chromosome number is 46.

**Discordance** The situation in which (1) one member of the pair has a certain qualitative trait and the other does not, or (2) the relatives have values of a quantitative trait that are at opposite ends of the distribution. See *concordance*.

**Disomy** See *uniparental disomy*.

**Disruption** A birth defect caused by destruction of tissue; may be caused by vascular occlusion, a teratogen, or rupture of the amniotic sac with entrapment.

**Dizygotic (DZ) twins** Twins produced by two separate ova, separately fertilized. Also called *fraternal twins*.

**DNA (deoxyribonucleic acid)** The molecule that encodes the genes responsible for the structure and function of living organisms and allows the transmission of genetic information from generation to generation.

**DNA methylation** In eukaryotes, the addition of a methyl residue to the 5-position of the pyrimidine ring of a cytosine base in DNA to form 5-methylcytosine.

**DNA polymerase** An enzyme that can synthesize a new DNA strand, using a previously synthesized DNA strand as a template.

**Domain** A region of the amino acid sequence of a protein that can be equated with a particular function.

**Dominant** A trait is dominant if it is phenotypically expressed in heterozygotes.

**Dominant negative** A disease-causing allele, or the effect of such an allele, that disrupts the function of a wild-type allele in the same cell.

**Donor splice site** The boundary between the 3′ end of an exon and the 5′ end of the next intron. Also called *5′ splice site*.

**Dosage compensation** As a consequence of X inactivation, the amount of product formed by the two copies of an X-linked gene in females is equivalent to the amount formed by the single gene in males. See *X inactivation*.

**Double heterozygote** An individual who is heterozygous at each of two different loci. Contrast with *compound heterozygote*.

**Double minutes** Very small accessory chromosomes, a form of gene amplification.

**Dyschronic expression** Expression of a gene at a time when it is not normally expressed.

**Dysmorphism** Morphological developmental abnormalities, as seen in many syndromes of genetic or environmental origin.

**Ecogenetic disorder** A disorder resulting from the interaction of a genetic predisposition to a specific disease with an environmental factor.

**Ectoderm** One of the three primary layers of the early embryo. Begins as the layer farthest from the yolk sac and ultimately gives rise to the nervous system, the skin, and neural crest derivatives such as craniofacial structures and melanocytes.

**Ectopic expression** Expression of a gene in places where it is not normally expressed.

**Embryonic stem cell** A cell derived from the inner cell mass that is self-renewing in culture and, when reintroduced into the inner cell mass of a blastocyst, can repopulate all the tissues of the embryo.

**Empiric risk** In human genetics, the probability that a familial trait will occur or recur in a family member, based on observed numbers of affected and unaffected individuals in family studies rather than on knowledge of the causative mechanism.

**Endoderm** One of the three primary layers of the early embryo. Ultimately gives rise to the gut, liver, and portions of the urogenital system.

**Enhancer** A DNA sequence that acts in *cis* (i.e., on the same chromosome) to increase transcription of a nearby gene. The enhancer may be upstream or downstream to the gene and may be in the same or the reverse orientation. Contrast with *silencer*.

**Enzymopathy** A metabolic disorder resulting from deficiency or abnormality of a specific enzyme.

**Epigenetic** The term that refers to any factor that can affect the phenotype without change in the genotype.

**Epistasis** The situation in which an allele of one gene can block the phenotypic expression of all alleles of another gene.

**Euchromatin** The major component of chromatin. It stains lightly with G banding, decondensing and becoming light-staining during interphase. Contrast with *heterochromatin*.

**Eugenics** Increasing the prevalence of desirable traits in a population by decreasing the frequency of deleterious alleles at relevant loci through controlled, selective breeding. The opposite is *dysgenics*.

**Eukaryote** A unicellular or multicellular organism in which the cells have a nucleus with a nuclear membrane and other specialized characteristics. See also *prokaryote*.

**Euploid** Any chromosome number that is an exact multiple of the number in a haploid gamete (n). Most somatic cells are diploid (2n). Contrast with *aneuploid*.

**Exon** A transcribed region of a gene that is present in mature messenger RNA.

**Expressed sequence tag (EST)** A short DNA sequence, derived by random sequencing of clones from a cDNA library, of sufficient length to uniquely identify a particular mRNA.

**Expressivity** The extent to which a genetic defect is expressed. If there is variable expressivity, the trait may vary in expression from mild to severe but is never completely unexpressed in individuals who have the corresponding genotype. Contrast with *penetrance*.

**Familial** Any trait that is more common in relatives of an affected individual than in the general population, whether the cause is genetic, environmental, or both.

**Fate** The structure or tissue into which a particular region of an embryo ordinarily and regularly develops. The embryonic *fate map* is a complete description of all the fates of all the different parts of the embryo.

**Fetoscopy** A technique for direct visualization of the fetus.

**FISH** Fluorescence in situ hybridization. See *in situ hybridization*.

**Fitness (f)** The probability of transmitting one's genes to the next generation as compared with the average probability for the population.

**Flanking sequence** A region of a gene preceding or following the transcribed region.

**Founder effect** A high frequency of a mutant gene in a population founded by a small ancestral group when one or more of the founders was a carrier of the mutant gene.

**Fragile site** Nonstaining gap in the chromatin of a metaphase chromosome, such as the fragile site at Xq27 in fragile X syndrome.

**Frameshift mutation** A mutation involving a deletion or insertion that is not an exact multiple of three base pairs and thus changes the reading frame of the gene downstream of the mutation.

**Gain-of-function mutation** A mutation associated with an increase in one or more of the normal functions of a protein. To be distinguished from *novel property mutations*.

**Gamete** A reproductive cell (ovum or sperm) with the haploid chromosome number.

**Gatekeeper genes** Tumor suppressor genes that directly regulate cell proliferation.

**Gene** A hereditary unit; in molecular terms, a sequence of chromosomal DNA that is required for the production of a functional product.

**Gene dosage** The number of copies of a particular gene in the genome.

**Gene family** A set of genes containing related exons, indicating that the genes have evolved from an ancestral gene by duplication and subsequent divergence.

**Gene flow** Gradual diffusion of genes from one population to another across a barrier. The barrier may be physical or cultural and may be breached by migration or mixing.

**Gene map** The characteristic arrangement of the genes on the chromosomes. Mapping genes to their chromosomal positions has been one purpose of the Human Genome Project.

**Gene pool** All the alleles present at a given locus or, more broadly, at all loci in the population.

**Gene therapy (gene transfer therapy)** Treatment of a disease by introduction of DNA sequences that will have a therapeutic benefit.

**Genetic** Determined by genes. Not to be confused with *congenital.*

**Genetic background** The total genotype within which a specific genotype is expressed.

**Genetic code** The 64 triplets of bases that specify the 20 amino acids found in proteins (see Table 3–1).

**Genetic counseling** The provision of information and assistance to affected individuals or family members at risk of a disorder that may be genetic, concerning the consequences of the disorder, the probability of developing or transmitting it, and the ways in which it may be prevented or ameliorated.

**Genetic disorder** A defect wholly or partly caused by genes.

**Genetic drift** Random fluctuation of gene frequencies in small populations.

**Genetic heterogeneity** The production of the same or similar phenotypes by different genetic mechanisms. See *allelic heterogeneity, clinical heterogeneity, locus heterogeneity.*

**Genetic lethal** A gene or genetically determined trait that leads to failure to reproduce, although not necessarily to early death.

**Genetic load** The sum total of death and defect caused by mutant genes.

**Genetic map** The relative positions of the genes on the chromosomes, as shown by linkage analysis. See *physical map* for comparison.

**Genetic marker** A locus that has readily classifiable alleles and can be used in genetic studies. It may be a gene or a restriction enzyme site, or any characteristic of DNA that allows different versions of a locus (or its product) to be distinguished one from another and followed through families. See *polymorphism.*

**Genetic screening** Testing on a population basis to identify individuals at risk of developing or of transmitting a specific disorder.

**Genocopy** A genotype that determines a phenotype closely similar to that determined by a different genotype.

**Genome** The complete DNA sequence, containing the entire genetic information, of a gamete, an individual, a population, or a species.

**Genomic DNA** The chromosomal DNA sequence of a gene or segment of a gene, including the DNA sequence of noncoding as well as coding regions. Also, DNA that has been isolated directly from cells or chromosomes or the cloned copies of all or part of such DNA.

**Genomics** The field of genetics concerned with structural and functional studies of the genome.

**Genotype** (1) The genetic constitution of an individual, as distinguished from the phenotype. (2) More specifically, the alleles present at one locus.

**Germline** The cell line from which gametes are derived.

**Germline mosaicism** In an individual, the presence of two or more genetically different types of germline cells, resulting from mutation during the proliferation and differentiation of the germline.

**Globin switching** Change in expression of the various globin genes during ontogeny.

**Haploid** The chromosome number of a normal gamete, with only one member of each chromosome pair. In humans, the haploid number is 23.

**Haploinsufficiency** A cause of genetic disease in which the contribution from a normal allele is insufficient to prevent disease, owing to a loss-of-function mutation at the other allele.

**Haplotype** A group of alleles in coupling at closely linked loci, usually inherited as a unit.

**Hardy-Weinberg law** The law that relates gene frequency to genotype frequency, used in population genetics to determine allele frequency and heterozygote frequency when the incidence of a disorder is known.

**Hemizygous** A term for the genotype of an individual with only one representative of a chromosome or chromosome segment, rather than the usual two; refers especially to X-linked genes in the male but also applies to genes on any chromosome segment that is deleted on the homologous chromosome.

**Heritability ($h^2$)** The fraction of total phenotypic variance of a quantitative trait that is due to genotypic differences. May be viewed as a statistical estimate of the hereditary contribution to a quantitative trait.

**Heterochromatin** Chromatin that stains darkly throughout the cell cycle, even in interphase. Generally thought to be late replicating and genetically inactive. Satellite DNA in regions such as centromeres, acrocentric short arms, and 1qh, 9qh, 16qh, and Yqh constitute *constitutive heterochromatin*, whereas the chromatin of the inactive X chromosome is referred to as *facultative heterochromatin.* Contrast with *euchromatin.*

**Heterogeneity** See *allelic heterogeneity, clinical heterogeneity, genetic heterogeneity, locus heterogeneity.*

**Heterokaryon** A cell with two separate nuclei, formed by fusion of two genetically different cells. Contrast with *homokaryon.*

**Heteromorphism** A normal morphological or staining variant of a chromosome.

**Heteroplasmy** The presence of more than one type of mitochondrial DNA in the mitochondria of a single individual. Contrast with *homoplasmy.*

**Heteroploid** Any chromosome number other than the normal.

**Heterozygote (heterozygous)** An individual or genotype with two different alleles at a given locus on a pair of homologous chromosomes.

**Histocompatibility** A host will accept a particular graft only if it is histocompatible—that is, if the graft contains no antigens that the host lacks.

**Histones** Proteins associated with DNA in the chromosomes that are rich in basic amino acids (lysine or arginine) and virtually invariant throughout eukaryote evolution.

**Holoenzyme** The functional compound formed by the binding of an apoenzyme and its appropriate coenzyme.

**Homeobox gene** A gene that contains a conserved 180 base-pair sequence in its coding region, termed a *homeobox*, encoding a protein motif known as the *homeodomain*. The 60 amino acid residues of the homeodomain is a DNA-binding motif, which is consistent with the role of homeodomain proteins in transcriptional regulation of genes involved in development. See *paired domain.*

**Homogeneously staining regions (HSRs)** Chromosome regions that stain uniformly and represent amplified copies of a DNA segment.

**Homokaryon** A cell derived by fusion of two genetically identical cells. Contrast with *heterokaryon.*

**Homologous chromosomes (homologs)** A pair of chromosomes, one inherited paternally, the other maternally, that pair with each other during meiosis I, undergo crossing over, and separate at anaphase I of meiosis. Homologous chromosomes are generally of similar size and shape when viewed under the microscope and contain the same loci, except for the two sex chromosomes in males (X and Y), which are only partially homologous (see *pseudoautosomal region*).

**Homologous genes (homologs)** Refers to genes in a single species, or in different species, that have overall similar DNA sequences, that may have related biochemical functions, and that arose from a common ancestral gene. Orthologous and parologous genes are types of homologous genes, but their meaning is more restricted.

**Homoplasmy** The presence of only one type of mitochondrial DNA in the mitochondria of a single individual. Contrast with *heteroplasmy.*

**Homozygote (homozygous)** An individual or genotype with identical alleles at a given locus on a pair of homologous chromosomes.

**Host** In molecular genetics, the organism in which a recombinant DNA molecule is isolated and grown; usually *Escherichia coli* or yeast.

**Housekeeping genes** Genes expressed in most or all cells because their products provide basic functions.

**Housekeeping proteins** Proteins expressed in virtually every cell that have fundamental roles in the maintenance of cell structure and function (versus *specialty* proteins).

**Human Genome Project** The major current research project, international in scope, to map and sequence the entire human genome and those of model organisms.

**Hybrid cell** A cell formed by the fusion of two cells of different origin in which the two nuclei have merged into one. Can be cloned to produce hybrid cell lines.

**Hybridization** In molecular biology, the bonding of two complementary single-stranded nucleic acid molecules according to base-pairing rules. In somatic cell genetics, fusion of two somatic cells, often from different organisms, to form a hybrid cell containing the genetic information of both parental cell types.

**Hydatidiform mole** An abnormality of the placenta in which it grows to resemble a hydatid cyst or bunch of grapes, associated with very abnormal fetal development. In a *complete mole*, the karyotype is 46,XX, representing duplication of the chromosomes of the sperm with no maternal contribution. A *partial mole* is triploid, usually with an extra paternal chromosome set.

**Identical by descent** Two individuals in a family who have the same allele(s) at a locus because they inherited the allele(s) from a common ancestor. See *coefficient of inbreeding.*

**Immunoglobulin gene superfamily** A family of evolutionarily related genes composed of human leukocyte antigen (HLA) class I and class II genes, immunoglobulin genes, T-cell receptor genes, and other genes encoding cell surface molecules.

**Imprinting** The phenomenon of different expression of alleles depending on the parent of origin. See *Prader-Willi syndrome* and *Angelman syndrome* in text for examples.

**Inborn error of metabolism** A genetically determined biochemical disorder in which a specific protein defect produces a metabolic block that may have pathological consequences.

**Inbreeding** The mating of closely related individuals. The progeny of close relatives are said to be *inbred.*

**Incompletely dominant** A trait that is inherited in a dominant manner but is more severe in a homozygote than in a heterozygote.

**Index case** An affected family member who is the first to draw attention to a pedigree of a genetic disorder. See *proband.*

**Induction** The determining of the fate of one region of an embryo by extracellular signals from a second, usually neighboring, region.

**In-frame deletion** A deletion that does not destroy the normal reading frame of the gene.

**Inner cell mass** A small group of cells within the preimplantation mammalian embryo that will become the primitive ectoderm (or epiblast) after implantation and, ultimately, will give rise to the embryo proper and not the placenta.

**Insert** In molecular biology, a fragment of foreign DNA cloned into a vector.

**Insertion** A chromosomal abnormality in which a DNA segment from one chromosome is inserted into a nonhomologous chromosome.

**In situ hybridization** Mapping a gene by molecular hybridization of a cloned DNA sequence, labeled by radioactivity or fluorescence, to a chromosome spread or cell nucleus on a slide.

**Intergenic complementation** The ability of cells from patients with similar phenotypes due to mutations in different genes to correct one another.

**Intergenic DNA** The untranscribed DNA of unknown function that makes up a large proportion of the total DNA in the genome.

**Interphase** The stage of the cell cycle between two successive mitoses.

**Intervening sequence** See *intron*.

**Intragenic (or interallelic) complementation** The ability of one mutant allele at a locus to correct for the loss of function associated with another allele at that locus, thus demonstrating that the mutations are not identical (see *complementation*).

**Intron** A segment of a gene that is initially transcribed but is then removed from within the primary RNA transcript by splicing together the sequences (exons) on either side of it.

**Inversion** A chromosomal rearrangement in which a segment of a chromosome is reversed end to end. If the centromere is included in the inversion, the inversion is *pericentric;* if not, it is *paracentric.*

**In vitro fertilization** A reproductive technology in which sperm are allowed to fertilize an egg in tissue culture and the fertilized eggs are then introduced back into the uterus to allow implantation.

**Isochromosome** An abnormal chromosome in which one arm is duplicated (forming two arms of equal length, with the same loci in reverse sequence) and the other arm is missing.

**Isolate** A subpopulation in which matings take place exclusively or usually with other members of the same subpopulation.

**Isolated case** An individual who is the only member of his or her kindred affected by a genetic disorder, either by chance or by new mutation. See also *sporadic*.

**Isotype** In immunology, refers to the five structurally and functionally different classes of immunoglobulin heavy chains, designated gamma, alpha, mu, delta, and epsilon, with corresponding immunoglobulins IgG, IgA, IgM, IgD, and IgE.

**Karyotype** The chromosome constitution of an individual. The term is also used for a photomicrograph of the chromosomes of an individual systematically arranged and for the process of preparing such a photomicrograph.

**kb (kilobase)** A unit of 1000 bases in a DNA or RNA sequence.

**Kindred** An extended family.

**Kinetochore** A structure at the centromere to which the spindle fibers are attached.

**Knockout mice** Mice in which a specific gene has been disrupted or "targeted" by recombinant DNA technology; used as models for investigation of the function and interactions of the normal counterparts of the disrupted genes.

**Library** In molecular biology, a collection of recombinant clones that contain a random sample of the DNA or RNA (as cDNA) of a tissue.

**Ligation** In molecular biology, the process of joining two double-stranded DNA molecules to form a recombinant DNA molecule, by means of phosphodiester bonds, using the enzyme DNA ligase.

**Lineage** The progeny of a cell, generally determined by experimentally labeling the cell so that all of its descendants can be identified. See *clone*.

**Linkage** Genes on the same chromosome are *linked* if they are transmitted together in meiosis more frequently than chance would allow. Compare with *synteny*.

**Linkage analysis** A statistical method in which the genotypes and phenotypes of parents and offspring in families are studied to determine whether two or more loci are assorting independently or exhibiting linkage during meiosis.

**Linkage disequilibrium** The occurrence of specific combinations of alleles in coupling phase at two or more linked loci more frequently than expected by chance.

**Linkage map** A chromosome map showing the relative positions of genes and other DNA markers on the chromosomes, as determined by linkage analysis.

**L1 family** A class of repetitive DNA made up of long interspersed sequences, up to 6 kb in length, occurring in several hundred thousand copies in the genome.

**Locus** The position occupied by a gene on a chromosome. Different forms of the gene (*alleles*) may occupy the locus.

**Locus control region (LCR)** A DNA domain, situated outside a cluster of structural genes, responsible for the appropriate expression of the genes within the cluster.

**Locus heterogeneity** The production of identical phenotypes by mutations at two or more different loci.

**Lod score** A statistical method that tests genetic marker data in families to determine whether two loci are linked. The lod score is the *l*ogarithm of the *od*ds in favor of linkage. By convention, a lod score of 3 (odds of 1000:1 in favor) is accepted as proof of linkage and a lod score of −2 (100:1 against) as proof that the loci are unlinked.

**Loops** Arrangement of chromatin, packaged as solenoids, attached to the chromosome scaffold. Thought to be a structural or functional unit, or both, of chromosomes.

**Loss-of-function mutation** A mutation associated with a reduction or a complete loss of one or more of the normal functions of a protein.

**Loss of heterozygosity (LOH)** Loss of a normal allele from a region of one chromosome of a pair, allowing a defective allele on the homologous chromosome to be clinically manifest. A feature of many cases of retinoblastoma, breast cancer, and other tumors due to mutation in a tumor-suppressor gene.

**Lyonization** Term used for the phenomenon of X inactivation, which was first described by the geneticist Mary Lyon. See *X inactivation*.

**Major histocompatibility complex (MHC)** The complex locus on chromosome 6p that includes the highly polymorphic human leukocyte antigen (HLA) genes.

**MHC restriction** An immunological phenomenon such that a T cell will only respond to an antigen if it is presented on the surface of a cell that shares the T cell's own MHC antigens.

**Male-to-male transmission** A pattern of inheritance of a trait from a father to all of his sons and none of his daughters (also referred to as *holandric* inheritance).

**Malformation syndrome** A recognizable pattern of dysmorphic features having a single cause, either genetic or environmental.

**Manifesting heterozygote** A female heterozygous for an X-linked disorder in whom, because of nonrandom X inactivation, the trait is expressed clinically with approximately the same degree of severity as in hemizygous affected males.

**Maternal inheritance** The transmission of genetic information only through the mother.

**Maternal serum screening** Laboratory test that relies on measuring the levels of particular substances, such as alpha-fetoprotein, human chorionic gonadotropin, and unconjugated estriol, in a pregnant woman's blood to screen for fetuses affected with certain trisomies or with neural tube defects.

**Meiosis** The type of cell division occurring in the germ cells, by which gametes containing the haploid chromosome number are produced from diploid cells. Two meiotic divisions occur: meiosis I and meiosis II. Reduction in chromosome number takes place during meiosis I.

**Mesoderm** The middle germ layer in the early embryo; the source of cells that go on to make bones, muscles, connective tissue, heart, hematopoietic system, kidney, and other organs.

**Messenger RNA (mRNA)** An RNA, transcribed from the DNA of a gene, that directs the sequence of amino acids of the encoded polypeptide.

**Metacentric** A type of chromosome with a central centromere and arms of apparently equal length.

**Metaphase** The stage of mitosis or meiosis in which the chromosomes have reached their maximal condensation and are lined up on the equatorial plane of the cell, attached to the spindle fibers. This is the stage at which chromosomes are most easily examined.

**Metastasis** Spread of malignant cells to other sites in the body.

**Methemoglobin** The oxidized form of hemoglobin, containing iron in the ferric rather than the ferrous state, that is incapable of binding oxygen.

**Microdeletion** A chromosomal deletion that is too small to be seen under the microscope. See also *contiguous gene syndrome*.

**Microsatellite marker** See *short tandem repeat polymorphism (STRP)*.

**Missense mutation** A mutation that changes a codon specific for one amino acid to specify another amino acid.

**Mitochondrial DNA (mtDNA)** The DNA in the circular chromosome of the mitochondria. Mitochondrial DNA is present in many copies per cell, is maternally inherited, and evolves 5 to 10 times as rapidly as genomic DNA.

**Mitochondrial inheritance** The inheritance of a trait encoded in the mitochondrial genome. Because the mitochondrial genome is strictly maternally inherited, mitochondrial inheritance occurs solely through the female line.

**Mitosis** The process of ordinary cell division, resulting in the formation of two cells genetically identical to the parent cell.

**Model-based linkage analysis** Linkage analysis that relies on assuming a particular mode of inheritance in order to infer when crossovers have occurred between two loci. Also referred to as *parametric linkage analysis*.

**Model-free linkage analysis** Linkage analysis that makes no assumptions as to the mode of inheritance. This form of analysis relies on determining whether the extent of allele sharing at any loci among related individuals who either do or do not share a disease or trait deviates significantly from what would be expected by chance alone. See *affected pedigree member method*. Also referred to as *nonparametric linkage analysis*.

**Modifier gene** A gene that alters the phenotype associated with mutations in a nonallelic gene.

**Monosomy** A chromosome constitution in which one member of a chromosome pair is missing, as in 45,X Turner syndrome.

**Monozygotic (MZ) twins** Twins derived from a single zygote and thus genetically identical. Also termed *identical twins*.

**Morphogen** A substance produced during development in a localized region of the organism that diffuses out to form a concentration gradient and directs cells into two or more specific developmental pathways depending on its concentration.

**Morphogenesis** The process whereby changes in cell shape, adhesion, movement, and number lead to three-dimensional structure.

**Mosaic** An individual or tissue with at least two cell lines differing in genotype or karyotype, derived from a single zygote. Not to be confused with *chimera*.

**Mosaic development** Embryological development in which different regions of the embryo develop independently from surrounding regions. See *regulative development*.

**Multifactorial inheritance** The type of nonmendelian inheritance shown by traits that are determined by a combination of multiple factors, genetic and environmental. Also termed *complex inheritance*.

**Multiplex** A pedigree in which there is more than one case of a particular disorder.

**Multipoint linkage analysis** Resolving the order of three or more loci by examining the genotypes of offspring of parents heterozygous at the loci and determining an order that would minimize the number of very unlikely double recombinations over a short interval.

**Mutagen** An agent that increases the spontaneous mutation rate by causing changes in DNA.

**Mutant** A gene that has been altered by mutation; also used to refer to a nonhuman organism carrying a mutant gene.

**Mutation** Any permanent heritable change in the sequence of genomic DNA.

**Mutation rate ($\mu$)** The frequency of mutation at a given locus, expressed as mutations per locus per gamete (or per generation, which is the same).

**Neoplasia** An abnormal growth produced by imbalance between normal cellular proliferation and normal cellular attrition. May be benign or malignant (cancer).

**Noncoding strand** See *antisense strand.*

**Nondisjunction** The failure of two members of a chromosome pair to disjoin during meiosis I, or two chromatids of a chromosome to disjoin during meiosis II or mitosis, so that both pass to one daughter cell and the other daughter cell receives neither.

**Nonsense mutation** A single-base substitution in DNA resulting in a chain-termination codon.

**Northern blotting** A technique analogous to Southern blotting, for detection of RNA molecules by hybridization to a complementary DNA probe.

**Novel property mutation** A mutation that confers a new property on the protein.

**Nuchal translucency** An ultrasonographic finding of an echo free space between the skin line and the soft tissue overlying the cervical spine in the subcutaneous tissue of the fetal neck. Associated with fetal aneuploidy.

**Nucleosome** The primary structural unit of chromatin, consisting of 146 base pairs of DNA wrapped twice around a core of eight histone molecules.

**Nucleotide** A molecule composed of a nitrogenous base, a 5-carbon sugar, and a phosphate group. A nucleic acid is a polymer of many nucleotides.

**Null allele** An allele that results either in the total absence of the gene product or in the total loss of function at the phenotypic level.

**Obligate heterozygote** An individual who may be clinically unaffected but on the basis of pedigree analysis must carry a specific mutant allele.

**Odds** A ratio of probabilities or risks. Often calculated as a ratio of the probability of an event occurring versus the probability of the event not occurring, as one way to assess the relative chance of the event. Odds can vary in value from 0 to infinity.

**Odds ratio** A comparison of the odds that individuals who share a particular factor (e.g., a genotype, an environmental exposure, or a drug) will have a disease or trait versus the odds for individuals who lack the factor. In individuals in whom the factor is present, the *odds* of being affected = (a/c). In individuals in whom the factor is absent, the *odds* of being affected = (b/d), and the odds ratio = (a/c)/(b/d) = ad/bc. See *relative risk.*

| | *Factor Present* | *Factor Absent* | *Total* |
|---|---|---|---|
| Affected | **a** | **b** | a + b |
| Unaffected | **c** | **d** | c + d |
| Total | a + c | b + d | a + b + c + d |

**Oligonucleotide** A short DNA molecule (usually 8 to 50 base pairs), synthesized for use as a probe or for use in the polymerase chain reaction.

**Oncogene** A dominantly acting gene involved in unregulated cell growth and proliferation, responsible for tumor development. Mutation, overexpression, or amplification of oncogenes in somatic cells may lead to neoplastic transformation. Contrast with *proto-oncogene* and with *tumor-suppressor gene.*

**Ontogeny** The developmental history of an organism.

**Open reading frame** The interval between the start and stop codons of a nucleotide sequence that encodes a protein.

**Orthologous** Refers to genes in different species that are similar in DNA sequence and also encode proteins that have the same function—at least at the biochemical level—in each species. Orthologous genes originate from the same gene in a common ancestor. Contrast with *paralogous.*

**p** In cytogenetics, the short arm of a chromosome (from the French *petit*). In population genetics, the frequency of the more common allele of a pair. In biochemistry, abbreviation of *protein* (e.g., p53 is a protein 53 kilodaltons in size).

**PACs (P1 artificial chromosomes)** Vectors capable of cloning DNA inserts 100 to 300 kb in size, used in high-resolution mapping and gene sequencing.

**Painting probe** See *chromosome painting probe.*

**Paired domain** A DNA-binding motif found in the members of a large class of mammalian transcription factors encoded by *PAX* genes. Named originally for the *Drosophila paired* gene in which it was first described.

**Palindrome** In molecular biology, a nucleotide sequence in which the 5′ to 3′ sequence of one strand of a segment of DNA is the same as that of its complementary strand. The sites of restriction enzymes are usually palindromes.

**Paralogous** Refers to two or more genes in a single species that are similar in DNA sequence and are likely to encode proteins with similar and perhaps overlapping, but not identical, functions. Paralogous genes are likely to have originated from a common ancestral gene. Example, $\alpha$- and $\beta$-globin genes.

**PCR** See *polymerase chain reaction.*

**Pedigree** In medical genetics, a family history of a hereditary condition, or a diagram of a family history indicating the family members, their relationship to the proband, and their status with respect to a particular hereditary condition.

**Penetrance** The fraction of individuals with a genotype known to cause a disease who have any signs or symptoms of the disease. Contrast with *expressivity.*

**Pharmacogenetics** The area of biochemical genetics concerned with drug responses and their genetically controlled variations.

**Pharmacogenomics** The application of genomic information or methods to pharmacogenetic problems.

**Phase** In an individual heterozygous at two syntenic loci, the designation of which allele at the first locus and which allele at the second locus are on the same chromosome. See *coupling* and *repulsion*.

**Phenocopy** A mimic of a phenotype that is usually determined by a specific genotype, produced instead by the interaction of some environmental factor with a normal genotype.

**Phenotype** The observed biochemical, physiological, and morphological characteristics of an individual, as determined by his or her genotype and the environment in which it is expressed. Also, in a more limited sense, the abnormalities resulting from a particular mutant gene.

**Philadelphia chromosome ($Ph^1$)** The structurally abnormal chromosome 22 that typically occurs in a proportion of the bone marrow cells in most patients with chronic myelogenous leukemia. The abnormality is a reciprocal translocation between the distal portion of 22q and the distal portion of 9q.

**Physical map** A map showing the order of genes and markers along a chromosome and their distances apart in units such as cytogenetic bands or base pairs. Physical mapping is performed by techniques such as radiation hybrid mapping, fluorescence in situ hybridization (FISH), and nucleotide sequencing, not by data from linkage analysis. See *genetic mapping* for comparison.

**Plasmids** Independently replicating, extrachromosomal circular DNA molecules in bacteria or yeast, used in molecular biology as vectors for cloned segments of DNA.

**Pleiotropy** Multiple phenotypic effects of a single gene or gene pair. The term is used particularly when the effects are not obviously related.

**Pluripotent** Describes an embryonic cell that is capable of giving rise to different types of differentiated tissues or structures depending on its location and environmental influences.

**Point mutation** A single nucleotide base-pair change in DNA.

**Polyadenylation site** In the synthesis of mature mRNA, a site at which a sequence of 20 to 200 adenosine residues (the polyA tail) is added to the 3′ end of an RNA transcript, aiding its transport out of the nucleus and, usually, its stability.

**Polygenic** Inheritance determined by many genes at different loci, with small additive effects. Not to be confused with *complex (multifactorial)* inheritance, in which environmental as well as genetic factors may be involved.

**Polymerase chain reaction (PCR)** The molecular genetic technique by which a short DNA or RNA sequence is amplified enormously by means of two flanking oligonucleotide primers used in repeated cycles of primer extension and DNA synthesis with DNA polymerase.

**Polymorphism** The occurrence together in a population of two or more alternative genotypes, each at a frequency greater than that which could be maintained by recurrent mutation alone. A locus is arbitrarily considered to be polymorphic if the rarer allele has a frequency of .01, so that the heterozygote frequency is at least .02. Any allele rarer than this is a *rare variant*.

**Polyploid** Any multiple of the basic haploid chromosome number other than the diploid number; thus, 3n, 4n, and so forth.

**Positional cloning** The molecular cloning of a gene on the basis of knowledge of its map position, without prior knowledge of the gene product.

**Preimplantation diagnosis** A type of prenatal diagnosis in which a cell is removed from a multicell embryo generated by in vitro fertilization and tested for the presence of a disease-causing mutation.

**Premutation** In triplet repeat disorders—for example, fragile X syndrome—a moderate expansion of the number of triplet repeats that has no phenotypic effect but is at increased risk of undergoing further expansion during meiosis and causing full expression of the disorder in the offspring.

**Primary constriction** See *centromere*.

**Primary structure** The amino acid sequence of a polypeptide.

**Primary transcript** The initial, unprocessed RNA transcript of a gene that is colinear with the genomic DNA, containing introns as well as exons.

**Primer** A short oligonucleotide designed to hybridize to a single-stranded DNA template and provide a free DNA end to which DNA polymerase can add bases and synthesize DNA complementary to the template.

**Private mutation** A very rare mutation, perhaps known in only a single family or single population.

**Proband** The affected family member through whom the family is ascertained. Also called the *propositus* or *index case*.

**Probe** In molecular genetics, a labeled DNA or RNA sequence used to detect the presence of a complementary sequence by molecular hybridization; or a reagent capable of recognizing a desired clone in a mixture of many DNA or RNA sequences. Also, the process of using such a molecule.

**Prokaryote** A simple unicellular organism, such as a bacterium, lacking a separate nucleus. See *eukaryote*.

**Promoter** A DNA sequence located in the 5′ end of a gene at which transcription is initiated.

**Prophase** The first stage of cell division, during which the chromosomes become visible as discrete structures and subsequently thicken and shorten. Prophase of the first meiotic division is further characterized by pairing (synapsis) of homologous chromosomes.

**Propositus** See *proband*.

**Proteomics** A field of biochemistry encompassing the comprehensive analysis and cataloging of the structure and function of all the proteins present in a given cell or tissue (the proteome). Parallels *genomics*, a similarly comprehensive approach to the analysis of DNA sequence and mRNA expression.

**Proto-oncogene** A normal gene involved in some aspect of cell division or proliferation that may become activated by mutation or other mechanism to become an oncogene.

**Pseudoautosomal region** Segment of the X and Y chromosome, located at the most distal portion of their respective p and q arms, at which crossing over occurs during male meiosis. Traits due to alleles at pseudoautosomal loci will appear to be inherited as autosomal traits despite the physical location of these loci on the sex chromosomes.

**Pseudodeficiency allele** A clinically benign allele that has a reduction in functional activity detected by in vitro assays but that has sufficient activity in vivo to prevent haploinsufficiency.

**Pseudogene** (1) An inactive gene within a gene family, derived by mutation of an ancestral active gene and frequently located within the same region of the chromosome as its functional counterpart (*nonprocessed pseudogene*); (2) a DNA copy of an mRNA, created by retrotransposition and inserted randomly in the genome (*processed pseudogene*). Processed pseudogenes are probably never functional.

**Pseudomosaicism** The occurrence of a single cytogenetically abnormal cell in a cytogenetic analysis of a chorionic villus sampling (CVS) or amniocentesis specimen. Generally considered artefactual and of no clinical significance.

**q** In cytogenetics, the long arm of a chromosome; in population genetics, the frequency of the less common allele of a pair.

**Qualitative trait** A trait in which an individual either has the trait or does not. Contrast with *quantitative trait*.

**Quantitative trait** A trait that is a measurable quantity that differs among different individuals, often following a normal distribution in the population. Contrast with *qualitative trait*.

**Radiation hybrid mapping** A gene mapping method that uses somatic cell hybridization to transfer small chromosomal fragments generated by x-rays into host cells.

**Random mating** Selection of a mate without regard to the genotype of the mate. In a randomly mating population, the frequencies of the various matings are determined solely by the frequencies of the genes concerned.

**Reading frame** One of the three possible ways of reading a nucleotide sequence as a series of triplets. An *open reading frame* contains no termination codons and thus is potentially translatable into protein.

**Rearrangement** Chromosome breakage followed by reconstitution in an abnormal combination. If *unbalanced*, the rearrangement can produce an abnormal phenotype.

**Recessive** A trait that is expressed only in homozygotes or hemizygotes.

**Reciprocal translocation** See *translocation*.

**Recombinant** An individual who has a new combination of alleles not found in either parent.

**Recombinant chromosome** A chromosome that results from exchange of reciprocal segments by crossing over between a homologous pair of parental chromosomes during meiosis.

**Recombinant DNA technology** Technology by which a DNA molecule is constructed in vitro from segments from more than one parental DNA molecule.

**Recombination** The formation of new combinations of alleles in coupling by crossing over between their loci.

**Recombination fraction ($\theta$)** The fraction of offspring of a parent heterozygous at two loci who have inherited a chromosome carrying a recombination between the loci.

**Recurrence risk** The probability that a genetic disorder present in one or more members of a family will recur in another member of the same or a subsequent generation.

**Reduction division** The first meiotic division, so called because at this stage the chromosome number per cell is reduced from diploid to haploid.

**Redundancy** The situation in which genes (often paralogous) have overlapping functions.

**Regulative development** A developmental stage during which removal or destruction of a particular region of the embryo is compensated for by other embryonic regions, thereby allowing normal development.

**Regulatory gene** A gene that codes for an RNA or protein molecule that regulates the expression of other genes.

**Regulatory region of a gene** A DNA segment, such as a promoter, enhancer, or locus-control region, within or near a gene that regulates the expression of the gene.

**Relative risk** A comparison of the *risk* for a disease or trait in individuals who share a particular factor (such as genotype, an environmental exposure, or a drug) versus the *risk* among individuals who lack the factor. The *risk* of being affected in individuals who have the factor = (a/a + c), the *risk* of being affected when the factor is absent = (b/b + d), and the relative risk = (a/a + c)/(b/b + d) = a(b + d)/b(a + c). Note that relative risk ≈ ad/bc, the odds ratio, when the disease is relatively rare (b < < d and a < < c). See *odds ratio*.

| | *Factor Present* | *Factor Absent* | *Total* |
|---|---|---|---|
| Affected | **a** | **b** | a + b |
| Unaffected | **c** | **d** | c + d |
| Total | a + c | b + d | a + b + c + d |

**Relative risk ratio ($\lambda_r$)** In complex disorders, the risk that a disease will occur in a relative of an affected person as compared with the risk for disease in any random person in the general population.

**Repetitive DNA (repeats)** DNA sequences that are present in multiple copies in the genome.

**Replication error positive** A phenotype of cancer cells in which loss of function of mismatch repair genes causes errors such as slipped mispairing to go unrepaired when microsatellite sequences are replicated. These errors lead to tissue mosaicism so that the cancer appears to contain more than two alleles at many short tandem repeat polymorphic loci.

**Restriction endonuclease (restriction enzyme)** An enzyme, derived from bacteria, that can recognize a specific sequence of DNA and cleave the DNA molecule within the recognition site or at some nearby site.

**Restriction fragment length polymorphism (RFLP)** A polymorphic difference in DNA sequence between individuals that can be recognized by restriction endonucleases. See *polymorphism.*

**Restriction map** A linear array of sites on DNA cleaved by various restriction endonucleases.

**Restriction site** A short sequence in DNA that can be recognized and cut by a specific restriction endonuclease.

**Retrovirus** A virus, with an RNA genome, that propagates by conversion of the RNA into DNA by the enzyme reverse transcriptase.

**Reverse transcriptase** An enzyme, RNA-dependent DNA polymerase, that catalyzes the synthesis of DNA on an RNA template.

**RFLP** See *restriction fragment length polymorphism.*

**Ribonucleic acid** See *RNA.*

**Ribosome** A cytoplasmic organelle composed of ribosomal RNA and protein, on which polypeptides are synthesized from messenger RNA.

**Ring chromosome** A structurally abnormal chromosome in which the telomere of each chromosome arm has been deleted and the broken arms have reunited in ring formation.

**Risk** The probability of an event occurring. Often calculated as the number of times the event occurs divided by the total number of opportunities there were for the event to occur. As with all probabilities, risk varies from 0 to 1.

**RNA (ribonucleic acid)** A nucleic acid formed upon a DNA template, containing ribose instead of deoxyribose. *Messenger RNA (mRNA)* is the template on which polypeptides are synthesized. *Transfer RNA (tRNA)*, in cooperation with the ribosomes, brings activated amino acids into position along the mRNA template. *Ribosomal RNA (rRNA)*, a component of the ribosomes, functions as a nonspecific site of polypeptide synthesis.

**RNA polymerase** An enzyme that synthesizes RNA on a DNA template.

**Robertsonian translocation** A translocation between two acrocentric chromosomes by fusion at or near the centromere, with loss of the short arms.

**Satellite DNA** DNA containing many tandem repeats of a short basic repeating unit. Not to be confused with *chromosomal satellites*, the chromatin at the distal end of the short arms of the acrocentric chromosomes.

**Scaffold** The nonhistone structure observed when histones are experimentally removed from chromosomes. Believed to represent a structural component of the nucleus and of chromosomes.

**Segmental aneusomy** Loss of a small segment from one chromosome of a pair, resulting in hemizygosity for genes in that segment on the homologous chromosome. See also *contiguous gene syndrome.*

**Segregation** In genetics, the disjunction of homologous chromosomes at meiosis.

**Segregation analysis** A statistical method that assesses the phenotypes of individuals in families to determine the most likely mode of inheritance of a disease or trait.

**Selection** In population genetics, the operation of forces that determine the relative fitness of a genotype in the population, thus affecting the frequency of the gene concerned.

**Sense strand** See *coding strand.*

**Sensitivity** In diagnostic tests, the frequency with which the test result is positive when the disorder is present.

**Sequence** (1) In genomics and molecular genetics, the order of nucleotides in a segment of DNA or RNA. (2) In clinical genetics, a recognizable pattern of dysmorphic features caused by a number of different etiologies. To be distinguished from *malformation syndromes.*

**Sequence-tagged site (STS)** A short DNA sequence that can be amplified and used to identify a specific location on the physical map.

**Sex chromatin** See *Barr body.*

**Sex chromosomes** The X and Y chromosomes.

**Sex-influenced** A trait that is not X-linked in its pattern of inheritance but is expressed differently, either in degree or in frequency, in males and females.

**Sex-limited** A trait that is expressed in only one sex, although the gene that determines the trait is not X-linked.

**Sex-linked** Old term for *X-linked*, now little used because formally it fails to distinguish between X- and Y-linkage.

**Short tandem repeat polymorphism (STRP)** A polymorphic locus consisting of a variable number of tandemly repeated bi-, tri-, or tetranucleotide units such as $(TG)_n$, $(CAA)_n$, or $(GATA)_n$; different numbers of units constitute the different alleles. Also termed a *microsatellite marker.*

**Sib, sibling** A brother or sister.

**Sibpair analysis** A form of model-free linkage analysis in which pairs of siblings either concordant or discordant for a phenotype or trait are analyzed at loci throughout the genome to determine whether there are any loci at which they share alleles significantly more or less than the expected average of 50 percent.

**Sibship** All the sibs in a family.

**Silencer** A DNA sequence that acts in *cis* (i.e., on the same chromosome) to decrease transcription of a nearby gene. The silencer may be upstream or downstream to the gene and may be in the same or the reverse orientation (contrast with *enhancer*).

**Silent allele** A mutant gene that has no detectable phenotypic effect.

**Simplex** In human genetics, the term used to describe a family history with only one member affected by a genetic disorder.

**Single-copy DNA** The type of DNA that makes up most of the genome.

**Single-gene disorder** A disorder due to one or a pair of mutant alleles at a single locus.

**Single nucleotide polymorphism (SNP)** A polymorphism in DNA sequence consisting of variation in a single base.

**Sister chromatid exchange** The exchange of segments of DNA between sister chromatids, either in the four-strand stage of meiosis or in mitosis. Occurs with particularly high frequency in patients with Bloom syndrome.

**SKY** See *spectral karyotyping*.

**Slipped mispairing** A mutational mechanism that occurs during DNA replication of sequences with repeats of one or more nucleotides, in which a repeat on one strand mispairs with a similar repeat on the complementary strand, generating a deletion or expansion of the number of repeats.

**SNP** See *single nucleotide polymorphism*.

**Solenoid** A fiber composed of compacted strings of nucleosomes, forming the fundamental unit of chromatin organization.

**Somatic cell genetics** The study of genetic phenomena in cultured somatic cells.

**Somatic mutation** A mutation occurring in a somatic cell rather than in the germline.

**Somatic rearrangement** Rearrangement of DNA sequences in the chromosomes of lymphocyte precursor cells, thus generating antibody and T-cell receptor diversity.

**Southern blotting** A technique, devised by the British biochemist Ed Southern, for preparation of a filter to which DNA has been transferred, following restriction enzyme digestion and gel electrophoresis to separate the DNA molecules by size. Specific DNA molecules can then be detected on the filter by their hybridization to labeled probes.

**Specialty proteins** Proteins, expressed in only one or a limited number of cell types, that have unique functions that contribute to the individuality of the cells in which they are expressed. Contrast with *housekeeping proteins*.

**Specification** The first stage of commitment in which a cell will follow its developmental program if explanted but can still be reprogrammed to a different fate if transplanted to a different part of the embryo.

**Specificity** In diagnostic tests, the frequency with which a test result is negative when the disease is absent.

**Spectral karyotyping (SKY)** A procedure that uses the fluorescence in situ hybridization (FISH) technique to stain each of the 24 human chromosomes distinctively.

**Splicing** The splicing out of introns and splicing together of exons in the generation of mature mRNA from the primary transcript.

**Sporadic** In medical genetics, a disease caused by a new mutation.

**Stem cell** A type of cell capable of both self-renewal and of proliferation and differentiation.

**Stop codon** See *termination codon*.

**Stratification** The situation in which a population contains a number of subgroups whose members have not freely and randomly mated with the members of other subgroups.

**Structural gene** A gene coding for any RNA or protein product.

**Structural protein** A protein that serves a structural role in the body, such as collagen.

**Submetacentric** A type of chromosome with arms of different lengths.

**Synapsis** Close pairing of homologous chromosomes in prophase of the first meiotic division.

**Syndrome** A characteristic pattern of anomalies, presumed to be causally related.

**Synteny** The physical presence together on the same chromosome of two or more gene loci, whether or not they are close enough together for linkage to be demonstrated.

**Tandem repeats** Two or more copies of the same (or very similar) DNA sequence arranged in a direct head-to-tail succession along a chromosome.

**TATA box** A consensus sequence in the promoter region of many genes that is located about 25 base pairs upstream from the start site of transcription and that determines the start site.

**T-cell antigen receptor (TCR)** Genetically coded receptor on the surface of T lymphocytes that specifically recognizes antigen molecules.

**Telomerase** A ribonucleoprotein reverse transcriptase that uses its own RNA template to add species-specific hexamers (such as TTAGGG in humans) to telomeres.

**Telomere** The end of each chromosome arm. Human telomeres end with tandem copies of the sequence $(TTAGGG)_n$, which is required for the proper replication of chromosome ends.

**Telophase** The stage of cell division that begins when the daughter chromosomes reach the poles of the dividing cell and that lasts until the two daughter cells take on the appearance of interphase cells.

**Teratogen** An agent that produces congenital malformations or increases their incidence.

**Termination codon** One of the three codons (UAG, UAA, and UGA) that terminate synthesis of a polypeptide. Also called a *stop codon*. (See Table 3–1.)

**Tertiary structure** Three-dimensional configuration.

**Transcription** The synthesis of a single-stranded RNA molecule from a DNA template in the cell nucleus, catalyzed by RNA polymerase.

**Transcription factor** One of a large class of proteins that regulate transcription by forming large complexes with other transcription factors and RNA polymerase; these complexes then bind to regulatory regions of genes to either promote or inhibit transcription.

**Transfection** Transfer of a gene into a cell, enabling the transfected cell to form a new gene product.

**Transfer RNA (tRNA)** See *RNA*.

**Transformation** A phenomenon in which certain cell lines, such as cancer cells, are able to grow indefinitely in culture.

**Transgenic mice** Mice that carry a foreign gene ("transgene") in their genome, produced by injection of oocytes with the foreign DNA. If the transgene has been incorporated into the germline, it may also be transmitted to the progeny.

**Transition mutation** Substitution of one purine for another purine or one pyrimidine for another pyrimidine.

**Translation** The synthesis of a polypeptide from its mRNA template.

**Translocation** The transfer of a segment of one chromosome to another chromosome. If two nonhomologous chromosomes exchange pieces, the translocation is *reciprocal*. See also *Robertsonian translocation*.

**Transversion** A mutation caused by substitution of a purine for a pyrimidine or vice versa.

**Triplet repeat (trinucleotide repeat) disorders** Diseases caused when the number of repeating units of a trinucleotide in a particular gene expands beyond a threshold and interferes with gene expression or function.

**Triploid** A cell with three copies of each chromosome, or an individual made up of such cells.

**Trisomy** The state of having three representatives of a given chromosome instead of the usual pair, as in trisomy 21 (Down syndrome).

**tRNA** Transfer RNA; see *RNA*.

**Tumor-suppressor gene** A normal gene involved in the regulation of cell proliferation. Recessive mutations can lead to tumor development, as in the retinoblastoma gene or the p53 gene. Contrast with *oncogene*.

**Two-hit model** The hypothesis that some forms of cancer can be initiated when both alleles of a tumor-suppressor gene become inactivated in the same cell

**Ultrasonography** A technique in which high-frequency sound waves are used to examine internal body structures; useful in prenatal diagnosis.

**Uniparental disomy** The presence in the karyotype of two copies of a specific chromosome, both inherited from one parent, with no representative of that chromosome from the other parent. If both homologs of the parental pair are present, the situation is *heterodisomy*; if one parental homolog is present in duplicate, the situation is *isodisomy*. See *Prader-Willi syndrome*, *Angelman syndrome*, in text.

**Vector** In molecular genetics, the DNA molecule into which a gene or DNA fragment has been cloned, capable of replicating in a specific host and thereby replicating the cloned DNA segment as well. Vectors include plasmids, bacteriophage lambda, cosmids, and both bacterial and yeast artificial chromosomes.

**VNTR (variable number of tandem repeats)** A type of DNA polymorphism created by a tandem arrangement of multiple copies of short DNA sequences. Highly polymorphic, used in linkage studies and in DNA "fingerprinting" for paternity testing and forensic medicine.

**Western blotting** A technique analogous to Southern blotting, used for detection of proteins, usually by immunological methods.

**Wild type** A term used to indicate the normal allele (often symbolized as +) or the normal phenotype.

**X;autosome translocation** Reciprocal translocation between an X chromosome and an autosome.

**X inactivation** Inactivation of genes on one X chromosome in somatic cells of female mammals, occurring early in embryonic life, at about the time of implantation. See *lyonization*.

**X linkage** The distinctive inheritance pattern of alleles at loci on the X chromosome that do not undergo recombination (crossing over) during male meiosis.

**Y linkage** Genes on the Y chromosome, or traits determined by such genes, are Y-linked.

**Yeast artificial chromosome (YAC)** A cloning vector composed of yeast chromosome telomeres and centromeres, into which very large DNA fragments (more than 1000 kb long) can be ligated.

**Zinc finger proteins** One class of transcription factor proteins containing loop-shaped tandem repeating segments that bind zinc atoms.

**Zygosity** The number of zygotes from which a multiple birth is derived. For example, twins may be either monozygotic (MZ) or dizygotic (DZ). To determine whether a certain pair of twins is MZ or DZ is to determine their zygosity.

**Zygote** A fertilized ovum.

# Answers to Problems

## *Chapter* 2 **Chromosomal Basis of Heredity**

1. (a) *A* and *a*. (b) i. At meiosis I. ii. At meiosis II.
2. Meiotic nondisjunction.
3. $(1/2)^{23} \times (1/2)^{23}$; you would be female.
4. (a) 23; 46. (b) 23; 23. (c) At fertilization; at S phase of the next cell cycle.

## *Chapter* 3 **The Human Genome: Structure and Function of Genes and Chromosomes**

1. There are several possible sequences because of the degeneracy of the genetic code. One possible sequence of the double-stranded DNA is
   5′AAA AGA CAT CAT TAT CTA 3′
   3′TTT TCT GTA GTA ATA GAT 5′
   RNA polymerase "reads" the bottom (3′ to 5′) strand. The sequence of the resulting mRNA would be
   5′AAA AGA CAU CAU UAU CUA 3′.
   The mutants represent the following kinds of mutations:
   Mutant 1: single nucleotide substitution in fifth codon; for example, UAU → UGU.
   Mutant 2: frameshift mutation, deletion in first nucleotide of third codon.
   Mutant 3: frameshift mutation, insertion of G between first and second codons.
   Mutant 4: in-frame deletion of three codons (nine nucleotides), beginning at the third base.
2. Chromosomes contain chromatin, consisting of nucleosomes. Chromosomes contain G-bands that contain several thousand kb pairs of DNA (or several million base pairs) and hundreds of genes, each containing (usually) both introns and exons. The exons are a series of codons, each of which is three base pairs in length.
3. Chromosome 5 contains about 200 million base pairs of DNA and approximately 3000 genes. Band 5p15 is about one tenth to one fifteenth of the total chromosome length and, therefore, can be estimated to contain approximately 10 to 20 million base pairs of DNA and approximately 200 genes. Even though these are gross estimates, the important concept to grasp is that chromosome bands potentially contain on the order of hundreds of genes.
4. Mutations in introns can influence RNA splicing, thus leading to an abnormally spliced mRNA (see Chapter 11). *Alu* or L1 sequences can be involved in abnormal recombination events between different copies of the repeat, thus deleting or rearranging genes. L1 repeats can also actively transpose around the genome, potentially inserting into a functional gene and disrupting its normal function. Locus control regions (LCRs) influence the proper expression of genes in time and space; deleting an LCR can thus disrupt normal expression of a gene(s) (see Chapter 11). Pseudogenes are, generally, nonfunctional copies of genes; thus, in most instances, mutations in a pseudogene would not be expected to contribute to disease.

## *Chapter* 4 **Tools of Human Molecular Genetics**

1. (a) Southern blot or polymerase chain reaction (PCR) of DNA obtained from chorionic villus sampling or amniotic fluid cell sample. In either case, Southern blot or PCR of another locus must be done simultaneously to make sure that failure to obtain a hybridization signal (Southern blot) or an amplified product (PCR) was caused by the deletion and not by technical difficulties with the DNA sample or the procedure used. (b) Northern blot. (c) Allele specific oligonucleotide analysis of a PCR product that spans the segment of DNA containing the base change. If the base change creates or destroys a restriction enzyme recognition site, you can use restriction digestion of the PCR product that spans the segment containing the mutation to determine whether the mutation is present.
2. The chief advantage of PCR is that much less DNA is required for an analysis than that required in Southern blotting. In addition, PCR is much faster and less expensive. Potential disadvantages include the fact that PCR can "see" only relatively short stretches of genomic DNA (in each assay), whereas Southern blotting can "examine" an entire

gene. PCR is also much more sensitive to contamination by extraneous DNA. In comparison with biochemical assays, PCR has the same advantage of speed. However, although biochemical assays can detect a range of mutations at a locus (including any unknown mutation that interferes with enzyme activity), PCR is best suited to examining specific, known mutations.

3. All except red blood cells. However, even samples of red blood cells or serum may contain enough DNA from contaminating white blood cells that testing could be done by PCR because PCR is so sensitive.

4. Establishes the gene responsible for a given disorder; provides opportunity to determine the molecular basis of a disorder, through extensive laboratory research; provides immediate tools for diagnosis and genetic counseling; could be used to design gene replacement therapy.

5. I would begin with the cDNA library because the cDNA would immediately provide a probe that could be used for Northern analysis of liver samples to examine the quantity and size of patients' mRNA as well as Southern analysis of all the exons in DNA obtained from the patients. Once I had the cDNA, electronic database search of human genomic sequence would give the exon/intron boundaries. This would allow the design of PCR primers that flank all the exons, to use to amplify each exon and intron/exon boundary to look for small mutations.

6. (a) A C > T transition converting an arginine codon to a stop, resulting in premature termination. (b) Oligonucleotides 2, 3, and 4 would be usable. Oligonucleotide 1 is specific for the mutant sequence, but the mismatch with the normal sequence would occur at the next to last base. It would be very difficult to establish hybridization conditions such that this oligonucleotide would hybridize stably to the mutant but not the normal sequence. Oligonucleotide 2 is specific for the normal sequence. By placing the base that is mutated in the center, it is easy to design conditions such that this oligonucleotide will form a stable duplex with the normal sequence but not the mutant. Oligonucleotide 3 is specific for the mutant sequence and would be an excellent discriminator between normal and mutant sequences. Oligonucleotide 4 is specific for the mutant sequence but would hybridize to the strand complementary to the one shown here and would serve to discriminate between normal and mutant. Oligonucleotide 5 is too short for there to be conditions that would allow discrimination between normal and mutant sequence.

## *Chapter* 5 Patterns of Single-Gene Inheritance

1. (b) Autosomal recessive; 1/4. (c) About 1/180, about 10 times population risk. (d) Calvin and Cathy are obligatory heterozygotes. Given that Calvin and Cathy are first cousins, it is also very likely that they inherited their mutant allele through Betty and Barbara from the same grandparent. Thus, Betty and Barbara are very likely to be carriers, but it is not obligatory. It is theoretically possible that Cathy inherited her CF allele from Bob and that Calvin inherited his from his father, Barbara's husband. DNA-based carrier testing will answer the question definitively.

2. (a) Heterozygous at each of two loci; for example, *A/a B/b*. (b) The parents (Gilbert and Gisele; Horace and Hedy) are all homozygous for the *same* recessive allele for congenital deafness.

3. Variable expressivity—d; Uniparental disomy—i; Consanguinity—j; Inbreeding—c; X-linked dominant inheritance—g; New mutation—e; Allelic heterogeneity—h; Locus heterogeneity—a; Homozygosity for an autosomal dominant trait—b; Pleiotropy—f.

4. (b) They are homozygous. (c) 100 percent; virtually zero if her partner is unaffected. (d) 50 percent; virtually zero if her partner is unaffected.

5. All are possible except (c), which is unlikely if the parents are completely unaffected.

6. (a) New mutation. (b) Mutation rate. (c) Mutation rate. (d) 50 percent.

## *Chapter* 6 Genetic Variation in Individuals: Mutation and Polymorphism

1. Assuming 40 years is one generation, 41 mutations/9 million alleles = $4.55 \times 10^{-6}$. Estimate is based on assumptions that ascertained cases result from new mutation, that the disease is fully penetrant, that all new mutants are liveborn (and ascertained), and that there is only a single locus at which mutations can lead to aniridia. If there are multiple loci, then the estimated rate is too high. If some mutations are not ascertained (because of lack of penetrance or death in utero), the estimated rate might be too low.

2. (a) An X-linked restriction fragment length polymorphism. (b) If the polymorphism is due to a point mutation, then individuals of different genotypes would have indistinguishable patterns with a different restriction enzyme. However, if the polymorphism is due to a 2-kb deletion/insertion, then the same polymorphism should be detected with

any restriction enzyme that cleaves on either side of the deletion/insertion.

3. One way of determining this is to reverse the question and ask instead what proportion of individuals would be *homozygous*. Then the proportion who are heterozygous is 1 minus the proportion who are homozygous. For each allele, the frequency of homozygotes would be $0.20 \times 0.20$, or 0.04. Thus, $5 \times 0.04$, or 20 percent, of individuals would be homozygous for allele 1 OR allele 2 OR . . . allele 5. Therefore, 80 percent of individuals would be heterozygous at this locus.

4. Yes; greater during subsequent pregnancies; disease can be prevented by using antibodies to Rh-D (RhoGAM) to clear the maternal circulation of Rh-positive blood cells before they can elicit a primary immune response; if the man were also Rh-negative, the child would have to be Rh negative, and no hemolytic disease would occur.

## *Chapter 7* Genetic Variation in Populations

1. (a) *a*, 0.1; *A*, 0.9. (b) Same. (c) $(0.18)^2$.

2. (a) 0.02. (b) $(0.04)^2$ or about 1 in 600 (homozygotes do not reproduce). (c) 0.0004. (d) 1/4.

3. Only (d) is in equilibrium. Selection for or against particular genotypes; nonrandom mating; recent migration.

4. (a) Abby has a 2/3 chance of being a carrier. Andrew has about a 1/150 chance of being a carrier. Therefore, their risk of having an affected child is $2/3 \times 1/150 \times 1/4$, or 1/900. (b) $2/3 \times 1/4 \times 1/4 = 1/24$. (c) $2/3 \times 1/22 \times 1/4 = 1/132$; $2/3 \times 1/4 \times 1/4 = 1/24$.

5. (a) Retinoblastoma, $q = 1/50{,}000$, $2pq = 1/25{,}000$; Friedreich's ataxia, $q = 1/158$, $2pq = 1/79$; choroideremia, $q = 1/25{,}000$, $2pq = 1/12{,}500$. (b) The autosomal dominant and X-linked disorders would increase rapidly, within one generation, to reach a new balance; the autosomal recessive would increase also but only very slowly, because the vast majority of the mutant alleles are not subject to selection.

6. Approximately 1/26 and 1/316.

7. Because the high incidence in Quebec appears to be due to a founder effect, most or all cases are descended from the one or more common founding ancestors; thus, the mutant alleles are expected to be relatively homogeneous. For Duchenne muscular dystrophy, because a large proportion of cases in each generation is the result of new mutation, the mutant alleles present in the population are heterogeneous. Color blindness is relatively common and is not a genetic lethal; thus, many mutant alleles are present in the population.

## *Chapter 8* Gene Mapping and the Human Genome Project

1. The *HD* and *MNSs* loci map far apart on chromosome 4 and are thus unlinked, even though syntenic.

2. For Huntington disease, yes, because all evidence suggests that only one or at most a few different premutations are responsible for all cases; premutations, as a result, only a few haplotypes, with CAG expansions that are above the normal mean but still within the normal range, contribute most of the expanded, disease-related alleles. For type 1 neurofibromatosis, we expect no linkage disequilibrium because approximately half of all cases result from new mutations, which occur on a variety of different haplotypes.

3. Fragment 1 is present in hybrids II, III, IV, and VII but absent in hybrids I, V, VI, and VIII. Fragment 2 cannot be mapped, because a mouse fragment of the same size is present in all hybrids, and the human and mouse fragments cannot be distinguished. Fragment 1 of the *Q* gene maps to chromosome 7.

4. The lod scores indicate that this polymorphism is closely linked to the polycystic kidney disease gene. The peak lod score, 25.85, occurs at 5 cM. The odds in favor of linkage at this distance compared with no linkage at all are $10^{25.85}$:1 (i.e., almost $10^{26}$:1). The data in the second study indicate that there is *no* linkage between the disease gene and the polymorphism in this family. Thus, there is genetic heterogeneity in this disorder, and linkage information can therefore be used for diagnosis only if there is previous evidence that the disease in that particular family is linked to the polymorphism.

5. Coppock's cataract seems to cosegregate with the "A" haplotype. There are no crossovers. A complete lod score analysis should be performed. In addition, one might examine the gamma crystallin gene itself for mutations in affected persons.

6. The phase in the mother is probably *B/WAS*, according to the genotype of the affected boy. This phase can be determined with only 95 percent certainty, because there is a 5 percent chance that a crossover occurred in the meiosis leading to the affected boy. On the basis of this information, there is a $(0.95 \times 0.95) + (0.05 \times 0.05)$ chance that the fetus (who is male) will be *unaffected*.

7. This surprising result (assuming paternity is as stated) indicates that the mother has inherited the *A* allele (and the *WAS* allele) from her mother—that is, her phase is *A*/*WAS*, not *B*/*WAS* as surmised in question 6. Thus, there must have been a crossover in the meiosis leading to the affected boy. To confirm this, one should examine polymorphisms on either side of this one on the X chromosome to make sure that the segregation patterns are consistent with a crossover. On the basis of this new information, there is now a 95 percent chance that the fetus in the current pregnancy is *affected*.

8. This question is for open discussion. Knowing the map position might suggest candidate genes for a disorder that maps to the same location. Knowing the map position might allow carrier detection or prenatal diagnosis by linked markers. A comparison of the human and mouse map in that region might point to possible animal models for the disease.

9. The region around *HPRT* is always retained because of the selection used; it therefore cannot be mapped by radiation hybrid methods that are based on *HPRT*. Use of another selectable marker, such as thymidine kinase on chromosome 17, would allow radiation hybrid mapping of the distal X chromosome around *HPRT*.

## *Chapter* 9 Principles of Clinical Cytogenetics

1. (a) Forty-six chromosomes, male; one of the chromosome 18s has a shorter long arm than is normal. (b) To determine whether the abnormality is *de novo* or inherited from a balanced carrier parent. (c) Forty-six chromosomes, male, only one normal 7 and one normal 18, plus a reciprocal translocation between chromosomes 7 and 18. This is a balanced karyotype. For meiotic pairing and segregation, see text, particularly Figure 9–12. (d) The $18q^-$ chromosome is the der(18) translocation chromosome, 18pter → 18q12::7q35 → 7qter. The boy's karyotype is unbalanced; he is monosomic for the distal long arm of 18 and is trisomic for the distal long arm of 7. Assuming that the human genome contains approximately 50,000 genes, one would predict that the boy is monosomic or trisomic for a few hundred genes.

2. (a) About 95 percent. (b) No increased risk.

3. Postzygotic nondisjunction, in an early mitotic division. Although the clinical course cannot be predicted with complete accuracy, it is likely that she will be somewhat less severely affected than would a nonmosaic trisomy 21 child.

4. (a) Abnormal phenotype, unless the marker is exceptionally small and restricted only to the centromeric sequences themselves. Gametes may be normal or abnormal; prenatal diagnosis indicated. (b) Abnormal phenotype (trisomy 13, see Chapter 10); will not reproduce. (c) Abnormal phenotype in proband and approximately 50 percent of offspring. (d) Normal phenotype, but risk for unbalanced offspring (see text). (e) Normal phenotype, but risk for unbalanced offspring (see text).

5. (a) Not indicated. (b) Fetal karyotyping indicated. At risk for trisomy 21, in particular. (c) Karyotype indicated for child to determine whether trisomy 21 or translocation Down syndrome. If translocation, then parental karyotypes are indicated. (d) Not indicated, unless other clinical findings might suggest a contiguous gene syndrome. (e) Karyotype indicated for the boys to rule out deletion or other chromosomal abnormality. If clinical findings indicate possibility of fragile X mental retardation, then a specific DNA diagnostic test would be indicated.

## *Chapter* 10 Clinical Cytogenetics: Disorders of the Autosomes and the Sex Chromosomes

1. Theoretically, X and XX gametes in equal proportions; expected XX, XY, XXX, and XXY offspring.

2. (a) To determine whether presence of an X-linked recessive disorder in the girl is due to a chromosome defect, such as an X;autosome translocation or 45,X Turner syndrome; to the presence of a condition (such as androgen insensitivity) allowing a female phenotype in an XY person; or to homozygosity or nonrandom X-inactivation in a 46,XX individual. See text. (b) The break disrupts one copy of the hemophilia A (*F8*) gene, while the normal X, as is usual with this type of translocation, is preferentially inactivated in most or all cells. See Figure 10–16.

3. No. XYY can result only from meiosis II nondisjunction in the male, whereas XXY can result from nondisjunction at meiosis I in the male or at either division in the female.

4. Translocation of Y chromosome material containing the sex-determining region (and the *SRY* gene) to the X chromosome or to an autosome.

5. 46,XY; androgen insensitivity (testicular feminization); the mother or child may be the result of a de novo mutation, but if the mother is heterozygous, the usual X-linked risks apply.

6. 46,XX; autosomal recessive; prenatal diagnosis possible; need for clinical attention in neonatal pe-

riod to determine sex and to forestall salt-losing crises.

7. (a) None; the short arms of all acrocentric chromosomes are believed to be identical and contain multiple copies of rRNA genes. (b) None if the deletion involves only heterochromatin (Yq12). A more proximal deletion might delete genes important in spermatogenesis (see Fig. 10–9). (c) Cri du chat syndrome, severity depending on the amount of DNA deleted. (d) Turner syndrome; the $Xq^-$ chromosome is preferentially inactivated in all cells (provided that the X-inactivation center is not deleted), thus reducing the potential severity of such a deletion.

   Different parts of the genome contain different density of genes. Thus, deletion of the same amount of DNA on different chromosomes might delete a vastly different number of genes, thus leading to different phenotypic expectations.

8. Question for discussion. See text for possible explanations.

9. (a) One percent risk is often quoted, but the risk is probably not greater than the population age-related risk. (b) Age-related risk is greater than 1 percent. (c) No increased risk if the niece with Down syndrome has trisomy 21. But if the niece carries a Robertsonian translocation, then the consultand may be a carrier and at high risk. (d) Ten to 15 percent. See text. (e) Only a few percent. See text. Woman's age-related risk may be relevant.

## *Chapter* 11 **Principles of Molecular Disease: Lessons from the Hemoglobinopathies**

1. The pedigree should contain the following information: (a) Hydrops fetalis is due to a total absence of $\alpha$ chains. (b) The parents each must have the genotype $\alpha\alpha$/--. (c) The $\alpha$- genotype is very common in some populations, including Melanesians. Parents with this genotype cannot transmit a --/-- genotype to their offspring.

2. Except in isolated populations, patients with $\beta$-thalassemia will often be genetic compounds because there are usually many alleles present in a population in which $\beta$-thalassemia is common. In such populations, the chance that a patient is a true homozygote of a single allele is greater than it would be in a population in which thalassemia is rare. In the latter group, more "private mutations" might be expected (ones found solely or almost solely in a single pedigree). A patient is more likely to have identical alleles if he or she belongs to a geographic isolate with a high frequency of a single or a few alleles or if his or her parents are consanguineous. See text in Chapter 7.

3. Three bands on the RNA blot could indicate, among other possibilities, that (a) one allele is producing two mRNAs, one normal in size and the other abnormal, and the other allele is producing one mRNA of abnormal size; (b) both alleles are making a normal-sized transcript and an abnormal transcript, but the aberrant ones are of different sizes; or (c) one allele is producing three mRNAs of different size, and the other allele is making no transcripts.

   Scenario (c) is highly improbable, if possible at all. Two mRNAs from a single allele could result from a splice defect that allows the normal mRNA to be made, but at reduced efficiency, while leading to the synthesis of another transcript of abnormal size that results from either the incorporation of intron sequences in the mRNA or the loss of exon sequences from the mRNA. In this case, the other abnormal band comes from the other allele. A larger band from the other allele could result from a splice defect or an insertion, whereas a smaller band could be due to a splice defect or a deletion. Hb E is caused by an allele from which both a normal and a shortened transcript are made (see Fig. 11–14); the normal mRNA makes up 40 percent of the total $\beta$-globin mRNA, producing only a mild anemia.

4. These two mutations affect different globin chains. The expected offspring are 1/4 normal, 1/4 Hb M Saskatoon heterozygotes with methemoglobinemia, 1/4 Hb M Boston heterozygotes with methemoglobinemia, and 1/4 double heterozygotes with four Hb types: normal, both types of Hb M, and a type with abnormalities in both chains. In the double heterozygotes, the clinical consequences are unknown—probably more severe methemoglobinemia.

5. $2/3 \times 2/3 \times 1/4 = 1/9$.

6. 1/4.

7. 8, 1, 2, 7, 10, 4, 9, 5, 6, and 3.

8. Exceptions to this rule can arise, for example, from splice site mutations that lead to the missplicing of an exon. The exon may be excluded from the mRNA, generating either an in-frame deletion of the protein sequence or causing a change in the reading frame, leading to the inclusion of different amino acids in the protein sequence.

9. Thr-Lys-Leu-Ala-Phe-Leu-Leu-Ser-Asn-Phe-Tyr-Stop.

## *Chapter* 12 The Molecular and Biochemical Basis of Genetic Disease

1. Three types of mutations that could explain a mutant protein that is 50 kD larger than the normal polypeptide are the following: (a) A mutation in the normal stop codon that allows translation to continue. (b) A splice mutation that results in the inclusion of intron sequences in the coding region. The intron sequences would have to be free of stop codons for sufficient length to allow the extra 50 kD of translation. (c) An insertion, with an open reading frame, into the coding sequence. For any of these, approximately 500 extra residues would be added to the protein if the average molecular weight of an amino acid is about 100. Five-hundred amino acids would be encoded by 1500 nucleotides.

2. A nucleotide substitution that changes one amino acid residue to another should be termed a *putative mutation* and, possibly, a *polymorphism*, unless (a) it has been demonstrated through a functional assay of the protein that the change impairs the function to a degree consistent with the phenotype of the patient or (b) instead of or in addition to a functional assay, it can be demonstrated that the nucleotide change is found *only* on mutant chromosomes, which can be identified by haplotype analysis in the population of patients and their parents, and *not* on normal chromosomes in this population. The fact that the nucleotide change is only rarely observed in the normal population and is found with significantly higher frequency in a mutant population is strong supportive evidence, but not proof, that the substitution is a mutation.

3. If Johnny has cystic fibrosis (CF), the chances are about 0.85 × 0.85, or 70 percent, that he has a previously described mutation that could be readily identified by DNA analysis. His parents are from northern Europe; therefore, the probability that he is homozygous for the ΔF508 mutation is 0.7 × 0.7, or 50 percent, because about 70 percent of CF carriers in northern Europe have this mutation. If he does not have the ΔF508 mutation, he could certainly still have CF because about 30 percent of the alleles (in the northern European population, at least) are not ΔF508. Steps to DNA diagnosis for CF include the following: (a) looking directly for the ΔF508 mutation; if not present, (b) looking for other mutations that are most likely; (c) then looking directly for other mutations based on probabilities suggested by the haplotype data; (d) if all efforts to identify a mutation fail (or if time does not allow), performing linkage analysis with polymorphic DNA markers closely linked to CF.

4. James may have a new mutation on the X chromosome because Joe inherited the same X chromosome from his mother, and in neither the mother nor Joe was the deletion present. If this is the case, there is no risk of recurrence. Alternatively, the mother may be a mosaic, and the mosaicism includes her germline. In this case, there is a definite risk that the mutant X could be inherited by another son or passed to a carrier daughter. About 5 to 15 percent of cases of this type appear to be due to maternal germline mosaicism. Thus, the risk is half of this figure for her male offspring, because the chance that a son will inherit the mutant X is 1/2 × 5 to 15 percent = 2.5 to 7.5 percent.

5. For DMD, as a classic X-linked recessive disease that is lethal in males, one third of cases are predicted to be new mutations. The large size of the gene is likely to account for the high mutation rate at this locus (i.e., it is a large target for mutation). The ethnic origin of the patient is unlikely to have any effect on either of these phenomena, although there is some evidence that the spectrum of mutations (point mutations versus deletions) may differ among different ethnic groups.

6. The limited number of amino acids that have been observed to substitute for glycine in collagen mutants reflects the nature of the genetic code. Single nucleotide substitutions at the three positions of the glycine codons allow only a limited number of missense mutations. See Table 3–1.

7. Two bands of G6PD on electrophoresis of a red-blood-cell lysate (see Table 12–8) indicate that the woman has a different *G6PD* allele on each X chromosome and that each allele is being expressed in her red-blood-cell population. However, no single cell expresses both alleles, because of X inactivation. Males have only a single X chromosome and thus express only one *G6PD* allele. A female with two bands could have two normal alleles with different electrophoretic mobility, one normal allele and one mutant allele with different electrophoretic mobility, or two mutant alleles with different electrophoretic mobility. Because the two common deficiency alleles ($A^-$ and $B^-$) migrate to the same position as the common normal activity alleles (*A* and *B*), the woman is unlikely to have a common deficiency allele at both loci. Apart from that, one cannot say much about the possible pathological significance of the two bands without measuring the enzymatic activity. If one of the alleles has low activity, then she would be at risk of hemolysis to the extent that the high activity allele is inactivated as a result of X inactivation.

8. The box in Chapter 12 entitled "Enzyme Deficiencies and Disease" lists the possible causes of loss of multiple enzyme activities: (a) They may share a cofactor whose synthesis or transport is defective. (b) They may share a subunit encoded by the mutant gene. (c) They may be processed by a common enzyme whose activity is critical to their becoming active. (d) They may normally be located in the same organelle, and a defect in the organelle's biological processes can affect all four enzymes. For example, they may not be imported normally into the organelle and may be degraded in the cytoplasm. Almost all enzymopathies are recessive (see text), and most genes are autosomal.

9. Haploinsufficiency. Thus, in some situations, the contributions of both alleles are required to provide a sufficient amount of protein to prevent disease. An example is provided by heterozygous carriers of low-density-lipoprotein (LDL) receptor deficiency.

10. This situation is well illustrated by diseases due to mutations in either mtDNA or in the nuclear genome that impair the function of the oxidative phosphorylation (OXPHOS) complex. Virtually all cells have mitochondria, and OXPHOS occurs in nearly all cells, yet defects in OXPHOS damage only a subset of organs, particularly the neuromuscular system with its high energy requirements.

11. One example is phenylketonuria, in which mental retardation is the only significant pathological effect of deficiency of phenylalanine hydroxylase, which is found not in the brain but solely in the liver and kidneys, organs that are unaffected by this biochemical defect. Hypercholesterolemia due to deficiency of the LDL receptor is another example. Although the LDL receptor is found in many cell types, the hepatic deficiency of it is primarily responsible for the increase in LDL-cholesterol levels in blood.

12. There are two defining characteristics of these alleles: (1) the hex A activity that they encode is sufficiently reduced to allow their detection in screening assays (when the other allele is a common Tay-Sachs mutation with virtually no activity); (2) their hex A activity is nevertheless adequate to prevent the accumulation of the natural substrate ($G_{M2}$ ganglioside). There are probably only a few substitutions in the hex A protein that would reduce activity to only a modest degree (i.e., without crippling the protein more substantially). Thus, the region of residues 247–249 appears to be relatively tolerant of substitutions, or at least of Trp for Arg. Substitutions that more dramatically alter the charge or bulk of the residues at these positions may well be disease-causing alleles.

## *Chapter* 13 The Treatment of Genetic Disease

1. Unresponsive patients may have mutations that drastically impair the synthesis of a functional gene product. Responsive patients may have mutations in the regulatory region of the gene. The effects of these mutations may be counteracted by the administration of interferon-$\gamma$ (IFN-$\gamma$). These mutations could be in the DNA binding site that responds to the IFN stimulus or in some other regulatory element that participates in the response to IFN-$\gamma$. Alternatively, responsive patients may produce a defective cytochrome-*b* polypeptide that retains a small degree of residual function. The production of more of this mutant protein, in response to IFN-$\gamma$, increases the oxidase activity slightly but significantly.

2. An enzyme that is normally intracellular can function extracellularly if the substrate is in equilibrium between the intracellular and extracellular fluids and if the product is either nonessential inside the cell or in a similar equilibrium state. Thus, enzymes with substrates and products that do not fit these criteria would not be suitable for this strategy. This approach may not work for phenylalanine hydroxylase because of its need for tetrahydrobiopterin. However, if tetrahydrobiopterin could diffuse freely across the polyethylene glycol layer around the enzyme, the administration of tetrahydrobiopterin orally may suffice. This strategy would not work for storage diseases because the substrate of the enzyme is trapped inside the lysosome. In Lesch-Nyhan syndrome, the most important pathological process is in the brain, and the enzyme in the extracellular fluid would not be able to cross the blood-brain barrier. Tay-Sachs disease could not be treated this way because of the nondiffusibility of the substrate from the lysosome.

3. Rhonda's mutations prevent the production of any low-density-lipoprotein (LDL) receptor. Thus, the combination of a bile acid binding resin and a drug (e.g., lovastatin) to inhibit cholesterol synthesis would have no effect in increasing the synthesis of LDL receptors. The boy must have one or two mutant alleles that produce a receptor with some residual function, and the increased expression of these mutant receptors on the surface of the hepatocyte reduces the plasma LDL-bound cholesterol.

4. Unresponsive patients probably have alleles that do not make any protein, that decrease its cellular abundance in some other way (e.g., make an unstable protein), or that disrupt the conformation of the protein so extensively that its pyridoxal-phosphate binding site has no affinity for the cofactor, even at high concentrations. The answer to the second part of this question is less straightforward. The answer given here is based on the generalization that most patients with a rare autosomal recessive disease are likely to have two different alleles, which assumes that there is no mutational hotspot in the gene and that the patients are not descended from a "founder" and are not members of an ethnic group in whom the disease has a high frequency. In this context, (a) Tom is likely to have two alleles that are responsive; (b) first cousins with the same recessive disease are likely to share only one allele, so that Allan is likely to have one responsive allele that he shares with Tom and another allele that is either unresponsive or that responds more poorly to the cofactor than Tom's other allele.

5. (a) You need both a promoter that will allow the synthesis of sufficient levels of the mRNA in the target tissue of choice and the phenylalanine hydroxylase cDNA. In reality, you also need a vector to deliver the "gene" into the cell, but this aspect of the problem has not been dealt with much in the text. (b) A phenylalanine hydroxylase "gene" will probably be effective in any tissue that had a good blood supply for the delivery of phenylalanine and an adequate source of the cofactor of the enzyme, tetrahydrobiopterin. The promoter would have to be capable of driving transcription in the target tissue chosen for the treatment. (c) Any mutation that severely reduces the abundance of the protein in the cell but has no effect on transcription. This group includes those mutations that impair translation or that render the protein highly unstable. The thalassemias include examples of all these types. (d) Liver cells are capable of making tetrahydrobiopterin, whereas other cells may not be. The target cell for the gene transfer should thus be capable of making this cofactor; otherwise, the enzyme will not function unless the cofactor is administered in large amounts. (e) Human phenylalanine hydroxylase probably exists as a homodimer or homotrimer. In patients whose alleles produce a mutant polypeptide (versus none at all), these alleles may manifest a dominant negative effect on the product of the transferred gene. This effect could be overcome by making a gene construct that produces more of the normal phenylalanine hydroxylase protein (thus diluting out the effect of the mutant polypeptide) or by transferring the gene into a cell type that does not normally express phenylalanine hydroxylase and that would therefore not be subject to the dominant negative effect.

## *Chapter* 14 Genetics of the Immune System

1. Association means that a *particular allele* (HLA-B27) is found more frequently in patients with the disease than would be expected from its allele frequency in the population. Linkage means that two *loci*, the *HLA-B* locus and the gene encoding the 21-hydroxylase enzyme, are located close to each other on the chromosome so that the recombination frequency between them is less than 50 percent; which alleles happen to be present at the two loci is irrelevant to whether or not the loci are linked.

2. (a) 1, monozygotic twin; 2, sib or dizygotic twin; 3, father, mother; 4, half-sib; 5, first cousin; 6, unrelated person. (b) The organ of a monozygotic twin might be genetically susceptible to the same problem that led the recipient to need a transplant.

3. Involves splicing and rearrangement of genomic DNA, whereas splicing of introns and exons involves RNA.

4. Because of allelic exclusion, expression is from only one of the two alleles in each cell. In this regard, this is more similar to expression of X-linked genes, although the mechanisms of allelic exclusion and X inactivation are quite different. For most other autosomal loci, other than those known to undergo genomic imprinting, both alleles are expressed.

5. Nonrandom inactivation presumably reflects the differential survival of the two cell populations (with one or the other X active) in B- or T-cell lineages. Cells with the mutant gene on the active X are presumably at a great selective disadvantage in the lineage in which the particular gene product plays a role. Thus, only cells with the normal allele on the active X survive. For autosomal forms, X inactivation is presumably random, because both types of cell populations have equally functional X-linked gene products.

## *Chapter* 15 Genetics of Disorders with Complex Inheritance

1. (a) Autosomal dominant with reduced penetrance. If it were truly multifactorial, the risk for more distantly related relatives would drop by more than 50 percent. (b) In dominant disease, you

would expect no increase in risk after an affected person has had two affected children, whereas in multifactorial inheritance, the risk after two affected children would be greater than after only one affected child because, with two affected, there is a greater likelihood that the parents are carrying a significant load of predisposing alleles at multiple loci; see text.

2. Male-to-male transmission can disprove X linkage; other criteria of multifactorial inheritance can be examined, as in text.

3. For autosomal recessive but not for multifactorial inheritance, there is almost no chance that a parent will be affected; for other criteria, see text.

## *Chapter* 16 Genetics and Cancer

1. Family history, careful examination of both parents' retinas, cytogenetic analysis if the tumor is associated with other malformations, mutation identification; advise parents of the risk, but point out that a future child could be examined immediately after birth and at short intervals for some time to make sure that if tumors develop, they are detected and treated early. The parents should be informed of the risk of disease in subsequent pregnancies, the availability of prenatal diagnosis, and the impact of the disease should it recur.

2. Colorectal cancer seems to require a number of sequential mutations in several genes, a process that may take longer than one (in hereditary) or two (in sporadic) mutations in the retinoblastoma gene. Age dependence may also reflect the number, timing, and rate of cell divisions in colon cells and in retinoblasts.

3. A cell line with i(17q) is monosomic for 17p and trisomic for 17q. Thus, formation of the isochromosome leads to loss of heterozygosity for genes on 17p. This may be particularly important if one or more tumor-suppressor genes (such as *TP53*) are present on 17p. In addition, a number of proto-oncogenes map to 17q. It is possible that increasing their dosage may confer a growth advantage on cells containing the i(17q).

4. The chief concern is the need to reduce radiation exposure to the lowest possible level because of the risk of cancer in children with this genetic defect.

5. Although most (>95 percent) of breast cancer appears to follow multifactorial inheritance, there are two known genes (*BRCA1* and *BRCA2*) and at least another suspected locus (*BRCA3*) in which mutations cause autosomal dominant premenopausal breast cancer that may be bilateral. The empiric risk figures are consistent with an overall multifactorial model with admixture of dominant forms of the disease with somewhat reduced lifetime penetrance. Direct mutation detection could be performed if desired by the probands in Wanda's and Wilma's families, and, if a mutation were found in *BRCA1* or *BRCA2*, a direct test for cancer risk could be offered to their relatives.

## *Chapter* 17 Genetic Aspects of Development

1. Specification and determination. Cells that have undergone specification will, when explanted, develop in the same way they would have developed if left in the embryo but, if transplanted, are competent for position-dependent development and will adopt the fate of the region in which the transplant occurred. Once determined, an embryonic tissue will follow its developmental program regardless of where it is transplanted.

2. A–3, B–2, C–4, D–1.

3. A paracrine signal is a diffusible substance released from one group of cells that elicits a response from a neighboring group of cells. A morphogen is a specialized type of paracrine signal that operates along a gradient, setting in motion different developmental programs depending on the concentration of the morphogen received by surrounding cells.

4. A–4, B–3, C–5, D–2, E–1.

5. Mature T or B cells that have somatically rearranged their T-cell receptor or immunoglobulin loci. This change is not epigenetic; it is a permanent alteration of the DNA sequence itself. Animals derived from a single nucleus from a mature T or B cell are incapable of mounting an appropriately broad immune response.

6. Consider issues of regulation versus simple capacity to carry out a biochemical reaction. Also, consider dominant negative effects of transcription factors, taking into account the frequent binary nature of such factors (DNA-binding and activation domains).

## *Chapter* 18 Prenatal Diagnosis

1. c, e, f, j, d, h, g, b, i, and a.

2. No, the child can have only Down syndrome or monosomy 21, which is almost always lethal. Thus, they should receive counseling and consider other alternatives for having children.

3. No, the problem could be maternal cell contamination.

4. The level of maternal serum alpha-fetoprotein (MSAFP) is typically elevated when the fetus

has an open neural tube defect. The levels of MSAFP and unconjugated estriol are usually reduced and the human chorionic gonadotrophin is usually elevated when the fetus has Down syndrome.

5. (a) Drop quickly to zero; very little effect. (b) Drop quickly to the level sustained by new mutations (about half). (c) Drop quickly to the level sustained by new mutations (very low).
6. (a) About 15 percent. (see Table 9–5.) (b) At least 50 percent are chromosomally abnormal. (c) No, prenatal diagnosis or karyotyping of the parents would be indicated only after three such abortions, provided that there are no other indications, such as advanced maternal age.
7. (a) Yes. The phase can be determined from analysis of her father, who transmitted a normal X chromosome to the woman. (b) Yes. If a male fetus received the grandpaternal X, it will be unaffected. If it received the grandmaternal X, it will be affected. This, of course, assumes no recombination in the transmitted chromosome and no gonadal mosaicism in the grandfather. (c) Deletion analysis.
8. Question for discussion. See text for examples and discussion.

## *Chapter* 19 **Genetic Counseling and Risk Assessment**

1. (a) Prior risk 1/4; posterior risk (two normal brothers) 1/10. (b) Zero.
2. (a) First, restrict your attention and conditional probability calculations to those women for whom we have conditional probability information that could alter their carrier risk. These individuals are: Lucy, who has an affected grandson and two unaffected grandsons; her daughter, Molly, who has an affected son; and Martha, who has two unaffected sons. Maud does not contribute any additional information because she has no sons. Write down an abbreviated pedigree (see below) and calculate all the possible prior probabilities. (This approach to Bayesian probability calculation is clearly described and explained in Hodge SE [1998] A simple, unified approach to bayesian risk calculations. J Genet Counseling 7:235–262.)

In *A*, Nathan is a new mutation with probability $\mu$.

In *B*, Molly is the new mutation—but because Lucy is NOT a carrier, Molly can only carry a new mutation and did not inherit the mutation, so her prior probability is $2\mu$ (NOT $4\mu$) because the new mutation could have occurred either on her paternal or her maternal X chromosome.

In *C*, Lucy is a carrier. As shown earlier in this chapter in the box describing the calculation for the probability that any female is a carrier of an X-linked lethal disorder, Lucy's prior probability = $4\mu$. Molly inherits the mutant gene, but Martha does not, so the probability her two sons would be unaffected is essentially 1.

In *D*, Lucy is a carrier as is Molly, but so is Martha, and yet she did not pass the mutant gene to her two sons.

(We do not consider all the other combinations of carrier states because they are so unlikely they can be ignored. For example, the possibility that Lucy is a mutation carrier but Molly does not inherit but then Nathan is *another* new mutation is vanishingly small because the joint probability of such an event would require TWO new mutations and would contain $\mu^2$ terms in the joint probability that are too small to contribute to the posterior probability.)

A

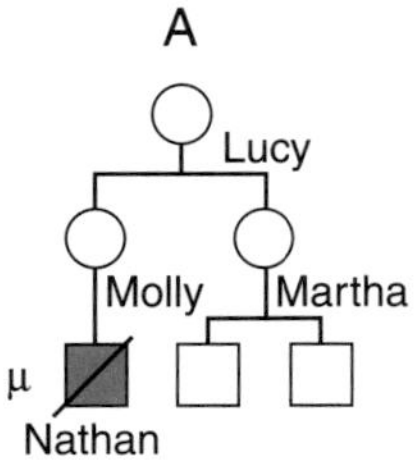


Prior
Nathan new mutation = $\mu$

Joint = $\mu$

B

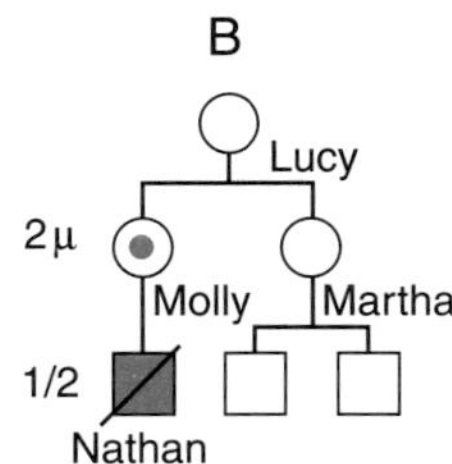


Prior
Molly new mutation = $2\mu$

Conditional
Nathan inherits = 1/2

Joint = $2\mu/2 = \mu$

C

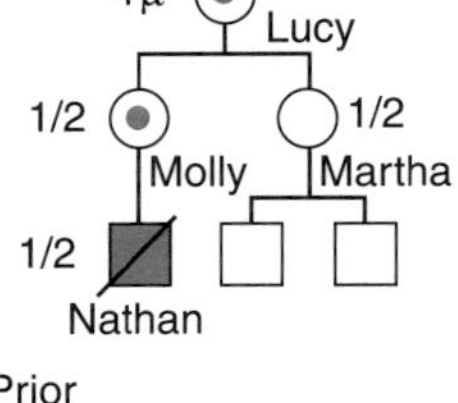


Prior
Lucy a carrier = $4\mu$

Conditional
Molly inherits = 1/2
Nathan inherits = 1/2
Martha does not inherit = 1/2

Joint = $4\mu/8 = \mu/2$

D

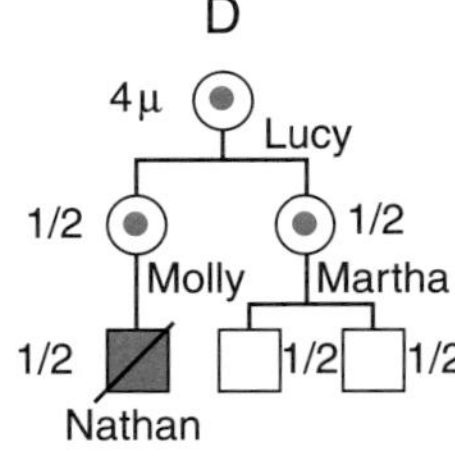


Prior
Lucy a carrier = $4\mu$

Conditional
Molly inherits = 1/2
Nathan inherits = 1/2
Martha inherits = 1/2
Two boys unaffected = 1/2 x 1/2

Joint = $4\mu/32 = \mu/8$

| | Both Carriers | Not Both Carriers |
|---|---|---|
| Prior risk for Ira and Margie | 4/9 | 5/9 |
| Conditional probability (3 normal children) | $(3/4)^3$ | 1 |
| Joint probability | $4/9 \times (3/4)^3 = 3/16 = .19$ | $5/9 = .56$ |
| Posterior probability | $.19/(.19 + .56) = \sim 1/4$ | $.56/.75 = \sim 3/4$ |

The conditional probabilities can then be calculated from these various joints.

For Molly, she is a carrier in situation *B*, *C*, and *D*, so her

$$\text{posterior probability of being a carrier} = \frac{\mu + \mu/2 + \mu/8}{\mu + \mu + \mu/2 + \mu/8} = 13/21$$

Similarly, Molly's mother Lucy, 5/21; Norma and Nancy, 13/42; Olive and Odette, 13/84; Martha, 1/21; Nora and Nellie, 1/42; Maud, 5/42; Naomi, 5/84.

(b) To have a 2 percent risk of having an affected son, a woman must have an 8 percent chance of being a carrier; thus, Martha, Nora, and Nellie would not qualify, because their carrier risk is less than 8 percent.

3. $(1/2)^{13}$; $(1/2)^{13} \times 2$. (The 2 arises because this is the chance of 13 consecutive male births *or* 13 consecutive female births, before any children are born.); 1/2. The probability of a boy is 1/2 for each pregnancy, regardless of how many previous boys were born (assuming there is straightforward chromosome segregation and no abnormality in sexual development that would alter the underlying 50 to 50 percent segregation of the X and Y chromosome during spermatogenesis).

4. (a) Use the first equation, $I = \mu + 1/2\text{H}$ to solve for H and substitute it for H in the second equation, $\text{H} = 2\mu + 1/2\text{H} + If$, solve for $I$, $I = 3\mu/(1 - \text{f})$. Substituting 0.7 for f, gives $I = 10\mu$; $\text{H} = 18\mu$;

| | Carrier | Noncarrier |
|---|---|---|
| Prior | $18\mu$ | $1 - 18\mu = \sim 1$ |
| Conditional | 1/2 | $\mu$ |
| Joint | $9\mu$ | $\mu$ |
| Posterior | $9\mu/(9\mu + \mu) = 0.9$ | $\mu/(9\mu + \mu) = 0.1$ |

90 percent; 45 percent.

(b) $3\mu$; $4\mu$. (c) 0.147.

5. Column B

__f__ Consultand

__h__ 2/3

__g__ Obligate heterozygote

__e__ Prior probability

__d__ Nonsense mutation in cystic fibrosis gene

__b__ Direct detection of a mutation by Southern blotting

__i__ Informative family

__a__ $4\mu$

__j__ First-degree relative

__c__ Linkage analysis

6. (a) The prior risk that either Ira or Margie is a cystic fibrosis carrier is 2/3; therefore, the probability that both are carriers is $2/3 \times 2/3 = 4/9$. (b) Their risk of having an affected child in any pregnancy is $1/4 \times 4/9 = 1/9$. (c) Bayesian analysis is carried out as above:

Thus, the chance that Ira's and Margie's next child will be affected is $1/4 \times 1/4 = 1/16$.

7. The child's prior probability of carrying a mutant myotonic dystrophy gene is 1/2. If it is assumed that he has a 1/2 chance of being asymptomatic even if he carries the mutant gene, then his chance of carrying it and showing no symptoms is 1/3. Testing is a complex issue. Many would feel that testing an asymptomatic child for an incurable illness with adult onset is improper because the child should be allowed to make that decision for himself or herself (see Chapter 20).

8. (a) Yes; autosomal recessive, autosomal dominant (new mutation), X-linked recessive, chromosomal disorder, or multifactorial. (b) This increases suspicion that the disorder is autosomal recessive. (c) This fact certainly supports the likelihood that the problem has a genetic explanation. The pedigree pattern would be consistent with autosomal recessive inheritance only if the sister's husband were carrying the same defect (possible if he is from the same village, for example). An X-linked recessive pattern (particularly if the affected children are all boys) or a chromosome defect ought to be considered. The mother and her son should receive a genetic evaluation appropriate to the clinical findings, such as karyotype, fragile X analysis, etc.

9. The woman is mistaken. She has a 1/2 risk of passing the mutant *NF1* gene to her offspring. The fact that she carries a new mutation only reduces the recurrence risk elsewhere in the family.

## *Chapter* 20 Genetics and Society

1. The first consideration is testing the boy for an incurable disease. Because the boy has symptoms and the family is seeking a diagnosis, this is *not* the same situation as described in problem 7 of Chapter 19, in which an asymptomatic child is being considered for myotonic dystrophy testing. However, because Huntington disease in a child is overwhelmingly the result of a trinucleotide expansion of an enlarged triplet repeat in one of the parents, usually the father, finding a markedly enlarged expansion in the child will automatically raise the possibility that one of the parents, probably the father, is a carrier of a repeat that is enlarged enough to cause adult-onset Huntington disease. Thus, by testing the child, one might inadvertently discover something about a parent's risk. Testing should therefore be carried out only after informed consent has been obtained from the parents. Other issues: (a) if one of the parents carries the *HD* gene, what do you do about testing the asymptomatic older sib? (b) Neither parent is currently symptomatic; what if neither parent carries an expanded *HD* allele, but the symptomatic child does carry an expanded allele?

2. Questions to consider in formulating your response are as follows: (a) Consider benefits of preventing disease by knowing a newborn's genotype at the $\beta$-globin locus. Can knowing the genotype help prevent pneumococcal sepsis? Other complications of sickle cell anemia? (b) Compare and contrast how sickle cell screening was introduced versus Tay-Sachs carrier screening with respect to community involvement and leadership. (c) Distinguish between *SS* homozygotes and *AS* heterozygotes. What harm might accrue from the identification of *SS* and *AS* individuals? What does identifying a newborn with *SS* or *AS* tell you about the genotypes of the parents and genetic risks for future offspring to the parents?

3. To justify screening, one must show that the good that comes from screening, the beneficence of the testing, outweighs the harm. Consider the issue of autonomy because implicit in the act of informing families that their child has a chromosomal abnormality is the fact that the child cannot decide whether she or he wants such testing later in life. One might argue that because abnormalities in learning and behavior occur in some individuals with sex chromosome anomalies, informing the parents and providing educational and psychological intervention before major problems arise might be beneficial. There is also, however, the concern about "the self-fulfilling prophecy," that telling parents there might be a problem increases the risk that there will be a problem by altering parental attitudes toward the child. There is a large amount of literature on this subject that would be worth investigating and reading.

   See, for instance,

   Bender BG, Harmon RJ, Linden MG, Robinson A (1995) Psychosocial adaptation of 39 adolescents with sex chromosome abnormalities. Pediatrics 96(2 Pt 1):302–308.

   Puck MH (1981) Some considerations bearing on the doctrine of self-fulfilling prophecy in sex chromosome aneuploidy. Am J Med Genet 9:129–137.

   Robinson A, Bender BG, Borelli JB, et al (1986) Sex chromosomal aneuploidy: Prospective and longitudinal studies. Birth Defects Orig Art Ser 22:23–71.

4. Factors to be considered are the incidence, which will affect the cost per true positive discovered, the ease or difficulty in making the diagnosis if no formal screening program is instituted, the harm and cost that would occur if deaf infants go unrecognized until they fail to develop verbal language, the efficacy of early treatment for infants identified through newborn screening, and the opportunity to provide genetic counseling for recurrence risks to the parents. With an incidence of bilateral sensorineural hearing loss of 1/350 to 1/500, "Universal newborn hearing screening is feasible, beneficial, and justified, as indicated by the frequency of the disease, the accuracy of screening tests, the ability to provide early intervention, the improved outcomes attributable to early amplification, and the recovery of all screening costs in the prevention of future intervention costs" (Mehl AL, Thomson V [1998] Newborn hearing screening: The great omission. Pediatrics 101:E4). In fact, newborn screening for deafness has been mandated in 10 states of the United States as of 1999. On the other hand, deaf individuals might have a different view of the situation, because some people in the deaf community do not view deafness as a disability to be corrected, but rather see it as a variation that helps to define their culture. It is estimated that 50 percent of severe congenital sensorineural deafness is attributable to genetic causes in the family, usually autosomal recessive forms of deafness. What implications and obligations, if any, does a positive test for deafness in a newborn impose on the states to pay for genetic counseling?

# Index

Note: Page numbers followed by the letter f refer to figures; those followed by t refer to tables.


A blood antigen, 88, 88t, 96t
*ABL-BCR* gene translocation, leukemia in, 318, 318f, 318t
ABO blood group system, 88, 88t, 96t
Abortion(s)
elective, 372
counseling on, 376–377
prenatal diagnosis and, 360, 393–394
spontaneous
chromosome abnormalities causing, 140t, 150–151, 151t
in consanguinity, 57
in Down syndrome, 158–159, 158t
in genetic defects, 353–354, 354f
in Turner syndrome, 174–175
Acetylation polymorphisms, 251
Acetylglucosaminidase deficiency, mucopolysaccharidoses in, 212, 213t, 214, 214f
Achondroplasia
assortative mating in, 101
fitness in, 102–103
heterozygous versus homozygous, 64
mutations in, 84, 85t, 86, 183
selection in, 102–103
Aciduria, methylmalonic, treatment of, 256f, 257t
Acquired immunodeficiency syndrome, resistance to, genetics of, 96–98, 97t, 107–108, 108f
Acrocentric chromosome, 137, 137f, 149
Acrodysostosis, zero fitness in, 102t
Adeno-associated viruses, as gene therapy vectors, 272–273
Adenomatous polyposis, of colon, 314t, 326–327, 327f
Adenosine deaminase deficiency
gene therapy for, 275
immunodeficiency in, 286t
replacement therapy for, 264, 264f
Adenoviruses, as gene therapy vectors, 272–273
Adoption, for disease recurrence prevention, 376
Adrenal hyperplasia, congenital
gonadal maldevelopment in, 176–177, 177f
HLA associations with, 280, 280t
population genetics of, 100t
treatment of, 257t
Affected pedigree member method, for gene mapping, 297
Affected sib pair method, for linkage analysis, 297–298
Agammaglobulinemia, 286t
Aganglionosis (Hirschsprung disease), 301–302, 302f
Age
maternal. *See* Maternal age.
of onset
late, recurrence risk determination in, 383–384, 384f
of single-gene defects, 55
paternal, mutation rate and, 86, 102
Aggregation, familial, 290–291, 291t
of quantitative traits, 294–295, 295f
AIDS (acquired immunodeficiency syndrome), resistance to, genetics of, 96–98, 97t, 107–108, 108f
Alcohol, teratogenic effects of, 338t
Alcohol dehydrogenase, polymorphism of, population variation in, 96t
Aldehyde dehydrogenase, polymorphism of, population variation in, 96t
Allele(s). *See also specific alleles.*
codominant, 53
common, polymorphism and, 87
definition of, 1, 5, 51, 87
distribution of. *See* Population genetics.
dominant, 53–54
in osteogenesis imperfecta, 234
fitness of. *See* Fitness.
frequency of
constant, exceptions to, 101–102
genotype frequency derivation from, 96
in genotype frequency calculation. *See* Hardy-Weinberg law.
stable, 103
HLA, 279–280, 279f
homozygosity for. *See* Homozygote(s).
in coupling *(cis)*, 122, 122f
in repulsion *(trans)*, 122, 122f
mutant, 51
of variable number of tandem repeats, 91–92, 92f
pseudodeficiency, in Tay-Sachs disease screening, 212
rare variants of, 87
recessive, 53–54
segregation of, in meiosis, 12
sharing of, among relatives, 291–292, 292f, 292t
stratification effects on, 100–101, 101t
wild-type, 51
Allele-specific oligonucleotides, 43–44, 44f, 46
Allelic exclusion, definition of, 281
Allelic heterogeneity. *See under* Heterogeneity.
Alpha$_1$-antitrypsin
deficiency of, 216–218, 218f
liver transplantation in, 268–269
Alpha$_1$-antitrypsin *(Continued)*
polymorphism of, 89–91, 89t, 91f, 96t
population genetics of, 100t
replacement of, 263–264
Alpha-fetoprotein measurement
in amniotic fluid, 362
in maternal blood, 364–365, 365f
Alpha-thalassemia. *See under* Thalassemia(s).
*Alu* family, in genome, 31
recombination among, 83f
Alzheimer disease, 234–236
age of onset of, 234
genetics of, 234–235
in Down syndrome, 158–159
incidence of, 234
inheritance of, 234–235, 303–304, 303t, 304f
pathogenesis of, 235–236, 236f, 237t, 238t
Ambiguous genitalia, 176–177, 177f
Amino acid(s), in protein synthesis, 23–24, 24t
Aminoacidopathies, 206–210, 207f, 208f, 209t. *See also* Phenylketonuria.
Aminopterin, for cell culture, 113
Amish community, founder effect in, 106, 106f
Amniocentesis, 362–363, 363f
complications of, 362–363
for chromosome analysis, 136, Color Insert following page 139
for cytogenetic studies, 369–372, 370f, 371t
in Down syndrome, 161–162
indications for, 361
sample preparation in, 369
Amniotic disruption sequence, 352, 352f
Amplification, gene, in cancer, 330, 331f
Amyloid deposition, in Alzheimer disease, 235, 236f, 237t
Analytical technique(s), 33–50
allele-specific oligonucleotide probes in, 43–44, 44f, 46
automated, 48–49
for nucleic acids, 41–44, 42f–44f
for prenatal diagnosis. *See* Prenatal diagnosis, methods of.
for proteins, 49, 49f
in situ hybridization as. *See* In situ hybridization.
libraries in, 34, 38f–40f, 39–41
molecular cloning in, 33, 35f
Northern blotting as, 34, 44, 46
polymerase chain reaction as. *See* Polymerase chain reaction.
restriction enzymes in, 33–35, 36f, 37t

Analytical technique(s) *(Continued)*
Sanger sequencing in, 48–49, 48f
Southern blotting as. *See* Southern blotting.
terminology of, 34
vectors in, 35–38, 37t, 38f, 39f
Western blotting as, 34, 49, 49f
Anaphase
of meiosis, 10, 11f
of mitosis, 6f, 7
Androgen insensitivity syndrome, 43, 43f, 172t, 176–178, 177f
Anemia(s)
Fanconi, 154t, 315t, 328
hemolytic, 88–89, 188t, 189–190, 190f, 191f, 252
in thalassemia. *See* Thalassemia(s).
sickle cell. *See* Sickle cell disease.
Anencephaly, 304–306, 305f, 306f, 307t, 385
Anesthesia, pharmacogenetics of, 250
Aneuploidy, 140–143, 142f
complicated, 142–143
definition of, 79, 140
in cancer, 330
incidence of, 150, 150t, 151t
of teratocarcinoma cells, 356
prenatal diagnosis of, ultrasonography in, 366–367, 367t
sex chromosome, 172–173, 173t
Aneusomy
in cancer, 330
segmental, 164, 164t
Angelman syndrome, 72–74, 74f, 74t, 164t
Aniridia, 85t, 337, 338t
Ankylosing spondylitis, HLA associations of, 280, 280t
Antibody(ies). *See* Immunoglobulin(s).
Anticodon(s), 24
Antigen(s)
blood group, 87–88, 88t
human leukocyte. *See* Human leukocyte antigens.
immunoglobulin response to, 281
Antigen presenting cells, 277, 278f
Antisense DNA strand, 22
Antitrypsin. *See* Alpha$_1$-antitrypsin.
Aortic stenosis, 307t
*APC* gene
mutations of, 314t, 326–327, 327f, 329, 329f
product of, 326–327, 327f
Apert syndrome, zero fitness in, 102t
Apheresis, in hypercholesterolemia, 262
Apolipoprotein E defects, in Alzheimer disease, 236, 236f, 237t, 238t, 303–304, 303t, 304f
Apoptosis
definition of, 5
failure of, 315t
in autoimmune lymphoproliferative syndrome, 328
in cancer, 312, 312f
in lymphoma, 318
in mitochondrial DNA diseases, 244–245
Argininosuccinate synthetase deficiency, diversion therapy for, 261, 261f
Arthrogryposes, 351
Artificial insemination, for disease recurrence prevention, 376
Aryl hydrocarbon hydroxylase, in carcinogen generation, 332
Ascertainment
bias of, 60, 291
population-based, 293
volunteer-based, 293
ASOs (allele-specific oligonucleotides), 43–44, 44f, 46
Association, 350
studies of, 297, 298–299
Assortative mating, 101
$\alpha_1$-AT. *See* Alpha$_1$-antitrypsin.
Ataxia
Friedreich, 239t, 243–244
spinocerebellar, 239t, 242, 243–244
Ataxia-telangiectasia
cancer in, 315t, 328
cytogenetics of, 154t
immunodeficiency in, 287t
Atelosteogenesis, zero fitness in, 102t
Atherosclerosis
coronary, 308–309
in hypercholesterolemia, 218–219, 221–222
Atrial septal defect, 307t
Autism, risk ratio for, 291t
Autoimmune disorder(s)
HLA associations of, 280, 280t
lymphoproliferative, 287t, 315t, 328
Autonomy
as ethical principle, 395
in morphogenesis, 345–346
Autosomal disorder(s). *See also specific disorders.*
deletion, 163–164, 164f
dominant, 61–65
cancer as, 314t–315t
characteristics of, 60, 66
epidemiology of, 61
homozygotes for, 63–64, 65f
male-to-male transmission of, 61
mutation rate in, 103
new mutations in, 61–62, 103
pedigree for, 61, 61f
phenotypic variability in, 62–63, 62f–64f
recessive, 315t
risk factors for, 60
selection against, 102–103, 102t
selection for, 397
sex-limited, 65, 66f
microdeletion, 164–165, 164t, 165f
recessive, 56–60
allele frequency and, 101–102
assortative mating and, 101
carrier frequency in, 56–57
consanguinity in, 57–59, 57f, 58f, 59t
founder effect in, 106, 106f, 107f
gene frequency in, 56–57
in genetic isolates, 58–59, 59t
inbreeding and, 58–59, 59t
pedigree for, 56, 56f
population genetics of, 103
rare, 58–59, 59t
segregation analysis of, 59–60
selection against, 103
selection for, 397
sex-influenced, 59
trisomy as. *See* Trisomy.
versus X-linked inheritance, 53
Autosomal inheritance. *See also* Autosomal disorder(s); *specific disorders.*
definition of, 53
dominant, 61–65, 61f–66f
recessive, 56–60, 56f–58f, 59t
Autosomes, definition of, 5
*AZF* gene mutations, 168
Azoospermia, Y-linked genes in, 167–168

B blood antigen, 88, 88t, 96t
B lymphocytes
Burkitt lymphoma of, 318–319
B lymphocytes *(Continued)*
immunoglobulin secretion from, 281
levels of, in immunodeficiency diseases, 286t–287t
Bacterial artificial chromosomes, 37–38, 37t, 127, 128f
Bacteriophage lambda, 37, 37t, 38f
Balanced rearrangement, of chromosomes, 143, 144f, 146–149, 151f, 152f
Banding, chromosome, 136–138
C, 137
classification system for, 136–137, 137f, 138f
fragile site viewing in, 138
G (Giemsa), 7–8, 7f, 8f, 137–138, 137f, 138f
high-resolution (prometaphase), 137–138, 138f
homogeneously staining regions in, 330
in cancer studies, 330
Q (quinacrine), 136
R (reverse), 136
high-resolution, 137–138, 138f
replication, 169, 170f
Barr bodies, 67, 67f, 169, 169f
in Klinefelter syndrome, 173
in trisomy X, 174
Base pair, 17
Bayesian analysis, in recurrence risk determination, 380, 380f
of hemophilia A, 380–382, 380f
of isolated X-linked disorders, 382–383, 383f, 384f
*BCHE* gene mutations, succinylcholine sensitivity in, 250
*BCL2* gene mutations, 318, 318t
Becker muscular dystrophy
clinical features of, 225
dystrophin detection in, 49, 49f
inheritance of, 49, 49f, 226
molecular analysis of, 228–229, 228f
pathology of, 225, 226f
prenatal diagnosis of, 229
Beckwith-Wiedemann syndrome, uniparental disomy in, 75
Behavioral disorders, in 47,XYY males, 174
Beneficence, as ethical principle, 395
Berg, Paul, 17
Beta-thalassemia. *See under* Thalassemia(s).
Bias
ascertainment, 60, 291
recall, 291
Bile acid–binding resins, in hypercholesterolemia, 261, 261f
Binomial theorem, in segregation analysis, 60
Biochemical genetics, definition of, 2
Biotinidase deficiency
enhancement therapy for, 262–263
prenatal treatment of, 257t
replacement therapy for, 260
Birth defects (dysmorphology), 350–353, 350f–353f
Birthmarks, development of, 355
Bivalent, in meiosis, 10
Blastocyst, development of, 340, 340f
Blindness, color, genotypes of, frequencies of, 98–99, 99t
Blood group system(s), 87–89
ABO, 88, 88t, 96t
Rh, 88–89
Bloom syndrome
cancer in, 315t, 328
cytogenetics of, 154, 154f, 154t
immunodeficiency in, 287t

BMD. *See* Becker muscular dystrophy.
Bone, collagen defect(s) in. *See also* Osteogenesis imperfecta.
  Ehlers-Danlos syndrome as, 55, 234, 235f
Bone marrow
  gene transfer into, 270–271
  in chromosome analysis, 136
  transplantation of
    in lysosomal storage diseases, 267–268, 267f, 268f
    in nonstorage diseases, 266–267
    in thalassemia, 196
*BRCA* genes, 325–326, 325f
  mutations of, 314t–315t
    in sporadic cancer, 329
    penetrance of, 326, 326f
  population genetics of, 101t
  products of, 321t, 325–326
  screening for, ethical issues in, 394
  structure of, 30, 30f
Breast cancer
  familial, 314t–315t, 325–326, 325f, 326f
  in Li-Fraumeni syndrome, 323–324, 324f
  population genetics of, 101t
  risk factors for, 326, 326f
  screening for, ethical issues in, 394
  tumor-suppressor gene mutations in, 321t
Burkitt lymphoma, 317–318, 318t
Butyrate therapy, for sickle cell disease, 265, 266f, 266t
Butyrylcholinesterase, defects of, succinylcholine sensitivity in, 250

C banding, 137
Café-au-lait spots, in neurofibromatosis, 62, 62f
CAG repeats. *See* Triplet repeat disorder(s).
Calcium abnormalities, in malignant hyperthermia, 250
Camptomelic dysplasia, sex reversal in, 176
Canavan disease, screening for, 392
Cancer, 311–333. *See also specific sites and types.*
  aneuploidy in, 330
  autosomal dominant inheritance of, 314t–315t, 321–328, 322f–328f, 324t
  autosomal recessive inheritance of, 315t
  biology of, 311–312, 312f
  chemically-induced, 331–332
  chromosome analysis in, 136
  clonal evolution in, 330, 331f
  cytogenetics of, 154–155, 330, 331f
  definition of, 311
  environmental factors in, 331–332
  familial, 313, 314t–315t
  forms of, 311–312
  gene amplification in, 330, 331f
  genetic basis of, 311–313, 312f, 314t–315t
  in chromosomal instability, 328
  in gene therapy, 273
  in tumor-suppressor gene mutations, 314t, 320–329, 321t, 322f–329f, 324t
  metastasis from, 311
  oncogenes in. *See* Oncogene(s).
  pathogenesis of, 312, 312f
  predisposition to, inheritance of, 54
  radiation-induced, 331
  somatic mutations in, 86
Cancer *(Continued)*
  sporadic
    oncogene activation in, 316–320, 316f–319f, 317t, 318t
    tumor-suppressor gene loss in, 328–329, 329f
  two-hit origin of, 320–321
Candidate gene, 131–132
Carcinogenesis, environmental factors in, 331–332
Carcinoma, definition of, 311
Carrier(s). *See also* Heterozygote(s); *specific diseases.*
  as prenatal diagnosis indication, 361, 362t
  definition of, 56
  dysgenetic effects of, 396–397
  frequency of, 56–57
  genetic counseling of, 378–379
  obligate, 380–382, 380f
  of inversions, 146–147
  of Robertsonian translocation, 149, 159–160
  of X-linked disorders, 382–383, 383f, 384f
  offspring disease risk and, 56
  recurrence risk and. *See* Recurrence risk determination.
  screening of, 392–393, 392t, 395
Case-control studies, of familial aggregation, 290–291
CAT (CCAAT) box, 25, 26f, 27
Cat-eye syndrome, microdeletion in, 164t, 165
β-Catenin, 326–327, 327f
CCAAT (CAT) box, 25, 26f, 27
*CCR5* deletion allele, in human immunodeficiency infection resistance, 96–98, 97t, 107–108, 108f
*CDH1* gene mutations, 314t
*CDK4* gene mutations, 314t
*CDKN2* gene mutations, 314t
cDNA (complementary DNA), 18, 19f, 34
Celiac disease, HLA associations of, 280t
Cell(s)
  autonomy of, 337
  culture of
    failure of, 370–371
    for cytogenetic analysis, 135
    for gene mapping, 111–113
    for prenatal diagnosis, 369
  division of. *See* Meiosis; Mitosis.
  nonautonomous, 337
  programmed death of. *See* Apoptosis.
  replacement of, in transplantation, 266
  senescence of, 112, 320
  transformation of, in culture, 112
Cell cycle, 5–8, 5f–9f
Cell lineage, 343
Centimorgans, as gene distance unit, 120–121, 126
Central dogma, of molecular biology, 18–22, 19f–21f
Centromere(s)
  absence of, in marker chromosomes, 145
  acrocentric, in translocation, 149
  appearance of, 7, 7f
  definition of, 5f, 6
  in dicentric chromosomes, 146
  position of, chromosome classification by, 137, 137f
  staining of, 137
Centrosomes, 6f, 7
CF. *See* Cystic fibrosis.
*CFTR* gene and protein, 130, 222–224, 223f, 223t
CG (CpG) islands, 27
Chain termination mutations, 82
Charcot-Marie-Tooth disease, 164t, 165
Checkpoints, in cell cycle, 5
Chédiak-Higashi syndrome, 287t
Chemical(s), cancer induced by, 331–332
Chemical individuality, definition of, 87
Chiasmata, in meiosis, 10
Children, genetic testing of, ethical issues in, 394–395
Chimera, 356
Chloride channel defects, in cystic fibrosis, 222–223, 223f
Cholesterol, excess of. *See* Hypercholesterolemia.
Cholinesterase defects, succinylcholine sensitivity in, 250
Choriocarcinoma, origin of, 151
Chorion frondosum, 364
Chorionic villi
  embryology of, 363–364, 363f
  hydatidiform mole of, 140, 151–153
  sampling of, 363f, 364
    for cytogenetic studies, 369–372, 370f, 371t
    indications for, 361
    sample preparation in, 369
Choroideremia, founder effect in, 106, 107f
Chromatids
  premature separation of, 142
  sister, 5, 5f, 6
    exchange of, 154, 154f
Chromatin
  condensed, 6, 8f, 9f
  decondensed, 6, 8f, 9f
  definition of, 4, 28
  sex (Barr body), 67, 67f, 169, 169f
  structure of, 28
Chromosome(s), 4–16, 148, 149f
  abnormalities of. *See* Chromosome abnormality(ies).
  adjacent-1 segregation in, 148, 149f
  adjacent-2 segregation in, 148, 149f
  alternate, 148, 149f
  analysis of. *See* Chromosome analysis.
  arms of, 7
  artificial, 37–38, 37t, 39f
    contigs of, 127, 128f, 129t
    transfer of, 273
  autosomes as, 5
  bacterial artificial, 37–38, 37t, 127, 128f
  complement of. *See* Karyotype(s).
  congression of, 7
  daughter, 7
  deficient segments in, 146–147, 147f
  definition of, 4
  deletion of. *See* Deletion(s).
  dicentric, 146
  disorders of. *See* Chromosome abnormality(ies).
  double minutes in, 330
  duplication of. *See* Duplication.
  extra structurally abnormal, 147f, 148–149
  gene assignment to. *See* Gene mapping.
  heteromorphisms in, 136
  homogeneously staining regions in, 330
  homologous, 5, 10, 118–119, 118f, 119f
  imbalance of, developmental abnormalities in, 338t
  in cell division. *See* Meiosis; Mitosis(es).
  in situ hybridization to, 46–48, 47f, 48f
  insertion in. *See* Insertion(s).
  instability of
    cancer in, 328
    syndromes of, 153–154, 154f, 154t
  interphase, 28, 28f

Chromosome(s) *(Continued)*
 inversion in, 146–147, 147f
 length of, 125, 125t
 marker, 144–145, 144f
 metaphase, 28, 28f, 29
 microdeletion of, autosomal disorders involving, 164–165, 164t, 165f
 mitochondrial, 29–30, 244
  disorders of, 77
 mutations of, 79–81, 79t
 number of, 5
  abnormal, 140–143, 142f
  in sperm, 13f
  reduction of, in meiosis, 12
 painting of, 47
 Philadelphia, 317, 318f
 possible number of combinations of, 10
 pseudodicentric. *See* Centromere(s).
 quadrivalent, 148, 149f
 rearrangement of, 143–149
  balanced, 143, 144f, 146–149, 151f, 152f
  unbalanced, 143–146, 144f, 145f
 ring, 144–145, 144f, 175–176
 segmental aneusomy of, 164, 164t
 segregation of, 6, 9, 9f
 sex. *See* Sex chromosome(s); X chromosome; Y chromosome.
 staining of, 7–8, 7f, 8f
 structure of, 27–30, 28f, 29f
 study of. *See* Cytogenetics.
 supernumerary, 144–145, 144f
 synapsis of, 10, 12f
 transfer of, gene mapping by, 112–115, 112f–116f, 114t
 translocation of. *See* Translocation(s).
 types of, 5
 with missing and duplicated arms (isochromosomes), 144f, 145–146, 145f
 yeast artificial, 37t, 38, 39f, 127, 128f
Chromosome abnormality(ies), 140–151. *See also specific disorders.*
 abbreviations for, 140, 141t
 definition of, 2
 genomic imprinting as, 72–75, 73f, 74t, 151, 152f
 in cancer, 154–155
 in live births, 150, 150t, 151t
 in parent, as prenatal diagnosis indication, 361
 in previous child, as prenatal diagnosis indication, 361
 incidence of, 140, 140t, 150–151, 150t, 151t
 instability as, 153–154, 154f, 154t
 mosaicism as. *See* Mosaicism.
 nomenclature of, 140, 141t
 numerical, 140–143, 142f
 prenatal diagnosis of. *See* Prenatal diagnosis.
 spontaneous abortion in, 353–354, 354f
 structural, 143–149, 144f
  balanced rearrangements as, 146–149, 147f, 148f
  unbalanced rearrangements as, 143–146, 145f
Chromosome analysis. *See also* Banding.
 applications of, 4
 culture for, 136
 identification in, 136–138, 137f, 138f
 in cancer, 330, 331f
 in situ hybridization in, 46–48, 47f, 48f, 138–139, Color Insert following page 139
Chromosome analysis *(Continued)*
 indications for, 135–136
 of amniotic fluid, 362–363
 prenatal, 369–371, 370f, 371t
 sample for, 135
Chromosome band(s). *See* Banding.
Chromosome spread, 7, 7f
Chronic granulomatous disease, 116, 117f, 287t
Chronic progressive external ophthalmoplegia, 245f, 246t, 248–249
Chymotrypsin, degradation of, 89
Cleft lip and/or palate, 293t, 307–308, 307t, 308t, 338t
Clinical genetics, definition of, 2
Clinodactyly, in Down syndrome, 158, 160f
Clones and cloning, 345
 definition of, 34, 337
 identification of, nucleic acid probes in, 34, 40–41, 41f
 molecular, 33, 35f
  libraries for. *See* Libraries.
 of animals, 356, 356f
 positional
  definition of, 128
  in cystic fibrosis, 129–130, 130f
  in Duchenne muscular dystrophy, 128–129
  in hereditary nonpolyposis colon cancer, 131
  in retinitis pigmentosa, 130–131
Closely linked marker method, for mutation detection, 385
Coagulation disorder(s), multifactorial inheritance of, 300–301
Codominant alleles, 53
Codon(s), 23, 24t
 anticodon binding to, 24
 mutations of, 82
 stop (nonsense), 23, 24
Coefficient of correlation, of physiological quantities, 295
Coefficient of inbreeding, 58, 58f, 59t
Cofactors
 in protein enhancement therapy, 262–263, 263f
 mutations affecting, 215–216, 216f
Collagen defect(s). *See also* Osteogenesis imperfecta.
 Ehlers-Danlos syndrome as, 55, 234, 235f
Colon
 cancer of. *See* Colorectal cancer.
 familial adenomatous polyposis of
  cancer in, 314t, 326–327, 327f
  genes of, in sporadic cancer, 329, 329f
 Hirschsprung disease of, 301–302, 302f
Color blindness
 genotypes of, frequencies of, 98–99, 99t
 inheritance of, 70, 70f
Colorectal cancer
 hereditary nonpolyposis, 315t, 327–328, 328f
  DNA repair defects in, 86–87
  genes of
   identification of, 131
   sporadic cancer in, 329, 329f
  tumor-suppressor gene mutations in, 321t, 327–328, 328f
 in familial adenomatous polyposis, 314t, 326–327, 327f
 somatic mutations in, 86
 sporadic, genes in, 329, 329f
Commitment, in development, 337
Comparative genome hybridization, 47, 47f
Competency, in embryonic induction, 337
Complement, deficiencies of, 287t
Complementary DNA, 18, 19f, 34
Complementation, 214
Complementation analysis, of mutations, 214–215
Complex inheritance. *See* Multifactorial disorder(s); Multifactorial inheritance.
Compound(s), genetic, phenylketonuria and, 208
Compound heterozygote, definition of, 52
Concordance, 290–292, 292f, 292t
Condensation, in cell cycle, 8, 9f
Conditional probability, definition of, 381
Confined placental mosaicism, 153
Congenital disorder(s). *See also specific disorders.*
 multifactorial inheritance of, 304–308, 304t, 305f, 306f, 307t, 308t
 versus genetic disorders, 55
Congression, of chromosomes, 7
Consanguinity, 57–59
 autosomal recessive disease in, 101
 definition of, 52, 53f, 57, 57f
 genetic counseling for, 385
 genetic isolates and, 58–59, 59t
 mating types in, 58, 58f, 59t
 measurement of, 57–58, 58f, 59t
 versus inbreeding, 59, 59t
Constant regions, of immunoglobulin chains, 281–283, 282f–284f
Constitutive heterochromatin, 137
Constriction, primary. *See* Centromere(s).
Consultand, definition of, 52, 375
Contig(s), of artificial chromosomes, 127, 128f, 129t
Contiguous gene syndromes, 54–55, 83, 164–165, 164t, 165f
Contraception, for disease recurrence prevention, 376
Cordocentesis, 364
Cornelia de Lange syndrome, 102t, 338t, 350, 351f
Coronary artery disease, 308–309
Correlation, of physiological quantities, 295–296
Cosmids, 37–38, 37t
Counseling. *See* Genetic counseling.
Coupling, alleles in, 122, 122f
Cousins. *See* Consanguinity.
Cowden disease, cancer in, 314t
CpG islands, 27
CREB-binding protein, defects of, 341, 342f, 343
Cri du chat syndrome, 163–164, 164f
Crick, Francis, 17
Crohn's disease, risk ratio for, 291t
Crossing over, 10, 12
 meiotic. *See* Recombination.
 unequal, 83–84, 84f, 144, 144f
  in contiguous gene syndromes, 165, 165f
Cryptic splice sites, in RNA, 196, 198f
Culture, cell. *See* Cell(s), culture of.
CVS. *See* Chorionic villi, sampling of.
Cystathionine synthase deficiency (homocystinuria), 215–216, 216f, 263
Cystic fibrosis, 222–225
 carrier frequency in, 56–57
 family studies in, 224–225
 gene of, 222–224, 223f, 223t
  isolation of, 130
  mutations in, 386–387
 genetics of, 223–225, 223t
 genotype-phenotype correlations in, 223t, 224

Cystic fibrosis *(Continued)*
heterozygote advantage in, 105
inheritance of, 56–57
linkage analysis of, 129–130, 130f
liver transplantation in, 268–269
pathophysiology of, 223
pedigree for, 126f
phenotypes of, 222
population genetics of, 96t, 100, 100t, 224, 396
prenatal diagnosis of, 224–225
screening for, 224, 392–393
treatment of, 225
uniparental disomy in, 75
Cystinosis, treatment of, 257
Cytochrome P450 gene mutations, cancer in, 331–332
Cytogenetics. *See also* Chromosome abnormality(ies); Chromosome analysis.
definition of, 2, 4
in prenatal diagnosis, 369–372, 370f, 371t
molecular, 138–139, Color Insert following page 139
of cancer, 154–155, 330
of hydatidiform moles, 151–153
of meiosis, 153
of mendelian disorders, 153–154, 154f
of ovarian teratoma, 151–153
Cytokine receptor gene, in human immunodeficiency infection resistance, 96–98, 97t, 107–108, 108f
Cytokinesis, 6f, 7
in meiosis, 10–11, 13f

Darwin, Charles, 396
Daughter chromosomes, 7
*DAX1* gene, in gonadal development, 176
*DAZ* gene mutations, 168
*DCC* gene product, 321t
Deafness
in mitochondrial disorders, 245f, 246t
progressive sensorineural, pedigree for, 61, 61f
Debrisoquin metabolism
cancer and, 332
polymorphism of, population variation in, 96t
Decondensation, in cell cycle, 8, 9f
Deformations, 351–352, 352f
Degenerate genetic code, 23
Deletion(s), 82–83, 143, 144f
autosomal disorders involving, 163–165, 164f, 164t, 165f
in Duchenne muscular dystrophy, 386, 386f
in hemoglobin Gun Hill, 191, 192f
in recombination, 83–84, 84f
interstitial, 143, 144f
large, 83
9p, gonadal maldevelopment in, 176
small, 83
terminal, 143, 144f
X chromosome, multiple, 116, 117f
Denaturation, in DNA analysis, 41, 41f
Denys-Drash syndrome, gonadal maldevelopment in, 176
Deoxyribonucleic acid. *See* DNA (deoxyribonucleic acid).
Depletion therapy, 260t, 262
Dermatan sulfate storage, in mucopolysaccharidoses, 212, 213t, 214, 214f
Determination, in development, 337
Determinism, genetic, 354–355
Developmental biology. *See also* Developmental genetics.
description of, 335, 336f, 337
disease and, 335–336, 338t
during fertilization to gastrulation, 339–341, 340f
of eye, 336–337, 339, 339f
program in, 337
Developmental genetics
cell migration and mixing in, 345–346
cellular differentiation in, 341, 342f, 343
clinical aspects of, 350f–354f, 350–355
definition of, 2
determinism in, 354–355
gene expression and, 341, 342f, 343
genome and, 341, 342f, 343
hierarchies of, 344, 345f–346f
*HOX* genes in, 346–347, 347f, 348f
models for, 336–337, 339, 339f, 339t
morphogenesis and, 345–346
of animal cloning, 356, 356f
of dysmorphology, 350–353, 351f–353f
of embryonic stem cells, 355–356, 355f
of reproduction, 353–354, 354f
of stem cells, 343–344, 343f
paracrine signals in, 347–348, 349f
potential applications of, 355–357, 355f, 356f
signaling pathway integration in, 348–349
stability of cell lineage and, 343
stochastic processes in, 354–355
Diabetes mellitus
HLA associations of, 280t
treatment of, 255–266, 255t
type 1
concordance of, in twins, 293, 293t
inheritance of, 302–303, 303t
risk ratio for, 291t
type 2, inheritance of, 302
Diakinesis, in meiosis, 10
Diaphragmatic hernia, prenatal treatment of, 257t
Dicentric chromosomes, 146
Dietary restriction, 258–260, 260t
Differentiation
definition of, 337
gene expression in, 341, 342f, 343
Digenic inheritance, of retinitis pigmentosa, 299–300, 300f
DiGeorge syndrome
immunodeficiency in, 286t
microdeletion in, 164t, 165
Diploid, definition of, 5
Diploidy, of hydatidiform mole, 151
Diplotene stage, of meiosis, 10
Discordance, definition of, 290
Disease association, studies of, 298–299
Disequilibrium, linkage, 124
in cystic fibrosis, 129–130, 130f
Disjunction, in meiosis, 10
Disomy, uniparental, 74, 75, 153
Disruptions, 351–352, 352f
Disulfide bond, of immunoglobulins, 281, 282f
Diversion therapy, 260t, 261, 261f
DMD. *See* Duchenne muscular dystrophy.
*DMPK* gene, expansion of, in myotonic dystrophy, 243
DNA (deoxyribonucleic acid)
amplification of, in cancer, 330, 331f
analysis of. *See* Analytical technique(s).
antisense, 22
DNA (deoxyribonucleic acid) *(Continued)*
binding domains of, 337
cellular compartmentalization of, 18
circular, plasmids as, 36–37, 37t, 40f
complementary, 18, 19f, 34
condensation of, 8, 9f
conjugated with protein, transfer of, 273
denaturation of, 41, 41f
double-stranded, 40–41, 41f
enzymatic cleavage of, 33–35, 36f, 37t
gene segments of. *See* Gene(s).
in chromatin, 28
in chromosome, 27–30, 28f, 29f
in genome, 4
in in situ hybridization, 46–48, 47f, 48f
in oncogene transformation, 316–317, 316f
lagging strand of, 319–320, 319f
liposome-packaged, transfer of, 273
methylation of, 82
in X inactivation, 169
microsatellite, instability of, 327
mitochondrial. *See* Mitochondrial DNA.
naked, transfer of, 273
polymorphism of. *See* Polymorphism(s).
proofreading of, 81
protein synthesis from, 18–22, 19f–21f. *See also* Gene expression.
proteins associated with, 27–28
recombinant
creation of, 35, 36f
definition of, 36
related sequences in, 31
repair of, errors in, 81, 86–87, 314t–315t, 328
repetitive, 30–31
replication of, 18, 19f
errors in, 81
origins of, 6
telomerase in, 318–320, 319f
samples of, collection of, 126
satellite, 31
sense, 22
single-copy (unique), 30–31
single-stranded, 40–41, 41f
structure of, 17–18, 18f, 19f
synthesis of, 5, 6
in Sanger technique, 48–49, 48f
transfer of. *See* Gene therapy.
DNA (deoxyribonucleic acid) fingerprinting, 92, 92f
DNA ligase, 35
DNA polymerase, in DNA analysis, 48–49, 48f
Domain, paired, 337
Dominant inheritance
autosomal, 61–65, 61f-66f
definition of, 53–54
of disorders. *See under* Autosomal disorder(s).
X-linked, 70–71, 71f
Dominant negative effect, definition of, 54
Dosage approach, to gene mapping, 115–116, 116f, 117f
Dosage compensation, in X inactivation, 67
Double minutes, in chromosomes, 330
Down syndrome (trisomy 21), 157–162, 338t
chromosome abnormalities in, 159–161, 160f, 161f
etiology of, 161
gene mapping in, 115, 116f
genetic counseling in, 378–379, 378f
historical perspective of, 157–158
in 21q21q translocation, 160

Down syndrome *(Continued)*
  incidence of, 157–158, 158t, 162
  karyotype of, 140, 142f
  mosaic, 160–161
  partial trisomy 21 in, 161
  phenotypes in, 158, 159f, 160f
  prenatal diagnosis of, 359, 360f, 364–365, 366
  risk factors for, 161–162
  Robertsonian translocation in, 159–160, 160f, 161f
  survival in, 158–159
*Drosophila melanogaster*, for genetic studies, 336, 339, 339t, 346–347
Drugs, adverse reactions to. *See* Pharmacogenetics.
Duchenne muscular dystrophy, 225–229
  as genetic lethal, 70
  carriers of, 68, 69f, 226, 229
  clinical features of, 225, 225f
  dystrophin detection in, 49, 49f
  gene of, 128–129, 226–227, 227f, 228f
  gene therapy for, 274–275
  genetics of, 225–229, 227f, 227t, 228f
  in females, 226, 227t
  inheritance of, 225–226, 227t
  maternal mosaicism in, 229
  molecular analysis of, 228–229, 228f
  mutations in
    deletion analysis of, 386, 386f
    rate of, 84, 85t
  pathology of, 225, 226f
  phenotypes of, 225, 225f
  population genetics of, 104t, 396
  prenatal diagnosis of, 229
  recurrence risk of, determination of, 382–383, 383f, 384f
  screening for, 392
  selection against, 103–104
  treatment of, 229
  with multiple X-linked disorders, 116, 117f
Duplication, 83–84, 84f, 144, 144f
  in inversion, 146–147, 147f
  in recombination, 83–84, 84f, 144, 144f
Dyschondrosteosis, 72, 72f
Dysgenics, 396–397
Dysmorphology, 350–353, 350f–353f
Dystrophin
  defects of. *See also* Becker muscular dystrophy; Duchenne muscular dystrophy.
    gene therapy for, 274–275
  detection of, 49, 49f
  function of, 227, 228f
  structure of, 226–227, 227f

Echocardiography, fetal, 367, 368t
Ecogenetic diseases, 218, 218f. *See also* Environmental factors; Smoking.
*Eco*RI restriction enzyme, 33, 35, 36f, 37t, 39, 39f
Ectopic gene expression, 182f, 183
Ectrodactyly, reduced penetrance in, 63, 64f
Edwards syndrome (trisomy 18), 162–163, 162f, 364–365
Ehlers-Danlos syndrome, 55, 234, 235f
Elastase
  degradation of, 89
  excess of, in alpha$_1$-antitrypsin deficiency, 216–218, 218f
Electrophoresis, in mutation rate estimation, 84
Ellis–van Creveld syndrome, founder effect in, 106, 106f
Embryo
  development of. *See* Developmental biology.
  stem cells of, 355–356, 355f
Emphysema
  alpha$_1$-antitrypsin replacement in, 263–264
  in alpha$_1$-antitrypsin polymorphism, 89–90, 89t, 255
  smoking and, 218, 218f, 255
Empiric recurrence risk, 384–385
Endothelial cells, gene transfer into, 272
Endothelins, defects of, in Hirschsprung disease, 301
Enhancers, 21, 27, 341
Environmental factors
  in cancer, 331–332
  in inheritance, 290–294, 292f, 292t
Enzyme(s). *See also specific enzymes and related diseases.*
  defects of, 204t, 206–218
    general concepts of, 217, 217f
  replacement of, 264–265, 265f
Epiblast, embryo formation from, 340, 340f, 341
Epigenetic regulation, 343
Epilepsy, concordance of, in twins, 293t
Epstein-Barr virus, in cell transformation, 112
Equilibrium, linkage, in cystic fibrosis, 129–130, 130f
Erythrocyte(s)
  antigens on. *See* Blood group system(s).
  sickling of. *See* Sickle cell disease.
Estriol, unconjugated, measurement of, in triple screen, 365
Ethical issue(s)
  in gene therapy, 274
  in testing, 393–396, 393t
    dilemmas in, 395
    dysgenics and, 396–397
    eugenics and, 396
    for disease predisposition, 394
    for Huntington disease, 241
    of children, 394–395
    prenatal, 372, 393–394
    principles of, 395
    privacy as, 395–396
Ethnic groups, 95, 96t
  disease(s) associated with, 100–101, 101t
    cleft lip and/or palate as, 308
    screening for, 392–393, 392t
    sickle cell, 189, 190, 191f
    Tay-Sachs disease as. *See* Tay-Sachs disease.
    thalassemia as. *See* Thalassemia(s).
  HLAs associated with, 279–280
  stratification of, 99–101, 100t, 101t
Eugenics, 396
Eukaryote, definition of, 18
Euploidy, definition of, 140
Exon(s)
  definition of, 20, 20f
  mutations of, in RNA, 198f, 199
Explantation, of embryonic tissue, 337
Expressed sequence tags, 132
Expression, gene. *See* Gene expression.
Expression vectors, in DNA analysis, 40
Expressivity, variable, 62
Extra structurally abnormal chromosomes, 144–145, 144f
Eye, development of, 336–337, 339, 339f

*f. See* Fitness.
F coefficient (of inbreeding), 58, 58f, 59t
Facial features
  in cri du chat syndrome, 163–164, 164f
  in Down syndrome, 158, 159f
  in trisomy 13, 163, 163f
  in trisomy 18, 162, 162f
Factor V Leiden, thrombosis due to, 300–301
Factor VIII
  defects in. *See* Hemophilia A.
  gene of, structure of, 20f
  replacement of, 263
Factor IX deficiency. *See* Hemophilia B.
Familial adenomatous polyposis, cancer in, 314t, 326–327, 327f
Familial aggregation, 290–291, 291t
  of quantitative traits, 294–295, 295f
Family(ies)
  cancer in, 313, 314t–315t
  disorders transmitted in. *See specific disorders.*
  suitable for gene mapping, 125–126, 126f
Family history
  importance of, 1
  of chromosome abnormality, chromosome analysis in, 136
  of genetic disease, as prenatal diagnosis indication, 361, 362t
  positive, 291
Fanconi anemia
  cancer in, 315t, 328
  cytogenetics of, 154t
Fate and fate map, in embryo, 337
Favism, 252
Feminization, testicular (androgen insensitivity syndrome), 43, 43f, 172t, 176–178, 177f
Fertility problems. *See* Infertility.
Fertilization, 14f, 15
  development after, 339–341, 340f
  in vitro, preimplantation genetic diagnosis for, 368–369, 376
  with two sperm, triploidy in, 140
Fetal alcohol syndrome, 338t
Fetal cells, in maternal blood, identification of, 369
Fetal hemoglobin. *See under* Hemoglobin(s).
Fibroblasts
  in chromosome analysis, 136
  in somatic cell studies, 112
Fingerprinting, DNA, 92, 92f
Fingerprints, development of, 355
Finland, genetic drift in, 106, 107f
First-degree relatives, definition of, 52, 53f
FISH (fluorescence in situ hybridization), 46–48, 47f, 48f
  fiber, 118
  in chromosome analysis, 138–139, Color Insert following page 139
  in gene mapping, 117–118, 117f
Fitness
  balance of, with mutation, 103
  definition of, 61, 102
  heterozygote advantage in, 104–105
  in hemophilia, 70
  in heterozygotes versus homozygotes, 104–105
  in X-linked recessive disorders, 103–104
  reduced, in autosomal dominant disorders, 62, 102–103, 102t
  zero, 102–103, 102t
Fluorescence in situ hybridization, 46–48, 47f, 48f
  in chromosome analysis, 138–139, Color Insert following page 139
  in gene mapping, 117–118, 117f

*FMR1* gene, loss of function of, in fragile X syndrome, 243
Folic acid, neural tube defects and, 306, 306f
Foot abnormalities
in trisomy 13, 163, 163f
in trisomy 18, 162–163, 162f
Founder effect, 106, 106f, 107f
Fragile sites, viewing of, 138
Fragile X syndrome, 239t, 242–243, 242f, 243f
cytogenetics of, 154t
genetic counseling in, 378–379
mutations in, 84
population genetics of, 104t
Frameshift mutation, 83
Frataxin defects, 244
Friedreich ataxia, 239t, 243–244
Fruitfly, for genetic studies, 336, 339, 339t, 346–347
Fryns syndrome, prenatal diagnosis of, 367t
Fumarylacetoacetase deficiency, founder effect in, 106
Function, simple gain of, 54

G (Giemsa) banding, 7–8, 7f, 8f, 137–138, 137f, 138f
$G_0$ phase, of cell cycle, 6
$G_1$ phase, of cell cycle, 5–6, 5f, 6f
$G_2$ phase, of cell cycle, 5–6, 5f, 6f
G proteins, defects of, in cancer, 317–318
Gain-of-function mutations, 182–183, 182f
Galactose-1-phosphate uridyltransferase deficiency, 256f, 257
Galactosemia, 256f, 257, 391
Galton, Francis, 396
Gamete(s)
balanced versus unbalanced chromosomes in, 146–147, 147f
chromosomes of, 5
genomic imprinting of, 72–75, 73f, 74t
nonrecombinant, 119–120
Gametogenesis, 12–15, 13f, 14f, 72
Gangliosidosis. *See* Tay-Sachs disease.
Gastrulation, abnormalities developing during, 341
Gaucher disease
bone marrow transplantation in, 268
enzyme replacement in, 264–265, 265f
Gender differences, in mutation, 85–86
Gene(s)
amplification of, in cancer, 330, 331f
arrangement of. *See* Genome.
candidate, 131–132
contiguous, defects of, 54–55, 83, 164–165, 164t, 165f
deficiency of, 21
definition of, 4, 20
distance between, measurement of, 120–121
families of, 21–22, 21f
heritability of, 296–297
housekeeping, 204–205, 341
interruption of, 20, 20f
locus for, 4
master, 341
mitochondrial, 29–30
modifier, 200, 205–206
mutations of. *See* Mutation(s).
number of, 4, 111, 132–133
organization of, 20–22, 20f, 21f
size of, 21
structure of, 20–22, 20f, 21f
wild-type, introduction of, 266
Gene expression, 25–27, 25f, 26f
ectopic, 182f, 183
example of, 25–27, 25f, 26f
heterochronic, 182f, 183
in cell fate, 344, 345f–346f
in cell lineage establishment, 343
in cell migration and mixing, 344–345
in cellular differentiation, 341, 342f, 343
in development, 341–349, 342f, 343f, 345f–349f
in identity development, 346–347, 347f, 348f
in morphogenesis, 345–346
in paracrine signal regulation, 347–348, 349f
in signaling pathway integration, 348–349
in stem cell differentiation, 343–344, 343f
modulation of, in disease treatment, 265, 266f, 266t
postadenylation in, 26f, 27
post-translational processing in, 24–25
RNA splicing in, 26f, 27
steps in, 22, 23f
transcription in, 22–23, 23f, 25–27, 25f, 26f
translation in, 23–24, 23f, 24t
variation in, clinical consequences of, 31–32
Gene flow, 107–108, 108f
Gene mapping, 4, 111–134
applications of, 125–132
approaches to, 111
artificial chromosome contigs in, 127, 128f, 129t
candidate gene approach to, 131–132
expressed sequence tags in, 132
for Human Genome Project, 1, 30, 132–133
genetic. *See also* Linkage analysis.
definition of, 111
versus physical, 125
high-resolution, 127
historical view of, 111
in adverse drug reaction studies, 252–253
in disease identification, 127–132
for cystic fibrosis, 129–130, 130f
for Duchenne muscular dystrophy, 128–129
for hereditary nonpolyposis colon cancer, 131
for retinitis pigmentosa, 130–131
for Tay-Sachs disease, 114, 114f, 114t
of complex traits, 297–299
physical, 111–118
chromosome transfer in, 112–115, 112f–116f, 114t
definition of, 111
fluorescence in situ hybridization in, 117–118, 117f
gene dosage in, 115–117, 116f, 117f
panels in, 113–114, 114f, 114t
radiation hybrids in, 115, 116f
somatic cell genetics in, 111–112
versus genetic, 125
positional cloning in, 128–131, 130f
suitable families for, 125–126, 126f
ten centimorgan limit in, 126
Gene pool, 97
deterioration of, dysgenics in, 396–397
improvement of, eugenics in, 396
small, genetic drift in, 105–107, 106f, 107f
Gene therapy, 269–275
compensating function of, 269–270, 271f
Gene therapy *(Continued)*
definition of, 269
ethical considerations in, 274
for adenosine deaminase deficiency, 275
for Duchenne muscular dystrophy, 274–275
for hemophilia B, 269, 274
for immunodeficiency, 285, 288
for severe combined immunodeficiency, 269, 274
goals of, 269, 271f
minimal requirements for, 270
nonviral vectors for, 273
pharmacologic effects of, 270, 271f
purposes of, 269–270, 271f
replacement function of, 270, 271f
risks of, 273–274
strategies for, 271f, 272
target cell for, 270–272
viral vectors for, 272–273
Genetic Alliance, 377
Genetic background, definition of, 200
Genetic code, 19, 23–24, 24t
degenerate, 23
Genetic compounds, phenylketonuria and, 208
Genetic counseling, 375–379
case management in, 377–379, 378f, 378t
counselor role in, 376
definition of, 2, 375
follow-up after, 378–379
for consanguinity, 385
for multifactorial traits, 309
for prenatal diagnosis, 360
for recurrence prevention, 376–377
indications for, 375, 375t
nondirective, 375–376
preassessment in, 378, 378f
process of, 375–376
psychological aspects of, 377
purpose of, 377
recurrence risk assessment for. *See* Recurrence risk determination.
support organizations recommended in, 377
Genetic disorder(s). *See also* Chromosome abnormality(ies); *specific disorders.*
classification of, 2
lethal. *See* Genetic lethal(s).
multifactorial. *See* Multifactorial disorder(s).
single-gene. *See* Single-gene defect(s).
treatment of. *See* Treatment; *specific diseases and treatments.*
versus congenital disorders, 55
Genetic diversity, 87, 95, 96t
Genetic drift, 104, 105–106, 106f, 107f
heterozygote advantage and, 104–105
Genetic lethal(s), 55
autosomal dominant, 102–103, 102t
Duchenne muscular dystrophy as, 70
in aneuploidy, 140
incontinentia pigmenti type 2 as, 71, 71f
osteogenesis imperfecta as, 76, 76f
recombinant 8 syndrome as, 147
X-linked, 104
Genetic markers, 118
Genetic polymorphism. *See* Polymorphism(s).
Genetic screening. *See* Screening.
Genetics
as medical specialty, 1
disciplines within, 1–2
population. *See* Population genetics.

Genetics *(Continued)*
  relevance of, 1
  somatic cell, 111–112
Genitalia
  embryology of, 166–167, 167f
  maldevelopment of, 176–178, 177f
Genocopy, definition of, 290
Genome
  components of, 4
  gene expression and, 341, 342f, 343
  modification of, transplantation for, 265–269, 267f, 268f
  mutations in, 79–80, 79t
  nuclear, mitochondrial interaction with, 248–249
  organization of, 17, 30–31, 30f. *See also* Chromosome(s); Gene(s).
  parameters of, 125, 125t
Genome scan, in linkage analysis, of complex traits, 297
Genomic imprinting, 72–75, 73f, 74t, 151, 152f
Genomic libraries, 38f, 39, 39f
Genomics, definition of, 2
Genotype(s)
  definition of, 51
  derivation of, from allele frequencies, 96
  distribution of. *See* Population genetics.
  frequency of, calculation of. *See* Hardy-Weinberg law.
  known, recurrence risk determination in, 379–380
  of X-linked disorders, frequencies of, 98–99, 99t
  versus phenotype, 205–206, 206t
Germ cells, formation of, 12–15, 13f, 14f
Germline
  mosaicism in, 76, 76f
  mutations in
    frequency of, 84–85, 85t
    gender differences in, 85–86
Giemsa banding, 7–8, 7f, 8f, 137–138, 137f, 138f
Globin(s). *See also* Hemoglobin(s); Hemoglobinopathy(ies).
  gene(s) of, 21–22, 21f
    expression of, 186–187, 186f, 187f
    α-globin gene as, 194–195, 194f, 195t. *See also* Thalassemia(s), α-.
    β-globin gene as
      expression of, 25–27, 25f, 26f, 186–187, 186f, 187f
      locus control region of, 187, 187f
      molecular studies of, 46
      population genetics of, 96t
      structure of, 20f, 25, 25f, 26f
    mutations of, sensitive versus insensitive area for, 186
  structure of, 185–186, 186f
  switching of, 186, 186f
Globoid cell leukodystrophy, bone marrow transplantation in, 268, 268f
Glucocerebrosidase deficiency
  bone marrow transplantation in, 268
  replacement therapy for, 264–265, 265f
Glucose-6-phosphate deficiency, pharmacogenetics of, 252
Glycosaminoglycan storage diseases (mucopolysaccharidoses), 212, 213t, 214, 214f
Glycosyltransferase gene, alleles of, in ABO blood group, 88
Gonads. *See* Ovary; Testis.
Gout, hypoxanthine guanine phosphoribosyltransferase defects in, 210
Graves disease, HLA associations of, 280t
Greig syndrome, 339t
Growth disorders, chromosome analysis in, 135
Gynecomastia, in Klinefelter syndrome, 173, 173f
Gyrate atrophy, population genetics of, 101t, 106–107, 107f

Hand, abnormalities of
  in Down syndrome, 158, 160f
  in split-hand syndrome, 63, 64f, 383, 384f
  in trisomy 13, 163, 163f
  in trisomy 18, 162, 162f
Haploid, definition of, 5
Haploinsufficiency
  definition of, 54
  in deletion, 143
Haplotype(s)
  definition of, 122
  of HLA, 279–280, 279f
Hardy-Weinberg law, 97–98, 98t
  applications of, 98
  assumptions of, 99, 99t
  factors disturbing, 99–108, 99t–102t, 106f–108f
HAT medium, for cell culture, 113
HD. *See* Huntington disease.
Heart disease
  congenital, 306–307, 307t
  in Down syndrome, 158
  prenatal diagnosis of, ultrasonography in, 367, 368t
Heavy chains, of immunoglobulins, 281–283, 282f–284f, 282t
Hedgehog gene, 348, 349f
Height
  heritability of, 296
  of parents versus children, 295–296, 295f
Heinz bodies, in thalassemia, 195f
Hematopoietic cells
  development of, 343–344, 343f
  malignancy of. *See also* Leukemia(s); Lymphoma(s).
    definition of, 311
  stem, transplantation of, 267
Heme, in ferric state, in methemoglobin, 191–192
Hemizygote(s), with respect to X-linked genes, 53
Hemochromatosis
  HLA associations of, 280, 280t
  inheritance of, 59
  screening for, 392
Hemoglobin(s), 189t
  A, 185, 185f
  anti-Lepore, 188t, 193, 193f
  Bart's, 194, 195t
  C, 188t, 190–191, 200
  Constant Spring, 189t, 195
  E, 188t, 193, 196, 199, 200
  embryology of, 185, 185f
  fetal, 185f, 186, 186f
    hereditary persistence of, 196, 199–201, 201f
    induction of, in sickle cell disease, 265, 266f, 266t
  function of, 185, 185f
  genes of, 21–22, 21f, 185–187, 185f–187f
  Gower, 185f
  Gun Hill, 188t, 191
  H, 194, 195t
  Hammersmith, 184t, 188t, 191
  Hispanic deletion, 199
Hemoglobin(s) *(Continued)*
  Hyde Park, 188t, 192
  in thalassemia. *See* Thalassemia(s).
  Kansas, 184t, 188t, 192, 192f
  Kempsey, 183, 184t, 188t, 192, 192f
  Lepore, 188t, 193, 193f, 196
  Miyada, 188t, 193, 193f
  Philly, 184t
  Portland, 185f
  reduced heme in (methemoglobin), 191–192
  S, 188t, 189–190, 190f, 200. *See also* Sickle cell disease.
  structure of, 185, 185f, 186f
  Tak, 188t, 193
  unstable, 191, 192f
  variant, 187–193, 188t, 189t
    with altered oxygen transport, 188t, 191–193, 192f
    with novel physical properties, 188t, 189–190, 190f–192f
    with thalassemia phenotypes, 188t–189t, 193, 193f
Hemoglobinopathy(ies), 184–185. *See also* Hemoglobin(s), variant; Sickle cell disease; Thalassemia(s).
  gene dosage in, 187
  globin structure in, 185–186, 186f
  mutations in, 184t, 187, 187f
Hemolysis and hemolytic anemia, 188t, 189–190, 190f, 191f. *See also* Sickle cell disease.
  in glucose-6-phosphate deficiency, 252
  in newborn, Rh blood group–induced, 88–89
Hemophilia A
  inheritance of, 65–66, 69, 69f
  mutation in, rate of, 85t
  population genetics of, 104, 104t
  recurrence risk determination for, 380–382, 380f
  sporadic, gene insertion in, 83
  transmission of, in uniparental disomy, 75
Hemophilia B
  gene therapy for, 269, 274
  mutations in
    paternal origin of, 86
    rate of, 85t
Heparan *N*-sulfatase deficiency, mucopolysaccharidoses in, 212, 213t, 214, 214f
Hepatocytes, gene transfer into, 271–272
Hereditary neuropathy with liability to pressure palsies, 164t
Hereditary nonpolyposis colon cancer. *See under* Colorectal cancer.
Heritability, 295–296
Hermaphroditism, 176
Hernia, diaphragmatic, prenatal treatment of, 257t
Heterochromatin, constitutive, 137
Heterochronic gene expression, 182f, 183
Heterogeneity, 55–56
  allelic, 55–56, 205, 206t
    in hyperphenylalaninemias, 208–209, 208f, 209t
    in Lesch-Nyhan disease, 210, 210f
    treatment and, 258
  clinical, 206t
  in hemoglobinopathies, 200
  locus, 55, 126, 205, 206t
    in hyperphenylalaninemias, 208–209, 208f, 209t
    treatment and, 258
  phenotypic, 206t
  treatment and, 258

Heterokaryon
complementation tests in, 215
definition of, 113
Heteromorphisms, in banding, 136
Heteroplasmy, in mitochondrial DNA mutations, 246t, 247–249, 248f
Heteroploidy, definition of, 140
Heterozygosity, loss of
in breast cancer, 329
in retinoblastoma, 323, 323f, 324t
Heterozygote(s). *See also specific diseases.*
assortative mating of, 101
autosomal dominant alleles in, selection against, 102–103, 102t
compound, 52
definition of, 52
dominant inheritance in, 53–54
for autosomal recessive disorders
coefficient of inbreeding for, 59, 59t
selection against, 103
for X-linked disorders, 68
haploinsufficiency in, 54
manifesting, 68
mating of, autosomal dominant disorders and, 63–64, 65f
screening of, 392–393, 392t
selection for, 104–105
Heterozygote advantage, definition of, 104–105
Hexosaminidase A deficiency. *See* Tay-Sachs disease.
High-density single nucleotide polymorphism map, 252–253
High-resolution (prometaphase) banding, 137–138, 138f
High-resolution gene mapping, 127
Highly discordant sib pair method, for linkage analysis, 298
Hirschsprung disease, 301–302, 302f
Histones, associated with DNA, 27–28, 28f
HLAs. *See* Human leukocyte antigens.
Hodgkin's lymphoma, tumor-suppressor gene mutations in, 328
Holoprosencephaly, 338t, 339t, 348, 349f
Holt-Oram syndrome, prenatal diagnosis of, 366f
Homeodomain, 337, 346
Homocystinuria
cofactor defects in, 215–216, 216f
enhancement therapy for, 263
Homogeneously staining regions, of chromosome, in cancer, 330
Homokaryon, definition of, 113
Homolog(s)
definition of, 5
in meiosis, 10
random assortment of, 12
recombination of, 118–119, 118f, 119f
Homoplasmy, in mitochondrial DNA mutations, 246t, 247–249, 248f
Homozygote(s). *See also specific diseases.*
allelic heterogeneity in, 56
assortative mating of, 101
definition of, 52
for autosomal dominant traits, 63–64, 65f
for autosomal recessive disorders, selection against, 103
for autosomal recessive traits, 56, 56f
for X-linked disorders, females as, 70, 70f
identical by descent, 58
in different populations, 59, 59t
recessive inheritance in, 53–54
Host, in DNA cloning, 34
Housekeeping genes and proteins, 204–205, 341
*HOX* genes, in development, 346–347, 347f, 348f
Human chorionic gonadotropin measurement, in triple screen, 365
Human genetics, definition of, 1
Human Genome Project, 1, 30, 132–133
ethical implications of, 393
pharmacogenomics and, 252–253
Human immunodeficiency virus infection, resistance to, genetics of, 96–98, 97t, 107–108, 108f
Human leukocyte antigens, 277–281
classes of, 277–279, 278f
disease associations of, 280–281, 280t
polymorphism of, 96t, 279–280, 279f, 279t
structure of, 277–278, 278f
T-cell antigen receptor and, 277, 278f, 284–285, 285f
Hunter syndrome, 213t, 214
Huntington disease, 240–241
age of onset of, 240, 240f
counseling on, 241
ethical issues in, 241
founder effect in, 106, 241
heterozygous versus homozygous, 64
inheritance of, 240–241, 241f
mutations in, 83–84
pedigree for, 126f
screening for, ethical issues in, 394
versus fragile X syndrome, 243
Hurler-Scheie syndrome, 213t, 214
Hurler syndrome, 213t, 214, 214f, 268
Hybridization
comparative genome, 47, 47f
definition of, 34
nucleic acid, 40–41, 41f
somatic cell, in gene mapping, 112–115, 112f–116f, 114t
Hydatidiform mole, 140, 151–153
Hydrops fetalis, in thalassemia, 194, 195t
3-Hydroxy-3-methylglutaryl coenzyme A reductase
in hypercholesterolemia, 219, 220f
inhibitors of, in hypercholesterolemia, 261f, 262
21-Hydroxylase deficiency, adrenal hyperplasia in, 176–177, 177f
Hyper IgM syndrome, 286t
Hyperammonemia, diversion therapy for, 261, 261f
Hypercholesterolemia, familial, 218–222, 309
atherosclerotic plaque formation in, 221–222
depletion therapy for, 260t, 262
diversion therapy for, 261, 261f
genetics of, 219, 219f
heterozygous, 64, 65f, 219, 219f
homozygous, 64, 65f, 219, 219f
inhibition therapy for, 260t, 261–262
pathophysiology of, 219, 220f, 221f
population genetics of, 96t, 101t
receptor mutations in, 219–222
Hyperornithinemia, founder effect in, 106, 107f
Hyperostosis syndrome, zero fitness in, 102t
Hyperphenylalaninemias. *See also* Phenylketonuria.
genetic heterogeneity of, 206t, 208–209, 208f, 209t
non-phenylketonuria, 208, 208t
Hyperthermia, malignant, 250
Hypogonadism, in Klinefelter syndrome, 173, 173f
Hypophosphatemic rickets, inheritance of, 71
Hypothyroidism, congenital, replacement therapy for, 260
Hypoxanthine, for cell culture, 113
Hypoxanthine guanine phosphoribosyltransferase
defects of, 210, 210f
gene of, structure of, 20f
in somatic cell hybridization, 113

I-cell disease, 215
ICF syndrome, cytogenetics of, 154, 154f
Ichthyosis, microdeletion in, 164t
Identical by descent, 58
Iduronate sulfatase deficiency, mucopolysaccharidoses in, 212, 213t, 214, 214f
Iduronidase deficiency, mucopolysaccharidoses in, 212, 213t, 214, 214f
Ileus, meconium, in cystic fibrosis, 222
Immune globulin, Rh, in pregnancy, 89
Immune response, definition of, 277
Immune system, 277–288
immunoglobulins in, 277–281, 278f, 281f–284f, 282t
major histocompatibility complex in, 277–281, 278f, 279f, 279t, 280t
single-gene disorders of, 285, 286t–287t, 288
T-cell antigen receptor in, 284–285, 285f
Immunoassay, for alpha-fetoprotein, 362
Immunodeficiency
bone marrow transplantation in, 266–267
severe combined, 285
adenosine deaminase replacement in, 264, 264f
gene therapy for, 269, 274, 275
Immunoglobulin(s), 281–284
classes (isotypes) of, 281–282, 282t
deficiencies of, 286t
definition of, 281
diversity of, 283–284
forms of, 281
genes of, 22, 282, 283f
levels of, in immunodeficiency diseases, 286t–287t
repertoire of, 281
somatic rearrangement of, 281–283, 284f
structure of, 281–282, 282f, 282t
Immunoglobulin gene superfamily, 22, 279
T-cell antigen receptor in, 277, 278f, 284–285, 285f
Implantation, 340, 340f
Imprinting, genomic, 72–75, 73f, 74t, 151, 152f
Imprinting center
defects of, 74
definition of, 72
In situ hybridization, 46–48, 47f, 48f
in chromosome analysis, 138–139, Color Insert following page 139
in gene mapping, 117–118, 117f
In vitro fertilization
for disease recurrence prevention, 376
preimplantation genetic diagnosis for, 368–369, 376
Inbreeding, 58–59, 58f, 59t. *See also* Consanguinity.
Incontinentia pigmenti type 2, male lethality in, 71, 71f
Index case, definition of, 52
Individuality, chemical, 87
Induction, embryonic, 337

Infertility
  chromosome analysis in, 136
  in cystic fibrosis, 222
  in Klinefelter syndrome, 173
  male, Y-linked genes in, 167–168
Inheritance
  atypical patterns of, 72–77, 73f–76f, 74t
  autosomal. *See* Autosomal inheritance.
  digenic, 299–300, 300f
  dominant. *See also* Autosomal inheritance.
    definition of, 53–54
    X-linked, 70–71, 71f
  maternal, 77, 247
  multifactorial. *See* Multifactorial disorder(s); Multifactorial inheritance; *specific disorders.*
  of grandparent genes, 118–119, 118f, 119f
  pseudoautosomal, 71–72, 72f
  recessive. *See also* Autosomal inheritance.
    definition of, 53–54
    of enzymopathies, 217
    X-linked, 68–70, 69f
  single-gene. *See* Single-gene defect(s).
  terminology of, 51–52
  X-linked. *See* X-linked inheritance.
Inhibition therapy, 260t, 261–262
Inner cell mass, embryo formation from, 340, 340f
Insemination, artificial, for disease recurrence prevention, 376
Insert, in DNA cloning, 34
Insertion(s), 82–83, 149
  in recombination, 83–84, 84f
  large, 83
  small, 83
Interphase
  chromosomes in, 28, 28f
  meiotic, 10–11, 13f
  mitotic, 5–6, 6f
Interstitial deletion, 143, 144f
Intron(s)
  definition of, 20–21, 20f
  mutations of, in RNA, 198f, 199
Inversion(s), 146–147, 147f
Ionizing radiation, cancer induced by, 331
Iron, oxidized, in methemoglobin, 191–192
Isochromosomes, 144f, 145–146, 145f
Isodisomy, definition of, 75
Isolate, definition of, 58–59
Isolated case, definition of, 52, 53f
Isoniazid, metabolism of, acetylation polymorphisms and, 251
Isotypes, of immunoglobulin(s), 281–282, 282t
Isotypic exclusion, definition of, 281

JAK3 deficiency, 286t
Joining segments, of immunoglobulin chains, 282–283, 283f, 284f
Joint probability, definition of, 381
Justice, as ethical principle, 395–396

Karyotype(s), 7–8, 7f–9f
  abnormal, 140, 140t, 141t
  definition of, 4, 8
  versus Barr body number, 169
  45,X. *See* Turner syndrome.
  XX male, 172t
Karyotype(s) *(Continued)*
  46,XX male, 167, 168f, 172t
  47,XXX (trisomy X), 172t, 173t, 174
  48,XXXX (tetrasomy X), 174
  49,XXXXX (pentasomy X), 174
  49,XXXXY, 174
  48,XXXY, 174
  47,XXY. *See* Klinefelter syndrome.
  48,XXYY, 174
  46,XY female, 167, 168f, 172t
  47,XYY, 172t, 173t, 174
Karyotyping
  in disease recurrence prevention, 376
  in Down syndrome, 159
  in neonatal death, 136
  prenatal, 369–372, 370f, 371t
  spectral, 47–48, 48f, 139, Color Insert following page 139
Kearns-Sayre syndrome, 245f, 246t, 249
Kidney
  cancer of, 314t
  hereditary papillary carcinoma of, 314t, 315–316
  polycystic disease of, 85t
  Wilms' tumor of, 86, 314t
Kilobase, definition of, 21
Kindred, definition of, 52, 53f
Kinetochore, definition of, 6
Klinefelter syndrome, 173–174, 173f
  clinical features of, 173t
  incidence of, 172t
Krabbe disease, bone marrow transplantation in, 268, 268f

L1 family, in genome, 31, 83
Lactase, polymorphism of, population variation in, 96t
Lagging strand, of DNA, 319–320, 319f
LDL (low-density lipoprotein)
  receptor for, defects in, 218–222, 219f–221f
  removal of, in hypercholesterolemia, 262
Leber's hereditary optic neuropathy, 245f, 246t, 247, 248f, 249
Leigh disease, 245f, 246t
Lentiviruses, as gene therapy vectors, 273
Lenz-Majewski hyperostosis syndrome, 102t
Leptotene stage, of meiosis, 10
Lesch-Nyhan syndrome, 210, 210f
Lethal(s), genetic. *See* Genetic lethal(s).
Leukemia(s)
  chronic myelogenous, 317, 318f, 318t
  in Fanconi anemia, 315t
  somatic mutations in, 86
  translocations in, 318t
Leukocyte adhesion deficiency, 287t
Leukocyte elastase, degradation of, 89
Leukodystrophy, globoid cell, bone marrow transplantation in, 268, 268f
Li-Fraumeni syndrome
  cancer in, 314t, 323–324, 324f
  tumor-suppressor gene mutations in, 321t
Libraries, 34, 38f–40f, 39–41
  complementary DNA, 39–40, 40f
  genomic, 38f, 39, 39f
  screening with, 40
Ligation, in DNA analysis, 34
Light chains, of immunoglobulins, 281–283, 282f–284f, 282t
Lineage, in development, 337
Linkage, definition of, 117–118, 117f
Linkage analysis, 118–125
  advantages of, 118
  definition of, 111
  detection of, 120–124, 122f, 123f, 123t
  distance in, physical versus genetic, 125, 125t
  genetic distance measurement in, 120–121
  in disease, 125–132
    cystic fibrosis and, 129–130, 130f
    Duchenne muscular dystrophy and, 128–129, 386, 386f, 387
    hereditary nonpolyposis colon cancer and, 131
    retinitis pigmentosa and, 130–131
  linkage equilibrium in, 124
  linkage maps in, 124
  lod scores in, 121–123, 122f, 123f, 123t
  model-based, 297
  model-free, 297–298
  multipoint, 124–125, 124f, 125f
  of complex traits, 297–298
  parametric, 297
  phase in, 122–123, 122f, 123f, 123t
  synteny and, 118–120, 118f–120f
Linkage disequilibrium, 124, 129–130, 130f
Linkage equilibrium, 124, 129–130, 130f
Lip, cleft, 293t, 307–308, 307t, 308t
Lipoprotein(s)
  excess of. *See* Hypercholesterolemia.
  low-density
    receptor for, defects in, 218–222, 219f–221f
    removal of, in hypercholesterolemia, 262
Liver
  cells of, gene transfer into, 271–272
  transplantation of, in metabolic diseases, 268–269
Lobster-claw malformation, reduced penetrance in, 63, 64f
Locus(i)
  definition of, 4
  distance between, measurement of, 120–121
  heterogeneity of, 126
  large numbers of, on linkage maps, 124
  linkage of, 119–122, 119f, 120f
Locus control regions, 27
  in gene structure, 21
  of $\beta$-globin gene, 187, 187f
Locus heterogeneity. *See under* Heterogeneity.
Lod score(s), 121–123, 122f, 123f, 123t
Logarithm of the odds. *See* Lod score(s).
Loops, in chromatin organization, 28, 28f
Loss-of-function mutations, 181–182, 182f
Loss of heterozygosity
  in breast cancer, 329
  in retinoblastoma, 323, 323f, 324t
Lung, cystic fibrosis affecting, 222–224
Lyase deficiency, diversion therapy for, 261, 261f
Lymphoblastoid cells, in chromosome analysis, 136
Lymphoid malignancy, definition of, 311
Lymphoma(s)
  Burkitt, 317–318, 318t
  follicular B-cell, 319, 319t
  in ataxia-telangiectasia, 315t
  in autoimmune lymphoproliferative disorder, 315t, 328
  somatic mutations in, 86
Lymphoproliferative syndrome, 287t, 315t

Lyon hypothesis, 66–67, 67f. *See also* X inactivation.
Lysosomal storage disease(s), 210–214, 211f, 211t, 212f, 213t, 214f. *See also specific diseases.*
  bone marrow transplantation in, 267–268, 267f, 268f
  enzyme replacement in, 264–265, 265f

M allele, of alpha$_1$-antitrypsin, 89–90, 89t
McKusick, Victor A., 51
Major histocompatibility complex, 277–281
  classes of, 277–279, 278f
  deficiency of, 286t
  disease associations of, 280–281, 280t, 302–303, 303t
  polymorphism of, 279–280, 279f, 279t
  structure of, 277–278, 278f
  T-cell antigen receptor and, 277, 278f, 284–285, 285f
Major histocompatibility complex restriction, 284
Malaria, resistance to, in sickle cell heterozygotes, 105, 190
Malformations, 350–352, 351f, 352f
Malignancy. *See* Cancer.
Malignant hyperthermia, 250
Manic-depressive disorder, risk ratio for, 291t
Manifesting heterozygote, definition of, 68
Mapping, gene. *See* Gene mapping.
Marker chromosomes, 144–145, 144f
Master genes, 341
Maternal age
  as chromosome analysis indication, 136
  as prenatal diagnosis indication, 359, 360f, 361
  chromosome abnormalities and, 140t
  Down syndrome and, 158, 158t, 159, 161–162
Maternal inheritance, 77
Mating
  assortative, 101
  consanguinous. *See* Consanguinity.
  of heterozygotes, autosomal dominant disorders and, 63–64, 65f
  random
    definition of, 99
    exceptions to, 99–101, 100t, 101t
Mean
  in normal distribution, 294, 294f
  regression to, 295f
Meckel-Gruber syndrome, prenatal diagnosis of, 367, 367t
Meconium ileus, in cystic fibrosis, 222
Medical genetics, definition of, 1–2
Medulloblastoma, chromosome analysis of, Color Insert following page 139
Meiosis, 9–12
  cytogenetics of, 153
  cytokinesis in, 10–11, 13f
  definition of, 5
  errors in
    Klinefelter syndrome and, 173
    trisomy X and, 174
  first division in (meiosis I), 9–10, 11f, 12f
    in oogenesis, 14f, 15
    in spermatogenesis, 13f
    nondisjunction in, 141, 142f
  genetic consequences of, 12
  homologous recombination in, 118–119, 118f, 119f
  in oogenesis, 12, 14–15, 14f
Meiosis *(Continued)*
  in spermatogenesis, 12–14, 13f
  inversion in, 146–147, 147f
  medical significance of, 15
  mutations in, 85–86
  nondisjunction in, 15, 140–143, 142f
  overview of, 9, 9f, 11f–14f
  second division in (meiosis II), 9f, 11–12, 11f
    in fertilization, 14f, 15
    in oogenesis, 14f, 15
    in spermatogenesis, 13–14, 13f
    nondisjunction in, 141, 142f
  sex chromosome pairing in, 166
  trisomy in, 159, 161
Melanoma, familial, 314t
MELAS (mitochondrial encephalomyopathy, lactic acidosis, and strokelike episodes), 245f, 246t, 249
*MEN* gene mutations, in multiple endocrine neoplasia, 313, 315
Mendelian disorders. *See* Single-gene defect(s).
*Mendelian Inheritance in Man*, 51
Meningomyelocele, 304–306, 305f, 306f
Mental retardation
  in cri du chat syndrome, 163
  in Down syndrome, 158
  in fragile X syndrome, 242
  in maternal phenylketonuria, 209–210
  in trisomy 13, 163
  in trisomy 18, 162
  X-linked, 172
MERRF (myoclonic epilepsy, ragged red fibers in muscle, ataxia, sensorineural deafness), 245f, 246t, 249
Mesonephric ducts, 167, 167f
Messenger RNA. *See under* RNA (ribonucleic acid).
*MET* gene mutations, in renal carcinoma, 314t, 315–316
Metabolic disorder(s). *See also specific disorders.*
  prenatal diagnosis of, 371, 371t
Metacentric chromosome, 137, 137f
Metaphase
  cell growth arrest during, for cytogenetic analysis, 135
  chromosomes in, 28, 28f, 29f
    normal banding patterns in, 136, 137f
  of meiosis, 10, 11f
  of mitosis, 6f, 7
Metastasis, from cancer, 311
Methemoglobins, 191–192
Methionine, codon specifying, 23–24
Methylation, of DNA, 82, 169
5,10-Methylenetetrahydrofolate reductase defects, neural tube defects in, 306, 306f
Methylmalonic aciduria, 184t, 256f, 257t
MHC. *See* Major histocompatibility complex.
Microdeletion, 54–55
  autosomal disorders involving, 164–165, 164t, 165f
Microsatellite markers, 92–93, 93f
Microtubules, in mitosis, 6f, 7
Migration
  gene expression during, 344–345
  gene flow in, 107–108, 108f
Minisatellite markers, 91–92, 92f
Miscarriage. *See* Abortion(s), spontaneous.
Missegregation mutations, 80
Missense mutation
  definition of, 82
  of mitochondrial DNA, 245
*MITF* gene mutations, 344, 345f–346f
Mitochondrial chromosomes, 29–30, 244
  disorders of, 77
Mitochondrial DNA, 29–30, 244–249
  deletions in, autosomally transmitted, 248–249
  diseases of, 77, 244–245
    diversity of, 245, 247f
    genetics of, 245, 246t, 247–249, 247f, 248f
    multifactorial, 249
    phenotypes of, 245f, 246t, 247f, 248f, 249
  functions of, 244–245
  inheritance of, 77, 247
  mutations of
    homoplasmy and heteroplasmy in, 246t, 247–249, 248f
    inheritance of, 247
  nuclear genome interactions with, 248–249
  structure of, 244, 245f
Mitochondrial DNA deletion syndrome, 248–249
Mitochondrial encephalomyopathy, lactic acidosis, and strokelike episodes (MELAS), 245f, 246t, 249
Mitosis
  definition of, 5
  interphase between, 5
  medical relevance of, 15
  nondisjunction in, 15
  process of, 6–8, 6f, 8f
Mitotic spindle, 7
*MLH* gene mutations of, 315t, 327
  products of, 321t
Model-based linkage analysis, 297
Model-free linkage analysis, 297–298
Modifier genes, 200, 205–206
Mole, hydatidiform, 140, 151–153
Molecular cloning, 33, 35f
Molecular genetics, definition of, 2
Mongolism. *See* Down syndrome (trisomy 21).
Monosomy
  comparative genome hybridization technique for, 47, 47f
  definition of, 140
  partial, in isochromosomes, 145
Monozyosity. *See* Twin(s), monozygotic (identical).
Morgan, Thomas Hunt, 121
Morphogen(s), 348, 349f
Morphogenesis, 337, 345–346
Mosaic development, 337, 340–341
Mosaicism, 75–76, 75f, 149–150
  confined placental, 153, 370, 370f
  definition of, 75, 75f
  germline, 76, 76f
  in Down syndrome, 160–161
  in Duchenne muscular dystrophy, 229
  in Klinefelter syndrome, 173–174
  in nondisjunction, 143
  in Turner syndrome, 175
  in X inactivation, 68, 69f
  of sex chromosomes, 172
  prenatal diagnosis of, 369–370, 370f
  somatic, 76
  true, 369
  versus pseudomosaicism, 149, 369–370
mRNA. *See* RNA (ribonucleic acid), messenger.
*MSH* genes
  mutations of, 315t, 327
    colon cancer in, 131
  products of, 321t

mtDNA. *See* Mitochondrial DNA.
Mu heavy chain deficiency, 286t
Mucopolysaccharidoses, 212, 213t, 214, 214f
Multifactorial disorder(s). *See also specific disorders.*
  Alzheimer disease as, 303–304, 303t, 304f
  cerebral venous thrombosis as, 300–301
  characteristics of, 289
  congenital malformations as, 304–308, 304t, 305f, 306f, 307t, 308t
  coronary artery disease as, 308–309
  definition of, 2
  developmental abnormalities in, 338t
  diabetes mellitus as, 302–303, 303t
  genetic counseling for, 309
  Hirschsprung disease as, 301–302, 302f
  incidence of, 289, 289t
  knowledge status for, 299
  mitochondrial DNA, 249
  population genetics of, 396–397
  prenatal diagnosis of, 367, 368f, 368t
  retinitis pigmentosa as, 299–300, 300f
  treatment of, 255–266, 255t
Multifactorial inheritance. *See also* Multifactorial disorder(s); *specific disorders.*
  characteristics of, 289
  definition of, 2
  genetic mapping of, 297–299
  qualitative trait(s) in, 289–294
    concordance as, 290–292, 292f, 292t
    familial aggregation of disease as, 290–291, 291t
    genetic versus environmental contributions to, 291–292, 291f, 292t
    twin studies of, 291–293, 293t
  quantitative traits in, 289, 293–297, 294f, 295f
Multiple births. *See* Twin(s).
Multiple endocrine neoplasia, 313, 314t, 315–316
Multiple sclerosis
  concordance of, in twins, 293t
  HLA associations of, 280t
  risk ratio for, 291t
Multipoint linkage analysis, 124–125, 124f, 125f
Muscular dystrophy. *See* Becker muscular dystrophy; Duchenne muscular dystrophy.
Mutagenesis screens, 336, 339t
Mutagens, definition of, 80
Mutant allele, definition of, 51
Mutation(s), 79–87. *See also specific genes.*
  autosomal dominant, selection against, 102–103, 102t
  autosomal recessive, selection against, 103
  chain termination, 82
  chromosome, 79–80, 79t
  cofactor dysfunction in, 215–216, 216f
  complementation analysis of, 214–215
  complementation in, 214
  definition of, 51, 52, 79–80
  deletions as. *See* Deletion(s).
  direct detection of, 385–387, 386f, 387f
  disease-causing, types of, 181–183, 182f
  dynamic, unstable, 236, 238, 239t, 240–244, 240f–244f
  ectopic gene expression and, 182f, 183
  fitness of. *See* Fitness.
  frameshift, 83
  gain-of-function, 182–183, 182f
  gender differences in, 85–86
  gene, 79–81, 79t
Mutation(s) *(Continued)*
  genome, 79–80, 79t
  genotype-phenotype relationship in, 205–206, 206t
  germline, 85–86
  heterochronic gene expression and, 182f, 183
  heterogenous clinical presentations of, 55–56
  "hotspots" of, 82
  in cancer, 311–313, 312f, 314t–315t. *See also specific genes.*
  in DNA repair, 81, 86–87
  in DNA replication errors, 81
  in enzymes, 204t, 206–218. *See also specific diseases.*
  in gene therapy, 273–274
  in oogenesis, 85–86
  in proteins, 181–183, 182f, 184t
    diseases due to, 203–204, 203t
    housekeeping, 204–205
    receptor, 218–222, 219f–221f
    specialty, 204–205
    structural, 225–234
    transport, 204t, 222–225, 223f, 223t
    treatment strategies targeted to, 262–265, 262t, 263f–265f
  in recombination, 83–84, 84f
  in spermatogenesis, 85–86
  insertions, 82–84, 84f
  lethal. *See* Genetic lethal(s).
  loss-of-function, 181–182, 182f
  missegregation, 80
  missense, 82, 245
  mitochondrial, 77, 244–249, 245f, 246t, 247f, 248t
  mosaicism in. *See* Mosaicism.
  new
    in autosomal dominant disorders, 61–62
    in neurofibromatosis, 63, 63f
    in X-linked disorders, 70, 71f
    paternal age and, 102
    rate of, 84–85, 85t
    zero fitness in, 102–103, 102t
  nomenclature of, 85
  nonsense, 82
  novel property, 182f, 183
  nucleotide substitutions as, 82
  origin of, 80–81, 80f
  pharmacogenetic diseases in, 249–253, 251f
  point, 82, 245
  rates of, 84–85, 85t
  RNA splicing, 82
    in thalassemia, 196, 197t, 198f, 199
  screening for, 336, 339t
  selection and. *See* Selection.
  selectively neutral, 87. *See also* Polymorphism(s).
  slipped mispairing in, 191, 192f
  somatic, 80, 86, 281–283, 284f
  studies of
    approach to, 46
    methods for. *See* Analytical technique(s).
  substitution in, 80, 80f
  transition in, 82
  transversion in, 82
  types of, 79–87, 79t, 84f, 85t
  unequal crossing over mechanism in, 83
  unstable, 236, 238, 239t, 240–244, 240f–244f
*MYC* gene, translocation of, Burkitt lymphoma in, 318–319
Myelomeningocele, recurrence risk determination for, 385
Myocardial infarction, 308–309
Myoclonic epilepsy, ragged red fibers in muscle, ataxia, sensorineural deafness (MERRF), 245f, 246t, 249
Myotonic dystrophy, 96t, 239t, 243, 244f

Narcolepsy, HLA associations of, 280t, 281
NARP (neuropathy, ataxia, retinitis pigmentosa, developmental delay, mental retardation, lactic acidemia), 245f, 246t
*NAT2* gene, polymorphisms of, 251
Natural killer cells, gene therapy effects on, 274
Neocentromeres, 145
Neonate(s). *See* Newborn(s).
Neoplasia. *See also* Cancer.
  definition of, 311
  pathogenesis of, 312, 312f
Neural crest, cell development from, 344, 345f
Neural tube defect(s), 304–306, 305f, 306f, 307t
  prenatal diagnosis of, 306, 361
    alpha-fetoprotein measurement in, 364–365, 365f
    amniocentesis in, 362
    triple screen in, 364–365
    ultrasonography in, 367, 368f, 368t
  recurrence risk determination for, 385
Neuroblastoma, prognosis of, 330, 331f
Neurodegenerative disease(s). *See also* Alzheimer disease; Triplet repeat disorder(s).
  of mitochondrial inheritance, 244–249, 245f, 246t, 247f, 248f
Neurofibrillary tangles, in Alzheimer disease, 235
Neurofibromatosis
  microdeletion in, 164t
  type 1
    cancer in, 314t
    linkage analysis of, 122–123
    mutations in, 84, 85t, 86
    phenotypic variation in, 62–63, 62f, 63f
    segmental, mosaicism in, 76
    tumor-suppressor gene mutations in, 321t, 325
  type 2, 314t, 321t
Neuroma(s), in multiple endocrine neoplasia, 313
Neuropathy, ataxia, retinitis pigmentosa, developmental delay, mental retardation, lactic acidemia (NARP), 245f, 246t
Neurotrophic factor, defects of, in Hirschsprung disease, 301
Nevoid basal cell carcinoma syndrome, 314t, 339t
Newborn(s)
  death of, chromosome analysis in, 135–136
  hemolytic disease of, 88–89
  hypothyroidism in, 260
  phenylketonuria screening in, 207
  screening of, 391–392, 391t
NF. *See* Neurofibromatosis.
*NF* genes, 321t, 325
Nondirective genetic counseling, 375–376
Nondisjunction
  in meiosis, 10, 15
    aneuploidy in, 140–143, 142f
  in mitosis, 15
  mosaicism in, 149
Nonrecombinant gametes, 119–120
Nonsense (stop) codons, 23, 24

Nonsense mutations, 82
Normal (gaussian) distribution, of physiological quantity, 294, 294f
Normal range, of physiological quantity, 294–295
Northern blotting, 34, 44, 46
Novel property mutations, 182f, 183
Nuchal translucency, fetal, ultrasonography of, 366
Nuclear genome, mitochondrial interaction with, 248–249
Nucleic acid(s). *See* DNA (deoxyribonucleic acid); RNA (ribonucleic acid).
Nucleic acid analysis, 34, 40–41, 41f
Nucleosome, definition of, 28, 28f
Nucleotides
  in DNA, 17–18, 18f, 19f
  substitution of, as mutation, 82

Obligate carriers, 380–382, 380f
Oligonucleotide(s)
  allele-specific, 43–44, 44f, 46
  as probes, 41
  definition of, 34
Oligospermia, Y-linked genes in, 167–168
Omenn syndrome, 285, 286t
Oncogene(s), 313–320
  abnormal expression of, 183
  activated
    hereditary syndromes due to, 313, 315–316
    in chromosome translocation, 317–318, 317t, 318f, 318t
    sporadic cancer due to, 316–320, 316f–319f, 317t, 318t
  definition of, 313
  telomerases as, 318–320, 319f
Oocyte(s), 14–15, 14f
Oogenesis
  cytogenetic studies of, 153
  mutations in, 85–86
Oogonia, 14–15, 14f
Ophthalmoplegia, chronic progressive external, 245f, 246t, 248–249
Optic cup, 336–337, 339f
Optic neuropathy, Leber's hereditary, 245f, 246t, 247, 248f, 249
Ornithine transcarbamylase deficiency
  population genetics of, 104t
  somatic mosaicism in, 76
Osteoarthritis, concordance of, in twins, 293t
Osteogenesis imperfecta, 229–234
  biochemical defects in, 230t
  genetics of, 230t, 233–234
  inheritance of, 230t
  lethal forms of, mosaicism in, 76, 76f
  molecular abnormalities in, 231, 233, 233f
  pathophysiology of, 231, 232f
  phenotypes of, 229, 230t, 231–233, 233f
  prenatal diagnosis of, 342, 367
  treatment of, 342
  versus normal collagen structure, 229–230, 231f, 232f
  zero fitness in, 102t
OTC (ornithine transcarbamylase) deficiency
  population genetics of, 104t
  somatic mosaicism in, 76
Ova, 14f, 15
  cytogenetics of, 153
  donated, for disease recurrence prevention, 376
  older, trisomy risk in, 161
Ovary
  embryology of, 166–167, 167f
  maldevelopment of, 176–177
  teratoma of, 151–152
Ovulation, 14f, 15
Oxidative phosphorylation enzymes, mitochondrial DNA diseases and, 244–245, 249
Oxygen transport, altered, variant hemoglobins and, 188t, 191–193, 192f
Oxyhemoglobin, 191–192

p53 protein
  defects of, in Li-Fraumeni syndrome, 324
  gene of. *See* *TP53* gene.
  tumor suppressor action of, 329
Pachytene stage, of meiosis, 10
Painting, of chromosomes, 47
Paired domain, 337
Palate, cleft, 293t, 307–308, 307t, 308t
Palindromes, in DNA sequences, 35
Pallister-Hall syndrome, 339t
Pancreas
  cancer of, in multiple endocrine neoplasia, 314t
  cystic fibrosis affecting, 222–224, 223t
Panel, in gene mapping, 113–114, 114f, 114t
Paracentric inversion, definition of, 146, 147f
Paracrine signals, in development, 347–348
Paramesonephric ducts, 167, 167f
Parametric linkage analysis, 297
Parent-of-origin effects, 151–153, 152f
Parkinson disease
  familial aggregation of, 291
  recurrence risk of, 383–384, 384f
Patau syndrome (trisomy 13), 163, 163f
Patent ductus arteriosus, 307t
Paternal age, mutation rate and, 86, 102
*PAX* genes
  in eye development, 336–337, 339, 339f
  mutations of, in Waardenburg syndrome, 344, 345f–346f
PCR. *See* Polymerase chain reaction.
Pearson syndrome, 246t, 249
Pedigree(s), 52, 52f, 53f
  in gene mapping, of complex traits, 297
  in genetic counseling, 378, 378f
  linkage analysis of, phase in, 122–123, 122f, 123f, 123t
  of autosomal dominant inheritance, 61, 61f, 63f, 65f, 66f
    mosaicism in, 76, 76f
  of autosomal recessive inheritance, 56, 56f, 57, 57f
  of consanguinity, 57, 57f
  of Li-Fraumeni syndrome, 324f
  of X-linked disorders, 69f–72f
    restriction fragment length polymorphisms as, 91f
  patterns of, factors affecting, 55
  phase-known, 123, 123t
  phase-unknown, 123, 123t
  segregation analysis of, 59–60
  X-linked
    in recurrence risk determination, 380–382, 380f
    phase of, 123, 123f
Penetrance
  incomplete, recurrence risk of, 383, 384f
  reduced, 62, 63
Pentasomy X, 174
Pericentric inversion, 146–147, 147f
Peutz-Jeghers syndrome, cancer in, 314t
Phagocytosis, disorders of, 287t
Pharmacogenetics, 249–253
  definition of, 249
  medical significance of, 252
  of acetylation, 251
  of acute intermittent porphyria, 251–252, 251f
  of anesthesia response, 250
  of glucose-6-phosphate deficiency, 252
Pharmacogenomics, 252–253
Phase, in linkage analysis, 122–123, 122f, 123f, 123t
Phenocopy, definition of, 290
Phenotype(s)
  clinical, treatment based on, 258, 259f
  codominant, 53
  definition of, 1, 51–52
  dominant, 53–54
  incompletely dominant, 53
  of ABO blood group, 88
  of autosomal dominant disorders, variability of, 62–63, 62f–64f
  of contiguous gene syndromes, 54–55
  of enzymopathies, 217
  quantitative, 294
  recessive, 53–54
  severe, recognition of, 257
  sex-limited, in autosomal disorders, 65, 66f
  total variance of, 294, 295
  versus genotype, 205–206, 206t
Phenylalanine, excess of. *See* Hyperphenylalaninemias; Phenylketonuria.
Phenylalanine hydroxylase, defects in, 207–209, 207f, 208f, 209t
Phenylketonuria, 206–210
  biochemical defects in, 206–207, 207f
  dietary restriction in, 259–260
  heterogeneity in, 208–209, 208f, 209t, 258
  heterozygote frequency of, 98
  maternal, 209–210
  mutation in, 182
  newborn screening for, 207
  pathophysiology of, 207
  population genetics of, 96t, 100t, 108
  screening for, 391
  tetrahydrobiopterin metabolic defects in, 206t, 207f, 209–210 treatment of, 257, 258
  variant, 206t, 208
Pheochromocytoma, in multiple endocrine neoplasia, 313, 314t, 315
Philadelphia chromosome, 317, 318f
Phosphorus-32, nucleic acid probe labeling with, 41
PKU. *See* Phenylketonuria.
Placenta
  development of, 363f, 364
  hydatidiform mole of, 140, 151–153
  mosaicism of, 153
  stem cells from, transplantation of, 267
Placental artery thrombosis, 300–301
Placode, in eye development, 336–337, 339f
Plaques, amyloid, in Alzheimer disease, 235, 236f, 237t
Plasmids, 36–37, 37t, 40f
Pleiotropy, 62, 343
Pluripotency
  definition of, 337
  of stem cells, 343, 343f, 355–356, 355f
  of teratocarcinoma cells, 355–356, 355f
*PMSL* gene mutations, 315t, 327

Point mutations
definition of, 82
of mitochondrial DNA, 245
Polarizing activity, zone of, 348
Polyadenylation, in gene transcription, 17, 22–23
Polycystic kidney disease, mutation in, 85t
Polydactyly, 338t, 347, 348f
postaxial, 339t
Polyethylene glycol–modified adenosine deaminase, 264
Polyglutamine defects, 239t, 240–242, 240f, 241f. *See also* Huntington disease.
Polymerase chain reaction, 33, 34f, 44–46, 45f
advantages of, 45–46
definition of, 34
in globin gene analysis, 46
in Tay-Sachs disease detection, 114, 114f
reverse transcriptase, 45
uses of, 45–46
Polymorphism(s), 87–93
balanced, 105
definition of, 51, 87
genetic, 87
in different populations, 96t. *See also* Population genetics.
medical significance of, 93
minisatellite and microsatellite, 91–93, 92f, 93f
of alpha$_1$-antitrypsin, 89–90, 89t
of blood group antigens, 87–89, 88t
of human leukocyte antigens, 279–280, 279f, 279t
restriction fragment length, 90–91, 90f, 91f
single nucleotide, 90–91, 91f
variable number of tandem repeats (VNTRs) as, 91–92, 92f
Polynucleotides, in DNA, 17–18, 18f, 19f
Polyposis, of colon, 314t, 326–327, 327f
Population-based ascertainment, 293
Population genetics, 95–109. *See also specific disorders.*
allele frequencies in, 95–97, 96t, 97t
assortative mating in, 101
consanguinity in. *See* Consanguinity.
constant allele frequency and, 101–102
definition of, 2, 95, 439
diversity in, 95, 96t
eugenics program and, 396
gene flow in, 107–108, 108f
genetic drift in, 104, 105–106, 106f, 107f
genotypes and, 96–97, 97t
Hardy-Weinberg law in, 97–98, 98t
factors disturbing, 99–108, 99t–102t, 106f–108f
of HLAs, 279–280
random mating principle in, 99
screening in. *See* Screening.
selection in. *See* Selection.
stratification in, 99–101, 100t, 101t
X-linked frequencies and, 98–99, 99t
Porphobilinogen deaminase deficiency, pharmacogenetics of, 251–252, 251f
Porphyria
acute intermittent, pharmacogenetics of, 251–252, 251f
variegate, founder effect in, 106
Position-dependent development, 337
Positional cloning, 128–131, 130f
Post-translational processing, in protein synthesis, 24–25
Posterior probability, definition of, 381
Prader-Willi syndrome, 72–74, 73f, 74t
chromosome analysis in, Color Insert following page 139
Prader-Willi syndrome *(Continued)*
microdeletion in, 164t
Precocious puberty, male-limited, 65, 66f
Pregnancy. *See also* Abortion(s); Prenatal diagnosis.
chromosome analysis in, 136
hydatidiform mole in, 140, 151–153
phenylketonuria in, 209–210
Rh incompatibility in, 88–89
Preimplantation
developmental biology of, 339–341, 340f
genetic diagnosis in, 368–369, 376
Premutations, in Huntington disease, 241
Prenatal diagnosis, 359–374. *See also specific diseases.*
ethical issues in, 372, 393–394
genetic counseling for, 360
historical background of, 359
impact of, on disease prevention and management, 372
indications for, 359–361, 360f, 362t
limitations of, 360
methods of, 360–367, 362t
cytogenetic, 369–372, 370f, 371t
emerging, 368–369
invasive, 361–364, 362t, 363f. *See also specific methods.*
noninvasive, 364–367, 365f, 366f, 367t, 368f, 368t
risks of, 360, 362
preimplantation, 368–369, 376
problems in, 369–371, 370f
purpose of, 359
screening in, 393
treatment based on, 256–257, 257t
unexpected adverse findings in, 371
Presenilin defects, in Alzheimer disease, 236, 236f, 237t
Primary constriction. *See* Centromere(s).
Primers, for polymerase chain reaction, 34
Primitive ectoderm, embryo formation from, 340, 340f
Prior probability, definition of, 381
Privacy, of genetic information, 395–396
Probability, in Bayesian analysis. *See* Bayesian analysis.
Proband
allele sharing with, 291–292, 292f, 292t
definition of, 52, 53f
in neurofibromatosis, 63, 63f
Probes
chromosome painting, 47
for DNA analysis, 34, 40–41, 41f
Procollagen defects. *See* Osteogenesis imperfecta.
Progress zone, teratogen effects on, 353, 353f
Prokaryote, definition of, 18
Prometaphase, of mitosis, 6f, 7–8, 8f
Prometaphase (high-resolution) banding, 137–138, 138f
Promoter(s), 20f, 21, 25–27, 341
Prophase
of meiosis, 10, 11f, 12f
of mitosis, 6f, 7
Propositus, definition of, 52
Protein(s)
analysis of, Western blotting in, 49, 49f
dietary, restriction of, 258–260
DNA conjugated with, transfer of, 273
enhancement of, in disease treatment, 262–263, 262t, 263f
housekeeping, mutations in, 204–205
mutations affecting. *See* Mutation(s), in proteins; *specific protein.*
primary abnormalities of, 183, 184t
Protein(s) *(Continued)*
receptor, mutations in, 218–222, 219f–221f
replacement of, in disease treatment, 262t, 263–265, 264f, 265f
secondary abnormalities of, 183, 184t
specialty, mutations in, 204–205
structural, mutations in, 225–234
synthesis of. *See also* Gene expression.
from DNA, 18–22, 19f–21f
post-translational processing in, 24–25
transport, mutations in, 204t, 222–225, 223f, 223t
Prothrombin defects, thrombosis due to, 300–301
Proto-oncogene(s), 311
activation of, 312–313, 312f
chromosome translocation in, 317–318, 317t, 318f, 318t
hereditary syndromes due to, 313, 315–316
sporadic cancer due to, 316–320, 316f–319f, 317t, 318t
function of, 317, 317f
Pseudoautosomal inheritance, 71–72, 72f
Pseudoautosomal region
genes, escape from X inactivation, 67
of sex chromosomes, 166, 166f
Pseudodicentric chromosomes. *See* Centromere(s).
Pseudogene(s), 22
Pseudohermaphroditism
female, 176–177, 177f
male, 176–178, 177f
Pseudomosaicism, 149, 369–370
Psoriasis
concordance of, in twins, 293t
HLA associations of, 280t
Psychological aspects, of genetic counseling, 377
*PTCH* gene mutations, 314t
*PTEN* gene mutations, 314t
Puberty, precocious, male-limited, 65, 66f
Purine metabolism, defects of, 210, 210f
Purine nucleoside phosphorylase deficiency, 286t, 440

Q (quinacrine) banding, 136
Qualitative traits, in inheritance, 289–293
Quantitative phenotype(s), 294
Quantitative traits, in inheritance, 293–297, 294f, 295f

R (reverse) banding, 136
high-resolution, 137–138, 138f
Radiation, cancer induced by, 331
Radiation hybrid mapping, 115, 116f
*RAG* gene defects, 286t
Random mating, 99–101, 100t, 101t
Range, normal, of physiological quantity, 294–295
Rare variants, of alleles, 87
*RAS* gene mutations, 317
in colon cancer, 329
*RB1* gene
mutations of, 314t, 320–323, 321t, 322f, 323f, 324t
product of, 321t, 323
Reading frame, of mRNA, 24
Recall bias, 291

Recessive inheritance
autosomal, 56f–58f, 56–60, 59t
definition of, 53–54
of enzymopathies, 217
X-linked, 68–70, 69f
Reciprocal translocation, 140, 148–149, 148f
Recombinant 8 syndrome, 147
Recombinase(s), in immunoglobulin rearrangement, 282–283, 284f
Recombinase activating gene defects, 286t
Recombination, 9
deletions in, 83–84, 84f
duplication in. *See* Duplication.
in meiosis, 118–119, 118f, 119f
Recurrence, prevention of, methods for, 376–377
Recurrence risk determination, for genetic disorder(s), 379–388
cystic fibrosis, 386–387
direct mutation detection in, 386–387, 386f, 387
Duchenne muscular dystrophy, 382–383, 383f, 384f, 386, 386f, 387
empiric, 384–385
in consanguinity, 385
isolated X-linked, 382–383, 383f, 384f
linkage analysis in, 387, 387f
molecular techniques applied to, 385–387, 386f
Parkinson disease, 384, 384f
single-gene, 379, 379f
thalassemia as, 387, 387f
with incomplete penetrance, 383, 384f
with known genotype, 379–380
with late age of onset, 383–384, 384f
with possible alternative genotypes, 380
with unidentified gene, 387–388
X-linked pedigrees in, 380–382, 380f
Red blood cell(s)
antigens on. *See* Blood group system(s).
sickling of. *See* Sickle cell disease.
Reduced penetrance
definition of, 62
in split-hand syndrome, 63, 64f
5$\alpha$-Reductase deficiency, in male pseudohermaphroditism, 177–178, 177f
Reduction division. *See* Meiosis, first division in (meiosis I).
Regression to mean, 295f
Regulative development, 337, 340
Reiter syndrome, HLA associations of, 280, 280t
Relative risk, of disease association, 298–299
Relative risk ratio
definition of, 290, 291t
versus relative risk, 298–299
Repetitive DNA, 30–31
Replacement therapy, 260, 260f, 260t
Replication banding, 169, 170f
Replication error positive phenotype, of DNA instability, 327–328, 328f
Reproduction. *See also* Infertility.
embryology of, 166–167, 167f
fitness for. *See* Fitness.
genetics of, 353–354, 354f
selection for or against. *See* Selection.
Reproductive compensation, 397
Repulsion, alleles in, 122, 122f
Restriction endonuclease(s), 33–35, 36f, 37t
Restriction fragment length polymorphisms, 90–91, 90f, 91f
*RET* gene mutations
heterogenous clinical presentations of, 55–56
*RET* gene mutations *(Continued)*
in Hirschsprung disease, 301–302, 302f
in multiple endocrine neoplasia, 313, 314t, 315–316
Retinitis pigmentosa
candidate gene for, 131
digenic, 299–300, 300f
gene mapping of, 120f, 130–131
heterogeneity in, 55
with multiple X-linked disorders, 116, 117f
Retinoblastoma
familial, 314t
mutations in, 85t, 86, 182
treatment of, 257
tumor-suppressor gene mutations in, 320–323, 321t, 322f, 323f, 324t
Retinoic acid embryopathy, 338t, 353
Retrotransposition, pseudogene formation in, 22, 31
Retroviruses, as gene therapy vectors, 272–273
Reverse transcriptase, 40, 40f
Reverse transcriptase polymerase chain reaction, 45
RFLPs (restriction fragment length polymorphisms), 90–91, 90f, 91f
Rh blood group system, 88–89
Rheumatoid arthritis
concordance of, in twins, 293t
HLA associations of, 280t
Ribonucleic acid. *See* RNA (ribonucleic acid).
Ribosomal RNA (ribonucleic acid), 19
Ribosomes, 19
Rickets, hypophosphatemic, inheritance of, 71
Ring chromosomes, 144–145, 144f
in Turner syndrome, 175–176
Risk, of disease recurrence. *See* Recurrence risk determination.
RNA (ribonucleic acid)
analysis of. *See also* Analytical technique(s).
Northern blotting test for, 44
reverse transcriptase polymerase chain reaction for, 45
in complementary DNA library creation, 40, 40f
messenger, 19
defective synthesis of, in thalassemia, 196, 197t, 198f, 199
in gene transcription, 22–23, 23f
nonfunctional, in thalassemia, 197t, 199
nonsense-mediated decay of, 82, 198f, 199
reading frame of, 24
ribosomal, 19
splicing of, 26f, 27, 198f
mutations related to, 82, 196, 197t, 198f, 199
structure of, 18, 19f
synthesis of, 18, 22, 23f
transfer, 19
RNA polymerase, action of, 22
RNA viruses, as gene therapy vectors, 272–273
Roberts syndrome, cytogenetics of, 154t
Robertsonian translocation, 149
in Down syndrome, 159–160, 160f, 161f
Robin sequence, 350
Rubenstein-Taybi syndrome, 338t, 341, 342f, 343, 351f
*RYR1* gene mutations, in malignant hyperthermia, 250
S allele, of alpha$_1$-antitrypsin, 89–90, 89t
S phase, of cell cycle, 5–6, 5f, 6f
*Saccharomyces cerevisiae*, in yeast artificial chromosome preparation, 37t, 38, 39f
Saethre-Chotzen syndrome, 339t
Sandhoff disease, 211
Sanfilippo syndrome, 213t, 214
Sanger sequencing technique, 48–49, 48f
Sarcoma
definition of, 311
in Li-Fraumeni syndrome, 324
Satellite(s), chromosomal, definition of, 137
Satellite DNAs, 31
Sau*3A* restriction enzyme, 39
Scaffold, in chromatin organization, 28, 28f
Scheie syndrome, 213t, 214
Schizophrenia
concordance of, in twins, 293t
risk ratio for, 291t
SCID. *See* Severe combined immunodeficiency.
Screening, 391–393. *See also specific disorders.*
definition of, 391
DNA libraries for, 40
ethical issues in. *See* Ethical issue(s).
maternal alpha-fetoprotein measurement in, 364–365
objective of, 391
of adults, 392
of children, 394–395
of heterozygotes, 392–393, 392t
of newborns, 391–392, 391t
prenatal, 393
privacy issues in, 395–396
triple screen in, 364–365
Second-degree relatives, definition of, 52, 53f
Secretase, in Alzheimer disease pathogenesis, 235, 236f
Segmental aneusomy, 164, 164t
Segregation, in reciprocal translocation, 148, 149f
Segregation analysis, 59–60
Selection, 102–105
against autosomal dominant mutations, 102–103, 102t
against autosomal recessive mutations, 103
against X-linked disorders, 70
against X-linked recessive mutations, 103–104, 104t
for heterozygotes, 104–105
neutral, 87. *See also* Polymorphism(s).
population deterioration and, 396–397
versus mutation, 103
Senescence
cellular, telomerase in, 320
in cell culture, 112
Sense DNA strand, 22
Sensorineural deafness
in mitochondrial disorders, 245f, 246t
progressive, pedigree for, 61, 61f
Sequences, 350, 351f
Severe combined immunodeficiency, 285
adenosine deaminase replacement in, 264, 264f
gene therapy for, 269, 274, 275
Sex
fetal
determination of
disorders of, 176–178, 177f
Y chromosome in, 166, 166f, 167, 168f
differentiation of, 165–167, 167f, 168f
selection of, ethical issues in, 394

Sex *(Continued)*
ultrasonographic determination of, 367
reversal of, in camptomelic dysplasia, 176
Sex chromatin (Barr body), 67, 67f, 169, 169f
Sex chromosome(s). *See also* X chromosome; Y chromosome.
abnormality(ies) of. *See also under* Karyotype(s).
clinical features of, 173, 173t
developmental, 176–178, 177f
hermaphroditism as, 176
incidence of, 172–173, 172t
Klinefelter syndrome as. *See* Klinefelter syndrome.
pseudohermaphroditism as, 176–178, 177f
sexual maldevelopment as, 176–178, 177f
trisomy X as, 172t, 173t, 174
Turner syndrome as. *See* Turner syndrome.
types of, 172–173, 172t
aneuploidy of, 172–173
definition of, 5
in sexual differentiation, 165–167, 167f, 168f
mosaicism of, 172
Sex-limited phenotypes, in autosomal disorders, 65, 66f
*SHH* (sonic hedgehog) gene, 348, 349f
Sib(s). *See also* Twin(s).
allele sharing by, 291–292, 292f, 292t
definition of, 52, 53f
diabetes mellitus risk in, 303t
in affected sib pair method, for linkage analysis, 297–298
in highly discordant sib pair method, for linkage analysis, 298
Sibship, definition of, 52
Sickle cell disease, 188t, 189–190, 190f, 191f
butyrate therapy for, 265, 266f, 266t
clinical features of, 189, 190f
concordance of, in twins, 293, 293t
epidemiology of, 189
heterozygote advantage in, 105
heterozygous, 189–190
inheritance of, 54
molecular pathology of, 189–190
mutation in, 183, 190, 191f
population genetics of, 96t, 100
screening for, 392
versus sickle cell trait, 189–190
Signaling pathways, integration of, in development, 348–349
Silencers, 21, 341
Simian crease, in Down syndrome, 158, 160f
Single nucleotide polymorphisms, 90–91, 91f
Single-copy (unique) DNA, 30–31
Single-gene defect(s), 51–78. *See also specific disorders.*
age of onset of, 55
autosomal. *See* Autosomal disorder(s); Autosomal inheritance.
cancer as, 313, 314t–315t, 321, 322f
contiguous gene, 54–55, 83, 164–165, 164t, 165f
cytogenetic abnormalities in, 153–154, 154f, 154t
definition of, 2, 52
developmental abnormalities in, 338t
epidemiology of, 51
family history of, as prenatal diagnosis indication, 361, 362t
Single-gene defect(s) *(Continued)*
genetic heterogeneity in, 55–56
genomic imprinting as, 72–75, 73f, 74t
in consanguinity, 57–58, 57f, 58f, 59t
segregation analysis of, 59–60
sex-influenced, 59
inheritance of
terminology of, 51–52, 52f, 53
types of, 53–56
mitochondrial, 77
mosaicism as, 75f, 75–76, 76f
of immune system, 285, 286t–287t, 288
pedigree patterns of, 55
prenatal diagnosis of, ultrasonography in, 367, 367t
recurrence risk determination for, 379, 379f
treatment of, 256–257, 256f, 257t
uniparental disomy as, 75
versus contiguous gene syndromes, 54–55
X-linked. *See* X-linked disorder(s); X-linked inheritance.
Sister chromatids, 5, 5f
exchange of, 154, 154f
*SKT11* gene mutations, 314t
SKY (spectral karyotyping), 47–48, 48f
Slipped mispairing, in deletion, 191, 192f
Smith-Magenis syndrome, 164t
Smoking
cancer in, 332
emphysema in, 218, 218f, 255
Smooth chorion, 364
Sodium benzoate, in urea cycle disorders, 261, 261f
Solenoid, in chromatin organization, 28, 28f
Somatic cells
definition of, 5
gene transfer into. *See* Gene therapy.
genetic studies of, 111–112
hybridization of, in gene mapping, 112–115, 112f–116f, 114t
life cycle of, 5–8, 5f–9f
mosaicism of, 76
mutations in, 80, 86
Sonic hedgehog gene, 348, 349f
Southern blotting, 34, 41–43, 42f, 43f
in globin gene analysis, 46
in restriction fragment length polymorphism, 90–91, 90f, 91f
*SOX9* gene mutations, in camptomelic dysplasia, 176
Specialty proteins, mutations in, 204–205
Specification, in development, 337
Spectral karyotyping, 47–48, 48f, 139, Color Insert following page 139
Sperm
chromosome analysis of, Color Insert following page 139
cytogenetics of, 153
Spermatids, 13–14, 13f
Spermatocyte(s), 13, 13f
in meiosis, 12f
Spermatogenesis
mutations in, 85–86
Y-linked genes in, 167–168
Spermatogonia, 13, 13f
Spina bifida, 304–306, 305f, 306f, 307t
Spinobulbar muscular atrophy, 241–242
Spinocerebellar ataxia, 239t, 242–244
Split-hand syndrome
recurrence risk of, 383, 384f
reduced penetrance in, 63, 64f
Sporadic case, definition of, 52
*SRY* gene, in sex determination, 167, 168f, 176
Staining, in chromosome analysis. *See* Banding.
Standard deviation, in normal distribution, 294, 294f
Statins, in hypercholesterolemia, 261f, 262
Stem cells, 343–344, 343f
embryonic, 355–356, 355f
gene transfer into, 270–271
transplantation of, 267
Sterilization, for disease recurrence prevention, 376
Steroid sulfatase, defects of, 68
Stickler syndrome, 350
Stillbirth
chromosome analysis in, 135–136
in genetic defects, 353–354, 354f
in neural tube defects, 304–306
Stochastic processes, in development, 354–355
Stomach cancer, familial, 314t
Stop (nonsense) codons, 23, 24
Storage diseases
lysosomal. *See* Lysosomal storage disease(s).
mucopolysaccharidoses as, 212, 213t, 214, 214f
Stratification, of population, 99–101, 100t, 101t
Submetacentric chromosome, 137, 137f
Succinylcholine sensitivity, in cholinesterase defects, 250
Supernumerary chromosomes, 144–145, 144f
Support organizations, for genetic disorders, 377
Synapsis, of chromosomes, 10
Synaptonemal complex, 10, 12f
Synpolydactyly, 338t, 347, 348f
Synteny, linkage analysis and, 118–120, 118f–120f
Systemic lupus erythematosus, concordance of, in twins, 293t

T lymphocytes
gene therapy effects on, 274
gene transfer to, in adenosine deaminase deficiency, 275
levels of, in immunodeficiency diseases, 286t–287t
TATA box, 25, 26f, 27
Tau protein deposition, in Alzheimer disease, 235, 236f
Tay-Sachs disease, 210–212
clinical features of, 210–212
gene mapping of, 114, 114f, 114t
heterozygote advantage in, 105
hexosaminidase A alleles in, 210–212, 211t, 212f
inheritance of, 58–59
population genetics of, 96t, 100, 100t, 101t, 212
screening for, 392
treatment of, 256f
T-cell antigen receptor, major histocompatibility complex interactions with, 277, 278f, 284–285, 285f
Telocentric chromosome, 137, 137f
Telomerases, as oncogenes, 318–320, 319f
Telomere(s)
absence of, in ring chromosomes, 145
definition of, 5f, 6
detection of, Color Insert following page 139

Telophase
of meiosis, 10, 11f
of mitosis, 6f, 7
Teratocarcinoma, pluripotent cells in, 355–356, 355f
Teratology, 338t, 352–353, 353f
Teratoma, ovarian, 151–152
Terminal deletion, 143, 144f
Testicular feminization (androgen insensitivity syndrome), 43, 43f, 172t, 177–178, 177f
Testis
embryology of, 166–167, 167f
maldevelopment of, 176–178
Testis-determining gene, 167, 168f
Testotoxicosis, familial, 65, 66f
Tetrad, in meiosis, 10
Tetrahydrobiopterin, metabolic defects of, 206t, 207f, 209–210
Tetraploidy
definition of, 140
incidence of, 150, 150t, 151t
Tetrasomy, partial, in isochromosomes, 145
Tetrasomy X, 174
Thalassemia(s), 193–201
$\alpha$-, 194–195
deletions in, 194–195, 194f, 195t
mutations in, 181–182
nondeletion forms of, 195
population genetics of, 101t
versus $\alpha$-thalassemia trait, 195
versus $\beta$-thalassemia, 195
$\beta^+$-, 196
$\beta$-, 195–201
anti-Lepore hemoglobin in, 193, 193f
bone marrow transplantation for, 266
hemoglobin E in, 193
hemoglobin Lepore in, 193, 193f
in infants, 196
linkage analysis in, 387, 387f
major, 195–196
minor, 196
molecular basis of, 46, 196, 197f, 197t, 198f, 199–201, 201f
mutations in, 182, 195–196, 195f
population genetics of, 100–101, 101t
screening for, 392
simple, 196, 197, 197t, 198f, 199
versus $\alpha$-thalassemia, 195
$\beta^0$-, 196
complex, 196, 199–201, 201f
$\delta\beta^0$-, 199–200, 201f
$\varepsilon\gamma\delta\beta^0$-, 199, 201f
$\gamma\delta\beta^0$-, 199, 201f
geographic distribution of, 194, 200
globin chain imbalance in, 193–194
mutations in, 181–182, 184t, 195–196, 195f
population genetics of, 100, 101t
versus hereditary persistence of fetal hemoglobin, 196
versus variant hemoglobinopathies, 188t-189t
Thalidomide, teratogenicity of, 353, 353f
Thanatophoric dysplasia, zero fitness in, 102t
Third-degree relatives, definition of, 52, 53f
Thrombosis, idiopathic central venous, 300–301
Thymidine, for cell culture, 113
Thymus, T-lymphocyte development in, 284
Thyroid cancer, in multiple endocrine neoplasia, 313, 314t, 315–316
Thyroiditis, subacute, HLA associations of, 280t
Total phenotypic variance, 294, 295
Townes-Brock syndrome, 339t
*TP53* gene
mutations of
in Li-Fraumeni syndrome, 323–324, 324f
in sporadic cancer, 328–329
product of, 321t
Transcription, 19, 22–23, 23f, 25–27, 25f, 26f
Transcription factors, 22
for globin gene, 25
mutations in, 341, 342f, 343, 344, 345f-346f
Transfer RNA (ribonucleic acid), 19
Transformation
DNA, of oncogenes, 316–317, 316f
in cell culture, 112
Transfusions, blood group compatibility in
ABO, 88
rh, 88–89
Transitions, in mutation, 82
Translation, 19, 23–24, 23f, 24t
Translocation(s)
balanced, detection of, Color Insert following page 139
cancer in, 311
oncogene activation in, 317–318, 317t, 318f, 318t
reciprocal, 140, 148–149, 148f
Robertsonian, 149
in Down syndrome, 159–160, 160f, 161f
unbalanced, detection of, Color Insert following page 139
X:autosome, 170–171
Transplantation, 265–269
bone marrow
in lysosomal storage diseases, 267–268, 267f, 268f
in nonstorage diseases, 266–267
embryonic tissue, 337
liver, in metabolic diseases, 268–269
problems with, 269
stem cell, 267
types of, 266
Transversion, in mutation, 82
Treatment. *See also specific diseases and treatments.*
genetic heterogeneity and, 258
long-term assessment of, 255t, 257–258
strategy(ies) for, 258–275, 259f, 260f
at protein level, 262–265, 262t, 263f–265f
gene expression modulation as, 265, 266f, 266t
gene therapy as. *See* Gene therapy.
in metabolic abnormalities, 258–262, 260t, 261f
levels of, 258, 259f
transplantation as, 265–269, 267f, 268f
Trinucleotide repeat disorders. *See* triplet repeat disorder(s).
Triple screen, in prenatal diagnosis, 364–365
Triplet repeat disorder(s), 236, 238–244
definition of, 238
examples of, 238, 239t
expansion in, 238, 242
features of, 238
Fragile X syndrome as, 239t, 242–243
Friedreich ataxia as, 239t, 243–244
Huntington disease as. *See* Huntington disease.
Triplet repeat disorder(s) *(Continued)*
inheritance of, 238
gender differences in, 86
myotonic dystrophy as, 96t, 239t, 243, 244f
of X chromosome. *See* Fragile X syndrome.
polyglutamine defects as, 239t, 240–242, 240f, 241f
slipped mispairing in, 238
spinal muscular atrophy as, 241–242
Triploidy
definition of, 140
incidence of, 150, 150t, 151t
of hydatidiform mole, 152
Trisomy
comparative genome hybridization technique for, 47, 47f
definition of, 140
incidence of, 150–151, 150t, 151t
partial, in isochromosomes, 145
Trisomy 13 (Patau syndrome), 163, 163f
Trisomy 18 (Edwards syndrome), 162–163, 162f, 364–365
Trisomy 21. *See* Down syndrome (trisomy 21).
"Trisomy rescue," 370
Trisomy X, 172t, 173t, 174
Trypsin, degradation of. *See* Alpha$_1$-antitrypsin.
Tumor(s). *See also* Cancer.
benign, 311
Tumor-suppressor genes, 321–329
caretaker type of, 320
definition of, 320
gatekeeper type of, 320
products of, 320, 321t
"two-hit" hypothesis and, 320–321
Turner syndrome, 174–176, 175f
clinical features of, 173t
incidence of, 172t, 174–175
Twin(s)
coronary artery disease risk in, 308
dizygotic
allele sharing by, 291, 292t
definition of, 292
disease concordance in, 292–293, 293t
in heritability studies, 296–297
monozygotic (identical)
abnormalities in, 354, 354f
allele sharing by, 291, 292t
definition of, 292
disease concordance in, 292, 293t
in heritability studies, 296–297
X inactivation in, 293
reared apart, genetic disease studies in, 293
studies of, 291–293, 292t, 293t
Twin-twin transfusion syndrome, prenatal treatment of, 257t
"Two-hit" hypothesis, of cancer, 320–321
Tyrosinemia, type I, founder effect in, 106

Ultrasonography, in prenatal diagnosis, 366–367, 366f, 367t, 368f, 368t
chromosome analysis after, 369
with maternal alpha-fetoprotein screen, 364–365
Unbalanced rearrangement, of chromosomes, 143–146, 145f
Uniparental disomy, 74, 75, 153

Urea cycle disorders, diversion therapy for, 261, 261f
Urinary tract obstruction, prenatal treatment of, 257t
Uveitis, HLA associations of, 280t

Variable expressivity, definition of, 62
Variable number of tandem repeats polymorphism, 91–92, 92f
Variable regions, of immunoglobulin chains, 281–283, 282f–284f, 282t
Variance
  in normal distribution, 294, 294f
  total phenotypic, 294, 295
Vas deferens, congenital bilateral absence of, in cystic fibrosis, 222
Vectors, in DNA analysis, 34–38, 37t, 38f, 39f, 40
Velocardiofacial syndrome, 164t, 165, 307, 338t
Ventricular septal defect, 307t
*VHL* gene product, 321t
Viruses, as gene therapy vectors, 272–273, 272f
Vitamin(s), replacement of
  in homocystinuria, 215–216
  in inborn errors, 262–263, 262t, 263f
Vitamin $B_{12}$, metabolism of, cofactor defects and, 216
VNTR (variable number of tandem repeat) polymorphism, 91–92, 92f
Volunteer-based ascertainment, 293
Von Hippel–Lindau disease, 314t, 321t
von Recklinghausen's disease. *See* Neurofibromatosis, type 1.

Waardenburg syndrome, 338t, 344, 345f–346f
Watson, James, 17
Western blotting, 34, 49, 49f
Wild-type allele, definition of, 51
Williams syndrome, microdeletion in, 164t
Wilms' tumor, 86, 314t
Wiskott-Aldrich syndrome, immunodeficiency in, 287t

X chromosome
  abnormalities of. *See also* Karyotype(s).
    incidence of, 150, 150t, 151t
  active versus inactive, 169–170
  definition of, 5
  fluorescence in situ hybridization study of, 139, 139f, Color Insert following page 139
  fragile site on. *See* Fragile X syndrome.
  genes of, 65
  ideogram of, 138, 138f
  inactivation of. *See* X inactivation.
  isochromosome of, 145
  pseudoautosomal region of, 67–68
  translocation of, with autosome, 170–171
X inactivation, 53, 66–68, 168–171
  dosage compensation in, 67
  escape from, 67–68, 169, 170f
    in dyschondrosteosis, 72, 72f
  functional mosaicism due to, 68, 69f
  in monozygotic twins, 293
  Lyon hypothesis for, 66–67, 67f
  mechanism of, 169, 169f, 170f
  nonrandom, 71, 169–171, 171f
  skewed, 68f
  unbalanced, 68
  variable expression of, 68
X inactivation center, 169, 171f
X-linked disorder(s), 65–71. *See also specific disorders.*
  androgen-insensitivity syndrome, 43, 43f
  dominant, 70–71, 71f
  family history of, as prenatal diagnosis indication, 361
  gene mapping of, 114–116, 115f, 117f
  gene therapy for, 274
  genotypes of, 65–66, 98–99, 99t
  in homozygous affected females, 70, 70f
  mosaicism in, 68, 69f, 76
  multiple, gene mapping of, 116, 117f
  new mutations in, 70
  of immune system, 286t
  pedigrees of
    in recurrence risk determination, 380–382, 380f
    phase of, 123, 123f
  phenotypes of, 65–66
  pseudoautosomal, 71–72, 72f
  recessive, 68–70, 69f
    selection against, 103–104
X-linked disorder(s) *(Continued)*
  recurrence risk of, determination of
    in isolated case, 382–383, 383f, 384f
    pedigrees in, 380–382, 380f
  sex selection in, 394
  unequal crossing over in, 83
  variable expression of, 68
  versus autosomal dominant disorders, 61
X-linked inheritance, 65–71
  definition of, 53
  dominant, 70–71, 71f
  recessive, 68–70, 69f
  versus autosomal inheritance, 53
  X inactivation in, 66–68, 67f, 69f
X-rays, in radiation hybrid preparation, 115, 116f
Xeroderma pigmentosum
  cancer in, 315t, 328
  cytogenetics of, 154t
  inheritance of, consanguinity and, 57
  mutations in, 215
*XIST* gene, in X inactivation, 169, 171f
XX and XY abnormalities. *See under* Karyotype(s).

Y chromosome
  abnormalities of, incidence of, 150, 150t, 151t
  definition of, 5
  in reproductive system embryology, 166–167, 167f
  in spermatogenesis, 167–168
  pseudoautosomal region of, 67–68
  sex-determining region of, 166, 166f, 167, 168f
  structure of, 166, 166f
Yeast artificial chromosomes, 37t, 38, 39f, 127, 128f

Z, in lod scores. *See* Lod score(s).
Z allele, of alpha$_1$-antitrypsin, 89–90, 89t
ZAP 70 kinase deficiency, 286t
Zone of polarizing activity, 348
Zygosity. *See also under* Twin(s).
  determination of, 292
Zygotene stage, of meiosis, 10, 12f